WITHDRAWN

Middleton's
ALLERGY
PRINCIPLES AND PRACTICE

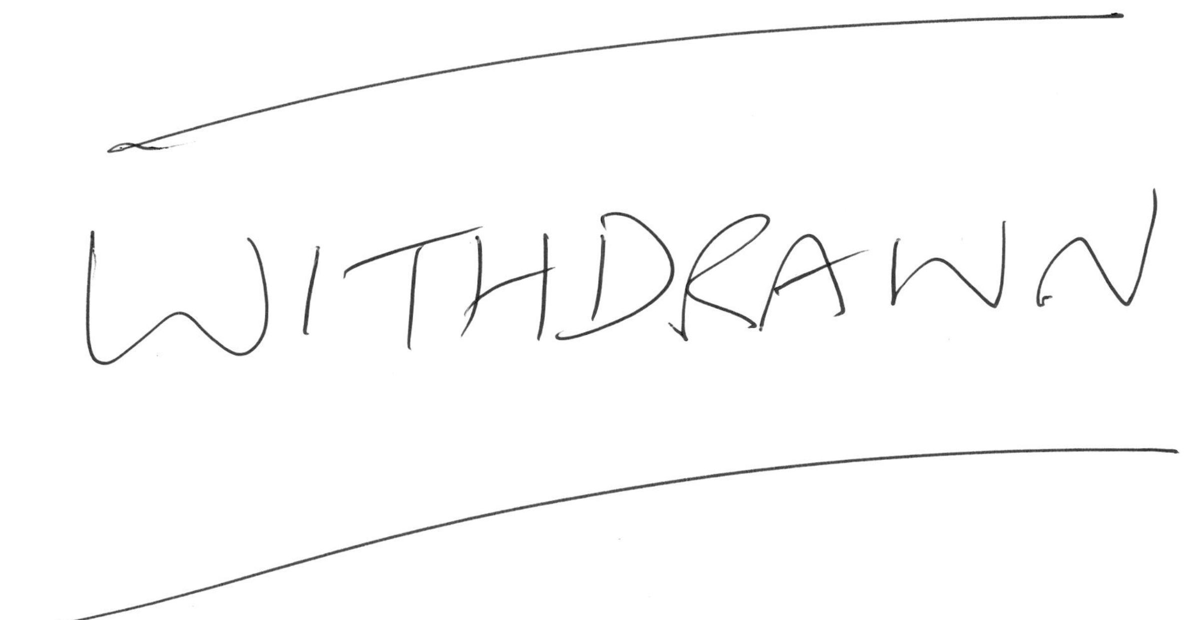

Middleton's

ALLERGY

PRINCIPLES AND PRACTICE

EIGHTH EDITION—VOLUME 2

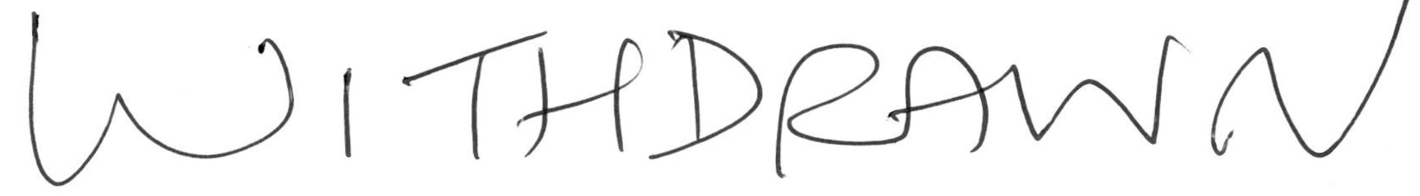

N. Franklin Adkinson, Jr., MD
Professor of Medicine
Division of Allergy and Clinical Immunology
Department of Medicine
Johns Hopkins University School of Medicine
Baltimore, Maryland, USA

Bruce S. Bochner, MD
Professor of Medicine and Director
Division of Allergy and Clinical Immunology
Department of Medicine
Johns Hopkins University School of Medicine
Baltimore, Maryland, USA

A. Wesley Burks, MD
Professor and Chair, Pediatrics
Physician-in-Chief
North Carolina Children's Hospital
University of North Carolina at Chapel Hill
Chapel Hill, North Carolina, USA

William W. Busse, MD
Professor of Medicine
Department of Medicine
Allergy, Pulmonary, and Critical Care Medicine
University of Wisconsin School of Medicine and Public Health
Madison, Wisconsin, USA

Stephen T. Holgate, MD, DSc, FMedSci
MRC Professor of Immunopharmacology
Clinical and Experimental Sciences
Faculty of Medicine
Southampton University and General Hospital
Southampton, United Kingdom

Robert F. Lemanske, Jr., MD
Professor of Pediatrics and Medicine
Head, Division of Pediatric Allergy, Immunology, and Rheumatology
University of Wisconsin School of Medicine and Public Health
Madison, Wisconsin, USA

Robyn E. O'Hehir, FRACP, PhD, FRCPath
Professor and Director
Department of Allergy, Immunology, and Respiratory Medicine
Alfred Hospital and Monash University
Melbourne, Victoria, Australia

ELSEVIER
SAUNDERS

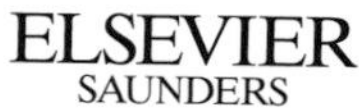

SAUNDERS

1600 John F. Kennedy Blvd.
Ste. 1800
Philadelphia, PA 19103-2899

MIDDLETON'S ALLERGY PRINCIPLES AND PRACTICE
Eighth Edition

Volume 1 PN 9996092240
Volume 2 PN 9996092305
Two-volume set ISBN: 978-0-323-08593-9

Notices

Knowledge and best practice in this field are constantly changing. As new research and experience broaden our understanding, changes in research methods, professional practices, or medical treatment may become necessary.

Practitioners and researchers must always rely on their own experience and knowledge in evaluating and using any information, methods, compounds, or experiments described herein. In using such information or methods they should be mindful of their own safety and the safety of others, including parties for whom they have a professional responsibility.

With respect to any drug or pharmaceutical products identified, readers are advised to check the most current information provided (i) on procedures featured or (ii) by the manufacturer of each product to be administered, to verify the recommended dose or formula, the method and duration of administration, and contraindications. It is the responsibility of practitioners, relying on their own experience and knowledge of their patients, to make diagnoses, to determine dosages and the best treatment for each individual patient, and to take all appropriate safety precautions.

To the fullest extent of the law, neither the Publisher nor the authors, contributors, or editors assume any liability for any injury and/or damage to persons or property as a matter of products liability, negligence or otherwise, or from any use or operation of any methods, products, instructions, or ideas contained in the material herein.

Library of Congress Cataloging-in-Publication Data

Middleton's allergy : principles and practice. —8th edition / N. Franklin Adkinson Jr. … [et al.].
p. ; cm.
Allergy
Includes bibliographical references and index.
ISBN 978-0-323-08593-9 (two-volume set : alk. paper)
I. Adkinson, N. Franklin, Jr. (Newton Franklin), 1943- II. Middleton, Elliott, Jr., 1925-1999.
III. Title: Allergy.
[DNLM: 1. Hypersensitivity. 2. Immunity. WD 300]
RC584
616.97—dc23

2013014886

Cover image adapted from Figure 21.2 in *Pathophysiology of Allergic Inflammation* by Peter J. Barnes.

Senior Content Strategist: Belinda Kuhn
Deputy Content Development Manager: Joanne Scott
Content Coordinator: Humayra Rahman Khan
Publishing Services Manager: Anne Altepeter
Project Manager: Louise King
Design Manager: Louis Forgione
Illustration Manager: Michael Carcel
Illustrator: Oxford Illustrators, Chartwell; Dartmouth Publishing, Inc.
Marketing Manager: Katie Alexo

Printed in China
Last digit is the print number: 9 8 7 6 5 4 3 2 1

Withdrawn

CONTENTS

Volume 1

Appendixes

PREFACE TO THE EIGHTH EDITION

With the publication of the eighth edition of *Middleton's Allergy: Principles and Practice*, the "beat goes on" for a textbook that was established nearly 40 years ago. Over these years, the book has continued to meet the educational needs of a diverse readership—students, trainees, investigators, and practitioners. Although there are new "verses" to the original "score" to reflect advances and discoveries over the past 4 decades, the basic "melody" to this textbook has been retained and builds on the success of the previous editions. The success over time for this textbook is an ongoing testimony to the insight, design, and wisdom of the founding editors: Elliott Middleton, Jr., Elliot F. Ellis, and Charles E. Reed. In 1978 they were academic leaders with expertise in the science and clinical practice of our specialty. Their visionary approach in the original design of this textbook recognized the need not only for a comprehensive textbook to codify state-of-the-art information on the ever-expanding and evolving science of allergic diseases and inflammation, but also to then translate this hard-won knowledge from research to clinical practice. This singular need and goal remain today the manifest vision of this undertaking.

It was their concept and design—one that has been adhered to in subsequent editions, including this eighth edition—that a comprehensive text should be built around two major informational foci. The first is the need to have a broad and comprehensive review and discussion of the underlying scientific basis that forms a foundation for allergic diseases (i.e., the *principles*). The second major component of the text builds upon and translates these scientific principles into discussions on the diagnosis and treatment of allergic diseases (i.e., the *practice*). It is the fondest hope of their successors, now seven in number, that the current eighth edition maintains the goals and standards so wisely established by Drs. Middleton, Ellis, and Reed.

In planning the eighth edition of *Middleton's Allergy*, a number of organizational changes were implemented. The ever-expanding knowledge of basic immunology fundamentals was applied to common diseases—including asthma, food allergies, and atopic dermatitis, for example—to add greater understanding of the pathogenesis and pathophysiology pathways of these disorders, which in turn would delineate more effectively treatment opportunities, both current and future. Although many examples of this approach are present in the eighth edition text, one of the most striking is the emergence since the last edition of new and lifesaving treatments for hereditary and acquired angioedemas. For years the fundamental defect in hereditary angioedema has been known, but it has taken a decade of exploration of its pathways to devise not just one, but several effective and safe treatments for patients with hereditary and, it is hoped, other forms of kinin-mediated angioedemas.

New technology continues to expand the identification and recognition of new aspects and "players" in the dynamic immune system network. Every attempt has been made to ensure that this advanced knowledge was included in this text, particularly as it may relate to allergic and immunologic diseases. In that spirit, the "overview" to immunity and how it works has been expanded to include chapters on both innate and adaptive immunity. Both of these components of immune responses are applicable to allergic diseases, and a broadened role for innate immune mechanisms is at the forefront of cutting-edge research. Other chapters covering the fundamental aspects of the immune system have been greatly expanded to reflect relevant advances, especially new insights about the roles of regulatory T cells in both sensitization and immunotherapy.

Advances in understanding of the origins and pathways of allergic diseases have accelerated tests of whether biologic therapies can be used to modulate, if not modify, human allergic and immunologic diseases. The rationale for these advances is often new pathways that may have direct and selective applicability to allergic reactions. To amplify more fully the seventh edition, three newly minted chapters were added: Immune Tolerance, Immunobiology of IgE and IgE Receptors, and Resolution of Allergic Inflammation. New findings expounded in these chapters hold promise of identifying novel potential targets for prevention and treatment of allergic disorders.

A separate section on aerobiology and allergens (Section B) has been added to the eighth edition to expand topics that are both unique and fundamental to the origins of a reaction to an environmental allergen: the structure and properties of foreign substances that become allergens, the host-environmental interactions leading to clinical disease, the role of air quality, and the standardization of allergen measurements in the assessment and management of allergic diseases. A new chapter, Particulate and Pollen Interactions, highlights how allergens and environmental particulates can and do interact to promote allergic sensitization.

New chapters have also been added to reflect advances of emerging fundamental and/or clinical importance, including: Respiratory Tract Mucosal Immunology, Ontogeny of Allergic Diseases and Asthma, Mouse Models of Allergic Airways Disease, Lung Imaging, and Gastrointestinal Mucosal Immunology. The topic of allergic bronchopulmonary aspergillosis and hypersensitivity pneumonitis receives new emphasis in this edition, reflecting the clear inclusion of these disorders within the clinical spectrum of allergy and immunology.

Asthma remains the predominant component of the section on the respiratory tract, and 10 chapters have undergone extensive revisions to reflect new information and clinical translation. The major advances in asthma pathogenesis are found in a newly authored chapter with subsequent chapters discussing diagnosis, treatment, and special aspects of asthma—occupational, exercise, and during pregnancy. Asthma is a heterogeneous disease and this is noted in many aspects, including onset, severity, and responsiveness to treatment. Heterogeneity is also reflected in asthma in terms of the ages of the patients affected. To recognize these critical distinctions, new chapters were delineated to deal with the unique aspects in the diagnosis and management of children and adults.

Systemic manifestations of allergic and immunologic disease are covered in Section G. In addition to comprehensive coverage of specific disorders (e.g., eosinophilia and eosinophil-related disorders), mastocytosis, drug allergy, human immunodeficiency virus, and anaphylaxis, chapters are devoted to diagnostic methods relevant for allergy evaluations, including recent advances such as component analysis. In the past 2 decades, research on food allergies has been unprecedented and has led to a greater recognition and appreciation of the scope of these allergic reactions and, more recently, of how to provide safe definitive prevention and treatments as alternatives to avoidance. Consequently, a new chapter on food allergy management has been added.

Finally, the section on therapeutics for allergic and immunologic diseases remains extensive and includes many new topics. This section has traditionally been a strength of the Middleton text and from our perspective continues to be so in the eighth edition. Control of allergic reactions by pharmacologic and immunologic means remains a main focus. An expanded discussion of immunotherapy includes a new chapter on sublingual immunotherapy to reflect its major advances and interest and its emerging clinical use. Two other chapters are now part of the Therapeutics section: Cytokine-Specific Therapy in Asthma and Complementary and Alternative Medicine. The use of biologics in allergic diseases is of considerable interest and reflects the culmination of applying knowledge from the basic biology of disease pathways to novel therapies for disease processes that may not be responsive to current treatment because of uniquely responsive subpopulations of patients.

The eighth edition continues to expand innovations of the seventh edition that brought widespread endorsement and acclaim. These include full-color coding and accenting, coordinated artwork with consistent format, an insistence on tabular and schematic graphical presentations wherever possible, summaries of important concepts for each chapter, and extensive referencing with an emphasis on recent findings. With this edition we also began the process of encouraging authors to conform their contributions to a common outline format so that there is some consistency in order of presentation within chapters. All of these features, plus other enhancements such as reference links and ability to extract figures as slide copy, are available on the searchable web version available to those who acquire the electronic format.

Along with the major content changes in the science and treatment of allergic diseases, the eighth edition of Middleton has seen changes in our editors. Dr. F. Estelle R. Simons has stepped down as an editor. We greatly miss her scholarship of allergic diseases but we are grateful that she and Dr. Cezmi A. Akdis have continued to author their very comprehensive and tour de force chapter Histamine and H_1-Antihistamines. Drs. Robyn E. O'Hehir and Wesley Burks are new and welcome additions as editors. They have brought special expertise in immunology/asthma and food allergy, respectively, as well as a fresh view to the overall direction of *Middleton's Allergy: Principles and Practice*. In addition, Dr. O'Hehir's acceptance means that we now have editors from three continents, which hopefully allows and encourages a fully global perspective.

The authorship for this text continues to expand in terms of geographic origin. The 215 contributing authors come from 17 countries on 5 continents. The Middleton text continues to evolve over time to become global in perspective, and editorial care has been exercised to ensure clear understanding of differences in practice norms, especially between the United States and Europe. Another continuing editorial policy is the systematic turnover of chapter authorship to ensure that fresh perspectives are aired and new voices can be heard, even when there is nothing fundamentally wrong with the "older" author. This sometimes results in perceived insults when authors are "dropped," but we believe the value of this principle continues to prove itself. Hence, in this edition, you will find new coauthorship in a majority of chapters, and totally new presentations in 43 of 102 chapters! We believe this newness alone is sufficient reason to acquire and engage the eighth edition—even for experienced clinicians and investigators.

In our opinion, the authors who have graciously contributed 102 chapters and two appendixes to the eighth edition have provided readers from all levels with comprehensive, evidence-based information and timely reviews of allergic diseases. They have "told the story" of the principles of our diseases as well as translated this information into practice for the most effective current care and treatment. It is impossible to sufficiently thank all of the authors for their wonderful and informative chapters. It has been our responsibility—and pleasure—to orchestrate their well-written chapters into a book that we hope will continue to effectively serve and meet the needs of our readership, from student to investigator to care provider.

This monumental cooperative effort among authors and editors could not have been undertaken without the superb support of our publishing staff at Elsevier, for whom we are especially grateful. Based in London, Joanne Scott and her associates Devika Ponnambalam and Humayra Rahman Khan arranged international conference calls, organized and documented our efforts and progress, and kept both authors and editors on track for an on-time completion. Belinda Kuhn, senior content strategist, and her predecessor, Sue Hodgson, oversaw the planning and evolution of the project over the past 4 years. Louise King in St. Louis managed the layout and proofing process, and numerous others at Elsevier did great service in artwork and design, publicity, and production. Mike Carcel, Louis Forgione, and Brett MacNaughton in Philadelphia managed the art line and cover and text design. It was a pleasure to work with this excellent multinational staff of professionals.

Lastly, a word about the future. Medical publishing is changing rapidly and we will change with it. The eighth edition will be published in print form and simultaneously issued in electronic format, as was true for the seventh edition. But the traditional 5-year cycle for completely new editions will be replaced by a continuously revised e-edition, which will allow all content to remain current. The details of this new era for the Middleton text are being finalized and should be available by the time of publication.

N. Franklin Adkinson, Jr.
Managing Editor
Bruce S. Bochner
A. Wesley Burks
William W. Busse
Stephen T. Holgate
Robert F. Lemanske, Jr.
Robyn E. O'Hehir

May 2013

PREFACE TO THE FIRST EDITION

Allergy, once a confusing subject for clinician and researcher alike, has emerged as a medical science in which immunology, physiology, and pharmacology interface uniquely. Our present state of knowledge is the culmination of the efforts of many workers over many decades of research in the clinic and laboratory. We want to acknowledge our incalculable debt to these investigators, both basic scientists and clinicians, who taught us not only fact but more importantly concepts and scientific method.

Several textbooks on allergy are already in existence. Why another one? We pondered this question for some time before embarking on what turned out to be, expectedly, a rather formidable task. It was our opinion that a truly comprehensive book about allergy should focus strongly not only on the exciting developments of the past decade or two in immunology but also provide in-depth coverage of equally pertinent new information on physiology and pharmacology, two areas of critical importance to the student of allergy. We have made no attempt to cover all of the subject matter considered to fall under the general rubric of clinical immunology and so do not include sections dealing with rheumatology, other connective tissue disorders, immunohematology, or tumor immunology, for example, since these subjects are well covered elsewhere.

The chapters dealing with immunology, pharmacology, and physiology appear at the beginning in the basic science section of the book to provide the necessary conceptual framework for the clinical science section, which deals with the variety of clinical states that fall within the purview of allergy and the allergist. The value of the clinical descriptions is vastly enhanced by a careful reading of the earlier chapters.

We were most fortunate in securing a truly outstanding "star-studded" cast of contributors who managed to find time in their already overcrowded schedules to help us write the book. We thank them all for their efforts and are grateful for the patient indulgence of a few who put up with some predictable editorial fussing meant to achieve proper balance and avoid excessive overlap.

Most of the chapters can be read as free-standing articles or monographs on that particular subject. This has led to a certain irreducible amount of duplication. By and large, there is consistency among chapters in which comparable material has been presented by different authors, but the reader will find occasional areas of controversy, a natural state of affairs in a rapidly growing field.

It is our opinion that some chapters in this book represent the most comprehensive summaries of the subject matter to be found in print. Thus Allergy: Principles and Practice serves not only as a textbook but as a reference book. Indeed, this was our intent, but original estimates for the length of the book were necessarily revised upward as it became clear that much excellent material could not properly be left out. The final product then turns out to be a book we hope will be useful to all students of allergy: practitioners, clinical investigators, other researchers, allergy trainees, and medical students.

The generous and unstinting help of many people in addition to the contributors made this book possible. Without the competent and devoted secretarial assistance of Marci Dame, Evelyn Beimers, Bonnie Barcy, Carol Speery, and Candace Anderson, the task could not have been accomplished. We thank our wives and families for their forbearance, while we were sequestered away from home for day and night weekend sessions during the planning and editing phases. From the beginning their support has been essential to the successful completion of our job. A number of colleagues, too numerous to name, provided help in critical reading of manuscripts. To these and others who were helpful in a variety of ways, we offer thanks.

We are saddened that two contributors died during the preparation of the book. Jane Harnett is the senior author of the chapter dealing with aspirin idiosyncrasy. Dr. Harnett compiled much of the information for the chapter and worked on the manuscript under extremely difficult circumstances up to within only a few days of her untimely death. She is remembered fondly and with respect by all those with whom she worked. Robert P. Orange, one of the most brilliant and creative investigators of his generation, died suddenly during the preparation of the book. No one can guess what additional important discoveries Dr. Orange would have made had he not died so prematurely.

We would like to record here our personal sorrow at the loss of these fine physicians. We hope that their representation in this textbook will help keep memories of them alive.

Elliott Middleton, Jr.
Charles E. Reed
Elliot F. Ellis

1978

WITHDRAWN

CONTRIBUTORS

Seema S. Aceves, MD, PhD
Associate Professor, Pediatrics and Medicine
Division of Allergy and Immunology, Departments of Pediatrics and Medicine
Director, Eosinophilic Gastrointestinal Disorders Clinic
University of California, San Diego
La Jolla, California, USA
Rady Children's Hospital
San Diego, California, USA
Gastrointestinal Mucosal Immunology

Ian M. Adcock, MD
Professor, National Heart and Lung Institute
Imperial College London
London, United Kingdom
Biology of Monocytes and Macrophages; Glucocorticosteroids

N. Franklin Adkinson, Jr., MD
Professor of Medicine
Division of Allergy and Clinical Immunology
Department of Medicine
Johns Hopkins University School of Medicine
Baltimore, Maryland, USA
Drug Allergy; Appendix B: Internet Resources for Allergy and Immunology Professionals

Cezmi A. Akdis, MD
Professor and Director, Swiss Institute of Allergy and Asthma Research
University of Zürich
Director, Christine Kühne–Center for Allergy Research and Education
President, European Academy of Allergy and Clinical Immunology
Zürich, Switzerland
Immune Tolerance; Histamine and H_1 Antihistamines

Mübeccel Akdis, PD, MD, PhD
Head of Immunodermatology, Swiss Institute of Allergy and Asthma Research
University of Zürich
Zürich, Switzerland
Immune Tolerance

Keith C. Allen, BSc
Medical Student
Medical Research Council Centre for Inflammation Research
Queen's Medical Research Institute
University of Edinburgh
Edinburgh, United Kingdom
Resolution of Allergic Inflammation

Andrea J. Apter, MD, MSc, MA
Professor of Medicine
Chief, Section of Allergy and Immunology
Division of Pulmonary, Allergy, and Critical Care Medicine
Perelman School of Medicine at the University of Pennsylvania
Philadelphia, Pennsylvania, USA
Adherence

Claus Bachert, MD, PhD
Professor of Medicine
Chief of Clinics
Head, Upper Airway Research Laboratory
Ear, Nose, and Throat Department
University Hospital Ghent
Ghent, Belgium
Rhinosinusitis and Nasal Polyps

Katherine J. Baines, PhD
Post-Doctoral Research Fellow
Department of Respiratory and Sleep Medicine
University of Newcastle
Hunter Medical Research Institute
Newcastle, New South Wales, Australia
Biology of Neutrophils

Mark Ballow, MD
Emeritus Professor of Pediatrics
Director, Allergy/Immunology Fellowship Training Program
Past Chief, Division of Allergy/Clinical Immunology and Pediatric Rheumatology
Women and Children's Hospital of Buffalo
SUNY Buffalo School of Medicine and Biomedical Sciences
Buffalo, New York, USA
Approach to the Patient with Recurrent Infections

Peter J. Barnes, FMedSci, FRS
Head of Respiratory Medicine
National Heart and Lung Institute
Imperial College London
London, United Kingdom
Pathophysiology of Allergic Inflammation

Neal P. Barney, MD
Professor, Department of Ophthalmology and Visual Sciences
Director of Cornea and External Disease Service
University of Wisconsin School of Medicine and Public Health
Madison, Wisconsin, USA
Allergic and Immunologic Diseases of the Eye

Fuad M. Baroody, MD, FACS
Professor of Surgery, Otolaryngology–Head and Neck Surgery and Pediatrics
Director, Pediatric Otolaryngology
The University of Chicago Medical Center
The Comer Children's Hospital
Chicago, Illinois, USA
Allergic and Nonallergic Rhinitis

Heidrun Behrendt, MD
Professor and Director Emeritus
Center of Allergy and Environment
Christine Kühne–Center for Allergy Research and Education
Munich, Germany
Particulate and Pollen Interactions

Bruce G. Bender, PhD
Professor of Pediatrics and Psychiatry
Head, Division of Pediatric Behavioral Health
National Jewish Health
Denver, Colorado, USA
Adherence

M. Cecilia Berin, PhD
Associate Professor of Pediatrics
Division of Allergy and Immunology
Jaffe Food Allergy Institute
Department of Pediatrics
Icahn School of Medicine at Mount Sinai
New York, New York, USA
Gastrointestinal Mucosal Immunology

Paul J. Bertics, PhD†
Kellett Professor of Biomolecular Chemistry
University of Wisconsin School of Medicine and Public Health
Madison, Wisconsin, USA
Signal Transduction

Thomas Bieber, MD, PhD, MDRA
Professor and Chair
Department of Dermatology and Allergy
University of Bonn
Bonn, Germany
Structure of the Skin and Cutaneous Immunology

Leonard Bielory, MD
Professor, Center of Environmental Prediction
Rutgers University
Attending, Robert Wood Johnson University Hospital
Director, STARx Allergy and Asthma Center
New Brunswick, New Jersey, USA
Unconventional Theories and Unproven Methods in Allergy

Judith Black, AO, MBBS, PhD
Professor and NHMRC Senior Principal Research Fellow, Discipline of Pharmacology
School of Medical Sciences and Woolcock Institute of Medical Research
The University of Sydney
Sydney, New South Wales, Australia
Noncontractile Functions of Airway Smooth Muscle

Bruce S. Bochner, MD
Professor of Medicine and Director
Division of Allergy and Clinical Immunology
Department of Medicine
Johns Hopkins University School of Medicine
Baltimore, Maryland, USA
Biology of Eosinophils; Appendix A: CD Molecules

Mark Boguniewicz, MD
Professor, Division of Allergy–Immunology
Department of Pediatrics, National Jewish Health
University of Colorado School of Medicine
Denver, Colorado, USA
Atopic Dermatitis

Larry Borish, MD
Professor of Medicine, Asthma and Allergic Disease Center Carter Immunology Center
University of Virginia Health System
Charlottesville, Virginia, USA
Cytokines in Allergic Inflammation

Louis-Philippe Boulet, MD, FRCPC, FCCP
Professor of Medicine, Department of Medicine
Laval University
Québec Heart and Lung Institute
Québec City, Québec, Canada
Diagnosis of Asthma in Adults

Jean Bousquet, MD
Professor of Pulmonology, Department of Allergology
Arnaud de Villeneuve Hospital
University Hospital of Montpellier
Montpellier, France
In Vivo Methods for the Study and Diagnosis of Allergy

Joshua A. Boyce, MD
Albert L. Sheffer Professor of Medicine in the Field of Allergic Diseases
Harvard Medical School
Jeff and Penny Vinik Center for Allergic Disease Research
Division of Rheumatology, Immunology, and Allergy
Brigham and Women's Hospital
Boston, Massachusetts, USA
Lipid Mediators of Hypersensitivity and Inflammation

†Deceased

Peter Bradding, BM, DM, FRCP
Professor of Respiratory Medicine
Institute for Lung Health
Department of Infection, Immunity, and Inflammation
University of Leicester
Leicester, United Kingdom
Biology of Mast Cells and Their Mediators

Christopher E. Brightling, MD, PhD, FCCP
Wellcome Senior Research Fellow
Clinical Professor in Respiratory Medicine
Institute for Lung Health
Department of Infection, Inflammation, and Immunity
University of Leicester
Glenfield Hospital
Leicester, United Kingdom
Lung Imaging; Cytokine-Specific Therapy in Asthma

David H. Broide, MB, ChB
Professor of Medicine
University of California, San Diego
La Jolla, California, USA
Cellular Adhesion in Inflammation

Simon G.A. Brown, MBBS, PhD, FACEM
Professor of Emergency Medicine
University of Western Australia
Royal Perth Hospital
Perth, Western Australia, Australia
Anaphylaxis

Rebecca H. Buckley, MD
J. Buren Sidbury Distinguished Professor of Pediatrics, Department of Pediatrics
Professor of Immunology, Department of Immunology
Duke University Medical Center
Durham, North Carolina, USA
Primary Immunodeficiency Diseases

Janette K. Burgess, PhD
Associate Professor and NHMRC Career Development Fellow, Discipline of Pharmacology
School of Medical Sciences and Woolcock Institute of Medical Research
The University of Sydney
Sydney, New South Wales, Australia
Noncontractile Functions of Airway Smooth Muscle

A. Wesley Burks, MD
Professor and Chair, Pediatrics
Physician-in-Chief
North Carolina Children's Hospital
University of North Carolina at Chapel Hill
Chapel Hill, North Carolina, USA
Reactions to Foods

Peter G.J. Burney, MD, FFPH, FMedSci
Professor, Department of Respiratory Epidemiology and Public Health
National Heart and Lung Institute
Imperial College London
London, United Kingdom
Epidemiology of Asthma and Allergic Airway Diseases

Robert K. Bush, MD
Professor Emeritus, Department of Medicine
Division of Allergy, Immunology, Pulmonary, and Critical Care Medicine
University of Wisconsin
Madison, Wisconsin, USA
Reactions to Food and Drug Additives

William W. Busse, MD
Professor of Medicine
Department of Medicine
Allergy, Pulmonary, and Critical Care Medicine
University of Wisconsin School of Medicine and Public Health
Madison, Wisconsin, USA
Management of Asthma in Adolescents and Adults

Jeroen Buters, PharmD
Associate Professor, Center of Allergy and Environment
Christine Kühne–Center for Allergy Research and Education
Munich, Germany
Particulate and Pollen Interactions

Lien Calus, MD
Resident in Otorhinolaryngology
Upper Airway Research Laboratory
Ear, Nose, and Throat Department
University Hospital Ghent
Ghent, Belgium
Rhinosinusitis and Nasal Polyps

Carlos A. Camargo, Jr., MD, PhD
Professor of Medicine
Harvard Medical School
Physician, Massachusetts General Hospital
Boston, Massachusetts, USA
Emergency Treatment and Approach to the Patient with Acute Asthma

Brendan J. Canning, PhD
Associate Professor of Medicine
Division of Allergy and Clinical Immunology, Department of Medicine
Johns Hopkins University School of Medicine
Baltimore, Maryland, USA
Neuronal Control of Airway Function in Allergy

Thomas B. Casale, MD
Professor of Medicine
Chief, Allergy/Immunology
Creighton University
Omaha, Nebraska, USA
Anti-Immunoglobulin E Therapy

Mario Castro, MD, MPH
Professor of Medicine and Pediatrics
Washington University School of Medicine
St. Louis, Missouri, USA
Lung Imaging

Gülfem E. Çelik, MD
Professor, Department of Immunology and Allergy
Ankara University School of Medicine
Ankara, Turkey
Drug Allergy

Christina Chambers, PhD, MPH
Professor, Departments of Pediatrics and Family and Preventive Medicine
University of California, San Diego
La Jolla, California, USA
Asthma and Allergic Diseases during Pregnancy

Javier Chinen, MD, PhD
Allergy and Immunology Specialist
Lake Houston Asthma, Allergy, and Immunology
Humble, Texas, USA
Adaptive Immunity

Anca Mirela Chiriac, MD
Allergologist, Department of Respiratory Medicine and Addictology
Arnaud de Villeneuve Hospital
University Hospital of Montpellier
Montpellier, France
In Vivo Methods for the Study and Diagnosis of Allergy

Sandra C. Christiansen, MD
Clinical Professor of Medicine, Department of Allergy
Kaiser Permanente Medical Center
San Diego, California, USA
University of California, San Diego
La Jolla, California, USA
Hereditary Angioedema and Bradykinin-Mediated Angioedema

Kian Fan Chung, MD, DSc, FRCP
Professor of Respiratory Medicine
Head of Experimental Studies
National Heart and Lung Institute
Imperial College London
Asthma Consortium Leader
Royal Brompton Hospital Biomedical Research Unit
London, United Kingdom
Biology of Monocytes and Macrophages; Glucocorticosteroids

Donald W. Cockcroft, BSc, MD, FRCP[C]
Professor of Respirology Medicine
Department of Medicine
University of Saskatchewan
Saskatoon, Saskatchewan, Canada
Bronchial Challenge Testing

Lauren Cohn, MD
Associate Professor, Section of Pulmonary and Critical Care Medicine
Department of Internal Medicine
Yale University School of Medicine
New Haven, Connecticut, USA
Biology of Lymphocytes

Ellen B. Cook, PhD
Senior Scientist, Department of Ophthalmology and Visual Sciences
University of Wisconsin School of Medicine and Public Health
Madison, Wisconsin, USA
Allergic and Immunologic Diseases of the Eye

Jonathan Corren, MD
Associate Clinical Professor of Medicine
David Geffen School of Medicine
University of California, Los Angeles
Los Angeles, California, USA
Allergic and Nonallergic Rhinitis

Adnan Custovic, MD, PhD
Professor of Allergy
University of Manchester
Manchester, United Kingdom
Allergen Control for Prevention and Management of Allergic Diseases

Pascal Demoly, MD, PhD
Professor of Respiratory Medicine
Department of Respiratory Medicine and Addictology
Arnaud de Villeneuve Hospital
University Hospital of Montpellier
Montpellier, France
In Vivo Methods for the Study and Diagnosis of Allergy

Dhananjay Desai, MBBS, MRCP
Specialist Registrar
Department of Infection, Inflammation, and Immunity
University of Leicester
Institute for Lung Health
Glenfield Hospital
Leicester, United Kingdom
Cytokine-Specific Therapy in Asthma

Graham Devereux, MA, MD, PhD
Professor, Royal Aberdeen Children's Hospital
Aberdeen, United Kingdom
Epidemiology of Asthma and Allergic Airway Diseases

Thomas Diepgen, MD
Professor and Chairman, Department of Clinical Social Medicine
Center of Occupational and Environmental Dermatology
Ruprecht Karl University of Heidelberg
Heidelberg, Germany
Contact Dermatitis

Myrna B. Dolovich, B Eng (Elec), P Eng
Professor, Department of Medicine
Michael DeGroote School of Medicine
Faculty of Health Sciences
McMaster University
Hamilton, Ontario, Canada
Aerosols and Aerosol Drug Delivery Systems

David A. Dorward, MBChB, BSc, MRCP
Clinical Research Fellow
Medical Research Council Centre for Inflammation Research
Queen's Medical Research Institute
University of Edinburgh
Edinburgh, United Kingdom
Resolution of Allergic Inflammation

Jo A. Douglass, FRACP, MD
Head, Department of Immunology and Allergy
Royal Melbourne Hospital
Clinical Professor
The University of Melbourne
Parkville, Victoria, Australia
Allergic Bronchopulmonary Aspergillosis and Hypersensitivity Pneumonitis

Stephen R. Durham, MA, MD, FRCP
Head, Section Allergy and Clinical Immunology
National Heart and Lung Institute
Imperial College School of Medicine
London, United Kingdom
Nasal Provocation Testing

Sandy R. Durrani, MD
Fellow, Department of Medicine, Allergy, Pulmonary, and Critical Care Medicine
University of Wisconsin School of Medicine and Public Health
Madison, Wisconsin, USA
Management of Asthma in Adolescents and Adults

Mark S. Dykewicz, MD
Professor of Internal Medicine
Director of Allergy and Immunology
Center for Human Genomics and Personalized Medicine
Wake Forest University School of Medicine
Winston-Salem, North Carolina, USA
Anticholinergic Therapies

Ronald Eccles, DSc
Director, Common Cold Centre
Cardiff School of Biosciences
Cardiff University
Cardiff, United Kingdom
The Nose and Control of Nasal Airflow

Alan M. Edwards, MA, MB, BChir
Clinical Assistant (Allergy) (retired)
The David Hide Asthma and Allergy Research Centre
St. Mary's Hospital
London, United Kingdom
The Chromones: Cromolyn Sodium and Nedocromil Sodium

Renata J.M. Engler, MD
Colonel, Medical Corps, US Army
Professor of Medicine and Pediatrics (Secondary)
Uniformed Services University of the Health Sciences
Director, Vaccine Healthcare Centers Network (Division, Military Vaccine Agency/US Public Health Command)
Walter Reed National Military Medical Center
Bethesda, Maryland, USA
Complementary and Alternative Medicine

Robert E. Esch, PhD
Chief Scientific Officer
Greer Laboratories, Inc.
Lenoir, North Carolina, USA
Preparation and Standardization of Allergen Extracts

Sean B. Fain, PhD
Associate Professor and Vice-Chair of Research in Medical Physics
Department of Medical Physics
University of Wisconsin School of Medicine and Public Health
Madison, Wisconsin, USA
Lung Imaging

Reuben Falkoff, MD, PhD
Clinical Physician, Department of Allergy
Kaiser Permanente Medical Center
San Diego, California, USA
Asthma and Allergic Diseases during Pregnancy

Matthew J. Fenton, PhD
Director, Division of Extramural Activities
National Institute of Allergy and Infectious Diseases
Bethesda, Maryland, USA
Innate Immunity

Thomas A. Fleisher, MD
Chief, Department of Laboratory Medicine
National Institutes of Health Clinical Center
National Institutes of Health
Bethesda, Maryland, USA
Adaptive Immunity

Joseph R. Fontana, MD
Chief Medical Officer and Lieutenant Commander
U.S. Public Health Service
Cardiovascular and Pulmonary Branch, National Heart, Lung, and Blood Institute
National Institutes of Health
Bethesda, Maryland, USA
Immunologic Nonasthmatic Diseases of the Lung

Michael M. Frank, MD
Samuel L. Katz Professor of Pediatrics
Medicine and Immunology
Department of Pediatrics
Duke University Medical Center
Durham, North Carolina, USA
Immune Complex–Mediated Diseases

Anthony J. Frew, MD, FRCP
Professor of Allergy and Respiratory Medicine
Department of Respiratory Medicine
Royal Sussex County Hospital
Brighton, United Kingdom
Sublingual Immunotherapy for Inhalant Allergens

Glenn T. Furuta, MD
Professor, Department of Pediatrics
University of Colorado School of Medicine
Director, Gastrointestinal Eosinophilic Diseases Program
Children's Hospital Colorado
National Jewish Health
Denver, Colorado, USA
Gastrointestinal Mucosal Immunology

Holger Garn, PhD
Head of Research, Institute of Laboratory Medicine and Pathobiochemistry–Molecular Diagnostics
Medical Faculty, Philipps University of Marburg, Biomedical Research Center
Marburg, Germany
Respiratory Tract Mucosal Immunology

Monica L. Gavala, PhD
Scientist, Department of Biomolecular Chemistry
University of Wisconsin
Madison, Wisconsin, USA
Signal Transduction

Philippe Gevaert, MD, PhD
Professor of Otorhinolaryngology
Head, Allergy Network
University Hospital Ghent
Ghent, Belgium
Rhinosinusitis and Nasal Polyps

Viviane Ghanim, MD
Research Fellow
Department of Internal Medicine
Division of Hematology and Hemostaseology
Medical University of Vienna
Vienna, Austria
Appendix A: CD Molecules

Peter G. Gibson, MBBS
Professor, Department of Respiratory and Sleep Medicine
University of Newcastle
Newcastle, New South Wales, Australia
Biology of Neutrophils

David B.K. Golden, MD
Associate Professor of Medicine, Division of Allergy and Clinical Immunology
Department of Medicine
Johns Hopkins University School of Medicine
Baltimore, Maryland, USA
Insect Allergy

Matthew J. Greenhawt, MD, MBA, MSc
Assistant Professor
Department of Internal Medicine
Division of Allergy and Clinical Immunology
University of Michigan Medical School
University of Michigan Health System
Ann Arbor, Michigan, USA
Adverse Reactions to Vaccines for Infectious Diseases

Anete S. Grumach, MD, PhD
Assistant Professor, Outpatient Group of Recurrent Infections
Head, Laboratory of Clinical Immunology
Faculty of Medicine ABC
São Paulo, Brazil
The Complement System

Theresa W. Guilbert, MD, MS
Associate Professor of Pediatrics
Division of Pediatric Pulmonary Medicine
University of Wisconsin–Madison
Madison, Wisconsin, USA
Diagnosis of Asthma in Infants and Children; Management of Asthma in Infants and Children

Sudhir Gupta, MD, PhD, MACP
Professor of Medicine
Pathology and Laboratory Medicine, and Microbiology and Molecular Genetics
Director, Programs in Primary Immunodeficiency and Aging
Chief, Basic and Clinical Immunology
University of California, Irvine
Irvine, California, USA
Molecular Biology and Genetic Engineering

Andrew J. Halayko, PhD
Professor and Canada Research Chair in Airway Cell and Molecular Biology
Departments of Physiology and Internal Medicine
Faculty of Medicine
University of Manitoba
Leader, Biology of Breathing Group
Manitoba Institute of Child Health
Winnipeg, Manitoba, Canada
Airway Smooth Muscle Function in Asthma: Extracellular Matrix and Airway Remodeling

Teal S. Hallstrand, MD, MPH
Associate Professor
Division of Pulmonary and Critical Care Medicine
University of Washington
Seattle, Washington, USA
Approach to the Patient with Exercise-Induced Bronchoconstriction

Robert G. Hamilton, PhD, D(ABMLI)
Professor of Medicine and Pathology, Division of Allergy and Clinical Immunology
Department of Medicine
Johns Hopkins University School of Medicine
Baltimore, Maryland, USA
Laboratory Tests for Allergic and Immunodeficiency Diseases

Hamida Hammad, PhD
Associate Professor of Medicine
Department of Molecular Biomedical Research
VIB–Ghent University
Ghent, Belgium
Antigen-Presenting Dendritic Cells

Trevor T. Hansel, MBBCh, FRCPath, PhD
Medical Director of Imperial Clinical Respiratory Research Unit
Centre for Respiratory Infection, St. Mary's Hospital
Imperial College London
London, United Kingdom
Nasal Provocation Testing

Catherine Hawrylowicz, PhD
Professor of Immune Regulation in Allergic Diseases
MRC/Asthma Centre in Allergic Mechanisms of Asthma
Department of Asthma, Allergy, and Respiratory Science
Guy's Hospital
King's College London
London, United Kingdom
Biology of Lymphocytes

Michelle L. Hernandez, MD
Assistant Professor, Department of Pediatrics
Division of Allergy, Immunology, Rheumatology, and Infectious Diseases
University of North Carolina School of Medicine
Chapel Hill, North Carolina, USA
Air Pollution: Indoor and Outdoor

C. Garren Hester, BS
Research Analyst, Department of Pediatrics
Duke University Medical Center
Durham, North Carolina, USA
Immune Complex–Mediated Diseases

Jeremy Hirota, PhD
Post-Doctoral Research Fellow, CIHR, MSFHR/Allergen, and IMPACT
UBC James Hogg Research Centre
St. Paul's Hospital
Vancouver, British Columbia, Canada
Airway Epithelial Cells

Stephen T. Holgate, MD, DSc, FMedSci
MRC Professor of Immunopharmacology, Clinical and Experimental Sciences
Faculty of Medicine
Southampton University and General Hospital
Southampton, United Kingdom
Asthma Pathogenesis; Allergic Bronchopulmonary Aspergillosis and Hypersensitivity Pneumonitis; The Chromones: Cromolyn Sodium and Nedocromil Sodium

John W. Holloway, PhD
Professor of Allergy and Respiratory Genetics
Faculty of Medicine
University of Southampton
Southampton, United Kingdom
Genetics and Epigenetics in Allergic Diseases and Asthma

Charles G. Irvin, PhD
Director, Vermont Lung Center
Professor, Medicine, Molecular Physiology, and Biophysics
College of Medicine
University of Vermont
Burlington, Vermont, USA
Development, Structure, and Physiology in Normal Lung and in Asthma

Richard S. Irwin, MD
Chair, Critical Care Operations
UMass Memorial Medical Center
Professor of Medicine and Nursing
University of Massachusetts Medical School
Worcester, Massachusetts, USA
Approach to the Patient with Chronic Cough

Elliot Israel, MD
Professor of Medicine, Department of Medicine
Harvard Medical School
Director, Pulmonary Clinical Research
Brigham and Women's Hospital
Boston, Massachusetts, USA
Pharmacogenomics of Asthma Therapies

Daniel J. Jackson, MD
Assistant Professor of Pediatrics
Division of Pediatric Allergy, Immunology, and Rheumatology
University of Wisconsin School of Medicine and Public Health
Madison, Wisconsin, USA
Diagnosis of Asthma in Infants and Children; Management of Asthma in Infants and Children

Peter K. Jeffery, PhD, DSc(Med), FRCPath
Emeritus Professor of Lung Pathology
Senior Research Investigator
Honorary Consultant Pathologist
Department of Gene Therapy
Royal Brompton Hospital
Imperial College London
London, United Kingdom
Pathology of Asthma

Diane F. Jelinek, PhD
Professor of Immunology
Chair, Department of Immunology
Mayo Clinic
Rochester, Minnesota, USA
Immunoglobulin Structure and Function

Richard B. Johnston, Jr., MD
Professor of Pediatrics
National Jewish Health and University of Colorado School of Medicine
Associate Dean for Research Development
University of Colorado School of Medicine
Denver, Colorado, USA
Innate Immunity

Stacie M. Jones, MD
Professor of Pediatrics and Physiology/Biophysics
Chief, Allergy and Immunology
Dr. and Mrs. Leeman King Chair in Pediatric Allergy
University of Arkansas for Medical Sciences
Arkansas Children's Hospital
Little Rock, Arkansas, USA
Food Allergy Management

H. William Kelly, PharmD
Professor Emeritus
Department of Pediatrics
University of New Mexico Health Sciences Center
Albuquerque, New Mexico, USA
Principles of Pharmacotherapeutics

John M. Kelso, MD
Clinical Professor of Pediatrics and Internal Medicine
University of California, San Diego School of Medicine
Staff Physician, Division of Allergy, Asthma, and Immunology
Scripps Clinic
San Diego, California, USA
Adverse Reactions to Vaccines for Infectious Diseases

Stephen F. Kemp, MD, FACP
Professor of Medicine and Pediatrics
Director, Allergy and Immunology Fellowship Program
The University of Mississippi Medical Center
Jackson, Mississippi, USA
Anaphylaxis

Hirohito Kita, MD
Professor of Medicine and Immunology
Departments of Medicine, Immunology, and Otorhinolaryngology
Mayo Clinic
Rochester, Minnesota, USA
Biology of Eosinophils

Amy D. Klion, MD
Clinical Investigator, Eosinophil Pathology Unit
Laboratory of Parasitic Diseases
National Institute of Allergy and Infectious Diseases
National Institutes of Health
Bethesda, Maryland, USA
Eosinophilia and Eosinophil-Related Disorders

Darryl Knight, MD
Professor and Head
School of Biomedical Sciences and Pharmacy
University of Newcastle
Callaghan, New South Wales, Australia
Airway Epithelial Cells

Marek L. Kowalski, MD, PhD
Professor and Chairman
Department of Immunology, Rheumatology, and Allergy
Chair of Clinical Immunology and Microbiology
Medical University of Lodz
Lodz, Poland
Hypersensitivity to Aspirin and Other Nonsteroidal Antiinflammatory Drugs

Cynthia J. Koziol-White, PhD
Postdoctoral Fellow
Pulmonary, Allergy, and Critical Care Division
Perelman School of Medicine at the University of Pennsylvania
Philadelphia, Pennsylvania, USA
Signal Transduction

Rakesh K. Kumar, MBBS, PhD, FRCPA(Hon)
Professor of Pathology
School of Medical Sciences
The University of New South Wales
Sydney, New South Wales, Australia
Pathology of Asthma

Gideon Lack, MD
Professor of Paediatric Allergy
King's College London
King's Health Partners
MRC & Asthma UK Centre in Allergic Mechanisms of Asthma, and the Department of Paediatric Allergy
Guy's and St. Thomas' NHS Foundation Trust
London, United Kingdom
Food Allergy Management

Bart N. Lambrecht, MD, PhD
Professor of Medicine and Department Director
Department of Molecular Biomedical Research, VIB–Ghent University
Department of Respiratory Medicine, University Hospital
Ghent, Belgium
Antigen-Presenting Dendritic Cells

Beth L. Laube, PhD
Professor of Pediatrics
Eudowood Division of Pediatric Respiratory Sciences
Johns Hopkins University School of Medicine
Baltimore, Maryland, USA
Aerosols and Aerosol Drug Delivery Systems

Heather K. Lehman, MD
Assistant Professor of Pediatrics, Division of Allergy/Clinical Immunology
Department of Pediatrics
Women and Children's Hospital of Buffalo
SUNY Buffalo School of Medicine and Biomedical Sciences
Buffalo, New York, USA
Approach to the Patient with Recurrent Infections

Robert F. Lemanske, Jr., MD
Professor of Pediatrics and Medicine
Head, Division of Pediatric Allergy, Immunology, and Rheumatology
University of Wisconsin School of Medicine and Public Health
Madison, Wisconsin, USA
Diagnosis of Asthma in Infants and Children; Management of Asthma in Infants and Children

Catherine Lemière, MD, MSc
Professor, Department of Medicine
University of Montréal
Montréal, Québec, Canada
Occupational Allergy and Asthma

Donald Y.M. Leung, MD, PhD
Edelstein Family Chair of Pediatric Allergy and Immunology
National Jewish Health
Professor, Department of Pediatrics
University of Colorado School of Medicine
Denver, Colorado, USA
Atopic Dermatitis

Ian P. Lewkowich, PhD
Assistant Professor
Division of Cellular and Molecular Immunology
Cincinnati Children's Hospital Medical Center
Cincinnati, Ohio, USA
Mouse Models of Allergic Airways Disease

James T. Li, MD, PhD
Professor of Medicine
Division of Allergy and Immunology
Mayo Clinic
Rochester, Minnesota, USA
Immunoglobulin Structure and Function

Xiu-Min Li, MS, MD
Professor, Department of Pediatrics
Division of Allergy and Immunology
Mount Sinai School of Medicine
New York, New York, USA
Complementary and Alternative Medicine

Phillip L. Lieberman, MD
Clinical Professor of Allergy and Immunology
Departments of Medicine and Pediatrics
University of Tennessee College of Medicine
Memphis, Tennessee, USA
Anaphylaxis

Andrew H. Liu, MD
Professor, Allergy and Immunology
Department of Pediatrics
National Jewish Health
University of Colorado School of Medicine
Denver, Colorado, USA
Innate Immunity

Clare Lloyd, PhD
Wellcome Senior Research Fellow in Basic Biomedical Science
Professor of Respiratory Immunology
Head of Leukocyte Biology Section
National Heart and Lung Institute
Faculty of Medicine, Imperial College London
London, United Kingdom
Mouse Models of Allergic Airways Disease

Christopher D. Lucas, BSc, MBChB
Clinical Lecturer
Medical Research Council Centre for Inflammation Research
Queen's Medical Research Institute
University of Edinburgh
Edinburgh, United Kingdom
Resolution of Allergic Inflammation

Andrew D. Luster, MD, PhD
Persis, Cyrus, and Marlow B. Harrison Professor of Medicine
Harvard Medical School
Chief, Division of Rheumatology, Allergy, and Immunology
Director, Center for Immunology and Inflammatory Diseases
Massachusetts General Hospital
Boston, Massachusetts, USA
Chemokines

Eric Macy, MS, MD, FAAAAI
Partner Physician, Department of Allergy
Kaiser Permanente Medical Center
Assistant Clinical Professor of Medicine
University of California, San Diego
La Jolla, California, USA
Asthma and Allergic Diseases during Pregnancy

J. Mark Madison, MD
Professor of Medicine and Microbiology and Physiological Systems
Department of Medicine
University of Massachusetts Medical School
Worcester, Massachusetts, USA
Approach to the Patient with Chronic Cough

Elizabeth C. Matsui, MD, MHS
Associate Professor of Pediatrics, Epidemiology, and Environmental Health Sciences
Division of Pediatric Allergy and Immunology
Johns Hopkins University School of Medicine
Baltimore, Maryland, USA
Epidemiology of Asthma and Allergic Airway Diseases

Michael H. Mellon, MD
Associate Clinical Professor of Pediatrics
Department of Allergy
University of California, San Diego
La Jolla, California, USA
Kaiser Permanente Medical Center
San Diego, California, USA
Asthma and Allergic Diseases during Pregnancy

Dean D. Metcalfe, MD
Chief, Laboratory of Allergic Diseases
National Institute of Allergy and Infectious Diseases
National Institutes of Health
Bethesda, Maryland, USA
Mastocytosis

Zamaneh Mikhak, MD
Assistant Professor of Medicine
Harvard Medical School
Assistant in Immunology, Medicine, and Pediatrics
Center for Immunology and Inflammatory Diseases
Division of Rheumatology, Allergy, and Immunology
Massachusetts General Hospital
Boston, Massachusetts, USA
Chemokines

E.N. Clare Mills, PhD
Professor of Molecular Allergology
Institute of Inflammation and Repair
Manchetser Institute of Biotechnology
The University of Manchester
Manchester, United Kingdom
Effect of the Food Matrix and Processing on the Allergenic Activity of Foods

Harold S. Nelson, MD
Professor of Medicine
National Jewish Health
University of Colorado School of Medicine
Denver, Colorado, USA
Injection Immunotherapy for Inhalant Allergens

Sarah K. Nicholas, MD
Clinical Instructor, Department of Pediatrics
Section of Allergy and Immunology
Baylor College of Medicine
Houston, Texas, USA
Human Immunodeficiency Virus and Allergic Disease

Rosemary L. Nixon, MPH, FACD, FAFOEM
Adjunct Clinical Associate Professor
Monash University
Clinical Associate Professor
University of Melbourne
Director, Occupational Dermatology Research and Education Centre
Skin and Cancer Foundation
Melbourne, Victoria, Australia
Contact Dermatitis

Anna Nowak-Węgrzyn, MD
Associate Professor, Department of Pediatrics
Jaffe Food Allergy Institute
Icahn School of Medicine at Mount Sinai
New York, New York, USA
Reactions to Foods

Paul M. O'Byrne, MB, FRCP(C), FRSC
E.J. Moran Campbell Professor and Chair
Department of Medicine
Michael G. DeGroote School of Medicine
McMaster University
Hamilton, Ontario, Canada
Inhaled β_2-Agonists

Hans C. Oettgen, MD, PhD
Associate Chief, Division of Immunology
Boston Children's Hospital
Professor of Pediatrics
Harvard Medical School
Boston, Massachusetts, USA
Immunobiology of IgE and IgE Receptors

Robyn E. O'Hehir, FRACP, PhD, FRCPath
Professor and Director
Department of Allergy, Immunology, and Respiratory Medicine
Alfred Hospital and Monash University
Melbourne, Victoria, Australia
Allergic Bronchopulmonary Aspergillosis and Hypersensitivity Pneumonitis; Sublingual Immunotherapy for Inhalant Allergens

Brian G. Oliver, PhD
NHMRC Career Development Fellow
Discipline of Pharmacology
School of Medical Sciences and Woolcock Institute of Medical Research
The University of Sydney
Sydney, New South Wales, Australia
Noncontractile Functions of Airway Smooth Muscle

Jordan S. Orange, MD, PhD
Chief, Section of Immunology, Allergy, and Rheumatology
Director, Center for Human Immunobiology
Texas Children's Hospital
Professor of Pediatrics, Pathology, and Immunology
Baylor College of Medicine
Houston, Texas, USA
Primary Immunodeficiency Diseases

Dennis R. Ownby, MD
Betty B. Wray Professor of Pediatrics
Professor of Internal Medicine
Chief, Division of Allergy, Immunology, and Rheumatology
Department of Pediatrics
Georgia Regents University
Augusta, Georgia, USA
Clinical Significance of Immunoglobulin E

C.P. Page, PhD
Professor of Pharmacology
Sackler Institute of Pulmonary Pharmacology
Institute of Pharmaceutical Science
School of Biomedical Science
Kings College London
London, United Kingdom
Theophylline and Phosphodiesterase Inhibitors

Reynold A. Panettieri, Jr., MD
Professor of Medicine
Chief, Asthma Section
Pulmonary, Allergy, and Critical Care Division
Perelman School of Medicine at the University of Pennsylvania
Philadelphia, Pennsylvania, USA
Noncontractile Functions of Airway Smooth Muscle

Hae-Sim Park, MD, PhD
Professor, Department of Allergy and Clinical Immunology
Ajou University School of Medicine
Suwon, South Korea
Hypersensitivity to Aspirin and Other Nonsteroidal Antiinflammatory Drugs

Mary E. Paul, MD
Associate Professor of Pediatrics
Baylor College of Medicine
Chief of Service, Retrovirology and Global Health
Texas Children's Hospital
Houston, Texas, USA
Human Immunodeficiency Virus and Allergic Disease

Ian D. Pavord, DM, FRCP
Consultant Physician and Honorary Professor of Medicine
Department of Respiratory Medicine, Thoracic Surgery, and Allergy
University Hospitals of Leicester NHS Trust
Glenfield Hospital
Leicester, United Kingdom
Cytokine-Specific Therapy in Asthma

Ruby Pawankar, MD, PhD, FAAAAI
Professor, Division of Allergy
Department of Pediatrics
Nippon Medical School
Tokyo, Japan
Allergic and Nonallergic Rhinitis

David B. Peden, MD
Harry S. Andrews Distinguished Professor of Pediatrics
Associate Chair for Research and Chief, Division of Pediatric Allergy, Immunology, Rheumatology, and Infectious Diseases
Director, Center for Environmental Medicine, Asthma, and Lung Biology
Senior Associate Dean for Translational Research
University of North Carolina at Chapel Hill
Chapel Hill, North Carolina, USA
Air Pollution: Indoor and Outdoor

R. Stokes Peebles, Jr., MD
Elizabeth and John Murray Professor of Medicine
Division of Allergy, Pulmonary, and Critical Care Medicine
Vanderbilt University Medical Center
Nashville, Tennessee, USA
Lipid Mediators of Hypersensitivity and Inflammation

Stephen P. Peters, MD, PhD
Professor of Internal Medicine, Pediatrics, and Translational Science
Associate Director, Center for Genomics and Personalized Medicine Research
Winston-Salem, North Carolina, USA
Anticholinergic Therapies

Werner J. Pichler, MD
Professor of Internal Medicine
Head of Allergology
Department of Rheumatology, Clinical Immunology, and Allergology
Bern University Hospital
Bern, Switzerland
Drug Allergy

Mark R. Pittelkow, MD
Professor
Departments of Dermatology and Biochemistry and Molecular Biology
Mayo Medical School
Consultant and Professor
Department of Dermatology
Mayo Clinic College of Medicine
Rochester, Minnesota, USA
Structure of the Skin and Cutaneous Immunology

Douglas A. Plager, PhD
Research Scientist
Mayo Clinic College of Medicine
Rochester, Minnesota, USA
Structure of the Skin and Cutaneous Immunology

Thomas A.E. Platts-Mills, MD, PhD, FRS
Professor and Division Chief
Department of Internal Medicine
University of Virginia Health Science Center
Charlottesville, Virginia, USA
Indoor Allergens

Susan L. Prescott, PhD, MD
Winthrop Professor, School of Paediatrics and Child Health
University of Western Australia
Paediatric Allergist and Immunologist
Princess Margaret Hospital
Perth, Western Australia, Australia
Ontogeny of Immune Development and Its Relationship to Allergic Diseases and Asthma

Benjamin A. Raby, MD, MPH
Associate Professor of Medicine
Harvard Medical School
Channing Division of Network Medicine and Division of Pulmonary and Critical Care Medicine
Director, Pulmonary Genetics Center
Brigham and Women's Hospital
Boston, Massachusetts, USA
Pharmacogenomics of Asthma Therapies

Hengameh H. Raissy, PharmD
Research Associate Professor
Pediatric Pulmonary
University of New Mexico School of Medicine
Albuquerque, New Mexico, USA
Principles of Pharmacotherapeutics

Cynthia S. Rand, PhD
Professor of Medicine and Director
Johns Hopkins Adherence Research Center
Department of Pulmonary and Critical Care Medicine
Johns Hopkins University School of Medicine
Baltimore, Maryland, USA
Adherence

Anuradha Ray, PhD
Professor of Medicine and Immunology
Departments of Medicine and Immunology
University of Pittsburgh School of Medicine
Pittsburgh, Pennsylvania, USA
Biology of Lymphocytes

Harald Renz, MD
Professor and Director
Institute of Laboratory Medicine and Pathobiochemistry, Molecular Diagnostics
Philipps University Marburg
University Hospital Giessen and Marburg GmbH
Marburg, Germany
Respiratory Tract Mucosal Immunology

Jonathan P. Richardson, PhD
Researcher, Division of Biomedical Sciences
St George's University of London
London, United Kingdom
The Structure and Function of Allergens

Johannes Ring, MD, PhD
Professor
Director and Chairman, Center of Allergy and Environment
Christine Kühne–Center for Allergy Research and Education
Munich, Germany
Particulate and Pollen Interactions

Clive Robinson, PhD, FHEA, FSB
Professor of Respiratory Cell Science
Division of Biomedical Sciences
St. George's University of London
London, United Kingdom
The Structure and Function of Allergens

Duncan F. Rogers, PhD, FSB
Reader, Section of Airway Disease
National Heart & Lung Institute
Imperial College London
London, United Kingdom
Airway Mucus and the Mucociliary System

Lanny J. Rosenwasser, MD
Dee Lyons/Missouri Chair in Pediatric Immunology Research
Children's Mercy Hospital and Clinics
Professor of Medicine and Pediatrics
University of Missouri–Kansas City School of Medicine
Kansas City, Missouri, USA
Cytokines in Allergic Inflammation

Adriano G. Rossi, BSc, PhD, DSc
Professor of Respiratory and Inflammation Pharmacology
Medical Research Council Centre for Inflammation Research
Queen's Medical Research Institute
University of Edinburgh
Edinburgh, United Kingdom
Resolution of Allergic Inflammation

Marc E. Rothenberg, MD, PhD
Professor of Pediatrics
Director, Division of Allergy and Immunology
Director, Cincinnati Center for Eosinophilic Disorders
Cincinnati Children's Hospital Medical Center
Cincinnati, Ohio, USA
Eosinophilic Gastrointestinal Disorders

Brian H. Rowe, MD, MSc, CCFP(EM)
Associate Dean, Clinical Research
Faculty of Medicine and Dentistry
Tier I Canada Research Chair in Evidence-Based Emergency Medicine
Professor, Department of Emergency Medicine
University of Alberta
Edmonton, Alberta, Canada
Emergency Treatment and Approach to the Patient with Acute Asthma

Sejal Saglani, MD
Clinical Senior Lecturer and Honorary Consultant
Leukocyte Biology and Respiratory Paediatrics
Imperial College London
London, United Kingdom
Mouse Models of Allergic Airways Disease

Sarbjit S. Saini, MD
Associate Professor of Medicine
Division of Allergy and Clinical Immunology
Johns Hopkins University School of Medicine
Baltimore, Maryland, USA
Urticaria and Angioedema

Hirohisa Saito, MD, PhD
Deputy Director
National Research Institute for Child Health and Development
Tokyo, Japan
Biology of Mast Cells and Their Mediators

Hugh A. Sampson, MD
Professor, Department of Pediatrics
Dean for Translational Biomedical Sciences
Icahn School of Medicine at Mount Sinai
New York, New York, USA
Reactions to Foods

Mario Sanchez-Borges, MD
Allergy and Clinical Immunology Department
Centro Medico–Docente La Trinidad
Caracas, Venezuela
Hypersensitivity to Aspirin and Other Nonsteroidal Antiinflammatory Drugs

Alessandra Sandrini, MD, PhD
Senior Clinical Fellow and Adjunct Senior Lecturer
Department of Allergy, Immunology, and Respiratory Medicine, and Department of Medicine
The Alfred Hospital and Monash University
Melbourne, Victoria, Australia
Allergic Bronchopulmonary Aspergillosis and Hypersensitivity Pneumonitis; Sublingual Immunotherapy for Inhalant Allergens

Guy W. Scadding, MA, MRCP
Clinical Research Fellow
Department of Allergy and Clinical Immunology
Imperial College London
London, United Kingdom
Nasal Provocation Testing

Michael Schatz, MD, MS
Staff Allergist, Department of Allergy
Kaiser Permanente Medical Center
San Diego, California, USA
Asthma and Allergic Diseases during Pregnancy

John T. Schroeder, PhD
Associate Professor of Medicine
Division of Allergy and Clinical Immunology
Johns Hopkins University School of Medicine
Baltimore, Maryland, USA
Biology of Basophils

Malcolm R. Sears, MB, FRACP, FRCPC
Professor and AstraZeneca Chair in Respiratory Epidemiology
Division of Respirology, Department of Medicine
Michael G. DeGroote School of Medicine
McMaster University
Hamilton, Ontario, Canada
Inhaled β_2-Agonists

Christine Seroogy, MD, FAAAAI
Associate Professor, Department of Pediatrics
University of Wisconsin
Madison, Wisconsin, USA
Ontogeny of Immune Development and Its Relationship to Allergic Diseases and Asthma

William T. Shearer, MD, PhD
Professor of Pediatrics and Immunology
Baylor College of Medicine
Member, Allergy and Immunology Service
Texas Children's Hospital
Houston, Texas, USA
Adaptive Immunity; Human Immunodeficiency Virus and Allergic Disease

James H. Shelhamer, MD
Deputy Chief and Senior Investigator
Critical Care Medicine Department, Clinical Center
National Institutes of Health
Bethesda, Maryland, USA
Immunologic Nonasthmatic Diseases of the Lung

Scott H. Sicherer, MD
Clinical Professor of Pediatrics
Chief, Division of Allergy and Immunology
Jaffe Food Allergy Institute
Department of Pediatrics
Mount Sinai School of Medicine
New York, New York, USA
Food Allergy Management

F. Estelle R. Simons, MD, FRCPC
Professor, Department of Pediatrics
Department of Immunology
University of Manitoba
Winnipeg, Manitoba, Canada
Histamine and H_1 Antihistamines

Jodie L. Simpson, PhD
Senior Research Fellow
Department of Respiratory and Sleep Medicine
School of Medicine and Public Health
The University of Newcastle
Newcastle, New South Wales, Australia
Biology of Neutrophils

Jay E. Slater, MD
Director, Division of Bacterial, Parasitic, and Allergenic Products
Office of Vaccines Research and Review
Center for Biologics Evaluation and Research
U.S. Food and Drug Administration
Rockville, Maryland, USA
Preparation and Standardization of Allergen Extracts

Peter D. Sly, MBBS, MD, DSc
Deputy Director
Queensland Children's Medical Research Institute
The University of Queensland
Brisbane, Queensland, Australia
Asthma Pathogenesis

Philip H. Smith, MD
Associate Professor, Pediatrics and Medicine, Division of Allergy and Immunology
Departments of Pediatrics and Medicine
Medical College of Georgia
Children's Hospital of Georgia
Georgia Regents University
Charlie Norwood Veterans Administration Medical Center
Augusta, Georgia, USA
Clinical Significance of Immunoglobulin E

Michael C. Sneller, MD
Medical Officer, Laboratory of Immunoregulation
National Institute of Allergy and Infectious Diseases
National Institutes of Health
Bethesda, Maryland, USA
Immunologic Nonasthmatic Diseases of the Lung

Domenico Spina, PhD
Reader in Pharmacology
Sackler Institute of Pulmonary Pharmacology
School of Biomedical Science
Kings College London
London, United Kingdom
Theophylline and Phosphodiesterase Inhibitors

P. Sriramarao, PhD
Professor and Associate Dean for Research
Department of Veterinary and Biomedical Sciences, and Division of Pulmonary, Allergy, Critical Care, and Sleep Medicine
Department of Medicine
University of Minnesota
St. Paul, Minnesota, USA
Cellular Adhesion in Inflammation

James L. Stahl, MS, PhD
Senior Scientist
Department of Ophthalmology and Visual Sciences
University of Wisconsin School of Medicine and Public Health
Madison, Wisconsin, USA
Allergic and Immunologic Diseases of the Eye

John W. Steinke, PhD
Associate Professor, Department of Medicine
Asthma and Allergic Diseases Center
Carter Center for Immunology Research
University of Virginia
Charlottesville, Virginia, USA
Cytokines in Allergic Inflammation

Geoffrey A. Stewart, BSC, PhD
Winthrop Professor
School of Pathology and Laboratory Medicine
The University of Western Australia
Perth, Western Australia, Australia
The Structure and Function of Allergens

Jeffrey R. Stokes, MD
Associate Professor of Medicine
Department of Medicine
Program Director, Allergy/Immunology
Creighton University
Omaha, Nebraska, USA
Anti-Immunoglobulin E Therapy

Kathleen E. Sullivan, MD, PhD
Professor of Pediatrics
The Children's Hospital of Philadelphia
Perelman School of Medicine at the University of Pennsylvania
Philadelphia, Pennsylvania, USA
The Complement System

Steve L. Taylor, PhD
Professor
Department of Food Science and Technology, Food Allergy Research, and Resource Program
University of Nebraska
Lincoln, Nebraska, USA
Reactions to Food and Drug Additives

Abba I. Terr, MD
Clinical Professor, Department of Medicine
University of California San Francisco Medical Center
San Francisco, California, USA
Unconventional Theories and Unproven Methods in Allergy

Euan Tovey, MSc, PhD
Associate Professor and Principal Research Fellow
Woolcock Institute of Medical Research
Sydney Medical School
University of Sydney
Sydney, New South Wales, Australia
Allergen Control for Prevention and Management of Allergic Diseases

Thai Tran, BSc(Hons), PhD
Assistant Professor
Department of Physiology
Yong Loo Lin School of Medicine
National University of Singapore
Singapore
Airway Smooth Muscle Function in Asthma: Extracellular Matrix and Airway Remodeling

Bradley J. Undem, PhD
Professor of Medicine, Department of Medicine
Division of Allergy and Clinical Immunology
Johns Hopkins University School of Medicine
Baltimore, Maryland, USA
Neuronal Control of Airway Function in Allergy

Peter Valent, MD
Professor
Department of Internal Medicine I
Division of Hematology and Hemostaseology
Scientific Director
Ludwig Boltzmann Cluster Oncology
Medical University of Vienna
Vienna, Austria
Appendix A: CD Molecules

Olivier Vandenplas, MD, PhD
Professor of Medicine
Department of Chest Medicine
Centre Hospitalier Universitaire de Mont-Godinne
Université Catholique de Louvain
Yvoir, Belgium
Occupational Allergy and Asthma

Stephan von Gunten, MD, PhD, MME
Research Group Leader
Institute of Pharmacology
University of Bern
Bern, Switzerland
Appendix A: CD Molecules

Richard W. Weber, MD
Professor of Medicine
National Jewish Health
University of Colorado School of Medicine
Denver, Colorado, USA
Aerobiology of Outdoor Allergens

Peter F. Weller, MD, FACP, FAAAAI
Professor of Medicine
Harvard Medical School
Professor of Immunology and Infectious Diseases
Harvard School of Public Health
Chief, Allergy and Inflammation Division
Chief, Infectious Diseases Division, Department of Medicine
Beth Israel Deaconess Medical Center
Boston, Massachusetts, USA
Eosinophilia and Eosinophil-Related Disorders

Sally E. Wenzel, MD
Professor of Medicine and Director
Pulmonary, Allergy, and Critical Care Medicine Division
University of Pittsburgh Asthma Institute at University of Pittsburgh Medical Center
Pittsburgh, Pennsylvania, USA
Antileukotriene Therapy in Asthma

Gregory J. Wiepz, PhD
Scientist
Department of Biomolecular Chemistry
University of Wisconsin
Madison, Wisconsin, USA
Signal Transduction

Marsha Wills-Karp, PhD
Professor of Environmental Health Sciences
Department of Environmental Health Sciences
Johns Hopkins Bloomberg School of Public Health
Baltimore, Maryland, USA
Mouse Models of Allergic Airways Disease

Robert A. Wood, MD
Professor of Pediatrics
Director, Pediatric Allergy and Immunology
Johns Hopkins University School of Medicine
Johns Hopkins Hospital
Baltimore, Maryland, USA
Oral Food Challenge Testing

Leman Yel, MD, FAAP, FAAAAI
Global Medical Director
Baxter Biosciences, Westlake Village
Emeritus Associate Professor of Clinical Medicine
Division of Basic and Clinical Immunology, Department of Medicine
University of California, Irvine
Irvine, California, USA
Molecular Biology and Genetic Engineering

Robert S. Zeiger, MD, PhD
Clinical Professor, Department of Pediatrics
University of California, San Diego
La Jolla, California, USA
Adjunct Physician Investigator
Kaiser Permanente Medical Center
San Diego, California, USA
Asthma and Allergic Diseases during Pregnancy

Jihui Zhang, PhD
Biological Project Manager
Drug Discovery Program
Division of Biomedical Sciences
St George's University of London
London, United Kingdom
The Structure and Function of Allergens

Bruce L. Zuraw, MD
Professor of Medicine
Department of Medicine
University of California, San Diego
Veterans Affairs San Diego Healthcare
La Jolla, California, USA
Hereditary Angioedema and Bradykinin-Mediated Angioedema

Withdrawn

SECTION F

Gastrointestinal Tract

67

Gastrointestinal Mucosal Immunology

M. CECILIA BERIN | GLENN T. FURUTA | SEEMA S. ACEVES

CONTENTS

SUMMARY OF IMPORTANT CONCEPTS

» Functions of the gastrointestinal tract include motility, immunologic regulation, and nutrient absorption.
» Gastrointestinal mucosal immunity is essential for tolerance and immune regulation to commensal and pathogenic microbiota.
» Symbiotic interactions between the GI immune system and the microbiome are required for proper GI mucosal development and function.
» Mucosal immunity comprises inductive and effector arms that involve both innate and adaptive immunity.
» Inductive sites include intraepithelial lymphocytes, lamina propria immune cells, Peyer patches, and mesenteric lymph nodes.
» The effector arm of mucosal immunity includes antimicrobial peptides, mast cells, phagocytes, cytotoxic and helper T cells, and B cells that produce neutralizing antibodies.

Introduction

The gastrointestinal (GI) tract has the unique characteristic of being the largest organ exposed to external antigens (Fig. 67-1). It is multifunctional and serves as a mucosal barrier, an absorptive surface, and a site of active immunity to foreign antigens. The normal structural and functional components of the gastrointestinal immune system are the focus of this chapter. From the protective layer of mucus to the specialized mucosal epithelium and the deeper immune aggregates, the GI tract requires precise regulation to balance immune reactions against foreign antigens while fostering the symbiotic, commensal microbiota. The innate and adaptive immune systems act in concert to hold the GI mucosal immune system in a state of tolerance to benign antigens while maintaining an appropriate capacity to respond to pathogenic insults.

Gastrointestinal Structure and Function

ESOPHAGUS

The esophagus functions as a muscular tube that coordinates food transit from the oral cavity to the stomach. The upper esophageal sphincter is the proximal boundary and the lower esophageal sphincter the distal boundary. After the mouth, the esophageal mucosa is the next mucosal barrier to contact antigens. Contact time is typically less than 10 seconds, but the exposure may be significant because foods have not undergone any digestive processing. The normal esophagus contains a baseline number of T cells and dendritic cells that likely participate in health and disease states.

Esophageal Development

The esophagus begins its development at human embryonic week 4 as a diverticulum of the primitive foregut that subsequently splits into the esophagus and trachea through the formation of the esophagotracheal septum. Although initially a ciliated epithelium, the esophageal epithelium loses its cilia and develops into a nonkeratinized, stratified squamous epithelium, a process that continues through birth.[1] Whereas the smooth muscle of the upper esophagus is derived from branchial arches 4, 5, and 6, the origin of the lower esophageal smooth muscle is from the mesenchyme and somites of the foregut. This derivation of the upper esophagus from branchial arches explains its innervation by the vagal and recurrent laryngeal nerves.

There is an intimate link between the mechanisms governing respiratory tract and esophageal development such that proper development of one is reliant on the other. Overactivation of β-catenin and its canonical downstream Wnt signaling pathway increases the abundant respiratory epithelium at the expense of esophageal mucosal development. Mutations in the sonic hedgehog, Wnt, and bmp-4 pathways result in a lack of adequate esophagotracheal separation and the presence of a resultant tracheoesophageal fistula. Mutations in a homeobox gene *Barx1* cause a radially mixed population of respiratory and esophageal cells (mucosa), with columnar ciliated epithelium on one surface and squamous epithelium on the other.[2]

Epithelium and Lamina Propria

Luminal regions of the human esophagus are composed of nonkeratinized squamous epithelium. This epithelium protects the body from swallowed materials as well as acid. Esophageal submucosal glands secrete bicarbonate and mucus, which augments these functions. Salivary mucins (e.g., MUC5b) are water soluble, thereby providing lubrication but not a viscoelastic protective barrier.[3]

The epithelium is composed of the stratum basale, which abuts the lamina propria and provides a constant renewal source of luminal epithelial cells; the stratum intermedium;

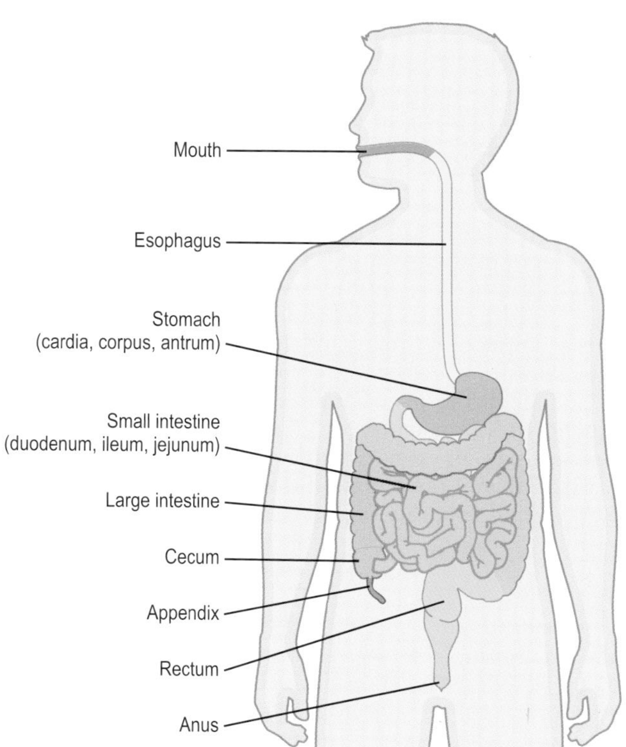

Figure 67-1 Overview of gastrointestinal organs.

and the stratum superficialis. Esophageal epithelial cells utilize desmosomes, adherens junctions, and tight junctions for intercellular attachment and to control intercellular permeability. Tight junction proteins belong to the families of claudins, occludins, and junctional adhesion molecules. Tight junction proteins such as zonula occludins protein 1 (zo-1) perform the additional function of linking claudins and occludins to the actin cytoskeleton. E-cadherin is a component of the adherens junction, which surrounds cell membranes and supports adhesion of tight junction proteins. Junctional proteins that are expressed in normal esophageal mucosae include claudins 1, 4, and 7.[4] Superficial cell layers express claudins 1 and 4, occludin, and zo-1, whereas intermediate and suprabasal layers express claudins 1 and 4 and occludin.[5] Functional loss of E-cadherin leads to decreased esophageal epithelial integrity and increased permeability.[6,7]

The lamina propria (LP) lies beneath the epithelium and is normally made up of a nonfibrotic, reticular network connecting the epithelium to the muscularis mucosa. Whereas the normal esophageal epithelium is usually devoid of eosinophils, the LP contains T and B cells, eosinophils, and mast cells.[8-10] In addition, lymphoid aggregates exist within the LP of the esophagus, but their role in antigen presentation and tolerance is unclear. Projections of the LP into the epidermal space are known as vascular papillae and can increase the contact surface area between the basal zone and the epithelium.

Esophageal Muscle

The most superficial layer of esophageal smooth muscle is the muscularis mucosa. The muscularis mucosal layer thickens from the proximal to the distal esophagus. The outer esophageal muscle layer, the muscularis propria, comprises two layers. Longitudinally oriented muscle fibers are external and concentric muscle fibers are internal. Actions of the proximal esophagus are coordinated by striated muscle, whereas actions of the mid- and distal esophagus are coordinated by smooth muscle.

STOMACH

The stomach is composed of at least three anatomically distinct sections—cardia, body (corpus, fundus), and antrum—each designed to initiate a stage of digestion. The stomach's primary function is to prepare ingested food products for digestion and absorption that will occur in the small intestine. This highly regulated function is a result of three closely related processes controlled by hormonal and neural mediators. The stomach initially acts mechanically and biochemically to disrupt large pieces of food and serves as a reservoir for residual *chyme,* the semisolid mass of partially digested foodstuffs. In a highly regulated manner, the stomach releases chyme into the small intestine.

Gastric Development

As with the esophagus, the stomach originates from the foregut, and by 20 weeks of development a fetus has a stomach comparable in appearance that of a term infant.[11] Acid-secreting parietal cells are functional as early as 19 weeks. Intrinsic factor is present by 12 weeks and pepsin by 21 weeks.

Cardia

The gastric cardia consists of a narrow strip of cells immediately distal to the gastroesophageal junction. Epithelia are primarily composed of mucous cells, thought to protect the esophagus from gastric acidity.

Corpus (Body or Fundus)

The corpus, which encompasses most of the stomach's surface area, participates in the mechanical breakdown of food through churning actions of rugal folds and in the biochemical breakdown initiated by secretion of acid and pepsin. A layer of secreted molecules that includes mucus, trefoil factors, bicarbonate, acid, defensins, and prostaglandins protects epithelial surfaces. The cellular interface is composed of columnar epithelia and a series of tightly packed tubular glands that contain acid-secreting parietal cells and pepsin-secreting chief cells. Underlying the epithelia are cells and molecules that form the structural and metabolic framework integral in supporting mucosal integrity. Resident cells include lymphocytes, endothelia, fibroblasts, myocytes, nerve cells, and a scattering of eosinophils. Distinctly absent are neutrophils. Structural features include a matrix of collagen intertwined between these resident cells.

Antrum

The remainder of the stomach is composed of the antrum; a smooth surface located just after the gastric body and just before the pyloricos. The antrum participates in two highly coordinated activities. First, it functions as a reservoir for chyme that has completed its initial digestive process in the gastric body. Second, in a highly regulated manner, the antrum releases chyme into the small intestine, where it will complete digestive and absorptive processes. To facilitate this process, the antrum contains a series of glands composed of mucous and endocrine cells.

TABLE 67-1 Structural Cells and Functions of Gastrointestinal Tract

Location	Structural Cells	Functions
Esophagus	Squamous epithelial cells	Motility Barrier
Cardia	Columnar epithelial cells Mucous cells Chief cells	Barrier Acid protection
Corpus (body, fundus)	Columnar epithelial cells D cells Chief cells	Mechanical food breakdown Acid and pepsin secretion
Antrum	Columnar epithelial cells Goblet cells Enterochromaffin cells Parietal (oxyntic) cells Chief cells D cells Mucous folveolar (pit) cells Chief cells	Complete digestion Chyme reservoir and release Mucus secretion Acid secretion Histamine release Prostaglandin E_2 secretion Pepsinogen secretion
Small Intestine	Absorptive columnar cells D cells Chief cells M cells Intraepithelial lymphocytes Goblet cells Crypt stem cells Paneth cells	Digestion Absorption Antigen processing and presentation
Colon	Columnar epithelial cells Crypt cells Goblet cells Endocrine cells Stem cells	Water absorption

RESIDENT CELLS

In addition to the columnar epithelia, GI mucosal surfaces are composed of various surface cells, including goblet, enterochromaffin, parietal, and chief cells (Table 67-1).

Parietal (Oxyntic) Cells

Parietal cells produce acid through the hydrogen-ATPase pump located in tubulovesicles near the apical surface of the cell. Three stimulatory and one inhibitory receptor are present on the basal surface of parietal cells. Muscarinic (M3) receptors are stimulated by parasympathetic vagal nerve–derived acetylcholine. Cholecystokinin (CCKB) receptors are stimulated by gastrin that is released from duodenal G cells following exposure to protein. Finally, gastrin and acetylcholine can stimulate production and release of histamine from enterochromaffin-like (ECL) cells. The end product of stimulation of these receptors is activation of the hydrogen-ATPase pump, leading to acid secretion and an intraluminal gastric pH of 2. The superiority of hydrogen-ATPase pump inhibitors (proton pump inhibitors) becomes clear because antagonism of all three stimulatory receptors on the basal surface would be required to inhibit acid secretion completely. Prostaglandin E_2 receptors are inhibitory to proton secretion. These receptors are stimulated by somatostatin that is produced by D cells located in the corpus, antral, and small intestinal mucosa. Whether or not lack of acid contributes to allergic diseases has not been determined, but some evidence suggests that host sensitization to specific food proteins may be increased in the absence of acid.[12]

Mucous Foveolar (Pit) Cells

Mucous cells continually secrete mucus that functions as a mechanical barrier, antimicrobial shield, and lubrication for foods. Mucus contains a number of structurally distinct glycoproteins, antimicrobial peptides, bicarbonate, and water that function to form a distinct separation of luminal contents from epithelial surface. Estimates in murine systems suggest that the thickness of mucus ranges from 100 to 200 μm. Whereas acetylcholine is the primary physiologic stimulant of mucus production, secretin and prostaglandins also can also stimulate secretion. Acid does not break down mucus, but pepsin, bile salts, ethanol, and nonsteroidal antiinflammatory drugs (NSAIDs) can penetrate the mucosal layer and cause mucosal injury.

Chief Cells

The primary function of chief cells is the synthesis and release of the proenzyme *pepsinogen.* Located throughout the gastric mucosa, as well as duodenum, chief cells produce pepsinogen in response to stimulation by acetylcholine, histamine, or cholecystekinin. Acid cleaves N-terminal amino acid sequences, which leaves the active enzyme pepsin to initiate protein digestion.

SMALL INTESTINE

The small intestine represents the largest portion of the GI tract. The small intestine's surface area, which is amplified by folds, villi and microvilli, is approximately the size of a tennis court. Its length, ranging from 6 to 10 m (20 to 30 ft), is separated from the stomach and colon by two sphincters, the pylorus and ileocecal valve. Each part of the intestinal tract represents a well-defined and anatomically separated microenvironment that functions to isolate digestive and immune processes and allow them to occur sequentially.

The small intestine consists of three components: the duodenum, jejunum, and ileum. The term *duodenum* refers to its length of 12 fingerbreadths, or about 25 cm (10 inches). The ampula of Vater enters the duodenum and brings the rich enzymatic contents of both the pancreas and the liver. Although the dividing point between the jejunum and ileum is not clear, morphologic features help distinguish these two sections. Compared with the ileum, the jejunum is thicker and contains larger folds *(valvulae conniventes)* that are thought to increase its absorptive surface. The ileum contains Peyer patches (PPs) and isolated lymphoid follicles (ILFs), which are the preferential site for antigen uptake (see later discussion on adaptive immunity).

Digestion and *absorption* are the most recognized functions of the small intestine. Release of pancreatic enzymes and bile into the small intestinal lumen initiates protein, carbohydrate, and fat absorption. In addition, minerals and vitamins are absorbed here through a number of well-defined transport systems. Whether deficiencies or excesses of these digestive processes are linked to allergic diatheses has not been determined.

The other major function of the small intestine is presentation and processing of antigenic material. It is uncertain how

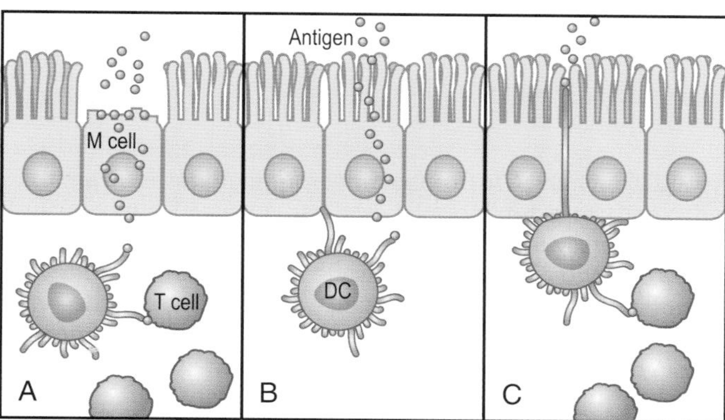

Figure 67-2 Uptake of antigens across epithelial surface. Antigens can cross the epithelial surface by at least three routes: **A,** passage through the M cells that overlie Peyer patches; **B,** transcellularly; or **C,** paracellularly through epithelia to underlying T cells or macrophages; and capture by dendritic cell (*DC*) processes that extend between epithelial cells.

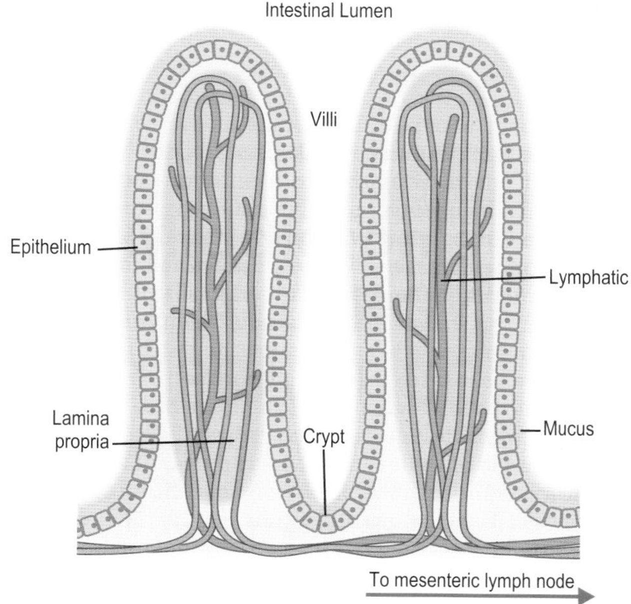

Figure 67-3 Lymphatic structures in the intestinal mucosa. Lymphatic vessels in the subepithelial space transport cells and mediators that regulate immunologic function.

the system defines which antigens will adhere to the apical epithelial surface and undergo processing. The following sections describe processes that define how mucosal surfaces are innately protected from and actively respond to antigens.

Mucosal surfaces are composed of villi and crypts (crypts of Lieberkuhn), which are spaced adjacent to each other with a 3:1 ratio of length (villi/crypt). The bulk of epithelia present on villous surfaces comprise absorptive columnar cells. Goblet cells, intraepithelial lymphocytes, and endocrine cells are also present. Crypts are also lined with stem cells, endocrine cells, and Paneth cells that serve to renew the villous epithelia and maintain epithelial health. Overlying lymphoid follicles and PPs is a single layer of columnar cells termed the follicle-associated epithelium (FAE). Centrally located within the FAE are specialized microfold (M) cells. M cells are different from absorptive epithelia; they do not contain microvilli or membrane-associated hydrolytic enzymes and contain less glycocalyx. M cells contain a characteristic feature, the invaginated subdomain within the basolateral membrane that forms an intraepithelial "pocket," which is thought to function in antigen processing and presentation (Fig. 67-2).

Underlying the epithelium is a robust set of immune cells, including lymphocytes, eosinophils, and mast cells. The submucosa is equipped with an efficient blood supply from the celiac and superior mesenteric arteries, venous drainage to the inferior vena cava, and a lymphatic system through the celiac and mesenteric nodes that permits communications with other mucosal surfaces (Figs. 67-3 and 67-4).

Development

The duodenum arises from the foregut, which by 20 weeks of age has well-developed villi and crypts and is structurally mature. The remainder of the small intestine arises from the midgut.[13]

COLON

The colon is derived from the midgut and hindgut. As with the rest of the GI tract, the colon begins and ends with a clearly demarcated boundaries; the proximal end begins with the ileocecal valve, and the distal side ends at the anal sphincter. The colon reaches a length of 1.5 m in adults and is divided into the cecum; ascending, transverse, descending, and sigmoid colon; and rectum.

The colon's primary function is to absorb water so that a formed stool can be expelled. With a remarkable absorptive capacity, the colon receives more than 1.5 L of fluid daily from the small intestine and excretes an average of 200 mL of excrement daily. In addition, the colon harbors the bulk of the intestinal microbiome. Bacteria ferment remaining stool components, and acetate, proprionate, and butyrate are created as byproducts.

Absorptive columnar epithelial cells line mucosal surfaces and are interspersed by crypts that contain goblet, endocrine, and stem cells. A layer of secreted molecules that includes mucus, trefoil factors and defensins protect epithelial surfaces. As in the rest of the GI tract, underlying cells and molecules form structural and metabolic frameworks integral to supporting mucosal integrity. Other cells include lymphocytes, endothelia, fibroblasts myocytes, endothelia, nerve cells, mast cells and a scattering of eosinophils. Neutrophils are distinctly absent.

Organization of Gastrointestinal Immune Tissue

The digestive tract mucosa from mouth to anus is variably populated with cells that participate in innate and adaptive immunity against foreign antigens. The mucosal immune system comprises intraepithelial lymphocytes, a dense population of resident immune cells in the LP, as well as organized lymphoid structures such as PPs, ILFs, and mesenteric lymph nodes that drain the small and large intestine (Fig. 67-4). The mucosal immune system can be further divided into effector

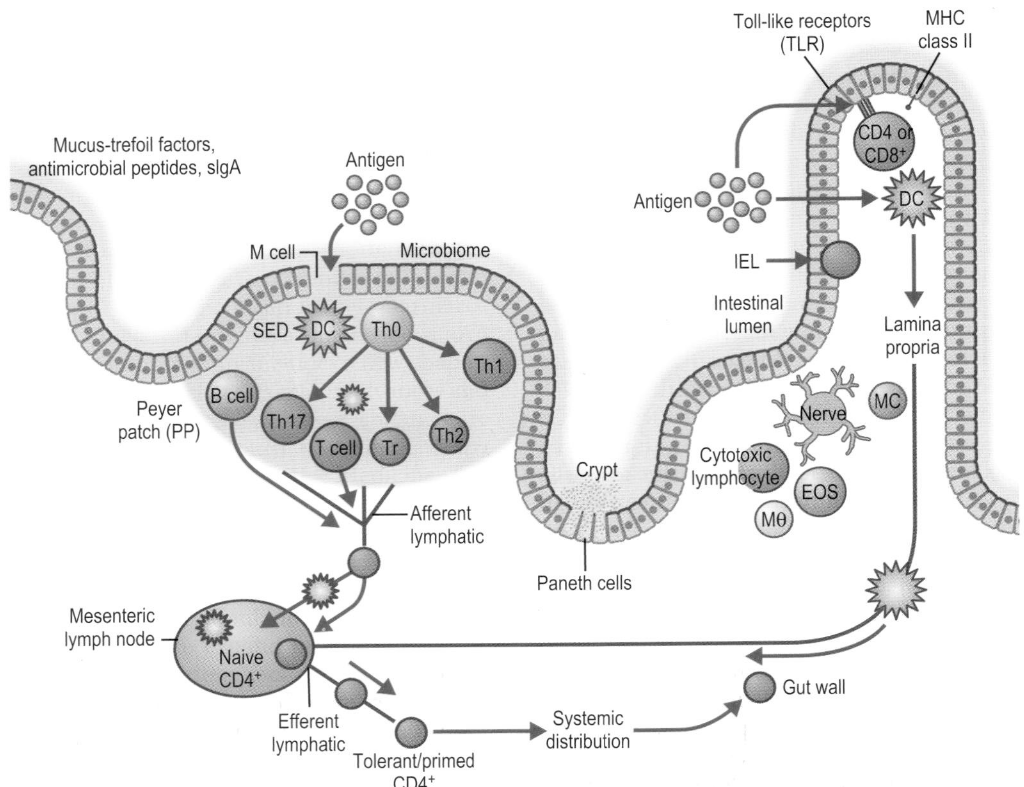

Figure 67-4 Intestinal mucosa overview. The epithelial surface is exposed to an abundant and diverse microbiome. To protect itself, it is coated with mucus that contains trefoil proteins, secretory IgA, and antimicrobial peptides. Antigens may pass through the epithelial surface and undergo processing in Peyer patches. Within the subepithelial dome *(SED)* reside a number of lymphocytes, including natural helper T (Th0) cells, which can differentiate into type 1 (Th1), type 2 (Th2), regulatory (Treg), or Th17 cells. Other resident cells include macrophages, cytotoxic lymphocytes, mast cells (*MC*), eosinophils (*EOS*), and dendritic cells (*DC*). *IEL,* Intraepithelial lymphocytes; *MHC,* major histocompatibility complex. *(Modified from Atkins D, Furuta GT. Mucosal immunology, eosinophilic esophagitis, and other intestinal inflammatory diseases. J Allergy Clin Immunol 2010;125[Suppl. 2]:255-61.)*

and inductive sites. The resident population of cells forms the effector arm of the mucosal immune system and comprises phagocytes that engulf and kill microbes; cytotoxic T cells that kill infected cells, B cells that produce neutralizing antibodies, and helper T cells that support these effector functions through production of cytokines.

Inductive sites of the GI tract are organized lymphoid structures that bring together naïve T cells, B cells, and antigen-presenting cells. These include the draining lymph nodes and specialized lymphoid structures within the GI mucosa. The latter include PPs in the small intestine and structurally similar lymphoid tissues in the rectum, as well as smaller ILFs and *cryptopatches* (precursor to intestinal lymphoid follicles) scattered throughout the intestine. After activation in these organized tissues, antigen-specific T and B cells hone in on effector sites of the GI mucosa.

Innate Immunity in Gastrointestinal Tract

The normal flora of the GI tract varies from mouth to anus. The oral cavity contains primarily streptococci. The stomach is largely sterile, as is the proximal small intestine. In contrast, the terminal ileum and colon contain about 10^{14} resident bacterial flora, representing more than 1000 species of anaerobes and aerobes. Close interactions between the microflora and the innate and adaptive immune systems forms a system of checks and balances for GI mucosal immune homeostasis.

ANTIMICROBIAL PEPTIDES

The innate immune system provides a functional host defense barrier and a bridge to the adaptive immune system. In the esophagus the first protective barrier is the mucous layer of mucin-2 and glycoproteins.[14] Goblet cells produce trefoil factors (TFFs) that are secreted into the mucous layer and are critical for immune defense and epithelial barrier function. TFFs are protease-resistant peptides throughout the GI tract that promote epithelial cell survival and migration. In multiple models of mucosal injury, recombinant TFF therapy can decrease the severity of epithelial injury and decrease the time to epithelial reconstitution.[15] The small intestine contains a mucous layer capable of neutralizing acid by actively secreting bicarbonate. In the small intestine the mucous layer contains both secretory immunoglobulin (sIgA) and antimicrobial peptides. Mucins play an important role in normal intestinal immune regulation, and mucin-2 deficiency causes spontaneous inflammation and cancer in murine models.[16,17]

In the GI tract, antimicrobial peptides help balance the appropriate bacterial load and diversity while controlling bacterial translocation. The small-molecule families of defensins (α and β), cathelicidins, and cryptidins are composed of antimicrobial peptides with bactericidal capacity. The defensin family includes human β-defensins (HBD) 1 and 2. The α-defensins comprise human neutrophil peptides (HNP) 1 to 6 and the cryptidins 1 to 6. Human LL-37 (cathelicidin) is another small antimicrobial peptide.

The α- and β-defensins and cathelicidins are normally expressed in the intestinal and colonic epithelial mucosa as well as in intestinal leukocytes. The significant difference in normal bacterial flora from mouth to anus is reflective of and maintained by the antibacterial spectrum of the antimicrobial peptides. HBD3 is expressed in the esophagus and oral cavity. HBD4 is expressed in the gastric antrum. Paneth cells express the α-defensins HD5 and HD6 as well as the antimicrobial enzymes phospholipase A_2 and lysozyme.[18] Generally, β-defensins are expressed throughout the intestine by epithelial cells. HBD1 is expressed in the epithelial cells of multiple gastrointestinal locations, including the small intestine and colon. In contrast, HBD2 is expressed only at low levels at baseline in the small intestine but can be upregulated in both the intestine and the stomach during inflammatory states. Normal human colonic mucosa expresses LL-37, and cathelicidin expression increases in response to bacterial CpG motifs.[19] Cryptidin 4, which has antibacterial activity against *Escherichia coli*, is not expressed in the small intestine but is expressed at high levels in the colon consistent with bacterial load being higher in the colon.

The importance of antimicrobial peptides in host defense has been shown by experimentally modulating their expression. For example, mice functionally deficient in Paneth cell α-defensins are susceptible to *Salmonella* infection, whereas transgenic expression of human defensin HD5 in mice is protective against *Salmonella* infection compared with wild-type littermate controls.[20,21] In addition to having antibacterial properties, the defensins and cathelicidins have chemotactic properties for neutrophils, dendritic cells, and memory T cells.[18,22,23]

TOLL-LIKE RECEPTORS AND NOD-LIKE RECEPTORS

Toll-like receptors (TLRs) were first characterized in the fruit fly *Drosophila melanogaster* as innate immune system, interleukin-1 (IL-1)–like receptors. Human TLRs 1 to 9 have since been well characterized. TLRs 1, 2, 4, 5, 6 are expressed on the cell surface. TLRs 3, 7, 8, 9 are expressed intracellularly and have ligands that are similar to host antigens and require endosomal internalization. TLRs and their signaling pathways are important for mucosal homeostasis and limit the penetration of commensal microbiota into the intestine and associated lymph nodes.[17] Generally, in healthy adults, TLRs are expressed ubiquitously in myeloid cells, leukocytes and epithelium.[24] However, in the gut, where the microflora is dense and diverse, TLR expression is regulated to avoid immune overreaction and to maintain GI homeostasis. TLR3 and TLR5 are expressed in intestinal epithelial cells. TLR2 and TLR4 are not typically expressed in the esophagus or small intestine, but both can be induced during disease states.[24,25]

As with the TLRs, the Nod-like receptors (NLRs) are pattern recognition receptors in the GI tract. They respond to bacterial and endogenous pathogen and damage-associated molecular patterns. Nod1 and Nod2 are cytosolic receptors that detect muropeptides derived from bacterial peptidoglycan and play a role in shaping the innate immune system, controlling the microflora and protecting against inflammation and cancer. Nods are expressed by epithelial cells, stromal cells, neutrophils, and dendritic cells. NLRP proteins interact with pyrin-containing proteins to form *inflammasomes* that cleave pro-IL-1β and pro-IL-18 into their mature forms by using the caspase-1 pathway. Activation of the caspase pathway leads to *pyroptosis,* a form of cell death that causes cellular release of mediators that instigate and propagate inflammatory pathways. NLRPs recognize both bacterial products (e.g., flagellin, toxins) and crystals (e.g., urea).[26]

In animal models, NLRs and the IL-1β pathway are important in innate gastrointestinal host defense. Nod signaling in the stromal compartment is required for formation of intestinal lymphoid follicles.[27] Interactions between Nods and the microbiome are also essential. For example, gram-negative bacteria induce Nod-dependent CCL20 and β-defensin secretion to promote development of intestinal lymphoid follicles from cryptopatches.[28] Nods are also required for appropriate microflora control. Nod2 deficiency increases bacterial load and decreases the clearance of bacteria from intestinal crypts.[29,30] In addition, mice deficient in Nod2 or transgenic for the Nod2 frame shift mutation have increased gut permeability, which also occurs in human Crohn disease; the etiology of increased permeability likely results from bacterial defection in response to increased T cell and TLR responses.[31] A complex interplay between the resident microflora and the innate and adaptive immune system is critical for controlling gut permeability, bacterial load, and inflammation.

INTESTINAL MICROBIOME

Several studies have evaluated the interaction among the normal commensal gut flora, the intestinal epithelium, and the mucosal immune system. A symbiotic relationship between the microbiome and gut immunity was first suggested by germ-free mice having very few immune cells and almost no IgA. Reconstitution with specific flora revealed that whereas mesenteric lymph nodes and PPs were genetically programmed, the development of isolated lymphoid follicles was dependent on gut flora. Despite the diversity of symbiotic bacteria, four phyla predominate in the human large intestine: Firmicutes, Bacteroidetes, Actinobacteria, and Proteobacteria. These symbionts and the mucosal epithelium have evolved in a mutually beneficial coexistence that can be altered to cause *dysbiosis.* The presence of microbiota is essential for proper epithelial rejuvenation. For example, when only half the usual microbiota are present, epithelial damage is increased but resultant epithelial cell proliferation is decreased.[32,33] Whether dysbiosis is a result of or a direct cause of local and systemic allergy or autoimmunity is unclear, but pathogenic states clearly are associated with distinct patterns of microbial dysbiosis. The microbiome also shapes adaptive immunity, including humoral and cellular immune responses.

The ability to raise mice under germ-free conditions and reconstitute such mice with a defined microbiota has highlighted the significant role the gut flora plays in the development of the mucosal immune system. For example, mice with lower levels of segmented filamentous bacteria (SFB) have reduced numbers of Th17 cells, which can be augmented by ingesting SFB. Reconstitution of mice with other organisms such as *Bacteroides fragilis* or *Clostridium* species show a preferential induction of regulatory T cells, demonstrating that the constituents of the microbiota can influence the effector/regulatory balance of the mucosal immune system.

INNATE IMMUNE CELLS

Eosinophils

The distribution of eosinophils in the GI tract varies from mouth to anus, with a general gradient of increasing baseline eosinophilia from proximal to distal. Eosinophils populate the fetal intestinal tract in early embryogenesis, and their intestinal accumulation is independent of bacterial colonization and presence of lymphocytes.[34,35] Whereas the normal esophageal epithelium is devoid of eosinophils, the lamina propria (LP) and muscularis mucosa normally have eosinophils.[10,36,37] The lower GI tract has significant numbers of eosinophils that traffic in a CCL-11 (eotaxin-1)–dependent manner.[35,37] Within the colonic LP, eosinophil numbers are relatively constant but are highest in the cecum and rectosigmoid.[37,38] Eosinophils are rarely found in the surface and crypt epithelium, and thus their presence in these locations may indicate a pathologic process.

The precise function of the eosinophil in the nondiseased GI tract is unknown, but models suggest that eosinophils may be recruited to sites of continual cell turnover and may regulate local immunity and tissue repair/remodeling.[39] With some parasitic infections, parasite expulsion on chronic or repeat infection can be dysregulated in the absence of eosinophils and IL-5.[40,41]

Mast Cells

The GI tract is one of the largest reservoirs of mast cells in the body. Mast cells are found in the human GI tract from the esophagus to the colon. The esophageal and colonic epithelium is normally entirely devoid of tryptase-positive cells, but tryptase-positive mast cells are found in varying numbers (14.5 to 17.6 per high-power field) through the colonic LP, and connective tissue mast cells (tryptase-chymase double-positive mast cells) predominate in the esophageal LP.[10,38]

During helminth infection in mice, mast cell mobilization from their normal location in the LP into the epithelium depends on intact notch signaling. Mast cell–deficient mice have delayed expulsion of *Trichinella spiralis* and *Strongyloides* as well as impaired helper T cell type 2 (Th2) responses.[42,43] Therefore, although GI mast cells are induced during immune responses to certain pathogens, their normal function in GI immune homeostasis remains unclear.

Innate lymphoid cells and Multifunctional IgA$^+$ Plasma Cells

Natural killer (NK) and lymphoid tissue inducer (LTi) cells were the first described members of the innate lymphoid cell family. LTi cells are required for lymph node formation during embryogenesis and produce IL-17 and IL-22. A group of cells that show mixed characteristics of NK and LTi cells has been more recently described. This population expresses CD56 and CD127 (the IL-7 receptor α chain) and produces IL-22. Additional innate lymphoid cells include natural helper cells, innate helper type 2 cells, and nuocytes, all of which produce the Th2 cytokines IL-5 and IL-13. These cells do not express lineage markers found on B, T, NK or NKT cells, mast cells, basophils, granulocytes, dendritic cells, or macrophages and are thus referred to as *lineage negative.* The precise relationship between these cell types is currently unclear, although the rapid and robust production of Th2 cytokines in response to IL-25 and IL-33 appears to be common to these populations. Through production of IL-5, innate lymphoid cells recruit eosinophils and are important for antihelminth immunity. In humans, these cells are found in the fetal gut as well as in the adult ileum.[44]

Natural helper (NH) cells were first described as being in visceral fat–associated lymphoid tissue. These cells express c-Kit, Sca-1, IL-2 receptor, IL-7 receptor, and IL-33 receptors as surface markers. They are dependent on IL-7, IL-2, and γ_c for their development and proliferation and on IL-25 and IL-33 to induce robust expression of IL-5 and IL-13. Rag2/γ_c-deficient mice (which lack lymphocytes completely) infected with the helminth *Nippostrongylus brasiliensis* have no IL-5 or IL-13 production as well as poor infection clearance that can be restored by adoptive transfer of NH cells.[45,46] Another population of IL-25–responsive, lineage-negative cells called "multipotent progenitor cells" exist in gut-associated lymphoid tissue (GALT) and have the potential to become mast cells and macrophages as well as promote Th2 responses and provide immunity to *Trichuris muris* infection.[47]

Mouse IgA$^+$ plasma cells have B cell and monocytic and dendritic cell markers.[48] A subset of polyreactive IgA-producing B cells also produce the antimicrobial agents tumor necrosis factor alpha (TNF-α) and inducible nitric oxide synthase, both of which are required to maintain homeostasis of gut microbiota. The acquisition of these lymphocytes depends on microbial stimulation and gut stroma, which indicates a symbiotic relationship between the microbiome and the gut immune system.

Macrophages

The GI mucosa is the largest reservoir of mononuclear phagocytes in the body. Macrophages regulate the inflammatory response to the normal flora, respond to pathogens, and scavenge debris and dead cells. Intestinal macrophages are derived from circulating monocytes. Once in intestinal tissue, macrophages have a life span of weeks to months. Resident macrophages are highly phagocytic and can ingest microbes and function as scavengers without generating an inflammatory response that could damage surrounding tissue. Innate signaling molecules such as MyD88 and TRIF adapter proteins are decreased or absent in intestinal macrophages, which explains the broad TLR nonresponsiveness of these cells despite TLR expression.[49] In the mouse, intestinal macrophages have regulatory activity through their production of IL-10 and retinoic acid,[50] but the same suppressive mechanisms have not yet been identified in human macrophages.

Despite their anergic phenotype, intestinal macrophages do participate in host defense through phagocytosis and microbial killing. They express an array of innate recognition receptors, including TLRs that allow microbial recognition; lipoprotein and phospholipid recognition receptors that facilitate uptake of apoptotic cells; and complement receptors. After uptake, intestinal macrophages efficiently kill microbes through mechanisms such as generation of reactive oxygen and nitrogen species and autophagy.

Denritic Cells

The intestinal lamina propria contains a dense network of dendritic cells that sample antigen and are responsible for the initiation of adaptive immune responses. Through their expression of TLRs and other pattern-recognition receptors, these resident cells also participate in innate immune responses. A subset of lamina propria DCs expressing the markers CD11c and CD103 express high levels of the flagellin sensor TLR5, but low levels of TLR4 in comparison to splenic DCs.[50a] TLR5 is necessary for detection of the pathogen *Salmonella typhimurium*. Activation of mucosal DCs through TLR5 leads to DC production of IL-23,[50b] and innate lymphoid cell expression of IL-17 and IL-22.[50c] These cytokines are important for antimicrobial defense in the intestine. Human intestinal DCs are also responsive to TLR3, TLR7, and TLR9 stimulation and therefore may play an important role in antiviral immunity.

Adaptive Immunity in Gastrointestinal Tract

Structural barriers as well as innate immune barriers limit the exposure of the mucosal immune system to antigenic material, but protein antigens penetrating through these barriers can be presented to T lymphocytes to generate an adaptive immune response. T cells reactive to exogenous antigens from food or flora are not deleted during thymic development as are self-reactive T cells, and therefore homeostatic mechanisms are necessary to suppress inappropriate immune reactivity to nonpathogenic material in the GI mucosa. Impairment of these homeostatic mechanisms can lead either to localized inflammation triggered by the microbial flora or food antigens or to systemic reactivity to food allergens.

ANTIGEN UPTAKE

The GI tract is exposed to a significant antigen burden derived from food and microbial flora. Different regions of the gut face different antigenic challenges, with a decreasing gradient of intact food allergens and an increasing microbial load from mouth to anus. The small intestine has been seen as the most relevant site of antigenic exposure because it is the site of nutrient absorption and therefore the most “leaky” from an electrophysiologic perspective. However, the epithelium of the mouth and esophagus has a dense network of antigen-presenting cells, and their presence indicates a readiness to absorb and present antigens.

Soluble and particulate antigens are handled by distinct mechanisms in the small intestine (see Fig. 67-2). Particulate antigens, such as viruses and bacteria, are preferentially taken up into the gut-associated lymphoid tissue (GALT), including PPs and ILFs. This results from the presence of specialized M cells in FAE overlying the PPs and ILFs (see earlier and Fig. 67-2). Antigens taken up by M cells are rapidly transported to the organized lymphoid tissue underneath, which includes a network of subepithelial dendritic cells in the PPs. Another mechanism of uptake of particulate antigens includes direct sampling by resident phagocytes that extend dendrites between enterocytes and can directly engulf bacteria from the intestinal lumen.[51]

Soluble antigens, including many food antigens, are not preferentially sampled by the M cells and are taken up primarily across enterocytes lining the intestinal villus. Under normal conditions, uptake of intact macromolecules occurs by a transcellular transport mechanism for depositing antigenic material across the basolateral surface of the epithelium. As a result, an immunologically significant quantity of food antigen reaches the systemic circulation intact after a meal.[52] When the person has been previously exposed to an antigen, uptake of that antigen can be modified by the presence of immunoglobulins. IgA primarily results in immune exclusion, whereas IgG and IgE can enhance uptake through epithelial expression of immunoglobulin receptors (FcRn[53] and CD23,[54] respectively).

ANTIGEN PRESENTATION

Antigen-presenting cells (APCs) in the GI tract include professional APCs such as dendritic cells (DCs), B cells, and macrophages, as well as nonprofessional APCs such as epithelial cells. DCs have the capacity to migrate to lymph nodes, where they can interact with naive T cells and induce an immune response. In the small and large intestine are two developmentally distinct CD11c$^+$ subsets.[55] One subset expresses the chemokine receptor CX_3CR1, extends dendrites into the small intestinal lumen, and is highly phagocytic and can efficiently capture antigen. This subset has also been described to be CD11b$^+$ and CD103$^-$. This CX_3CR1^+ subset does not migrate to the draining mesenteric lymph node (MLN) and is therefore likely to play a role in recall responses rather than in initiation of immune responses. The second subset of CD11c$^+$ cells expresses the marker CD103. Despite having a low level of antigen capture relative to CX_3CR1^+ cells, these cells are more efficient at antigen presentation and transport their cargo to the MLN for presentation to naïve T cells.[56] Therefore, the initiation of immune responses to soluble antigens depends on the CD103$^+$ DC subset. Within the PPs, subepithelial DCs migrate to T cell areas of the PP on appropriate stimulation, such as in response to adjuvant. A number of DC subsets are in the PPs and can be differentiated by their surface markers, such as CD11b, CD8α, and CCR6.[57,58] There is evidence the different DC phenotypes are specialized to respond to specific inflammatory stimuli or microbial challenges.

Within the stratified epithelium of the oral and esophageal mucosa are subsets of DCs that are distinct from those in the lower GI tract and bear greater similarity to those described in the skin. These include the Langerhans cells found in the most superficial epithelial layers, interstitial DCs, and langerin$^+$ interstitial DCs.[59] It is well known from studies on sublingual vaccination or immunotherapy that oral DCs acquire and present antigen to T cells and can generate either tolerance or protective immunity, depending on the context of antigen administration. Whether esophageal DCs can acquire and present ingested food antigens in vivo is unknown.

Mononuclear phagocytes without migratory activity in the GI mucosa interact with resident T cells of the LP and participate in the reactivation of memory T cells. Local activation of effector T cells may be a key part of the nonmigrating CX_3CR1^+ phagocytes of the small intestine that express major histocompatibility complex class II (MHC II) as well as process and present acquired antigens. CD11c$^-$ macrophages of the mouth and small intestine can also present antigen to T cells and preferentially induce the development of regulatory T cells (Tregs) through an IL-10– and retinoic acid–dependent mechanism. Epithelial cells of the GI tract are also capable of presenting antigen to T cells. Epithelial cells induce the expansion of CD8$^+$ T cells with regulatory activity through a CD1d-dependent mechanism.[60] During inflammatory states, epithelial cells of the esophagus and small intestine upregulate MHC II and can activate CD4$^+$ T cells[61,62] (see Fig. 67-4).

ADAPTIVE IMMUNITY TO FOOD ANTIGENS: IMMUNE TOLERANCE

The average daily protein intake in young children in the United States is greater than 50 g.[63] Although the majority of protein is digested and absorbed as amino acids or immunologically inert peptides, intact antigen can be readily detected in the blood after a meal in healthy volunteers. The immune system is not ignorant of these proteins, as shown by the presence of food-specific IgG and IgA antibodies in the serum of healthy individuals.[64]

The clinical tolerance to these exogenous proteins is thought to result from an active regulatory immune response termed *oral tolerance.* Wells and Osborne[65] first described oral tolerance in 1911, when they found that guinea pigs could not be induced to undergo anaphylaxis to proteins that were already present in the diet.[65] Subsequent studies showed that oral administration of antigen resulted in the generation of CD4$^+$ and CD8$^+$ T cells with regulatory or suppressive activity in mice and humans.[66] Transfer of CD4$^+$ or CD8$^+$ T cells from fed mice to naïve mice could transfer tolerance in an antigen-specific manner. Although CD8$^+$ T cells are not required for oral tolerance, they are capable of mediating tolerance, as shown by intragastric administration of MHC class I–specific epitopes of ovalbumin.[67] Deletion of peripherally induced forkhead box P3 protein (FOXP3$^+$) CD4$^+$ CD25$^+$ Tregs can reverse oral tolerance.[68] These Tregs are distinct from thymus-derived natural Tregs bearing the same markers that suppress autoimmunity.

Although immune tolerance can be generated at sites other than the GI tract (such as the airways), DCs migrating from the small intestinal LP are uniquely specialized to program responder T cells to develop into Tregs. Migratory CD103$^+$ DCs isolated from the MLN of mice or humans induce Tregs with gut-homing capacity through a mechanism dependent on retinoic acid and TGF-β.[69] Inhibition of DC migration to the lymph node or surgical ablation of the MLN abolishes the development of oral tolerance in mice.[70] These newly induced Tregs then migrate to the LP, where they are further expanded by resident DCs before seeding the periphery and suppressing systemic antigen-specific immunity through TGF-β–dependent mechanisms.[68] There is evidence that the liver can also participate in the induction of oral tolerance mediated through plasmacytoid DCs that induce the deletion of antigen-specific CD8$^+$ T cells.[71] The relative role of the MLN versus the liver in the induction of tolerance may depend on the nature of the antigen and how it is handled after breaching the intestinal epithelial barrier. Immune tolerance can be induced through the airways or by the sublingual route. Thus, multiple sites along the GI tract likely contribute to the development of clinical tolerance to food antigens.

ADAPTIVE IMMUNITY TO MICROBIAL ANTIGENS: IMMUNE EXCLUSION

The gastrointestinal immune system is exposed to a significant microbial antigen burden. The density of organisms is highest in the large intestine, but the mouth, esophagus, and small intestine also contain a normal commensal flora. As outlined earlier, the GI tract is generally seen as being hyporesponsive to signaling through the TLRs. However, the innate and adaptive immune system work in a coordinated manner to keep the flora compartmentalized to the GI mucosa. In the absence of signaling through MyD88 and TRIF, the downstream signaling molecules of the TLRs, there is a compensatory systemic antibody response against the intestinal flora that protects against systemic dissemination of bacteria.[72] Mice lacking both innate signaling and immunoglobulin production develop failure to thrive and protein-losing enteropathy triggered by the gut flora.

Commensal bacteria are normally sampled by the mucosal immune system and carried by migratory DCs to the draining MLN, where they induce an IgA response partially dependent on T cell help.[73] T cell–independent IgA class switching has also been documented in the intestinal LP.[74] In the absence of an intact MLN, flora can breach the mucosal compartment and be found systemically.[73] IgA induced by the flora is secreted into the intestinal lumen by epithelial cells expressing the polymeric immunoglobulin receptor (pIgR). Although the body expends considerable energy in IgA production, IgA deficiency is associated with a relatively mild phenotype, and humans with IgA deficiency can be asymptomatic. This may be caused by the overlapping functions of the innate and acquired immune systems in containing the intestinal flora.

The normal T cell response to the commensal flora is not as well defined as the IgA response. The generation of a commensal flora–triggered IL-17 and interferon-γ (IFN-γ) response from T cells is associated with pathology in inflammatory bowel disease. There are conflicting data on the role of the commensal flora in the development of intestinal Tregs. Although germ-free mice have no deficit in Treg populations in the gut,[75] microbial colonization is associated with an expansion of Tregs in the large intestine, and blockade of IL-10 during this induction allows the development of IL-17– and IFN-γ–secreting T cells in the large intestine.[76] FOXP3$^+$ Tregs are also significant providers of T cell help for IgA responses to the gut flora.[77]

In the presence of normal innate and adaptive immune responses within the gastrointestinal mucosal immune system, the systemic immune system is kept ignorant of the commensal flora. This is in contrast to the normal immune response to food antigens, in which active immune tolerance is observed systemically. Unique immune regulatory mechanisms have been generated to maintain homeostasis in the face of antigenic challenges from dietary and microbial antigens.

Conclusion

The mucosal immune system uses several strategies to prevent inappropriate immune reactivity to harmless antigens derived from the food and microbiota. These include structural, chemical, and immunologic barriers to prevent the uptake of intact antigens from the gut lumen. Furthermore, the immune milieu characterized by immuno-regulatory cytokines (such as TGF-β and IL-10) and other tolerogenic factors promote the development of a regulatory adaptive immune response to antigens that do penetrate beyond the epithelium. Factors that perturb these homeostatic mechanisms of immune tolerance likely contribute to immune-mediated diseases of the gastrointestinal tract, including inflammatory bowel disease or food allergy.

REFERENCES

Gastrointestinal Structure and Function

1. Kuo B, Urma D. Esophagus: anatomy and development. GI Motility online, 2006. Available at http://www.nature.com/gimo/contents/pt1/full/gimo6.html (accessed 2006)
2. Woo J, Miletich I, Kim BM, Sharpe PT, Shivdasani RA. Barx1-mediated inhibition of Wnt signaling in the mouse thoracic foregut controls tracheo-esophageal septation and epithelial differentiation. PLoS One 2011;6: e22493.
3. Kuo B, Urma D. Esophageal mucosal defense mechanisms. GI Motility online, 2006. Available at http://www.nature.com/gimo/contents/pt1/full/gimo6.html (accessed 2006)
4. Lioni M, Brafford P, Andi C, et al. Dysregulation of claudin-7 leads to loss of E-cadherin expression and the increased invasion of esophageal squamous cell carcinoma cells. Am J Pathol 2007;170:709-21.
5. Oshima T, Koseki J, Chen X, Matsumoto T, Miwa H. Acid modulates the squamous epithelial barrier function by modulating the localization of claudins in the superficial layers. Lab Invest 2012;92:22-31.
6. Jovov B, Que J, Tobey NA, et al. Role of E-cadherin in the pathogenesis of gastroesophageal reflux disease. Am J Gastroenterol 2011; 106:1039-47.
7. Tobey NA, Argote CM, Hosseini SS, Orlando RC. Calcium-switch technique and junctional permeability in native rabbit esophageal epithelium. Am J Physiol Gastrointest Liver Physiol 2004;286:G1042-9.
8. Lucendo AJ, Navarro M, Comas C, et al. Immunophenotypic characterization and quantification of the epithelial inflammatory infiltrate in eosinophilic esophagitis through stereology: an analysis of the cellular mechanisms of the disease and the immunologic capacity of the esophagus. Am J Surg Pathol 2007;31:598-606.
9. Vicario M, Blanchard D, Stringer KF, et al. Local B cells and IgE production in the oesophageal mucosa in eosinophilic oesophagitis. Gut 2010; 59:12-20.
10. Aceves SS, Chen D, Newbury RO, et al. Mast cells infiltrate the esophageal smooth muscle in patients with eosinophilic esophagitis, express TGF-β1, and increase esophageal smooth muscle contraction. J Allergy Clin Immunol 2010;126:1198-204 e4.
11. Thapar N, Roberts DJ. Stomach and duodenum: anatomy, embryology, and congenital abnormalities. In: Kleinman R, Goulet, O-J, Mieli-Vergani G, editors. Walker's pediatric gastrointestinal disease. 5th ed. Hamilton, Ontario, Canada: BC Decker; 2008. p. 117-26.
12. Untersmayr E, Bakos M, Schöll I, et al. Anti-ulcer drugs promote IgE formation toward dietary antigens in adult patients. FASEB J 2005;19:656-8.
13. DeSanta Barbara P. The intestine: anatomy and embryology. In: Kleinman R, Goulet O-J, Mieli-Vergani G, editors. Walker's pediatric gastrointestinal disease. 5th ed. Hamilton, Ontario, Canada: BC Decker; 2008. p. 207-16.

Innate Immunity in Gastrointestinal Tract

14. Atkins D, Furuta GT. Mucosal immunology, eosinophilic esophagitis, and other intestinal inflammatory diseases. J Allergy Clin Immunol 2010;125(Suppl. 2):255-61.
15. Peterson DE, Barder NP, Akhmadullina LI, et al. Phase II, randomized, double-blind, placebo-controlled study of recombinant human intestinal trefoil factor oral spray for prevention of oral mucositis in patients with colorectal cancer who are receiving fluorouracil-based chemotherapy. J Clin Oncol 2009;27: 4333-8.
16. Johansson ME, Phillipson J, Petersson M, et al. The inner of the two Muc2 mucin-dependent mucus layers in colon is devoid of bacteria. Proc Natl Acad Sci USA 2008;105: 15064-9.
17. Marques R, Boneca IG. Expression and functional importance of innate immune receptors by intestinal epithelial cells. Cell Mol Life Sci 2011;68:3661-73.
18. Cunliffe RN, Mahida YR. Expression and regulation of antimicrobial peptides in the gastrointestinal tract. J Leukoc Biol 2004;75:49-58.
19. Koon HW, Shih DQ, Chen J, et al. Cathelicidin signaling via the Toll-like receptor protects against colitis in mice. Gastroenterology 2011; 141:1852-63.e1-3.
20. Wilson CL, Quellette AJ, Satchnell DP, et al. Regulation of intestinal alpha-defensin activation by the metalloproteinase matrilysin in innate host defense. Science 1999;286(5437): 113-7.
21. Salzman NH, Ghosh D, Huttner KM, Paterson Y, Bevins CL. Protection against enteric salmonellosis in transgenic mice expressing a human intestinal defensin. Nature 2003;422(6931): 522-6.
22. De Yang, Chen Q, Schmidt AP, et al. LL-37, the neutrophil granule– and epithelial cell–derived cathelicidin, utilizes formyl peptide receptor-like 1 (FPRL1) as a receptor to chemoattract human peripheral blood neutrophils, monocytes, and T cells. J Exp Med 2000;192:1069-74.
23. Durr M, Peschel A. Chemokines meet defensins: the merging concepts of chemoattractants and antimicrobial peptides in host defense. Infect Immun 2002;70:6515-7.
24. Testro AG, Visvanathan K. Toll-like receptors and their role in gastrointestinal disease. J Gastroenterol Hepatol 2009;24:943-54.
25. Mulder DJ, Lobo D, Mak N, Justinich CJ. Expression of Toll-like receptors 2 and 3 on esophageal epithelial cell lines and on eosinophils during esophagitis. Dig Dis Sci 2012;57: 630-42.
26. Werts C, Rubino S, Ling A, Girardin SE, Philpott DJ. Nod-like receptors in intestinal homeostasis, inflammation, and cancer. J Leukoc Biol 2011; 90:471-82.
27. Bouskra D, Brézillon C, Bérard M, et al. Lymphoid tissue genesis induced by commensals through NOD1 regulates intestinal homeostasis. Nature 2008;456(7221):507-10.
28. Eberl G, Lochner M. The development of intestinal lymphoid tissues at the interface of self and microbiota. Mucosal Immunol 2009;2: 478-85.
29. Petnicki-Ocwieja T, Hrncir T, Liu YJ, et al. Nod2 is required for the regulation of commensal microbiota in the intestine. Proc Natl Acad Sci USA 2009;106:15813-8.
30. Rehman A, Sina C, Gavrilova O, et al. Nod2 is essential for temporal development of intestinal microbial communities. Gut 2011;60:1354-62.
31. Barreau F, Madre C, Meinzer U, et al. Nod2 regulates the host response towards microflora by modulating T cell function and epithelial permeability in mouse Peyer's patches. Gut 2010;59:207-17.
32. Pull SL, Doherty JM, Mills JC, Gordon JI, Strappenbeck TS. Activated macrophages are an adaptive element of the colonic epithelial progenitor niche necessary for regenerative responses to injury. Proc Natl Acad Sci USA 2005;102:99-104.
33. Moens E, Veldhoen M. Epithelial barrier biology: good fences make good neighbours. Immunology 2012;135:1-8.
34. Carlens J, Wahl B, Ballmaier M, et al. Common gamma-chain-dependent signals confer selective survival of eosinophils in the murine small intestine. J Immunol 2009;183:5600-7.
35. Mishra A, Hogan SP, Lee JJ, Foster PS, Rothenberg ME. Fundamental signals that regulate eosinophil homing to the gastrointestinal tract. J Clin Invest 1999;103:1719-27.
36. Aceves SS, Newbury RO, Dohil R, Bastian JF, Broide DH. Esophageal remodeling in pediatric eosinophilic esophagitis. J Allergy Clin Immunol 2007;119:206-12.
37. DeBrosse CW, Case JW, Putnam PE, Collins MH, Rothenberg ME. Quantity and distribution of eosinophils in the gastrointestinal tract of children. Pediatr Dev Pathol 2006;9:210-8.
38. Saad AG. Normal quantity and distribution of mast cells and eosinophils in the pediatric colon. Pediatr Dev Pathol 2011;14:294-300.
39. Lee JJ, Jacobsen EA, McGarry MP, Schleimer RP, Lee NA. Eosinophils in health and disease: the LIAR hypothesis. Clin Exp Allergy 2010;40: 563-75.
40. Vallance BA, Blennerhassett PA, Deng Y, et al. IL-5 contributes to worm expulsion and muscle hypercontractility in a primary *T. spiralis* infection. Am J Physiol 1999;277(2 Pt 1):G400-8.
41. Svensson M, Bell L, Little MC, et al. Accumulation of eosinophils in intestine-draining mesenteric lymph nodes occurs after *Trichuris muris* infection. Parasite Immunol 2011;33:1-11.
42. Lawrence CE, Paterson YY, Wright SH, Knight PA, Miller HR. Mouse mast cell protease-1 is required for the enteropathy induced by gastrointestinal helminth infection in the mouse. Gastroenterology 2004;127:155-65.
43. Sasaki Y, Yoshimoto T, Maruyama H, et al. IL-18 with IL-2 protects against *Strongyloides venezuelensis* infection by activating mucosal mast cell–dependent type 2 innate immunity. J Exp Med 2005;202:607-16.
44. Mjösberg JM, Trifari S, Crellin NK, et al. Human IL-25- and IL-33-responsive type 2 innate lymphoid cells are defined by expression of CRTH2 and CD161. Nat Immunol 2011;12: 1055-62.
45. Moro K, Ymada T, Tanabe M, et al. Innate production of T(H)2 cytokines by adipose tissue-associated c-Kit(+)Sca-1(+) lymphoid cells. Nature 2010;463(7280):540-4.
46. Koyasu S, Moro K. Type 2 innate immune responses and the natural helper cell. Immunology 2011;132:475-81.
47. Saenz SA, Siracusa MC, Perriqoue JG, et al. IL25 elicits a multipotent progenitor cell population that promotes T(H)2 cytokine responses. Nature 2010;464(7293):1362-6.
48. Fritz JH, Rojas OL, Simard N, et al. Acquisition of a multifunctional IgA+ plasma cell phenotype in the gut. Nature 2012;481(7380):199-203.
49. Smythies LE, Sellers M, Clements RH, et al. Human intestinal macrophages display profound inflammatory anergy despite avid

phagocytic and bacteriocidal activity. J Clin Invest 2005;115:66-75.
50. Denning TL, Wang YC, Patel SR, Williams IR, Pulendran B. Lamina propria macrophages and dendritic cells differentially induce regulatory and interleukin 17–producing T cell responses. Nat Immunol 2007;8:1086-94.
50a. Uematsu S, Jang MH, Chevrier N, et al. Detection of pathogenic intestinal bacteria by Toll-like receptor 5 on intestinal CD11c+ lamina propria cells. Nat Immunol 2006;7:868-74.
50b. Kinnebrew MA, Buffie CG, Diehl GE, et al. Interleukin 23 production by intestinal CD103(+)CD11b(+) dendritic cells in response to bacterial flagellin enhances mucosal innate immune defense. Immunity 2012;36:276-87.
50c. Van Maele L, Carnoy C, Cayet D, et al. TLR5 signaling stimulates the innate production of IL-17 and IL-22 by CD3(neg)CD127+ immune cells in spleen and mucosa. J Immunol 2010;185:1177-85.

Adaptive Immunity in Gastrointestinal Tract

51. Rescigno M, Urbano M, Valzasina B, et al. Dendritic cells express tight junction proteins and penetrate gut epithelial monolayers to sample bacteria. Nat Immunol 2001;2:361-7.
52. Husby S, Jensenius JC, Svehag SE. Passage of undegraded dietary antigen into the blood of healthy adults: quantification, estimation of size distribution, and relation of uptake to levels of specific antibodies. Scand J Immunol 1985;22:83-92.
53. Yoshida M, Matsuda A, Kuo TT, et al. IgG transport across mucosal barriers by neonatal Fc receptor for IgG and mucosal immunity. Springer Semin Immunopathol 2006;28:397-403.
54. Li H, Nowak-Wegrzyn A, Charlop-Powers Z, et al. Transcytosis of IgE-antigen complexes by CD23a in human intestinal epithelial cells and its role in food allergy. Gastroenterology 2006;131:47-58.
55. Bogunovic M, Ginhoux F, Helft J, et al. Origin of the lamina propria dendritic cell network. Immunity 2009;31:513-25.
56. Schulz O, Jaensson E, Persson EK, et al. Intestinal CD103[+], but not CX3CR1[+], antigen sampling cells migrate in lymph and serve classical dendritic cell functions. J Exp Med 2009;206:3101-14.
57. Kelsall B. Recent progress in understanding the phenotype and function of intestinal dendritic cells and macrophages. Mucosal Immunol 2008;1:460-9.
58. Salazar-Gonzalez RM, Neiss JH, Zammit DJ, et al. CCR6-mediated dendritic cell activation of pathogen-specific T cells in Peyer's patches. Immunity 2006;24:623-32.
59. Nudel I, Einekave M, Furmanov K, et al. Dendritic cells in distinct oral mucosal tissues engage different mechanisms to prime CD8[+] T cells. J Immunol 2011;186:891-900.
60. Allez M, Brimnes J, Dotan I, Mayer L. Expansion of CD8[+] T cells with regulatory function after interaction with intestinal epithelial cells. Gastroenterology 2002;123:1516-26.
61. Dotan I, Allez M, Nakazawa A, et al. Intestinal epithelial cells from inflammatory bowel disease patients preferentially stimulate CD4+ T cells to proliferate and secrete interferon-gamma. Am J Physiol Gastrointest Liver Physiol 2007;292:G1630-40.
62. Mulder DJ, Pooni A, Mak N, et al. Antigen presentation and MHC class II expression by human esophageal epithelial cells: role in eosinophilic esophagitis. Am J Pathol 2011;178:744-53.
63. Fulgoni 3rd VL. Current protein intake in America: analysis of the National Health and Nutrition Examination Survey, 2003-2004. Am J Clin Nutr 2008;87:1554S-7S.
64. Husby S, Oxelius VA, Teisner B, Jensenius JC, Svehag SE. Humoral immunity to dietary antigens in healthy adults: occurrence, isotype and IgG subclass distribution of serum antibodies to protein antigens. Int Arch Allergy Appl Immunol 1985;77:416-22.
65. Wells HG, Osborne TB. The biological reactions of the vegetable proteins. I. Anaphylaxis. J Infect Dis 1911;8:66-124.
66. Weiner HL, da Cunha AP, Quintana F, Wu H. Oral tolerance. Immunol Rev 2011;241:241-59.
67. Arnaboldi PM, Roth-Walter F, Mayer L. Suppression of Th1 and Th17, but not Th2, responses in a CD8(+) T cell–mediated model of oral tolerance. Mucosal Immunol 2009;2:427-38.
68. Hadis U, Wahl B, Schulz O, et al. Intestinal tolerance requires gut homing and expansion of FoxP3[+] regulatory T cells in the lamina propria. Immunity 2011;34:237-46.
69. Jaensson E, Uronen-Hansson H, Pabst O, et al. Small intestinal CD103[+] dendritic cells display unique functional properties that are conserved between mice and humans. J Exp Med 2008;205:2139-49.
70. Worbs T, Bode U, Yan S, et al. Oral tolerance originates in the intestinal immune system and relies on antigen carriage by dendritic cells. J Exp Med 2006;203:519-27.
71. Goubier A, Dubois B, Gheit H, et al. Plasmacytoid dendritic cells mediate oral tolerance. Immunity 2008;29:464-75.
72. Slack E, Hapfelmeier S, Stecher B, et al. Innate and adaptive immunity cooperate flexibly to maintain host-microbiota mutualism. Science 2009;325(5940):617-20.
73. Macpherson AJ, Uhr T. Induction of protective IgA by intestinal dendritic cells carrying commensal bacteria. Science 2004;303(5664):1662-5.
74. He B, Xu W, Santini PA, et al. Intestinal bacteria trigger T cell–independent immunoglobulin A(2) class switching by inducing epithelial-cell secretion of the cytokine APRIL. Immunity 2007;26:812-26.
75. Chinen T, Volchkov PY, Chervonsky AV, Rudensky AY. A critical role for regulatory T cell–mediated control of inflammation in the absence of commensal microbiota. J Exp Med 2010;207:2323-30.
76. Geuking MB, Cahenzli J, Lawson MA, et al. Intestinal bacterial colonization induces mutualistic regulatory T cell responses. Immunity 2011;34:794-806.
77. Cong Y, Feng T, Fujihashi K, Schoeb TR, Elson O. A dominant, coordinated T regulatory cell–IgA response to the intestinal microbiota. Proc Natl Acad Sci USA 2009;106:19256-61.

68

Eosinophilic Gastrointestinal Disorders

MARC E. ROTHENBERG

CONTENTS

SUMMARY OF IMPORTANT CONCEPTS

» Eosinophils are constituents of the gastrointestinal tract at baseline, meaning their mere presence is not pathognomonic for a particular disease.
» Eosinophilic gastrointestinal disorders consist of eosinophilic esophagitis, eosinophilic gastritis, eosinophilic enteritis, and eosinophilic colitis, as well as eosinophilic gastroenteritis (involving a combination of GI segments).
» Eosinophilic gastrointestinal disorders are primarily food allergen–driven diseases associated with helper T cell type 2 cytokines.
» Therapy for eosinophilic gastrointestinal disorders consists of a combination of approaches, including allergen avoidance, elemental diets, and antiinflammatory agents.

Introduction

Eosinophilic gastrointestinal disorders (EGID) are defined as disorders that selectively affect the gastrointestinal (GI) tract with eosinophil-rich inflammation in the absence of known causes for eosinophilia (e.g., drug reactions, parasitic infections, malignancy). These disorders are being increasingly recognized and include eosinophilic esophagitis (EoE), eosinophilic gastritis, eosinophilic gastroenteritis, eosinophilic enteritis, and eosinophilic colitis. Eosinophils are integral members of the GI mucosal immune system, and EGID are primarily polygenic allergic disorders involving mechanisms that fall between pure immunoglobulin E (IgE)–mediated and delayed helper T cell type 2 (Th2) responses. Studies have identified a contributory role for allergens, the cytokines interleukin-5 (IL-5) and IL-13, and the eotaxin family of chemokines, and the findings provide a rationale for disease-specific therapy.

Overview of Disorders

Eosinophil accumulation in the GI tract is a common feature of many GI disorders, including classic IgE-mediated food allergy, eosinophilic gastroenteritis, allergic colitis, EoE, inflammatory bowel disease (IBD), and gastroesophageal reflux disease (GERD).[1] In IBD, eosinophils usually represent only a small percentage of the infiltrating leukocytes, but their level has been proposed to be a negative prognostic indicator. The EGID, including EoE, eosinophilic gastritis, eosinophilic gastroenteritis, eosinophilic enteritis, and eosinophilic colitis, are defined as disorders that primarily affect the GI tract, with eosinophil-rich inflammation in the absence of known causes for eosinophilia, such as drug reactions, parasitic infections, connective tissue diseases, and malignancy (Box 68-1).

Patients with EGID have a variety of problems, including failure to thrive, abdominal pain, irritability, gastric dysmotility, vomiting, diarrhea, and dysphagia. These diseases can have a significant impact on quality of life, often resulting in school and work absenteeism, and are associated with multiple food allergies that dramatically alter lifestyle because of extensive dietary restrictions.[2-4] Evidence is accumulating that supports the concept that EGID arise secondarily to the interplay of genetic and environmental factors. Notably, about 10% of patients with EGID have an immediate family member affected by the disorder.[5] Additionally, several lines of evidence support an allergic etiology: about 75% of patients with EGID are atopic[6]; disease activity can sometimes be reversed by instituting an allergen-free diet;[7] histologic evidence suggests mast cell activation and degranulation; and Th2 cytokines are overexpressed after allergen stimulation.[8] Models of EGID support a potential allergic etiology for these disorders.[1] Although patients with EGID usually have food-specific IgE, only a minority have food-induced anaphylactic responses. Thus, EGID have properties that fall between pure IgE-mediated food allergy and cellular-mediated hypersensitivity disorders (e.g., celiac disease) (Fig. 68-1).

The incidence of primary EGID has not been rigorously calculated, but a mini-epidemic of these diseases (especially EoE) has been noted over the last decade. For example, EoE is a global health problem now reported in Australia, Brazil, England, Italy, Israel,[9] Japan, Spain, and Switzerland. One study revealed a 0.4% (~4:1000) prevalence of EoE in a random sample of Swedish adults,[10] and EoE occurred in about 1:1000 children in the Cincinnati metropolitan area over a 10-year period.[5] Epidemiologic results indicate that EGID is increasing in incidence and prevalence and may have a combined prevalence even higher than pediatric IBD.

BOX 68-1 CLASSIFICATION OF EOSINOPHILIC GASTROINTESTINAL DISORDERS

EOSINOPHILIC ESOPHAGITIS

Primary

- Atopic
- Nonatopic
- Familial

Secondary

- Eosinophilic disorders
  - Eosinophilic gastroenteritis
  - Hypereosinophilic syndrome
- Noneosinophilic disorders
  - Iatrogenic
  - Infection
  - Gastroesophageal reflux disease
  - Esophageal leiomyomatosis
  - Connective tissue disease (scleroderma)

EOSINOPHILIC GASTRITIS AND GASTROENTERITIS

Primary (Mucosal, Muscularis, and Serosal Forms)

- Atopic
- Nonatopic
- Familial

Secondary

- Eosinophilic disorders
  - Hypereosinophilic syndrome
- Noneosinophilic disorders
  - Celiac disease
  - Connective tissue disease (scleroderma)
  - Iatrogenic
  - Infection
  - Inflammatory bowel disease
  - Vasculitis (Churg-Strauss syndrome)

EOSINOPHILIC COLITIS

Primary Eosinophilic Colitis (also Allergic Colitis of Infancy)

- Atopic
- Nonatopic

Secondary

- Eosinophilic disorders
  - Eosinophilic gastroenteritis
  - Hypereosinophilic syndrome
- Noneosinophilic disorders
  - Celiac disease
  - Connective tissue disease (scleroderma)
  - Iatrogenic
  - Infection
  - Inflammatory bowel disease
  - Vasculitis (Churg-Strauss syndrome)

From Rothenberg ME. Eosinophilic gastrointestinal disorders (EGID). J Allergy Clin Immunol 2004;113:11-28. © 2004, with permission from the American Academy of Allergy, Asthma, and Immunology.

In more than 50% of patients, EGID occur independent of peripheral blood eosinophilia, indicating the potential significance of GI-specific mechanisms for regulating eosinophil levels; indeed, the author's work has demonstrated the importance of the eotaxin pathway in this process. However, some patients with EGID (typically those with eosinophilic gastritis) have substantially elevated levels of peripheral blood eosinophils and meet the diagnostic criteria for hypereosinophilic syndrome (HES)[11]; this syndrome is defined by sustained, severe peripheral blood eosinophilia (>1500 cells/mm^3) and the presence of end-organ involvement, in the absence of known causes for eosinophilia.[12] Notably, although HES frequently involves the GI tract, the other end organs typically associated with HES (e.g., heart, skin) are infrequently involved in EGID. A subset of patients with HES have a microdeletion on chromosome 4 that generates an activated tyrosine kinase susceptible to imatinib mesylate therapy. This microdeletion is being investigated, along with other genetic events in EGID patients, especially those with significant circulating eosinophilia.

GASTROINTESTINAL EOSINOPHILS UNDER HOMEOSTATIC HEALTHY STATES

Eosinophils are present at low levels in numerous tissues. In biopsy and autopsy specimens, the only organs that normally demonstrate tissue eosinophils at substantial levels are GI tract, spleen, lymph nodes, and thymus. In the healthy pediatric GI tract, eosinophil levels progressively increase from the proximal to the distal intestine.[13] Table 68-1 lists the level of eosinophils in the GI tract in apparently normal endoscopic biopsies. Preliminary evidence suggests that morphologic degranulation may be observed in the GI tract, but it remains possible that this is an artifact related to tissue processing.

A search for eosinophils throughout the GI tract of conventional healthy mice (i.e. untreated mice maintained under pathogen-free conditions) has revealed that these cells are normally present in the lamina propria of the stomach, small intestine, cecum, and colon.[14] Unlike intestinal lymphocytes and mast cells, eosinophils are not normally present in Peyer patches or intraepithelial locations, although they frequently infiltrate these regions in EGID.[1] Fetal mice have eosinophils located in similar regions and in similar concentrations to adult mice,[14] which indicates that eosinophil homing into the GI tract occurs independent of endogenous flora. Indeed, germ-free mice[14] and mice deficient in innate signaling responses (MYD88 deficient) have normal levels of GI eosinophils. These data suggest that eosinophils respond to distinct stimuli compared with other intestinal leukocytes; constitutive expression of eotaxin-1 provides the unique signal that promotes localization of murine eosinophils into the GI tract at baseline. Tissue-dwelling eosinophils have distinct cytokine expression patterns under inflammatory or noninflammatory conditions, with esophageal eosinophils from patients with EoE expressing relatively high levels of Th2 cytokines.

PROINFLAMMATORY ROLE OF EOSINOPHILS

Eosinophils are pleiotropic cells that respond to a variety of triggers. In vitro studies show that eosinophil granule constituents are toxic to a variety of tissues, including intestinal epithelium. Eosinophil granules contain a crystalloid core composed of major basic proteins MBP-1 and MBP-2 as well as a matrix composed of eosinophil cationic protein (ECP), eosinophil-derived neurotoxin (EDN), and eosinophil peroxidase (EPX). These cationic proteins share certain proinflammatory properties but differ in other ways. For example, MBP, EPX, and ECP

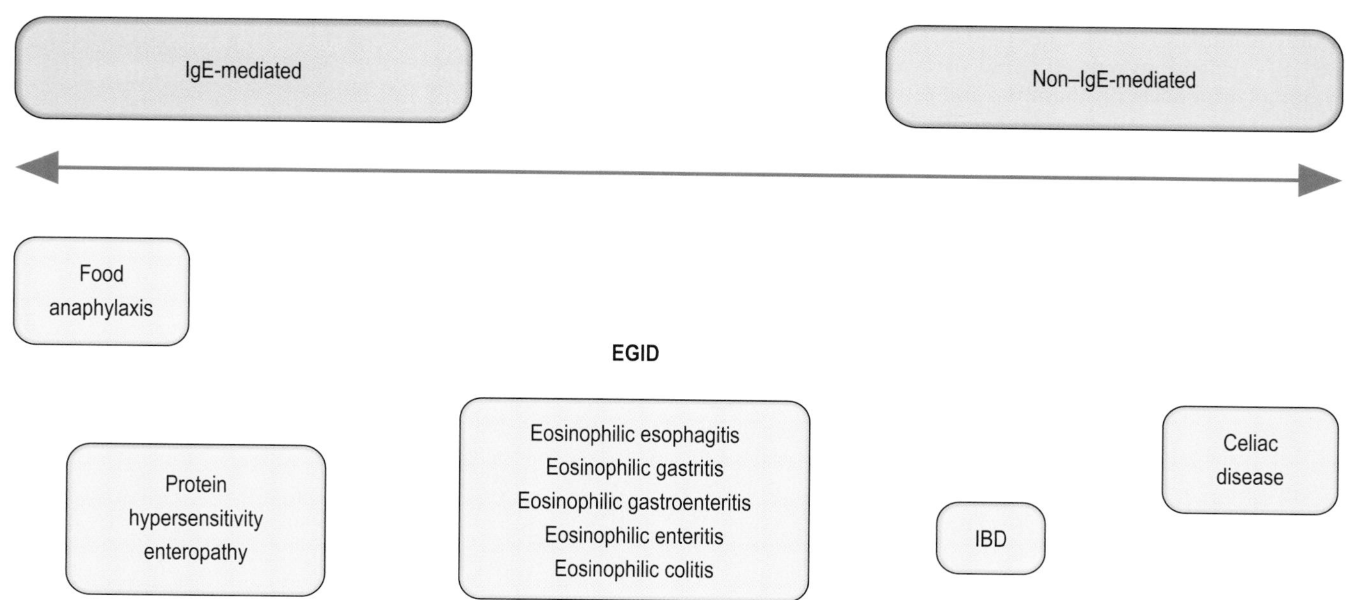

Figure 68-1 The spectrum of gastrointestinal inflammatory disorders involving eosinophils. Gastrointestinal eosinophils accumulate in a variety of disorders, with variable dependence on immunoglobulin E (*IgE*) ranging from predominant IgE dependence (food anaphylaxis) to non-IgE dependence (celiac disease). Primary eosinophilic gastrointestinal disorders (*EGID*) are in the middle of the spectrum and have some overlap with pure protein hypersensitivity disorders and inflammatory bowel disease (*IBD*). *(From Rothenberg ME, Mishra A, Brandt EB, et al. Gastrointestinal eosinophils in health and disease. Adv Immunol 2001;78:291-328.)*

TABLE 68-1 Gastrointestinal Eosinophil Levels in Normal Pediatric Endoscopy Biopsies*

Gastrointestinal Segment	LAMINA PROPRIA		VILLOUS LAMINA PROPRIA		SURFACE EPITHELIUM		CRYPT/GLANDULAR EPITHELIUM	
	Mean	Max	Mean	Max	Mean	Max	Mean	Max
Esophagus	N/A	N/A	N/A	N/A	0.03 ± 0.10	1	N/A	N/A
Antrum	1.9 ± 1.3	8	N/A	N/A	0.0	0	0.02 ± 0.04	1
Fundus	2.1 ± 2.4	11	N/A	N/A	0.0	0	0.008 ± 0.03	1
Duodenum	9.6 ± 5.3	26	2.1 ± 1.4	9	0.06 ± 0.09	2	0.26 ± 0.36	6
Ileum	12.4 ± 5.4	28	4.8 ± 2.8	15	0.47 ± 0.25	4	0.80 ± 0.51	4
Ascending colon	20.3 ± 8.2	50	N/A	N/A	0.29 ± 0.25	3	1.4 ± 1.2	11
Transverse colon	16.3 ± 5.6	42	N/A	N/A	0.22 ± 0.39	4	0.77 ± 0.61	4
Rectum	8.3 ± 5.9	32	N/A	N/A	0.15 ± 0.13	2	1.2 ± 1.1	9

From Debrosse CW, Case JW, Putnam PE, et al. Quantity and distribution of eosinophils in the gastrointestinal tract of children. Pediatr Dev Pathol 2006;9:210-8.
N/A, Not applicable.
*Values indicate cells/hpf ± SD, the mean number of eosinophils per high-power field plus or minus the standard deviation, for each anatomic region of the GI tract and each region of the mucosa.

have cytotoxic effects on epithelium at concentrations similar to those in biologic fluids from patients with eosinophilia. Also, ECP and EDN belong to the ribonuclease A superfamily and possess antiviral and ribonuclease activity. Circulating levels of EDN are elevated in patients with EoE and can distinguish patients with active and inactive disease.[15] MBP triggers degranulation of mast cells and basophils.

Triggering of eosinophils by engagement of receptors for cytokines, immunoglobulins, and complement can lead to the generation of a wide range of inflammatory cytokines, including IL-1, -3, -4, -5, and -13; granulocyte-macrophage colony-stimulating factor (GM-CSF); transforming growth factors (TGFs); tumor necrosis factor-α (TNF-α); RANTES (CCL5); macrophage inflammatory protein 1α (MIP-1α, a.k.a. CCL3), vascular endothelial cell growth factor (VEGF); and eotaxin-1 (CCL-11). Although mostly found in modest quantities per eosinophil compared with other cells, these cytokines have the potential to modulate multiple aspects of the immune response. In fact, eosinophil-derived TGF-β is linked with epithelial growth, fibrosis, and tissue remodeling. Additionally, eosinophils can "catapult" their mitochondrial DNA in response to activation, thus resulting in DNA nets that may have a role in trapping intestinal pathogens.[16] Eosinophils express major histocompatibility complex (MHC) class II molecules and relevant costimulatory molecules (CD28, CD40, CD80 [B7-1], CD86 [B7-2]) and secrete an array of cytokines capable of promoting lymphocyte proliferation and activation and Th1 or Th2 polarization (IL-2, -4, -6, -12, -10). Further eosinophil-mediated damage is caused by toxic hydrogen peroxide and halide acids generated by EPX and by superoxide generated by the respiratory burst oxidase enzyme pathway in eosinophils. Clinical investigations demonstrate extracellular deposition of MBP and ECP in the small bowel of patients with eosinophilic gastroenteritis and a correlation between the level of eosinophils and disease severity.

Electron microscopy studies have revealed ultrastructural changes in the secondary granules (indicative of eosinophil degranulation and mediator release) in duodenal samples from patients with eosinophilic gastroenteritis. Furthermore, Charcot-Leyden crystals, remnants of eosinophil degranulation, are often found on microscopic examination of stool obtained from patients with eosinophilic gastroenteritis.

Clinical Evaluation

Patients with EGID present with a variety of clinical problems, most often failure to thrive, abdominal pain, irritability, gastric dysmotility, vomiting, diarrhea, dysphagia, microcytic anemia, and hypoproteinemia. A diagnostic evaluation for EGID should be performed on all patients with these refractory problems, especially in individuals with a strong history of allergic diseases, peripheral blood eosinophilia, or a family history of EGID. Depending on the intestinal segment involved, the frequency of specific symptoms varies. For example, abdominal pain and dysphagia are most common in eosinophilic gastroenteritis and EoE, respectively. However, there are no pathognomonic symptoms or blood tests for diagnosing EGID. Although blood eosinophil counts are generally in the normal range in most patients, above-normal levels can distinguish patients with active versus inactive EoE.[15] If EGID are suspected on the basis of clinical presentation or evaluation of endoscopic biopsies, additional testing should be considered to rule out another primary disease process, such as drug hypersensitivity, collagen vascular disease, malignancy, or infection.

The evaluation for EGID starts with a comprehensive history and physical examination, followed by diagnostic testing (Box 68-2). Evaluation for intestinal parasites by examination of stool samples, intestinal aspirates obtained during colonoscopy, or specific blood antibody titers should be performed, especially when patients have high-risk exposure (e.g., foreign travel, living on a farm, drinking well water). For example, the common dog hookworm *Ancylostoma caninum*, as detected on endoscopy, can cause eosinophilic enteritis, suggesting that other occult infections may be involved in pathogenesis of EGID. As a precaution, before using systemic immunosuppression for EGID, infection with *Strongyloides stercoralis* should be ruled out because it can become life-threatening with immunosuppression. Measuring total IgE levels can be useful in stratifying patients with atopic variants of EGID or suggesting further consideration for occult parasitic infections. Skin-prick testing to a panel of food allergens and aeroallergens helps to identify sensitization to specific allergens. Indeed, patients with the atopic variant of EGID have evidence of IgE sensitization to a mean of 14 different foods. Cutaneous hypersensitivity testing (skin patch testing) for specific food antigens may be helpful in further identifying allergic variants of EoE.

BOX 68-2 DIAGNOSTIC WORKUP FOR EOSINOPHILIC GASTROINTESTINAL DISORDERS

GENERAL

- Complete blood count and differential
- Total IgE
- Erythrocyte sedimentation rate
- Skin-prick testing
- Infection workup (stool and colonic aspirate analysis)
- Upper and lower gastrointestinal endoscopy with biopsies
- (pH probe, skin patch testing, tests for specific IgE)

IN THE PRESENCE OF HYPEREOSINOPHILIA

- Bone marrow analysis
- Serum tryptase
- Serum vitamin B_{12}
- Echocardiogram
- Genetic analysis for *FIP1L1-PDGFRA* fusion gene
- (Evaluation and biopsy of any other potentially involved tissue)

From Rothenberg ME. Eosinophilic gastrointestinal disorders (EGID). J Allergy Clin Immunol 2004;113:11-28. © 2004, with permission from the American Academy of Allergy, Asthma, and Immunology.

The diagnosis of EGID depends on the microscopic evaluation of endoscopic biopsy samples, with careful attention being given to the quantity, location, and characteristics of the eosinophilic inflammation. Patients with EGID often present with a clear history and positive biopsy results for the disease but have a variety of endoscopic findings. The endoscopic appearance of the GI tract may look normal, so microscopic evaluation of biopsy samples is essential. Furthermore, the disease is characterized by patchy involvement, necessitating the analysis of multiple endoscopic biopsies from each intestinal segment. Because no widely accepted diagnostic criteria have been established for EGID, the diagnosis depends on the expertise of the physicians involved in the evaluation of the biopsy samples. Although the normal esophagus is devoid of eosinophils, the rest of the GI tract contains readily detectable eosinophils.[13] Thus, differentiation of EGID from the normal condition relies on several factors, including (1) eosinophil quantification, with comparison to normal values at each medical center; (2) location of eosinophils, such as their presence in abnormal positions (e.g., intraepithelial and intestinal crypt regions); (3) associated pathologic abnormalities (e.g., epithelial hyperplasia in EoE); and (4) the absence of pathologic features suggestive of other primary disorders (e.g., neutrophilia and granulomas associated with IBD, vasculitis associated with Churg-Strauss syndrome). The normal level of GI eosinophils in pediatric patients has recently been reported, but with no agreement on the application of these quantitative threshold levels to the diagnosis of EGID.[13] Given the lack of firm diagnostic criteria, patients often suffer from symptoms for an extended time (mean of 4 years) before a true diagnosis of EGID is established.

EVALUATION FOR HYPEREOSINOPHILIC SYNDROME

The term *hypereosinophilic syndrome* was introduced in 1968 to designate patients with marked eosinophilia. Diagnostic criteria formulated in 1975 for HES include (1) persistent eosinophilia of at least 1500 cells/mm^3 for a minimum of 6 months, (2) lack of known causes for eosinophilia (e.g., parasitic or allergic triggers), and (3) symptoms and signs of organ system involvement. These criteria were modified in 2006 to remove the requirement of 6 months of sustained eosinophilia because this may not be clinically possible or advisable.[11] On the basis of these revised diagnostic criteria, patients with EGID and blood eosinophil counts greater than 1500/mm^3 meet the diagnostic criteria. However, patients with EGID generally do not have the high risk of life-threatening complications associated with classic HES—cardiomyopathy or central nervous system involvement. Notably, any disease that results in prolonged and marked eosinophilia can be associated with endomyocardial disease. For example, endomyocardial disease can occur during helminth infections and in various malignancies associated with marked eosinophilia.

Thus, patients with marked eosinophilia are at risk for the development of cardiac disease regardless of the underlying etiology of the eosinophilia. In patients with EGID and peripheral blood eosinophilia, routine surveillance of the cardiorespiratory system is warranted (e.g., echocardiography, plethysmography). In patients with EGID, the diagnosis of HES should always be considered, especially if they develop extra-GI manifestations (e.g., splenomegaly; cutaneous, cardiac, or respiratory system involvement/pathology). Thus, additional diagnostic testing for HES should be considered, including bone marrow analysis (searching for evidence of myelodysplasia), serum mast cell tryptase and vitamin B_{12} levels (both moderately elevated in classic HES), and genetic analysis for the presence of the *FIP1L1-PDGFRA* fusion event (see Box 68-2), as well as other fusion events, including genes such as *PDGFRB* and *FGFR1*.[17]

Eosinophilic Esophagitis

The esophagus is normally devoid of eosinophils, so the finding of esophageal eosinophils denotes pathology.[2,18] It is now appreciated that eosinophil infiltration in the esophagus accompanies many disorders, such as EoE, eosinophilic gastroenteritis, GERD, recurrent vomiting, parasitic and fungal infections, IBD, HES, esophageal leiomyomatosis, myeloproliferative disorders, carcinomatosis, periarteritis, allergic vasculitis, scleroderma, pemphigus vegetans, and drug injury.[1] Eosinophil-associated esophageal disorders are classified into primary and secondary. The *primary* subtype includes the atopic, nonatopic, and familial variants; the *secondary* subtype is divided into two groups, systemic eosinophilic disorders (HES) and noneosinophilic disorders (see Box 68-1). Of note, primary EoE has also been called *idiopathic EoE* or *allergic esophagitis*. The familial form of EoE is seen in 5% to 10% of patients.[5] The sibling recurrence risk ratio has been estimated to be more than 50-fold.[19,20]

ETIOLOGY

The etiology of EoE is poorly understood, but food allergy has been implicated. In fact, the majority of patients have evidence of food allergen and aeroallergen sensitization, as defined by skin-prick and allergen-specific IgE tests; however, only a minority have a history of food anaphylaxis. It has also been suggested that esophageal eosinophilic inflammation is mechanistically linked to pulmonary inflammation, on the basis of the induction of experimental EoE by repeated delivery of specific allergens or the Th2 cytokine IL-13 to the lung of mice.[21-23] Increased eosinophil accumulation in the esophagus of patients with seasonal allergic rhinitis (e.g., grass hypersensitivity) and a strong relationship between atopy and EoE have been shown. Indeed, patients with EoE typically report seasonal variations in their symptoms. In addition to eosinophils, T cells and mast cells are elevated in esophageal mucosal biopsies, suggesting chronic Th2-associated inflammation.[24] Elevated TGF-β, produced by eosinophils and mast cells, has been shown to contribute to tissue remodeling and smooth muscle dysfunction.[25,26] Exposure to antigen through an epicutaneous route primes for marked eosinophilic inflammation in the esophagus, triggered by a single airway antigen challenge.[27] IL-5 is required for this eosinophilic inflammation, indicating a Th2-dependent mechanism. Consistent with this view, overexpression of IL-5 induces EoE, and neutralization of IL-5 completely blocks allergen-induced or IL-13–induced EoE in mice.[22,23,28]

A landmark advance in EoE research was a genome-wide microarray profile analysis of esophageal tissue.[20] Investigators compared gene transcript expression in the esophageal tissue of patients with EoE, patients with chronic esophagitis (typical of GERD), and normal individuals. A remarkable dysregulated expression of about 1% of the entire human genome identified an EoE genetic signature. In pediatric patients with EoE, eotaxin-3 was the most overexpressed gene, and levels of overexpression correlated with disease severity. Furthermore, a single-nucleotide polymorphism (SNP) in the eotaxin-3 gene was overrepresented in patients with EoE compared with normal individuals. The same investigators demonstrated that mice with a genetic ablation of the eotaxin receptor (CCR3) were protected from the development of experimental EoE. Eotaxin-3 (a gene found in humans but not in mice) is induced by the Th2 cytokine IL-13. These data have been replicated in a number of studies,[29-31] and the overexpression of eotaxin-3 alone has a predictive value of 89% in diagnosing EoE in a single biopsy.[32]

These results strongly implicate eotaxin-3 in the pathoetiology of EoE and offer a molecular connection between Th2 inflammation and the development of EoE. The molecular basis for the specific dysregulation of eotaxin-3 (and not other eotaxin chemokines) is now under active investigation. The first genome-wide association study has linked EoE to genetic locus region 5q22, which harbors the gene for thymic stromal lymphopoeitin (TSLP) protein; TSLP has a known role in processes germane to EoE, such as polarization of Th2 immunity and induction of eotaxins.[33,34] Additionally, genetic variants in TSLP and its receptor have been associated with EoE susceptibility.[35]

CLINICAL AND DIAGNOSTIC STUDIES

Patients with primary EoE typically present with feeding disorders, vomiting, epigastric or chest pain, dysphagia, and food impactions; these symptoms generally occur in chronologic order with patient age (Fig. 68-2), such that adult EoE is primarily characterized by dysphagia and food impactions.[5] In a study of 26 adult patients with EoE, all had dysphagia, 11 had food impaction, and 19 of those 26 patients responded well to EoE treatment.[36] Patients with EoE are predominantly males and have relatively high levels of eosinophils (>15 eosinophils/high-power field [hpf])[1] in the esophageal mucosa, extensive epithelial hyperplasia, and a high rate of atopic disease compared with patients with GERD.[37]

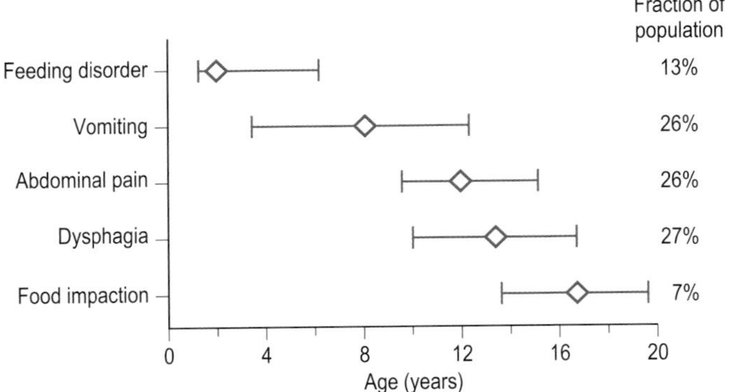

Figure 68-2 Presenting symptoms of eosinophilic esophagitis (EoE) vary according to age. Population-based data from 103 individuals under age 20 years with EoE indicate distinct presenting symptoms across various pediatric ages (median and interquartile range; $P < 0.001$, Kruskal-Wallis test).[5] The column on the right side of the chart specifies the fractional representation of each presenting symptom within the population. *(From Noel RJ, Rothenberg ME. Eosinophilic esophagitis. Curr Opin Pediatr 2005;17:690-4.)*

Table 68-2 outlines the distinguishing features between GERD and EoE. Identifying the number and location of eosinophils is helpful when trying to differentiate EoE from GERD. Up to 7 eosinophils/hpf (400×) is most indicative of GERD; 7 to 15/hpf likely represents a combination of GERD and food allergy; and more than 15/hpf is characteristic of EoE.[1] Eosinophil levels greater than 5/hpf have been associated with long-term sequelae.[38,39] Differential expression of eotaxin-3 occurs only in EoE and is absent in non-EoE disorders.[20] The anatomic location of eosinophils to both the proximal and the distal esophagus denotes EoE, whereas the accumulation of eosinophils mainly in the distal esophagus is characteristic of GERD.

Esophageal biopsy specimens from patients with EoE have thickened mucosa with basal layer hyperplasia and papillary lengthening. EoE has been associated with esophageal dysmotility, and although the etiology of the motor disturbances is unclear, eosinophil activation and degranulation is possible. Esophageal ultrasound has revealed the presence of a dysfunctional muscularis mucosa in patients with EoE, providing a possible explanation for the impaired esophageal dysmotility. Radiographic and endoscopic studies have shown many findings, including strictures, mucosal rings, ulcerations, whitish papules, and polyps. On endoscopy, it is common to visualize linear creases oriented longitudinally (furrowing; Fig. 68-3). Another common endoscopic feature of EoE is the presence of white mucosal exudates that correspond to sites of eosinophilic accumulation (Fig. 68-4).

Assessment of EoE includes an extensive allergy evaluation for food allergen and aeroallergen sensitization either by skin-prick tests or measurement of allergen-specific IgE in serum and the exclusion of GERD as well as other causes of eosinophils in the esophagus. Evaluation of food protein sensitization by delayed skin patch testing may increase the likelihood of identifying food allergy compared with evaluation by skin-prick testing alone.

It has been reported that more than 75% of patients with EoE have significantly improved endoscopic findings after dietary elimination of allergy-triggering foods identified on the basis of skin-prick and atopic patch testing. The presence of GERD does not exclude the diagnosis of EoE or food allergy;

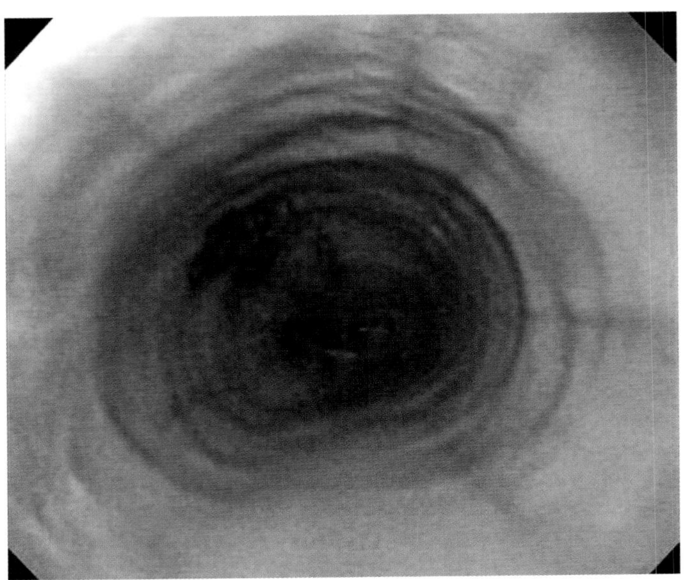

Figure 68-3 Esophageal furrowing in a patient with eosinophilic esophagitis. On endoscopy, it is common to visualize linear creases oriented longitudinally.

TABLE 68-2 Comparison of Eosinophilic Esophagitis (EoE) and Gastroesophageal Reflux Disease (GERD)

Characteristic Features	EoE	GERD
CLINICAL		
Prevalence	≈1 : 1000	≈1 : 10
Prevalence of atopy	Very high	Normal
Prevalence of food sensitization	Very high	Normal
Gender preference	Male	None
Abdominal pain and vomiting	Common	Common
Food impaction	Common	Uncommon
INVESTIGATIVE FINDINGS		
pH probe/impedence study	Normal	Abnormal
Endoscopic furrowing	Very common	Occasional
HISTOPATHOLOGY/PATHOGENESIS		
Involvement of proximal esophagus	Yes	No
Involvement of distal esophagus	Yes	Yes
Epithelial hyperplasia	Severely increased	Increased
Eosinophil levels in mucosa	>15/hpf	0-7/hpf
Elevated eotaxin-3 level	Yes	No
TREATMENT		
H_2-antihistamines	Not helpful	Helpful
Proton pump inhibitors	Sometimes helpful (but eosinophil levels remain >15/hpf)	Helpful
Glucocorticoids	Helpful	Not helpful
Specific food antigen elimination	Sometimes helpful	Not helpful
Elemental diet	Helpful	Not helpful

Modified from Rothenberg ME. Eosinophilic gastrointestinal disorders (EGID). J Allergy Clin Immunol 2004;113:11-18. © 2004, with permission from the American Academy of Allergy, Asthma, and Immunology.

hpf, High-power field.

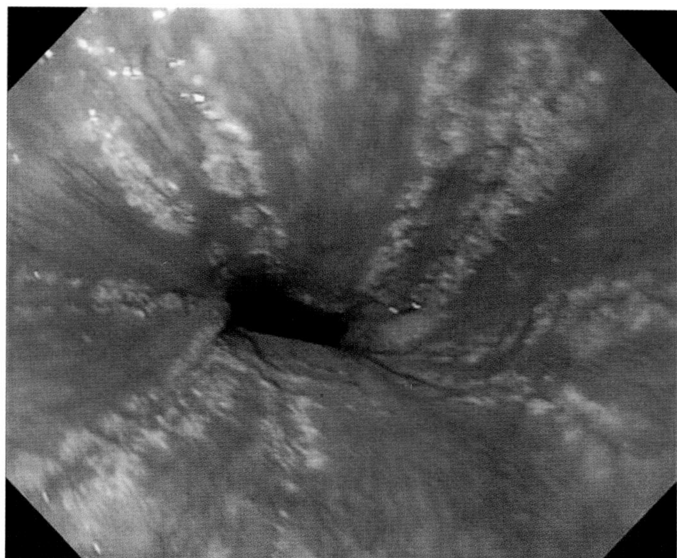

Figure 68-4 Esophageal white exudates in a patient with eosinophilic esophagitis, corresponding to sites of eosinophilic accumulation. These common white exudates can be confused with *Candida* esophagitis; however, microscopic analysis typically demonstrates eosinophilic microabscesses and eosinophilic surface labeling.

therefore, food allergy evaluation should be conducted in these patients.

TREATMENT

A trial of specific food allergen and aeroallergen avoidance is often indicated for patients with atopic EoE. If results are unsatisfactory or avoidance is difficult for practical reasons (e.g., when the patient is sensitized to many allergens), a diet consisting of an elemental (amino acid–based) formula or avoidance of the most common allergic foods (cow's milk, soy, wheat, egg, peanut/tree nuts, seafood/shellfish) is advocated.[40] In patients with primary EoE (allergic or nonallergic subtypes), dietary therapy frequently leads to reduction in symptoms and the number of eosinophils in the esophagus. Patients receiving elemental diets frequently require placement of a gastrostomy tube to achieve adequate caloric support.

Systemic or topical glucocorticoids have also been used with satisfactory results in patients with EoE. Systemic glucocorticoids are used for acute exacerbations, and topical glucocorticoids are used to provide long-term control. The efficacy of continuing corticosteroids and food elimination therapy for EoE has been shown. For administering fluticasone topical steroids, using a metered-dose inhaler without a spacer is recommended. Alternatively, a slurry of budesonide (in the form used for nebulizers) with sucralose (Splenda) is also recommended.[37,41] The patient is instructed to swallow the dose to promote deposition on the esophageal mucosa. EoE in patients unable to use inhalers may be successfully managed by using an oral suspension of budesonide. In a placebo-controlled, double-blind trial, swallowed topical fluticasone was effective in inducing EoE remission, as indicated by reductions in eosinophil, mast cell, and CD8 T cell levels, as well as epithelial hyperplasia.[42] Half of the patients responded to topical glucocorticoids, and 10% responded to placebo. In another study of topical fluticasone, all 19 of the treated patients with EoE had decreased symptoms and esophageal eosinophil counts.[36] In a controlled study of topical budesonide, within only 3 weeks, more than 85% of patients responded to therapy. In the author's practice, fluticasone dipropionate is the drug most used and is prescribed at a wide range of dosages on the basis of disease severity and level of response. In controlled blinded-label studies, topical fluticasone lowers levels of eosinophils and mast cells in the proximal and distal esophagus in adults and children.[42,43]

The toxicity associated with inhaled or oral glucocorticoids (e.g., adrenal suppression) is unlikely with swallowed fluticasone or budesonide because these drugs undergo first-pass metabolism in the liver after GI absorption. However, patients do rarely develop esophageal candidiasis, which is treatable with antifungal therapy. In addition, in multiple trials, including a randomized controlled trial, humanized anti–IL-5 monoclonal antibody therapy was helpful in reducing esophageal eosinophil levels; larger-scale trials are currently under way.[44-47] Another recent study showed the promising effect of anti–human IL-13 antibody in an animal model of IL-13–induced airway and esophageal eosinophilia.[48] A new approach is to target the sialic acid–binding immunoglobulin-like lectin F (Siglec-F), an inhibitory receptor expressed on eosinophils, because Siglec-F inhibition was useful in a mouse model of EoE.[49] Also, even if GERD is not present, neutralizing gastric acidity with proton pump inhibitors may improve symptoms and the degree of esophageal pathology.

PROGNOSIS

It appears that EoE requires prolonged treatment, similar to allergic asthma. The natural history of EoE has not been fully delineated; however, results of a 15-year follow up study of esophageal eosinophilia indicate that the vast majority of patients have ongoing symptoms from childhood into adulthood.[39] Children with EoE may have a parent with a longstanding history of esophageal strictures. Examination of esophageal biopsy slides from such parents has revealed that some have longstanding EoE. Symptoms occur in chronologic order; feeding problems, vomiting, abdominal pain, dysphagia, and food impactions occur with increasing age (see Fig. 68-2).[5] Thus, if left untreated, chronic EoE will likely develop into progressive esophageal scarring and dysfunction. The risk for developing Barrett esophagitis, especially in patients with coexisting EoE and GERD, has not been determined but is certainly of concern. Additionally, patients with EoE are at increased risk for developing other forms of EGID[6]; thus, routine surveillance of the entire GI tract by endoscopy and consideration of esophageal dilation as therapy are warranted.

Eosinophilic Gastritis and Gastroenteritis

In contrast to the esophagus, the stomach and intestine have readily detectable baseline eosinophils under healthy conditions. Making the diagnosis of eosinophilic gastritis, enteritis, and gastroenteritis is therefore even more complex than making the diagnosis of EoE. In this chapter, eosinophilic gastritis, enteritis, and gastroenteritis are grouped together because they are clinically similar and a paucity of information is available concerning their pathogenesis; however, they likely are distinct entities in most patients.

Eosinophilic gastritis and gastroenteritis are characterized by the selective infiltration of eosinophils in the stomach and small intestine, with variable involvement of the esophagus and large intestine. Many disorders are accompanied by eosinophil infiltration in the stomach, including parasitic and bacterial infections (e.g., *Helicobacter pylori*), IBD, HES, myeloproliferative disorders, periarteritis, allergic vasculitis, scleroderma, drug injury, and drug hypersensitivity. As with EoE, these disorders are classified into primary and secondary. The primary subtype includes the atopic, nonatopic, and familial variants, and the secondary subtype is divided into two groups, systemic eosinophilic disorders (HES) and noneosinophilic disorders (see Box 68-1). Primary eosinophilic enteritis, gastritis, and gastroenteritis have also been called *idiopathic* or *allergic gastroenteropathy*. The familial form has not been well characterized but is seen in about 10% of the author's patients. Primary eosinophilic gastroenteritis encompasses multiple disease entities subcategorized into three types on the basis of the level of histologic involvement: mucosal, muscularis, and serosal. As any of the three layers of the GI tract can be involved, endoscopic biopsy can be normal in patients with the muscularis or serosal subtypes.

ETIOLOGY

Although eosinophilic gastritis and gastroenteritis are idiopathic, it has been suggested that an allergic mechanism occurs in at least a subset of patients. Indeed, elevated total IgE and food-specific IgE have been detected in the majority of patients. On the other hand, syndromes with focal erosive gastritis, enteritis, and occasionally esophagitis with prominent eosinophilia, such as dietary (food) protein–induced enterocolitis and dietary protein enteropathy, are characterized by negative skin tests and absent specific IgE. Most patients have positive skin tests to a variety of food antigens but do not have typical anaphylactic reactions, consistent with a delayed type of food hypersensitivity syndrome.

Indeed, experimental murine induction of eosinophilic gastroenteritis (involving the esophagus, stomach, and intestine) is accomplished by oral allergen administration (in the form of enteric-coated allergen beads) to sensitized mice.[50] Notably, the mice developed eosinophil-associated GI dysfunction, including gastromegaly, delayed food transit, and weight loss, all strongly dependent on the chemokine eotaxin-1.[51] Ultrastructural analysis of intestinal tissue suggested that the eosinophils were mediating axonal necrosis; the same finding has been reported in patients with intestinal eosinophilia associated with IBD. Notably, mast cells are also increased in EGID, and a recent murine model of oral allergen–induced diarrhea has indicated that mast cells have a critical role in the pathogenesis of allergic diarrhea in EGID.[52]

Data from clinical studies suggest that patients with eosinophilic gastroenteritis have increased secretion of IL-4 and IL-5 by peripheral blood T cells. Furthermore, T cells derived from the lamina propria of the duodenum of patients with EGID preferentially secrete Th2 cytokines (especially IL-13) when stimulated with milk proteins. IgA deficiency has also been associated with eosinophilic gastroenteritis, possibly related to the associated increased rate of atopy or to an occult GI infection. Eosinophilic gastroenteritis and the dietary protein–induced syndromes (enterocolitis, enteropathy, colitis) may represent a continuum of EGID with similar underlying immunopathogenic mechanisms. In addition, eosinophilic gastroenteritis can frequently be associated with protein-losing enteropathy.[53] Eosinophilic enteritis has been reported in patients with systemic lupus erythematosus, although the pathologic association is unknown.

CLINICAL AND DIAGNOSTIC STUDIES

In general, eosinophilic gastritis and gastroenteritis present with a constellation of symptoms that are related to the degree and area of the GI tract affected. However, even patients with isolated eosinophilic enteritis (e.g., duodenitis) can have a range of GI symptoms. The mucosal form of eosinophilic gastroenteritis, the most common variant, is characterized by vomiting, abdominal pain that can mimic acute appendicitis, diarrhea, blood loss in stools, iron deficiency anemia, malabsorption, protein-losing enteropathy, and failure to thrive.[53] The muscularis form is characterized by infiltration of eosinophils predominantly in the muscularis layer, leading to thickening of the bowel wall, which may result in symptoms of GI obstruction mimicking pyloric stenosis or other causes of gastric outlet obstruction. The serosal form occurs in a minority of patients with eosinophilic gastroenteritis, characterized by exudative ascites with higher peripheral eosinophil counts compared with the other forms.

No standards exist for diagnosing eosinophilic gastritis or gastroenteritis. The following findings support the diagnosis: (1) presence of elevated eosinophils in biopsy specimens from the GI tract wall (compared with normal levels as shown in Table 68-1); (2) infiltration of eosinophils within intestinal crypts and gastric glands; (3) lack of involvement of other organs; and (4) exclusion of other causes of eosinophilia (e.g., infections, IBD). A recent study has suggested that eosinophil levels >30 eosinophils/hpf differentiate eosinophilic gastritis from normal adult controls.[54] Histologic analysis of the small bowel from patients with these disorders reveals extracellular deposition of eosinophil granule constituents; immunohistochemical analysis reveals elevated extracellular MBP and ECP. Patients with eosinophilic gastritis can have micronodules or polyposis noted on endoscopy, and these lesions often contain marked aggregates of lymphocytes and eosinophils. Food allergy and peripheral eosinophilia are not required for diagnosis.

TREATMENT

Eliminating the dietary intake of foods implicated by skin-prick tests (or measurement of allergen-specific IgE levels) has variable effects in patients with eosinophilic gastritis and gastroenteritis, but complete resolution is generally achieved with amino acid–based elemental diets.[53] Once disease remission has been obtained by dietary modification, the specific food groups are slowly reintroduced, at about 3-week intervals for each food group, and endoscopy is performed every 3 months to identify either sustained remission or disease flare-up. Drugs such as cromoglycate, montelukast, ketotifen, suplatast tosilate, mycophenolate mofetil (inosine monophosphate dehydrogenase inhibitor), and "alternative Chinese medicines" have been advocated, but these are generally unsuccessful in the author's experience. However, successful long-term remission of eosinophilic gastroenteritis after montelukast treatment has been reported. In the author's institution, an appropriate therapeutic approach includes a trial of food elimination if sensitization to food is found by skin-prick tests or measurement of specific IgE levels.

If no sensitization is found or if specific food avoidance is not feasible, elemental formula feedings are instituted.

The management of EGID, in addition to an elemental diet as previously mentioned, includes systemic and topical steroids, noncorticosteroid therapy, management of other EGID complications (e.g., iron deficiency anemia), and management of therapeutic toxicity. Antiinflammatory drugs (systemic or topical steroids) are the main therapy if diet restriction is not feasible or has failed to improve the disease. For systemic steroid therapy, a course of 2 to 6 weeks with relatively low doses seems to work better than a 7-day course of burst glucocorticoids. Several forms of topical glucocorticoids are designed to deliver drugs to specific GI tract segments; for example, budesonide tablets (Entocort EC) deliver the drug to the ileum and proximal colon. As with treatment for asthma, topical steroids have a better benefit-to-risk effect than systemic steroids. Anti–IL-5 and anti-IgE therapies are being studied, and anti-IgE appears to have some value.[45-47,55] In patients with severe disease (i.e., refractory to or dependent on glucocorticoid therapy), intravenous alimentation or immunosuppressive antimetabolite therapy with azathioprine or 6-mercaptopurine are alternatives. Also, even if GERD is not present, neutralization of gastric acidity with proton pump inhibitors may improve symptoms and the degree of esophageal and gastric pathology.

PROGNOSIS

The natural history of eosinophilic gastritis, enteritis, and gastroenteritis has not been well documented; however, these diseases wax and wane chronically. Because the GI segments involved may vary over time, regular endoscopic evaluation is needed. In patients with food antigen–induced disease, abnormal levels of circulating IgE and eosinophils often serve as markers for tissue involvement. Because these diseases can often be a manifestation of another primary disease process, routine surveillance of cardiopulmonary systems is recommended. When the disease presents in infancy and specific food sensitization can be identified, there is a high likelihood of disease remission by late childhood.

Eosinophilic Colitis

Eosinophils accumulate in the colon of patients with a variety of disorders, including eosinophilic gastroenteritis, allergic colitis of infancy, infections (e.g., pinworms, dog hookworms), drug reactions, vasculitis (e.g., Churg-Strauss syndrome), and IBD.[2] Allergic colitis in infancy, also known as dietary protein–induced proctocolitis of infancy syndrome, is the most common cause of bloody stools in the first year of life. Similar to other EGID, these disorders are classified into primary and secondary subtypes (see Box 68-1). The primary subtype includes the atopic and nonatopic variants; the secondary subtype is divided into systemic eosinophilic disorders (HES) and noneosinophilic disorders.

ETIOLOGY

In contrast to other EGID, eosinophilic colitis is usually a non-IgE–associated disease. Some studies point to a T lymphocyte–mediated process, but the exact immunologic mechanisms responsible for this condition have not been identified.[2] In a murine model of oral antigen–induced diarrhea associated with colonic inflammation, colonic T cells transferred from antigen-challenged mice to naïve mice caused the disease by a STAT6-dependent mechanism. Allergic colitis of infancy might be an early expression of protein-induced enteropathy or protein-induced enterocolitis syndrome. Cow's milk and soy proteins are the foods most frequently implicated in allergic colitis of infancy, but other food proteins can also provoke the disease. Interestingly, this condition may occur more often in infants exclusively breastfed and can even occur in infants fed with protein hydrolysate formulas.

CLINICAL AND DIAGNOSTIC STUDIES

Eosinophilic colitis is associated with a variety of symptoms that depend on the degree and location of tissue involvement. Although diarrhea is a classic symptom, other symptoms that can occur independent of diarrhea include abdominal pain, weight loss, and anorexia. There is a bimodal age distribution, with the infantile form presenting at a mean age at diagnosis of about 60 days and the other form presenting during adolescence and early adulthood. In infants, bloody diarrhea precedes diagnosis by several weeks, and anemia from blood loss may be seen. The majority of infants affected do not have constitutional symptoms and are otherwise healthy. As evaluated by endoscopic examination, patchy erythema, loss of vascularity, and lymphonodular hyperplasia are mostly localized to the rectum but might extend to the entire colon.[2] Histologic examination often reveals that the overall architecture of the mucosa is well preserved; however, there are focal aggregates of eosinophils in the lamina propria, crypt epithelium, and muscularis mucosa, and multinucleated giant cells are occasionally present in the submucosa. No single test is the "gold standard" for diagnosis, but finding peripheral blood eosinophilia or eosinophils in the stool suggests eosinophilic colitis.

TREATMENT

Treatment of eosinophilic colitis varies primarily depending on the disease subtype. For example, eosinophilic colitis of infancy is generally a benign disease. On withdrawal of the offending protein trigger from the diet, the gross blood in the stools usually resolves within 72 hours, although occult blood loss may persist longer. Treatment of eosinophilic colitis in older individuals usually requires medical management because IgE-associated triggers are rarely identified. Drugs such as cromoglycate, montelukast, and histamine receptor antagonists are generally unsuccessful in the author's experience. Antiinflammatory drugs, including aminosalicylates and systemic or topical glucocorticoids, are typically used and appear to be efficacious, but they have not been evaluated in careful clinical trials. Although several forms of topical glucocorticoids are designed to deliver drugs to the distal colon and rectum, eosinophilic colitis usually also involves the proximal colon. As with other EGID, in severe cases (i.e., patients refractory to or dependent on systemic glucocorticoid therapy), alternatives include intravenous alimentation or immunosuppressive antimetabolite therapy with azathioprine or 6-mercaptopurine.

PROGNOSIS

When eosinophilic colitis presents in the first year of life, the prognosis is good, and the vast majority of patients are able to tolerate the culprit food(s) by 1 to 3 years of age. Although several studies have found an association between allergic colitis and later development of IBD, this association is controversial. The prognosis for eosinophilic colitis that develops later in life is more guarded than the infantile subtype. Similar to eosinophilic gastroenteritis, the natural history has not been documented, and this disease is considered to be a chronic waxing-and-waning disorder. Because eosinophilic colitis can often be a manifestation of other primary disease processes, routine surveillance of cardiopulmonary systems and regular upper and lower GI endoscopy is recommended.

Conclusion

In a variety of medical conditions, eosinophils accumulate in numerous locations in the body and can often account for the majority of the cellular inflammatory infiltrate, as in primary EGID and HES. EGID are being recognized more frequently, and the recent mini-epidemic of EoE in the pediatric population has led to the establishment of patient-founded support/advocacy groups such as the American Partnership for Eosinophilic Disorders (www.APFED.org) and the Campaign Urging Research for Eosinophilic Disease (CURED, www.curedfoundation.org). EGID have strong genetic and allergic components and share clinical and immunopathogenic features with asthma. EGID are associated with a variety of nonspecific, common GI symptoms, which makes their diagnosis completely dependent on microscopic examination of GI biopsy samples, generally obtained during endoscopic evaluation.

Clinical and experimental models show that eosinophils promote potent proinflammatory effects mediated by their ability to release their cytotoxic secondary granule constituents and a variety of lipid mediators and cytokines (Fig. 68-5). During Th2-associated GI inflammatory conditions, eosinophil

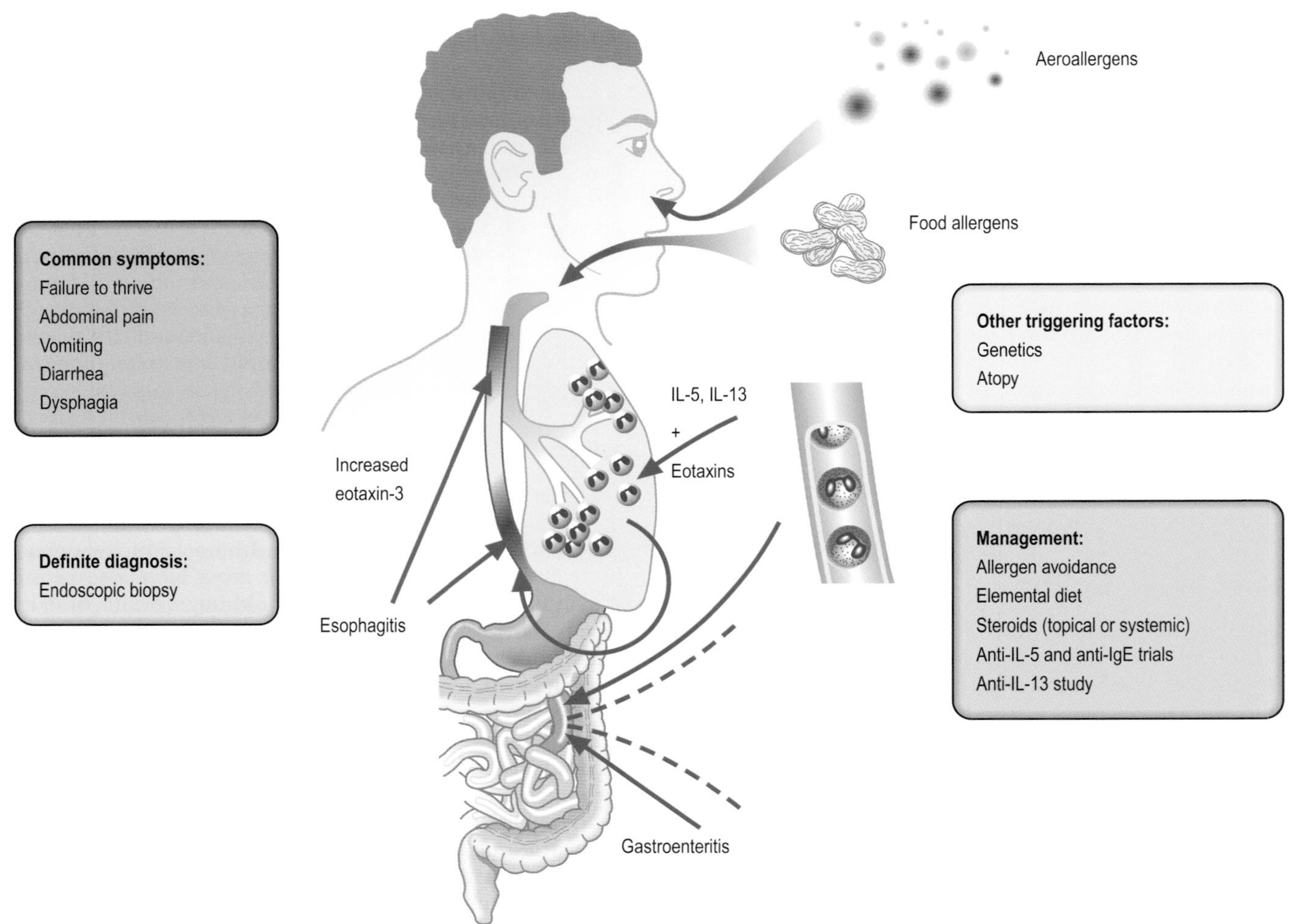

Figure 68-5 Summary of pathogenesis and treatment strategies for eosinophilic gastrointestinal disorders (EGID) and hypereosinophilic syndrome (HES). Pathologic increases in eosinophils occur in EGID, a series of disorders strongly associated with food and aeroallergen sensitization. EGID are generally tissue-specific problems, whereas HES tends to involve the heart, lungs, and skin; however, there can be overlap, especially when EGID are accompanied by marked blood eosinophilia. Although EGID may simultaneously involve multiple GI segments, as in eosinophilic gastroenteritis, specific regions of the GI tract may be selectively involved, as in eosinophilic esophagitis (EoE), a disease mechanistically linked with eosinophilic airway inflammation (asthma). The cytokines IL-5, IL-13, and eotaxins likely play an important role in various manifestations of EGID. Clinical intervention strategies for EGID thus include allergen avoidance and therapy with anti–IL-5 and anti–IL-13 humanized antibodies, CCR3 antagonists, and imatinib mesylate. This figure also lists common symptoms of EGID, triggering factors, diagnosis, and management. *(From Rothenberg ME. Eosinophilic gastrointestinal disorders [EGID]. J Allergy Clin Immunol 2004;113:11-18. © 2004, with permission from the American Academy of Allergy, Asthma, and Immunology.)*

levels are elevated in the lamina propria in an eotaxin chemokine family–dependent manner. Furthermore, following mucosal allergen challenge, eosinophils accumulate under the regulation of IL-5, IL-13, and eotaxin-3/CCR3 in the esophagus, an organ normally devoid of eosinophils. Eosinophil accumulation in the esophagus can be experimentally induced by aeroallergen or IL-13 delivery to the lung, thereby establishing a primary link between pulmonary and esophageal eosinophilic inflammation.

On the basis of these and other results, a variety of new therapeutic approaches are now underway for EGID, including treatment with humanized anti–IL-5, the tyrosine kinase inhibitor imatinib mesylate, CCR3 antagonists, and IL-4/IL-13 inhibitors. Early results of a phase I/II trial of anti–IL-5 therapy using mepolizumab for EoE are encouraging, but more studies are needed.[45-47] Imatinib mesylate and other tyrosine kinase inhibitors may be helpful not only for certain myeloproliferative forms of HES, but also for mast cell–induced problems associated with EGID, because these agents inhibit stem cell factor (formerly called c-kit ligand), a tyrosine kinase required for normal mast cell growth and development.[56,57]

Although much has been learned regarding the GI eosinophil and EGID, knowledge is sparse compared with other cell types and GI diseases that may be even less common (e.g., IBD). It is anticipated that a better understanding of the pathogenesis and treatment of EGID will emerge by combining comprehensive clinical and research approaches involving experts in the fields of allergy, gastroenterology, nutrition, and pathology.

Acknowledgments

The author would like to thank the numerous colleagues who have contributed to the body of information presented in this review, including Drs. Simon Hogan, Anil Mishra, Philip Putnam, Amal Assa'ad, Margaret Collins, James Franciosi, Sean Jameson, Bridget Buckmeier Butz, and Glenn Furuta. The author is grateful to Shawna Hottinger for editorial assistance and for Dr. Jonathan Kushner for the endoscopic images. This work was supported in part by the NIH/NIAID R01 AI42242 and AI45898 and the kind support of the CURED Foundation, Buckeye Foundation, and Food Allergy Research & Education (formerly FAI and FAAN).

REFERENCES

Overview of Disorders

1. Rothenberg ME, Mishra A, Collins MH, et al. Pathogenesis and clinical features of eosinophilic esophagitis. J Allergy Clin Immunol 2001;108:891-4.
2. Rothenberg ME. Eosinophilic gastrointestinal disorders (EGID). J Allergy Clin Immunol 2004; 113:11-28.
3. Franciosi JP, Hommel KA, Debrosse CW, et al. Quality of life in paediatric eosinophilic oesophagitis: what is important to patients? Child Care Health Dev 2012;38:477-83.
4. Ingerski LM, Modi AC, Hood KK, et al. Health-related quality of life across pediatric chronic conditions. J Pediatr 2010;156:639-44.
5. Noel RJ, Putnam PE, Rothenberg ME. Eosinophilic esophagitis. N Engl J Med 2004;351: 940-1.
6. Assa'ad AH, Putnam PE, Collins MH, et al. Pediatric patients with eosinophilic esophagitis: an 8-year follow-up. J Allergy Clin Immunol 2007;119:731-8.
7. Liacouras CA. Eosinophilic esophagitis: treatment in 2005. Curr Opin Gastroenterol 2006;22: 147-52.
8. Yamazaki K, Murray JA, Arora AS, et al. Allergen-specific in vitro cytokine production in adult patients with eosinophilic esophagitis. Dig Dis Sci 2006;51:1934-41.
9. Shitrit AB, Reinus C, Zeides S, et al. Eosinophilic esophagitis. Isr Med Assoc J 2006;8:587.
10. Ronkainen J, Talley NJ, Aro P, et al. Prevalence of eosinophilia and eosinophilic esophagitis in adults in the community: a random population based study (Kalixanda). Gastroenterology 2006;130:A575.
11. Klion AD, Bochner BS, Gleich GJ, et al. Approaches to the treatment of hypereosinophilic syndromes: a workshop summary report. J Allergy Clin Immunol 2006;117:1292-302.
12. Assa'ad AH, Spicer RL, Nelson DP, et al. Hypereosinophilic syndromes. Chem Immunol 2000;76:208-29.
13. Debrosse CW, Case JW, Putnam PE, et al. Quantity and distribution of eosinophils in the gastrointestinal tract of children. Pediatr Dev Pathol 2006;9:210-8.
14. Mishra A, Hogan SP, Lee JJ, et al. Fundamental signals that regulate eosinophil homing to the gastrointestinal tract. J Clin Invest 1999;103: 1719-27.
15. Konikoff MR, Blanchard C, Kirby C, et al. Potential of blood eosinophils, eosinophil-derived neurotoxin, and eotaxin-3 as biomarkers of eosinophilic esophagitis. Clin Gastroenterol Hepatol 2006;4:1328-36.
16. Yousefi S, Gold JA, Andina N, et al. Catapult-like release of mitochondrial DNA by eosinophils contributes to antibacterial defense. Nat Med 2008;14:949-53.

Clinical Evaluation

17. Gotlib J. World Health Organization–defined eosinophilic disorders: 2011 update on diagnosis, risk stratification, and management. Am J Hematol 2011;86:677-88.

Eosinophilic Esophagitis

18. Rothenberg ME, Mishra A, Brandt EB, et al. Gastrointestinal eosinophils. Immunol Rev 2001;179:139-55.
19. Blanchard C, Wang N, Rothenberg ME. Eosinophilic esophagitis: pathogenesis, genetics, and therapy. J Allergy Clin Immunol 2006;118: 1054-9.
20. Blanchard C, Wang N, Stringer KF, et al. Eotaxin-3 and a uniquely conserved gene-expression profile in eosinophilic esophagitis. J Clin Invest 2006;116:536-47.
21. Mishra A, Hogan SP, Brandt EB, et al. An etiological role for aeroallergens and eosinophils in experimental esophagitis. J Clin Invest 2001; 107:83-90.
22. Mishra A, Rothenberg ME. Intratracheal IL-13 induces eosinophilic esophagitis by an IL-5, eotaxin-1, and STAT6-dependent mechanism. Gastroenterology 2003;125:1419-27.
23. Zuo L, Fulkerson PC, Finkelman FD, et al. IL-13 induces esophageal remodeling and gene expression by an eosinophil-independent, IL-13Rα2-inhibited pathway. J Immunol 2010; 185:660-9.
24. Abonia JP, Blanchard C, Butz BB, et al. Involvement of mast cells in eosinophilic esophagitis. J Allergy Clin Immunol 2010;126:140-9.
25. Aceves SS, Chen D, Newbury RO, et al. Mast cells infiltrate the esophageal smooth muscle in patients with eosinophilic esophagitis, express TGF-β1, and increase esophageal smooth muscle contraction. J Allergy Clin Immunol 2010;126:1198-204.e4.
26. Mishra A, Wang M, Pemmaraju VR, et al. Esophageal remodeling develops as a consequence of tissue specific IL-5-induced eosinophilia. Gastroenterology 2008;134:204-14.
27. Akei HS, Mishra A, Blanchard C, et al. Epicutaneous antigen exposure primes for experimental eosinophilic esophagitis in mice. Gastroenterology 2005;129:985-94.
28. Mishra A, Hogan SP, Brandt EB, et al. Interleukin-5 promotes eosinophil trafficking to the esophagus. J Immunol 2002;168:2464-9.
29. Lucendo AJ, De Rezende L, Comas C, Caballero T, Bellón T. Treatment with topical steroids downregulates IL-5, eotaxin-1/CCL11, and eotaxin-3/CCL26 gene expression in eosinophilic esophagitis. Am J Gastroenterol 2008; 103:2184-93.
30. Blanchard C, Mingler MK, Vicario M, et al. IL-13 involvement in eosinophilic esophagitis: transcriptome analysis and reversibility with glucocorticoids. J Allergy Clin Immunol 2007; 120:1292-300.
31. Bhattacharya B, Carlsten J, Sabo E, et al. Increased expression of eotaxin-3 distinguishes between eosinophilic esophagitis and gastroesophageal reflux disease. Hum Pathol 2007;38: 1744-53.
32. Blanchard C, Stucke EM, Rodriguez-Jimenez B, et al. A striking local esophageal cytokine expression profile in eosinophilic esophagitis. J Allergy Clin Immunol 2011;127:208-17, 217.e1-7.
33. Rothenberg ME, Spergel JM, Sherrill JD, et al. Common variants at 5q22 associate with

pediatric eosinophilic esophagitis. Nat Genet 2010;42:289-91.

34. Sherrill JD, Rothenberg ME. Genetic dissection of eosinophilic esophagitis provides insight into disease pathogenesis and treatment strategies. J Allergy Clin Immunol 2011;128:23-32, quiz 33-4.
35. Sherrill JD, Gao PS, Stucke EM, et al. Variants of thymic stromal lymphopoietin and its receptor associate with eosinophilic esophagitis. J Allergy Clin Immunol 2010;126:160-5.e3.
36. Remedios M, Campbell C, Jones DM, et al. Eosinophilic esophagitis in adults: clinical, endoscopic, histologic findings, and response to treatment with fluticasone propionate. Gastrointest Endosc 2006;63:3-12.
37. Liacouras CA, Furuta GT, Hirano I, et al. Eosinophilic esophagitis: updated consensus recommendations for children and adults. J Allergy Clin Immunol 2011;128:3-20.e6; quiz 21-2.
38. DeBrosse CW, Collins MH, Buckmeier Butz BK, et al. Identification, epidemiology, and chronicity of pediatric esophageal eosinophilia, 1982-1999. J Allergy Clin Immunol 2010;126:112-9.
39. DeBrosse CW, Franciosi JP, King EC, et al. Long-term outcomes in pediatric-onset esophageal eosinophilia. J Allergy Clin Immunol 2011; 128:132-8.
40. Kagalwalla AF, Sentongo TA, Ritz S, et al. Effect of six-food elimination diet on clinical and histologic outcomes in eosinophilic esophagitis. Clin Gastroenterol Hepatol 2006;4: 1097-102.
41. Dohil R, Newbury R, Fox L, Bastian J, Aceves S. Oral viscous budesonide is effective in children with eosinophilic esophagitis in a randomized, placebo-controlled trial. Gastroenterology 2010; 139:418-29.
42. Konikoff MR, Noel RJ, Blanchard C, et al. A randomized double-blind placebo-controlled trial of fluticasone propionate for pediatric eosinophilic esophagitis. Gastroenterology 2006;131:1381-91.
43. Straumann A, Conus S, Degen L, et al. Budesonide is effective in adolescent and adult patients with active eosinophilic esophagitis. Gastroenterology 2010;139:1526-37, 1537.e1.
44. Stein ML, Collins MH, Villanueva JM, et al. Anti-interleukin-5 (mepolizumab) therapy for eosinophilic esophagitis. J Allergy Clin Immunol 2007;118:1312-9.
45. Assa'ad AH, Gupta SK, Collins MH, et al. An antibody against IL-5 reduces numbers of esophageal intraepithelial eosinophils in children with eosinophilic esophagitis. Gastroenterology 2011;141:1593-604.
46. Abonia JP, Rothenberg ME. Eosinophilic esophagitis: rapidly advancing insights. Annu Rev Med 2012;63:421-34.
47. Spergel JM, Rothenberg ME, Collins MH, et al. Reslizumab in children and adolescents with eosinophilic esophagitis: results of a double-blind, randomized, placebo-controlled trial. J Allergy Clin Immunol 2012;129:456-63.
48. Blanchard C, Mishra A, Saito-Akei H, et al. Inhibition of human interleukin-13-induced respiratory and oesophageal inflammation by anti-human-interleukin-13 antibody (CAT-354). Clin Exp Allergy 2005;35:1096-103.
49. Rubinstein E, Cho JY, Rosenthal P, et al. Siglec-F inhibition reduces esophageal eosinophilia and angiogenesis in a mouse mode of eosinophilic esophagitis. J Pediatr Gastroenterol Nutr 2011; 53:409-16.

Eosinophilic Gastritis and Gastroenteritis

50. Hogan S, Mishra E, Brandt E, et al. A critical role for eotaxin in experimental oral antigen-induced eosinophilic gastrointestinal allergy. Proc Nat Acad Sci USA 2000;97:6681-6.
51. Hogan SP, Mishra A, Brandt EB, et al. A pathological function for eotaxin and eosinophils in eosinophilic gastrointestinal inflammation. Nat Immunol 2001;2:353-60.
52. Brandt EB, Strait RT, Hershko D, et al. Mast cells are required for experimental oral allergen-induced diarrhea. J Clin Invest 2003;112: 1666-77.
53. Chehade M, Magid MS, Mofidi S, et al. Allergic eosinophilic gastroenteritis with protein-losing enteropathy: intestinal pathology, clinical course, and long-term follow-up. J Pediatr Gastroenterol Nutr 2006;42:516-21.
54. Lwin T, Melton SD, Genta RM. Eosinophilic gastritis: histopathological characterization and quantification of the normal gastric eosinophil content. Mod Pathol 2011;24:556-63.
55. Foroughi S, Foster B, Kim N, et al. Anti-IgE treatment of eosinophil-associated gastrointestinal disorders. J Allergy Clin Immunol 2007; 120:594-601.

Conclusion

56. Rothenberg ME, Mishra A, Brandt EB, et al. Gastrointestinal eosinophils in health and disease. Adv Immunol 2001;78:291-328.
57. Noel RJ, Rothenberg ME. Eosinophilic esophagitis. Curr Opin Pediatr 2005;17:690-4.

SECTION G

Systemic Disease

69 Clinical Significance of Immunoglobulin E

PHILIP H. SMITH | DENNIS R. OWNBY

CONTENTS

SUMMARY OF IMPORTANT CONCEPTS

» Immunoglobulin E (IgE) is evolutionarily highly conserved and appears to have evolved to provide a means for rapidly responding to certain types of stimuli, primarily internal and external parasites.

» Normal serum concentrations of IgE are typically low (average, 25 kU/L [60 ng/mL]) and vary greatly among individuals.

» IgE antibody-antigen interactions can initiate potent biologically amplified reactions capable of causing life-threatening symptoms in minutes.

» Many disease processes can cause alterations of serum IgE concentrations that appear to reflect the overall balance of immune regulation.

» Serum IgE concentrations tend to be greater in persons with allergic diseases and those with asthma, but the degree of increase is neither consistent nor large enough to be diagnostically valuable.

Introduction

Of the five isotypes of human immunoglobulin, immunoglobulin E (IgE) is present in the smallest quantities, contributing only 0.002% of circulating immunoglobulins. Serum concentrations of IgE are typically reported as nanograms (ng) or international units (IU) per volume of serum (e.g., IU/mL, kIU/L), and 1 IU is equal to 2.4 ng of protein. Evolutionarily, IgE is conserved and found in all mammals, including monotremes. Of all immunoglobulin isotypes, IgE has the highest affinity for antigens and for its receptors.[1] The tremendous biologic amplification linked to IgE and its receptors is shown by the fact that even low (ng/mL) concentrations of cell surface IgE can cause life-threatening reactions within minutes of allergen exposure in highly sensitive individuals. IgE-mediated immunity and inflammatory reactions are thought of primarily in terms of immediate or type I allergic reactions and as part of the immune response to parasites, but research suggests that IgE is involved in a variety of inflammatory processes in humans.[1-3] This chapter reviews the many biologic properties of IgE that are expressed in human health and disease.

IgE concentrations can be altered by disease processes through four mechanisms. First, total serum IgE levels can reflect nonspecific changes in protein production or catabolism. Second, total serum IgE concentrations can reflect the balance or overall regulation of the immune system. Third, in some diseases, factors specifically stimulate IgE production. Fourth, some diseases may result directly from the production of IgE antibodies specific for certain allergens. All of these mechanisms can quickly alter serum levels of IgE, which has the shortest half-life of all immunoglobulin isotypes: 1 to 5 days in humans and 12 hours in mice.[1]

IgE synthesis and IgE-mediated release of cytokines and chemokines are discussed in other chapters. Chapters 3, 11, and 23 present the basic immunologic mechanisms that regulate IgE production and mediator release, and Chapters 14 and 15 discuss the effects of the mediators. The details of the laboratory methods for measuring IgE antibodies are presented in Chapter 74.

The research efforts of many scientists eventually revealed that human allergic disease results from the formation of antibodies belonging to a unique immunoglobulin isotype: IgE. In 1921, the collaboration of Otto Prausnitz and Heinz Küstner produced a critical discovery. Küstner, who had been highly allergic to fish since childhood, began his medical career as an assistant to Prausnitz, who suffered from grass pollen hay fever. During the course of their investigations, they demonstrated that when Küstner's serum was injected into Prausnitz's skin, the immediate sensitivity to fish was transferred to the site. They concluded that a serum component was responsible for transferring the specific sensitivity. The technique of passively transferring allergic sensitivity became known as the Prausnitz-Küstner (PK) reaction or test. The substance that transferred the sensitivity was called the *reagin*, and sera containing reagins were called *reaginic*. It was not until 1966 that two groups of investigators identified reagin as a unique immunoglobulin isotype, IgE (see Chapter 23).

Normal Immunoglobulin E Production

IgE antibody production is normally highly regulated, resulting in minimal IgE concentrations in body fluids.[2] Most of the

IgE-producing plasma cells are found in the lymphoid tissue associated with the gastrointestinal and respiratory tracts. The highest concentrations of IgE-producing plasma cells have been found in the tonsils and adenoids. Like other immunoglobulin isotypes, the IgE molecule is composed of two light and two heavy chains. The heavy chain of IgE contains four constant domains (Cε1 through Cε4), rather than the three found in other immunoglobulins (e.g., IgG). Most IgE produced in the body is bound to a high-affinity receptor (FcεRI) that is expressed mainly on mast cells and basophils. Other cells, such as B cells and airway smooth muscle cells, have lower-affinity IgE receptors (e.g., FcεRII [CD23])[3] (see Chapter 23).

ONTOGENY OF IMMUNOGLOBULIN E PRODUCTION

IgE production has been observed as early as 11 weeks in human fetal tissue cultures, but determination of how early in gestation a fetus becomes capable of producing IgE antibodies is complicated by a low rate of diffusion of maternal IgE into the amniotic fluid. Germline transcripts for the ε chain of IgE are detectable as early as 7 to 10 weeks, and B cells primed to undergo class switching for IgE production can produce IgE by 20 weeks' gestation.[4] Normally, in developed countries, little IgE is produced until after birth. Limited IgE production apparently correlates with limited fetal antigenic exposure. In developed countries, less than 1% of cord serum samples contain detectable IgE antibodies to common allergens, and some of the detected allergen-specific IgE may be of maternal origin, but allergen-specific IgE rarely has been demonstrated in cord serum when IgE antibodies to the same allergen were not detectable in the mother's serum. Most studies have failed to find fetal IgE production in the absence of maternal production.[5]

In developed countries, serum IgE concentrations gradually increase after birth and reach maximum values between the ages of 10 and 15 years.[6,7] Figure 69-1 shows the changes with age of serum IgE concentrations in cohorts of allergic and nonallergic children who were studied by Lindberg and Arroyave.[7]

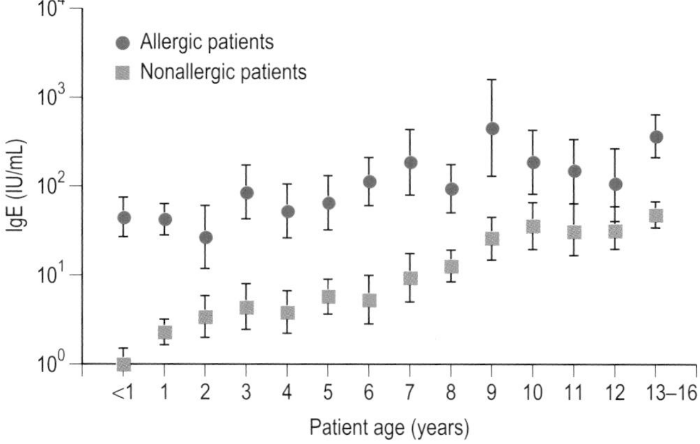

Figure 69-1 The geometric means plus or minus the 95% confidence intervals of immunoglobulin E (IgE) levels are compared from allergic and nonallergic children of various ages. Significant differences ($P < .05$) were observed at all ages, except at 11 and 12 years of age. *(Reproduced with permission from Lindberg RE, Arroyave C. Levels of IgE in serum from normal children and allergic children as measured by an enzyme immunoassay. J Allergy Clin Immunol 1986;78:614-8.)*

After reaching maximum values in the early teens, IgE levels decline throughout adulthood.[6,7] The rate of IgE decline in adults has varied in different studies, with sex and smoking contributing to the observed differences.[6] Basal serum IgE levels appear to be under genetic control, but the precise mode of genetic control has remained elusive (see Chapter 23). In children, no significant gender difference has been found in mean serum IgE concentrations, but men have significantly higher mean IgE concentrations than women.[6,7] The gender difference found in adults in some studies may partially result from different rates of smoking by men and women and from differences in IgE changes with age.[8]

NORMAL SERUM IMMUNOGLOBULIN E CONCENTRATIONS

Serum IgE concentrations vary widely. Figure 69-2 shows the frequency distribution of serum IgE levels in a sample population of 2743 white Anglo-Americans older than 6 years of age living in Tucson, Arizona.[6] Plotting the IgE frequencies on an arithmetic scale demonstrates a highly skewed distribution. Replotting the data on a logarithmic scale approximates a normal distribution.[6] The skewed distribution of IgE values in most populations does not allow the use of parametric statistical tests leading to the more common use of logarithmically transformed IgE values in most research studies comparing IgE values in different populations and the use of the geometric mean to describe the central tendency of IgE values from a population. When 95% confidence intervals are calculated using the logarithmically transformed data, the upper limits of normal are relatively high compared with the geometric mean. The high upper limits of normal and broad overlap between IgE concentrations in atopic and nonatopic people limit the diagnostic value of total serum IgE measurements for detecting allergic disease.

Serum IgE levels are also influenced by age, genetic predisposition, race, immune status, season of the year, medications, and some disease processes. Racial factors seem to be important in controlling IgE levels, although it is often difficult to separate racial and genetic factors from environmental effects.[9] In a study of blacks and whites living in the United States, Grundbacher and Massie[9] found consistently higher IgE serum levels in blacks in all age groups. Studies of other racial and ethnic groups suggest that normal total serum IgE levels vary widely, presumably because of genetic differences and differences in environmental exposures. Polymorphisms of CCL11 (i.e., eotaxin) also appear to be associated with total IgE, with one nucleotide eotaxin polymorphism variant associated with increases in African American families and other polymorphism variants associated with lower total IgE levels in whites.[10] Racial norms for IgE have not been established.

Total serum IgE levels may vary twofold to fourfold annually in sensitive patients in response to pollen seasons. The maximum IgE levels are usually reached 4 to 6 weeks after the peak of the pollen season, followed by a gradual decline until the onset of the next pollen season.

Questions have arisen about "undetectable" or "absent" serum IgE levels. Most clinical assays for total IgE have a lower limit of detection of 2 to 5 IU/mL. Concentrations of less than 2 IU/mL are reported as undetectable. Some have speculated that undetectable concentrations of IgE might be related to autoimmune disease or recurrent infections. In a

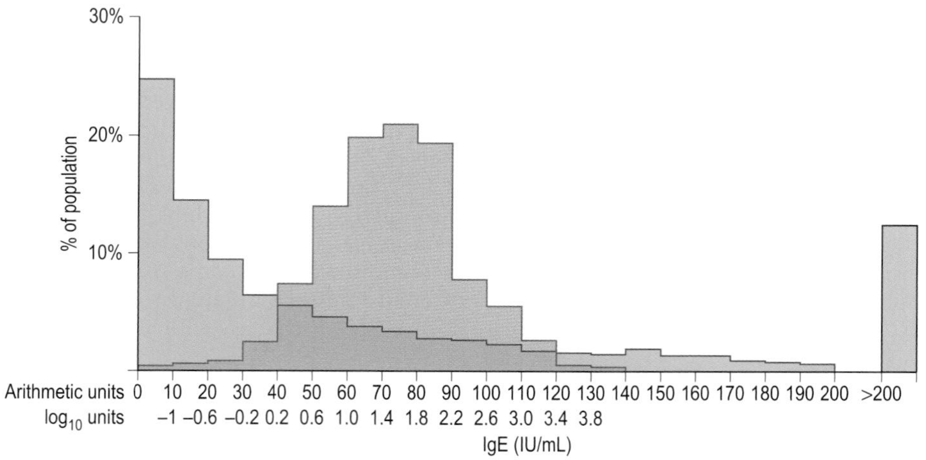

Figure 69-2 Arithmetic (*aqua-blue*) versus logarithmic (*light red*) distributions of total serum immunoglobulin E (IgE) in a community population sample. Before logarithmic conversion, the distribution is skewed, with almost 40% of values at 20 IU/mL or less. Normalization occurs after logarithmic conversion with a geometric mean level of 32.1 IU/mL. *(Reproduced with permission from Barbee RA, Halonen M, Lebowitz M, Burrows B. Distribution of IgE in a community population sample: Correlations with age, sex, and allergen skin test reactivity. J Allergy Clin Immunol 1981;68:106-11.)*

BOX 69-1 CONDITIONS ASSOCIATED WITH UNUSUALLY HIGH SERUM IMMUNOGLOBULIN E CONCENTRATIONS (≥500 IU/mL)

Allergic bronchopulmonary mycosis
Allergic fungal sinusitis
Atopic dermatitis
Human immunodeficiency virus (HIV) infection
Hyperimmunoglobulin E (hyper-IgE) syndrome
Immunoglobulin E myeloma
Kimura disease
Lymphoma
Netherton syndrome
Systemic helminthic parasitosis
Tuberculosis

population-based study of 626 healthy women, Levin and colleagues found that 3.4% had serum IgE concentrations of less than 2 IU/mL.[11] When a more sensitive assay was used, IgE was measurable in all of the women with a geometric mean IgE level of 1.2 IU/mL. Compared with the women with higher IgE levels, the women with low levels were less likely to have physician-diagnosed sinusitis or asthma. A low serum IgE level may also indicate low levels of other serum proteins, including other classes of immunoglobulins, as occur in patients with common variable immunodeficiency. Box 69-1 lists several conditions for which unusually high serum IgE concentrations have been reported.

IMMUNOGLOBULIN E IN OTHER BODY FLUIDS

Total and some allergen-specific IgE levels have been reported in nasal and bronchial washings, nasal polyp tissue, intestinal fluids, feces, saliva, breast milk, urine, tears, middle ear effusions, aqueous humor, and cerebrospinal fluid, typically at concentrations of less than 1% of the serum concentration. In a few instances, investigators have demonstrated allergen-specific IgE in certain body fluids when the specific IgE antibodies were not demonstrable in serum. Even though local production of IgE in tissues has been shown in individuals in whom circulating IgE of the same specificity could not be demonstrated, the clinical significance of local production has not been well established.[12,13]

Immunoglobulin E in Allergic Disease

Total serum IgE levels are related to the probability of an individual having detectable allergen-specific IgE to common allergens. In a study of a large adult population, subjects with total serum IgE concentrations in the highest quintile (>66 IU/mL) were 37 times more likely to have IgE antibodies specific for one or more common allergens.[8] In a 5-year follow-up study of 223 working adults, geometric mean IgE levels were higher in skin test–positive than skin test–negative individuals initially (30.1 versus 97.0 IU/mL) and at follow-up (24.9 versus 92.9).[14] Initial IgE levels were also significantly higher in those whose skin test results converted from negative to positive compared with those whose skin test results remained negative (92.3 versus 30.1 IU/mL, $P < .003$).[14]

Many studies have shown that total serum IgE concentrations tend to be higher in adults and children with allergic diseases compared with nonallergic individuals, but despite these suggestive relationships, the diagnostic value of total serum IgE concentrations is limited. A large study by Wittig and cowokers[15] calculated the diagnostic sensitivity and specificity of total serum IgE determinations using three cutoff levels for 570 asthmatic and 244 rhinitic individuals. When the highest cutoff level of 320 IU/mL was used, the specificity of the IgE test was 98% for the rhinitic and asthmatic groups, but the sensitivity was only 55% for individuals with asthma and 30% for those with rhinitis. When the cutoff level was reduced to 100 IU/mL, the sensitivity increased to 78% and 60% for the asthmatic and rhinitic groups, respectively, but with a reduction in specificity to 80% for both groups.[15] Marsh and colleagues[16] calculated that the optimal total serum IgE level for discriminating between allergic and nonallergic adults was 100 IU/mL; however, this cutoff misclassified approximately 20% of each group. Collectively, these and other studies have shown that measurement of total serum IgE concentrations is of limited value as a screening test for allergic disease.

IMMUNOGLOBULIN E AND RISK OF ASTHMA

Burrows and associates[17] reported that rates of asthma in a population-based sample of people older than 6 years of age highly correlated with serum IgE levels. For this study, serum IgE levels were expressed as standardized *z* scores adjusted for age and gender. None of the persons with the lowest *z* scores (<1.46 standard deviations below the mean) had asthma, regardless of age. The relationship between the rates of self-reported asthma and the total serum IgE concentrations was stronger than the relationship between asthma rates and skin test reactivity to a battery of common allergens.[17] The rates of self-reported rhinitis were more closely related to skin test reactivity than to serum IgE concentrations.

Similar findings were reported by Sunyer and associates[18] from a study of more than 1600 Spanish adults between the ages of 20 and 44 years. For total serum IgE concentrations of 100 IU/mL or higher, the odds ratio for asthma was 4.7 compared with those with lower IgE levels. Even after persons with positive test results for allergen-specific IgE antibodies were excluded, the association between IgE levels of 100 IU/mL or higher and asthma persisted, with an odds ratio of 18, suggesting a relationship beyond that related to allergic sensitivity.[18] These investigators also found an association between a history of wheezing and bronchial hyperresponsiveness to methacholine without attacks of asthma and total IgE levels, with an odds ratio of 5, which persisted (odds ratio = 5.9) after excluding those with detectable allergen-specific IgE levels.[18] These results are consistent with studies demonstrating significantly increased numbers of mast cells and macrophages bearing high-affinity IgE receptors (FcεRI) in bronchial biopsies from allergic and nonallergic asthmatics.[13]

In a study of 1037 children from New Zealand, Sears and colleagues[19] found that diagnosed asthma was strongly related to serum IgE levels ($P < .0001$ for trend). None of the children with IgE levels less than 32 IU/mL had asthma, whereas 36% of those with IgE levels of at least 1000 IU/mL had asthma. Airway hyperresponsiveness to methacholine was also highly correlated with serum IgE levels ($P < .0001$), and the correlation persisted even after excluding children with asthma ($P < .0001$) or all children with histories of wheezing, rhinitis, or eczema ($P < .0001$).[19] Additional analysis of this study found that when lung function and serum IgE levels were considered, other diagnoses and symptoms explained little of the variation in methacholine responsiveness.[20] One study reported that there was a correlation between serum IgE and methacholine responsiveness in European-American children but not among African-American children.[21] In this study, serum IgE levels were significantly different between European-American children with and without asthma, although not between African-American children with and without asthma. These differences were not altered by adjusting for the child's gender, parental education, parental smoking, or maternal smoking during pregnancy.[21] These studies suggest an association between serum IgE levels and asthma that is separate from the association between serum IgE levels and allergen-specific IgE antibodies.

In contrast to earlier studies, a consortium-based study of the genetics of asthma involving analysis of DNA from almost 27,000 individuals found six genetic polymorphisms associated with asthma, and none of them was significantly associated with IgE levels.[22] The locus for the class II human leukocyte antigen DR (*HLA-DR*) was found to have a significant genome-wide association with IgE, whereas other loci strongly associated with IgE levels were not associated with asthma. The estimated population attributable risk fraction for the combined actions of the loci related to asthma was 38% (95% confidence interval [CI], 24% to 44%) for childhood-onset asthma.[22] These findings suggest that the association between IgE and asthma is more likely related to environmental exposures affecting asthma risk and IgE levels than to common genetic influences.

The anti-human IgE monoclonal antibody, omalizumab, has been approved for treatment of allergic asthma in individuals 12 years old and older.[23] The package insert indicates that IgE levels cannot be measured accurately after treatment with omalizumab has commenced, however, at least one common commercial assay continues to produce accurate results in sera from individuals receiving omalizumab.[24] In most studies total IgE levels increase for several months after the initiation of omalizumab therapy and then decline to very low levels.

One of the few allergic diseases in which total serum IgE levels are of clinical value is allergic bronchopulmonary aspergillosis (ABPA)[25] (see Chapter 61). An elevated serum IgE level (>416 IU/mL [1000 ng/mL]) is one of the diagnostic criteria for this condition, and the level of IgE can be used to follow the course of the disease. When the disease is successfully treated with glucocorticoids, the serum IgE level falls, and disease exacerbations often are heralded by an increase in serum IgE concentrations. There appears to be an association between disease activity and levels of anti-*Aspergillus* IgE antibodies. Several studies have suggested that treatment of ABPA with omalizumab is effective in controlling the disease while using significantly lower doses of oral corticosteroids.[25]

Many physicians assume that treating allergic patients with oral corticosteroids can reduce serum total serum IgE concentrations, but a study of 10 adults with allergic asthma demonstrated that 20 mg of oral prednisone given twice daily resulted in increased IgE concentrations in all 10 individuals (medians: 242.5 IU/mL before prednisone and 384.5 IU/mL after prednisone).[26] The increase in IgE was polyclonal, as shown by measurements of IgE specific to different allergens. Serum IgG levels were unchanged.

A gross elevation of serum IgE may also be helpful in distinguishing tropical pulmonary eosinophilia from some other causes of pulmonary symptoms associated with eosinophilia, such as Churg-Strauss syndrome and Wegener granulomatosis (i.e., granulomatosis with polyangiitis).[25]

IMMUNOGLOBULIN E AND LUNG FUNCTION

Evaluation of the relationship between total serum IgE levels and lung function is complicated by the associations between asthma and IgE concentrations and between cigarette smoking and IgE concentrations.[27] Several studies have suggested that higher total serum IgE levels are associated with a more rapid decline in lung function with advancing age. Sherrill and coworkers evaluated the relationship between total serum IgE levels and the decline in forced expiratory volume in 1 second (FEV_1) in 1533 adults older than 35 years of age as part of the Tucson Epidemiological Study of Airways Obstructive Disease.[28] Subjects had been observed over an interval of up to 20 years. A significant inverse association was found between IgE levels and lung function. This association was independent of smoking and asthma status, and it was statistically distinct from age, except in current smokers older than 55 years of age. The effect was small in nonasthmatic subjects but larger in current and never-smoking asthmatic subjects.[28]

Somewhat different results came from a study in the United Kingdom of individuals 65 years old or older who were evaluated for pulmonary function, methacholine responsiveness, skin test reactivity to common allergens, and total serum IgE levels and then were followed for 4 years.[29] For the 212 subjects who completed the study, multivariable analysis demonstrated that male gender was the most important predictor of FEV_1 decline. Methacholine responsiveness also tended to be associated with FEV_1 decline. When the analysis was restricted to individual categories by smoking status, age was the only significant factor in never-smokers, whereas skin test reactivity and methacholine responsiveness were significant predictors of accelerated FEV_1 decline in former and current smokers combined.[29] There is conflicting information concerning an inverse relationship between IgE levels and FEV_1 in smokers, but there does not appear to be a significant relationship between IgE levels and the rate of decline of FEV_1.[30,31]

In a study of the genetics of asthma and atopy, total serum IgE levels were found to be different among current-, previous-, and never-smoking individuals after considering gender, personal or family history of asthma, and socio-occupational class.[32] In this study, there was also evidence that passive exposure to environmental tobacco smoke was associated with increased IgE levels in women who were first-degree relatives of asthmatics.[32] Some studies have found correlations between total serum IgE concentrations and exhaled nitric oxide levels in patients with asthma,[33,34] but other studies suggest the relationship is with allergic sensitization.[35]

IMMUNOGLOBULIN E IN CORD BLOOD

Because IgE is not normally transferred across the placenta to the infant, the IgE concentration in cord blood is thought to indicate an infant's basal predisposition to IgE production. If this is true, cord blood IgE concentrations should be a useful indicator of a child's risk of developing allergic disease. The predictive value of cord blood has been widely debated, but it appears to be modest.[36] Several early studies suggested that cord blood IgE was a useful marker of allergic risk, but subsequent studies have failed to show strong associations between cord blood IgE concentrations and allergic risk during childhood. There have also been conflicting reports about the extent to which cord blood IgE concentrations are influenced by maternal and paternal allergy. Although early studies were hampered by the imprecision of assays for measuring IgE at concentrations of less than 1 IU/mL, newer assays can measure even lower concentrations in sera much more precisely and reproducibly.

One of the more difficult problems is distinguishing when a cord blood IgE concentration has been elevated by maternal blood admixture during delivery. Most studies suggest that admixture of maternal and fetal blood is a relatively uncommon event, occurring in less than 5% of cases, but many studies have shown highly significant correlations between maternal and cord blood IgE concentrations, raising the question of admixture or maternal influences controlling maternal and fetal IgE production.[37] There have been conflicting reports concerning the effect of gestational age and other influences (Box 69-2) on IgE concentrations, but two very large studies encompassing 5305 and 6401 cord blood samples failed to find any effect of gestational age within the range of 34 to 42 weeks' gestation.[38]

BOX 69-2 FACTORS EVALUATED FOR EFFECT ON CONCENTRATION OF IMMUNOGLOBULIN E IN CORD BLOOD

FACTORS ASSOCIATED WITH INCREASED LEVELS

- Maternal atopy
- Atopy in first-degree relatives
- Elevated maternal immunoglobulin E (IgE) levels
- Male gender
- Black or Hispanic ethnicity
- Progesterone administration to the pregnant mother
- Maternal parasitosis
- Maternal smoking

FACTORS NOT AFFECTING LEVELS

- Prenatal oral contraceptives
- Albuterol administration
- Pregnancy diet
- Maternal smoking
- Gestational age of 34 to 42 weeks
- Type of delivery (e.g., spontaneous, cesarean section, vacuum extraction)
- Maternal use of corticosteroids

FACTORS ASSOCIATED WITH DECREASED LEVELS

- Maternal hepatitis B carrier status
- Maternal alcohol consumption

DETECTION OF ALLERGEN-SPECIFIC IMMUNOGLOBULIN E

Factors Affecting Immunoglobulin E Levels

The discovery that reaginic antibodies were limited to the IgE isotype soon led to immunoassays for measuring the quantities of allergen-specific IgE antibodies (see Chapter 74). The first allergen-specific IgE immunoassays using radioisotopes were relatively imprecise, and a scoring system of 0 to 4+ was used to indicate the range from undetectable through increasing quantities of IgE. Attempts to increase the sensitivity of the assays led to modifying the procedures for counting radioactivity in samples and the addition of classes to produce a modified scoring system. Unfortunately, these changes in counting and scoring did not change the analytic sensitivity of the assay, and the net result of the changes was an increase in sensitivity and a corresponding decrease in specificity. Current assays for allergen-specific IgE are based on enzyme labels, and the newer assays can accurately measure specific IgE in terms of mass units of IgE per volume.

The clinical value of knowing the mass units of allergen-specific IgE has been well documented in studies showing the predictive value of food-specific IgE antibody levels and positive results for food challenges.[39] Information on the relationship between inhalant allergy-specific IgE and symptoms is not as robust. Some studies have shown relationships between allergen-specific IgE levels and measures of lung function and inflammation.[35,40] The strongest relationships have been found between the total amount of allergen-specific IgE (i.e., sum of all specific

IgE measurements performed) measured and the levels of exhaled nitric oxide.

Specific IgE concentrations vary according to a person's age, the degree and duration of the most recent allergen exposure, the degree and duration of exposure to cross-reactive allergens, and immunotherapy. Specific IgE levels are typically highest in school-age children and young adults, whereas specific IgE may be difficult to detect in infants because of the very low IgE concentrations present. Allergen-specific IgE concentrations also usually rise as a result of pollen exposure. The levels of specific IgE typically peak approximately 4 weeks after a seasonal pollen exposure and then gradually fall to a nadir before the next pollen season. These seasonal changes are not usually of sufficient magnitude to shift an assay result from negative to positive, but the change may shift a borderline sample result to positive. Similarly, IgE antibody levels rise after insect stings in some individuals, irrespective of whether the sting provoked allergic symptoms. A general trend of declining allergen-specific IgE concentrations with time has been documented with insect venom and drug-specific IgE. IgE levels also tend to decline during allergen immunotherapy, but part of the decline observed in some studies might have been the result of IgG antibody formation blocking the detection of IgE antibodies.

Indications for Measuring Specific Immunoglobulin E Antibodies

The association between the presence of detectable allergen-specific IgE (determined by positive skin test results or IgE antibody measurements) with allergic symptoms is inconsistent.[41,42] Allergic symptoms were evaluated in a group of individuals with positive skin-prick test results for grass pollen, and the same individuals underwent nasal challenges with grass pollen and kept symptom diaries during the next grass pollen season. Among those with positive skin-prick test results, only 68% had nasal symptoms with challenge, and only 64% had symptoms correlating with pollen counts, suggesting that more than 30% of those with positive skin-prick test results for grass were asymptomatic when naturally exposed to grass pollen in the air.[43]

Results were similar in a cross-sectional study of 2295 Dutch adults between 20 and 70 years of age, who were questioned about nasal symptoms and tested by skin-prick and in vitro tests for IgE antibodies to nine common allergens. Associations between nasal symptoms after indoor and outdoor allergen exposures and positive test results for specific IgE antibodies were highly significant but far from absolute. In individuals with indoor-only, outdoor-only, and combined indoor and outdoor symptoms, the prevalences of at least one positive skin-prick test result were 39.1%, 43.7%, and 55.4%, respectively, but 15.5% of those without any nasal symptoms had at least one positive skin-prick test result.[44] In the pioneering work of Settipane and colleagues,[45] students beginning their first year of college were skin tested and their symptoms followed. Of the 1243 students evaluated as freshmen, 989 were reassessed 3 years later as seniors. A total of 614 had no histories of allergic symptoms as freshmen, but 108 of them had at least one positive skin-prick test result in response to a panel of 15 common allergens, and 19 of these students had developed rhinitis symptoms. The more strongly reactive the skin test response, the greater the risk that symptoms would develop.[45] Even when the students were followed for 23 years, the risk of developing allergic symptoms was still greater among those initially having positive skin test results.

Numerous theories have been advanced to explain the lack of symptoms in some sensitized individuals. Differences in the levels of allergen-specific IgE antibodies, differences in the affinity of some specific IgE antibodies for allergen, and the presence or absence of antibodies of other isotypes specific for the same allergen epitopes have been proposed.[41] Because of the inconsistent relationship between allergic sensitization determined by the presence of detectable allergen-specific IgE and symptoms, the results of tests for allergen-specific IgE are clinically valuable only when considered in the context of a patient's history.

After the clinical decision has been made to test for allergen-specific IgE, the physician must determine whether in vivo or in vitro tests are in the patient's best interests. Box 69-3 compares the relative advantages of skin tests and in vitro immunoassays. When an individual is highly sensitive, both skin tests and immunoassays are likely to detect IgE specific to the provoking allergens. In some highly sensitive individuals, the most compelling advantage of in vitro assays is their freedom from the risk of an anaphylactic reaction. In vitro assays are also more convenient when it is difficult to withdraw an interfering medication or when a patient's skin is not normally reactive to histamine. Some individuals may have medical problems that can interfere with skin testing, including hospitalized patients on pressors, those with severe burns or other extensive skin diseases, and those with nonhemolytic transfusion reactions. In some very uncooperative individuals, such as mentally impaired adults, skin testing may be hazardous to the patient and the person attempting to perform the tests. In some circumstances, it may be more convenient to transport a serum sample than to transport the patient for testing. When individuals with very high levels of total IgE from parasitic disease are tested, in vitro analysis may be more reliable.

Despite the advantages, two major concerns limit the use of in vitro tests for allergen-specific IgE in the United States. First, in most cases, in vitro tests are not as sensitive as skin tests for detecting allergen-specific IgE. Second, on a per test basis, skin tests have lower time and reagent costs. Efforts to reduce the cost of laboratory tests for allergen-specific IgE have included development of screening tests using multiple allergens in a

BOX 69-3 RELATIVE ADVANTAGES OF IMMUNOASSAYS AND SKIN TESTS FOR ALLERGEN-SPECIFIC IMMUNOGLOBULIN E

IMMUNOASSAYS

- Lack of risk for allergic reaction
- Results unaffected by drugs
- Results unaffected by condition of skin
- Greater patient convenience (special expertise not required)
- Easier-to-document quality control
- Immunoglobulin E (IgE) level predictive of disease (especially for food allergy)
- Well standardized and reproducible

SKIN TESTS

- Greater sensitivity
- Wider selection of allergens
- Results immediately available
- Less time and reagent expense per test

single test and discussions of the maximum number of tests needed for diagnosis.[42]

Detection of cross-reactive IgE antibodies is a potential problem with in vitro tests.[46] Many individuals allergic to pollens have detectable IgE antibodies to foods, and 20% to 30% of those with food-specific IgE antibodies do not report symptoms related to foods. Many of the pollen-food cross-reactions may result from profilin, a highly conserved molecule among plants. Cross-reactive antibodies between foods and latex allergens also complicate the interpretation of in vitro tests for latex specific IgE antibodies.

Immunoglobulin E in Infectious and Parasitic Disease

Serum IgE levels have been measured in many infectious and parasitic diseases. The changes observed with some infections appear to be the result of IgE antibodies specific for the infectious agent, whereas in other diseases, changes in IgE appear to be nonspecific or may indicate a difference in individual susceptibility to infection. Some of the diseases associated with unusually high or low IgE concentrations are listed in Box 69-1.

VIRAL INFECTIONS

Welliver and colleagues[47] were the first to report that IgE specific for the respiratory syncytial virus (RSV) was highly associated with wheezing and other signs of lower respiratory tract involvement during primary RSV infections in children. Peak IgE-RSV titers during acute infection were also significantly associated with the risk of recurrent wheezing episodes during a 4-year follow-up study.[47] The role of RSV infection in allergic disease remains a focus of intense research, but it has been difficult to reproduce Welliver's original findings.[48] Later research suggests that IgE antibodies are formed in some individuals after viral infections and immunizations. The role of these IgE antibodies in relation to vaccine effectiveness and adverse reactions needs further investigation.[49]

Studies evaluating changes in serum IgE concentrations during viral infections have produced variable results. Studies of mononucleosis related to Epstein-Barr virus infection have found an initial rise in IgE concentration for 7 to 10 days, followed by a decline and then a return to baseline levels over a course of weeks to months. The mean serum IgE level at initial presentation of measles was 258 IU/mL for 182 Peruvian children, compared with a mean of only 82.5 IU/mL during the second week after the appearance of the skin rash in children without complications. IgE levels in children with measles-related pneumonia were similar to those with uncomplicated disease, whereas children who developed measles encephalitis had the highest mean levels (540 IU/mL) in the first week after the onset of rash and a slower decline in their IgE levels.

Skoner and coworkers[50] reported that experimentally induced rhinovirus infections in adults with allergic rhinitis acutely produced a highly significant increase in total serum IgE levels ($P < .000008$ compared with baseline, and $P < .0001$ compared with convalescent samples), whereas no significant change in IgE levels was found in nonallergic adults. Serum IgG, IgA, and IgM levels did not change significantly in allergic or nonallergic individuals.

Another interesting association between IgE and infectious agents is found with human retroviruses. Increased serum IgE concentrations have been reported in patients with human immunodeficiency virus type 1 (HIV-1) infections, and in contrast to patients with many other diseases with elevated IgE levels, patients with acquired immunodeficiency syndrome (AIDS) have a remarkably high incidence of allergic reactions to drugs and to environmental allergens.[51] The factors associated with elevated IgE levels in HIV-1 disease are not completely understood. A stepwise regression analysis of data from a study of serum HIV-1 status of intravenous drug users and homosexual men found that the factors related to IgE levels were HIV-1 status ($P < .0009$), intravenous drug use ($P < .014$), $CD8^+$ cell counts ($P < .0001$), plasma level of vitamin E ($P < .006$), and alcohol intake ($P < .047$). These five variables accounted for 71% of the variation in total serum IgE.[51] The relationship between the progression of HIV-1 infection and IgE levels has varied among studies, but increasing levels of IgE in HIV-1 infection appears to be a poor prognostic sign.[52] In children with HIV-1 infection, there was an association between elevated IgE and secondary infections.[53]

BACTERIAL INFECTIONS

The production of IgE specific for common bacteria has been examined. IgE specific for *Staphylococcus aureus* exotoxins is usually found in patients with hyperimmunoglobulinemia E with recurrent infection syndrome (see Chapter 72). Older studies of IgE specific to *S. aureus* were sometimes difficult to interpret because of the ability of some *Staphylococcus* cell wall components to bind IgE nonspecifically. Later studies using relatively pure staphylococcal toxins have shown that anti-staphylococcal toxin IgE may be related to various allergic diseases, especially nasal polyps and chronic rhinosinusitis[54] (see Chapter 43).

Children develop IgE antibodies specific for pertussis and tetanus toxoids after immunization. However, these antibodies do not appear to have major clinical significance.[55,56]

YEASTS AND FUNGI

Some individuals form IgE antibodies specific for yeasts or fungi. IgE antibodies specific for individual antigens in *Candida albicans* infection can be detected, and the levels of these antibodies may be increased in individuals with atopic dermatitis.[57] Others have reported that IgE antibodies to the yeast *Pityrosporum ovale* are found in people with atopic dermatitis of the head, face, and neck. Sensitivity to *Trichophyton* organisms has been associated with asthma in patients with *Trichophyton* infections, and their asthma symptoms have been reduced after treating cutaneous infections.[58]

IMMUNOGLOBULIN E AND PARASITIC DISEASES

Increased IgE levels typically occur during helminth parasitic infections. There seems to be an association between increasing levels of tissue invasion and increasing levels of IgE. The increased IgE concentrations are the result of parasite-specific and nonspecific polyclonal IgE production. One mechanism proposed to explain the increase in total IgE levels is the secretion by parasites of factors that stimulate production of interleukin-4 (IL-4) or interleukin-13 (IL-13), or both, leading to increased IgE levels. Total serum IgE levels typically fall after successful treatment of the parasitized individual.[59,60]

The hypothesis that IgE is at least partially protective in parasitic disease is widely debated.[61] Some studies strongly support a protective role for IgE antibodies, whereas other studies show no protective effect. After controlling for water contact and levels of antilarval antigen antibodies of other isotypes, a study of schistosomiasis showed that antilarval antigen IgE levels were significantly related to a reduced risk of reinfection after treatment. In other studies of *Ascaris* and malaria, antiparasite IgE levels were related to the risk of reinfection.

The apparent inverse relationship between parasitic and allergic disease has been investigated. Lynch and colleagues[62] examined the effects of antihelminth treatment on IL-4 production, IgE levels, and skin test reactivity among children living in a tropical slum area where infections with *Ascaris lumbricoides* (roundworm) and *Trichuris trichiura* (whipworm) were common. Although a controlled study was not possible, the investigators could compare the results in children who underwent 22 months of treatment to children in the same area whose parents declined treatment. As expected, serum levels of IL-4, total IgE levels, and blood eosinophilia declined in treated children, whereas levels in untreated children increased. In contrast to the fall in total serum IgE levels, treated children were more likely to be skin test positive to house dust extract at the end of the study than at the beginning (17% versus 68%, $P < .001$).

Patients frequently complain that they are allergic to mosquito bites based on the redness and itching of the local acute and late phase reactions after bites. IgE specific for mosquito saliva allergens and allergic reactions from mosquito bites have been reported.[63] Another blood-sucking insect that provokes an IgE response is the kissing bug (*Triatoma* species). IgE antibodies specific for *Triatoma* antigens have been demonstrated, and *Triatoma*-induced anaphylaxis has been reported.[64] Bed bugs (*Cimex* species) have been commonly reported in Western countries. Bites of bed bugs can provoke allergic reactions, and because bed bugs and kissing bugs feed at night, the bites of these insects should be considered in the differential diagnosis of nighttime urticaria and anaphylaxis. The intense itching produced in humans by some ectoparasites, including scabies (*Sarcoptes scabiei*) and chiggers (*Trombicula* species), suggests that IgE antibodies, mast cells, and basophils play a role in the response to these skin infestations.

Immunoglobulin E in Nonatopic Diseases

Some studies have examined IgE antibody levels in nonallergic diseases. Current understanding of the clinical importance of IgE in most of these nonallergic diseases is limited, as is our understanding of the underlying mechanisms (Box 69-4).

NEOPLASTIC DISEASE

The most direct relationship between IgE and neoplastic disease occurs with IgE myeloma. IgE myelomas are rare, with only 40 cases reported since the initial description by Johansson and Bennich in 1967. The low frequency of IgE myelomas presumably reflects the small number of IgE-producing cells normally present in the body. Some IgE myelomas might have been missed because the quantity of IgE produced by the myeloma might have been less than that detectable by routine screening tests for myelomas, or they might have been misclassified as

BOX 69-4 NONALLERGIC DISEASES ASSOCIATED WITH ALTERED TOTAL SERUM IMMUNOGLOBULIN E LEVELS

INCREASED LEVELS (≥500 IU/mL)

Parasitic Diseases

- Ascariasis
- Visceral larva migrans
- Capillariasis
- Paragonimiasis
- Fascioliasis
- Schistosomiasis
- Hookworm
- Trichinosis
- Filariasis
- Strongyloidiasis
- Echinococcosis
- Onchocerciasis
- Malaria

Infections

- Allergic bronchopulmonary mycosis
- Systemic candidiasis
- Coccidioidomycosis
- Leprosy
- Epstein-Barr virus mononucleosis
- Cytomegalovirus mononucleosis
- Viral respiratory infections
- Human immunodeficiency virus (HIV) type 1 infections
- Pertussis

Cutaneous Diseases

- Alopecia areata
- Bullous pemphigoid
- Chronic acral dermatitis
- Streptococcal erythema nodosum

Other Diseases and Disorders

- Nephrotic syndrome
- Drug-induced interstitial nephritis
- Liver disease
- Cystic fibrosis
- Kawasaki disease
- Infantile polyarteritis nodosa
- Primary pulmonary hemosiderosis
- Guillain-Barré syndrome
- Burns
- Rheumatoid arthritis
- Bone marrow transplantation
- Cigarette smoking
- Alcoholism

Neoplastic Diseases

- Hodgkin disease
- Immunoglobulin E (IgE) myeloma
- Bronchial carcinoma

Immunodeficiency Diseases

- Wiskott-Aldrich syndrome
- Hyper-IgE syndrome
- Thymic hypoplasia (DiGeorge syndrome)
- Cellular immunodeficiency with immunoglobulins (Nezelof syndrome)
- Selective IgA deficiency

Medications

- Enfuvirtide
- Pholcodine

DECREASED LEVELS (<5 IU/mL)

- Familial IgE deficiency and recurrent sinopulmonary infections
- Human T cell lymphotropic virus type 1 infections
- Primary biliary cirrhosis

light-chain disease. IgE concentrations at the time of diagnosis ranged from 0.6 to 63 g/L. Symptoms of IgE myeloma are indistinguishable from those of other myelomas, although average survival time is shorter than with other myelomas.

Other links between IgE and neoplasia have been investigated.[1] The strongest association has been between allergic sensitization and gliomas.[65] The anergy exhibited with some lymphoid malignancies such as Hodgkin disease has been associated with increased serum IgE levels. High IgE concentrations in Hodgkin disease have been particularly associated with a nodular sclerotic histologic pattern, and IgE levels usually fall with successful treatment.

Studies of forms of cancer other than Hodgkin disease have not revealed consistent patterns of IgE elevation associated with the cancer or the response to therapy. Although some studies have examined whether allergy is protective against cancer, no consensus has emerged. A Swedish study evaluated total and allergen-specific IgE in relation to cancer in more than 70,000 individuals and found no association.

The relationship of serum IgE levels to the prognosis of cancer patients has been evaluated. Larger quantities of allergen-specific IgE were associated with a poorer prognosis for patients with bronchial carcinoma. IgE levels above the geometric mean for age were a poor prognostic sign for women with primary breast cancer but only if the patient's tumor displayed estrogen receptors. In some animal tumor models, antitumor antigen IgE antibodies have been protective against tumor growth.

The anticancer effects of tumor antigen–specific IgE and IgE of other antigen specificities are being evaluated.[1] In some model systems, the unique properties of IgE, especially related to the ability to attract and activate eosinophils, appear to have important antitumor effects.

TRANSPLANTATION

Increases in serum IgE levels from sevenfold to 2000-fold have been reported in patients after bone marrow transplantation. Initially, the increased IgE levels were thought to result from graft-versus-host disease, but subsequent studies showed that IgE levels also increased in patients who did not have graft-versus-host disease. Increased IgE concentrations do not seem to result from the myeloablative or immunosuppressive therapy used in patients with neoplasia, because increased IgE levels have also been observed in immunodeficient children in whom bone marrow was transplanted without myeloablative therapy.

Many cases of new-onset allergic sensitization and disease after solid organ (e.g., kidney, liver, lung) transplantation have been reported.[66,67] They may be partially related to the specific immunosuppressive drugs used to prevent rejection.

RENAL AND LIVER DISEASE

Total serum IgE levels are elevated in patients with nephrotic syndrome associated with different forms of glomerulonephritis, including minimal change disease, IgM nephropathy, focal glomerulosclerosis, and membranous glomerulonephritis.[67a] High IgE levels in adults and children with nephrotic syndrome are associated with a decreased response to steroid therapy. With adequate therapy, IgE concentrations decline, but no reason has been found for this association.

Increased levels of IgE have also been reported for patients with liver disease, but it is unclear whether this is related to liver disease in general or the particular cause of liver disease. In one study of 52 patients with liver cirrhosis, only alcoholic patients with cirrhosis had elevated IgE levels compared with controls or patients with cirrhosis related to hepatitis B or C or other causes.

Environmental Exposures and Immunoglobulin E

CIGARETTE SMOKING

Multiple studies have evaluated the relationships between cigarette smoking and serum IgE levels. Most studies have found increased serum IgE concentrations in smokers compared with nonsmokers and intermediate concentrations in ex-smokers, although a few studies found no difference. The effect of smoking on serum IgE levels is usually greater in men than in women. In addition to having increased serum IgE levels, smokers do not exhibit the normal age-related decline in serum IgE levels. In some studies, the degree of serum IgE increase in smokers is not related to the intensity or duration of smoking,[8] but other studies have found higher IgE levels with increasing pack-years of smoking after controlling for other variables such as atopic status. There appears to be a relationship between the duration of smoking cessation and decline in IgE levels. Studies have shown that smoking workers are at increased risk for allergic sensitivity to certain occupational allergens.[68]

The results of various studies on the relationship of passive smoking with allergy have been conflicting. Some have shown an increase in the prevalence of allergic sensitization, whereas others have not found differences.[68a] In one controlled challenge, tobacco smoke exposure increased allergen-specific IgE production.[69] The effect of tobacco exposure on total IgE appears to be linked to the expression of a CD14 polymorphism. Increases in asthma severity and total IgE levels vary according to ethnicity.[70]

Total IgE levels are increased in atopic and nonatopic alcoholics. The usual association between cytokines and IgE production does not appear to apply to alcoholics, who have a lower ratio of IL-4 to interferon-γ and no relationship between IgE concentrations and IL-10, IL-12, or IL-13 levels.[71] However, in another study, sensitization to pollen correlated with greater alcohol intake.[72]

DIESEL EXHAUST

Many epidemiologic studies have suggested that the prevalence of allergic disease, especially asthma, has been increasing in developed countries over the past 30 years.[72a,72b] One factor contributing to this trend is air pollution, especially airborne concentrations of diesel exhaust particles. In vivo and in vitro studies showed a direct effect of diesel exhaust particles on IgE production in mice. Diaz-Sanchez and colleagues[73] performed nasal challenges in 11 healthy, nonsmoking adults with various quantities of diesel exhaust particles and found that the particles acted as an adjuvant for IgE production. Diaz-Sanchez and coworkers[74] demonstrated that the increased IgE concentrations were associated with an increase in intranasal cytokine production, including IL-4, IL-5, IL-6, and IL-10. These studies suggest that exposure to diesel exhaust particles and perhaps to other air pollutants may alter local nasal IgE production.

ANIMAL EXPOSURE

The hygiene hypothesis has been used to explain the increase in allergic disease in Western countries over the past few decades. Meta-analyses of the data from many studies show a relatively consistent effect of animal exposure on allergic sensitization and the risk of allergic disease and, in some studies, total serum IgE levels.[75,76] It appears that exposure to indoor dogs and cats during pregnancy reduces cord blood IgE levels and that the effect of animal exposure during the first year of life may persist at least until 18 years of age.[77]

Summary

IgE is an evolutionarily highly conserved isotype in mammals that has many unique effector functions. IgE is most frequently associated with allergic disease, but IgE antibodies are involved in many other types of immune functions. Even though total IgE concentrations are often elevated in allergic individuals, measures of total IgE levels are not useful in the diagnosis of allergic diseases because of the wide range of normal concentrations. With a serum half-life of 2 to 5 days, serum IgE concentrations can change in days or weeks as a result of changes in the balance of helper T cell type 1, helper T cell type 2, and regulatory T cell immune functions. These changes can result from a wide variety of exposures, including allergens, viral infections, medications, and tumors. Measurements of allergen-specific IgE are useful in the diagnosis of allergic disease when they are interpreted in the context of an individual's medical history.

REFERENCES

Introduction

1. Jensen-Jarolim E, Achatz G, Turner MC, et al. AllergoOncology: the role of IgE-mediated allergy in cancer. Allergy 2008;63:1255-66.
2. Burton OT, Oettgen HC. Beyond immediate hypersensitivity: evolving roles for IgE antibodies in immune homeostasis and allergic diseases. Immunol Rev 2011;242:128-43.
3. Rosenwasser LJ. Mechanisms of IgE inflammation. Curr Allergy Asthma Rep 2011;11:178-83.

Normal Immunoglobulin E Production

4. Lima JO, Zhang L, Atkinson TP, et al. Early expression of iepsilon, CD23 (FcepsilonRII), IL-4Ralpha, and IgE in the human fetus. J Allergy Clin Immunol 2000;106:911-7.
5. Bertino E, Bisson C, Martano C, et al. Relationship between maternal- and fetal-specific IgE. Pediatr Allergy Immunol 2006;17:484-8.
6. Barbee RA, Halonen M, Lebowitz M, Burrows B. Distribution of IgE in a community population sample: correlations with age, sex, and allergen skin test reactivity. J Allergy Clin Immunol 1981;68:106-11.
7. Lindberg RE, Arroyave C. Levels of IgE in serum from normal children and allergic children as measured by an enzyme immunoassay. J Allergy Clin Immunol 1986;78:614-8.
8. Omenaas E, Bakke P, Elsayed S, Hanoa R, Gulsvik A. Total and specific serum IgE levels in adults: Relationship to sex, age and environmental factors. Clin Exp Allergy 1994;24:530-9.
9. Grundbacher FJ, Massie FS. Levels of immunoglobulin G, M, A, and E at various ages in allergic and nonallergic black and white individuals. J Allergy Clin Immunol 1985;75:651-8.
10. Raby BA, Van Steen K, Lazarus R, et al. Eotaxin polymorphisms and serum total IgE levels in children with asthma. J Allergy Clin Immunol 2007;117:298-305.
11. Levin TA, Ownby DR, Smith PH, et al. Relationship between extremely low total serum IgE levels and rhinosinusitis. Ann Allergy Asthma Immunol 2006;97:650-2.
12. Vicario M, Blanchard C, Stringer KF, et al. Local B cells and IgE production in the oesophageal mucosa in eosinophilic oesophagitis. Gut 2010;59:12-20.
13. Forester JP, Calabria CW. Local production of IgE in the respiratory mucosa and the concept of entopy: does allergy exist in nonallergic rhinitis? Ann Allergy Asthma Immunol 2010;105:249-55.

Immunoglobulin E in Allergic Disease

14. Oryszczyn M-P, Annesi I, Neukirch F, Doré M-F, Kauffmann F. Longitudinal observations of serum IgE and skin prick test response. Am J Respir Crit Care Med 1995;151:663-8.
15. Wittig HG, Belloit J, De Fillippi I, Royal G. Age-related serum immunoglobulin E levels in healthy subjects and in patients with allergic disease. J Allergy Clin Immunol 1980;66:305-13.
16. Marsh DG, Bias WB, Ishizaka K. Genetic control of basal serum immunoglobulin E level and its effect on specific reaginic sensitivity. Proc Natl Acad Sci USA 1974;71:3588-92.
17. Burrows B, Martinez FD, Halonen M, Barbee RA, Cline MG. Association of asthma with serum IgE levels and skin-test reactivity to allergens. N Engl J Med 1989;320:271-7.
18. Sunyer J, Antó JM, Castellsagué J, Soriano JB, Roca J, The Spanish Group of the European Study of Asthma. Total serum IgE is associated with asthma independently of specific IgE levels. Eur Respir J 1996;9:1880-4.
19. Sears MR, Burrows B, Flannery EM, et al. Relation between airway responsiveness and serum IgE in children with asthma and in apparently normal children. N Engl J Med 1991;325:1067-71.
20. Burrows B, Sears MR, Flannery EM, Herbison GP, Holdaway MD. Relationships of bronchial responsiveness assessed by methacholine to serum IgE, lung function, symptoms, and diagnoses in 11-year-old New Zealand children. J Allergy Clin Immunol 1992;90:376-85.
21. Joseph CLM, Ownby DR, Peterson EL, Johnson CC. Racial differences in physiologic parameters related to asthma among middle-class children. Chest 2000;117:1336-44.
22. Moffatt MF, Gut IG, Demenais F, et al. A large-scale, consortium-based genomewide association study of asthma. N Engl J Med 2010;363:1211-21.
23. Rosenwasser LJ, Nash DB. Incorporating omalizumab in asthma treatment guidelines: consensus panel recommendations. Pharm Ther 2003;28:400-10.
24. Hamilton RG. Accuracy of US Food and Drug Administration-cleared IgE antibody assays in the presence of anti-IgE (omalizumab). J Allergy Clin Immunol 2006;117:759-66.
25. Kousha M, Tadi R, Soubani AO. Pulmonary aspergillosis: a clinical review. Eur Respir Rev 2011;20:156-74.
26. Zieg G, Lack G, Harbeck RJ, Gelfand EW, Leung DY. In vivo effects of glucocorticoids on IgE production. J Allergy Clin Immunol 1994;94(Pt 1):222-30.
27. Villar T, Holgate ST. IgE, smoking and lung function. Clin Exp Allergy 1994;24:508-10.
28. Sherrill DL, Lebowitz MD, Halonen M, Barbee RA, Burrows B. Longitudinal evaluation of the association between pulmonary function and total serum IgE. Am J Respir Crit Care Med 1995;152:98-102.
29. Tracey M, Villar A, Dow L, et al. The influence of increased bronchial responsiveness, atopy, and serum IgE on decline in FEV1. Am J Respir Crit Care Med 1995;151:656-62.
30. Burrows B, Lebowitz MD, Barbee RA, Knudson RJ, Halonen M. Interactions of smoking and immunologic factors in relation to airways obstruction. Chest 1983;84:657-61.
31. Vollmer WM, Buist AS, Johnson LR, McCamant LE, Halonen M. Relationship between serum IgE and cross-sectional and longitudinal FEV1 in two cohort studies. Chest 1986;90:416-23.
32. Oryszczyn M-P, Annesi-Maesano I, Charpin D, et al. Relationship of active and passive smoking to total IgE in adults of the epidemiological study of the genetics and evnironment of asthma, bronchial hyperresponsiveness, and atopy (EGEA). Am J Respir Crit Care Med 2000;161:1241-6.
33. Simpson A, Custovic A, Pipis S, et al. Exhaled nitric oxide, sensitization, and exposure to allergens in patients with asthma who are not taking inhaled steroids. Am J Respir Crit Care Med 1999;160:45-9.
34. Saito J, Inoue K, Sugawara A, et al. Exhaled nitric oxide as a marker of airway inflammation for an epidemiologic study in school children. J Allergy Clin Immunol 2004;114:512-6.
35. Malinovschi A, Janson C, Holmkvist T, et al. IgE sensitization in relation to flow-independent nitric oxide exchange parameters. Respir Res 2006;7:92-9.
36. Shah PS, Wegienka G, Havstad S, et al. The relationship between cord blood immunoglobulin E levels and allergy-related outcomes in young

adults. Ann Allergy Asthma Immunol 2011;106: 245-51.
37. Bonnelykke K, Pipper CB, Bisgaard H. Transfer of maternal IgE can be a common cause of increased IgE levels in cord blood. J Allergy Clin Immunol 2010;126:657-63.
38. Bergmann RL, Schulz J, Günther S, et al. Determinants of cord-blood IgE concentrations in 6401 German neonates. Allergy 1995;50: 65-71.
39. Sicherer SH, Leung DY. Advances in allergic skin disease, anaphylaxis, and hypersensitivity reactions to foods, drugs, and insects in 2010. J Allergy Clin Immunol 2011;127:326-35.
40. Choi SY, Sohn MH, Yum HY, Kwon BC, Kim KE. Correlation between inhalant allergen-specific IgE and pulmonary function in children with asthma. Pediatr Pulmonol 2005;39:150-5.
41. Bosquet J, Anto JM, Bachert C, et al. Factors responsible for differences between asymptomatic subjects and patients presenting an IgE sensitization to allergens. A GA^{2}LEN Project. Allergy 2006;61:671-80.
42. Bernstein IL, Li JT, Bernstein DI, et al. Allergy diagnostic testing: an updated practice parameter. Ann Allergy Asthma Immunol 2008; 100(Suppl 3):S1-148.
43. Nelson HS, Oppenheimer J, Buchmeier A, Kordash TR, Freshwater LL. An assessment of the role of intradermal skin testing in the diagnosis of clinically relevant allergy to timothy grass. J Allergy Clin Immunol 1996;97: 1193-201.
44. Droste JHJ, Kerkhof M, deMonchy JGR, Schouten JP, Rijcken B; The Dutch ECRHS Group. Association of skin test reactivity, specific IgE, total IgE, and eosinophils with nasal symptoms in a community-based population study. J Allergy Clin Immunol 1996;97: 922-32.
45. Settipane RJ, Hagy GW, Settipane GA. Long-term risk factors for developing asthma and allergic rhinitis: a 23 year follow up study of college students. Allergy Asthma Proc 1994;15: 21-5.
46. Aalberse RC, Crameri R. IgE-binding epitopes: a reappraisal. Allergy 2011;66:1261-74.

Immunoglobulin E in Infectious and Parasitic Disease

47. Welliver RC, Sun M, Rinaldo D, Ogra PL. Predictive value of respiratory syncytial virus-specific IgE responses for recurrent wheezing following bronchiolitis. J Pediatr 1986;109: 776-80.
48. Domachowske JB, Rosenberg HF. Respiratory syncytial virus infections: immune response, immunopathogenesis, and treatment. Clin Microbiol Rev 1999;12:298-309.
49. Smith-Norowitz TA, Wong D, Kusonruksa M, et al. Long term persistence of IgE anti-influenza virus antibodies in pediatric and adult serum post vaccination with influenza virus vaccine. Int J Med Sci 2011;8:239-44.
50. Skoner DP, Doyle WJ, Tanner EP, Kiss J, Fireman P. Effect of rhinovirus 39 (RV-39) infection on immune and inflammatory parameters in allergic and non-allergic subjects. Clin Exp Allergy 1995;25:561-7.
51. Miguez-Burbano MJ, Shor-Posner G, Fletcher MA, et al. Immunoglobulin E levels in relationship to HIV-1 disease, route of infection, and vitamin E status. Allergy 1995;50:157-61.
52. Israäel-Biet D, Labrousse F, Tourani J-M, et al. Elevation of IgE in HIV-infected subjects: a marker of poor prognosis. J Allergy Clin Immunol 1992;89:68-75.
53. Ellaurie M, Rubinstein A, Rosenstreich DL. IgE levels in pediatric HIV-1 infection. Ann Allergy Asthma Immunol 1995;75:332-6.
54. Lee JH, Lin YT, Yang YH, Wang LC, Chiang BL. Increased levels of serum-specific immunoglobulin E to staphylococcal enterotoxin A and B in patients with allergic rhinitis and bronchial asthma. Int Arch Allergy Immunol 2005;138: 305-11.
55. Mayorga C, Torres MJ, Corzo JL, et al. Immediate allergy to tetanus toxoid vaccine: determination of immunoglobulin E and immunoglobulin G antibodies to allergenic proteins. Ann Allergy Asthma Immunol 2003;90:238-43.
56. Martin-Muñoz MF, Pereira MJ, Posadas S, et al. Anaphylactic reaction to dipheria-tetanus vaccine in a child: specific IgE/IgG determinations and cross-reactivity studies. Vaccine 2002;20:3409-12.
57. Ito K, Ishiguro A, Kanbe T, Tanaka K, Torii S. Characterization of IgE-binding epitopes on *Candida albicans* enolase. Clin Exp Allergy 1995;25:529-35.
58. Platts-Mills TAE, Call RS, Deuell BA, Karlsson G, Ward GW. The association of hypersensitivity diseases with dermatophyte infections. Clin Exp Allergy 1992;22:427-8.
59. Yazdanbakhsh M, Sacks DL. Why does immunity to parasites take so long to develop? Nat Rev Immunol 2010;10:80-1.
60. Friberg IM, Bradley JE, Jackson JA. Macroparasites, innate immunity and immunoregulation: developing natural models. Trends Parasitol 2010;26:540-9.
61. Watanabe N, Bruschi F, Korenaga M. IgE: a question of protective immunity in *Trichinella spiralis* infection. Trends Parasitol 2005;21:175-8.
62. Lynch NR, Hagel I, Perez M, et al. Effect of anthelmintic treatment on the allergic reactivity of children in a tropical slum. J Allergy Clin Immunol 1993;92:404-11.
63. Peng Z, Yang M, Simons FER. Measurement of mosquito *Aedes vexans* salivary gland-specific IgE and IgG antibodies and the distribution of these antibodies in human sera. Ann Allergy 1995;74:259-64.
64. Rohr AS, Marshall NA, Saxon A. Successful immunotherapy for *Triatoma protracta*-induced anaphylaxis. J Allergy Clin Immunol 1984;73: 369-75.

Immunoglobulin E in Nonatopic Diseases

65. Calboli FC, Cox DG, Buring JE, et al. Prediagnostic plasma IgE levels and risk of adult glioma in four prospective cohort studies. J Natl Cancer Inst 2011;103:1588-95.
66. Atkins D, Malka-Rais J. Food allergy: transfused and transplanted. Curr Allergy Asthma Rep 2010;10:250-7.
67. Gruber S, Tiringer K, Dehlink E, et al. Allergic sensitization in kidney-transplanted patients prevails under tacrolimus treatment. Clin Exp Allergy 2011;41:1125-32.
67a. Abdel-Hafez M, Shimada M, Lee PY, Johnson RJ, Garin EH. Idiopathic nephrotic syndrome and atopy: is there a common link? Am J Kidney Dis 2009;54:945-53.

Environmental Exposures and Immunoglobulin E

68. Nielsen GD, Olsen O, Larsen ST, et al. IgE-mediated sensitization, rhinitis and asthma from occupational exposures. Smoking as a model for airborne adjuvants? Toxicology 2005; 216:87-105.
68a. Havstad SL, Johnson CC, Zoratti EM, et al. Tobacco smoke exposure and allergic sensitization in children: a propensity score analysis. Respirology 2012;17:1068-72.
69. Diaz-Sanchez D, Rumold R, Gong Jr H. Challenge with environmental tobacco smoke exacerbates allergic airway disease in human beings. J Allergy Clin Immunol 2006;118:441-6.
70. Choudhury S, Avila PC, Nazario S, et al. CD14 tobacco gene-environment interaction modifies asthma severity and immunoglobulin E levels in Latinos with asthma. Am J Respir Crit Care Med 2007;172:173-82.
71. Dominguez-Santala MJ, Vidal C, Vinuela J, Perez LF, Gonzalez-Quintella A. Increased serum IgE in alcoholics: relationship with Th1/Th2 cytokine production by stimulated blood mononuclear cells. Alcohol Clin Exp Res 2001; 25:1198-205.
72. Gonzalez-Quintella A, Gude F, Boquete O, et al. Association of alcohol consumption with total serum immunoglobulin E levels and allergic sensitization in an adult population-based survey. Clin Exp Allergy 2003;33:199-205.
72a. Akinbami LJ, Moorman JE, Bailey C, et al. Trends in asthma prevalence, health care use, and mortality in the United States, 2001-2010. NCHS Data Brief May 2012, No. 94, pp 1-8.
72b. Bach J-F. The effect of infections on susceptiblility to autoimmune and allergic diseases. N Engl J Med 2002;347:911-20.
73. Diaz-Sanchez D, Dotson AR, Takenaka H, Saxon A. Diesel exhaust particles induce local IgE production *in vivo* and alter the pattern of IgE messenger RNA isoforms. J Clin Invest 1994;94: 1417-25.
74. Diaz-Sanchez D, Tsien A, Casillas A, Dotson AR, Saxon A. Enhanced nasal cytokine production in human beings after in vivo challenge with diesel exhaust particles. J Allergy Clin Immunol 1996;98:114-23.
75. Tse K, Horner AA. Defining a role for ambient TLR ligand exposures in the genesis and prevention of allergic disease. Semin Immunopathol 2008;30:53-62.
76. Takkouche B, Gonzáles-Barcala F-J, Etminan M, FitzGerald M. Exposure to furry pets and the risk of asthma and allergic rhinitis: a meta-analysis. Allergy 2008;63:857-64.
77. Wegienka G, Johnson CC, Havstad S, Ownby DR, Zoratti EM. Indoor pet exposure and the outcomes of total IgE and sensitization at age 18 years. J Allergy Clin Immunol 2010;126: 274-9.

70

In Vivo Methods for the Study and Diagnosis of Allergy

ANCA MIRELA CHIRIAC | JEAN BOUSQUET | PASCAL DEMOLY

CONTENTS

SUMMARY OF IMPORTANT CONCEPTS

» Immediate-reading skin tests address type I hypersensitivity and can confirm sensitization to a specific allergen. They represent the primary diagnostic tool of immunoglobulin E (IgE)-mediated diseases.

» The value of skin tests relies on technically correct methodology (i.e., use of negative and positive controls, standardized allergen extracts whenever possible, positivity criteria) and on accurate interpretation in the context of the clinical history and physical examination findings, because sensitization is not always clinically relevant.

» Performing skin tests enables the clinician to confirm or refute sensitization and atopy, which has important prognostic and therapeutic implications.

» In addition to their diagnostic value, skin tests are used in the standardization of allergen extracts and in pharmacologic, immunotherapy, and epidemiologic studies.

Introduction

Since the recognition that immunoglobulin E (IgE)-mediated allergic diseases are caused by exposure to allergens, it has been a common practice to establish the presence or absence of sensitization by reexposure of the individual to the allergen. Skin tests have been the primary tool for investigation in allergy since their introduction in 1865 by Blackley.[1] The intracutaneous test proposed by Mantoux in 1908[2] was rapidly applied to investigation of immediate hypersensitivity diseases. Some years later, Lewis and Grant[3] described the prick test. Without major modifications, these methods have been refined and further validated.

Skin tests can provide useful confirmatory evidence of sensitization to a specific allergen. The selection and number of allergens should be based on the history provided by the patient. Skin tests are simple, quick to perform, low cost, and highly sensitive, which explains their key position in allergy diagnosis. However, when improperly performed, skin tests can lead to falsely positive or negative results. The main limitation of the skin test is that a positive reaction does not necessarily mean that patients will experience symptoms, because patients can have allergen-specific IgE without clinical symptoms. Skin tests are also used to help understand the pathophysiology of the allergic response, to evaluate the mechanisms of action of antiallergic treatments, to analyze general or specific population sensitization profiles in epidemiologic and pharmacologic studies, and to standardize allergen extracts.

Pathophysiology of the Skin Response

The IgE-mediated allergic response in the skin results immediately in a wheal and flare reaction that depends on proinflammatory and neurogenic mediators (i.e., immediate reaction). It is irregularly followed by a late phase reaction (LPR) starting 1 to 2 hours later, peaking at 6 to 12 hours, and resolving in approximately 24 to 48 hours. The LPR is represented by an erythematous inflammatory reaction.

IMMEDIATE REACTION

The immediate reaction is essentially induced by mast cell degranulation after allergen challenge.[4] Histamine and tryptase release begins about 5 minutes after allergen injection and peaks at 30 minutes.[5] The injection of histamine into the skin by prick or intradermal techniques mimics the allergen-induced wheal and flare reaction. Histamine is the major, but not exclusive, mediator of the wheal and flare reaction. The size of the wheal usually does not correlate with the concentration of histamine released, and some patients show no significant histamine release during the immediate phase as assessed by the microdialysis technique.[6] Neurogenic and cellular components of inflammation participate in the immediate reaction. In humans, substance P[7] and, to a lesser extent, neurokinin A or calcitonin gene–related peptide (CGRP) produce dose-related wheal and flare reactions. CGRP also induces a slow-onset, intense vasodilation in skin; vasodilation persists for several hours and is associated with leucocyte infiltration.[7] More than any other mediator, histamine can trigger the release of substance P by axonal reflexes, and this neurogenic mediator may further enhance the immediate reaction by causing additional histamine release from cutaneous mast cells (i.e., positive feedback loop).[7] Nitric oxide[8] and corticotropin-releasing hormone[9] may also be involved.

LATE-PHASE REACTION

The LPR occurring after allergen challenge is mechanistically related to IgE but not IgG antibodies (e.g., Arthus type III reaction).[10] Granulocyte accumulation in the developing LPR is accompanied by altered expression of adhesion molecules on local vascular endothelium.[11] The cell inflammatory infiltrate has been extensively characterized in the skin LPR.[12] However, the same cellular pattern may be found after an immediate wheal and flare response that does not lead to a macroscopic LPR.

The mechanisms of the erythematous inflammatory LPR are not completely characterized. Mast cells appear to initiate the release of chemotactic mediators and cytokines that attract inflammatory cells to the site of the allergic reaction. The release of mast cell vasoactive mediators increases vascular permeability, which enables migration of inflammatory cells and exposure of these cells to chemoattractant factors. Histamine accounts for only a limited portion of the LPR.[13] Lymphocytes, predominantly $CD4^+$ T cells,[14] play a key role in the generation and regulation of the LPR by the generation and release of cytokines.[15] These findings are in contrast to delayed hypersensitivity, in which $CD8^+$ T cells are significant participants.[16] Eosinophils are activated during cutaneous LPRs[17] and produce cytotoxic proteins.[18] These cells can perpetuate inflammation because they can release a chemokine called *regulated on activation, normal T cell expressed and secreted* (RANTES) and interleukin-4 (IL-4).

Mediators recovered from skin blister fluids after allergen challenge during the LPR include histamine, kallikrein, thromboxane B_2, prostaglandin D_2 (PGD_2), leukotriene C_4 (LTC_4), and small amounts of platelet-activating factor (PAF). Development of localized macroscopic inflammatory responses after their injection into the skin indicates their potential involvement in IgE-dependent LPR cutaneous responses. Several mediators that can activate the coagulation, fibrinolytic, and bradykinin pathways may also play a role.[19]

The use of pharmacologic inhibitors has provided additional insight regarding the pathophysiology of allergen skin tests. Prednisone inhibits the appearance of inflammatory mediators and the influx of eosinophils and basophils associated with the cutaneous LPR.[20] In contrast, various treatment results have been obtained with cyclooxygenase inhibitors; for example, misoprostol, a PGE_2 analog, reduces the cutaneous LPR.[21]

Techniques of Skin Tests

METHODS OF SKIN TESTING

Prick-puncture and intradermal tests are routinely used for skin testing. In the prick-puncture method, antigen is placed on the skin and introduced into the epidermis with a variety of devices.[22] In the intradermal method, the antigen is injected into the dermis using a hypodermic syringe and needle (Fig. 70-1). Before initiating any skin test procedure, some precautions should be taken (Box 70-1).

Prick-Puncture Tests

First described by Lewis and Grant in 1924,[3] the prick-puncture test became widespread in the 1970s after it was modified by Pepys.[23] The modified prick test is performed by placing a small drop of each test extract and control solution on the volar surface of the forearm (or occasionally on the back). The drops are placed 2 cm or more apart to avoid false-positive reactions.[22] A 23- to 26-gauge, disposable hypodermic needle is passed through the drop and inserted into the epidermal surface at a low angle with the bevel facing up. The needle tip is then gently lifted upward to elevate a small portion of the epidermis

BOX 70-1 SKIN TESTING PRECAUTIONS

1. Never perform skin tests unless a physician is immediately available to treat systemic reactions.
2. Have emergency equipment, including epinephrine, readily available.
3. Be careful with patients with current allergic symptoms.
4. Determine the potency and stability of the allergen extracts used.
5. Be certain that the test concentrations are appropriate.
6. Include a positive and a negative control solution.
7. Perform tests in normal skin.
8. Evaluate the patient for dermographism.
9. Determine and record medications taken by the patient and time of last dose.
10. Record the reactions at the proper time.

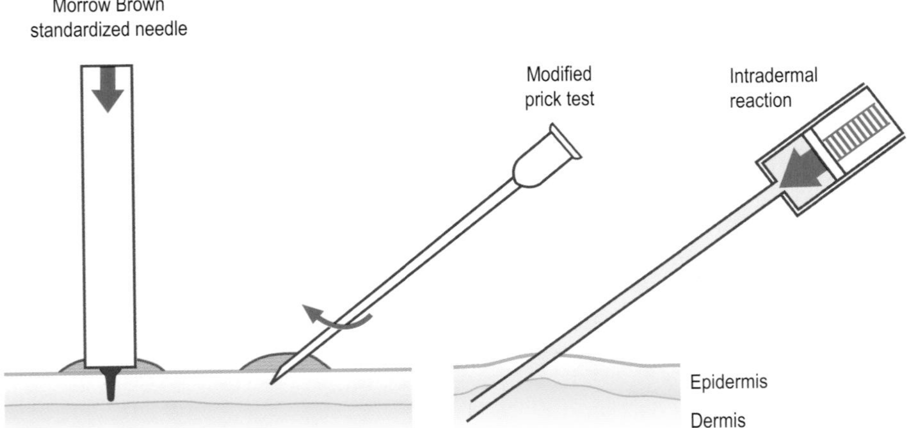

Figure 70-1 Common methods of skin testing.

without inducing bleeding. The needle is withdrawn and the solution gently wiped away with a paper tissue approximately 1 minute later. A separate needle must be used for each test to avoid mixing the solutions. Using the same needle or lancet wiped with dry cotton wool[24] or cotton moistened with 75% ethanol[25] between tests produces an unacceptable number of false-positive results.

The Occupational Safety and Health Administration (OSHA) of the U.S. Department of Labor has provided information alerting its personnel on the risk of exposure to bloodborne pathogens when technicians performing the testing inadvertently prick themselves with the device while wiping it between tests.[26] Smearing test solutions to adjacent test sites must be avoided. Some common errors in prick testing are listed in Box 70-2.

Other prick-puncture test methods in which the test instrument is inserted perpendicular to the skin have been proposed to decrease the variability of the prick procedure by different investigators.[22] The most popular instruments are the Morrow Brown standardized needle, the Pricker, the Stallerpointe, and the Phazet. Puncture tests also can be performed with a bifurcated smallpox vaccination needle or with other devices, some of which are commonly used in the United States (e.g., DermaPik, Duo Tip Test[27]). In another variant of prick testing, a drop of extract is carried from the bottle with the lancet and the skin is pricked; application of extract and the puncture occur in one step. Opinions concerning these methods vary according to the skill, experience, and preference of the nurse or physician, but among trained investigators, they are highly reproducible.

One study[28] compared devices commonly used in Europe: a 23-gauge intravenous needle, the ALK Lancet; the Stallergenes (STG) Prick Lancet; and the Stallerpointe. The intravenous needle and the two metal lancets yielded equivalent results and proved to be superior to the Stallerpointe in terms of sensitivity (96% to 100% for the metal devices versus 20% to 57% for Stallerpointe) and interpatient and intrapatient reproducibility and acceptability.

Skin prick testing can be carried out with multiheaded devices that permit several tests to be performed with one application. These devices, which are mostly marketed and distributed in the United States, may minimize technician time, increase efficiency, and be more acceptable to children. In a head-to-head prospective study comparing the performance of eight skin test devices (i.e., four single-headed and four multiheaded devices) on the arms and back of each subject, all devices except the multiheaded Greer Track had sensitivities between 86% and 97% and specificities of 98% or greater.[29] Single-headed devices produced larger reactions on the arm, whereas similar-sized reactions using multiheaded devices occurred on the back. Multiheaded devices demonstrated significant intradevice variability and were more painful than single-headed devices. Devices such as the Multi-Test or the Combion test are not strictly prick test devices because their needles are long enough to penetrate through the dermis. The wheal reaction induced by the Multi-Test varies more than the reactions with other prick test methods, and the flare cannot be studied.[22]

Regardless of the technique used, performing skin testing with food extracts usually leads to poor results because of enzymatic degradation of the relevant proteins contained within the extracts. In a proposed alternative,[30] the prick-prick test, the same device is used to prick fresh food and then the skin.

The prick-puncture test appears to be safe. Systemic reactions after testing with inhalant allergens, although anecdotal, have been reported.[31] The overall rate of generalized reactions with fresh food was 0.52% in one pediatric study[32] and 0.26% in another pediatric and adult study.[33] The high incidence in the former report was questioned because of concerns regarding duplication of the tests (which increases local antigen load). The same group later reported the results of a prospective study[34] that revealed a lower risk (0.12%) for generalized allergic reactions in a population of 5908 children investigated with skin prick tests for inhalant and food allergens. Possible risk factors for adverse reactions during skin testing were suggested: low age and active eczema for generalized allergic reactions; female gender and multiple skin prick tests performed on a single patient for vasovagal reactions. No fatalities have been reported.

No report or case study regarding nosocomial infections resulting from skin prick test procedures has been published. However, even if no methicillin-resistant *Staphylococcus aureus* or vancomycin-resistant enterococci were observed in field samples,[35] nosocomial infections may become a concern if skin tests are performed on subjects who are pathogen carriers. Skin bacteria such as *Staphylococcus epidermidis* can survive in allergen extracts for as long as 21 days.

Intradermal Tests

Intradermal tests described by Mantoux in 1908 are still used in clinical practice.[2] The allergen extract is injected intracutaneously from a 0.5- or 1.0-mL tuberculin syringe through a 26- or 27-gauge needle. Before injection, all bubbles are carefully eliminated to avoid splash reactions that could be misinterpreted. The syringe is placed at an angle of less than 45 degrees to the skin with the bevel of the needle facing up, and penetration of the needle should not be deeper than the superficial layers of the skin to avoid the subepidermal capillary bed of the skin. A volume of approximately 0.02 to 0.05 mL is gently injected to produce a small, superficial bleb approximately 2 to 4 mm in diameter (Fig. 70-2). Some common errors in intradermal testing are listed in Box 70-3.

Intradermal tests can elicit pain, which may be reduced by the use of a topical anesthetic cream such as the eutectic mixture of local anesthetics (EMLA), which reduces the flare but not the wheal responses.[36] They can provoke a low rate of untoward, large local (immediate and late) and systemic reactions, with an incidence ranging from 0.02% to 1.4% of the tested patients.[22] Some fatalities have been reported.[37] Although intradermal tests may be performed by a nurse or a technician, a physician should always be nearby. A waiting period of 20 minutes in the office of the physician is recommended before the patient is released, and this period may be extended for high-risk patients.[22]

BOX 70-2 COMMON ERRORS IN PRICK TESTING

1. Tests are placed too close together (<2 cm), and overlapping reactions cannot be separated visually.
2. Induction of bleeding can lead to false-positive results.
3. Insufficient penetration of skin by puncture instrument can lead to false-negative results; this occurs more frequently with plastic devices.
4. Allergen solutions can spread during the test or when the solution is wiped away.

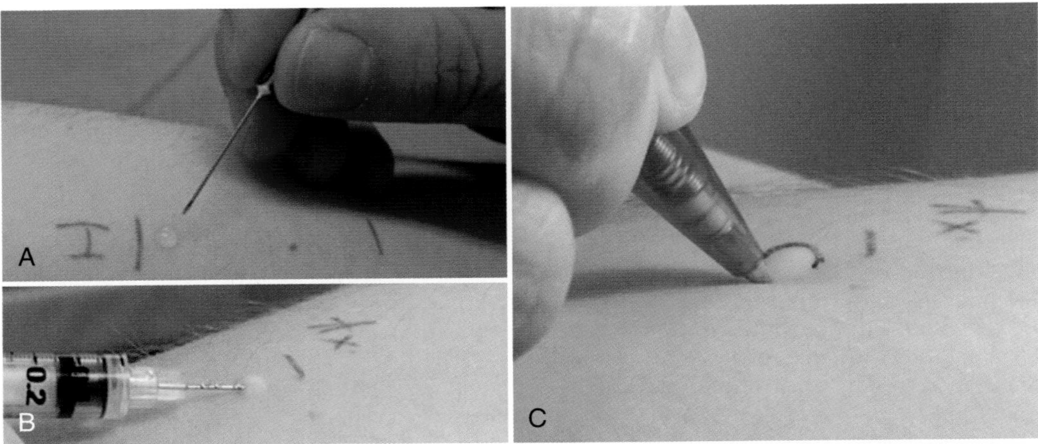

Figure 70-2 Methods of skin testing. **A,** Prick-puncture test. **B,** For the intradermal test, a volume of approximately 0.02 to 0.05 mL of allergen extract is injected intracutaneously to produce a small superficial bleb (2 to 4 mm in diameter). **C,** The size of skin tests may be outlined with a pen to obtain a permanent record.

BOX 70-3 COMMON ERRORS IN INTRADERMAL TESTING

1. Test sites are too close together, and false-positive results can be observed.
2. Volume injected is too large (>0.1 mL).
3. High concentration of allergen can lead to false-positive results.
4. Splash reaction is caused by air injection.
5. Subcutaneous injection leads to a false-negative test (i.e., no bleb formed).
6. Intracutaneous bleeding site is read as a positive test result.
7. Too many tests performed at the same time may induce systemic reactions.

TABLE 70-1 Relative Advantages of Prick and Intradermal Tests

Advantages	Prick Test	Intradermal Test
Simplicity	+++	++
Speed	++++	++
Interpretation of positive and negative reactions	++++	++
Discomfort	+	+++
False-positive reactions	Rare	Possible
False-negative reactions	Possible	Rare
Reproducibility	+++	++++
Sensitivity	+++	++++
Specificity	++++	+++
Detection of IgE antibodies	Yes	Yes
Safety	++++	++
Testing of infants	Yes	Difficult

+, Mild; ++, moderate; +++, high; ++++, very high.

Particular care should be taken in patients treated with β-blocking agents, which may increase the risk of fatal systemic reactions. Performing prick-puncture tests before intradermal tests and using serial tenfold dilutions of the usual test concentration, especially in patients with histories of anaphylaxis, are useful ways to minimize untoward adverse local and systemic reactions.[38] In case of a generalized anaphylactic reaction, a rubber tourniquet should be placed above the test site on the arm and a 1 : 1000 aqueous epinephrine (adrenaline) solution administered intramuscularly, preferentially in the lateral thigh (i.e., vastus lateralis).[39] Because of the risk of infectious bacterial or viral diseases, allergy testing of multiple patients must not be performed with a common intradermal skin test syringe.

The starting dose of solutions in patients with a preceding negative prick test result should range between 100-fold and 1000-fold dilutions of the concentrated extract used for prick-puncture testing.[22,40] With potent standardized allergen extracts (i.e., 100,000 allergy units [AU] per milliliter], the range of starting intradermal skin tests in patients with a negative prick-puncture test result is between 10 and 100 AU. For less potent allergen extracts of 10,000-AU concentrations, the range is between 100 and 1000 AU.

Comparison of Prick-Puncture and Intradermal Tests

The value of prick-puncture tests is limited because low-potency extracts can induce false-negative results. The concentration of allergen extract required to elicit a positive reaction with intradermal testing is 1000 to 30,000 times smaller than that necessary for a positive prick-puncture test. With standardized or potent extracts, the prick-puncture test appears to have several advantages over the intradermal test (Table 70-1), including economy of time, patient comfort, safety, and a steeper dose-response curve, which is more useful in titrated skin testing. Prick testing also uses extracts in 50% glycerin, which results in greater stability. The intradermal testing procedure cannot use this diluent because it results in irritant or false-positive responses. Prick-puncture tests are considered to be less sensitive, less reproducible, but more specific than intradermal tests. However, it is questionable whether the increased sensitivity of intradermal tests at the concentrations customarily used is clinically necessary or it only increases the chance of a false-positive response.[41] Prick-puncture testing correlates better with symptoms.[42] Based on these observations, skin prick-puncture tests are recommended as the primary test for the diagnosis of IgE-mediated allergic diseases and for research purposes by the European Academy of Allergy and Clinical Immunology[43] and the U.S. Joint Council of Allergy Asthma and Immunology.[40]

NEGATIVE AND POSITIVE CONTROL SOLUTIONS

Because of variability in cutaneous reactivity, it is necessary to include negative and positive controls in every skin test evaluation. The negative control solutions are the diluents used to preserve the allergen extracts. All negative controls should be totally negative. The rare dermographic patient develops wheal and erythema reactions to the negative control. The negative control also detects traumatic reactivity induced by the skin test device (the wheal may approach a diameter of 3 mm with some devices) or the technique of the tester.[40] Although any reaction at a negative control test site makes interpreting allergen sites more difficult, these responses are essential in accurately assessing the presence or absence of true allergic sensitization.[40]

Positive control solutions are used to detect suppression by medications or diseases, to detect exceptional patients who are poorly reactive to histamine, and to determine variations in technician performance or the potency of the testing reagent. For many years in the United States, the only available positive control for prick-puncture testing was histamine phosphate, which was used at a concentration of 5.43 mmol/L (or 2.7 mg/mL, equivalent to 1 mg/mL of histamine base). Wheal diameters with this preparation range from 2 to 7 mm. However, a tenfold greater concentration may be more appropriate, producing a mean wheal size between 5 and 8 mm. A 10-mg/mL histamine dihydrochloride control is available currently and preferred as positive control for prick-puncture skin tests.[40] For the intradermal test, the concentration routinely used is 0.0543 mmol/L. The mean wheal size elicited is 10 to 12 mm. Mast cell secretagogues such as codeine phosphate (9% solution) may also be used as positive controls.

GRADING OF SKIN TESTS

Measurement

Skin tests should be read at the peak of their reaction and in a standard manner.[40,43] Whatever method is used, the immediate skin test induces a response that reaches a peak in 8 to 10 minutes for histamine, 10 to 15 minutes for mast cell secretagogues, and 15 to 20 minutes for allergens. Late phase reactions are not often recorded, because their exact clinical significance is unknown.[22,40] When the reactions are mature, the size of each reaction is measured with a millimeter rule. The longest and smallest diameters of the wheal or erythema are measured. Because the reactions are often oval or irregular in shape, the diameters are measured at right angles to each other. Both diameters are recorded, summed, and divided by 2. The longest diameter is the optimal measurement.[44] To obtain a permanent record, the size of the reaction may be outlined with a pen, blotted onto cellophane tape, and stored on paper. The area of the cutaneous response may be estimated by planimetry or by weighing the excised tape with a precision balance, or it may be scanned by a computer and the surface areas measured using commercially available software. Ultrasonic measurements permit assessment of other parameters, such as the wheal thickness and wheal volume, which can improve the distinction between different tests when performing the end-point titration. Quantification also may be done by laser Doppler flowmetry determination of blood flow in the wheal and erythema. The erythematous reaction of the LPR may be evaluated by thermography.[22]

Measuring and recording the reaction site is important because of the great degree of variability in scoring and interpreting skin test results.[45] To standardize allergy testing records, the Immunotherapy Committee of the American Academy of Allergy, Asthma, and Clinical Immunology and the Joint Task Force on Practice Parameters[40] developed a skin test form for reporting all important information.

Criteria for Positivity

Evaluation of the wheal or erythema is used to assess the positivity of skin tests. The positive control should optimally show a wheal diameter that is 3 mm or larger.[46] Pepys[23] suggested that when control sites of the prick-puncture test are completely negative, small wheals of 1 to 2 mm with flare and itching are likely to represent a positive immunologic response and the presence of specific IgE antibodies. Although significant in immunologic terms, small positive reactions do not necessarily indicate the presence of a clinically relevant allergy. Reactions to prick-puncture tests are regarded as indicative of clinical allergy if they are greater than 3 mm in wheal diameter (i.e., wheal area of 7 mm^2) and greater than 10 mm in flare diameter.[47] Another criterion is the ratio of the size of the wheal induced by the allergen compared with the positive control. Any degree of positive response, with appropriate positive and negative controls, indicates the presence of allergic sensitization to a particular allergen but not necessarily the presence of allergic disease. Correlating skin test results with the clinical history is essential in interpreting the clinical significance of the testing procedure.

Grading Systems

Several grading systems have been proposed. For prick-puncture tests, the sizes of the wheal and erythema often are not taken into consideration, although a grading system based on the relation between the reactions induced by allergen and the histamine reference (5.43 mmol/L) has been used in Scandinavia for many years.[42] Because of the log/log relationship between changes in skin prick-puncture test response and allergen concentrations, only large differences in skin sensitivity are detected using a fixed concentration of allergen, and only a threshold dilution titration skin test using serial dilutions can give more information.[22] End-point titrations (estimated as the concentration of allergen giving a wheal size comparable to that of a positive control solution) have been performed, but they should be replaced by methods based on parallel-line bioassay or on medial slope.[42]

For intradermal tests, one of the most widely used grading systems was derived from studies reported by Norman and colleagues.[48] Although a single concentration of a specific extract may be used for testing and grading reaction positivity, more information is obtained through skin testing using the threshold dilution technique, which is performed by employing a threefold or tenfold dilution series. The grading of the reaction may be studied using the wheal or the erythema, or both.[22] The size of a wheal for a single allergen dose is not accurate because identical reactions may be observed for tests performed with allergenic extracts whose potency differs by 100-fold. Several methods of evaluation have therefore been proposed. The least dilution required for a 1+ or 2+ reaction is considered the end point.[22,48] Other investigators have considered the titer end point to be the dilution of extract that gives a wheal identical to the histamine-positive control. Norman and colleagues[48] introduced the midpoint method by establishing a dose-response curve and determining the dose of allergen extract producing a wheal 7 mm in diameter. They found that the midpoint skin test result correlated with serum IgE levels, leukocyte histamine release, provocative challenges, and symptoms.

Van Metre and coworkers[49] examined the effect of immunotherapy with ragweed extracts on skin sensitivity and did not detect an effect using the end-point titration but did detect a significant reduction in sensitivity with midpoint skin tests. Turkeltaub and colleagues[50] used the erythema's diameter, not the wheal's diameter, because the slope of the regression line of the former was steeper. Overall, for routine diagnosis of allergy, a single allergen concentration is usually sufficient, but for research purposes, more sophisticated techniques are required. Studies indicate that the LPR is also a measure of IgE sensitivity, but its grading has not been standardized.[22]

NUMBER OF SKIN TESTS AND FREQUENCY OF SKIN TESTING

Number of Skin Tests

The number of skin tests varies according to the age of the patient (i.e., fewer prick-puncture tests needed in infants for food allergens, house-dust mites, indoor molds, indoor insects, and animal danders versus pollens[40]); the geographic location of the patient; and the history of the allergic disease (e.g., persistent versus intermittent symptoms, clear causative factors). A large, multicenter, open-label study involving 3034 allergic subjects[51] indicated sensitization rates were comparable for the most frequent inhalant allergens across Europe. On the basis of identified sensitization patterns, a standardized prick testing core panel that included 18 inhalant allergens was proposed for implementation in European allergy centers. Depending on the country,[52] 2 to 9 allergens of 18 were sufficient to identify 95% of sensitized subjects, whereas 4 to 13 allergens were required to identify 100% of sensitized subjects. The number and the type of allergens correlated strongly with the country, and local allergens were often of relevance.

Frequency of Skin Testing

Skin tests may be repeated for a variety of reasons,[40] including the age of the patient (i.e., allergic children acquire new sensitivities, beginning with foods and indoor allergens and followed by pollens and outdoor molds); the patient's exposure to new allergens (e.g., acquisition of a new pet, geographic relocation) or increase in symptoms; and venom immunotherapy. Routine repeat skin testing is not recommended for nonvenom allergen immunotherapy.

OTHER SKIN TEST METHODS

Passive Transfer Test

Historically, the serum passive transfer test reaction was used to demonstrate the presence of reagins. After the discovery of IgE in 1967, the need for this test diminished greatly. It is now strictly contraindicated because of the unacceptable potential risks of injecting serum containing several infectious agents (e.g., HIV, hepatitis viruses).

Skin Window Techniques and Derived Methods

The skin window technique proposed by Rebuck and Crowley in 1955[53] was modified by Dunsky and Zweiman,[54] who developed the skin chamber technique.

Factors That Affect Skin Tests

ALLERGENIC EXTRACTS

Skin responses to allergens depend on several variables. The quality of the allergen extract is of major importance. Some false-negative reactions are caused by the lack of allergens in nonstandardized extracts. Although many years ago skin test materials were often made directly in hospital laboratories or in physicians' offices by extracting allergenic raw materials, this practice cannot be recommended. When possible, physicians should use allergen extracts standardized using biologic methods and labeled in biologic units.[40] Allergen extracts should be marketed only if their potency, composition, and stability have been documented as extracts from a single source material or mixtures of related, cross-reacting allergens, such as grass pollen, deciduous tree pollen, related ragweed pollen, and related mite allergen extracts. Mixtures of unrelated allergens should be avoided because their use may result in false-negative responses due to overdiluted allergenic epitopes in some mixes[40] or enzymatic degradation by proteases. For marketing, the relative amounts of each component of the mixture and stability data should be indicated on the label.

Variations in the quality and potency of commercial extracts, which may be related or not to the differences between the U.S. and the European standardization systems, are particularly found in extracts for mites, animal danders, molds, and pollens.[46] In addition to problems related to standardization, some extracts (e.g., hymenoptera venoms) can induce false-positive reactions by nonimmunologic mechanisms. Preservatives used in allergen extracts also may be irritants; thimerosal can elicit a wheal and flare reaction in nonsensitized subjects.[55]

Because of the difficulties in preparing consistently standardized extracts from natural raw material, new technologies have been tried. Starting from allergen-encoding cDNAs, large amounts of highly pure allergens with a high batch-to-batch consistency can be produced that satisfy the quality requirements of medicinal products manufactured by recombinant DNA technology. Recombinant allergens (rAllergens) used for in vivo diagnoses should have the same IgE binding activity as their natural counterparts.[43] The rAllergens of various pollens, molds, mites, bee venom, latex, and celery have been used for skin testing in more than 1500 allergic and control individuals.[56] Skin prick tests and intradermal tests with rAllergens have proved to be highly specific and safe. Although the diagnostic sensitivity of single rAllergens usually is lower than those obtained with allergen extracts, it can be increased by using rAllergen panels covering the most important allergenic structures in a given complex allergen extract. Alt a 1 allergen in its natural or recombinant form is sufficient for a reliable diagnosis of *Alternaria alternata* sensitization, inducing a skin prick reactivity comparable with that produced by *A. alternata* extract.[57] This type of approach with rAllergens may be of great importance for the diagnosis of allergy to unstable allergen extracts such as fruits and cross-reacting allergens.

For skin testing with fresh foods, thermal denaturation of allergen structure by cooking has been well established.[58]

Fresh seasonal fruits are not always available throughout the year, and it is common practice to perform skin testing by using frozen aliquots of these fruits. The validity of this method has been confirmed in two studies,[59,60] which were conducted on 23 birch-allergic patients with oral allergy syndrome and 48 fruit-allergic patients. Skin testing with frozen fruits from the Rosaceae and Curcubitaceae families proved to be a reliable alternative, with a performance similar to that of fresh fruits.

AREA OF THE BODY

The site of skin testing may affect the results.[22,40] The middle and upper back areas are more reactive than the lower back. The back as a whole is more reactive than the forearm, and this differential effect is more pronounced for allergen extracts than for histamine solutions. The antecubital fossa is the most reactive portion of the arm, and the wrist is the least reactive. The ulnar side of the arm is more reactive than the radial side. Tests should not be placed in areas 5 cm from the wrist or 3 cm from the antecubital fossae. However, some investigators[29] have not been able to demonstrate any significant differences between the upper and lower arm nor between the upper and lower back.

AGE

Skin reactions vary with age.[22] Infants react predominantly with a large erythematous flare and a small wheal. Using prick-puncture test, it has been observed that a significant wheal was detectable after 3 months of age in most infants tested with histamine, codeine phosphate, or allergen extracts. It is therefore possible to perform skin tests to diagnose allergic disorders in infancy, but the size of the wheal is often reduced, and criteria of positivity should always compare the size of the wheal induced by allergen extracts with that elicited by positive control solutions. Skin test wheals increase in size from infancy to adulthood and then often decline after the age of 50.

GENDER

Overall, there have been no clear-cut differences in skin test reactivity based on gender. However, some findings demonstrated a higher prick test response to histamine in male than in female subjects.[61] Women displayed the weakest histamine wheal capacity during the first day of the menstrual cycle and a second minimum around the twentieth day and the strongest allergen wheal capacity at midcycle.[62] The clinical significance of these findings is unclear.

RACE

The wheal capacity in response to histamine is significantly greater in healthy, nonatopic black subjects with darkly pigmented skin than it is in whites with light skin pigmentation.[22] The flare is always difficult to measure in subjects whose skin is pigmented.

CIRCADIAN RHYTHMS AND SEASONAL VARIATIONS

The circadian variation of skin reactivity is minimal and does not affect the clinical interpretation of skin tests.[22] Seasonal variations in skin test sensitivity related to specific IgE antibody synthesis have been demonstrated in cases of pollen and house-dust mite allergy. For example, skin sensitivity for tree pollen allergy[63] increases after the pollen season and then declines until the next season. This may be clinically relevant for patients with a low level of sensitization or for allergen extracts that have weak potency. Ultraviolet B radiation significantly reduces wheal intensities.[64]

PATHOLOGIC CONDITIONS

Eczema diminishes skin reactivity to histamine,[65] but this finding is not consistently observed. It has been anecdotally reported that the stress provoked by playing video games or by frequently ringing mobile phones enhances allergen-induced skin wheal responses and leads to a concomitant increased release of substance P, vasoactive intestinal peptide, and nerve growth factor.[66] It seems reasonable not to perform skin tests in areas where a skin lesion may interfere with skin reactivity. Patients with chronic renal failure or on regular hemodialysis treatment usually have decreased skin reactivity, and the texture of their skin makes testing difficult.[22] Some patients with cancer have decreased skin reactivity, and the effect is more pronounced on the flare than on the wheal.[67] Patients with spinal cord injuries[22] or peripheral nerve abnormalities such as diabetic neuropathy have decreased flare reactivity.

DRUGS

Some drugs can interfere with the performance of skin tests and can modulate the wheal or the flare, complicating interpretation of skin tests. Other drugs used in allergic or asthmatic patients do not modify the cutaneous responsiveness, and they can be continued.[22] Table 70-2 outlines the inhibitory effects of therapeutic drugs on skin tests and the delay of suppression of such treatments before performing skin tests. However, it is not reasonable to consider the suppression of antidepressant treatment in psychiatric disorders without consulting the prescribing doctor.

Antihistamines

The H_1 antihistamines inhibit the wheal and flare response to histamine, allergen, and mast cell secretagogues. The duration of the inhibitory effect is linked to the pharmacokinetics of the drug and its active metabolites. First-generation H_1 antihistamines reduce skin reactivity for up to 24 hours or slightly longer. Ketotifen, another first-generation H_1 antihistamine, suppresses skin test responses for more than 5 days. The second-generation H_1 antihistamines azelastine, bilastine, cetirizine, desloratadine, ebastine, fexofenadine, levocetirizine, loratadine, mizolastine, and rupatadine may suppress skin responses for 3 to 7 days. Tachyphylaxis, as defined by a reduction of the inhibitory effects on skin tests, developed with first-generation H_1 antihistamines but not with the second-generation H_1 antihistamines. Some H_1 antihistamines, such as cetirizine, inhibit skin tests more than others do, and this effect correlates with relief of allergic rhinitis symptoms.[68] For other antihistamines, such as loratadine, blunting of skin test reactivity to allergen or histamine is not necessarily predictive of the clinical efficacy of these drugs in seasonal allergic rhinitis treatment.[69]

Topical H_1 antihistamines such as levocabastine may suppress skin tests as these medications can be measured in plasma

TABLE 70-2 Inhibitory Effect of Drugs on IgE-Mediated Skin Tests

Drugs	Degree	SUPPRESSION Duration (days)	SUPPRESSION Clinical Significance*
H_1 antihistamines			
Azelastine	++++	3-10	Yes
Bilastine	++++	3-10	Yes
Cetirizine	++++	3-10	Yes
Chlorpheniramine	++	1-3	Yes
Clemastine	+++	1-10	Yes
Cyproheptadine	0 to +	1-8	Yes
Desloratadine	++++	3-10	Yes
Diphenhydramine	0 to +	1-3	Yes
Doxepin	++	3-11	Yes
Ebastine	++++	3-10	Yes
Hydroxyzine	+++	1-10	Yes
Ketotifen	++++	>5	Yes
Levocabastine	Possible		Yes
Levocetirizine	++++	3-10	Yes
Loratadine	++++	3-10	Yes
Mequitazine	++++	3-10	Yes
Mizolastine	++++	3-10	Yes
Promethazine	++	1-3	Yes
Tripelennamine	0 to +	1-3	Yes
H_2 antihistamines			
Cimetidine	0 to +		No
Ranitidine	+		No
Imipramines	++++	>10	Yes
Phenothiazines	++		Yes
Corticosteroids			
Systemic, short term	0		
Systemic, long term	Possible		Yes
Inhaled	0		
Topical skin	0 to ++		Yes
Theophylline	0 to +		No
Cromolyn	0		
β_2-Agonists			
Inhaled	0 to +		No
Oral, injection	0 to ++		No
Formoterol	Unknown		
Salmeterol	Unknown		
Dopamine	+		
Clonidine	++		
Montelukast	0		
Allergen immunotherapy	0 to ++		No

+, Mild; ++, moderate; +++, high; ++++, very high.
*Clinical significance for skin testing.

within 1 to 2 hours of administration of single doses of nasal spray and eye drops. A single dose of azelastine nasal spray does not significantly alter the wheal and flare response to histamine, but if multiple doses are used, the drug should be discontinued for at least 48 hours before skin testing.[70]

H_2 antihistamines used alone have a limited inhibitory effect on skin tests. Studies on the coadministration of H_1 and H_2 antihistamines have produced conflicting results, with some indicating enhancement of the inhibitory effect. Discontinuing H_2 antagonists on the day of testing is probably sufficient to prevent significant suppression of skin tests.

Imipramines, Phenothiazines, and Tranquilizers

Tricyclic antidepressants exert a potent and sustained reduction in skin responses to histamine. This effect may last for a few weeks. Tranquilizers and antiemetic agents of the phenothiazine class have H_1 antihistaminic activity and can abrogate skin test responses. Topical doxepin hydrochloride abolishes skin reactivity after 1 to 3 days of therapy and for up to 11 days after its discontinuation.

Corticosteroids

Short-term (<1 week) administration of corticosteroids used at therapeutic doses in asthmatic patients does not modify cutaneous reactivity to histamine, compound 48/80, or allergen. Long-term corticosteroid therapy does not alter histamine-induced vascular reactivity in skin but affects cutaneous mast cell responses and modifies the skin texture, which makes interpretation of immediate skin tests difficult in some cases. However, it has been shown that allergen-induced skin tests can be accurately performed in asthmatic patients receiving long-term oral corticosteroid treatment.[71] The effects of inhaled corticosteroids have not been directly evaluated, but because therapeutic doses produce fewer systemic effects than oral steroids, their potential for interference is predictably insignificant. In contrast, the application of topical dermal corticosteroids for 1 week reduces the immediate and the late phase skin reaction induced by allergen.

Other Immunomodulators

Few data are available regarding the effect of other immunomodulating agents, including biologicals, on skin testing. During omalizumab treatment in asthmatic allergic patients, the size of allergen-induced early phase and late phase skin responses dereases.[72] Theophylline slightly reduces skin tests, but its administration does not need to be stopped before skin testing.

Short-acting, inhaled β_2-agonists in doses approved for the treatment of asthma do not usually inhibit allergen-induced skin tests. Oral terbutaline can decrease the allergen-induced wheal, but this inhibitory effect has little significance in clinical practice. For long-acting, inhaled β_2-agonists, such as formoterol and salmeterol, definitive results are lacking. Conversely, β-blocking agents such as propranolol can significantly increase skin histamine reactivity.

Inhaled cromolyn and nedocromil do not alter the skin wheal response to skin tests with allergens or degranulating agents, and neither does cutaneously applied sodium cromoglycate.[73] Dopamine and clonidine can decrease skin test reactivity, whereas this effect has not been observed with nifedipine and montelukast. Angiotensin-converting enzyme inhibitors moderately increase skin reactivity to allergen, histamine, codeine, and bradykinin. Topical pimecrolimus does not seem to modify skin reactivity.[74]

Allergen Immunotherapy

A decreased wheal and flare reaction has been observed in patients undergoing allergen immunotherapy with inhalant allergens,[22] sublingual latex extract,[75] oral peanut extract,[76] or Hymenoptera venoms and in professional beekeepers who are spontaneously desensitized. However, these effects were seen mostly when skin tests were carried out using several dilutions. Allergen immunotherapy with pollen extracts, including treatment delivered by the sublingual route, induces a decreased late phase reaction.[77]

Interpretation of Skin Tests

POSITIVE SKIN TESTS IN A POPULATION WITHOUT CLINICAL ALLERGY

A positive skin test response confirms the presence of allergic sensitization but not the presence of allergic disease. Allergic sensitization with no correlative allergic disease is a common finding, occurring in 8% to 30% of the population when using a local standard panel of aeroallergens. In some cases, the presence of irritants or nonspecific mast cell secretagogues may explain positive responses with concentrated extracts, especially when they are used by the intradermal route. As assessed by the pan-European prick test study, among inhalant allergen sensitizations in Europe, grass had the highest rate of clinical relevance (88.4%) and plane tree had the lowest (59.9%). For all other allergens, more than 60% of recorded sensitizations were clinically relevant.[78] However, positive skin test results for asymptomatic subjects may foreshadow the subsequent onset of allergic symptoms. Prospective studies have shown that 30% to 60% of sensitized-only individuals subsequently develop allergic symptoms that can be attributed to exposure to allergens that previously elicited positive skin test responses.[79,80]

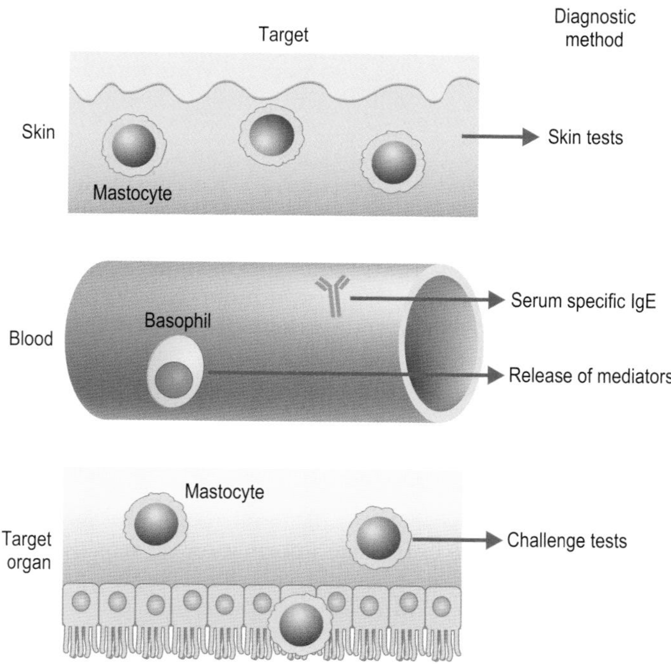

Figure 70-3 Differences between in vivo and in vitro tests used in the diagnosis of IgE-mediated allergic diseases.

FALSE-POSITIVE AND NEGATIVE SKIN TESTS

False-positive and false-negative skin test results may reflect improper technique or material.[22] False-positive results may be provoked by impurities, contaminants, and nonspecific mast cell secretagogues in the extract, as well as by dermatographism, respiratory syncytial virus infection (RSV), and nonspecific enhancement from a nearby strong reaction. RSV exposure increased wheal and flare responses to histamine and allergens and increased de novo positive responses to allergens in individuals with negative responses at baseline.[81]

False-negative skin test results can be caused by extracts of poor initial potency or subsequent loss of potency[42]; drugs modulating the allergic reaction; diseases attenuating the skin response; decreased reactivity of the skin in infants and elderly patients; improper technique (e.g., no or weak puncture); ultraviolet radiation exposure; a too-short or too-long time interval from the reaction; organ allergy; non–IgE-mediated mechanism; and infections, such as those by helminths. Antihelminthic treatment of infected children can increase their skin test reactivity to mite extracts.[82] The use of positive control solutions may help to clarify some of the false-negative results, because reactions are decreased or abolished in patients with weakly reactive skin. A positive intracutaneous test preceded by a negative prick-puncture test may denote clinical allergy in a less-sensitive patient or the presence of an IgE reagin that cannot be detected by prick-puncture tests.[40]

After a systemic reaction induced by hymenoptera sting, a refractory period of up to 6 weeks was found by Goldberg and colleagues.[83] They suggested that an early evaluation might be performed, but in this case, only positive skin test results should be taken into account. If an early evaluation yields negative results, a retest at 4 to 6 weeks is mandatory. In the absence of further studies, this observation has been applied to the exploration of other supposedly IgE-mediated reactions.

CORRELATION WITH OTHER DIAGNOSTIC TESTS USED FOR ALLERGY DIAGNOSIS

Many tests have been proposed for the diagnosis of IgE-mediated allergic diseases, but their results do not have the same significance as those of skin tests (Fig. 70-3).

In Vitro Tests

Comparisons between the titration of specific IgE depend on the quality and standardization of allergens used in both tests and to a lesser extent on the method of skin testing used.[42] Using standardized extracts, the percentage agreement between in vitro allergen-specific IgE tests and skin prick-puncture tests is between 85% and 95%, depending on the allergens being evaluated.[22,84] Typically, skin tests are more sensitive but less specific than in vitro allergen-specific IgE tests.[85]

In Vivo Tests

When both methods of skin testing are compared with bronchial, nasal, or oral challenges, prick-puncture tests are more specific but less sensitive than intradermal tests.[43] When there is a suggestive history and strongly positive skin test results, the correlation between skin tests and bronchial or nasal challenges is highly significant. Poor correlations often are observed with nonstandardized allergenic extracts or when there is a discrepancy between the history and skin test responses. Conjunctival provocative test results may be positive in rhinitis sufferers with negative skin test results,[86] and this suggests local IgE production.

DIAGNOSTIC VALUE OF SKIN TESTS

The position papers on skin tests from the European Academy of Allergy and Clinical Immunology[43] and the U.S. Joint Council of Allergy, Asthma, and Immunology[40] agree that when properly performed, prick-puncture tests are considered to be the most convenient and least expensive screening method for detecting allergic reactions in most patients. However, until the diagnostic efficacy of prick-puncture tests is fully established with standardized allergens and methods, negative prick-puncture results may be confirmed by more sensitive intradermal techniques, especially for drugs and stinging insect venoms. Even after false-positive and false-negative results have been eliminated, the proper interpretation of test results requires a thorough knowledge of the history and physical findings. A positive skin test result alone does not confirm definite clinical sensitivity to an allergen.

With inhalant allergens, the skin prick test is the cheapest and most effective method to diagnose respiratory allergies. Skin prick tests give immediate information on sensitivity to individual allergens and should therefore be the primary method clinicians use to assess respiratory allergic diseases. Positive skin test results with a medical history that suggests clinical sensitivity strongly incriminate the allergen as a contributor to the disease process. For example, Crobach and colleagues[84] demonstrated (with reference to experts' diagnosis) that the predictive value of the clinical history alone for the diagnosis of allergic rhinitis was 82% to 85% for intermittent seasonal allergens (and at least 77% for persistent allergens), and the rate increased to between 97% and 99% when skin prick tests (or specific IgE tests) were performed. Conversely, a negative skin test result with a negative history favors a nonallergic disorder. Interpretation of skin tests that do not correlate with the clinical history is more difficult, and in these situations, measurements of allergen-specific IgE and provocative challenges are of interest. For example, Wood and colleagues[87] demonstrated that in patients with negative skin prick and RAST test results to cat allergens in the context of cat exposure, the negative predictive value of both tests were almost identical (72% to 75%) for the diagnosis of cat allergy. Intradermal tests added little to the diagnosis evaluation. The wheal size appears to have diagnostic value. In a potentially allergic population undergoing skin prick testing using standardized extracts, a 6-mm skin prick wheal differentiated individuals who were cat allergic from those who were not.[88]

Particular caution should be used when interpreting skin test results for foods. Skin test specificity and sensitivity values are, respectively, 30% to 70% and 20% to 60% for food allergens and 70% to 95% and 80% to 97% for inhalant allergens. The differences may reflect numerous cross-reactions between food and inhalant allergens that have no clinical significance or food protein instability. Sensitivity increases up to 90% when prick-prick tests[30] with fresh foods are used.[89] A study comparing the wheal diameters with commercial extracts and fresh foods in children with suspected food allergy showed a higher concordance between a positive prick test and a positive challenge with fresh foods (91.7%) compared with commercial extracts (58.8%).[89] As with inhalant allergens, the wheal size has diagnostic value. In a study that evaluated subjects with histories of peanut allergy by skin prick tests, antigen-specific IgE assays, and challenges, the positive predictive value for a clinical allergy was 94.4% for a wheal diameter of at least 8 mm, with a specificity of 98.5%.[90] However, this approach does not apply to all allergens and all countries. Skin test results and antigen-specific IgE values should not be used to validate a diagnosis of wheat allergy because the specificity and predictive values are much lower.[91] Skin tests with commercial food allergen extracts are much less reliable than skin tests with inhalant allergens, and only a fraction of patients with positive results for food skin tests react during a food challenge.[22,91] These observations suggest that many patients having IgE antibodies to foods do not react or have lost their clinical sensitivities. With food extracts, prick-puncture tests seem to be more reliable than intradermal tests, because the latter can induce many false-positive reactions. The molecular characterization of major food allergens and the production of recombinant allergens make it possible to obtain high-quality reagents for skin and antigen-specific IgE tests.

Skin tests with venoms provide useful confirmatory evidence of an IgE response. Skin prick-puncture tests with venoms (at 100 to 300 μg/mL) can be used to evaluate sting-sensitive patients,[92] although intradermal tests are preferred. At the concentration of 1 μg/mL, about 30% of patients with systemic reactions have negative intradermal test results,[93] and one fourth of nonallergic subjects have positive results because of mast cell degranulating compounds contained in venoms.

Latex allergy can be confirmed by skin prick tests with commercially prepared natural rubber latex standardized for allergen content.[94] In one study,[95] the diagnostic sensitivity of different latex extracts ranged from 90% to 98%, and the specificity was 100%. Moreover, the size of the skin prick test response may reflect the severity of latex-induced clinical allergic responses.[95] Sensitization as assessed by skin prick test (and in vitro IgE testing) may disappear after cessation of exposure,[96] but there are few data on whether this loss of skin sensitization serves as a guarantee for tolerance upon allergen challenge.

The value of skin tests varies for diagnosing drug hypersensitivity.[97] The diagnosis is often difficult because patients may be allergic to one of the drug metabolites, there is a lack of standardization, and non–IgE-dependent mechanisms may be involved. With a few major exceptions, skin tests for drug allergies have poor predictive values, and the concentrations used are not all validated. The European Network for Drug Allergy and the Drug Allergy Interest Group of the European Academy of Allergy and Clinical Immunology have undertaken the task of standardizing skin test concentrations for systemically administered drugs based on the available literature.

In patients with histories of anaphylactic shock after injection of a muscle relaxant, the sensitivity of the skin tests performed within a brief period is more than 95%.[98] In penicillin allergy, the haptens used are benzylpenicilloyl-poly-L-lysine (PPL), a mixture of minor determinants (MDM) and penicillin G, amoxicillin, ampicillin, and any other relevant β-lactam.[99,100] Preliminary results regarding the good negative predictive value of skin testing with radiocontrast media and gadolinium contrast agents that were evaluated in small case series[101,102] await confirmation in larger series.

The position papers on skin testing from the Joint Practice Parameter of the American Academy of Allergy, Asthma, and Immunology and the American College of Allergy, Asthma, and Immunology[40] and from the European Academy of Allergology and Clinical Immunology[43] agree that for occupational sensitizers, skin tests are often unreliable in detecting industrial sensitization, with the exception of high-molecular-weight compounds such as natural rubber latex, enzymes, and flour. Moreover, although a positive skin test result may indicate clinical sensitization, there are subjects with positive results who do not exhibit any symptoms when they are exposed to these allergens.

In bronchopulmonary aspergillosis, skin tests (mainly intradermal) with *Aspergillus fumigatus* antigen offer a diagnostic tool that can produce immediate and late phase reactions. However, because some patients with *Aspergillus*-induced asthma or aspergilloma may also have biphasic skin responses, positive skin test results are not pathognomonic of bronchopulmonary aspergillosis. Recombinant allergens can be used for testing.[103]

Skin Tests Used for Nondiagnostic Purposes

STANDARDIZATION OF ALLERGENS

Skin tests are largely used in the standardization of allergen extracts for the evaluation of the biologic activity of an allergen standard and for the calibration of the potency of a new batch against a standard.[42] Many methods have been proposed, but two are more popular than others. The U.S. standardization system is based on the evaluation of the erythema[40] induced by intradermal skin tests, whereas the Nordic standardization system[104] is based on the evaluation of the wheal induced by skin prick-puncture tests. An extract should contain stable and definite amounts of all clinically relevant allergens representing the allergic population.

PHARMACOLOGIC STUDIES

Most pharmacologic studies examine variations in the early but not late phase reaction. The intradermal skin tests and prick-puncture tests can be used. The most common measure of skin tests, the wheal size, does not appear to be accurate enough for the purpose of pharmacologic studies. End-point titration should be replaced by methods based on parallel-line bioassay or median slope estimating the change in concentration needed to obtain the same wheal response before and after treatment.[42] However, more sophisticated techniques can also be employed.[22]

These tests must be carefully performed, and factors that may modify their interpretation should be rigorously checked. Ideally, the same trained investigator should perform the entire study by using lyophilized extracts from the same batch that are freshly reconstituted with an appropriate diluent at recommended time intervals. Skin window techniques may be used to assess the mechanism of action of drugs, but they are usually performed on very small numbers of patients.[22]

IMMUNOTHERAPY STUDIES

Demonstrating allergen sensitization before starting allergen immunotherapy is mandatory. Skin sensitivity to venom decreases during venom immunotherapy,[22] and it has been suggested that the treatment may be stopped when skin tests or specific IgE assays are negative; however, anaphylaxis may occur in patients with negative skin test results. Routine repeat skin testing is not recommended for nonvenom allergen immunotherapy.

EPIDEMIOLOGIC STUDIES

Skin tests have been used in epidemiologic studies to assess the prevalence of skin positivity to common allergens in the general population[105] and how it compares with the prevalence and severity of symptomatic allergic or respiratory diseases, for long-term studies of the development of sensitization and natural desensitization and the factors that influence both, and to explore the interactions between genetic susceptibility and environment.[106] Because many methods can be used, the precise method should be described to facilitate comparisons of studies from different geographic regions. The descriptions should include the test method used, the positivity criteria chosen, the site of the body on which tests were applied, the time of the year when the tests were done, and the quality of the allergen extracts.[43]

Skin prick-puncture tests are preferable to intradermal skin tests because of their safety, better specificity, and lower cost. The cutoff limit (i.e., size of the skin test) and the number of positive skin tests (as an indicator of atopy) should also be established. Other methods, such as ImmunoCAP, are also used to characterize the atopic status in epidemiologic studies.[107] Cross-sectional studies have shown that age, gender, and smoking may affect the results of skin prick tests. Outcomes of longitudinal epidemiologic studies of a working population surveyed 5 years apart suggest the prevalence of positive skin prick test results has significantly increased over time.[108] Skin test reactivities to common aeroallergens (i.e., house-dust mites, mixed grass pollen, mixed tree pollen, and ragweed) are significant independent predictors of subsequent decline of lung function among middle-aged and older men with no history of asthma.[109]

Conclusions

When properly performed, skin tests represent the major tool for the diagnosis of IgE-mediated diseases and are of particular importance in fields such as allergen standardization, pharmacology, and epidemiology. Although it is relatively easy to perform the tests, accurate interpretation requires investigators and clinician specialists to be experienced in the technical aspects and nuances of the testing procedures and in interpreting the observed findings in the context of the clinical history and physical examination findings. A major challenge of practitioners working in the allergy field is to create awareness, especially among primary care physicians, of the value of skin tests. Performing skin tests enables the clinician to confirm or refute sensitization and atopy, which has important prognostic implications for development of comorbid diseases such as asthma. After allergic sensitization and relevant diseases have been established, proper education regarding allergen avoidance and the prescribing of appropriate medical therapy (including allergen immunotherapy) can be safely and appropriately instituted.

REFERENCES

Introduction

1. Blackley C. Hay fever: its causes, treatment and effective prevention; experimental researches. 2nd ed. London: Baillieres, Tindal & Cox; 1880.
2. Mantoux C. Intradermoréaction de la tuberculose. CR Acad Sci 1908;147:355.
3. Lewis T, Grant R. Vascular reactions of the skin to injury. Part II. The liberation of a histamine-like substance in injured skin, the underlying cause of factitious urticaria and of wheals produced by burning; and observations upon the nervous control of certain skin reactions. Heart 1924;209:1924.

Pathophysiology of the Skin Response

4. Friedman MM, Kaliner M. Ultrastructural changes in human skin mast cells during antigen-induced degranulation in vivo. J Allergy Clin Immunol 1988;82:998-1005.
5. Shalit M, Schwartz LB, von-Allmen C, et al. Release of histamine and tryptase during continuous and interrupted cutaneous challenge with allergen in humans. J Allergy Clin Immunol 1990;86:117-25.
6. Horsmanheimo L, Harvima IT, Harvima RJ, et al. Histamine release in skin monitored with the microdialysis technique does not correlate with the weal size induced by cow allergen. Br J Dermatol 1996;134:94-100.
7. Foreman JC. Substance P and calcitonin gene-related peptide: effects on mast cells and in human skin. Int Arch Allergy Appl Immunol 1987;82:366-71.
8. Wallengren J, Larsson B. Nitric oxide participates in prick test and irritant patch test reactions in human skin. Arch Dermatol Res 2001;293:121-25.
9. Theoharides TC, Singh LK, Boucher W, et al. Corticotropin-releasing hormone induces skin mast cell degranulation and increased vascular permeability, a possible explanation for its proinflammatory effect. Endocrinology 1998; 139:403-13.
10. Frew AJ, Kay AB. Failure to detect deposition of complement and immunoglobulin in allergen-induced late-phase skin reaction in atopic subjects. Clin Exp Immunol 1991;85: 70-4.
11. Leung DY, Pober JS, Cotran RS. Expression of endothelial-leukocyte adhesion molecule-1 in elicited late phase allergic reactions. J Clin Invest 1991;87:1805-9.
12. Reshef A, Kagey-Sobotka A, Adkinson Jr N, Lichtenstein LM, Norman PS. The pattern and kinetics in human skin of erythema and mediators during the acute and late-phase response (LPR). J Allergy Clin Immunol 1989;84: 678-87.
13. Gronneberg R, Dahlen SE. Interactions between histamine and prostanoids in IgE-dependent, late cutaneous reactions in man. J Allergy Clin Immunol 1990;85:843-52.
14. Frew AJ, Kay AB. The relationship between infiltrating CD4$^+$ lymphocytes, activated eosinophils, and the magnitude of the allergen-induced late phase cutaneous reaction in man. J Immunol 1988;141:4158-64.
15. Vowels BR, Rook AH, Cassin M, Zweiman B. Expression of interleukin-4 and interleukin-5 mRNA in developing cutaneous late-phase reactions. J Allergy Clin Immunol 1995;96: 92-6.
16. Tsicopoulos A, Hamid Q, Haczku A, et al. Kinetics of cell infiltration and cytokine messenger RNA expression after intradermal challenge with allergen and tuberculin in the same atopic individuals. J Allergy Clin Immunol 1994;94:764-72.
17. Werfel S, Massey W, Lichtenstein LM, Bochner BS. Preferential recruitment of activated, memory T lymphocytes into skin chamber fluids during human cutaneous late-phase allergic reactions. J Allergy Clin Immunol 1995;96:57-65.
18. Leiferman KM, Fujisawa T, Gray BH, Gleich GJ. Extracellular deposition of eosinophil and neutrophil granule proteins in the IgE-mediated cutaneous late phase reaction. Lab Invest 1990;62:579-89.
19. Dor PJ, Vervloet D, Sapene M, et al. Induction of late cutaneous reaction by kallikrein injection: comparison with allergic-like late response to compound 48/80. J Allergy Clin Immunol 1983;71:363-70.
20. Charlesworth EN, Kagey-Sobotka A, Schleimer RP, Norman PS, Lichtenstein LM. Prednisone inhibits the appearance of inflammatory mediators and the influx of eosinophils and basophils associated with the cutaneous late-phase response to allergen. J Immunol 1991;146: 671-6.
21. Alam R, Dejarnatt A, Stafford S, et al. Selective inhibition of the cutaneous late but not immediate allergic response to antigens by misoprostol, a PGE analog. Results of a double-blind, placebo-controlled randomized study. Am Rev Respir Dis 1993;148:1066-70.

Techniques of Skin Tests

22. Demoly P, Piette V, Bousquet J. In vivo methods for study of allergy: skin tests, techniques and interpretation. In: Adkinson Jr NF, Yunginger JW, Busse WW, et al. editors. Allergy: principles and practice. 6th ed. New York: Mosby; 2003, p. 631-55.
23. Pepys J. Skin testing. Br J Hosp Med 1975;14: 412-25.
24. Piette V, Bourret E, Bousquet J, Demoly P. Prick tests to aeroallergens: is it possible to simply wipe the device between tests? Allergy 2002;57: 940-2.
25. Kupczyk M, Kuprys I, Gorski P, Kuna P. Not one lancet for multiple SPT. Allergy 2001;56:256-7.
26. Occupation Safety and Health Administration. Hazard information bulletin. Washington, D.C.: Occupation Safety and Health Administration; 1995.
27. Nelson HS, Lahr J, Buchmeier A, McCormick D. Evaluation of devices for skin prick testing. J Allergy Clin Immunol 1998;101:153-6.
28. Masse MS, Granger Vallée A, Chiriac A, et al. Comparison of five techniques of skin prick tests used routinely in Europe. Allergy 2011; 66:1415-9.
29. Carr WW, Martin B, Howard RS, Cox L, Borish L. Immunotherapy Committee of the American Academy of Allergy, Asthma and Immunology. Comparison of test devices for skin prick testing. J Allergy Clin Immunol 2005;116:341-6.
30. Dreborg S. Food allergy in pollen-sensitive patients. Ann Allergy 1988;61:41-6.
31. Liccardi G, D'Amato G, Canonica GW, et al. Systemic reactions from skin testing: literature review. J Investig Allergol Clin Immunol 2006; 16:75-8.
32. Devenney I, Fälth-Magnusson K. Skin prick tests may give generalized allergic reactions in infants. Ann Allergy Asthma Immunol 2000; 85:457-60.
33. Codreanu F, Moneret-Vautrin DA, Morisset M, et al. The risk of systemic reactions to skin prick-tests using food allergens: CICBAA data and literature review. Eur Ann Allergy Clin Immunol 2006;38:52-4.
34. Norrman G, Fälth-Magnusson K. Adverse reactions to skin prick testing in children—prevalence and possible risk factors. Pediatr Allergy Immunol 2009;20:273-8.
35. Veillette M, Cormier Y, Duchaine C. Survival of *Staphylococcus* and other bacteria in skin prick test antigens solutions. Am J Infect Control 2009;37:606-8.
36. Sicherer SH, Eggleston PA. EMLA cream for pain reduction in diagnostic allergy skin testing: effects on wheal and flare responses. Ann Allergy Asthma Immunol 1997;78:64-8.
37. Lockey RF, Benedict LM, Turkeltaub PC, Bukantz SC. Fatalities from immunotherapy (IT) and skin testing (ST). J Allergy Clin Immunol 1987;79:660-77.
38. Co-Minh HB, Bousquet PJ, Fontaine C, Kvedariene V, Demoly P. Systemic reactions during skin tests with β-lactams: a risk factor analysis. J Allergy Clin Immunol 2006;117: 466-8.
39. Lieberman P. Anaphylaxis. Med Clin North Am 2006;90:77-95.
40. Bernstein IL, Li JT, Bernstein DI, Hamilton R, et al. American Academy of Allergy, Asthma and Immunology; American College of Allergy, Asthma and Immunology. Allergy diagnostic testing: an updated practice parameter. Ann Allergy Asthma Immunol 2008;100:S1-148.
41. Wood RA, Phipatanakul W, Hamilton RG, Eggleston PA. A comparison of skin prick tests, intradermal skin tests, and RASTs in the diagnosis of cat allergy. J Allergy Clin Immunol 1999;103:773-9.
42. Dreborg S, Backman A, Basomba A, et al. Skin tests used in type I allergy testing. Position paper of the European Academy of Allergy and Clinical Immunology. Allergy 1989;44:1-69.
43. Position paper: Allergen standardization and skin tests. The European Academy of Allergology and Clinical Immunology. Allergy 1993; 48:48-82.
44. Konstantinou GN, Bousquet PJ, Zuberbier T, Papadopoulos NG. The longest wheal diameter is the optimal measurement for the evaluation of skin prick tests. Int Arch Allergy Immunol 2010;151:343-5.
45. McCann WA, Ownby DR. The reproducibility of the allergy skin test scoring and interpretation by board-certified/board-eligible allergists. Ann Allergy Asthma Immunol 2002;89: 368-71.
46. Bousquet J, Heinzerling L, Bachert C, et al. Practical guide to skin prick tests in allergy to aeroallergens. Allergy 2012;67:18-24.
47. Adinoff AD, Rosloniec DM, McCall LL, Nelson HS. Immediate skin test reactivity to Food and Drug Administration–approved standardized extracts. J Allergy Clin Immunol 1990;86: 766-74.
48. Norman P, Lichtenstein L, Ishizaka K. Diagnostic tests in ragweed hay fever. A comparison of direct skin tests, IgE antibody measurements, and basophil histamine release. J Allergy Clin Immunol 1973;52:210-24.

49. Van-Metre Jr TE, Adkinson Jr N, Kagey-Sobotka A, et al. Immunotherapy decreases skin sensitivity to ragweed extract: demonstration by midpoint skin test titration. J Allergy Clin Immunol 1990;86:587-8.
50. Turkeltaub PC, Rastogi SC, Baer H, Anderson MC, Norman PS. A standardized quantitative skin-test assay of allergen potency and stability: studies on the allergen dose-response curve and effect of wheal, erythema, and patient selection on assay results. J Allergy Clin Immunol 1982;70:343-52.
51. Heinzerling LM, Burbach GJ, Edenharter G, et al. GA(2)LEN skin test study. I: GA(2)LEN harmonization of skin prick testing: novel sensitization patterns for inhalant allergens in Europe. Allergy 2009;64:1498-506.
52. Bousquet PJ, Burbach G, Heinzerling LM, et al. GA2LEN skin test study III: minimum battery of test inhalent allergens needed in epidemiological studies in patients. Allergy 2009;64:1656-62.
53. Rebuck JW, Crowley JH. A method of studying leukocyte function in vivo. Ann N Y Acad Sci 1955;59:757-61.
54. Dunsky EH, Zweiman B. The direct demonstration of histamine release in allergic reactions in the skin using a skin chamber technique. J Allergy Clin Immunol 1978;62:127-30.

Factors That Affect Skin Tests

55. Guerin B, Tioulong S. Analysis of the nonimmunological activity of allergen extracts in cutaneous tests. Clin Allergy 1979;9:283-91.
56. Schmid-Grendelmeier P, Crameri R. Recombinant allergens for skin testing. Int Arch Allergy Immunol 2001;125:96-111.
57. Asturias JA, Ibarrola I, Ferrer A, et al. Diagnosis of *Alternaria alternata* sensitization with natural and recombinant Alt a 1 allergens. J Allergy Clin Immunol 2005;115:1210-7.
58. Mills EN, Mackie AR. The impact of processing on allergenicity of food. Curr Opin Allergy Clin Immunol 2008;8:249-53.
59. Bégin P, Des Roches A, Nguyen M, et al. Freezing does not alter antigenic properties of fresh fruits for skin testing in patients with birch tree pollen-induced oral allergy syndrome. J Allergy Clin Immunol 2011;127:1624-6.
60. Garriga T, Guilarte M, Luengo O, et al. Frozen fruit skin prick test for the diagnosis of fruit allergy. Asian Pac J Allergy Immunol 2010;28:275-8.
61. Bordignon V, Burastero SE. Age, gender and reactivity to allergens independently influence skin reactivity to histamine. J Investig Allergol Clin Immunol 2006;16:129-35.
62. Kirmaz C, Yuksel H, Mete N, Bayrak P, Baytur YB. Is the menstrual cycle affecting the skin prick test reactivity? Asian Pac J Allergy Immunol 2004;22:197-203.
63. Sin BA, Inceoglu O, Mungan D, et al. Is it important to perform pollen skin tests in the season? Ann Allergy Asthma Immunol 2001;86:382-6.
64. Vocks E, Stander K, Rakoski J, Ring J. Suppression of immediate-type hypersensitivity elicitation in the skin prick test by ultraviolet B irradiation. Photodermatol Photoimmunol Photomed 1999;15:236-40.
65. Uehara M. Reduced histamine reaction in atopic dermatitis. Arch Dermatol 1982;118:244-5.
66. Kimata H. Enhancement of allergic skin wheal responses in patients with atopic eczema/dermatitis syndrome by playing video games or by a frequently ringing mobile phone. Eur J Clin Invest 2003;33:513-7.
67. Bousquet J, Pujol JL, Barneon G, et al. Skin test reactivity in patients suffering from lung and breast cancer. J Allergy Clin Immunol 1991;87:1066-72.
68. Purohit A, Duvernelle C, Melac M, Pauli G, Frossard N. Twenty-four hours of activity of cetirizine and fexofenadine in the skin. Ann Allergy Asthma Immunol 2001;86:387-92.
69. Persi L, Demoly P, Harris AG, et al. Comparison between nasal provocation tests and skin tests in patients treated with loratadine and cetirizine. J Allergy Clin Immunol 1999;103:591-4.
70. Pearlman DS, Grossman J, Meltzer EO. Histamine skin test reactivity following single and multiple doses of azelastine nasal spray in patients with seasonal allergic rhinitis. Ann Allergy Asthma Immunol 2003;91:258-62.
71. Des Roches A, Paradis L, Bougeard YH, et al. Long-term oral corticosteroid therapy does not alter the results of immediate-type allergy skin prick tests. J Allergy Clin Immunol 1996;98:522-7.
72. Ong YE, Menzies-Gow A, Barkans J, et al. Anti-IgE (omalizumab) inhibits late-phase reactions and inflammatory cells after repeat skin allergen challenge. J Allergy Clin Immunol 2005;116:558-64.
73. Vieira Dos Santos R, Magerl M, Martus P, et al. Topical sodium cromoglycate relieves allergen- and histamine-induced dermal pruritus. Br J Dermatol 2010;162:674-6.
74. Weissenbacher S, Traidl-Hoffmann C, Eyerich K, et al. Modulation of atopy patch test and skin prick test by pretreatment with 1% pimecrolimus cream. Int Arch Allergy Immunol 2006;140:239-44.
75. Nettis E, Colanardi MC, Soccio AL, et al. Double-blind, placebo-controlled study of sublingual immunotherapy in patients with latex-induced urticaria: a 12-month study. Br J Dermatol 2007;156:674-81.
76. Varshney P, Jones SM, Scurlock AM, et al. A randomized controlled study of peanut oral immunotherapy: clinical desensitization and modulation of the allergic response. J Allergy Clin Immunol 2011;127:654-60.
77. Parker Jr WA, Whisman BA, Apaliski SJ, Reid MJ. The relationships between late cutaneous responses and specific antibody responses with outcome of immunotherapy for seasonal allergic rhinitis. J Allergy Clin Immunol 1989;84:667-77.

Interpretation of Skin Tests

78. Burbach GJ, Heinzerling LM, Edenharter G, et al. GA(2)LEN skin test study II: clinical relevance of inhalant allergen sensitizations in Europe. Allergy 2009;64:1507-15.
79. Bodtger U, Poulsen LK, Malling HJ. Asymptomatic skin sensitization to birch predicts later development of birch pollen allergy in adults: a 3-year follow-up study. J Allergy Clin Immunol 2003;111:149-54.
80. Pastorello EA, Incorvaia C, Ortolani C, et al. Studies on the relationship between the level of specific IgE antibodies and the clinical expression of allergy: I. Definition of levels distinguishing patients with symptomatic from patients with asymptomatic allergy to common aeroallergens. J Allergy Clin Immunol 1995;96:580-7.
81. Skoner DP, Gentile DA, Angelini B, Doyle WJ. Allergy skin test responses during experimental infection with respiratory syncytial virus. Ann Allergy Asthma Immunol 2006;96:834-9.
82. van den Biggelaar AH, Rodrigues LC, van Ree R, et al. Long-term treatment of intestinal helminths increases mite skin-test reactivity in Gabonese schoolchildren. J Infect Dis 2004;189:892-900.
83. Goldberg A, Confino-Cohen R. Timing of venom skin tests and IgE determinations after insect sting anaphylaxis. J Allergy Clin Immunol 1997;100:182-4.
84. Crobach MJJS, Hermans JO, Kaptein AA, et al. The diagnosis of allergic rhinitis: how to combine the medical history with the results of radioallergosorbent tests and skin prick tests. Scand J Prim Health Care 1998;16:30-6.
85. van-der-Zee JS, de-Groot H, van-Swieten P, et al. Discrepancies between the skin test and IgE antibody assays: study of histamine release, complement activation in vitro, and occurrence of allergen-specific IgG. J Allergy Clin Immunol 1988;82:270-81.
86. Leonardi A, Fregona IA, Gismondi M, et al. Correlation between conjunctival provocation test (CPT) and systemic allergometric tests in allergic conjunctivitis. Eye (Lond) 1990;4:760-4.
87. Wood RA, Phipatanakul W, Hamilton RG, Eggleston PA. A comparison of skin prick tests, intradermal skin tests, and RASTs in the diagnosis of cat allergy. J Allergy Clin Immunol 1999;103:773-9.
88. Zarei M, Remer CF, Kaplan MS, et al. Optimal skin prick wheal size for diagnosis of cat allergy. Ann Allergy Asthma Immunol 2004;92:604-10.
89. Rance F, Juchet A, Bremont F, Dutau G. Correlations between skin prick tests using commercial extracts and fresh foods, specific IgE, and food challenges. Allergy 1997;52:1031-5.
90. Roberts G, Lack G. Diagnosing peanut allergy with skin prick and specific IgE testing. J Allergy Clin Immunol 2005;115:1291-6.
91. Scibilia J, Pastorello EA, Zisa G, et al. Wheat allergy: a double-blind, placebo-controlled study in adults. J Allergy Clin Immunol 2006;117:433-9.
92. Harries MG, Kemeny DM, Youlten LJ, Mills MM, Lessof MH. Skin and radioallergosorbent tests in patients with sensitivity to bee and wasp venom. Clin Allergy 1984;14:407-12.
93. Golden DB, Kagey-Sobotka A, Norman PS, Hamilton RG, Lichtenstein LM. Insect sting allergy with negative venom skin test responses. J Allergy Clin Immunol 2001;107:897-901.
94. Turjanmaa K, Palosuo T, Alenius H, et al. Latex allergy diagnosis: in vivo and in vitro standardization of a natural rubber latex extract. Allergy 1997;52:41-50.
95. Blanco C, Carrillo T, Ortega N, et al. Comparison of skin-prick test and specific IgE determination for the diagnosis of latex allergy. Clin Exp Allergy 1999;29:133-4.
96. Merget R, van Kampen V, Sucker K, et al. The German experience 10 years after the latex allergy epidemic: need for further preventive measures in healthcare employees with latex allergy. Int Arch Occup Environ Health 2010;83:895-903.
97. Brockow K, Romano A, Blanca M, et al. General considerations for skin test procedures in the diagnosis of drug hypersensitivity. Allergy 2002;57:45-51.

98. Mertes PM, Laxenaire MC, Lienhart A, et al. Working Group for the SFAR; ENDA; EAACI Interest Group on Drug Hypersensitivity. Reducing the risk of anaphylaxis during anaesthesia: guidelines for clinical practice. J Invest Allergol Clin Immunol 2005;15:91-101.
99. Torres MJ, Blanca M, Fernandez J, et al. ENDA; EAACI Interest Group on Drug Hypersensitivity. Diagnosis of immediate allergic reactions to beta-lactam antibiotics. Allergy 2003;58: 961-72.
100. Romano A, Blanca M, Torres MJ, et al. ENDA; EAACI. Diagnosis of nonimmediate reactions to beta-lactam antibiotics. Allergy 2004;59: 1153-60.
101. Caimmi S, Benyahia B, Suau D, et al. Clinical value of negative skin tests to iodinated contrast media. Clin Exp Allergy 2010;40:805-10.
102. Chiriac AM, Audurier Y, Bousquet PJ, Demoly P. Clinical value of negative skin tests to gadolinium contrast agents. Allergy 2011;66: 1504-6.
103. Moser M, Crameri R, Brust E, Suter M, Menz G. Diagnostic value of recombinant *Aspergillus fumigatus* allergen I/a for skin testing and serology. J Allergy Clin Immunol 1994;93:1-11.

Skin Tests Used for Nondiagnostic Purposes

104. Nordic Council on Medicines. Registration of allergen preparations. 2nd ed. NLN publication no 23. Uppsala: Nordiska Läkemedelsnämnden; 1989.
105. The International Study of Asthma and Allergies in Childhood Steering Committee. Worldwide variation in prevalence of symptoms of asthma, allergic rhinoconjunctivitis, and atopic eczema: ISAAC. Lancet 1998;351:1225-32.
106. Postma DS, Bleecker ER, Amelung PJ, et al. Genetic susceptibility to asthma-bronchial hyperresponsiveness coinherited with a major gene for atopy. N Engl J Med 1995;333: 894-900.
107. Tschopp JM, Sistek D, Schindler C, et al. Current allergic asthma and rhinitis: diagnostic efficiency of three commonly used atopic markers (IgE, skin prick tests, and Phadiatop). Results from 8329 randomized adults from the SAPALDIA Study. Swiss Study on Air Pollution and Lung Diseases in Adults. Allergy 1998;53: 608-13.
108. Oryszczyn MP, Annesi I, Neukirch F, et al. Longitudinal observations of serum IgE and skin prick test response. Am J Respir Crit Care Med 1995;151:663-8.
109. Gottlieb DJ, Sparrow D, O'Connor GT, Weiss ST. Skin test reactivity to common aeroallergens and decline of lung function. The Normative Aging Study. Am J Respir Crit Care Med 1996;153:561-6.

71

Approach to the Patient with Recurrent Infections

MARK BALLOW | HEATHER K. LEHMAN

CONTENTS

SUMMARY OF IMPORTANT CONCEPTS

» Medical history is important for determining whether there are potential common risk factors (e.g., passive smoking, day care, atopy, anatomic defects) for frequent infections.
» Patients with antibody deficiency disorders are usually well until 7 to 9 months of age because of maternal immunoglobulin G (IgG) antibodies placentally derived during the third trimester of pregnancy.
» The response to antimicrobial treatment, frequency, duration, and severity are important factors to consider.
» Gastrointestinal and autoimmune disturbances are common in patients with immunodeficiency.
» Recurrent skin infections are usually associated with phagocytic defects in host defense.
» The pathogen responsible for the infection may yield important information about the nature of the underlying defect in host defense.
» Obtaining an extensive family history is important because many of the immunodeficiency disorders are X-linked and heritable.
» Findings of a comprehensive physical examination often reflect significant aspects of the medical history and can inform the diagnosis of a specific immunodeficiency.
» Although the absence of lymphoid tissue (e.g., tonsils) on physical examination is an important finding for diagnosing an immunodeficiency disorder, the presence of lymphoid tissue (e.g., hepatosplenomegaly) does not exclude an underlying immunodeficiency.

Introduction

Immunodeficiency diseases are relatively uncommon in the general population; nevertheless, it is important for physicians to understand immune defenses and to be able to recognize these diseases. Evaluation of a patient with frequent infections requires a careful history and physical examination directed at finding clues that may help to categorize the nature of the underlying immunodeficiency.[1] In this chapter, we focus on the basic principles of the immune system as related to the signs and symptoms of immunodeficiency diseases.

The human host defense system has evolved to protect individuals from invasion by microorganisms. Primary immunodeficiencies usually result from genetic defects that interfere with phagocytic function or lymphocyte development and function or that lead to absent or nonfunctional serum proteins or small-molecule components of the immune system. These disorders are rare, with the exception of immunoglobulin A (IgA) deficiency, which occurs with a frequency of approximately 1 case per 500 to 700 in Caucasians. The estimated range of prevalence for other primary immunodeficiencies is 1 case per 10,000 to 200,000 people, depending on the specific diagnosis.[2] Advances in newborn screening may place the incidence of severe combined immunodeficiency disease (SCID) much higher (1 case per 30,000 neonates) compared with previous estimates of 1 case per 300,000 neonates.[3] More than 185 genetic defects that result in immunodeficiency have been identified.[4] Defects involving B cell immunity are the most common immune abnormalities, accounting for more than 50% of the recognized causes of primary immunodeficiency. Combined humoral and cellular deficiencies constitute 20% to 30% of all cases, followed by phagocytic defects at a rate of about 18% and complement deficiencies at 2%.[2]

The Medical History in Immunodeficiency

Differentiation of frequent infections due to common risk factors such as child care attendance or passive smoking from primary immune dysfunction should be based on a detailed history and physical examination, usually followed by appropriate laboratory studies. Early diagnosis and treatment can improve the quality of life for patients and lifesaving treatments and genetic counseling can be initiated early in the course of the disease.

Normal young children may have four to six upper respiratory tract infections per year for the first 3 to 5 years of life. Children attending child care facilities or those with school-aged siblings at home can have even more frequent infections due to increased exposure to infectious agents. Typically, children with an intact immune system and no other predisposing factors handle these infections well, with rapid resolution of bacterial infections using appropriate antibiotics. Several nonimmunologic factors contribute to the risk of infections during

BOX 71-1 FACTORS THAT CONTRIBUTE TO THE RISK OF RECURRENT INFECTIONS

Atopy or allergic disease
Day care attendance
School-age siblings
Second-hand tobacco smoke exposure
Gastroesophageal reflux
Anatomic abnormalities of upper or lower airways
Foreign body
Cystic fibrosis
Immotile cilia syndrome

BOX 71-2 CRITICAL ELEMENTS OF THE MEDICAL HISTORY

Age at onset
- 4-5 months (combined T/B cell immunodeficiency, phagocytic disorder)
- 7-9 months (B cell immunodeficiency)

History of recurrent infections
- Sites of infection
- Types of infection

Gastrointestinal symptoms
Autoimmune diseases
Family history
Adverse reaction to vaccines

childhood (Box 71-1). Passive tobacco smoke inhalation in the home is associated with an increased number of infections, and it is a contributing factor to allergy and asthma symptoms. Atopy affects 20% to 25% of children and causes chronic inflammation of the airways that can mimic recurrent or chronic upper respiratory infections.

Individuals with anatomic defects can present with recurrent or chronic infections. Foreign bodies should be considered when the infections are chronic and localized to one anatomic site, such as one ear canal or one nostril. Children with recurrent or chronic sinusitis with documented anatomic defects of the sinuses causing poor drainage frequently have favorable outcomes with corrective surgery. Gastroesophageal reflux is frequently associated with asthma symptoms, but it sometimes can be confused with bronchitis or lead to aspiration and recurrent pneumonia. Children with recurrent sinopulmonary infections, especially when accompanied by symptoms such as malabsorption or nasal polyps, should be evaluated for possible cystic fibrosis. Recurrent sinopulmonary infections with situs inversus may indicate immotile cilia (i.e., Kartagener syndrome).

The approach to the patient with recurrent infection begins with the medical history. Box 71-2 outlines several of the critical elements of the history.

AGE AT ONSET

Typically, the younger the age at onset of infections, the more severe is the underlying immunodeficiency. For example, patients with SCID, who lack function of T and B cell immunity usually begin having infections by 4 to 5 months of age. In contrast, patients with only B cell deficiencies are usually well until 7 to 9 months of age, by which time placentally derived maternal IgG decreases to below protective levels in the infant, resulting in increased susceptibility to infection.

TABLE 71-1 Sites of Infection

Infection	Associated Pathology
Otitis media, recurrent mastoiditis	B cell deficiency
Sinusitis	B cell deficiency
Pneumonia bronchiectasis	B cell deficiency
Meningitis	B cell deficiency
Sepsis	B cell deficiency, complement pathway defect, neutropenia
Skin infections	B cell deficiency, neutrophil or phagocyte defects
Gingivitis or stomatitis	Neutrophil or phagocyte defects
Organ abscesses	Neutrophil or phagocyte defects
Lymphadenitis	Neutrophil or phagocyte defects

INFECTIONS

Sites of Infection

The frequency, duration, severity, and complications of an illness and the response to antimicrobial treatment should be considered in differentiating an infectious process from a noninfectious condition such as allergy. Bacterial infections should be documented with appropriate cultures. The sites of infection are important in determining the significance of the patient's recurrent infections. Recurrent pharyngitis (e.g., due to group A *Streptococcus*) is not typically a serious or significant site of infection. The sites of infection in a patient may also provide insights into the immunobiology of the specific immunologic defect (Table 71-1). For example, patients with persistent or recurrent gingivitis may have a phagocytic defect or neutropenia. Skin infections are a characteristic feature in patients with phagocytic abnormalities and may also be seen in patients with antibody immunodeficiency. Recurrent septicemia suggests a defect in opsonization: an inability to generate specific IgG antibody or a lack of the nonspecific opsonins of the classic, alternative, or late complement pathway components. Poor wound healing can suggest a leukocyte adhesion deficiency (LAD), as can umbilical cord separation delayed beyond 6 to 8 weeks of age in neonates.

Microbiology of Infections

The type of organism responsible for the patient's infections often yields important information about the nature of the defect in host defense (Table 71-2). For example, recurrent viral, fungal, mycobacterial, or protozoal infections suggest T cell defects. *Mycobacterium avium-intracellulare* and *Pneumocystis jiroveci* are typical opportunistic infections seen in patients with severe T cell defects. Patients with CD40 ligand deficiency (and CD40 deficiency), which is associated with elevated serum levels of IgM, have infections with opportunistic pathogens such as cytomegalovirus (CMV), herpes simplex, *P. jiroveci*, *Cryptococcus*, and cholangitis due to *Cryptosporidium*, indicating that they have a T cell deficiency.[5] Infection with *Candida* species can provide clues to the type of underlying immunodeficiency. Systemic or disseminated candidiasis usually is associated with disorders of phagocytosis and neutropenic conditions, although patients with central lines are especially prone to *Candida*

TABLE 71-2 Microbiology of Infections

Organism	Associated Pathology
BACTERIA	
Mycobacteria *Mycobacterium avium-intracellulare*	T cell deficiency, NK cell defect, IL-12/IFN-γ pathway defects
Enteric bacterial organisms *Campylobacter* *Salmonella* species *Clostridium difficile*	B cell immunodeficiency
Encapsulated organisms *Streptococcus pneumoniae* *Hemophilus influenza* *Neisseria* species	B cell or complement deficiency
Catalase-positive organisms *Staphylococcus aureus* *Burkholderia cepacia* *Klebsiella* *Serratia*	Neutrophil and phagocyte defects (CGD)
VIRUSES	
Herpesvirus, varicella, CMV	T cell deficiency, IL-12 and IFN-γ pathway defects, NK cell defects
Epstein-Barr virus	XLP
HPV	T cell, WHIM syndrome
Enteroviruses (e.g., echovirus, coxsackievirus)	B cell deficiency
Rotavirus	B cell deficiency
FUNGI	
Candida	T cell deficiency
Aspergillus	T cell or phagocyte defects
PARASITES	
Giardia lamblia	B cell deficiency
Toxoplasma gondii	T cell deficiency
OPPORTUNISTIC INFECTIONS	
Pneumocystis jiroveci	T cell deficiency
Cryptosporidium	T cell deficiency

CGD, Chronic granulomatous disease; *HPV*, human papillomavirus; *IFN*, interferon; *IL*, interleukin; *NK*, natural killer; *WHIM*, warts, hypogammaglobulinemia, bacterial infections, and myelokathesis; *XLP*, X-linked lymphoproliferative disease.

sepsis. Cutaneous candidiasis is not uncommon in infants because of infected articles such as pacifiers or in patients with a secondary immunodeficiency, as in HIV, diabetes, long-term use of antibiotics, or chemotherapy. Mucocutaneous candidiasis is common in patients with a primary T cell deficiency.

Helper T type 17 (Th17) cells are important in protecting against superficial *Candida* infections in patients with chronic mucocutaneous candidiasis. Patients with autosomal dominant hyper-IgE syndrome (HIES), which is characterized by eczema, mucocutaneous candidiasis, *Staphylococcus aureus* skin infections, and pneumatocele formation, have mutations in the transcription factor encoding STAT3. This leads to decreased interleukin-17 (IL-17)-producing T cells.[6] Patients with autoimmune polyendocrinopathy, candidiasis, and ectodermal dystrophy (APECED) syndrome, who also have problems with candidiasis, have autoantibodies to the Th17 cytokines, such as IL-17 and IL-22.[7] Mutations in *CARD9* and *CLEC7A* (formerly designated Dectin-1) are associated with chronic mucocutaneous candidiasis.[8] CLEC7A and CARD9 are part of the signaling pathway leading to Th17 cell differentiation and the production of cytokines (e.g., IL-17A, IL-17F, IL-22) that are important in the host defense to mucosal *Candida* infections.[9] Other patients with mucocutaneous candidiasis have been described that have mutations in the IL-17 receptor and the gene that produces IL-17F.[10]

In contrast, recurrent sinopulmonary infections with encapsulated invasive bacteria, such as *Streptococcus pneumoniae* and *Haemophilus influenzae* (type b and nontypable), suggest an antibody deficiency disorder. Within the category of antibody deficiency disorders, certain infections are characteristic of specific diseases. Patients with IgA deficiency or common variable immunodeficiency (CVID) frequently have protracted gastrointestinal symptoms as a result of *Giardia lamblia* infestation; other pathogens are shown in Table 71-2. Patients with X-linked agammaglobulinemia (XLA [Bruton disease]) have an increased susceptibility to infections with enteroviruses (i.e., echovirus and coxsackievirus), which can lead to meningoencephalitis. Arthritis of the large joints in these patients can be caused by *Ureaplasma urealyticum* and *Mycoplasma. S. pneumoniae* is a pathogen most commonly associated with humoral immunodeficiency, and in patients with abnormalities of the innate immune system, such as mutations in *IRAK4* and *MYD88*.[11] With increasing age of individuals with IRAK4 and MYD88 deficiencies, infections with *S. pneumoniae* are less of a problem because of maturation of the adaptive immune system.

A child presenting with lymphadenitis or recurrent abscesses due to low-virulence, gram-negative organisms such as *Escherichia coli*, *Serratia*, or *Klebsiella* may have an abnormality in phagocytic function. Infections with unusual pathogens such as *Staphylococcus epidermidis, Pseudomonas*, or *Burkholderia cepacia* can also suggest a phagocytic disorder such as chronic granulomatous disease. Patients with a phagocytic defect typically have a history of recurrent skin infections with catalase-positive *S. aureus* and recurrent gingivitis, underscoring the importance of effective phagocytosis and intracellular superoxide-mediated killing in controlling these infections.[12] *Aspergillus* or other fungal organisms can cause infection in patients with phagocytic abnormalities.

Recurrent *Neisseria* infection is a hallmark presentation of patients with congenital deficiencies affecting the late complement components (i.e., C5, C6, C7, C8, and C9) and properdin deficiency.[13] Atypical mycobacterial, *Salmonella*, or severe herpesvirus infection may suggest a defect in the interferon-γ/interleukin-12 (IFN-γ/IL-12) cytokine pathway in the form of cytokine production defects or receptor defects.[14] Patients with recessive mutations in *IL12B* or *IL12RB1* have increased susceptibility to mycobacterial disease early in life because of impairment of the IL-12–dependent production of IFN-γ. Infection with atypical mycobacteria may be seen in patients with ectodermal dysplasia who have defects in the nuclear factor-κB (NF-κB) pathway (i.e., NF-κB essential modulator [NEMO]) and natural killer (NK) cell function. Patients with X-linked lymphoproliferative disease (XLP) may develop a fulminant infectious mononucleosis after infection with Epstein-Barr virus. In cellular deficiencies with a significant NK cell defect, recurrent infections with herpesvirus occur. Patients with mutations in *UNC93B* and *TLR3* present with childhood herpes simplex virus type 1 (HSV-1) disease, most frequently encephalitis from impairment in the production of antiviral interferons in the central nervous system.[15]

TABLE 71-3 Gastrointestinal Disturbances

Disease or Disorder	Associated Pathology
Malabsorption, chronic diarrhea	
Failure to thrive	T cell or IPEX
Lactose intolerance	CVID, IgA deficiency
Celiac disease	CVID, IgA deficiency
Bacterial overgrowth in small bowel	CVID, IgA deficiency
Parasites	CVID, IgA deficiency
Inflammatory bowel disease	B cell deficiency (CVID, IgA deficiency)
Nodular lymphoid hyperplasia	B cell deficiency (CVID, IgA deficiency)
Atrophic gastritis or achlorhydria	CVID
Gastric carcinoma	CVID
Pancreatic insufficiency	Neutrophil defect

CVID, Common variable immunodeficiency; *IgA*, immunoglobulin A; *IPEX*, immune dysregulation, polyendocrinopathy, enteropathy, X-linked syndrome.

TABLE 71-4 Autoimmune Disorders

Disorders	Associated Pathology
Rheumatic disease	
Lupus erythematosus	Early complement component deficiency, CVID
Hemolytic-uremic syndrome	Factor H deficiency
Glomerulonephritis	C3 deficiency, ALPS, CVID
Autoimmune endocrinopathies	CVID, IgA deficiency, APECED, IPEX
Autoimmune neuropathies	
Guillain-Barré syndrome	ALPS
Autoimmune hematologic diseases	
Hemolytic anemia	CVID, ALPS, Wiskott-Aldrich syndrome
Thrombocytopenia	CVID, ALPS
Autoimmune neutropenia	CVID, ALPS, Wiskott-Aldrich syndrome, type 1 hyper-IgM syndrome

ALPS, Autoimmune lymphoproliferative disease; *APECED*, autoimmune polyendocrinopathy candidiasis, ectodermal dystrophy syndrome; *C3*, third component of complement; *CVID*, common variable immunodeficiency; *IPEX*, immune dysregulation, polyendocrinopathy, enteropathy, X-linked syndrome.

The warts, hypogammaglobulinemia, bacterial infections, and myelokathesis syndrome (WHIM syndrome) is an autosomal dominant disorder with mutations in the gene encoding for the chemokine receptor CXCR4.[16] Patients typically have herpes simplex or human papillomavirus (HPV)-related diseases, which manifest as treatment-refractory cutaneous warts and HPV involvement of the genital tract.[17] Patients with mutations in the dedicator of cytokinesis 8 gene (*DOCK8*) have cutaneous viral infections caused by herpes simplex, human papillomavirus, molluscum contagiosum virus, and varicella zoster virus.[18]

GASTROINTESTINAL DISTURBANCES

Many patients with primary immunodeficiency disorders have symptoms and clinical findings of the gastrointestinal tract (Table 71-3). In a survey of 248 patients with CVID, 21% had significant gastrointestinal disease.[19] Liver disease occurred in an additional 12%. Bacterial overgrowth in the small bowel, including infections with *Yersinia* and *Campylobacter*, parasitic infestations with organisms such as *Giardia lamblia*, and chronic viral enteritis caused by enteroviruses and CMV are relatively common in patients with B or T cell immune defects. Patients with the X-linked syndrome of immune dysregulation, polyendocrinopathy, and enteropathy (IPEX), a genetic defect of the Forkhead box protein 3 (FOXP3) transcription factor, which is essential for the development of regulatory T cells, often present with watery diarrhea that can lead to failure to thrive.[20]

AUTOIMMUNE DISEASE

Patients lacking one of the early complement components (e.g., C1, C2, C4) often present with a lupus-like illness[13] that has the typical features of systemic lupus erythematosus (SLE) but produces serology-negative results (i.e., anti-DNA antibodies are absent and the antinuclear antibody [ANA] is present in low titer). Significant renal disease and systemic vasculitis can occur in patients who lack an early complement component but have no other evidence of SLE or autoimmunity. Homozygous factor H deficiency may present as hemolytic uremic syndrome. Likewise, deficiencies of late complement components may occasionally be associated with vasculitis or other lupus-like illnesses. Less frequently, patients with late complement component deficiencies have developed Raynaud disease, scleroderma, or dermatomyositis. Deficiencies of the third component of complement are associated with recurrent infections and an increased incidence of lupus-like illness, including glomerulonephritis.

Immunodeficiencies of T and B cells are associated with autoimmune disease (Table 71-4). Patients with XLA have a higher occurrence of juvenile rheumatoid arthritis, sensorineural hearing loss, and a dermatomyositis-like syndrome. The latter disorder has been associated with enteroviral infections. Approximately 20% to 30% of patients with CVID have autoimmune disease. The most common autoimmune manifestations are hematologic, such as idiopathic thrombocytopenic purpura and hemolytic anemia. In one study, 11% of CVID patients had a cytopenia that developed before or concurrent with the diagnosis of CVID. Rheumatologic diseases (1% to 10%), inflammatory bowl–like disease or celiac disease (6% to 10%), or autoimmune endocrinopathies also occur in patients with CVID.[21] The elevated levels of factors important in B cell maturation and survival (i.e., BAFF and APRIL) may have some role in the development of autoimmune diseases in CVID patients.[22] Those CVID patients (7% to 10%) who have a mutation in the transmembrane activator and calcium-modulating ligand interactor gene (*TACI*) have an increased incidence of autoimmunity.[23] One half the CVID patients with granulomatous disease have had autoimmune disease and a decrease in the proportion of switched memory B cells.[24]

Organ-specific autoimmunity of the endocrine glands (i.e., parathyroid [89%], adrenal [60%], gonads [45%], pancreas, and thyroid) is seen in patients with APECED syndrome.[25]

Nonendocrine autoimmune manifestations in these patients include alopecia, pernicious anemia, chronic hepatitis, and vitiligo. This autosomal recessive disorder is associated with genetic mutations of a nuclear transcription factor that functions in the thymus to regulate central tolerance, the autoimmune regulator (*AIRE*).[26] The most common autoimmune disease in patients with IPEX syndrome is early-onset, insulin-dependent diabetes, but other autoimmune endocrinopathies or hematologic autoimmune disease can occur.[20] In patients with CD40 ligand defects (e.g., X-linked hyper-IgM syndrome) inflammatory bowel disease, seronegative arthritis, and chronic neutropenia occur. A Coombs-positive autoimmune hemolytic anemia, autoimmune neutropenia, and immune thrombocytopenia are the most common autoimmune diseases in patients with autoimmune lymphoproliferative disease (ALPS),[27] a disease characterized by massive splenomegaly and lymphadenopathy. ALPS is caused by a defect in lymphocyte apoptosis, most frequently resulting from mutations in the tumor necrosis factor (TNF) receptor gene (*TNFRSF6*), which encodes FAS (CD95).[28] Gene mutations encoding the FAS ligand and caspases 8 and 10 have also been described.[28] Autoimmune disease has been reported in 40% of patients with the Wiskott-Aldrich syndrome, who most commonly have autoimmune hemolytic anemia and thrombocytopenia.[29]

MALIGNANCIES

Individuals with certain immunodeficiency disorders are more susceptible to malignancies, especially those with abnormalities of T cell function and DNA repair.[30] In some cases, malignancy may result from abnormal or reduced clearance of viruses due to abnormalities of T cell function. XLP caused by mutations in the SRC homology 2 domain–containing gene 1A (*SH2D1A*), which encodes the signaling lymphocytic activation molecule (SLAM)-associated protein (SAP), is characterized by fulminant infectious mononucleosis, hypogammaglobulinemia, and non-Hodgkin B cell lymphoma. Patients with XLP due to a mutation in the X-linked inhibitor of apoptosis gene (*XIAP*) do not develop lymphoma. In both types of XLP, the uncontrolled expansion of Epstein-Barr virus–infected B cells, NK T cells, reactive CD8$^+$ T cells, and macrophages can lead to hemophagocytic lymphohistiocytosis (HLH). Individuals with autosomal recessive-HIES can develop malignancies such as squamous cell carcinoma, cutaneous T cell leukemia, and lymphoma during adulthood. Patients with CVID have an increased incidence of lymphoma and gastric cancer; the latter cancer may be related to *Helicobacter pylori* infection.

FAMILY HISTORY

Because many of the immunodeficiency diseases are inherited as an autosomal recessive or an X-linked disorder, obtaining a detailed family history is important (Box 71-3). Consanguinity raises the possibility of an autosomal recessive disorder. CVID and IgA deficiency are familial conditions and are often seen in a setting of other family members with autoimmune disorders. In any family in which the mother's brother died of recurrent infection in early childhood, the first serious bacterial infection in her son should alert the astute clinician to suspect an X-linked immunodeficiency in the boy.

BOX 71-3 FAMILY HISTORY

- Consanguinity of the parents
- History of a sibling dying early in life of infections
- Family history of an X-linked or autosomal recessive inheritance of a primary immunodeficiency

ADVERSE REACTIONS TO VACCINES OR TRANSFUSIONS

An adverse reaction to a vaccine or transfusion may indicate an underlying immunodeficiency. For example, paralytic polio occurs in patients with B cell deficiency and SCID who received live-attenuated oral polio vaccine. Disseminated mycobacterial disease after bacillus Calmette-Guérin vaccine immunization can be seen in interferon-γ– and IL-12–related immunodeficiencies. Anaphylaxis to a transfusion of blood and some blood products can occur in patients with IgA deficiency because of the development of IgE antibodies to IgA.

The American Academy of Pediatrics and the Advisory Committee on Immunization Practices of the Centers for Disease Control and Prevention have published recommended contraindications to vaccination in patients with primary immunodeficiency,[31] which are based on documented development of vaccine-strain disease in immunodeficient patients and on theoretical risk. The current disease-specific recommendations are summarized in Table 71-5.

Physical Examination

The physical examination may give the clinician important clues to the cause of the defect in host defense that underlies

TABLE 71-5 Vaccine Contraindications and Precautions in Patients with Primary Immunodeficiency

Vaccine Type	When to Avoid Vaccination
Live virus vaccines	T and B cell deficiency
Oral polio vaccine	
Varicella vaccine*	
MMR vaccine*	
Intranasal influenza vaccine	
Rotavirus vaccine	
Smallpox vaccine	
Yellow fever vaccine	
Herpes zoster vaccine	
Live bacterial vaccines	T and B cell deficiency, CGD, LAD, IFN-γ pathway or NEMO defects
BCG vaccine	
Oral *Salmonella typhi* vaccine	

Data from Pickering LK, Baker CJ, Kimberlin DW, Long SS, editors. Red book: 2009 report of the Committee on Infectious Diseases. 28th ed. Elk Grove Village, Ill: American Academy of Pediatrics; 2009; National Center for Immunization and Respiratory Diseases, Centers for Disease Control and Prevention (CDC). General recommendations on immunization—recommendations of the Advisory Committee on Immunization Practices (ACIP). MMWR Recomm Rep 2011;60:2.

BCG, Bacillus Calmette-Guérin vaccine; *CGD*, chronic granulomatous disease; *IFN*, interferon; *LAD*, leukocyte adhesion deficiency; *MMR*, measles, mumps, rubella; *NEMO*, nuclear factor-κB essential modulator.

*Measles and varicella vaccinations may be considered in some B cell deficiencies.

recurrent infections. Digital clubbing or a loud pulmonic heart sound with a right ventricular heave indicates pulmonary hypertension, which implies that serious pulmonary damage has occurred. The examination can reveal physical signs that reflect the patient's previous infectious history, and some severe immunodeficiency syndromes are associated with specific physical abnormalities or dysmorphisms. Table 71-6 outlines areas of the physical examination deserving special attention.

GROWTH PARAMETERS

Onset of recurrent infections during the first 6 months of life is frequently accompanied by growth failure and delayed maturation. Children with significant T cell impairment tend to grow poorly and often suffer from failure to thrive during their first years of life. Normal or near-normal height and weight do not, however, exclude the possibility of a significant defect in host defense.

DYSMORPHISMS

Developmental embryologic abnormalities of the thymus result in atresia or dysplasia, conditions that underlie a T cell immunodeficiency (e.g., DiGeorge anomaly). Developmental abnormalities often give rise to defects in other structures formed from the third and fourth branchial pouches, including the thymus and parathyroid glands, the mandible and related structures, and the great blood vessels and the heart. Neonatal tetany, congenital heart disease, and facial abnormalities, including hypoplastic mandible, high arched palate, shortened philtrum, small mouth, and low-set, posteriorly rotated ears, are frequently recognized before the immunodeficiency manifests. Conotruncal abnormalities of the heart include tetralogy of Fallot, ventricular septal defect, atrial septal defect, and pulmonic artery atresia or stenosis. The expression of DiGeorge anomaly varies, but some patients have profound T cell immunodeficiency without significant hypoparathyroidism or cardiac anomalies. Approximately 80% to 90% of the patients have a deletion at 22q11.2, whereas other patients (1% to 2%) have a deletion at chromosome 10p14. Some patients have mutations in the *TBX1* gene (22q11.21).[32]

Cartilage-hair hypoplasia is associated with defects in bone formation and immune abnormalities. Because of the physical findings of short-limbed dwarfism and abnormal hair, these children can be identified early in infancy on the basis of their appearance, before the clinical manifestation of their immune defects.

Dysmorphic features, especially of the face, can be seen in other types of immunodeficiency. Defects in NF-κB regulation (i.e., NEMO defect) are associated with ectodermal dysplasia characterized by conical teeth; fine, sparse hair; and frontal bossing.[33] Ming and Stiehm[34] have reviewed the genetic syndromic abnormalities associated with immunodeficiencies.

EVALUATION OF THE SKIN AND MUCOUS MEMBRANES

Infections of the skin and mucous membranes without sinopulmonary infections may indicate a primary immunodeficiency of the phagocytic system. For example, the congenital neutropenic disorders are characterized by a reduction in the absolute neutrophil count that enhances the susceptibility of patients to bacterial skin infections, deep tissue infections, sepsis, and fever.[35] Patients with CD40 ligand and CD40 deficiency may also have neutropenia. Patients with LAD have a leukocytosis associated with poor wound healing, skin infections, and severe periodontal disease.[36]

The skin and oral mucosa can give valuable clues to the diagnosis of the underlying disease process. For example, patients with Wiskott-Aldrich syndrome present with recurrent infections, intractable eczema, and petechiae. Candidiasis of the skin or mucous membranes may indicate T cell deficiency. Patients with ataxia-telangiectasia have recurrent infections, cerebellar ataxia, and telangiectasia of the skin, which are readily observed on physical examination. These small-vessel abnormalities over the bulbar conjunctivae, bridge of the nose, the ears, and antecubital fossae tend to occur in late childhood, usually several years after the onset of ataxia and infectious problems. A form of skin disease resembling severe atopic dermatitis is common in individuals with HIES. Additional clinical findings include craniosynostosis, coarse facies, and skeletal and dental abnormalities.[37]

Various types of rashes can be seen in patients with immunodeficiencies. Boys with XLA can develop a dermatomyositis-like rash, with livedo reticularis, muscle weakness, neurologic symptoms, and developmental failure or regression resulting from chronic infection with an enterovirus. A lupus-like malar rash with negative or low-titer ANAs may occur in deficiencies of the early components of the classic complement pathway. Erythroderma in a patient with failure to thrive, eosinophilia, hepatosplenomegaly, and recurrent infections may suggest Omenn syndrome. Silvery hair, pale skin, and photophobia are seen in children with Chédiak-Higashi syndrome.[38] Griscelli syndrome patients have characteristic clinical findings of the skin and hair, including large melanin clumps in the hair shaft and abnormal skin melanocytes.[39] A related disease, Hermansky-Pudlak syndrome, is characterized by oculocutaneous albinism, severe thrombasthenia, and immunodeficiency.[40] Candidiasis of the skin or mucous membranes may be an important indication of T cell deficiency in patients with APECED[25] or IPEX syndromes.[41]

EAR, NOSE, MOUTH, AND THROAT EVALUATION

Recurrent otitis media is a common problem in pediatrics and among persons with antibody deficiency. In studies of children with recurrent otitis media, however, this complaint has not been a reliable indicator of immunodeficiency. Increased exposure to viral and bacterial pathogens because of day care attendance or school-age siblings may contribute to the risk of recurrent otitis media (see Box 71-1).

Examination of the nose and pharynx for the clinical signs of sinusitis is important. Children and adults with antibody deficiency frequently have recurrent infections of the paranasal sinuses. However, the clinical diagnosis of sinusitis is frequently overlooked in children. Pharyngitis does not indicate underlying immune defects, but absence of tonsillar tissue is a significant physical finding, particularly in the child with recurrent upper respiratory infection, and it should raise the suspicion of Bruton disease (i.e., XLA). Chronic periodontitis is common among patients with neutrophil abnormalities. Severe gingivostomatitis, often with dental erosions, occurs in patients with LAD.[42]

TABLE 71-6 Physical Examination of Patients with Recurrent Infection

Diagnosis and Physical Findings	Associated Pathology
GROWTH FAILURE	
SCID	T/B cell combined deficiency
DYSMORPHISMS	
Micrognathia, short philtrum, ear anomalies	T cell deficiency (DiGeorge anomaly)
Short-limbed dwarfism	T cell deficiency (cartilage-hair hypoplasia)
Hypertelorism, epicanthal folds, flat nasal bridge	ICF syndrome
Ectodermal dysplasia	NEMO defect
Coarse facies	HIES
SKIN AND ORAL MUCOSA	
Rashes	
Lupus-like malar rash	Early complement pathway defect
Dermatomyositis rash	Bruton disease (XLA)
Erythroderma	Omenn syndrome
Eczema	Wiskott-Aldrich, hyper-IgE syndrome
Petechiae	Wiskott-Aldrich syndrome
Pyoderma, abscesses	Neutrophil or B cell defects
Poor wound healing	LAD
Candidiasis	T cell or T/B cell combined deficiency, APECED, IPEX, CMC
Telangiectasia	Ataxia-telangiectasia
Delayed umbilical cord separation	Neutrophil adhesion defect
Abnormal hair	Cartilage-hair hypoplasia, NEMO defect, Chediak-Higashi syndrome, Griscelli syndrome
EARS, NOSE, THROAT, AND MOUTH	
Chronic otitis media	B cell deficiency; mannose-binding lectin deficiency
Dull tympanic membranes	
Poor light reflex	
Scarring	
Perforations of the tympanic membrane	
Sinusitis	B cell deficiency
Purulent nasal discharge	
Purulent post-pharyngeal exudate	
Pharyngeal cobblestoning	
Dentition, gums	NEMO defect
Conical teeth	NEMO defect
Peridonditis	LAD, neutropenia
RESPIRATORY TRACT	
Digital clubbing	Defect in any immune component
Rales	Defect in any immune component
Wheezing	B cell (IgA) deficiency
CARDIAC SYSTEM	
Heart murmur (conotruncal abnormalities)	DiGeorge anomaly
LYMPHATIC SYSTEM	
Absent tonsils, lymph nodes	Bruton disease (XLA), T/B cell combined deficiencies
Diffuse lymphoid hyperplasia	CVID, CGD, HIV infection, ALPS, XLP
Lymphadenitis	CGD
MUSCULOSKELETAL SYSTEM	
Arthralgia, arthritis	B cell deficiency
Dermatomyositis	B cell or complement deficiency
Lupus-like syndrome	Complement (early classic pathway), CVID or IgA deficiency
Short-limb dwarfism	Cartilage-hair syndrome
Craniosynostosis	Hyper-IgE syndrome
NEUROLOGIC SYSTEM	
Ataxia	Ataxia-telangiectasia
Enteroviral meningoencephalitis	B cell deficiency (Bruton disease [XLA])
Neuropathies	Chediak-Higashi and Griscelli syndromes
Pernicious anemia	CVID

ALPS, Autoimmune lymphoproliferative disease; *APECED*, autoimmune polyendocrinopathy candidiasis, ectodermal dystrophy syndrome; *CGD*, chronic granulomatous disease; *CMC*, chronic mucocutaneous candidiasis; *CVID*, common variable immunodeficiency; *HIES*, hyperimmunoglobulin E (hyper-IgE) syndrome; *HIV*, human immunodeficiency virus; *ICF*, immunodeficiency, centromere instability, and facial anomalies; *Ig*, immunoglobulin; *LAD*, leukocyte adhesion deficiency; *NEMO*, nuclear factor-κB (NF-κB) essential modulator; *SCID*, severe combined immunodeficiency disease; *XLA*, X-linked agammaglobulinemia; *XLP*, X-linked lymphoproliferative disease.

PULMONARY EXAMINATION

Examination of the chest of the patient with recurrent infections should include careful auscultation for rales or rhonchi. Digital clubbing is an important indicator of significant lung disease, and it necessitates a thorough workup; it is rarely seen in uncomplicated asthma. In patients with chronic lung disease, especially in patients with a B cell immunodeficiency, baseline, high-resolution computed tomography (CT) of the chest is recommended. Periodic pulmonary function testing to determine the diffusing capacity of the lung for carbon monoxide (DLCO) is important even if patients are not symptomatic. The most common abnormality is obstructive changes, although restrictive changes and diminished carbon monoxide diffusion also occur, especially in patients with bronchiectasis or pulmonary granuloma.[43] In retrospective review of patients with CVID, 84% of patients had pneumonia at least once before receiving intravenous immune globulin (IVIG) therapy; after treatment over 6.6 years, the number of patients experiencing pneumonia dramatically decreased (22%).[44] However, Kainulainen and colleagues[45] reported that despite adequate immunoglobulin replacement therapy in patients with primary hypogammaglobulinemia, pulmonary disease might still develop and might be silent and progress asymptomatically. Subclinical infections can lead to ongoing pulmonary damage. In a study of patients with XLA, Quartier and coworkers reported that IVIG replacement therapy with trough levels of more than 500 mg/dL prevented severe acute bacterial pneumonia, but it did not prevent chronic lung disease. Studies by Orange and colleagues[46] and Chapel and associates[21] suggested that trough IgG levels of more than 850 mg/dL may be required to prevent chronic lung diseases. In patients with CVID or XLA, increased IVIG doses per kilogram are associated with less decline in lung function over time.[47] The serum IgG level before diagnosis may not predict an association with severe pneumonia or other severe infections,[21] and the serum IgG may not be the only important factor in the development of progressive pulmonary disease.

Lymphoid interstitial pneumonia (LIP) occurs in approximately 10% of patients with CVID. The clinical course can vary, but a progressive course can lead to lymphoma. If the disease is confirmed by high-resolution CT of the chest, a biopsy is recommended to determine lymphocyte clonality. Noncaseating granulomas occur in 10% to 18% of patients with CVID and are often mistaken for sarcoid tissue; many of these patients also have autoimmune disease.[48] Treatment of granulomatous lung disease in CVID patients include low-dose corticosteroids, cyclosporine or anti-TNF monoclonal antibodies.[49] CVID patients may develop a combination of granuloma nodules and LIP with granulomatous-lymphocytic interstitial lung disease (GLILD).[50] Wheat and colleagues[51] reported that human herpesvirus 8 infection was associated with GLILD. Patients with GLILD have a poorer prognosis, are T cell deficient, and develop B cell lymphoproliferative disease.[50] Mucosal-associated lymphoid lymphomas (MALT) have also occurred in CVID patients.

CARDIOVASCULAR EXAMINATION

The cardiovascular examination may provide an indication of DiGeorge anomaly. Conotruncal cardiac defects such as tetralogy of Fallot, micrognathia, and ear anomalies may be associated with congenital absence of the thymus and hypoparathyroidism. Physical findings of pulmonary hypertension may be observed in immunodeficient patients with chronic lung disease resulting from repeated infections.

EVALUATION OF THE LYMPHORETICULAR SYSTEM

Examination of the lymphatic system for hepatosplenomegaly and for the presence or absence of lymphoid tissue is important for a patient with suspected immunodeficiency. Patients with SCID or infantile XLA do not have palpable lymphoid tissue or visible tonsils. However, the presence of lymphoid tissue can be misleading; adult patients with CVID may have enlarged lymphoid tissue and hepatosplenomegaly. Tissue hypertrophy occurs because the reticuloendothelial system undergoes hyperplasia in the absence of opsonic antibody. Draining abscesses of the lymph nodes suggest a phagocyte defect.

Two other groups of patients present with perturbations of lymphoid proliferation. The autosomal recessive hyper-IgM syndromes caused by genetic mutations producing activation-induced cytidine deaminase (AID) deficiency and uracil-*N*-glycosylate (UNG) deficiency have profound lymphoid hyperplasia (66% of patients) with massive germinal centers, leading to prominent cervical lymphadenopathy and tonsillar hypertrophy. ALPS patients usually present before age 5 with a chronic, nonmalignant lymphadenopathy and massive splenomegaly, and they have increased circulating double-negative ($CD4^-/CD8^-$) α/β^+ receptor T cells. Patients are at significantly higher risk for lymphoma.[52]

NEUROLOGIC EXAMINATION

Abnormalities of the neuromuscular system may be the first indicator of ataxia-telangiectasia. The serum alpha fetoprotein level is elevated in these children. The onset of overt immunodeficiency varies, usually occurring after the onset of neurologic disease but occasionally preceding it.[53] Flaccid paralysis after live poliomyelitis vaccination suggests combined immunodeficiency or antibody defects. Adults with CVID occasionally develop pernicious anemia, and delayed diagnosis and prompt treatment may lead to neurologic defects. Neurologic symptoms are also seen in Chédiak-Higashi syndrome. Patients may have cognitive impairment, nystagmus, and cerebellar, spinal, and peripheral neuropathies.[38] Patients with Griscelli syndrome have clinical neurologic manifestations that include seizures, ataxia, and oculomotor and reflex abnormalities. Patients with DiGeorge anomaly have developmental issues that may manifest later as school problems.

MUSCULOSKELETAL EVALUATION

Patients with immunodeficiency may have arthritis because of joint infection or aseptic inflammation. Children with antibody deficiency and some of those with deficiencies of the complement system have an increased incidence of septic arthritis with pyogenic bacteria. Children and adults with deficiencies of the early classic complement pathway often present with arthritis, frequently in conjunction with dermal vasculitis. Patients with XLA have an increased incidence of arthritis (25% to 35%) from infection with a mycoplasmal organism (e.g., *Ureaplasma urealyticum*). Patients with XLA and other B cell abnormalities may present with dermatomyositis, arthralgia, or overt arthritis. Patients with cartilage-hair syndrome (i.e., short-limbed dwarfism with metaphyseal or spondyloepiphyseal dysplasia) and adenosine deaminase deficiency (i.e., rib-end cupping and flaring) also have skeletal abnormalities. Craniosynostosis is seen in patients with HIES.

Laboratory Tests for Screening Patients with Recurrent Infections

The history and physical examination may lead the physician evaluating a patient with recurrent infection in an appropriate direction to identify which of the recognized abnormalities in immune function best fits the findings and to confirm the diagnosis with pertinent laboratory studies. The Joint Task Force of the American Academy of Allergy, Asthma, and Immunology (AAAAI) and American College of Allergy, Asthma, and Immunology (ACAAI) developed the practice parameters for the diagnosis and management of primary immunodeficiency disorders. These criteria were established to help physicians formulate a diagnosis using simple, objective guidelines and definitions. Several lay organizations, including the Jeffrey Modell Foundation (http://www.geneticalliance.org/organization/jeffrey-modell-foundation) and the Immune Deficiency Foundation (http://www.primaryimmune.org), have raised public awareness about primary immunodeficiencies. Application of basic screening tests enables the clinician to determine the need for more detailed laboratory testing and referral to a clinical immunologist. Reports in the early 1980s indicated that there was an appreciable delay (about 10 years) between the onset of recurrent infections and recognition of an immunodeficiency. When this problem was reexamined for patients with CVID, an improvement was observed, but there was still a delay in diagnosis of 4 to 6 years.[19]

EVALUATION OF INNATE IMMUNE DISORDERS

Box 71-4 shows the screening tests for the disorders of the innate immune system. The white blood cell count and differential count are used to calculate the absolute neutrophil count to exclude neutropenia, and the peripheral blood smear is used to evaluate leukocyte morphology. For example, in Chédiak-Higashi syndrome, the leukocytes have very large granules. Evaluation of the complement system is most easily accomplished by obtaining a total hemolytic complement (CH_{50}) assay.[13] In patients with congenital complement deficiency, the CH_{50} is not measurable. If a deficiency of early components of the alternative pathway is suspected, an alternative pathway CH_{50} (AP_{50}) assay using rabbit erythrocytes is required. A C3 or C4 assessment is most useful for evaluating patients with vasculitis or complement consumption caused by immune complex diseases such as SLE. A nitroblue tetrazolium test or dihydrorhodamine assay by flow cytometry is useful for screening defects of neutrophil oxidative metabolism such as chronic granulomatous disease. Assays for chemotactic defects or for opsonic or phagocytic disorders require specialized laboratories. In the patient with delayed separation of the umbilical cord, infections with poor localization of leukocytes at infected foci, or poor wound healing, flow cytometry using monoclonal antibodies to evaluate expression of CD11/CD18 and CD15a (i.e., selectin ligand sialyl-Lewis X [sLe^x]), the leukocyte adhesion glycoprotein on the cell surface of monocytes, is diagnostic. Several research laboratories assay for Toll-like receptor (TLR) function and their signaling pathway components, an approach that has led to the description of novel innate immune defects.[8,15,18,54]

BOX 71-4 SCREENING TESTS FOR INNATE DEFENSE FACTORS

SCREENING TESTS

- Absolute granulocyte count, cell morphology
- Serum total hemolytic complement (CH_{50}), alternative pathway hemolytic activity (AP_{50})
- Nitroblue tetrazolium (NBT) test or flow cytometry using dihydrorhodamine dye test
- Flow cytometry for leukocyte adhesion molecules (CD11/CD18 and CD15a)

ADVANCED TESTING

- Phagocytic assays
- Chemotaxis assays
- Analysis of Toll-like receptor pathways
- Molecular analysis for specific defects

EVALUATION OF T CELL IMMUNITY

The evaluation of patients with suspected T cell immunodeficiency is outlined in Box 71-5. The finding of a total lymphocyte count below 1500/mm^3 in an adult or below 4000/mm^3 in an infant should raise the suspicion of T cell immunodeficiency. Delayed-type hypersensitivity skin testing may be used for screening cellular immunity, but standardized reagents are not available. In vitro analysis of lymphocyte subsets using flow cytometry testing can be helpful. A fluorescent in situ hybridization (FISH) assay for chromosomal abnormalities such as deletions at 22q11.2 is helpful in patients with possible DiGeorge anomaly. Chromosome analysis is used to diagnose the syndrome of immunodeficiency, centromere instability, and facial anomalies (ICF). Alpha fetoprotein levels are raised in patients with ataxia-telangiectasia. Patients with Wiskott-Aldrich syndrome have thrombocytopenia and small platelets. Additional

BOX 71-5 SCREENING TESTS FOR T CELL IMMUNITY

SCREENING TESTS

- Newborn screening for TREC analysis (not available in all states)
- Absolute lymphocyte count
- Chest radiograph for thymus shadow in newborns
- Delayed skin hypersensitivity to recall antigens
- Quantification of T cell subsets

ADVANCED TESTING

- Lymphocyte proliferative responses to mitogens, antigens, and allogeneic cells in MLC
- Lymphocyte-mediated cytotoxicity: NK and ADCC activity
- Production of cytokines
- Functional response to cytokines
- Signal transduction studies
- Molecular analysis for specific defects

ADCC, Antibody-dependent cellular cytotoxicity; *MLC*, mixed lymphocyte culture; *NK*, natural killer; *TREC*, T cell receptor excision circles.

BOX 71-6 SCREENING TESTS FOR B CELL IMMUNE FUNCTION

SCREENING TESTS

- Quantitative serum immunoglobulins
- Specific antibodies to vaccine responses
  - Tetanus, diphtheria (IgG1)
  - Pneumococcal and meningococcal polysaccharides (IgG2)
  - Viral respiratory pathogens (IgG1 and IgG3)
  - Other vaccines: hepatitis B, influenza, MMR, polio (killed vaccine)
- Isohemagglutinins (IgM antibodies to A and B blood group antigens)
- B cell quantitation by flow cytometry

ADVANCED TESTING

- In vitro B cell immunoglobulin production
- Regulation of immunoglobulin synthesis
- CD40 ligand-CD40 interactions
- B-cell subsets: non-switched and switched memory B cells
- Molecular analysis for gene deletions or mutations

IgG, Immunoglobulin G; *MMR*, measles, mumps, rubella vaccine.

testing of T cell function may be required, including in vitro lymphocyte proliferation assays for mitogens such as phytohemagglutinin and concanavalin A, antigens such as tetanus or *Candida* proteins, or allogeneic cells in mixed lymphocyte culture. More advanced analysis for NK cell function, cytokine production, or signaling pathways may be needed. Identification of genetic mutations for many immunodeficiency disorders can be extremely helpful in making the diagnosis.[55]

EVALUATION FOR B CELL IMMUNODEFICIENCY

Box 71-6 outlines an approach to the evaluation of patients with suspected B cell deficiency. Serum immunoglobulin concentrations should be measured by quantitative techniques (e.g., nephelometry). Values for children must be compared with normal-for-age laboratory values. Immunoelectrophoresis (IEP) is semiquantitative and should not be used to evaluate a patient with suspected antibody deficiency. IEP should be used only to examine serum for paraproteins, such as those found in Waldenström macroglobulinemia or multiple myeloma. IgG subclass quantitation may be helpful, although there is continuing debate about the utility of these measurements. To determine the clinical significance of an IgG subclass deficiency, the physician also need to obtain a detailed history, perform a complete physical examination, and measure functional or specific antibodies.[56]

Patients may have normal total values of serum immunoglobulins and IgG subclasses but fail to make specific antibodies to bacterial or common viral pathogens. The assessment of specific antibody formation after vaccine administration is therefore an important part of the laboratory evaluation of patients with suspected B cell deficiency. Isohemagglutinins are naturally occurring IgM antibodies to ABO blood group substances. By 1 year of age, 70% of infants have positive isohemagglutinin titers, depending on their blood type. Responses to protein antigens usually fall in the IgG1 subclass, whereas the immune response to the polysaccharide antigens resides within the IgG2 subclass. With the conjugated vaccines for *H. influenzae* type b and pneumococcal polysaccharides, antibody responses occur primarily in the IgG1 rather than IgG2 subclass. These conjugate vaccines therefore may not be helpful in the functional evaluation of an IgG2 subclass deficiency or a selective polysaccharide antibody deficiency. Fortunately, the vaccine for pneumococcal polysaccharide antigens is still available for evaluating patients for a selective or antigen-specific antibody deficiency. The response to killed influenza vaccine can also help these determinations.

Because many of these patients have recurrent upper respiratory tract infections, their serum can be tested for the presence of antibodies to common respiratory viral agents such as influenza A and B, mycoplasma, respiratory syncytial virus, adenovirus, and the parainfluenza viruses. These antibodies fall into the IgG1 and IgG3 subclasses. Molecular analysis for genetic abnormalities, especially those that involve the early stages of B cell maturation in patients who present without B cells (e.g., XLA), can aid diagnostic evaluations.[55]

Conclusions

The immune evaluation of patients with recurrent infections requires a medical history, physical examination, and appropriate tests for screening immune function. Although discussed as separate entities, the complement, phagocytic, and T cell and B cell immune systems all work in concert to achieve their common goal, the protection of the host from antigenic substances and microorganisms. As Dr. Robert A. Good pointed out, these experiments of nature have opened doors to a greater understanding of the pathophysiology of the immune system: "The road to progress in clinical medicine is a two-way street, with traffic from [the] laboratory bench to bedside and [back from the] bedside to [the] laboratory bench being of greatest significance." From these doors will emerge new concepts of other diseases affecting other organ systems and new approaches in the therapy of a wide range of clinical disorders in humans.

Acknowledgments

The authors wish to acknowledge the secretarial assistance of Michele Bauer.

REFERENCES

Introduction

1. Bonilla FA, Bernstein IL, Khan DA, et al. Practice parameter for the diagnosis and management of primary immunodeficiency. Ann Allergy Asthma Immunol 2005;94(Suppl. 1):S1-63.
2. Stiehm ER, Ochs HD, Winkelstein JA, editors. Immunologic disorders in infants and children. 5th ed. Philadelphia: WB Saunders; 2004. p. 292-296.
3. Jongco AM, Isabelle J, Vogel G, et al. Newborn screening for severe combined immunodeficiency in New York State. J Clin Immunol 2011;31(Suppl. 1):S2.
4. Al-Herz W, Bousfiha A, Casanova J-L, et al. Primary immunodeficiency diseases: an update on the classification from the International Union of Immunological Societies Expert Committee for Primary Immunodeficiency. Frontiers in Immunology 2011;2:54-86.

The Medical History in Immunodeficiency

5. Ferrari S, Plebani A. Cross-talk between CD40 and CD40L: lessons from primary immune deficiencies. Curr Opin Allergy Clin Immunol 2002;2:489-94.
6. Milner J, Brenchley JM, Lawrence A, et al. Impaired Th17 cell differentiation in subjects with autosomal dominant hyper IgE syndrome. Nature 2008;452:773-6.

7. Puel A, Döffinger R, Natividad A, et al. Autoantibodies against IL-17A, IL-17F, and IL-22 in patients with chronic mucocutaneous candidiasis and autoimmune polyendocrine syndrome type I. J Exp Med 2010;207:291-7.
8. Ferwerda B, Ferwerda G, Plantinga TS, et al. Human dectin-1 deficiency and mucocutaneous fungal infections. N Engl J Med 2009;361:1760-7.
9. Palm NW, Medzhitov R. Antifungal defence turns 17. Nat Immunol 2007;8:549-51.
10. Puel A, Cyppowyj A, Bustamante J, et al. Chronic mucocutaneous candidiasis in humans with inborn errors of interleukin-17 immunity. Science 2011;332:65-8.
11. Von Bernuth H, Picard C, Jin Z, et al. Pyogenic bacterial infections in humans with MyD88 deficiency. Science 2008;321:691-6.
12. Segal BH, Leto TL, Gallin JI, Malech HL, Holland SM. Genetic, biochemical, and clinical features of chronic granulomatous disease. Medicine (Baltimore) 2000;79:170-200.
13. Wen L, Atkinson JP, Giclas PC. Clinical and laboratory evaluation of complement deficiency. J Allergy Clin Immunol 2004;113:585-93.
14. Dupuis S, Doffinger R, Picard C, et al. Human interferon-gamma-mediated immunity is a genetically controlled continuous trait that determines the outcome of mycobacterial invasion. Immunol Rev 2000;178:129-37.
15. Zhang SY, Jouanguy E, Ugolini S, et al. TLR3 deficiency in patients with herpes simplex encephalitis. Science 2007;317:1522-7.
16. Hernandez PA, Gorlin RJ, Lukens JN, et al. Mutations in the chemokine receptor gene CXCR4 are associated with WHIM syndrome, a combined immunodeficiency disease. Nat Genet 2003;34:70-4.
17. Gorlin RJ, Gelb B, Diaz GA, et al. WHIM syndrome, an autosomal dominant disorder: clinical haematological and molecular studies. Am J Med Genet 2000;91:368-76.
18. Zhang Q, Davis J, Lamborn IT, et al. Combined immunodeficiency associated with DOCK8 mutations. N Engl J Med 2009;361:2046-55.
19. Cunningham-Rundles C, Bodian C. Common variable immunodeficiency: clinical and immunological features of 248 patients. Clin Immunol 1999;92:34-48.
20. Levy-Lahad E, Wildin RS. Neonatal diabetes mellitus, enteropathy, thrombocytopenia, and endocrinopathy: further evidence for an X-linked lethal syndrome. J Pediatr 2001;138:577-80.
21. Chapel H, Lucas M, Lee M, et al. Common variable immunodeficiency disorders: division into distinct clinical phenotypes. Blood 2008;112:277-86.
22. Knight AK, Radigan L, Marron T, et al. High serum levels of BAFF, APRIL, and TACI in common variable immunodeficiency. Clin Immunol 2007;124:182-9.
23. Zhang L, Radigan L, Satzer U, et al. Transmembrane activator and calcium-modulating cyclophilin ligand interactor mutations in common variable immunodeficiency: clinical and immunologic outcomes in heterozygotes. J Allergy Clin Immunol 2007;120:1178-85.
24. Wehr C, Kivioja T, Schmitt C, et al. The EUROclass trials: defining subgroups in common variable immunodeficiency. Blood 2008;111:77-85.
25. Lilac D. New perspectives on the immunology of chronic mucocutaneous candidiasis. Curr Opin Infect Dis 2002;15:143-7.
26. Su MA, Anderson MS. AIRE: an update. Curr Opin Immunol 2004;16:746-52.
27. Sneller MC, Wang J, Dale JK, et al. Clinical, immunologic and genetic features of an autoimmune lymphoproliferative syndrome associated with abnormal lymphocyte apoptosis. Blood 1997;89:1341-8.
28. Bleesing JJH, Straus SE, Fleisher TA. Autoimmune lymphoproliferative syndrome: a human disorder of abnormal lymphocyte survival. Pediatr Clin North Am 2000;47:1291-310.
29. Sullivan KE, Mullen CA, Blaese RM, Winkelstein JA. A multi-institutional survey of the Wiskott-Aldrich syndrome. J Pediatr 1994;125:876-85.
30. Rezaei N, Hedayat M, Aghamohammadi A, Nichols KE. Primary immunodeficiency diseases associated with increased susceptibility to viral infections and malignancies. J Allergy Clin Immunol 2011;127:1329-41.
31. Kroger AT, Sumaya CV, Pickering LK, Atkinson WL. General recommendations on immunization: recommendations of the Advisory Committee on Immunization Practices (ACIP). MMWR Morb Mortal Wkly Rep 2011;60:1-64.

Physical Examination

32. Yagi H, Furutani Y, Hamada H, et al. Role of TBX1 in human del22q11.2 syndrome. Lancet 2003;362:1366-73.
33. Wisniewski SA, Kobielak A, Trzeciak WH, Kobielak K. Recent advances in understanding of the molecular basis of anhidrotic ectodermal dysplasia: discovery of a ligand, ectodysplasin A and its two receptors. J Appl Genet 2002;43:97-107.
34. Ming JE, Stiehm ER. Genetic syndromic immunodeficiencies with antibody defects. Immunol Allergy Clin North Am 2008;28:715-36.
35. Badolato R, Fontana S, Notarangelo LD, Savoldi G. Congenital neutropenia: advances in diagnosis and treatment. Curr Opin Allergy Clin Immunol 2004;4:513-21.
36. Rosenzweig SD, Holland SM. Phagocyte immunodeficiencies and their infections. J Allergy Clin Immunol 2004;113:620-6.
37. Grimbacher B, Holland SM, Gallin JI, et al. Hyper-IgE syndrome with recurrent infections: an autosomal dominant multisystem disorder. N Engl J Med 1999;340:692-702.
38. Introne W, Boissy RE, Gahl WA. Clinical, molecular, and cell biological aspects of Chediak-Higashi syndrome. Mol Genet Metab 1999;68:283-303.
39. Sanal O, Ersoy F, Tezcan I, et al. Griscelli disease: genotype-phenotype correlation in an array of clinical heterogeneity. J Clin Immunol 2002;22:237-43.
40. Clark R, Griffiths GM. Lytic granules, secretory lysosomes and disease. Curr Opin Immunol 2003;15:516-21.
41. Torgerson TR, Oats HD. Immune dysregulation, polyendocrinopathy, enteropathy, X-linked syndrome: a model of immune dysregulation. Curr Opin Allergy Clin Immunol 2002;2:481-7.
42. Etzion IA, Tonetti M. Leukocyte adhesion deficiency II: from A to almost Z. Immunol Rev 2000;178:138-47.
43. Touw CML, van de Ven AA, de Jong PA, et al. Detection of pulmonary complications in common variable immunodeficiency. Pediatr Allergy Immunol 2010;21:793-805.
44. Busse PJ, Razvi S, Cunningham-Rundles C. Efficacy of intravenous immunoglobulin in the prevention of pneumonia in patients with common variable immunodeficiency. J Allergy Clin Immunol 2002;109:1001-4.
45. Kainulainen L, Varpula M, Liippo K, et al. Pulmonary abnormalities in patients with primary hypogammaglobulinemia. J Allergy Clin Immunol 1999;104:1031-6.
46. Orange JS, Grossman WJ, Navickis RJ, Wilkes MM. Impact of trough IgG on pneumonia incidence in primary immunodeficiency: a meta-analysis of clinical studies. Clin Immunol 2010;137:21-30.
47. Chen Y, Stirling RG, Paul E, et al. Longitudinal decline in lung function in patients with primary immunoglobulin deficiencies. J Allergy Clin Immunol 2011;127:1414-7.
48. Mechanic LJ, Dikman S, Cunningham-Rundles C. Granulomatous disease in common variable immunodeficiency. Ann Intern Med 1997;127:613-7.
49. Thatayatikom A, Thatayatikom S, White AJ. Infliximab treatment for severe granulomatous disease in common variable immunodeficiency: a case report and review of the literature. Ann Allergy Asthma Immunol 2005;95:293-300.
50. Bates CA, Ellison MC, Lynch DA, et al. Granulomatous-lymphocytic lung disease shortens survival in common variable immunodeficiency. J Allergy Clin Immunol 2004;114:415-21.
51. Wheat WH, Cool CD, Morimoto Y, et al. Possible role of human herpesvirus 8 in the lymphoproliferative disorders in common variable immunodeficiency. J Exp Med 2005;202:479-84.
52. Straus SE, Jaffe ES, Puck JM, et al. The development of lymphomas in families with autoimmune lymphoproliferative syndrome with germline Fas mutations and defective lymphocyte apoptosis. Blood 2001;98:194-200.
53. Nowak-Wegrzyn A, Crawford TO, Winkelstein JA, et al. Immunodeficiency and infections in ataxia-telangiectasia. J Pediatr 2004;144:505-11.

Laboratory Tests for Screening Patients with Recurrent Infections

54. Picard C, Puel A, Bonnet M, et al. Pyogenic bacterial infections in hymans with IRAK-4 deficiency. Science 2003;299:2076-9.
55. Lehman HK, Hernandez-Trujillo VP, Ballow M. The use of commercially available genetic tests in immunodeficiency disorders. Ann Allergy Asthma Immunol 2008;101:212-8.
56. Ballow M. Primary immunodeficiency disorders: Antibody deficiency. J Allergy Clin Immunol 2002;109:581-91.

72 Primary Immunodeficiency Diseases

REBECCA H. BUCKLEY | JORDAN S. ORANGE

CONTENTS

SUMMARY OF IMPORTANT CONCEPTS

- More than 180 genetically determined immunodeficiency diseases have been recognized, and the molecular basis is known for more than 80% of them.
- Patients with primary immunodeficiency diseases usually look overtly normal, with rare exceptions. They typically are identified as immunodeficient only when they present with opportunistic or recurrent infections, and often not even then. Until 2010, no screening was available for any of these conditions at any time during life anywhere in the world. Since 2010, newborn screening for severe combined immunodeficiency (SCID) has been approved by the U.S. Department of Health and Human Services and implemented in a number of states. The allergist-immunologist will play an important role in the evaluation of infants identified by this screening.
- The allergist-immunologist should not hesitate to test for these conditions if such testing is indicated as part of a general workup. Screening tests are not expensive. Early recognition is key to optimal therapy.
- Once immunocompromise or a specific immunodeficiency disease is recognized to be part of the clinical picture, investigation using all of the currently available and evolving immunologic and molecular methods is indicated, to fully define the underlying defect and to enable selection of the most effective therapy.
- The allergist-immunologist should endeavor to determine the underlying molecular defect in patients with these conditions, in order to provide appropriate genetic counseling to them and their families.

Introduction

Approaches for diagnosing and treating primary immunodeficiency diseases change frequently, because new conditions are recognized at a rapidly increasing rate. Immunodeficiency disorders can manifest as presumed allergic disorders accompanied by repeated infections. It is important that allergy and immunology specialists be current on the expanding knowledge about these diseases, because patients with such conditions frequently are referred to them by primary care physicians. Correct and prompt diagnosis is important for appropriate and timely treatment.[1] The allergist-immunologist often also serves as a genetic counselor for patients with a primary immunodeficiency disorder and their family members.

Since Bruton discovered agammaglobulinemia in 1952,[2] more than 180 other primary immunodeficiency syndromes have been described.[3] These disorders may involve one or more components of the immune system, including T, B, and natural killer (NK) lymphocytes; phagocytic cells; and complement proteins. Most defects stem from recessive mutations in genes on either the X chromosome or autosomal chromosomes (Table 72-1). Mutations in more than 200 individual genes have been identified as resulting in primary immunodeficiency diseases. The conditions discussed in this chapter do not include all of the known primary immunodeficiency syndromes; the ones selected were chosen because of new information about them, their relative importance, or their connections to allergic diseases. For a more comprehensive listing, readers are referred to specific print[3] and online resources, including the Resource of Asian Primary Immunodeficiency Diseases (RAPID) and the Immunodeficiency Resource (IDR) (available at http://rapid.rcai.riken.jp/RAPID/browseByPIDGenes and http://bioinf.uta.fi/idr/index.shtml, respectively).

Immunodeficiency diseases are characterized by unusual susceptibility to infection, but they also may have associated autoimmune or allergic manifestations. Knowledge of the particular infectious agents involved and the anatomic sites most often affected in a given patient can provide clues to the most likely type of defect. Patients with B cell, phagocytic cell, or complement defects have recurrent infections with encapsulated bacterial pathogens. By contrast, patients with T cell defects have problems with common and opportunistic infections with viral and fungal agents. In these children, failure to thrive also becomes evident shortly after these problems develop. Excessive use of antibiotics has altered the textbook presentation of many of these conditions; consequently, patients often go undiagnosed until they become seriously ill. Because antibiotics can mask infection susceptibility, allergic or autoimmune problems may be the presenting illnesses.[4] Some immunodeficiency diseases are accompanied by excessive production of immunoglobulin E (IgE) antibodies or of autoantibodies. Malignancy also is increased in patients with primary immunodeficiency, particularly in conditions involving deficiencies of B or T cell function.[5]

The true incidence and prevalence of genetically determined immunodeficiencies diseases are unknown, because until recently, screening for any of these disorders at birth or during infancy, childhood, or adulthood did not occur anywhere in the

TABLE 72-1 Locations of Faulty Genes in Primary Immunodeficiency Diseases

Chromosomal Locus	Disease
1q21	MCH class II antigen deficiency caused by RFX5 mutation*
1q22-q25	SCID due to CD3 ζ chain deficiency*
1q23	ALPS type 1b caused by deficiency of Fas ligand (CD178)*
1q25	Chronic granulomatous disease (CGD) caused by gp67^{phox} deficiency*
1q31-q32	SCID due to CD45 deficiency*
1q42-q43	Chédiak-Higashi syndrome*
2p11	κ Chain deficiency*
2p12	CD8 deficiency due to CD8 antigen α polypeptide deficiency*
2q12	CD8^{+} lymphocytopenia caused by ZAP-70 deficiency*
2q33	Autosomal recessive CVID due to ICOS deficiency*
2q33-q34	ALPS types IIa and IIb caused by deficiencies of caspase 10 or 8*
2q35	CID with microcephaly due to Cernunnos deficiency*
5p13	SCID or Omenn syndrome due to IL-7 receptor α chain deficiency*
5q31.1-q33.1	IL-12 p40 deficiency*
6p21.3	MHC class I antigen defects caused by TAP 1, TAP 2, or Tapasin deficiencies*
6p21.3	(?)Common variable immunodeficiency and selective IgA deficiency
6q23-q24	IFN-γ receptor 1 deficiency due to α chain deficiency*
7q11.23	CGD caused by gp47^{phox} deficiency*
8q21	Nijmegen breakage syndrome due to mutations in *Nibrin**
9p13	Cartilage-hair hypoplasia due to deficiency of RNA component of mitochondrial RNA-processing endoribonuclease*
10p13	SCID (Athabascan, radiation-sensitive) due to mutations in the *Artemis* gene*
10p13	DiGeorge syndrome/velocardiofacial syndrome
10q23.2-q23.33	Agammaglobulinemia due to BLNK deficiency*
10q23-q24	ALPS type 1a due to CD95 (Fas) deficiency*
11p13	IL-2 receptor α chain deficiency*
11p13	SCID or Omenn syndrome caused by RAG-1 or RAG-2 deficiencies*
11q14.3-q21	LAD-2 due to deficiency of sialyl Lewis X
11q22.3	Ataxia-telangiectasia (AT), attributable to *AT* mutation, causing deficiency of DNA-dependent kinase*
11q23	SCID or non-SCID due toCD3 γ, δ, or ε chain deficiencies*
12	Hyper-IgM syndrome cause by deficiency of uracil-DNA glycosylase*
12p13	Hyper-IgM caused by deficiency of activation-induced cytidine deaminase (AICDA)*
12q12	IRAK4 deficiency*
13q	MHC class II antigen deficiency caused by RFXAP deficiency*
13q33-q34	Ligase 4 deficiency
14q13.1	Purine nucleoside phosphorylase (PNP) deficiency*
14q32.3	Immunoglobulin heavy-chain deletion*
15q21	Griscelli syndrome due to myosin VA or Rab27a deficiencies*
16p11.2	CVID due to CD19 deficiency*
16p13	MHC class II antigen deficiency caused by CIITA deficiency*
17p11.2	CVID or IgA deficiency due to TACI deficiency*
16q24	CGD caused by gp22^{phox} deficiency*
17q11-q12	Human nude defect due to FOXN1 deficiency*
19p12	MHC class II antigen deficiency caused by RFXANK deficiency*
19p13.1	IL-12 receptor β chain deficiency*
19p13.1	SCID caused by Janus kinase 3 (Jak3) deficiency*
19p13.2	Agammaglobulinemia caused by mutations in Igα gene*
20q12-q13.2	Hyper-IgM syndrome due to CD40 deficiency
20q13.2-q13.11	SCID caused by adenosine deaminase (ADA) deficiency*
21q22.1-q22.2	IFN-γ receptor 2 deficiency due to β chain deficiency*
21q22.3	APCED due to AIRE deficiency*

Continued

TABLE 72-1 Locations of Faulty Genes in Primary Immunodeficiency Diseases—cont'd

Chromosomal Locus	Disease
21q22.3	Leukocyte adhesion deficiency type 1 (LAD-1), caused by CD18 deficiency*
22q11.2	Agammaglobulinemia caused by mutations in λ5 surrogate light chain gene*
22q11.2	DiGeorge/velocardiofacial syndrome
22q13.1-q13.3	CVID due to BAFF-R deficiency
Xp21.1	CGD caused by gp91^{phox} deficiency*
Xp11.22	Wiskott-Aldrich syndrome, caused by Wiskott-Aldrich syndrome protein (WASp) deficiency*
Xp11.23	IPEX due to Foxp3 deficiency*
Xp11.3-p21.1	Properdin deficiency*
Xq13.1-q13.3	X-linked SCID caused by common γ chain (γc) deficiency*
Xq22	X-linked agammaglobulinemia, caused by Bruton tyrosine kinase (Btk) deficiency*
Xq25-26	X-linked lymphoproliferative syndrome, caused by mutations in the *SH2D1A* gene*
Xq26	Immunodeficiency with hyper-IgM caused by CD154 (CD40 ligand) deficiency*
Xq26	Hypogammaglobulinemia with growth hormone deficiency due to mutation of ELF-4 (ETS-related transcription factor 4)
Xq28	Anhidrotic ectodermal dysplasia with immunodeficiency caused by mutations in the nuclear factor-κB essential modulator (NEMO)*

AIRE, Autoimmune regulator; *ALPS*, autoimmune lymphoproliferative syndrome; *APCED*, autoimmune polyendocrinopathy–candidiasis–ectodermal dystrophy; *BLNK*, B cell linker adaptor protein; *CGD*, chronic granulomatous disease; *CVID*, common variable immunodeficiency; *ICOS*, inducible [T cell] costimulator; *IFN*, interferon; *IgA*, *IgM*, immunoglobulins A, M; *IL*, interleukin; *MHC*, major histocompatibility complex; *SCID*, severe combined immunodeficiency; *TACI*, transmembrane activator, calcium modulator, and cyclophilin ligand interactor.
*Gene cloned and sequenced; gene product known.

world. B cell defects appear to outnumber those affecting T cells, phagocytic cells, or complement proteins.[3] Selective IgA deficiency is the most common, with reported incidence rates ranging from 1 in 333 to 1 in 700. Primary immunodeficiency is diagnosed more often in childhood, when it occurs predominantly in males, than in adult life, when it occurs slightly more often in females.

Until 1993, insight into the fundamental problems underlying a majority of these conditions was largely lacking. Such defects have mostly now been mapped to specific chromosomal locations, and the fundamental biologic errors have been identified in more than 150 conditions. In 2011, a committee of the World Health Organization (WHO) published an updated classification of primary immunodeficiency diseases.[3] Table 72-1 lists numerous conditions for which the molecular basis is already known. Discovery of mutated genes that cause primary immunodeficiencies has significantly advanced the current understanding of the pathogenesis of these diseases and of the functions of normal gene products. Seemingly identical clinical conditions, however, are caused by mutations in different immune system genes, which means that certain conditions formerly considered to represent single diseases are now considered specific syndromes. Severe combined immunodeficiency (SCID) is now known to be caused by mutations in at least 13 different genes. Hyper-IgM syndrome can result from mutations in any of 6 different genes. Omenn syndrome can be caused by mutations in at least 3 different genes. Common variable immunodeficiency (CVID) can be caused by mutations in any of at least 10 different genes, although the molecular basis for CVID in more than 90% of the patients is unknown and is likely to be diverse.[6] To make matters even more complicated, the phenotypic presentation of mutations in a single gene can differ within the same family, as dictated by the mutation's location and type of mutation, as well as other genetic factors and environmental influences (Table 72-2).[7]

Antibody Deficiency Syndromes

Antibody deficiencies are more common than defects affecting cellular functions or the complement proteins.

X-LINKED AGAMMAGLOBULINEMIA

Discovered by Colonel Ogden Bruton in 1952, X-linked agammaglobulinemia (XLA) was the first recognized human host defect involving the immune system.[2]

Epidemiology. The incidence and prevalence of XLA are unknown because general population screening for the disorder is not done. XLA may be present even when the family history is negative, because one third of X-linked mutations are new mutations in the patient.

Pathogenesis and Etiology. In 1993, two groups of investigators independently and almost simultaneously discovered the mutated gene in XLA.[3,6,7] The intracellular signaling tyrosine kinase was named "Bruton tyrosine kinase" (Btk) in honor of Dr. Bruton. Btk is a member of the tec family of cytoplasmic tyrosine kinases, which includes Lck, Fyn, and Lyn, and is found in many types of hematopoietic cells.[8,9] Btk is expressed at high levels in all B lineage cells, including pre-B cells. It has not been detected in any cells of T lineage but has been found in cells of the myeloid series.[9] Thus far, all males with known XLA (by family history) have had low or undetectable Btk mRNA and kinase activity (Fig. 72-1). Many different mutations of the human *Btk* gene (more than 550) have been described, and the mutations encompass most parts of the coding portions of the gene, but no clear correlation has been found between mutation location and clinical phenotype. Female carriers of XLA can be identified by the presence of either nonrandom X chromosome inactivation in their B cells or the mutated gene

TABLE 72-2 **Mutated Immune System Genes with Variable Phenotypic Expression***

Mutated Gene	Normal Gene Product	Classic Syndrome	Variant Syndrome(s)
RAG1	Recombinase-activating gene product 1 (RAG-1)	SCID	1. Omenn syndrome 2. Oligoclonal γ/δ T cells, autoimmune disease, and CMV infection
BTK	Bruton tyrosine kinase	Agammaglobulinemia	Polysaccharide antibody deficiency
WASP	Wiskott-Aldrich syndrome protein (WASp)	Wiskott-Aldrich syndrome	X-linked thrombocytopenia
SH2D1A	Slam-associated protein (SAP)	Fatal infectious mononucleosis	1. Common variable immunodeficiency 2. Hemophagocytic lymphohistiocytosis
CD3E	CD3ε chain	SCID	Moderate susceptibility to infection
IL2RG	IL-2 receptor γ (common γ chain [γc])	SCID	Moderate combined immunodeficiency*
ADA	Adenosine deaminase	SCID	Moderate combined immunodeficiency
JAK3	Jak3	SCID	Moderate combined immunodeficiency

From Buckley RH. Variable phenotypic expression of mutations in genes of the immune system. J Clin Invest 2005;115:2974-6.

CMV, Cytomegalovirus; *Jak3,* Janus kinase 3; *NEMO,* nuclear factor-κB essential modulator; *SCID,* severe combined immunodeficiency.

*Data from Hanson EP, Monaco-Shawver L, Solt LA, et al. Hypomorphic NEMO mutation database and reconstitution system identifies phenotypic and immunologic diversity. J Allergy Clin Immunol 2008;112:1169-77.

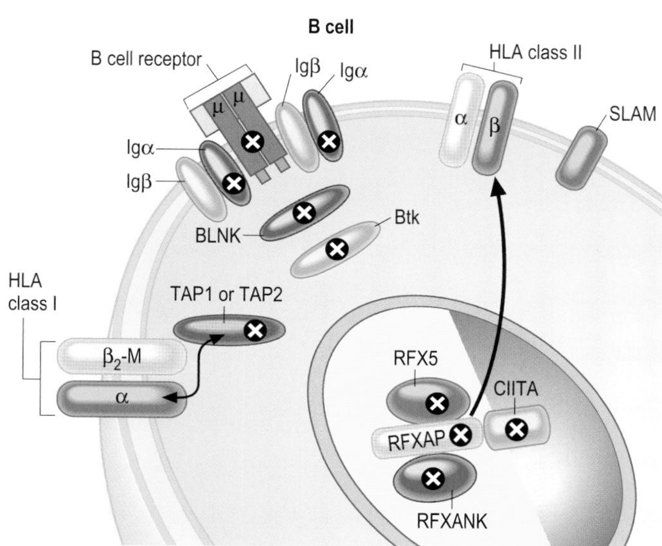

Figure 72-1 Locations of mutant proteins in B cells and activated CD4+ T cells identified in primary immunodeficiency diseases. Each mutant protein is identified by a white **x**. *BLNK,* B cell linker adaptor protein; *Btk,* Bruton tyrosine kinase; *HLA,* human leukocyte antigen; Igα, Igβ, immunoglobulins α and β [signaling molecules]; *$β_2M$,* $β_2$-microglobulin; *SLAM,* signaling lymphocyte activation molecule; *TAP1, TAP2,* transporter of processed antigen types 1 and 2. *RFX5, RXANK, RFXAP,* and *CIITA* are transcription factors. *(From Buckley RH. Primary immunodeficiency diseases due to defects in lymphocytes. N Engl J Med 2000;343:1317.)*

(if known in the family).[10] Prenatal diagnosis of affected or nonaffected male fetuses also has been accomplished by detection of the mutated gene in chorionic villus or amniocentesis samples. Btk also is expressed in cells of myeloid lineage, and in boys with XLA, intermittent neutropenia can occur, particularly at onset of an acute infection. It is conceivable that Btk is one of several signaling molecules participating in myeloid maturation and that neutropenia would be observed in XLA only when rapid production of myeloid cells is needed. XLA has been reported in association with growth hormone deficiency, and this association may involve mutations in the *ELF4* (ETS-related transcription factor 4) gene on the X chromosome.[11] With XLA, sensorineural hearing loss can be caused by deletion mutations affecting both *Btk* and the *TIMM8A* gene, which is on the X chromosome.[12]

Clinical Features. Most patients with XLA or other antibody deficiency syndromes are identified after having recurrent infections with encapsulated bacterial pathogens. Protected by passive immunity from maternally transmitted IgG antibodies, boys with XLA usually remain well during the first few months of life, although they may have mucous membrane infections (e.g., conjunctivitis, otitis) because of the lack of secretory IgA antibodies. Thereafter, boys with XLA are highly susceptible to infections with encapsulated organisms such as pneumococci, streptococci, and *Haemophilus influenzae.* They also may experience infections with other high-grade pathogens such as meningococci, staphylococci, *Pseudomonas* organisms, and various species of *Mycoplasma.* Because patients with XLA have a profound deficiency of antibodies of all isotypes, the infections may be systemic (e.g., meningitis or septicemia) or involve mucous membrane surfaces (sinusitis, pneumonia, otitis, conjunctivitis, or gastrointestinal and urinary tract infections), joints (septic arthritis), or skin (cellulitis or abscesses). The tonsils, adenoids, and peripheral lymph nodes are very small because of the absence of germinal centers. The structures and contents of the thymus and thymus-dependent areas of peripheral lymphoid tissues are normal. Growth and development usually are normal despite chronic or recurrent bacterial infections, unless bronchiectasis or persistent enteroviral infections develop.[13] Fungal infections are not usually a problem, and *Pneumocystis jirovecii* pneumonia is rare. Except for those due to hepatitis viruses and enteroviruses, viral infections usually are handled normally. Various echoviruses and coxsackieviruses also can cause chronic, progressive and, eventually, fatal central nervous system infections in patients with XLA.[13] Septic arthritis and joint inflammation similar to that in rheumatoid arthritis also may be features. *Ureaplasma urealyticum* organisms and viral agents such as echoviruses, coxsackieviruses, and adenoviruses have been identified even in joint fluid of patients on intravenous immunoglobulin (IVIG) replacement therapy.

Evaluation and Diagnosis. With XLA, concentrations of all serum immunoglobulins are extremely low. Because antibody formation is profoundly impaired in XLA, it can be distinguished from transient hypogammaglobulinemia of infancy or from protein-losing states by testing for antibodies to blood group substances and to vaccine antigens (e.g., diphtheria, tetanus, *H. influenzae,* pneumococci).

Flow cytometry detects few, if any, circulating B cells in patients with XLA. Some bone marrow precursor B cells can be found, but those cells are strongly biased to a fetal-like repertoire of *VDJ* gene usage. Circulating T cells and natural killer (NK) cells are relatively increased, and the percentages of the helper and cytotoxic subsets are normal in most patients. T cell functions are normal in Bruton's disease.

Treatment and Prognosis. The overall prognosis for patients with XLA is reasonably good if IVIG replacement therapy is instituted early, and in the absence of polio, other persistent enteroviral infections, arthritis, or lymphoreticular malignancy (an incidence as high as 6% has been reported). In a majority of patients, systemic infection can be prevented by administration of IVIG at a dose of 400-800 mg/kg every 3 to 4 weeks.[10] Despite receiving this therapy, some patients develop persistent enteroviral infections or crippling sinopulmonary disease, because no effective means exists for replacing secretory IgA at the mucosal surface. Chronic antibiotic therapy in addition to IVIG infusions can be effective for management of pansinusitis or bronchiectasis in patients with XLA.

AUTOSOMAL RECESSIVE AGAMMAGLOBULINEMIA

Autosomal recessive mutations in the genes encoding immunoglobulin heavy or light chains or their associated signaling molecules lead to agammaglobulinemia or hypogammaglobulinemia, which resembles XLA phenotypically (see Table 72-1 and Fig. 72-1). Mutations in μ chain,[14] λ5/14.1 (surrogate light chain),[15] Igα (B cell antigen receptor signaling molecule)[16] and Igβ,[17] and B cell linker (*BLNK*) genes[18] are responsible for absence of circulating B cells. As alluded to earlier, a rare autosomal dominant mutation of the *LRRC8A* gene also has been identified.[19]

COMMON VARIABLE IMMUNODEFICIENCY

Epidemiology. CVID may have many clinical aspects similar to those of XLA. Age at onset of infections, however, may be later than in XLA. The true incidence and prevalence of CVID are unknown, but it generally is considered to be more common than XLA. The sexes are almost equally affected in CVID.

Pathogenesis and Etiology. Because CVID occurs in first-degree relatives of patients with selective IgA deficiency (A Def), and some patients with A Def later become panhypogammaglobulinemic, it has long been suspected that CVID and A Def have a common genetic basis. The high incidence rates of abnormal immunoglobulin concentrations, autoantibodies, autoimmune disease, and malignancy in families of patients with both disorders also suggest a shared hereditary influence. Patients with either A Def or CVID exhibit a high incidence of C4-A gene deletions and C2 rare gene alleles in the class III major histocompatibility complex (MHC) region, which suggests the presence of a susceptibility gene in this region on chromosome 6.[20] A small number of HLA haplotypes is shared by persons affected with CVID and A Def, and at least one of two particular haplotypes was present in 77% of those affected.[20] The association with HLA also was borne out in a genome-wide association study (GWAS) whereby more than 100 unique exonic duplications and deletions were identified in patients with CVID.[6] Most CVID cases are sporadic or follow an autosomal dominant pattern of inheritance for which the underlying genetic defect(s) have not been discovered. In male patients who have a clinical presentation of CVID, however, the *SH2D1A, Btk,* and *CD154* genes should be evaluated. Both males and females with a clinical presentation of CVID should be evaluated for mutations in the *AIDCA,* uracil DNA deglyosylase *(UNG),* and *CD40* genes. Seven presumed single-gene causes of this syndrome are discussed next.

Inducible Costimulator Deficiency in Autosomal Recessive Common Variable Immunodeficiency

In the Black Forest region of Germany, some patients with CVID have an autosomal recessive pattern of inheritance and lack the inducible costimulator (ICOS), a surface protein on activated T cells.[21] Binding of ICOS to its ligand induces a significant increase in T cell proliferation and cytokine production, especially of interleukin (IL)-10, which has been implicated in the differentiation of B cells to plasma cells. Nine patients from six families had identical homozygous large genomic deletions of the *ICOS* gene, suggesting a founder effect. No examples of ICOS deficiency have been found in the United States.

Patients with a clinical presentation of CVID can have mutations involving intermediates in B cell signaling and developmental pathways. Specifically, defects in CD19, CD81,[22] CD20,[23] CD27, B cell–activating factor of the tumor necrosis factor (TNF) family receptor (BAFF-R) and transmembrane activator, calcium modulator, and cyclophilin ligand interactor (TACI) genes have been identified.[24,25] BAFF and APRIL serve as ligands for BAFF-R, TACI, and B cell maturation antigen (BCMA). Patients with mutations in genes encoding BAFF-R or TACI may lack the necessary B cell signaling for proper maturation and generation of a diverse antibody repertoire. Patients with CD19, CD20, and CD81 deficiency have impaired signaling after B cell receptor ligation, whereas CD27 deficiency results in a specific deficit in memory B cells.

Clinical Features. Patients with CVID generally have the same kinds of infections with the same bacterial etiologic agents as in patients with X-linked or other B cell–negative agammaglobulinemias. In CVID, tonsils and lymph nodes are either normal in size or enlarged, and splenomegaly occurs in approximately 25%. In addition, a tendency toward autoantibody formation and autoimmunity has been described.[26] Other reported manifestations include lymphoid interstitial pneumonia, pseudolymphoma, amyloidosis, and noncaseating granulomas of the lungs, spleen, skin, and liver. Women in their 50s and 60s with CVID have a 438-fold increased risk for lymphoma formation.[27] CVID has been variably associated with a spruelike syndrome, nodular follicular lymphoid hyperplasia of the intestine, colitis, small bowel lymphoma, gastric atrophy, achlorhydria, thymoma, alopecia areata, hemolytic anemia, and pernicious anemia. Several cases of lupus erythematosus converting to CVID have been reported. These patients have frequent thyroid abnormalities, vitiligo, keratoconjunctivitis sicca, and arthritis. Frequent complications include giardiasis (seen more often with CVID than with XLA), bronchiectasis, gastric carcinoma, lymphoreticular malignancy, and cholelithiasis.

Evaluation and Diagnosis. Serum immunoglobulin and antibody deficiencies in CVID may be as profound as those in XLA, but CVID is defined by concentrations of IgG and at least one other serum immunoglobulin of more than 2 standard deviations (SD) below the age-specific mean in the presence of circulating B cells but an impaired ability to generate specific antibody (typically measured by failed IgG response to vaccine antigen challenge). Although a majority of patients with CVID have lymphoid cortical follicles, blood B cells do not differentiate into immunoglobulin-producing cells. T cells usually are present in normal percentages, but T cell function may be depressed.

Treatment and Prognosis. Treatment for CVID is essentially the same as for XLA.[28] Although rare, anaphylactic reactions can be caused by IgE antibodies to IgA; therefore, caution is warranted in initiating therapy with IVIG preparations containing IgA.[29] The prognosis for patients with CVID is reasonably good, although life expectancy declines if lymphoproliferation, severe autoimmune disease, or malignancy develop.[30]

SELECTIVE IMMUNOGLOBULIN A DEFICIENCY

Epidemiology. Isolated absence or near-absence (i.e., with levels less than 10 mg/dL) of serum and secretory IgA is believed to be the most common immunodeficiency disorder. Among a group of blood donors, A Def frequency was 1 in 333.[31]

Pathogenesis and Etiology. The basic defect leading to A Def is unknown. The occurrence of A Def in both males and females and in families is consistent with autosomal inheritance; in many families, this appears to be dominant with variable expressivity. Treatments with phenytoin, D-penicillamine, sulfasalazine, or gold compounds may facilitate expression of this defect. As already noted, A Def occurs in pedigrees with patients with CVID, and molecular genetic studies suggest that the susceptibility genes for these two defects may reside in the MHC class III region as an allelic condition on chromosome 6.[20] A recent GWAS has further defined specific genetic associations with A Def, such as linkages with *IFIH1* and *CLEC16A*, which have both been associated with autoimmune conditions.[6]

Clinical Features. Although A Def can occur in apparently healthy persons,[31] it is commonly associated with ill health. Infections associated with A Def are predominantly in the respiratory, gastrointestinal, and urogenital tracts. The bacterial agents responsible are essentially the same as in other types of antibody deficiency syndromes. There is no clear evidence that patients with A Def have an undue susceptibility to viral agents. Like CVID, A Def frequently is associated with autoimmune diseases. As with CVID, incidence of malignancy is increased with A Def.

Evaluation and Diagnosis. In patients with A Def, serum concentrations of other immunoglobulins usually are normal, although IgG2 subclass may be deficient and IgM (often monomeric) may be elevated. As many as 44% of patients with selective IgA deficiency have antibodies to IgA in the sera.[31] Several patients with A Def have had severe or fatal anaphylactic reactions after intravenous administration of blood products containing IgA, and the reactions may have been caused by anti-IgA antibodies (particularly IgE anti-IgA antibodies).[29] For this reason, patients with this disorder should receive washed normal donor erythrocytes or blood products from other persons with A Def. A high incidence of autoantibodies also has been noted.

Treatment and Prognosis. Currently there is no treatment for A Def beyond the vigorous treatment of specific infections with appropriate antimicrobial agents. IVIG (99% IgG) is not indicated, because most patients with this disorder make IgG antibodies normally.[28] In some affected children the defect disappears with time, although in adults it usually persists. In some patients, A Def evolves into CVID.

IMMUNOGLOBULIN G SUBCLASS DEFICIENCY

Epidemiology. Patients can have deficiencies of one or more subclasses of IgG despite having normal total IgG serum concentrations.

Pathogenesis and Etiology. IgG subclass protein deficiency can occur in the absence of documented broad antibody deficiencies; some persons who totally lack IgG1, IgG2, IgG4, or IgA1 because of heavy-chain gene deletions are completely asymptomatic and produce antibodies normally.[32] Children with low IgG2 subclass levels and history of frequent infections can have broader and more varied patterns of immunologic dysfunction than healthy children with low IgG2 levels, and the variation may be indicative of CVID development.[33]

Clinical Features. IgG2 deficiency is suspected if patients have repeat problems with encapsulated bacterial pathogens, because a majority of the antipolysaccharide antibody molecules are of the IgG2 isotype. Numerous healthy children, however, have low levels of IgG2 but normal responses to polysaccharide antigens upon immunization.

Evaluation and Diagnosis. IgG subclass measurement is not very helpful in the general assessment of immune function. Such assays provide no information about the patient's capacity to produce specific antibodies to protein, polysaccharide, or viral antigens. Moreover, measurements reported for different subclasses can vary in different commercial laboratories even when aliquots of the same serum sample are tested. Thus, when low IgG subclass levels are reported, the clinician should consider the following question: What is the patient's capacity to make specific antibodies to protein and polysaccharide antigens?

Treatment and Prognosis. IVIG should not be given to IgG subclass–deficient patients unless they are shown to have a deficiency of antibodies to a broad array of antigens.[28]

TRANSIENT HYPOGAMMAGLOBULINEMIA OF INFANCY

Epidemiology. Transient hypogammaglobulinemia of infancy does not appear to be a common entity: In a 12-year study, only 11 cases among more than 10,000 patients were noted.[34] However, the disorder can be associated with somewhat sluggish complete vaccine-specific antibody responses as well as elevated B cell counts.[35]

Pathogenesis and Etiology. Transient hypogammaglobulinemia of infancy has been found in pedigrees of patients with other immune defects, including CVID and severe combined immunodeficiency disorders (i.e., SCIDs).

Clinical Features. Patients diagnosed with this condition usually are infants who have recurrent upper respiratory infections.

Evaluation and Diagnosis. Unlike patients with XLA or CVID, patients with transient hypogammaglobulinemia of infancy can synthesize antibodies to human type A and B erythrocytes and to diphtheria and tetanus toxoids.[34] Often these antibodies are found in normal titer when the infant is 6 to 11 months of age, long before immunoglobulin concentrations become normal.

Treatment and Prognosis. IVIG therapy generally is not indicated in transient hypogammaglobulinemia of infancy[28] because of the risk of inducing antiallotype antibodies. In addition, passively administered IgG antibodies could suppress endogenous antibody formation to infectious agents in the same manner that RhoGAM suppresses anti-D antibodies in Rh-negative mothers delivering Rh-positive infants.

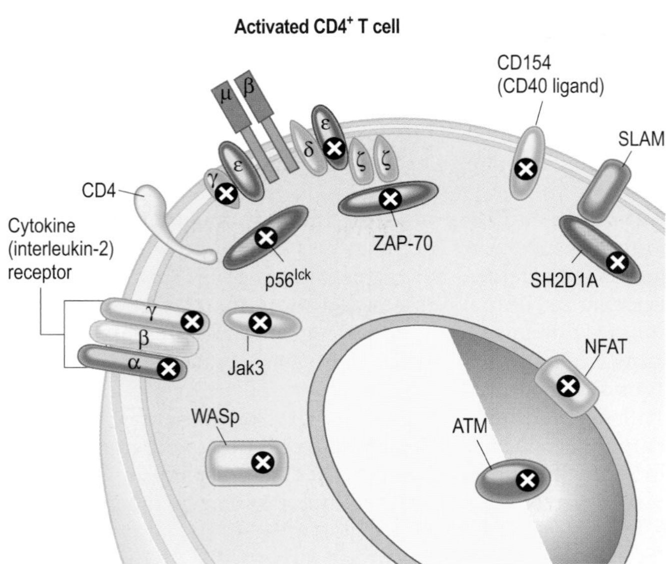

Figure 72-2 Locations of mutant proteins in B cells and activated CD4+ T cells identified in primary immunodeficiency diseases. Each mutant protein is identified by a white **x**. *ATM,* Ataxia-telangiectasia mutation; *Jak3,* Janus kinase 3; *NFAT,* nuclear factor of activated T cells; *SH2D1A,* SLAM-associated protein; *SLAM,* signaling lymphocyte activation molecule; *WASp,* Wiskott-Aldrich syndrome protein; *ZAP-70,* zeta-associated protein 70. *(From Buckley RH: Primary immunodeficiency diseases due to defects in lymphocytes. N Engl J Med 2000;343:1317.)*

IMMUNODEFICIENCY WITH THYMOMA

Patients who have immunodeficiency with thymoma are adults who almost simultaneously develop recurrent infections, panhypogammaglobulinemia, deficits in cell-mediated immunity, and benign thymoma.[3,36] Patients also may have eosinophilia or eosinopenia, aregenerative or hemolytic anemia, agranulocytosis, thrombocytopenia, or pancytopenia. Antibody formation is poor, and progressive lymphopenia develops, although percentages of B lymphocytes usually are normal. The thymomas are predominantly of the spindle cell variety, although other types of benign and malignant thymic tumors also have been seen.

X-LINKED IMMUNODEFICIENCY WITH HYPERIMMUNOGLOBULINEMIA M: HIGM1

Epidemiology. The incidence and prevalence of hyperimmunoglobulinemia M syndrome are unknown, but the condition generally is considered to be less common than CVID. The hyper-IgM syndrome is genetically diverse, with at least six mutated genes identified among persons presenting clinically with this condition.

Pathogenesis and Etiology. X-linked hyper IgM, also known as HIGM1, formerly was classified as a B cell defect, because only IgM is produced. Normal numbers of B lymphocytes, however, usually are present in the circulation of affected patients, and the B cells can synthesize IgM, IgA, and IgG normally when cocultured with an activated T cell line.[37] The abnormal gene in X-linked hyper-IgM syndrome is localized to Xq26.[38] The gene product is a T cell surface molecule known as CD154 (or CD40 ligand [CD40L]), which interacts with CD40 molecules on B cells[38] (Fig. 72-2). CD154 is a type II integral membrane glycoprotein with significant sequence homology to TNF (making it a TNF superfamily member); it is found only on activated T cells, primarily of the CD4 phenotype. Most mutations are in the TNF homology domain located in the carboxyl-terminal (C-terminal) region. Mutations in *CD154* result in a lack of signaling between activated T cells and B cells. Cross-linking of CD40 on either normal or HIGM1 B cells with a monoclonal antibody to CD40 or with soluble CD154 in the presence of cytokines (IL-2, IL-4, or IL-10) causes the B cells to undergo proliferation and isotype switching and to secrete various types of immunoglobulins. In vivo, because of the lack of CD154 on T cells, HIGM1 B cells fail to undergo isotype switching and produce only IgM. The lack of stimulation of CD40 also results in failure of B cells to upregulate CD80 and CD86 or to become IgD-CD27+ memory B cells. CD80 and CD86 are important costimulatory molecules that interact with CD28/cytotoxic T lymphocyte–associated protein 4 (CTLA-4) on T cells. The lack of interaction between these molecules results in a propensity for tolerogenic T cell signaling.

Another X-linked cause of hyper-IgM syndrome is NEMO deficiency; certain mutations in the *NEMO* gene can abrogate CD40 signals in B cells,[39] as discussed in greater detail further on. Typically, but not always, these patients have abnormal skin, hair, and facial features characteristic of ectodermal dysplasia.[40]

Clinical Features. Because they lack IgG, IgA, and IgE antibodies, patients with the various types of hyper-IgM syndrome resemble those with XLA in their susceptibility to encapsulated bacterial infections.[41] The likelihood of autoantibody formation

TABLE 72-3 Hyper-IgM (HIGM) Syndrome Molecular Subtypes: Clinical Features

HIGM Type	PJ Pneumonia	Neutropenia	Lymphadenopathy	Early Death
HIGM1 (CD40L [CD154] def)	Yes	Yes	No	Yes
NEMO	No	No	No	Yes
HIGM2 (AICDA def), UNG def	No	No	Yes	No
HIGM3 (CD40 def)	Yes	Yes	No	Unknown
HIGM4 (molecular defect unknown)	No	No	Yes	No

AICDA, Activation-induced cytidine deaminase; *CD40L*, CD40 ligand; *def*, defect/deficiency; *IgM*, immunoglobulin M; *NEMO*, nuclear factor-κB essential modulator; *PJ*, *Pneumocystis jirovecii*; *UNG*, uracil-DNA glycosylase.

is increased as well.[41] Hemolytic anemia and thrombocytopenia may occur, and transient, persistent, or cyclic neutropenia is common. In HIGM1, patients frequently have an initial presentation of *P. jirovecii* pneumonia, which may be caused by coexistent neutropenia or by T cell malfunctioning. In addition, the incidence of malignancy is increased.[41] Lymph node histologic features are abnormal, showing only abortive germinal center formation and a severe depletion and phenotypic abnormalities of follicular dendritic cells.

Evaluation and Diagnosis. Concentrations of serum IgG, IgA, and IgE are very low, whereas serum IgM concentration is either normal or elevated and polyclonal. Low-molecular-weight IgM molecules are present in some patients. When $CD4^+$ T cells from patients with HIGM1 are stimulated with phorbol myristate acetate and ionomycin in vitro, the cells fail to upregulate the CD40L on their surfaces.

Treatment and Prognosis. Because the prognosis is not good for many patients with HIGM1, the treatment of choice is bone marrow transplantation.[42] Otherwise, the treatment for this condition is the same as for agammaglobulinemia: monthly IVIG infusions.[28] Patient neutropenia is responsive to granulocyte colony-stimulating factor (G-CSF) treatment.

AUTOSOMAL RECESSIVE HYPERIMMUNOGLOBULINEMIA M

Unlike B cells in the HIGM1 condition, B cells from patients with autosomal recessive hyper-IgM syndrome are not able to switch from IgM-secreting to IgG-, IgA-, or IgE-secreting cells, even when cocultured with monoclonal antibodies to CD40 and a variety of cytokines.[43] Thus, in these patients, the condition truly is a B cell defect. Discussed next are three autosomal hyper-IgM defects for which the molecular basis is known. It is likely, however, that this syndrome can be caused by at least one more autosomal recessive molecular defect, as yet undefined.

Autosomal Recessive Hyper-Immunoglobulin M Due to Activation-Dependent Cytidine Deaminase Deficiency: HIGM2

Pathogenesis and Etiology. Patients with the HIGM2 form of hyper-IgM syndrome have mutations in a gene on chromosomal segment 12p13 that encodes an activation-induced cytidine deaminase (AICDA), an RNA- and DNA-editing enzyme specifically expressed in germinal center B cells.[44,45] A deficiency of AICDA results in impaired terminal differentiation of B cells and failed isotype switching. A lack of immunoglobulin gene somatic hypermutation also has been noted. B cells from these patients constitutively produce large quantities of IgM in vitro.

Clinical Features and Diagnosis. Patients have profoundly decreased serum IgG, IgA, and IgE concentrations and marked susceptibility to bacterial infections. In contrast with patients with HIGM1, however, they have markedly elevated serum IgM concentrations. Unlike those with HIGM1, patients with this defect have lymphoid hyperplasia because they do have germinal centers, albeit defective ones (Table 72-3).

Autosomal Recessive Hyper-IgM Syndrome Due to Uracil-DNA Glycosylase Deficiency: HIGM4

Pathogenesis and Etiology. In targeted DNA, AICDA deaminates cytosine into uracil, and subsequently uracil is removed by uracil-DNA glycosylase (UNG). Three patients with hyper-IgM syndrome were found to have mutations in the gene encoding UNG.[46] In this form of the disorder, designated HIGM4, B cells have profoundly impaired class switch recombination and a partial defect in somatic hypermutation.

Clinical Features. The clinical and immunologic characteristics are similar to those in patients with AICDA deficiency.

Autosomal Recessive Hyper-IgM Syndrome Due to CD40 Deficiency: HIGM3

Pathogenesis and Etiology. CD40, encoded by a gene on chromosome 20, is a type I integral membrane glycoprotein belonging to the TNF and nerve growth factor receptor superfamily. It is expressed on B cells, macrophages, and dendritic cells. It interacts with CD40L on activated $CD4^+$ T cells. Ligation of CD40 leads to activation of nuclear factor of κB (NF-κB) light chain enhancer in B cells, which in turn promotes the production of AICDA and UNG to enable B cell functioning. Three patients with autosomal recessive hyper-IgM syndrome in which CD40 was not expressed on B cell surfaces, designated HIGM3, have been identified.[47]

Clinical Features. Affected patients have clinical presentations similar to those in patients with X-linked hyper-IgM syndrome (see Table 72-3).

Treatment and Prognosis. The treatment for all autosomal recessive forms of hyper-IgM syndrome is monthly infusions of IVIG. The prognosis is better in these types than in HIGM1 because the defect is limited to B cells.

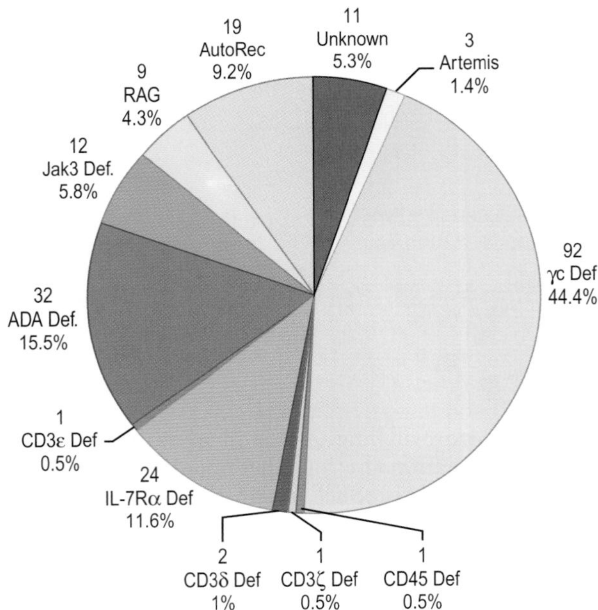

Figure 72-3 Relative frequencies of the different genetic types of severe combined immunodeficiency (SCID) among 207 patients seen consecutively at a single institution over 4 decades (RHB, unpublished data). *ADA,* Adenosine deaminase; *AutoRec,* autosomal recessive; *Def,* deficiency; *IL-7Rα,* interleukin-7 receptor α; *Jak3,* Janus kinase 3; *RAG,* recombinase-activating gene [protein].

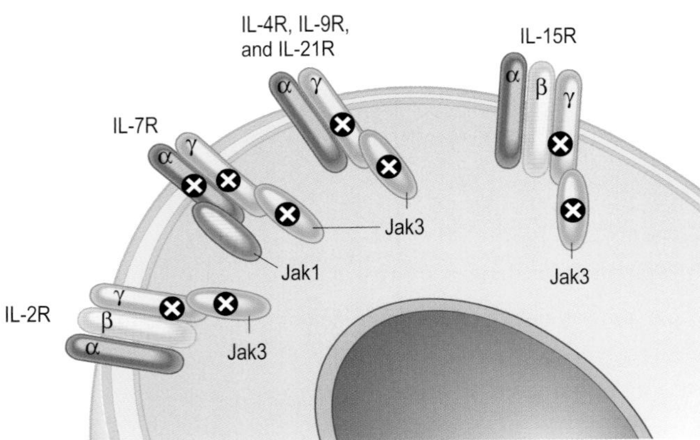

Figure 72-4 Diagram showing that Janus kinase 3 (*Jak3*) is the major signal transducer for the common γ (γc) chain shared by multiple cytokine (interleukin [*IL*]) receptors. Mutations in the gene encoding Jak3 result in a form of autosomal recessive severe combined immunodeficiency (SCID) that mimics the X-linked form (SCID-X1) phenotypically. *(Reprinted from Buckley RH. Primary cellular immunodeficiencies. J Allergy Clin Immunol 2002;109:747-57.)*

SEVERE COMBINED IMMUNODEFICIENCY DISEASE

SCID is a fatal syndrome characterized by profound deficiencies of T and B cell function.[48,49] Since the initial description of SCID in 1950,[50] it has become evident that the genetic origins of SCID are quite diverse.[48] X-linked SCID (SCID-X1) is the most common form and accounts for approximately 46% of U.S. cases.[48] Figure 72-3 shows the frequency of the various genetic forms of SCID as encountered in clinical practice by one of us (RHB, unpublished data) over the past 4 decades.

Epidemiology. Until very recently, the incidence of this syndrome was unknown. In January of 2010, the U.S. Department of Health and Human Services (DHHS) Advisory Committee on Heritable Disorders of Newborns and Children unanimously approved a recommendation that SCID and other severe T cell defects be added to the routine newborn screening panel, and the DHHS Secretary approved this recommendation in May of 2010.[51] Data from several pilot studies conducted in the past 3 years suggest an incidence of SCID of approximately 1 in 40,000 births.

X-linked Severe Combined Immunodeficiency

Pathogenesis and Etiology. The abnormal gene in X-linked SCID (i.e., SCID-X1) was mapped by restriction fragment length polymorphism (RFLP) analysis to the Xq13 region and later identified as encoding a common γ (γc) chain shared by several cytokine receptors, including those for IL-2, IL-4, IL-7, IL-9, IL-15, and IL-21[52,53] (Fig. 72-4). Mutations in the *IL2RG* gene result in faulty signaling through several cytokine receptors, which explains how multiple cell types can be affected by a mutation in a single gene (see Fig. 72-4). Among the first 136 patients studied, 95 distinct mutations spanning all eight *IL2RG* exons were identified, and most mutations consisted of changes to one or a few nucleotides (Fig. 72-5). These mutations resulted in abnormal γc chains in two thirds of cases and absent γc protein in the remainder. Carriers of SCID-X1 can be detected by the presence of nonrandom X chromosome inactivation in T, B, and NK lymphocytes or by mutation analysis if a family member's mutation is known. As more patients are studied, it is likely that atypical SCID-X1 cases will be found. The pathogenesis and etiology of the other molecular types of SCID are discussed further on.

Clinical Features—All Types. Regardless of the underlying molecular defect, affected infants present within the first few months of life with frequent episodes of diarrhea, pneumonia, otitis, sepsis, and cutaneous infections. Growth initially may appear normal, but extreme wasting usually develops after infections and diarrhea begin. Persistent infections with opportunistic organisms such as *Candida albicans, P. jirovecii,* varicella-zoster virus (including vaccine-derived), adenovirus, parainfluenza 3, herpesviruses, cytomegalovirus, Epstein-Barr virus (EBV), and bacille Calmette-Guérin (BCG) lead to death. These infants also lack the ability to reject foreign tissue and are therefore at risk for graft-versus-host disease. This condition can result from maternal T cells that cross into the fetal circulation while the infant with SCID is in utero or from T lymphocytes in nonirradiated blood products or allogeneic bone marrow.[42] Typically, infants with SCID have a very small thymus (usually weighing less than 1 g), which fails to descend from the neck, contains few thymocytes, and lacks corticomedullary distinction and Hassall's corpuscles. Nevertheless, the tiny epithelial thymuses are capable of supporting normal T cell development.[54] In patients with SCID, thymus-dependent areas of the spleen are depleted of lymphocytes, and lymph nodes, tonsils, adenoids, and Peyer's patches are absent or extremely underdeveloped.

Evaluation and Diagnosis—All Types. In normal persons, 70% of circulating lymphocytes are T cells. Because infants with

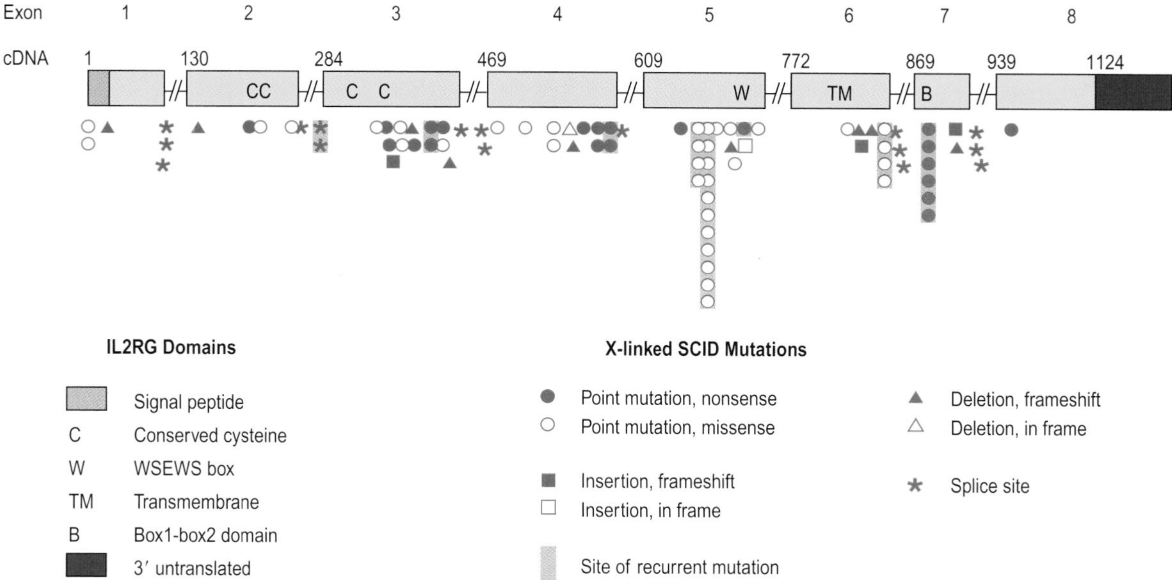

Figure 72-5 *IL2RG* complementary DNA (*cDNA*) map showing exons, cDNA numbers corresponding to the first coding nucleotide of each exon, protein domains, and sites of mutations found in 87 unrelated families with X-linked severe combined immunodeficiency (SCID). Identical mutations found in unrelated patients are surrounded by *shaded boxes. (From Puck JM, Pepper AE, Henthorn PS, et al: Mutation analysis of* IL2RG *in human X-linked severe combined immunodeficiency. Blood 1997;89:1970.)*

all molecular types of SCID lack T cells from birth, they are invariably lymphopenic.[48,55] Their lymphocytes have an absence of proliferative responses to mitogens, antigens, and allogeneic cells in vitro, even in samples collected in utero or from the cord blood. Therefore physicians caring for infants need to be aware of the normal ranges for the absolute lymphocyte count in infancy.[56] For infants with values below these ranges, flow cytometry and T cell functional studies are indicated.[48,55] At 6 to 7 months of age, when most cases of SCID have been diagnosed, normal infants have a high absolute lymphocyte count, and any count below 4000/μL is lymphopenic.[56] Serum immunoglobulin concentrations are diminished to absent, and no antibody formation occurs after immunization. Despite the uniformly profound lack of T or B cell function, patients with SCID-X1 have elevated percentages of B cells.[48,55] However, these B cells do not produce immunoglobulin normally, even after T cell reconstitution by bone marrow transplantation, because they still have the 6 abnormal cytokine receptors on their surfaces. By contrast, all infants with SCID, except those with transplacentally acquired maternal T cells, have few or no T cells, and NK cells and NK function usually are very low or totally lacking in patients with SCID-X1 (Box 72-1 and Table 72-4).[48,55] The extremely small thymuses present in all molecular types are not visible roentgenographically, so a chest radiograph can be a major diagnostic aid.

BOX 72-1 THIRTEEN ABNORMAL GENES IN SEVERE COMBINED IMMUNODEFICIENCY DISEASE

CYTOKINE RECEPTOR GENES

IL2RG
JAK3—Janus kinase 3 gene
IL7RA

ANTIGEN RECEPTOR GENES

RAG1
RAG2
DCLRE1C—Artemis gene
LIG4—ligase 4 gene
PRKDC
CD3D—CD3δ gene
CD3E—CD3ε gene
CD247—CD3ζ gene

OTHER GENES

ADA
CD45

ADA, Adenosine deaminase; *DCLRE1C*, DNA cross-link repair 1C; *IL2RG*, interleukin-2 receptor γ; *PRKDC*, protein kinase, DNA-activated, catalytic polypeptide; *RAG1*, *RAG2*, recombinase-activating genes 1 and 2.

Treatment and Prognosis—All Types. SCID is a pediatric emergency.[55,48] Replacement therapy with IVIG is indicated and also is frequently needed after curative therapy.[28] Unless bone marrow transplantation from HLA-identical or haploidentical donors can be performed, death usually occurs before the patient's first birthday. Transplantation in the first 3.5 months of life offers a greater than 94% chance of survival[54,57] (Fig. 72-6). Therefore early diagnosis is essential. Data from recent studies indicate that the immune reconstitution resulting from stem cell transplants is due to thymic education of the transplanted donor stem cells. The thymic output appears to occur sooner and to a greater degree in infants who undergo transplantation during the neonatal period.[54] Currently, more than 600 patients with SCID worldwide are living as a result of successful bone marrow transplantation.[42,55,58-61]

More than a decade ago, a normal γc complementary DNA (cDNA) was successfully transduced into autologous marrow stem cells of nine infants with SCID-X1 by retroviral gene

TABLE 72-4 Severe Combined Immunodeficiency (SCID) Lymphocyte Phenotypes

Phenotype	Associated Deficiency Phenotype
$T^-B^+NK^-$	γc-deficient Jak3-deficient
$T^-B^+NK^+$	IL-7Rα–deficient CD3δ-deficient CD3ε-deficient CD3ζ-deficient CD45-deficient
$T^-B^-NK^-$	ADA-deficient
$T^-B^-NK^+$	RAG-1/RAG-2–deficient Artemis-deficient Ligase 4–deficient

ADA, Adenosine deaminase; *IL-7Rα*, interleukin-7 receptor alpha [chain]; *Jak3*, Janus kinase 3; *NK*, natural killer [cell]; *RAG-1*, *RAG-2*, recombinase-activating gene proteins 1, 2.

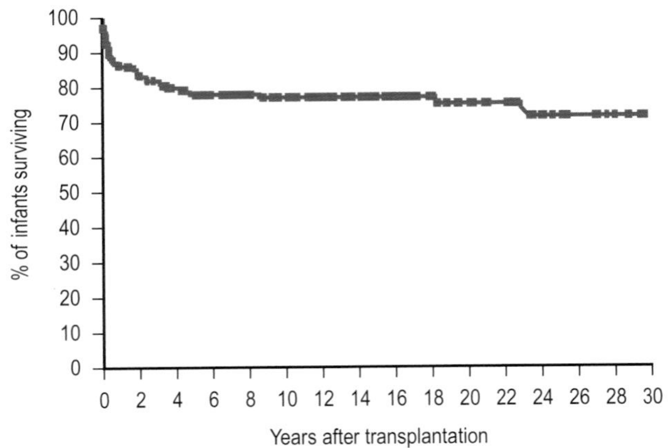

Figure 72-6 Kaplan-Meier survival curve for 169 consecutive infants with severe combined immunodeficiency (SCID) who received marrow transplants at Duke University Medical Center from human leukocyte antigen (HLA)-identical (17) or haploidentical (152) donors without pretransplantation chemoablation and without posttransplantation graft-versus-host disease prophylaxis. Deaths occurred from viral infections present at the time of diagnosis in three fourths of those who did not survive. Forty-nine of 52 (94%) infants who received transplants before they were 3½ months of age survived for periods of 4 months to 31 years after transplantation.

transfer, and after reinfusion of the stem cells, T, B, and NK cell defects were fully corrected.[62] Unfortunately, leukemias or lymphoma developed because of insertional oncogenesis in 5 of 20 patients so treated.[63,64] A decade after treatment, T cells are the only lineage demonstrating sustained correction among survivors.[65,66] The serious adverse events necessitated a halt in the initial clinical trials, but subsequently, intense study of the basis for the events, as well as possible prevention mechanisms, has been undertaken.

AUTOSOMAL RECESSIVE SEVERE COMBINED IMMUNODEFICIENCY DISEASE

Autosomal recessive SCID, the first form of SCID to be described, was reported by Swiss workers in 1950.[50] Autosomal recessive inheritance is less common in the United States than in Europe.[48,67] Mutated genes on autosomal chromosomes have been identified in 12 genetic types of SCID: adenosine deaminase (ADA) deficiency, Janus kinase 3 (Jak3) deficiency, IL-7 receptor α chain (IL-7Rα) deficiency, recombinase-activating gene (RAG-1 or RAG-2) protein deficiencies, Artemis deficiency, ligase 4 deficiency, DNA-PKcs (DNA-dependent protein kinase, catalytic subunit), CD3 δ, ε, and ζ chain deficiencies, and CD45 deficiency (see Box 72-1).[48,67] Each of these molecular types of SCID has a characteristic lymphocyte phenotype (see Table 72-4).

Autosomal Recessive Severe Combined Immunodeficiency Disease Caused by Adenosine Deaminase Deficiency

Epidemiology. Absence of the enzyme ADA has been observed in approximately 16% of patients with SCID (see Fig. 72-3).[48,55,68]

Pathogenesis and Etiology. The gene encoding ADA has been mapped to chromosomal region 20q13-ter.[69] ADA deficiency mutations result in pronounced accumulations of adenosine, 2′-deoxyadenosine, and 2′-*O*-methyladenosine.[69] The latter two metabolites directly or indirectly lead to apoptosis of thymocytes and circulating lymphocytes, which causes the immunodeficiency.

Clinical Features. Patients with ADA deficiency have the same clinical problems of susceptibility to opportunistic bacterial, viral, and parasitic diseases as described earlier for SCID-X1 and also are at risk for development of graft-versus-host disease from allogeneic T cells in blood products or bone marrow given for treatment. Distinguishing features of ADA deficiency include the presence of rib cage abnormalities similar to a rachitic rosary and multiple skeletal abnormalities of chondroosseous dysplasia, which can be seen by radiographic examination and occur predominantly at costochondral junctions, at apophyses of the iliac bones, and in vertebral bodies.[69]

Evaluation and Diagnosis. Patients with ADA deficiency usually have a much more profound lymphopenia than infants with other types of SCID: Mean absolute lymphocyte counts typically are less than 500/μL, and T, B, and NK cells are essentially absent (see Table 72-4).[48,55] However, NK function may be normal,[48,55] and after bone marrow transplantation without pretransplantation chemotherapy, B cell function can develop even without donor B cells. ADA deficiency primarily affects T cell function, which is absent, as in all of the other forms of SCID. Milder forms of this condition occur and are characterized by delayed diagnosis of immunodeficiency, even to adulthood.

Treatment and Prognosis. As with other types of SCID, ADA deficiency can be cured by HLA-identical or haploidentical T cell–depleted bone marrow transplantation.[42,48,55,57] In a study of more than 100 ADA-deficient patients, enzyme replacement therapy with polyethylene glycol (PEG)–modified bovine ADA (PEG-ADA), administered subcutaneously once weekly, resulted in both clinical and immunologic improvement.[70] Immunocompetence was not near the level induced with bone marrow transplantation, however.[71] PEG-ADA therapy should not be initiated if bone marrow transplantation is contemplated, because it will confer graft rejection capability upon the infant. Immune reconstitution has been accomplished by gene therapy in at least 20 patients with ADA-deficient SCID who did not receive PEG-ADA concomitantly and who underwent low-dose busulfan preconditioning.[72]

Autosomal Recessive Severe Combined Immunodeficiency Disease Caused by Janus Kinase 3 Deficiency

Pathogenesis and Etiology. Because Jak3 is the only signaling molecule known to be associated with γc, *JAK3* was a candidate gene for autosomal recessive SCID (see Fig. 72-4). To date, more than 30 patients who lack Jak3 have been identified.[48,73,74] Like patients with SCID-X1, they have very low or no NK cell activity.[48]

Clinical Features. Like all patients with SCID, those with Jak3 deficiency are susceptible to infection and to graft-versus-host disease from allogeneic T cells.

Evaluation and Diagnosis. In Jak3-deficient SCIDs, lymphocyte characteristics most closely resemble those in X-linked SCID, such as an elevated percentage of B cells and very low percentages of T and NK cells (see Table 72-4).[48,74]

Treatment and Prognosis. Infants with Jak3-deficient SCID fail to develop NK cells even after successful T cell reconstitution by nonablative transplantation of haploidentical stem cells.[42] Despite having high numbers of B cells, these patients also cannot develop normal B cell function after transplantation unless they have donor B cell engraftment; lifelong immunoglobulin replacement therapy may therefore be necessary.[28] Failure to develop NK cell or B cell function is believed to be due to the defective function of the multiple cytokine receptors that share γ on the host cells (see Fig. 72-4).

Autosomal Recessive Severe Combined Immunodeficiency Caused by Interleukin 7 Receptor α Chain Deficiency

Pathogenesis and Etiology. Mice with mutated genes for either the α chain of the IL-7 receptor or of IL-7 itself are profoundly deficient in T and B cell function but have NK cell function. Thus, infants who had $T^-B^+NK^+$ SCID but not γc or Jak3 deficiency were screened for mutations in the IL7R α chain and IL-7 genes. Mutations in the IL-7Rα gene on chromosome 5p13 have been found in 24 of the first author's patients, making IL-7Rα deficiency the third most common type of SCID (see Fig. 72-3).[75,48] The lymphocyte phenotype in patients with IL-7Rα–deficient SCID is $T^-B^+NK^+$ (see Table 72-4), which suggests that the T cell but not the NK cell defect in SCID-X1 and Jak3-deficient SCID results from an inability to signal through the IL-7 receptor (see Fig. 72-4). Because these patients acquire normal B cell function after nonablative haploidentical bone marrow stem cell transplantation without donor B cells, the B cell defect in SCID-X1 probably is not due to failure of IL-7 signaling.

Autosomal Recessive Severe Combined Immunodeficiency Caused by Recombination-Activating Gene Product Deficiencies

Infants with autosomal recessive SCID caused by RAG-1 or RAG-2 protein deficiencies resemble all other infants with SCID in their infection susceptibility and complete absence of T or B cell function. Their lymphocyte phenotype, however, differs from that in patients with SCID caused by γc, Jak3, IL-7Rα, or ADA deficiencies in that they lack both B and T lymphocytes and have primarily NK cells in their circulation (see Table 72-4).[48] This pattern indicates a possible problem with antigen receptor gene rearrangement, and many infants with this lymphocyte phenotype have mutations in the genes encoding RAG-1 or RAG-2.[76-78]

Patients with Omenn syndrome also have mutations in *RAG1* or *RAG2* genes, which leads to partial and impaired V(D)J recombinational activity.[77,78] Omenn syndrome is characterized by the development soon after birth of a generalized erythroderma and desquamation, diarrhea, hepatosplenomegaly, and hypereosinophilia, with markedly elevated serum IgE levels. These clinical features are caused by circulating activated, oligoclonal T lymphocytes that do not respond normally to antigens in vitro. Circulating B cells are not found, and lymph node architecture is abnormal because of a lack of germinal centers. The condition is fatal unless corrected by bone marrow transplantation.[42]

Autosomal Recessive Severe Combined Immunodeficiency Caused by Deficiencies of the Artemis Gene Product

SCID also can result from mutations in the Artemis gene, on chromosome 10p, which encodes a novel V(D)J recombination/DNA repair factor that belongs to the metallo-β-lactamase superfamily.[78,79] A deficiency of this factor results in an inability to repair DNA after double-stranded cuts have been made by RAG-1 or RAG-2 in rearranging antigen receptor genes from their germline configuration. Similar to RAG-1/RAG-2–deficient SCID, this defect results in another form of $T^-B^-NK^+$ SCID (see Table 72-4), also called Athabascan SCID. Patients with Athabscan SCID exhibit increased radiation sensitivity in both skin fibroblasts and bone marrow cells.[78,79]

Autosomal Recessive Severe Combined Immunodeficiency Caused by Deficiencies of Ligase 4

Another cause of radiation-sensitive $T^-B^-NK^+$ SCID (see Box 72-1 and Table 72-4) is mutation in the ligase 4 gene (*LIG4*).[80] The *LIG4* gene product is necessary for catalyzing the ligation step in the nonhomologous end joining (NHEJ) pathway of DNA double-strand break (DSB) repair. Sequencing analysis of the *LIG4* gene in a female Turkish infant with $T^-B^-NK^+$ SCID who was not microcephalic and who had normal development revealed a homozygous deletion of three nucleotides, CAA, at nucleotide position 5333-5335 (National Center for Biotechnology Information [NCBI] designation AF479264). *LIG4* transcripts were present, but the absence of detectable ligase 4 suggested that the mutation affects protein stability. The mutations in *LIG4* that had been previously reported were hypomorphic and resulted in radiosensitivity and leukemia in two patients and in pancytopenia, microcephaly, and developmental and growth delay, collectively called the LIG4 syndrome, in eight other patients.[81]

Autosomal Recessive Severe Combined Immunodeficiency Caused by a Mutation in the Gene Encoding DNA-Dependent Protein Kinase, Catalytic Subunit

Another cause of radiation-sensitive $T^-B^-NK^+$ SCID is a mutation in the gene *PRKDC,* which encodes DNA-dependent protein kinase, catalytic subunit (DNA-PKcs).[82] For many years it was known that mutations in *PRKDC* cause murine SCID, but such mutations were not found in humans with SCID until 2009. Van der Berg and colleagues[82] reported the case of a girl diagnosed with $T^-B^-NK^+$ SCID when she was 5 months of age whose parents, of Turkish origin, were first-degree relatives. She was found to have a missense mutation in the *PRKDC* gene that did not interfere with DNA-PKcs protein expression, kinase activity, or DNA end-binding capacity, but did affect the quality of coding joins (with long stretches of P nucleotides) and overall end-joining activity.

Autosomal Recessive Severe Combined Immunodeficiency Caused by CD45 Deficiency

Another molecular defect causing T⁻B⁺NK⁺ SCID (see Box 72-1 and Table 72-4) is a mutation in the gene encoding the common leukocyte surface protein CD45.[83,84] This hematopoietic cell–specific transmembrane protein tyrosine phosphatase functions to regulate Src kinases required for T and B cell antigen receptor signal transduction. A 2-month-old male infant with SCID had a very low number of T cells but a normal number of B and NK cells. A large deletion was found at one CD45 allele, and a point mutation causing an alteration of the intervening sequence 13 donor splice site was identified at the other allele.[83] A second case of SCID due to CD45 deficiency has been reported,[84] but in both of these cases the patient is deceased. As recently reported by one of us (RHB and associates), a third example of this defect caused by uniparental disomy was successfully treated with a nonablated, T cell–depleted haploidentical parental bone marrow stem cell transplant.[85]

Autosomal Recessive Severe Combined Immunodeficiency Caused by Mutations in Genes Encoding Chains of the CD3 Complex

In 2003, Dadi and colleagues[86] reported that mutations in the gene encoding the δ chain of the CD3 complex cause SCID. Later, de Saint Basile and coworkers[87] studied three families with fetuses or infants who had SCID of unknown molecular type. All had the T⁻B⁺NK⁺ lymphocyte phenotype (see Table 72-4): They had no T cells but did have phenotypically normal B cells and NK cells—the same phenotype as in the SCID infants reported by Dadi's group.[86] Mutations in CD3δ chain were found in only two of the families. In the third family, a homozygous mutation in *CD3E*, the CD3ε gene, created a premature stop codon near the start of the extracellular domain, which resulted in the absence of CD3 expression. More recently, mutations in the CD3 ζ chain gene were found to also result in T⁻B⁺NK⁺ SCID (see Table 72-4).[88]

Hypomorphic mutations in the CD3ε gene had been previously reported in a 4-year-old boy who had recurrent *H. influenzae* pneumonia early in life but later became healthy.[89] His T cells had low expression of the CD3 complex but did respond to antigens. Defective expression of the T cell receptor (TCR) CD3 complex also was reported in two brothers in a Spanish family with mutations in the CD3γ gene (*CD3G*).[90] One of the siblings died at age 31 months with autoimmune hemolytic anemia and viral pneumonia, but the other was healthy. Both had very low expression of CD3 on their T cells but were capable of making antigen-specific responses and had IgG2 subclass deficiency.

SEVERE COMBINED IMMUNODEFICIENCY WITH LEUKOPENIA (RETICULAR DYSGENESIS)

In 1947, identical-twin male infants who exhibited a total lack of both lymphocytes and granulocytes in their peripheral blood and bone marrow were described. In a subsequent study of eight infants with this defect, seven died between 3 and 119 days of age from overwhelming infections; the eighth achieved complete immunologic reconstitution after a bone marrow transplant. In all affected infants who died, the thymus glands weighed less than 1 g, Hassall's corpuscles were absent, and few or no thymocytes were seen. Autosomal recessive mutations in the adenylate kinase 2 gene (*AK2*) have been identified as causing reticular dysgenesis.[91,92]

OTHER COMBINED IMMUNODEFICIENCIES

The term *combined immunodeficiency* (CID) is used to distinguish conditions marked by low but not absent T cell function from SCID. Three examples follow.

Purine Nucleoside Phosphorylase Deficiency

Epidemiology. More than 40 patients with CID have been identified as having purine nucleoside phosphorylase (PNP) deficiency.[93,69]

Pathogenesis and Etiology. The gene encoding PNP has been mapped to chromosomal locus 14q13.1 and has been cloned and sequenced. A variety of mutations in *PNP* cause deficiency of the protein.[69] Unlike in ADA deficiency, in PNP deficiency serum and urinary uric acid are deficient because PNP is needed to form the urate precursors hypoxanthine and xanthine.

Clinical Features. Some patients present with severe atopic disease, including anaphylactic reactions to foods. Two thirds of patients have neurologic abnormalities ranging from spasticity to mental retardation. One third of patients develop an autoimmune disease, most commonly autoimmune hemolytic anemia. Deaths have occurred from generalized vaccinia, varicella, lymphosarcoma, and graft-versus-host disease mediated by T cells from nonirradiated allogeneic blood or bone marrow.

Evaluation and Diagnosis. Most patients have elevated IgE and normal or elevated concentrations of all other serum immunoglobulins. PNP-deficient patients are as profoundly lymphopenic as those with ADA deficiency, with absolute lymphocyte counts usually less than 500/μL. Other abnormalities include a profound deficiency of T cells and of T cell subsets but an increased percentage of NK cells. T cell function is low but not absent and is variable with time.

Treatment and Prognosis. PNP deficiency is invariably fatal in childhood unless immunologic reconstitution can be achieved. Bone marrow transplantation is the treatment of choice but has thus far been successful in only a few patients.[42,94,95]

Ataxia-Telangiectasia

Ataxia-telangiectasia is a complex combined immunodeficiency syndrome with associated neurologic, endocrinologic, hepatic, and cutaneous abnormalities.[96]

Epidemiology. The incidence and prevalence of this condition are unknown, but it is thought to be rare. Inheritance of ataxia-telangiectasia follows an autosomal recessive pattern.

Pathogenesis and Etiology. The mutated gene responsible for this defect, *ATM* (ataxia-telangiectasia mutation), was mapped by restriction fragment length polymorphism analysis to the long arm of chromosome 11 (11q22-23) and was cloned.[96,97]

The gene product is related to phosphatidylinositol-3 kinase, an enzyme involved in signal transduction and glucose transport, and is thought to be involved in mitogenic signal transduction, meiotic recombination, and cell cycle control.[96] Cells from patients as well as from heterozygous carriers have increased sensitivity to ionizing radiation, defective DNA repair, and frequent chromosomal abnormalities. In more than 50% of the cases, the sites of chromosomal breakage involve genes that encode the T cell receptor on chromosome 7 and the immunoglobulin heavy chains on chromosome 14, most likely accounting for the combined T and B cell abnormalities seen. These rearrangements may be clonal and may either be stable or undergo malignant transformation.

Clinical Features. The most prominent features are progressive cerebellar ataxia, oculocutaneous telangiectasias, chronic sinopulmonary disease, a high incidence of malignancy, and variable humoral and cellular immunodeficiency. The ataxia typically becomes evident shortly after the child begins to walk and progresses until he or she is confined to a wheelchair, usually by the age of 10 to 12 years. The telangiectasias develop between 3 and 6 years of age. Recurrent sinopulmonary infections, usually bacterial, occur in approximately 80% of patients. Fatal varicella was observed in one patient. Transfusion-associated graft-versus-host disease also has been reported. The malignancies reported in this condition usually have been lymphoreticular, but adenocarcinoma and other forms also have been seen. An increased incidence of malignancy also is seen in unaffected relatives.

Evaluation and Diagnosis. Between 50% to 80% of affected patients have selective IgA deficiency. IgE concentrations are usually low, and IgM may be of the low-molecular-weight variety. IgG2 or total IgG may be decreased. Specific antibody titers may be decreased or normal. There is impaired (but not absent) cell-mediated immunity in vivo, and in vitro tests of lymphocyte function have generally shown moderately depressed proliferative responses to T and B cell mitogens. The percentages of $CD3^+$ and $CD4^+$ T cells are only modestly low, the number of $CD8^+$ T cells usually is normal or increased, and γ/δ T cell receptor–positive cell counts may be elevated. The thymus is hypoplastic, exhibits poor organization, and is lacking in Hassall's corpuscles. Radiation sensitivity can be demonstrated in cell lines in vitro.

Treatment and Prognosis. No satisfactory definitive treatment has been found.[96] The prognosis is exceedingly poor for patients with this condition, though some have reached adulthood. The most common causes of death are lymphoreticular malignancy and progressive neurologic disease.

Immunodeficiency with Thrombocytopenia and Eczema: Wiskott-Aldrich Syndrome

Epidemiology. Wiskott-Aldrich syndrome is an X-linked recessive syndrome characterized by atopic eczema, thrombocytopenic purpura with normal-appearing megakaryocytes but small defective platelets, and undue susceptibility to infection. The incidence and prevalence of this condition are unknown, but the condition is believed to be very rare.

Pathogenesis and Etiology. The mutated gene responsible for this defect was mapped to Xp11.22-11.23 and isolated in 1994 by Derry and coworkers.[98] Expression is limited to lymphocytic and megakaryocytic lineages.[98] The gene product, a 501-amino-acid proline-rich protein that lacks a hydrophobic transmembrane domain, was designated Wiskott-Aldrich syndrome protein (WASp). WASp interacts with more than 20 different proteins and functions as a signaling adaptor, but also participates in specialized modifications of the actin cytoskeletion in immune cells.[99] As such, WASp is considered an actin nucleation factor, which facilitates the addition of a single monomer of actin to an existing filament. This modification is essential for cell motility, changes in cell shape, and reorientation of certain cell surface receptors, which can be instrumental in forming the immunologic synapse. WASp is limited to expression in hematopoietic cells.

A large and varied number of mutations in the *WASP* gene may cause Wiskott-Aldrich syndrome, and the site of mutation has some correlation with severity of infection and susceptibility (see Fig. 72-1).[100] C-terminal truncations tend to result in severe phenotypes with greatly shortened patient survival, whereas amino-terminal (N-terminal) missense mutations often result in milder disease. The latter can initially manifest and persist as thrombocyopenia only (so-called X-linked thrombocytopenia), but the median duration of serious event–free survival is approximately 9 years. Certain unusual missense mutations in the middle of the protein can result in a neutropenia-only phenotype, labeled X-linked neutropenia.[101]

Carriers of *WASP* mutations can be identified by their having nonrandom X chromosome inactivation in several hematopoietic cell lineages or a mutated gene (if known in the family). Prenatal diagnosis of Wiskott-Aldrich syndrome also can be made if the family mutation is known. In one case, the syndrome was diagnosed in a girl was attributed to an X-linked defect of nonrandom X chromosome inactivation.[102] Characteristic diagnostic features of Wiskott-Aldrich syndrome include platelet counts below 70,000/μL and small platelets. Automated blood counting machines in clinical laboratories typically exclude small volume platelets from measurements, thereby artificially inflating mean platelet volume.

Clinical Features. Patients usually present during infancy with either prolonged bleeding from the circumcision site, bloody diarrhea, or excessive bruising. Atopic dermatitis and recurrent infections usually also develop during the first year of life. Asthma and other atopic diseases may also be seen. In younger patients, infections are usually those produced by pneumococci and other encapsulated bacteria, which result in otitis media, pneumonia, meningitis, or sepsis. Later, infections with opportunistic agents such as *P. jirovecii* and the herpesviruses typically become more problematic. Autoimmune cytopenias are common in patients who live beyond infancy. Vasculitis is a major problem in many older children with Wiskott-Aldrich syndrome. Survival beyond the teens is rare in the more severe forms of the syndrome without bone marrow transplantation; infections and bleeding may cause death, and a 12% incidence of fatal malignancy has been reported in patients with this condition.

Evaluation and Diagnosis. Patients with Wiskott-Aldrich syndrome have impaired humoral immune responses to polysaccharide antigens, as evidenced by absent or greatly diminished isohemagglutinins and poor or absent antibody responses to polysaccharide antigens.[103] In addition, antibody titers to protein antigens fall with time, and anamnestic responses are often poor or absent. Other abnormalities include an accelerated rate of synthesis as well as hypercatabolism of albumin, IgG, IgA, and IgM, which results in highly variable immunoglobulin concentrations. Most often serum IgM is low, IgA and IgE are elevated, and IgG concentration is normal or slightly low, with normal IgG2 levels. Percentages of $CD3^-$, $CD4^-$, and CD8-bearing T cells are moderately reduced, but NK cells are increased. Lymphocyte responses to mitogens are moderately depressed as is NK-cell-mediated cytolytic function.[104,105]

Treatment and Prognosis. In numerous patients with Wiskott-Aldrich syndrome, complete correction of both the platelet and the immunologic abnormalities has been achieved with HLA-identical sibling bone marrow transplants after preconditioning with irradiation or busulfan and cyclophosphamide.[42] Success has been minimal with use of T cell–depleted haploidentical stem cell transplants in Wiskott-Aldrich syndrome, but correction of the defect has been accomplished with use of matched related or matched unrelated donor (MUD) transplants when attempted in children younger than 5 years of age.[106] Based on success in in vitro transfection studies,[107] the first gene therapy trials for this condition were performed and initially were successful.[108] Insertional oncogenesis occurred with use of retroviral vectors, however, so additional studies are under way using modified lentiviral gene transfer vectors.[109]

The most common cause of death in patients with Wiskott-Aldrich syndrome currently is Epstein-Barr virus (EBV)-induced lymphoreticular malignancy. It has been hypothesized that development of such lesions is due in part to a deficiency of NK cell cytolytic function, which can be partially restored by administration of IL-2.[110]

T CELL ACTIVATION DEFECTS

These defects are characterized by normal or elevated numbers of blood T cells that appear phenotypically normal but fail to proliferate or produce cytokines normally in response to stimulation with mitogens, antigens, or other signals delivered to the TCR because of defective signal transduction from the TCR to intracellular metabolic pathways[111] (Fig. 72-7). This condition can be caused by mutations in genes for a variety of cell surface molecules or signal transduction molecules. These patients have problems similar to those of other T cell–deficient persons, and some with severe T cell activation defects may resemble patients with SCID clinically. Two examples are described next.

Defective Ca^{2+} Release–Activated Ca^{2+} Channels

Two male infants born to consanguineous parents had SCID-like infection susceptibility despite phenotypically normal blood lymphocytes. However, their T cells were unable to produce IL-2, interferon (IFN)-γ, IL-4, and TNF-α.[112] This problem was subsequently shown to be secondary to defective store-operated Ca^{2+} entry and Ca^{2+} release–activated Ca^{2+} (CRAC) channel function. The molecular defect responsible for this condition was recently discovered.[113] The two infants were found to be homozygous for a single missense mutation in the gene encoding a novel protein called Orai1. This protein contains four putative transmembrane segments. Expression of wild-type Orai1 in SCID T cells restored store-operated Ca^{2+} influx and the CRAC current. Orai1 may be an essential component or regulator of the CRAC channel complex.

ζ Chain–Associated Protein 70 Deficiency

Epidemiology. Most persons with ζ chain–associated protein 70 (ZAP-70) deficiency are Mennonites.[111,114] However, ZAP-70 deficiency has been associated with at least three other ethnicities and/or races.

Pathogenesis and Etiology. This condition is attributable to mutations in the gene encoding ZAP-70, a non-src family protein tyrosine kinase important in T cell signaling[111] (see Fig. 72-7). The gene is on chromosome 2 at position q12. ZAP-70 has an essential role in both positive and negative selection in the thymus. Numbers of $CD4^+$ T cells are normal, possibly because thymocytes can use the other member of the same tyrosine kinase family, Syk, to facilitate positive selection of $CD4^+$ cells. In addition, a stronger association of Lck with $CD4^+$ than with $CD8^+$ cells has been documented. Syk levels are four times higher in thymocytes than in peripheral T cells, which possibly accounts for the lack of normal responses by the $CD4^+$ blood T cells.

Clinical Features. Patients with $CD8^+$ lymphocytopenia caused by ZAP-70 deficiency present during infancy with severe, recurrent, sometimes fatal infections; however, they usually live longer and exhibit clinical (infectious) manifestations beginning at a later age than for patients with SCID.[111]

Evaluation and Diagnosis. These patients have normal, low, or elevated serum immunoglobulin concentrations and normal or elevated numbers of circulating $CD4^+$ T lymphocytes but essentially no $CD8^+$ cells. Their $CD4^+$ T cells fail to respond normally to mitogens or to allogeneic cells in vitro or to generate cytotoxic T lymphocytes. By contrast, NK activity is normal. The thymus of one patient exhibited normal architecture, with normal numbers of $CD4^+CD8^+$ (double-positive) thymocytes but an absence of $CD8^+$ (single-positive) thymocytes.

Treatment and Prognosis. The prognosis for individuals with this condition is poor unless successful immune reconstitution can be achieved through bone marrow transplantation. One of us (RHB) has corrected the defect in one such patient with a nonablated HLA-identical related donor transplant. Success with nonablated haploidentical transplants, however, has been more problematic.

DEFECTIVE EXPRESSION OF MAJOR HISTOCOMPATIBILITY COMPLEX ANTIGENS

Major Histocompatibility Complex Class I Antigen Deficiency

An isolated deficiency of MHC class I antigens is rare, and the resulting immunodeficiency is much milder than that in SCID; therefore, age at presentation is later, and clinical illness primarily relates to sinus and lung infections.[115] Sera from affected patients contain normal quantities of β_2-microglobulin, but class I MHC antigens are not detected on any cells in the body. There is a deficiency of $CD8^+$ but not $CD4^+$ T cells. Mutations have been found in two genes within the MHC locus on chromosome 6 that encode the peptide transporter proteins, TAP1 and TAP2 (see Box 72-1 and Fig. 72-1).[115-117] These proteins

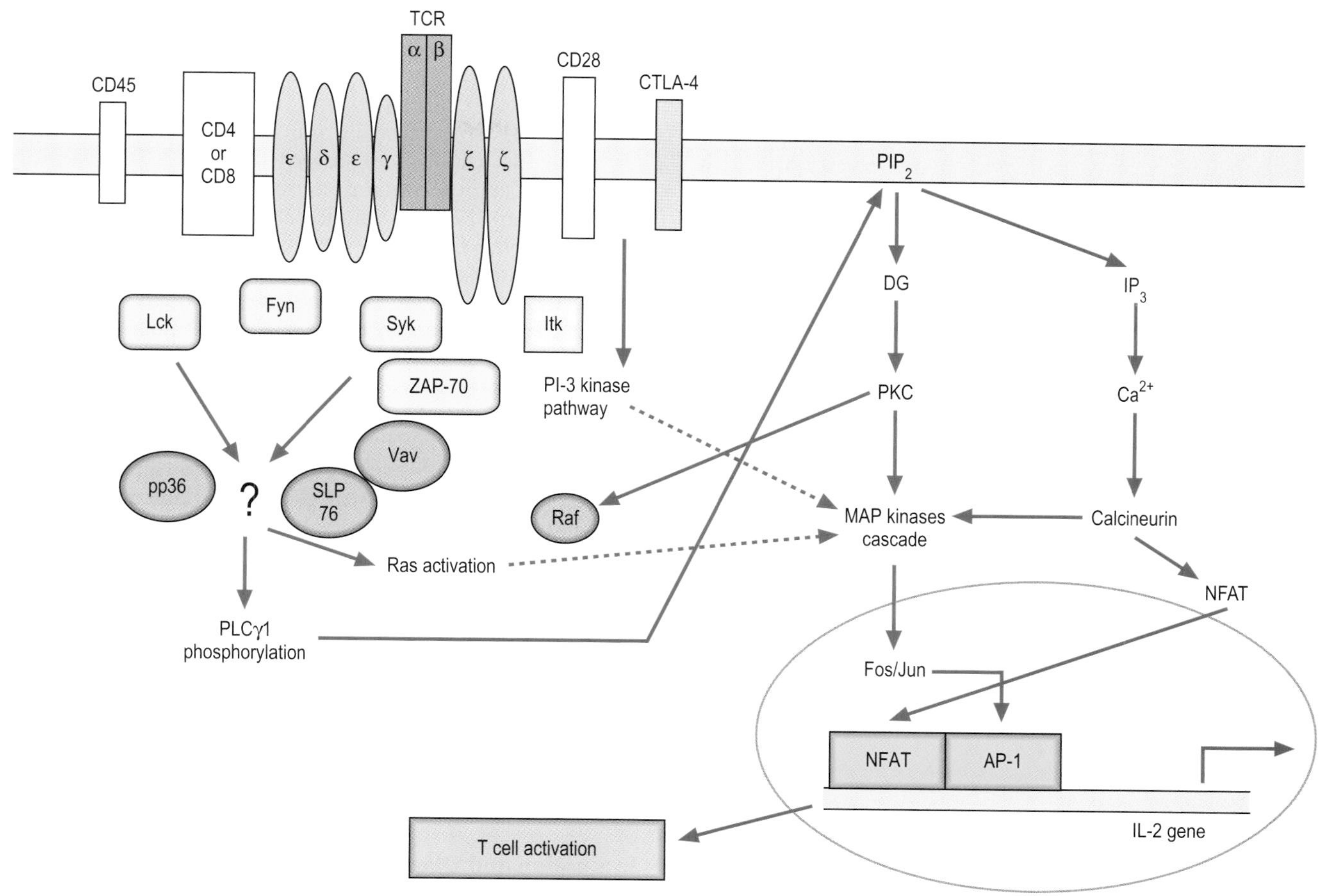

Figure 72-7 T cell signal transduction pathway. The T cell receptor (*TCR*) spans the plasma membrane in association with CD3 γ, δ, ε, and ζ and CD4 or CD8, CD28, and CD45. Cytoplasmic protein tyrosine kinases (PTKs) associated with the TCR are activated on antigen binding to the TCR. These PTKs include Lck, Fyn, zeta-associated protein 70 (*ZAP-70*), and Syk. PTK activation results in the phosphorylation of phospholipase Cγ 1 and the activation of other signaling molecules. Distal signaling events, including protein kinase C (*PKC*) activation and Ca^{2+} mobilization, result in the transcription of genes encoding interleukin (IL)-2 and other proteins, culminating in T cell activation, differentiation, and proliferation. Ionomycin and phorbol myristate acetate (PMA) can be used to mimic distal signaling events. Mutations in the gene encoding ZAP-70 result in greatly impaired T cell activation, in addition to abnormal thymic selection resulting in CD8 deficiency. *AP-1*, Activator protein 1; *CTLA-4*, cytotoxic T lymphocyte–associated protein 4; *DG*, diacyl glycerol; *IP₃*, inositol trisphosphate; *MAP*, mitogen-activated protein; *NFAT*, nuclear factor of activated T cells; *PI-3*, phosphatidylinositol-3; *PIP₂*, phosphatidyl inositol-bisphosphate; *PLCγ1*, phospholipase Cγ1; *SLP 76*, SH2 domain–containing leukocyte protein of 76 kD [lymphocyte cytosolic protein 2]. *(Modified from Elder ME. Severe combined immunodeficiency due to a defect in the tyrosine kinase ZAP-70. Pediatr Res 1996;39:744.)*

normally transport peptide antigens from the cytoplasm across the Golgi apparatus membrane to associate with the α chain of MHC class I molecules and β_2-microglobulin. The complex then moves to the cell surface; however, if the assembly of the complex cannot be completed because of a lack of peptide antigen, the MHC class I complex is destroyed in the cytoplasm. Clinically, patients have unusual granulomatous skin lesions that are rich in NK cells and can be physically deforming. Formation of such lesions is believed to be the result of some form of autoreactivity, because NK cells typically are restrained by killer cell immunoglobulin-like receptors (KIRs) that transmit an inhibitory signal after recognizing MHC class I.

Major Histocompatibility Complex Class II Antigen Deficiency

Epidemiology. Many persons affected with MHC class II antigen deficiency, inherited as an autosomal recessive trait, are of North African descent. More than 70 patients have been identified.

Pathogenesis and Etiology. Four different molecular defects resulting in impaired expression of MHC class II antigens have been identified (see Table 72-1 and Fig. 72-1).[118] One is a mutation in the gene on the long arm of chromosome 1 (1q) that encodes the protein RFX5, a subunit of RFX, a multiprotein complex that binds the X-box motif of MHC II promoters.[119] A second antigen deficiency is caused by mutations in a gene on 13q that encodes a second 36-kD subunit of the RFX complex, called RFX-associated protein (RFXAP).[120] The most common cause of MHC class II defects are mutations in *RFXANK*, the gene encoding a third subunit of RFX.[121] The fourth defect is a mutation in the gene on chromosome 16p13 that encodes a novel MHC class II transactivator (CIITA), a non–DNA-binding coactivator that controls the cell type specificity and inducibility of MHC II expression.[122] All of these defects cause impaired coordinate expression of MHC class II molecules on the surface of B cells and macrophages.[118]

Clinical Features. These patients present in infancy with persistent diarrhea often associated with cryptosporidiosis; bacterial pneumonia; *P. jirovecii*; septicemia; and viral or monilial infections. Nevertheless, the immunodeficiency is not as severe as in SCID, as evidenced by a failure to develop "BCG-osis" or graft-versus-host disease from nonirradiated blood transfusions.[118]

Evaluation and Diagnosis. MHC class II–deficient patients have a very low number of $CD4^+$ T cells but normal or elevated numbers of $CD8^+$ T cells. Lymphopenia is of only moderate severity. The MHC class II antigens, HLA-DP, -DQ, and -DR, are undetectable on blood B cells and monocytes. Patients have impaired antigen-specific responses caused by the absence of these antigen-presenting molecules. In addition, MHC antigen–deficient B cells fail to stimulate allogeneic cells in mixed leukocyte culture. Lymphocytes respond normally to mitogens but not to antigens. The thymus and other lymphoid organs are severely hypoplastic. The lack of class II molecules results in abnormal thymic selection, since recognition of HLA molecules by thymocytes is central to both positive and negative selection. The lack of normal selection results in circulating $CD4^+$ T cells that have altered CDR3 profiles. The associated defects of both B and T cell immunity and of HLA expression emphasize the important biologic role for HLA determinants in effective immune cell cooperation.

Treatment and Prognosis. The prognosis is poor. Bone marrow transplantation is the treatment of choice, but the rate of success has been very low.[42]

NUCLEAR FACTOR-κB ESSENTIAL MODULATOR DEFICIENCY

Epidemiology. Nuclear factor-κB essential modulator (NEMO) deficiency is a syndrome involving a diverse array of immunologic defects and frequently is characterized by the presence of anhidrotic ectodermal dysplasia (EDA with immunodeficiency [EAD-ID]).[39,123] It is considered to be rare, but population data on incidence or prevalence are lacking.

Pathogenesis and Etiology. The condition results from hypomorphic mutations (partial loss of function) in the *IKBKG* gene at position 28q on the X chromosome. *IKBKG* encodes NEMO (also called IKKγ, the IκB kinase γ subunit), which is a regulatory protein that serves as a scaffold for two kinases necessary for activation of the transcription factor NF-κB. Activation of NF-κB by proinflammatory stimuli or ligation of innate danger-sensing receptors, such as Toll-like receptors, leads to increased expression of genes involved in inflammation, including TNF-α and IL-12. B cells from NEMO-deficient patients fail to undergo class switch recombination, because TNF superfamily receptors, which include CD40, require NF-κB to function. Signaling through NEMO and NF-κB also is necessary for signaling of the ectodysplasin receptor, which is a TNF superfamily receptor required for normal development of ectodermal tissues. Many types of mutations in NEMO interrupt the activation of NF-κB downstream of this receptor and cause ectodermal dysplasia. Germline loss-of-function mutations cause the X-linked dominant condition incontinentia pigmenti in females, and inheritance of large deletion mutations in NEMO is lethal to male fetuses. A similar but less common syndrome, EDA-ID, occurs secondary to hypermorphic mutations in the *NFKBIA* gene encoding the inhibitor of NF-κB (IκB).[124] EDA-ID has been inherited as an autosomal dominant condition, and the mutations interrupt NEMO function because IκB is a target of the kinase complex directed by NEMO. The mutated IκB cannot be phosphorylated and thus serves a persistent inhibitory function in the NF-κB activation pathway. Although patients with EDA-ID are far fewer in number, they do phenocopy NEMO deficiency.

Clinical Features. The ectodermal dysplasia in NEMO deficiency is characterized by frontal bossing, fine sparse hair, oligodontia, conical incisors, hypopigmentation, and hypohidrosis due to deficient eccrine sweat glands. The presence of ectodermal dysplasia is not required for diagnosis, however, and at least one third of patients have immunodeficiency without obvious signs of ectodermal dysplasia.[40] Because the disease-causing mutations in NEMO deficiency are hypomorphic, numerous clinical and immunologic associations between genotypes and particular phenotypes exist (Table 72-5). For example, mutations affecting the NEMO leucine zipper tend not to cause ectodermal dysplasia but do result in immunodeficiency.[40] The variety in associations probably results from individual molecular interactions of the NEMO protein with components of particular signaling pathways.

Evaluation and Diagnosis. The immunodeficiency in NEMO deficiency is variable (see Table 72-5), with most patients showing impaired antibody responses to polysaccharide antigens.[40] Some patients present with hyper IgM syndrome as a consequence of interrupted CD40 function. Generally, these patients possess mutations affecting the extreme C terminus of the NEMO protein. A major immunologic abnormality in NEMO deficiency is interruption of innate immunity, and a majority of patients have defective functions of Toll-like receptors that help detect pathogen-associated molecular patterns and initiate inflammatory responses. As a result, affected patients incur more substantial bacterial infections than patients with antibody deficiency only.

Treatment and Prognosis. Because of the diverse abnormalities in NEMO deficiency, the disease typically is quite severe. Since the diagnosis was established in 2000, approximately one-third of diagnosed patients have died. Despite this, there have been therapeutic successes in NEMO deficiency. Patients benefit from a multifaceted approach, including immunoglobulin replacement as well as prophylactic antibiotics to protect against atypical mycobacteria, *P. jirovecii*, and pyogenic bacterial infections. Mycobacterial infection in patients with NEMO deficiency is very difficult to treat and typically requires extended multidrug regimens that are of limited success.[125,40] In addition, susceptibility to DNA viral infections also has been observed; specific antiviral prophylaxis can therefore be helpful in patients with a history of exposure or infection. Cytokine therapies also have been used in NEMO deficiency: IFN-γ may have had some utility in mycobacterial disease, and IL-2 may improve defective NK cell functions.[125,126] Stem cell transplantation has been performed for NEMO deficiency and has been successful,

TABLE 72-5 Clinical and Immunologic Features in NEMO Deficiency

Functional/Clinical Category	Frequency (% of Patients Affected)
Ectodermal dysplasia	77
Osteopetrosis	8
Lymphedema	8
Small for gestational age	14
Autoimmune/inflammatory disease	24
Death	36
Infection susceptibility	98
Bacterial infection	87
Mycobacterial infection	44
Pneumocystis pneumonia	8
DNA virus infection	21
Meningitis or encephalitis	21
Pneumonia	31
Sepsis/bacteremia	33
Abscess	30
Hyper-IgM	15
Hypogammaglobulinemia	59
Hyper-IgA	37
Hyper-IgD	40
Specific antibody deficiency	64
Pneumococcal antibody deficiency	81
Deficient B cell costimulation/CD40 signaling	94
Deficient TNF response	82
Deficient IL-1 response	86
Deficient TLR response	64
Deficient NK cell function	100

Adapted from Hanson EP, Monaco-Shawver L, Solt LA, et al. Hypomorphic NEMO mutation database and reconstitution system identifies phenotypic and immunologic diversity. J Allergy Clin Immunol 2008;112:1169-77.

IgA, IgG, IgM, Immunoglobulins A, G, M; *IL,* interleukin; *NEMO,* nuclear factor-κB essential modulator; *NK,* natural killer; *TLR,* Toll-like receptor; *TNF,* tumor necrosis factor.

especially in the case of an HLA-matched sibling donor, but failures have been more common than might be expected.[127] Thus caution is necessary in considering transplantation.

CD8 DEFICIENCY DUE TO A MUTATION IN THE CD8α GENE

Another cause for CD8 deficiency, in addition to ZAP-70 deficiency and MHC class I antigen deficiency, was discovered in a 25-year-old Spanish man with a history of recurrent respiratory infections since childhood. Immunoglobulins and antibodies were normal, as were T cell proliferation and NK cell function. However, the man had a complete absence of $CD8^+$ T cells. Molecular studies revealed a missense mutation in both alleles of the immunoglobulin domain of the CD8α gene in the patient and in two of his sisters.[128,129]

CARTILAGE-HAIR HYPOPLASIA

Epidemiology. In 1965, an unusual form of short-limbed dwarfism with frequent and severe infections, termed cartilage-hair hypoplasia (CHH), was reported among the Pennsylvania Amish; non-Amish cases have since been described.

Pathogenesis and Etiology. CHH is an autosomal recessive condition, and the defective gene was mapped to chromosomal region 9p21-p13 in Amish and Finnish families. Numerous mutations have been found in the untranslated *RMRP* gene that cosegregates with the CHH phenotype.[130] The gene product, endoribonuclease RNase MRP (RNA component of mitochondrial RNA-processing endoribonuclease), consists of an RNA molecule bound to several proteins. It has at least two functions: cleavage of RNA in mitochondrial DNA synthesis and nucleolar cleaving of pre-RNA. Mutations in *RMRP* cause CHH by disrupting a function of RNase MRP RNA that affects multiple organ systems.[130]

Clinical Features. Patients with CHH have short, pudgy hands with redundant skin, metaphyseal chondrodysplasia, hyperextensible joints of hands and feet but an inability to extend the elbows completely, and fine, sparse light hair and eyebrows. As seen with radiography, the bones have scalloping and sclerotic or cystic changes in the metaphyses. In contrast with ADA deficiency, in which the predominant changes are in the apophyses of the iliac bones, the ribs, and vertebral bodies, the chondrodysplasia in CHH is principally in the limbs. Severe and often fatal varicella infections, progressive vaccinia, and vaccine-associated poliomyelitis have occurred in patients with CHH. Associated conditions include deficient erythrogenesis, Hirschsprung disease, and an increased risk of malignancies. Patients with milder types of immune deficiency have lived to adulthood, some even to old age.

Evaluation and Diagnosis. Three patterns of immune dysfunction have been identified: defective antibody-mediated immunity, defective cellular immunity (most common form), and SCID. However, NK cells are increased in number and function.

Treatment and Prognosis. Bone marrow transplantation has resulted in immunologic reconstitution in some CHH patients with the SCID phenotype.[55]

HYPERIMMUNOGLOBULINEMIA E SYNDROME

The hyperimmunoglobulinemia E (hyper-IgE) syndrome is a relatively rare primary immunodeficiency syndrome characterized by recurrent severe staphylococcal abscesses of the skin (Fig. 72-8), lungs, and viscera and greatly elevated levels of serum IgE.[131,132] Both dominant and recessive forms have been reported.

Autosomal Dominant Hyper-IgE Syndrome

Epidemiology. In 1972, two young boys were reported as having hyper-IgE syndrome.[131] Early observations suggested that the condition was characterized by autosomal dominant inheritance: Eight families in a Duke series of 42 patients had more than 1 affected member, usually members of successive generations,[132] as did five families among the 30 patients in a

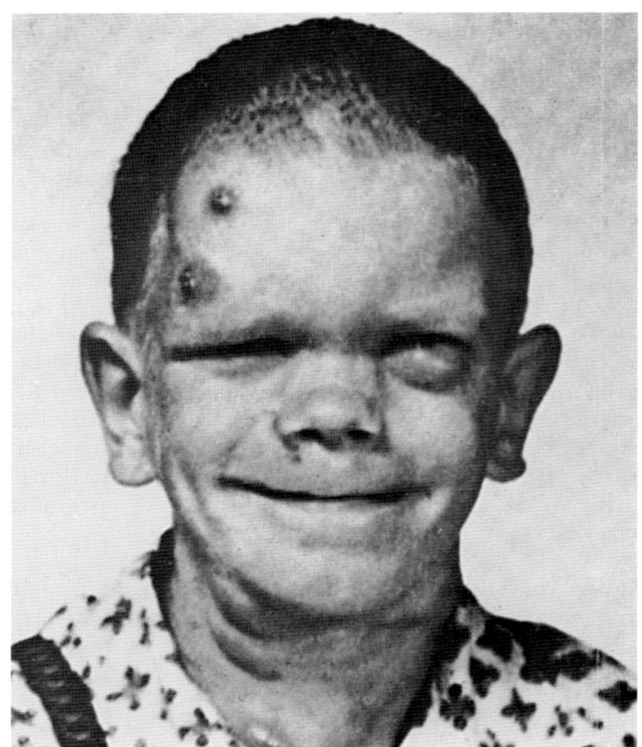

Figure 72-8 Patient with hyper-immunoglobulinemia E (hyper-IgE) syndrome with characteristic coarse facial features. Multiple abscesses of the face and neck are evident. *(From Buckley RH, Wray BB, Belmaker EZ. Extreme hyperimmunoglobulinemia E and undue susceptibility to infection. Pediatrics 1972;49:59.)*

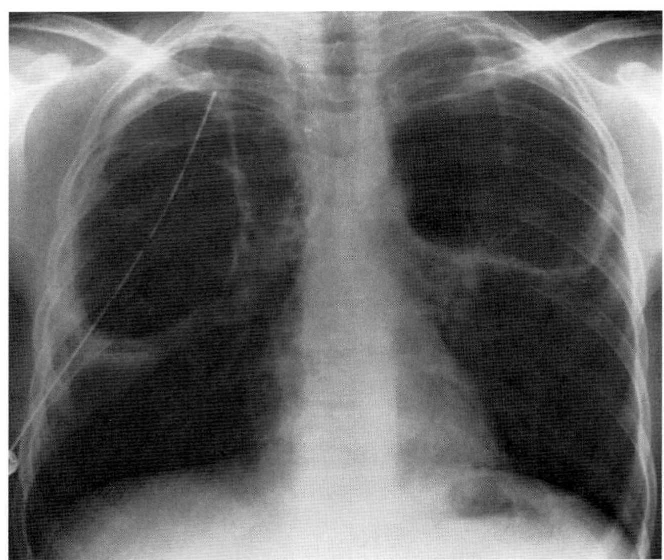

Figure 72-9 Chest roentgenogram of a 12-year-old boy with hyper-immunoglobulinemia E (hyper-IgE) syndrome. Giant pneumatoceles were present for more than 1 year. A putrid abscess caused by *Enterobacter cloacae* necessitated chest tube insertion on the right. Left cyst required emergency excision because of massive hemoptysis and was found to contain an aspergilloma.

National Institutes of Health (NIH) series.[133] Members of both sexes and several races have been affected.

Pathogenesis and Etiology. Autosomal dominant hyper-IgE syndrome is almost always caused by dominant negative heterozygous mutations in the gene encoding the STAT3 (signal transducer and activator of transcription 3) protein.[134,135] STAT3 is a member of a family of six highly conserved proteins that transmit signals from cell surface receptor complexes to the nucleus, bind to each other and to other proteins, and bind to DNA and turn on or off specific genes. STAT3 is a key mediator for many pathways, including those of the immune system, cancer, wound healing, and vascular remodeling, and it is expressed widely in most tissue types. Precisely how mutations in this gene cause all of the features of this condition is not entirely clear, but affected patients lack Th17 T cells.[136] IL-17 has an evolving role in immunology and is the subject of much study. Mice that lack IL-17 have a propensity to candidal and extracellular bacterial infections. In addition, IL-17 is thought to be involved in antimicrobial peptide expression and neutrophil recruitment. Thus the absence of IL-17 in this syndrome may help explain some of the infection susceptibility.

Clinical Features. Patients with autosomal dominant hyper-IgE syndrome have a history of staphylococcal abscesses involving the skin, lungs, joints, and other sites from infancy onward. Persistent pneumatoceles develop as a result of recurrent pneumonias (Fig. 72-9 and Table 72-6). Pruritic dermatitis that is not typical atopic eczema occurs but does not always persist. Respiratory tract allergic symptoms are usually absent. Patients with this syndrome look very different from their nonaffected family members: Coarse or distinct facial features are typical.[131,133] Among the reported characteristics were a prominent forehead, deep-set eyes, a broad nasal bridge, a wide fleshy nasal tip, mild prognathism, and facial asymmetry and hemihypertrophy. Grimbacher and associates have reported that the mean nasal interalar distance in these patients was above the 98th percentile ($P < .001$). These features were present in all patients in the study by the age of 16 years.[133] High incidence rates for scoliosis and hyperextensible joints also were noted. In this group of patients, 72% had primary teeth that either failed to shed or were delayed in shedding because of lack of root resorption.[133] Unexplained osteopenia also is present in most cases of autosomal dominant hyper-IgE syndrome, and affected patients have problems with recurrent fractures from even minor trauma.[132,133]

TABLE 72-6 Distinctive Features of the Two Major Types of Hyper-IgE Syndrome

Features Present in the Autosomal Dominant Hyper-IgE Syndrome Missing in the Autosomal Recessive Form	Features Present in the Autosomal Recessive Hyper-IgE Syndrome Missing in the Autosomal Dominant Form
Unusual facial features	Severe skin viral infections
Pneumatoceles	Frequent neurologic complications
Osteopenia with fractures	Severe allergies
Delayed shedding of baby teeth	T cell proliferation defects
	Early death

hyper-IgE, Hyper-immunoglobulinemia E.

Evaluation and Diagnosis. Laboratory features of the syndrome include exceptionally high serum IgE (2000 to 130,000 IU/mL); elevated serum IgD; normal concentrations of IgG, IgA, and IgM; pronounced blood and sputum eosinophilia; abnormally low anamnestic antibody responses to booster immunizations; and poor antibody-mediated and cell-mediated responses to neoantigens. Percentages of blood lymphocytes are normal except for a decreased percentage of T cells with the memory (CD45RO) phenotype. It is possible that this decrease is related to impaired anamnestic antibody responses, impaired antigen-specific T cell responses, and abnormal mixed leukocyte responses. Paradoxically, B cells from these patients do not produce as much IgE as normal or atopic B cells do when they are cultured with IL-4 and anti-CD40 in vitro.[137] The latter finding indicates that the B cells may have already been exposed to IL-4 in vivo. Most patients have normal lymphocyte-proliferative responses to mitogens but very low or absent responses to antigens or allogeneic cells from family members. Blood, sputum, and histologic sections of lymph nodes, spleen, and lung cysts have striking eosinophilia. In a postmortem examination of one patient, Hassall's corpuscles and normal thymic architecture were observed. Phagocytic cell ingestion, metabolism, killing, and total hemolytic complement activity have been normal in all patients. Variable defects of mononuclear or polymorphonuclear chemotaxis have been present in some but not all patients and are therefore not the basic problem in this syndrome.[132]

Treatment and Prognosis. The most effective management for the autosomal dominant condition is long-term therapy with a penicillinase-resistant penicillin or cephalosporin, with the addition of other antibiotics or antifungal agents as required for specific infections, and appropriate thoracic surgery for superinfected pneumatocoeles or those persisting beyond 6 months.[132] Neither IFN-γ therapy nor bone marrow transplantation is of any clinical benefit. The prognosis is good if the diagnosis is made early and appropriate doses of antistaphylococcal antibiotic therapy are rendered continuously. Three patients are known to have died of lymphoreticular malignancy, and three have had cryptococcal meningitis.

Autosomal Recessive Hyper-IgE Syndrome

Epidemiology. Renner and associates first described this syndrome in 2004 in 13 patients.[138] Five years later, Zhang and coworkers[139] reported 11 additional cases in patients who had been diagnosed as having combined immunodeficiency but in whom clinical findings were very similar to those in the initially reported series and who had mutations in the gene encoding the dedicator of cytokinesis 8 (DOCK8). One month later, Engelhardt and colleagues[140] described 21 patients diagnosed with autosomal recessive hyper-IgE syndrome who had mutations in the DOCK8 gene. Many of the latter patients also were included in the paper by Zhang and coworkers.[139] Of the 33 distinct patients reported, 25 were from Turkey, 2 each were from Mexico and Iran, and one each was from Lebanon, Oman, Italy, and Ireland. Thus this condition is not likely to be seen in the United States with any significant frequency.

Pathogenesis and Etiology. With the exception of one patient, who had a mutation in the gene encoding Tyk2,[141] all of the other reported patients with autosomal recessive hyper-IgE syndrome had mutations in the gene encoding DOCK8, which is on chromosome 9.[139,140] DOCK8 is a member of the 11-member DOCK protein family.[140] DOCK8 is likely to function as a guanine exchange factor (GEF) for the Rho guanosine triphosphatases (Rho-GTPases) Cdc42 and Rac1. GTPase activation induces dynamic filamentous actin rearrangements and lamellipodia formation, leading to cell growth, migration, and adhesion. DOCK8 may be important for the formation of the immunologic synapse that leads to T cell activation, proliferation, and differentiation.[140]

Clinical Features. A large majority of patients with autosomal recessive hyper-IgE syndrome have severe atopic dermatitis, asthma, and food allergies. They also can have recurrent skin viral infections, including severe herpes simplex, herpes zoster, molluscum contagiosum, and papillomavirus skin infections (see Table 72-6). In addition, patients can have abscesses, candidiasis, upper respiratory infections, and pneumonia. Neurologic problems, including strokes, meningitis, and aneurysms, are prominent. Malignancies also are common. Patients do not have pneumatoceles, a history of fractures, unusual facial features, or delayed shedding of the baby teeth, as seen with the autosomal dominant form of the hyper-IgE syndrome (see Table 72-6).

Evaluation and Diagnosis. Most patients with autosomal recessive hyper-IgE syndrome have severe atopy with anaphylaxis, elevated serum IgE levels, and eosinophilia. They also have lymphopenia with low T cell numbers and function and low serum IgM levels and exhibit variable IgG antibody responses.

Treatment and Prognosis. The prognosis with the autosomal recessive form of the hyper-IgE syndrome is much poorer than with the autosomal dominant form, and most patients die early (see Table 72-6). The treatment of choice is allogeneic bone marrow transplantation.[140]

THYMIC HYPOPLASIA: DIGEORGE SYNDROME

Epidemiology. DiGeorge syndrome occurs in both males and females and is relatively more common than other T cell immunodeficiencies.

Pathogenesis and Etiology. Dysmorphogenesis of the third and fourth pharyngeal pouches during early embryogenesis leads to hypoplasia or aplasia of the thymus and parathyroid glands.[142] Many patients have microdeletions of specific DNA sequences from 22q11.2 (the DiGeorge chromosomal region), where several candidate genes have been identified.[142] The T-box transcription factor 1 (TBX1) can be mutated in isolation and recapitulate the syndrome.[143] Another chromosomal deletion associated with DiGeorge and velocardiofacial syndromes has been identified on 10p13.[144]

Clinical Features. The diagnosis can be suspected with hypocalcemic seizures or recognition of a characteristic cardiac defect during the neonatal period. A variable degree of hypoplasia is more frequent than total aplasia of the thymus and parathyroid glands. As a result, a majority of children with DiGeorge syndrome have "partial" DiGeorge syndrome and have little trouble with life-threatening infections, grow normally, and are mostly affected by cognitive developmental abnormalities.[145] The small percentage with immunologically severe (complete) DiGeorge syndrome may resemble patients with SCID in their susceptibility to infections with opportunistic pathogens (i.e., fungi, viruses, and *P. jirovecii*) and to graft-versus-host disease (GVHD) from nonirradiated blood transfusions.

Evaluation and Diagnosis. Patients with DiGeorge syndrome usually are only mildly lymphopenic.[145] However, they do have variable reductions in the proportion of T cells, which result in a relative increase in the proportion of B cells. B cell function is impaired only when helper T cells are needed. Immunoglobulin concentrations are usually normal, though sometimes IgE is elevated and IgA is low. Total $CD3^+$ T cells are decreased among blood lymphocytes, but usually the proportions of $CD4^+$ and $CD8^+$ cells are normal. The ratio of naïve to memory T cells is reduced, whereas in healthy young children the ratio normally is relatively high. Blood lymphocyte responses after mitogen stimulation are absent, reduced, or normal, depending on the degree of thymic deficiency, and such variability suggests that the T lymphocytes that are present are intrinsically normal.

Treatment and Prognosis. No immunologic treatment is needed for the partial form of DiGeorge syndrome. Patients with immunologically severe (complete) DiGeorge syndrome have experienced successful immunologic reconstitution after transplantation of unrelated donor mature thymic tissue explants.[146]

Diseases of Immune Dysregulation

X-LINKED LYMPHOPROLIFERATIVE DISEASE

Epidemiology. X-linked lymphoproliferative disease (XLP), or Duncan disease, is caused by a recessive trait and characterized by an abnormal immune response to infection with EBV, which results in (usually) fatal malignant or nonmalignant immune cell proliferation or in immunodeficiency syndromes.[147]

Pathogenesis and Etiology. The defective gene in XLP was localized to the Xq26-q27 region, cloned, and identified as *SH2D1A*.[148,149] This form of XLP is now referred to as XLP-1. *SH2D1A* is expressed in many tissues involved in immune system functioning. The gene encodes a novel T cell–specific adaptor protein composed of a single SH2 domain. It functions as an inhibitory adaptor protein for a high affinity self-ligand called signaling lymphocyte activation molecule (SLAM), which is present on the surfaces of T and B cells. The adaptor protein, called SAP (for SLAM-associated protein) or SH2D1A, normally inhibits signal transduction by SLAM, so that T cell proliferation does not continue unchecked in response to EBV and possibly other types of infections. Inboys who have mutations in *SH2D1A,* this signaling fails to occur. SH2D1A also associates with 2B4 on NK cells,[150] a receptor capable of providing an activation signal after ligation by CD48, which is induced on EBV-infected B cells. In patients with SAP-deficient XLP, ligation of 2B4 on NK cells fails to initiate cytotoxicity. Nevertheless, CD2- or CD16-induced cytotoxicity of SAP-deficient NK cells is similar to that of normal NK cells. Thus selective impairment of 2B4-mediated NK cell activation may contribute to the immunopathology of XLP.[150] Patients with XLP also lack NK T cells, which raises the possibility that this specialized T cell population has roles in immune regulation and defense against EBV.

Clinical Features. Affected boys are apparently healthy until they acquire infectious mononucleosis. XLP-1 has three major phenotypes: fulminant infectious mononucleosis (50%), B cell lymphomas (20%), and hypogammaglobulinemia (30%). The mononucleosis is fatal primarily because of extensive liver necrosis caused by polyclonally activated $CD8^+$ cytotoxic T cells that recognize EBV-infected autologous B cells. The mean age at presentation is under 5 years.

Evaluation and Diagnosis. In most patients surviving the primary infection, lymphomas or hypogammaglobulinemia develops subsequently. In addition, NK function is markedly depressed.[150] Patients with mutations in *SH2D1A* may present as having common variable immunodeficiency, even without antecedent EBV infection. Although *SH2D1A* mutations are infrequent among large cohorts of patients with CVID, male siblings in one arm of two separate pedigrees with *SH2D1A* mutations had only CVID, whereas in another arm of each pedigree, male siblings presented with fulminant infectious mononucleosis.[151] The finding of *SH2D1A* mutations in both arms of each family indicates that XLP must be considered in male patients with CVID. Systemic vasculitis, hypogammaglobulinemia, and hemophagocytic lymphohistiocytosis can occur with XLP.

Treatment and Prognosis

Approximately one half of the limited number of patients with XLP given HLA-identical related or unrelated unfractionated bone marrow transplants are currently surviving, without any signs of the disease.[42]

OTHER FORMS OF X-LINKED LYMPHOPROLIFERATIVE DISEASE

A second molecular cause of XLP, also referred to as XLP-2, has been identified. The product of the responsible gene, *XIAP* (also known as *BIRC4*), is the X-linked inhibitor of apoptosis[152] The clinical presentations and immunologic defects of XLP-1 and XLP-2 are more similar than not, but patients with XLP-1 have a high incidence of lymphoma, whereas patients with XLP-2 are far more likely to present with recurrent fevers, cytopenias, and splenomegaly.[153]

An autosomal recessive syndrome similar to XLP-1 and XLP-2 has been recently identified in two girls from a consanguineous Turkish family. They possessed missense mutations in the inducible T cell kinase (IKT) gene and suffered from fatal EBV infection–driven lymphoproliferation.[154]

Immune Dysregulation, Polyendocrinopathy, Enteropathy, X-linked (IPEX) Syndrome

Epidemiology. Immune dysregulation, polyendocrinopathy, enteropathy, X-linked (IPEX) syndrome is an X-linked recessive immunologic disorder characterized by multisystem autoimmunity.

Pathogenesis and Etiology. The condition is due to mutations in the forkhead box P3 gene (*FOXP3*) at Xp11.23, which encodes a forkhead domain-containing protein, Foxp3.[155] Foxp3 is expressed predominantly in the $CD4^+CD25^{high}$ subset of regulatory T cells (Tregs), and studies in mutant mice indicate that Foxp3 is essential for the development of Tregs.

Clinical Features. Infants with IPEX syndrome most commonly present with early-onset type 1 diabetes mellitus, moderate to severe recurrent infections caused by *Enterococcus* and *Staphylococcus* spp., and severe enteropathy with watery and often bloody diarrhea associated with eosinophilic inflammation and an eczematous dermatitis.

Evaluation and Diagnosis. The number and phenotype of $CD4^{+}CD25^{high}$ T cells appear to be normal in patients with IPEX syndrome, but either Foxp3 is lacking in these cells or a mutant Foxp3 protein associated with abnormal regulatory function is present.[156] The findings suggest that Foxp3 has a key role in maintaining self-tolerance and preventing autoimmune and allergic diseases.

Treatment and Prognosis. Because IPEX syndrome can be both extreme and severe in its clinical presentation, immunosuppression is the main therapeutic option. A variety of agents have been used, but particular success has been achieved with siroliumus. In patients with severe symptoms, allogeneic stem cell transplantation has been performed successfully in some instances.[157]

Autoimmune Polyendocrinopathy–Candidiasis–Ectodermal Dysplasia

Patients with autoimmune polyendocrinopathy–candidiasis–ectodermal dysplasia (APECED) present with chronic mucocutaneous candidiasis and polyendocrinopathy, usually involving the parathyroid or adrenal glands and less frequently affecting the thyroid, liver, and skin. APECED, also called autoimmune polyendocrinopathy syndrome type I (APS1), is due to a mutation in the autoimmune regulator (*AIRE*) gene.[158] The gene product, AIRE, is expressed at high levels in purified human thymic medullary stromal cells and is thought to regulate the cell surface expression of tissue-specific proteins such as insulin and thyroglobulin. Expression of these self-proteins allows for the negative selection of autoreactive T cells during their development. Failure of negative selection results in organ-specific autoimmune destruction. The overall significance of AIRE in establishing and maintaining T cell self-tolerance is not well understood. The susceptibility to chronic candidal infections has been hypothesized to be due to preferential generation of autoantibodies directed against IL-17,[159,160] which is a central factor in anticandidal immunity. The reason for preferential generation of these particular autoantibodies is unclear, but it may relate to a role for AIRE in innate signaling after *Candida* recognition.[161]

Chronic Mucocutaneous Candidiasis

Epidemiology. Chronic mucocutaneous candidiasis (CMC) represents the chronic infection of mucous membranes and skin by the fungal pathogen *Candida*. The incidence and prevalence of this condition are unknown.

Pathogenesis and Etiology. The number of gene defects known to result in the CMC phenotype is growing. Two autosomal recessive forms are due to mutations in genes that encode the IL-17A or IL-17F cytokines.[160] Patients with APECED syndrome have autoantibodies directed against IL-17A or IL-17F cytokines. An autosomal dominant form of CMC is due to particular *STAT1* gene mutations.[162] The mutations lead to aberrant T helper cell subset 17 (Th17) responses but differ clinically from autosomal recessive loss-of-function STAT1 mutations that lead to other infection susceptibilities, such as to atypical mycobacteria. Patients with homozygous CARD9 mutations have a more severe fungal susceptibility than typical patients with CMC. Two patients have had fungal sepsis in addition to CMC, and dermatophyte infections also were present.[163]

Clinical Features. Although oral candidiasis can occur in normal infants, patients with CMC are chronically affected and remain so well beyond the first year of life. Susceptibility to candidal infection occurs in a variety of T cell deficiencies, but patients with CMC generally do not have other infectious difficulties characteristic of T cell defects. These patients do not have clinically apparent infections with other yeasts or fungal pathogens.

Evaluation and Diagnosis. Some patients with CMC exhibit decreased *Candida*-induced lymphocyte proliferation, but many do not. More recent studies suggest that symptoms are caused by impairments in the IL-17 cytokine pathway of Th-17 cells, and that this cytokine is required for *Candida* control.

Treatment and Prognosis. Although CMC can be quite bothersome, the infections are limited to mucosal surfaces and therefore can be treated directly. Once treatment is stopped, however, the infection returns. Consequently, continual prophylaxis with topical or systemic antifungal agents is frequently used.

Autoimmune Lymphoproliferative Syndrome

Epidemiology. The incidence and prevalence of autoimmune lymphoproliferative syndrome (ALPS) are unknown.

Pathogenesis and Etiology. The most frequent genetic causes of ALPS are germline-dominant, heterozygous mutations in the *TNFRSF6* (TNF receptor superfamily member 6) gene (in ALPS type Ia), which encodes CD95 (also known as Fas), a mediator of apoptosis. Somatic mutations in the gene also have been found. Other causes are mutations in genes encoding either the CD95 ligand (in ALPS type Ib), caspase 10 (in ALPS type IIa), or caspase 8 (in ALPS type IIb). These causative mechanisms of ALPS underscore the critical role of cell surface receptor–mediated apoptosis in eliminating redundant proliferating lymphocytes with autoreactive and oncogenic potential.

Clinical Features. ALPS is a disorder of apoptosis in which the inability of lymphocytes to die leads to nonmalignant massive lymphadenopathy, hypersplenism, and autoimmune cytopenias of childhood onset.[164]

Penetrance and range of disease manifestations in ALPS are highly variable, even among family members who share the same dominant *TNFRSF6* mutation.[164]

Evaluation and Diagnosis. Consistent immunologic findings include polyclonal hypergammaglobulinemia and an expansion of T cells lacking either CD4 or CD8 on their surfaces (i.e., double-negative T cells).

Treatment and Prognosis. Although most episodes of cytopenias respond to courses of conventional immunomodulatory agents, massive splenomegaly may require splenectomy and/or ongoing immunosuppressive treatment. Major determinants of morbidity and mortality in ALPS are the severity of the autoimmune disease, hypersplenism, and the development of Hodgkin or non-Hodgkin lymphoma.

Disorders of Phagocytic Cells

CHRONIC GRANULOMATOUS DISEASE

In approximately 65% of patients with chronic granulomatous disease (CGD), an X-linked (X-CGD) mode of inheritance has been documented; in the remainder, autosomal recessive (AR-CGD) inheritance.[165,166]

Epidemiology. X-CGD is characterized by defective intracellular killing of bacteria and fungi.[165,166] The true incidence of this condition is unknown, but it is estimated to occur at a frequency of 1 in 500,000 births.[165,166]

Pathogenesis and Etiology. The defect in X-CGD is attributable to mutations in the gene that encodes the heavy chain of the cytochrome *b245* heterodimer.[166,167] The heavy chain of cytochrome *b245* heterodimer is a glycoprotein of 91 kD and is referred to as gp91^{phox} (for phagocyte oxidase); this chain does not contain the cytochrome activity.[167] The gene encoding gp91^{phox} is at Xp21.1 on the short arm of the X chromosome.[167]

Clinical Features. During infancy, patients with CGD begin to have infections with catalase-positive organisms, such as *Staphylococcus aureus, Serratia marcescens, Pseudomonas,* and *Salmonella* spp., but not with catalase-negative organisms, such as *Streptococcus pneumoniae* or *Haemophilus influenzae.*[168] Several recent cases of infection with *Granulibacter bethesdensis* also have been described.[169,170] Abscess formation is characteristic, with lesions developing in the skin, lymph nodes, liver, lungs, or other viscera. These abscesses often require surgical drainage. Osteomyelitis caused by bacteria (particularly *S. marcescens*) and by fungi (especially *Aspergillus* spp.) is more frequent in this condition than in any other form of immunodeficiency. Ineffective destruction of phagocytized organisms and compensatory responses by lymphoid cells lead to formation of granulomatous lesions, especially in the liver and gastrointestinal and urinary tracts.[165,166]

Evaluation and Diagnosis. Neutrophil counts are normal or elevated, and the chemotactic, adherence, and phagocytic functions of these cells are normal. The immunologic defect in CGD lies solely in the inability of the phagocyte to kill ingested organisms.[165,166] During normal phagocytosis, a "respiratory burst" occurs in which nicotinamide adenine dinucleotide phosphate ($NADP^+$) is converted to NADPH, which is then moved from the cytosol to an electron transport chain in the cell membrane driven by NADPH oxidase. A 66-kD flavoprotein appears to be the receptor for NADPH in the membrane, and it is linked to cytochrome *b245,* the terminal component of the electron transport chain. Cytochrome *b245* is capable of directly reducing molecular oxygen to superoxide. Superoxide then dismutates to hydrogen peroxide, which is directly toxic to microorganisms or interacts with a chloride ion to produce hypochlorite. Defects exist in this electron transport chain in all forms of CGD, with the defect in the X-linked type due to the inability of cytochrome *b245* to reduce molecular oxygen to superoxide.

A diagnosis of CGD is made if the patient's neutrophils are unable to generate superoxide ions after phagocytosis or phorbol myristate acetate (PMA) stimulation. Currently the most accurate and accessible means of determining this is by a respiratory burst assay that involves flow cytometry.[171]

Treatment and Prognosis. When CGD was first described, it usually was fatal in early childhood. Aggressive treatment with antibiotics, especially trimethoprim-sulfamethoxazole, antistaphylococcal antibiotics, and aminoglycosides, has reduced the frequency and severity of bacterial infections.[168] Fungal infections, especially with *Aspergillus* spp., have been a more common cause of death. Prophylaxis with itraconazole can be very effective in preventing *Aspergillus* infections,[172] but if there is a breakthrough infection, voriconazole or posaconazole should be substituted in treatment doses. Once *Aspergillus* infections are brought under control with the latter therapy, chronic therapy with the imidazole antifungals is very effective in preventing recurrences. A double-blind placebo-controlled study of the efficacy and safety of subcutaneous injections of IFN-γ three times a week in preventing serious infections was conducted in 128 patients with CGD. It showed a significant reduction in the number of infections necessitating hospitalization in those patients who received IFN-γ subcutaneously compared with placebo.[173] Nevertheless, this therapy is not uniformly prescribed, particularly in Europe. Bone marrow transplantation has been problematic in patients with CGD because they often have chronic indolent bacterial or fungal infections that are difficult to control when the necessary pretransplantation chemotherapy is given.[42] If an HLA-identical sibling or matched unrelated donor is available, an unfractionated marrow transplant can be curative.[174] Gene therapy using retroviral vector–based delivery into autologous stem cells also has been attempted in CGD.[175] The treated patients ultimately experienced malignant transformations, however, so this therapy has not been continued.

AUTOSOMAL RECESSIVE CHRONIC GRANULOMATOUS DISEASE

Pathogenesis and Etiology. As in X-CGD, the molecular defects in the three forms of AR-CGD lie solely in the inability of the phagocyte to kill ingested organisms.[165,166] In the autosomal forms, defects exist in different components of the electron transport chain. Approximately 5% of patients with AR-CGD have a defect in the 22-kD subunit (p22^{phox}), or light chain, of the cytochrome *b245* heterodimer, which is encoded by a gene mapped to chromosomal locus 16q24.[165] However, in a majority of patients with AR-CGD, cytochrome *b245* is intact.[165] Evaluation of cytochrome-positive patients with AR-CGD led to the identification of cytosolic proteins that participate in the respiratory burst. A majority (25% of all patients with CGD) lack a 47-kD phosphoprotein (p47^{phox}) encoded by a gene on chromosome 7 at position q11.23, but in approximately 5% of patients a 65-kD protein (p67^{phox}) encoded by a gene on chromosome 1 at position q25 is missing.[165]

Clinical Features. Patients with autosomal recessive forms of CGD (AR-CGD) have infectious processes similar to those in patients with X-CGD: suppurative adenopathy, pneumonia, cutaneous and visceral abscesses, and osteomyelitis caused by infections with catalase-positive bacteria or fungi.

Evaluation and Diagnosis. As in X-CGD, a diagnosis of AR-CGD is made by demonstration of an inability of patient neutrophils to undergo a respiratory burst after phagocytosis or PMA stimulation, as measured by a flow cytometry dye reduction test.[171] Unlike those with X-CGD, however, carriers of AR-CGD cannot be detected by the flow cytometry method. Delineation of the specific molecular abnormality in any given patient with AR-CGD requires molecular techniques.[166]

Treatment and Prognosis. The treatment and prognosis for AR-CGD are the same as for X-CGD.

LEUKOCYTE ADHESION DEFICIENCY TYPES 1 AND 2

Leukocyte Adhesion Deficiency 1

Pathogenesis and Etiology. Leukocyte adhesion deficiency type 1 (LAD-1) is attributable to mutations in a gene on chromosome 21 at position q22.3 that encodes CD18, a 95-kD β subunit shared by three adhesive heterodimers: LFA-1 on B, T, and NK lymphocytes; complement receptor type 3 (CR3) on neutrophils, monocytes, macrophages, eosinophils, and NK cells; and p150,95 (another complement receptor) (see Chapter 8).[176] The α chains of these three molecules (encoded by genes on chromosome 16) are not expressed because of the abnormal β chain.

Clinical Features. Patients with LAD-1 have histories of delayed separation of the umbilical cord, omphalitis, gingivitis, recurrent skin infections, repeated otitis media, pneumonia, septicemia, ileocolitis, peritonitis, perianal fistulas, and impaired wound healing.[176] Life-threatening bacterial and fungal infections account for the high mortality. No increased susceptibility to viral infection or malignancy has been documented.

Evaluation and Diagnosis. Blood neutrophil counts usually are significantly elevated even when no infection is present because the cells are unable to adhere to vascular endothelium and migrate out of the intravascular compartment. All cytotoxic lymphocyte functions are considerably impaired because of a lack of the adhesion protein LFA-1; deficiency of LFA-1 also interferes with immune cell interaction and immune recognition. Deficiencies of these glycoproteins can be screened for by flow cytometry of blood leukocytes with monoclonal antibodies to CD18 or to CD11a, b, or c.

Treatment and Prognosis. Beyond good antibiotic treatment of infections, no effective treatment of LAD-1 is available other than stem cell transplantation, which can be curative. The prognosis without specific treatment is poor.

Leukocyte Adhesion Deficiency Type 2

Epidemiology. Leukocyte adhesion deficiency type 2 (LAD-2) was discovered in two unrelated Israeli boys, 3 and 5 years of age, each the offspring of consanguineous parents. The condition is very rare.

Pathogenesis and Etiology. LAD-2 is attributable to the absence of neutrophil sialyl-Lewis^X, a ligand of E-selectin on vascular endothelium.[176] It was postulated that a general defect in fucose metabolism is the basis for LAD-2 because the genes for the red blood cell H antigen and for the secretor status encode distinctα1,2-fucosyltransferases and the synthesis of sialyl-Lewis^X requires anα1,3-fucosyltransferase. Missense mutations in the guanosine diphosphate (GDP)-fucose transporter cDNA were subsequently found in three patients with LAD-2, which confirmed that GDP-fucose transporter deficiency is a cause of LAD-2.[177]

Clinical Features. Both boys had severe mental retardation, short stature, a distinctive facial appearance, and the Bombay (hh) blood phenotype, and both were secretor- and Lewis-negative. Like patients with LAD-1, they both had had recurrent severe bacterial infections, including pneumonia, peridontitis, otitis media, and localized cellulitis, but pus formation was absent at sites of recurrent cellulitis.

Evaluation and Diagnosis

Similar to patients with LAD-1, the patients with LAD-2 had infections accompanied by a marked intravascular leukocytosis (with counts of 30,000 to 150,000 cells/μL). In vitro studies revealed a pronounced defect in neutrophil motility. Flow cytometry demonstrated an absence of CD15 on neutrophils.

Treatment and Prognosis. The treatment and prognosis are the same as for LAD-1.

CHÉDIAK-HIGASHI SYNDROME

Pathogenesis and Etiology. The fundamental defect in Chédiak-Higashi syndrome, inherited as an autosomal recessive trait, was found to be caused by mutations in a gene on human chromosome 1 at position q42-43.[178] This gene is similar to the one mutated in the murine *beige* defect.[178] The gene is postulated to function with other genes as components of a vesicle membrane–associated signal transduction complex that regulates intracellular protein trafficking.[178]

Clinical Features. Chédiak-Higashi syndrome is characterized by oculocutaneous albinism and susceptibility to recurrent respiratory tract and other types of infections.[179] In approximately 85% of affected patients, an "accelerated phase" of the disease is seen, with fever, jaundice, hepatosplenomegaly, lymphadenopathy, pancytopenia, bleeding diathesis, and neurologic changes. Chédiak-Higashi has substantial overlap with Hermansky-Pudlak syndrome type 2 and Griscelli syndrome type 2, which are due to mutations of *AP3* and *RAB27A* genes, respectively. All three conditions result in some degree of oculocutaneous albinism, impaired phagocytes, and defective cytotoxic lymphocyte functions. All can develop an accelerated phase.

Evaluation and Diagnosis. The characteristic feature of the disease is giant lysosomal granules, not only in neutrophils but also in most of the other cells of the body, including melanocytes, neural Schwann cells, renal tubular cells, gastric mucosa, pneumatocytes, hepatocytes, cutaneous Langerhans cells, and adrenal cells.[179] The granules in neutrophils stain positive for peroxidase, acid phosphatase, and esterase. The abnormal lysosomes are unable to fuse with phagosomes, so ingested bacteria cannot be lysed normally. An additional feature of the disease is nearly complete absence of cytotoxic T lymphocyte and NK cell activity, as a result of abnormal lysosomal granule function.[179]

Treatment and Prognosis. Once the accelerated phase begins, the disease usually is fatal within 30 months unless successful treatment with an unfractionated HLA-identical bone marrow transplant after cytoreductive conditioning can be accomplished.[42]

Defects of Innate Immunity

INTERFERON-γ RECEPTOR TYPE 1 AND TYPE 2 MUTATIONS

A 2.5-month-old Tunisian female infant had fatal idiopathic disseminated BCG infection,[180] and four children from Malta had disseminated atypical mycobacterial infection in the absence of a recognized immunodeficiency.[181] Consanguinity was a factor in all five families. All of the patients had defective upregulation of TNF-α production by their blood macrophages in response to stimulation with IFN-γ. Furthermore, all lacked expression of IFN-γRs on their blood monocytes or lymphocytes, and each was found to have a mutation in the gene on chromosomal region 6q22-q23 that encodes IFN-γR1. Patients with mutations in the IFN-γR2 also have been identified.[181] Of interest, these patients do not appear to be susceptible to infection with agents other than mycobacteria. Th1 responses appear to be normal. The susceptibility of these children to mycobacterial infections indicates that IFN-γ is obligatory for efficient macrophage antimycobacterial activity.[181]

INTERLEUKIN-12 RECEPTOR β1 MUTATIONS

IL-12 is produced by activated antigen-presenting cells (dendritic cells, macrophages). It promotes the development of Th1 responses and is a powerful inducer of IFN-γ production by T and NK cells.[181] T and NK cells from seven unrelated patients who had severe recurrent mycobacterial and *Salmonella* infections failed to produce IFN-γ when stimulated with IL-12.[182,183] The patients were otherwise healthy. They were found to have missense mutations in the IL-12 receptor β1 chain in the extracellular domain, which results in unresponsiveness to IL-12.[182,183]

GERMLINE STAT1 MUTATION

Interferons induce the formation of two transcriptional activators: γ-activating factor (GAF) and interferon-stimulated γ factor 3 (ISGF3). A natural heterozygous germline *STAT1* mutation associated with susceptibility to mycobacterial but not viral disease was found in two unrelated patients with unexplained mycobacterial disease.[184] This mutation impaired the nuclear accumulation of GAF but not of ISGF3 in cells stimulated by interferons, which implies that the antimycobacterial but not the antiviral effects of human interferons are mediated by GAF. More recently, two patients have been identified with homozygous *STAT1* mutations who developed both post–BCG vaccination disseminated disease and lethal viral infections. The mutations in these patients caused a lack of formation of both GAF and ISGF3.[185] These mutations of *STAT1* are in contrast with the autosomal dominant variants associated with fungal disease described above.

INTERLEUKIN-1 RECEPTOR–ASSOCIATED KINASE 4 DEFICIENCY AND MYELOID DIFFERENTIATION FACTOR 88

Members of the interleukin-1 receptor (IL-1R) and the Toll-like receptor superfamily share an intracytoplasmic Toll–IL-1 receptor (TIR) domain, which mediates recruitment of the interleukin-1 receptor–associated kinase (IRAK) complex via TIR-containing adaptor molecules.[186] Three unrelated, otherwise healthy children with recurrent pyogenic infections due to pneumococci and staphylococci exhibited normal immunocompetence by standard immune studies. Titers of antipneumococcal antibodies were normal. Their blood and fibroblast cells, however, did not activate nuclear factor-κB (NK-κB) and mitogen-activated protein kinase (MAPK) and failed to induce downstream cytokines in response to any of the known ligands of TIR-bearing receptors. They each were found to have an inherited deficiency of IRAK-4. Thus the TIR-IRAK signaling pathway appears to be crucial for protective immunity against specific bacteria but is redundant against most other microorganisms.[186] More than 50 cases of IRAK4 deficiency have now been documented, and a commonality among cases is susceptibility to pyogenic bacterial infection with pneumococci and *Pseudomonas*.[187] The pneumococcal infections have the potential to be invasive (even as a presenting feature) and are associated with poor clinical outcomes. Severe viral and fungal infections are atypical. The myeloid differentiation factor 88 (MYD88) is an effective phenocopy of IRAK4 deficiency.[187] Although discovered later than IRAK4 deficiency, MYD88 is an upstream adaptor for IRAK4 and links it to TLRs, which results in a very similar immunologic defect and clinical syndrome.

NATURAL KILLER CELL DEFICIENCY

NK cells are the major lymphocytes of the innate immune system. NK cells recognize virally infected and malignant cells and mediate their elimination. Persons with absence or functional deficiencies of NK cells are rare, and they typically exhibit susceptibility to the herpesviruses (including varicella-zoster virus [VZV], herpes simplex virus [HSV], cytomegalovirus [CMV], and EBV) as well as papillomaviruses.[188] A number of gene defects have been associated with these isolated abnormalities in NK cells. Autosomal recessive CD16 gene mutations have been described in three separate families and they altered the first immunoglobulin-like domain of this important NK cell activation receptor. Patients with these mutations have functionally impaired NK cells and exhibit clinical susceptibility to herpesviruses. Autosomal dominant deficiency of NK cells occurs in persons with mutations in the GATA2 transcription factor.[189] These patients also have low numbers of monocytes. They have extreme susceptibility to human papillomavirus as well as mycobacteria—the latter presumably from the monocytic defect. Finally, autosomal recessive mutations in the *MCM4* gene have been identified in a cohort of consanguineous Irish who exhibited growth failure and susceptibility to herpesviruses. These patients possessed the immature CD56bright minor subset but lacked the major mature CD56dim subset of NK cells. The reason why *MCM4*, which encodes a DNA helicase, would interfere with NK cell development remains unclear.

Other cases of NK cell deficiencies have been identified, and molecular explanations are pending. As part of their treatment, patients should be maintained on antiviral prophylaxis, and allogeneic stem cell transplantation has been successful in certain cases.[190]

Complement Component Deficiencies

Inherited deficiencies in almost all of the complement proteins have been discovered.[191] Complete deficiencies of complement proteins are rare, and such rarity attests to their importance in host defense. All but one of these proteins are encoded by genes on autosomal chromosomes; the gene encoding properdin is on the X chromosome.[192] Complete deficiencies of the complement proteins (except properdin) require homozygous mutations and are therefore autosomal recessive traits. Heterozygosity for complement protein deficiencies, which is relatively common, is not associated with a higher incidence of infections than that found in the general population, but combinations of such heterozygosities may be seen with increased frequency in autoimmune disease.[193] Complement protein deficiencies can be divided into those that involve the alternative pathway, the classical pathway, or late components of complement.[191]

Patients with deficiencies in either the classical pathway or later components tend to do relatively well except when stressed by septicemia or any infection with a high-grade pathogen. By contrast, patients deficient in alternative pathway factors tend to have more frequent and severe infections, particularly early in life, because the alternative pathway is very important for host defense during the first exposure to an infectious agent. After patients develop antibodies to the infectious agents, they become partially protected. A high incidence of autoimmune disease also is seen in patients with inherited complement deficiencies, possibly because of inadequate removal of immune complexes from the circulation secondary to a lack of opsonins derived from the complement pathway. These circulating immune complexes may then localize in the kidneys and other tissues, where they causing inflammatory reactions.[191] The complement pathways are described in detail in Chapter 8.

C1q, C1r, C1s, C2, AND C4 DEFICIENCIES

Deficiencies of the classical pathway complement proteins C1q, C1r, C1s, C2, and C4 tend to result in less infection susceptibility than deficiencies of the alternative pathway.[191] Each of the classical pathway component deficiencies, however, may be associated with an increased susceptibility to infections with encapsulated bacteria. The most common inherited complement deficiency is an absence of C2, which affects approximately 1 in 10,000 individuals. Clinically normal persons with C2 deficiency have been described, but some have had recurrent septicemia, meningitis, or osteomyelitis.

Patients with any of the classical pathway component deficiencies may have symptoms resembling those of discoid lupus or systemic lupus erythematosus (SLE). In patients with the SLE-like syndrome, disease begins at an early age, with pronounced photosensitivity and a low but clinically significant incidence of renal disease. Antinuclear antibody titers may be negative. Patients with C2 or C4 deficiency also have increased incidence rates of dermatomyositis, vasculitis, cold urticaria, inflammatory bowel disease, Hodgkin's disease, and Henoch-Schönlein purpura.[191]

C3 DEFICIENCY

In general, alternative pathway defects lead to recurrent infections, such as pneumonia, otitis media, and sinusitis, caused by high-grade encapsulated pathogens. One example is C3 deficiency, which leads to abnormal classical pathway activation as well. C3 deficiency is a rare disorder caused by either hypercatabolism or hyposynthesis of C3. Patients with hypercatabolism lack C3b inactivator (factor I deficiency). The consequence is lack of control of the alternative complement pathway convertase, so that C3b is not converted to C3bi. The enzyme PC3bBb acts to deplete native C3, and whatever C3 antigen remains is in the form of C3b. C3 deficiency often is associated with repeated infections of both low- and high-grade pathogens.[191] Deficiency of factor H, the cofactor for factor I and C4b inactivator, manifests similarly but affects C4 as well as C3.

Properdin deficiency is an X-linked disorder that should be suspected in male patients with recurrent systemic meningococcal disease or recurrent pyogenic infections. Properdin is a glycoprotein that upregulates the alternative pathway of complement by stabilizing the C3b-Bb complex. More than 50 cases of properdin deficiency have been recorded in patients of various ethnic origins. On the basis of immunochemical and functional measurements of properdin, three subtypes of properdin deficiency are recognized: type I (total deficiency), type II (partial deficiency), and type III, caused by a dysfunctional molecule. Various point mutations have been found in the properdin gene at Xp11.3-p21.1 in patients with type I and type II properdin deficiency.[192]

DEFICIENCIES OF TERMINAL COMPLEMENT COMPONENTS

Hereditary deficiency of one of the terminal complement components (C5, C6, C7, or C8) may be present in healthy persons or may be associated with an increased incidence of infection or autoimmune disease. Deficiencies of these late complement components lead to a high incidence of disseminated neisserial infections. Opsonization of neisserial organisms appears to be inadequate for their elimination because C3—the principal opsonin generated by complement—is normal in these patients; lysis is required for the destruction of these organisms. Patients with C5 deficiency have been reported to have SLE and associated Raynaud's phenomenon, arthritis, diffuse membranoproliferative glomerulonephritis, recurrent pneumococcal pneumonia, and disseminated gonococcal infection. Deficiencies of C6, C7, or C8 have been associated with recurrent meningococcal meningitis or disseminated gonococcal infection. C7 and C8 deficiencies also may be associated with rheumatic diseases such as SLE or rheumatoid arthritis.[191]

Evaluation and Diagnosis. A diagnosis of a congenital complement deficiency should be considered in any patient presenting with a history of recurrent infections with encapsulated bacterial pathogens, with or without the concomitant presence of an autoimmune disease. The diagnosis of deficient terminal complement components should be suspected in any patient with recurrent neisserial infections. Total hemolytic complement determination (CH50) may be used as a screening procedure for all inherited complement protein deficiencies; in patients with complement protein deficiencies CH50 levels are extremely low or nondetectable. Individual complement components should be specifically quantified in specialized (usually research) laboratories.

Treatment and Prognosis. No specific treatment is available for complement component deficiencies. Acute infections are treated with antibiotics; long-term management of these disorders often includes prophylactic antibiotics. Complement components cannot yet be replaced. All of the complement protein and regulator genes have been sequenced, and many have been cloned.

INTRAUTERINE DIAGNOSIS AND CARRIER DETECTION OF PRIMARY IMMUNODEFICIENCY DISEASES

Intrauterine diagnoses of ADA and PNP deficiencies can be made by enzyme analysis on amnion cells (fresh or cultured) obtained before 20 weeks of gestation.[69] In immunodeficiency disorders for which the defective gene has been cloned and cDNA probes are available, if the mutation in the family is known, a diagnosis can be made by mutational analysis of chorionic villus samples obtained during the first trimester.

When the mutation is not known, diagnosis of SCID or other severe T cell deficiencies, MHC class I or II antigen deficiencies, CGD, or Wiskott-Aldrich syndrome (by platelet size) can be made using appropriate tests of phenotype or function on small samples of blood obtained by fetoscopy at 18 to 22 weeks of gestation. This is technically difficult, however, and is not widely available.

Carriers of ADA and PNP deficiency can be detected by quantitative enzyme analyses of blood samples. Carriers of X-linked agammaglobulinemia, X-linked SCID, or the Wiskott-Aldrich syndrome can be identified by mutation analysis if the mutation is known or with use of techniques designed to detect nonrandom X chromosome inactivation in one or more blood cell lineages.

Approach to Treatment of Primary Immunodeficiency Disorders

The principal modes of therapy for the primary immunodeficiency disorders include protective isolation, use of antibiotics for eradicating or preventing bacterial and fungal infections, and attempted replacement of missing humoral or cellular immunologic functions. Because of the complexities of immunodeficiency diseases and their treatment, all patients with an immunodeficiency disease should be evaluated in centers with the capability for detailed studies of immune function before therapy is selected or begun.

ANTIBODY DEFICIENCY DISORDERS

Judicious use of antibiotics and regular administration of antibodies are the only treatments that have proved effective for antibody deficiency disorders. Concomitant antibiotic prophylaxis as an adjunct therapy also is perceived as effective. Patients with agammaglobulinemia, hyper-IgM syndrome, CVID, Wiskott-Aldrich syndrome, and all forms of SCID are candidates for immunoglobulin replacement therapy.[28] Anaphylactic reactions caused by IgE antibodies (in the patient) to IgA (in the IVIG preparation) are rare but may occur in patients with CVID whose serum lacks IgA.[29] If anti-IgA antibodies are detected, IVIG therapy may still be possible with use of IVIG containing almost no IgA.[28]

Immunoglobulin replacement therapy is contraindicated in patients with selective absence of serum and secretory IgA because of the high frequency of anti-IgA antibodies[29,31] and because these patients usually have normal quantities of IgG antibodies.[28] IVIG also should not be given to infants with transient hypogammaglobulinemia because it could suppress their innate capacity to form antibodies. The use of immunoglobulin therapy is not indicated for patients with IgG subclass deficiencies unless they have convincing defects in antibody-forming capacity, because these patients are best treated by managing comorbid conditions and/or using antibiotic prophylaxis, which is perceived as an effective intervention in many of the milder antibody deficiencies. It is futile to give immunoglobulin therapy to patients who have low IgG associated with protein-losing states, such as the nephrotic syndrome, intestinal lymphangiectasia, or other protein-losing enteropathies, because the administered IgG will be extremely short-lived, and antibody production in these patients usually is adequate despite the low serum level of IgG.[28]

CELLULAR IMMUNODEFICIENCY DISORDERS

Immunoreconstitution with bone marrow cells that are MHC-compatible or haploidentical with the recipient cells is the treatment of choice for most severe cellular defects. With complete DiGeorge syndrome, however, cultured mature thymic tissue explants have successfully reconstituted immune function in several patients.[146]

Graft-versus-host disease is the major risk in recipients of bone marrow or cord blood transplants. the development of techniques to deplete all postthymic T cells from donor marrow has, however, permitted the safe and successful use of haploidentical (half-matched) bone marrow cells without pretransplantation chemoablation or posttransplantation GVHD immunosuppressive drugs for the correction of Scid[55,58-60] (see Fig. 72-6). More than 500 infants with SCID who lacked an HLA-identical donor have been treated with T cell–depleted haploidentical parental bone marrow, with usually little or no graft-versus-host disease; 61% to 96% survive with successful immune reconstitution.[55,58-61] Patients with less severe forms of cellular immunodeficiency reject such grafts unless they undergo chemoablation before transplantation.[42] Several patients with Wiskott-Aldrich syndrome and other forms of partial cellular immunodeficiency have been treated successfully with unfractionated HLA-identical or matched unrelated bone marrow transplants after immunosuppression.[42] in view of the success of gene therapy in ADA deficiency,[72] it is hoped that modifications in the viral vectors used to insert the normal gene into the DNA of patients with X-linked SCID, CGD, and Wiskott-Aldrich syndrome will be able to prevent the insertional oncogenesis seen in the first trials.[64,194]

REFERENCES

Introduction

1. Buckley RH. Primary immunodeficiency or not? Making the correct diagnosis. J Allergy Clin Immunol 2006;117:756-8.
2. Bruton OC. Agammaglobulinemia. Pediatrics 1952;9:722-8.
3. Al-Herz W, Bousfiha A, Casanova JL, et al. Primary immunodeficiency diseases: an update on the classification from the International Union of Immunological Societies Expert Committee for Primary Immunodeficiency. Front Immunol 2011;2:54.
4. Torgerson TR. Immune dysregulation in primary immunodeficiency disorders. Immunol Allergy Clin North Am 2008;28:315-ix.
5. Rezaei N, Hedayat M, Aghamohammadi A, Nichols KE. Primary immunodeficiency diseases associated with increased susceptibility to viral infections and malignancies. J Allergy Clin Immunol 2011;127:1329-41.
6. Orange JS, Glessner JT, Resnick E, et al. Genome-wide association identifies diverse causes of common variable immunodeficiency. J Allergy Clin Immunol 2011;127:1360-7.
7. Buckley RH. Variable phenotypic expression of mutations in genes of the immune system. J Clin Invest 2005;115:2974-6.

Antibody Deficiency Syndromes

8. Vetrie D, Vorechovsky I, Sideras P, et al. The gene involved in X-linked agammaglobulinaemia is a member of the src family of protein-tyrosine kinases. Nature 1993; 361:226-33.
9. Tsukada S, Saffran DC, Rawlings DJ, et al. Deficient expression of a B cell cytoplasmic tyrosine kinase in human X-linked agammaglobulinemia. Cell 1993;72:279-90.
10. Smith CI, Satterthwaite AB, Witte ON. X-linked agammaglobulinemia: a disease of Btk tyrosine kinase. In: Ochs HD, Smith CI, Puck JM, editors. Primary immunodeficiency diseases: a molecular and genetic approach. 2nd ed. New York: Oxford University Press; 2007. p. 279-303.
11. Stewart DM, Tian L, Notarangelo LD, Nelson DL. X-linked hypogammaglobulinemia and isolated growth hormone deficiency: an update. Immunol Res 2008;40:262-70.
12. Sediva A, Smith CI, Asplund AC, et al. Contiguous X-chromosome deletion syndrome encompassing the BTK, TIMM8A, TAF7L, and DRP2 genes. J Clin Immunol 2007;27:640-6.
13. Wilfert CM, Buckley RH, Mohanakumar T, et al. Persistent and fatal central nervous system echovirus infections in patients with agammaglobulinemia. N Engl J Med 1977;296: 1485-9.
14. Yel L, Minegishi Y, Coustan-Smith E, et al. Mutations in the mu heavy chain gene in patients with agammaglobulinemia. N Engl J Med 1996;335:1486-93.
15. Minegishi Y, Coustan-Smith E, Wang YH, et al. Mutations in the human lambda 5/14.1 gene result in B cell deficiency and agammaglobulinemia. J Exp Med 1998;187:71-7.
16. Minegishi Y, Coustan-Smith E, Rapalus L, et al. Mutations in Igalpha (CD79a) result in a complete block in B-cell development. J Clin Invest 1999;104:1115-21.
17. Dobbs AK, Yang T, Farmer D, et al. Cutting edge: a hypomorphic mutation in Igbeta (CD79b) in a patient with immunodeficiency and a leaky defect in B cell development. J Immunol 2007;179:2055-9.
18. Minegishi Y, Rohrer J, Coustan-Smith E, et al. An essential role for BLNK in human B cell development. Science 1999;286:1954-7.
19. Sawada A, Takihara Y, Kim JY, et al. A congenital mutation of the novel gene LRRC8 causes agammaglobulinemia in humans. J Clin Invest 2003;112:1707-13.
20. Schroeder HW, Zhu Z, March RE, et al. Susceptibility locus for IgA deficiency and common variable immunodeficiency in the HLA-DR3, -B8, -A1 haplotypes. Mol Med 1998;4:72-86.
21. Grimbacher B, Hutloff A, Schlesier M, et al. Homozygous loss of ICOS is associated with adult-onset common variable immunodeficiency. Nat Immunol 2003;4:261-8.
22. van Zelm MC, Smet J, Adams B, et al. CD81 gene defect in humans disrupts CD19 complex formation and leads to antibody deficiency. J Clin Invest 2010;120:1265-74.
23. Kuijpers TW, Bende RJ, Baars PA, et al. CD20 deficiency in humans results in impaired T cell-independent antibody responses. J Clin Invest 2010;120:214-22.
24. van Zelm MC, Reisli I, van der Burg M, et al. An antibody-deficiency syndrome due to mutations in the CD19 gene. N Engl J Med 2006;354:1901-12.
25. Salzer U, Chapel HM, Webster AD, et al. Mutations in TNFRSF13B encoding TACI are associated with common variable immunodeficiency in humans. Nat Genet 2005;37:820-8.
26. Agarwal S, Cunningham-Rundles C. Autoimmunity in common variable immunodeficiency. Curr Allergy Asthma Rep 2009;9: 347-52.
27. Cunningham-Rundles C, Cooper DL, Duffy TP, Strauchen J. Lymphomas of mucosal-associated lymphoid tissue in common variable immunodeficiency. Am J Hematol 2002;69:171-8.
28. Orange JS, Hossny EM, Weiler CR, et al. Use of intravenous immunoglobulin in human disease: a review of evidence by members of the Primary Immunodeficiency Committee of the American Academy of Allergy, Asthma and Immunology. J Allergy Clin Immunol 2006;117(4 Suppl):S525-53.
29. Burks AW, Sampson HA, Buckley RH. Anaphylactic reactions after gamma globulin administration in patients with hypogammaglobulinemia. N Engl J Med 1986;314:560-4.
30. Chapel H, Cunningham-Rundles C. Update in understanding common variable immunodeficiency disorders (CVIDs) and the management of patients with these conditions. Br J Haematol 2009;145:709-27.
31. Clark JA, Callicoat PA, Brenner NA. Selective IgA deficiency in blood donors. Am J Clin Pathol 1983;80:210-3.
32. Lefranc MP, Hammarstrom L, Smith CI, Lefranc G. Gene deletions in the human immunoglobulin heavy chain constant region locus: molecular and immunological analysis. Immunol Rev 1991;2:265-81.
33. Shackelford PG, Granoff DM, Polmar SH, et al. Subnormal serum concentrations of IgG2 in children with frequent infections associated with varied patters of immunologic dysfunction. J Pediatr 1990;116:529-38.
34. Tiller Jr TL, Buckley RH. Transient hypogammaglobulinemia of infancy: review of the literature, clinical and immunologic features of 11 new cases, and long-term follow- up. J Pediatr 1978;92:347-53.
35. Dorsey MJ, Orange JS. Impaired specific antibody response and increased B-cell population in transient hypogammaglobulinemia of infancy. Ann Allergy Asthma Immunol 2006; 97:590-5.
36. Agarwal S, Cunningham-Rundles C. Thymoma and immunodeficiency (Good syndrome): a report of 2 unusual cases and review of the literature. Ann Allergy Asthma Immunol 2007; 98:185-90.
37. Mayer L, Swan SP, Thompson C. Evidence for a defect in "switch" T cells in patients with immunodeficiency and hyperimmunoglobulinemia M. N Engl J Med 1986;314:409-13.
38. Allen RC, Armitage RJ, Conley ME, et al. CD40 ligand gene defects responsible for X-linked hyper IgM syndrome. Science 1993; 259:990-3.
39. Jain A, Ma CA, Liu S, et al. Specific missense mutations in NEMO result in hyper-IgM syndrome with hypohydrotic ectodermal dysplasia. Nat Immunol 2001;2:223-8.
40. Hanson EP, Monaco-Shawver L, Solt LA, et al. Hypomorphic nuclear factor-kappaB essential modulator mutation database and reconstitution system identifies phenotypic and immunologic diversity. J Allergy Clin Immunol 2008;122:1169-77.
41. Levy J, Espanol-Boren T, Thomas C, et al. Clinical spectrum of X-linked hyper IgM syndrome. J Pediatr 1997;131:47-54.
42. Buckley RH, Fischer A. Bone marrow transplantation for primary immunodeficiency diseases. In: Ochs HD, Smith CI, Puck JM, editors. Primary immunodeficiency diseases: a molecular and genetic approach. 2nd ed. New York: Oxford University Press; 2007. p. 669-87.
43. Durandy A, Revy P, Fischer A. Autosomal hyper-IgM syndromes caused by an intrinsic B cell defect. In: Ochs HD, Smith CI, Puck JM, editors. Primary immunodeficiency diseases: a molecular and genetic approach. 2nd ed. New York: Oxford University Press; 2007. p. 269-78.
44. Revy P, Muto T, Levy Y, et al. Activation-induced cytidine deaminase (AID) deficiency causes the autosomal recessive form of the hyper-IgM syndrome (HIGM2). Cell 2000;102: 565-75.
45. Minegishi Y, Lavoie A, Cunningham-Rundles C, et al. Mutations in activation-induced cytidine deaminase in patients with hyper IgM syndrome. Clin Immunol 2000;97:203-10.
46. Imai K, Catalan N, Plebani A, et al. Hyper-IgM syndrome type 4 with a B lymphocyte-intrinsic selective deficiency in Ig class-switch recombination. J Clin Invest 2003;112:136-42.
47. Ferrari S, Giliani S, Insalaco A, et al. Mutations of CD40 gene cause an autosomal recessive form of immunodeficiency with hyper IgM. Proc Natl Acad Sci U S A 2001;98:12614-9.
48. Buckley RH. Molecular defects in human severe combined immunodeficiency and approaches to immune reconstitution. Annu Rev Immunol 2004;22:625-55.
49. Buckley RH. Primary immunodeficiency diseases due to defects in lymphocytes. N Engl J Med 2000;343:1313-24.
50. Glanzmann E, Riniker P. Essentielle lymphocytophtose. Ein neues krankeitsbild aus der Sauglingspathologie. Ann Paediatr 1950;174: 1-5.
51. Buckley R. The long quest for neonatal screening for SCID. J Allergy Clin Immunol 2012; 129:597-604.

52. Noguchi M, Yi H, Rosenblatt HM, et al. Interleukin-2 receptor gamma chain mutation results in X-linked severe combined immunodeficiency in humans. Cell 1993;73:147-57.
53. Vosshenrich CA, Di Santo JP. Cytokines: IL-21 joins the gamma(c)-dependent network? Curr Biol 2001;11:R175-7.
54. Myers LA, Patel DD, Puck JM, Buckley RH. Hematopoietic stem cell transplantation for severe combined immunodeficiency in the neonatal period leads to superior thymic output and improved survival. Blood 2002;99:872-8.
55. Buckley RH, Schiff SE, Schiff RI, et al. Hematopoietic stem cell transplantation for the treatment of severe combined immunodeficiency. N Engl J Med 1999;340:508-16.
56. Altman PL. Blood leukocyte values: man. In: Dittmer DS, editor. Blood and other body fluids. Washington, D.C.: Federation of American Societies for Experimental Biology; 1961, p. 125-6.
57. Buckley RH. Transplantation of hematopoietic stem cells in human severe combined immunodeficiency: longterm outcomes. Immunol Res 2011;49:25-43.
58. Sarzotti-Kelsoe M, Win CM, Parrott RE, et al. Thymic output, T-cell diversity, and T-cell function in long-term human SCID chimeras. Blood 2009;114:1445-53.
59. Railey MD, LoKhnygina Y, Buckley RH. Long term clinical outcome of patients with severe combined immunodeficiency who received related donor bone marrow transplants without pre-transplant chemotherapy or post-transplant GVHD prophylaxis. J Pediatr 2009;155:834-40.
60. Buckley RH. Transplantation of hematopoietic stem cells in human severe combined immunodeficiency: long term outcomes. Immunol Res 2011;49:25-43.
61. Gennery AR, Slatter MA, Grandin L, et al. Transplantation of hematopoietic stem cells and long-term survival for primary immunodeficiencies in Europe: entering a new century, do we do better? J Allergy Clin Immunol 2010;126:602-10.
62. Hacein-Bey-Abina S, Le Deist F, Carlier F, et al. Sustained correction of X-linked severe combined immunodeficiency by ex vivo gene therapy. N Engl J Med 2002;346:1185-93.
63. Hacein-Bey-Abina S, Garrigue A, Wang GP, et al. Insertional oncogenesis in 4 patients after retrovirus-mediated gene therapy of SCID-X1. J Clin Invest 2008;118:3132-42.
64. Howe SJ, Mansour MR, Schwarzwaelder K, et al. Insertional mutagenesis combined with acquired somatic mutations causes leukemogenesis following gene therapy of SCID-X1 patients. J Clin Invest 2008;118:3143-50.
65. Hacein-Bey-Abina S, Hauer J, Lim A, et al. Efficacy of gene therapy for X-linked severe combined immunodeficiency. N Engl J Med 2010;363:355-64.
66. Gaspar HB, Cooray S, Gilmour KC, et al. Long-term persistence of a polyclonal T cell repertoire after gene therapy for X-linked severe combined immunodeficiency. Sci Transl Med 2011;3:97ra79.
67. Buckley RH. The multiple causes of human SCID. J Clin Invest 2004;114:1409-11.
68. Buckley RH, Schiff RI, Schiff SE, et al. Human severe combined immunodeficiency (SCID): genetic, phenotypic and functional diversity in 108 infants. J Pediatr 1997;130:378-87.
69. Hirschhorn R, Candotti F. Immunodeficiency due to defects of purine metabolism. In: Ochs HD, Smith CI, Puck JM, editors. Primary immunodeficiency diseases: a molecular and genetic approach. 2nd ed. New York: Oxford University Press; 2007. p. 169-96.
70. Hershfield MS, Buckley RH, Greenberg ML, et al. Treatment of adenosine deaminase deficiency with polyethylene glycol-modified adenosine deaminase (PEG-ADA). N Engl J Med 1987;316:589-96.
71. Chan B, Wara D, Bastian J, et al. Long-term efficacy of enzyme replacement therapy for adenosine deaminase (ADA)-deficient severe combined immunodeficiency (SCID). Clin Immunol 2005;117:133-43.
72. Aiuti A, Cattaneo F, Galimberti S, et al. Gene therapy for immunodeficiency due to adenosine deaminase deficiency. N Engl J Med 2009;360:447-58.
73. Russell SM, Tayebi N, Nakajima H, et al. Mutation of Jak3 in a patient with SCID: Essential role of Jak3 in lymphoid development. Science 1995;270:797-800.
74. Roberts JL, Lengi A, Brown SM, et al. Janus kinase 3 (JAK3) deficiency: clinical, immunologic and molecular analyses of 10 patients and outcomes of stem cell transplantation. Blood 2004;103:209-18.
75. Puel A, Ziegler SF, Buckley RH, Leonard WJ. Defective IL7R expression in T(−)B(+)NK(+) severe combined immunodeficiency. Nat Genet 1998;20:394-7.
76. Schwarz K, Gauss GH, Ludwig L, et al. RAG mutations in human B cell-negative SCID. Science 1996;274:97-9.
77. Corneo B, Moshous D, Gungor T, et al. Identical mutations in RAG1 or RAG2 genes leading to defective V(D)J recombinase activity can cause either T−B− severe combined immune deficiency or Omenn syndrome. Blood 2001;97:2772-6.
78. de Villartay J-P, Schwarz K, Villa A. V(D)J recombination defects. In: Ochs HD, Smith CI, Puck JM, editors. Primary immunodeficiency diseases: a molecular and genetic approach. 2nd ed. New York: Oxford University Press; 2007, p. 153-68.
79. Moshous D, Callebaut I, de Chasseval R, et al. Artemis, a novel DNA double-strand break repair/V(D)J recombination protein, is mutated in human severe combined immune deficiency. Cell 2001;105:177-86.
80. van der Burg M, van Veelen LR, Verkaik NS, et al. A new type of radiosensitive T−B−NK+ severe combined immunodeficiency caused by a LIG4 mutation. J Clin Invest 2006;116:137-45.
81. Buck D, Moshous D, de Chasseval R, et al. Severe combined immunodeficiency and microcephaly in siblings with hypomorphic mutations in DNA ligase IV. Eur J Immunol 2006;36:224-35.
82. van der Burg M, Ijspeert H, Verkaik NS, et al. A DNA-PKcs mutation in a radiosensitive T−B− SCID patient inhibits Artemis activation and nonhomologous end-joining. J Clin Invest 2009;119:91-8.
83. Kung C, Pingel JT, Heikinheimo M, et al. Mutations in the tyrosine phosphatase CD45 gene in a child with severe combined immunodeficiency disease. Nat Med 2000;6:343-5.
84. Tchilian EZ, Wallace DL, Wells RS, et al. A deletion in the gene encoding the CD45 antigen in a patient with SCID. J Immunol 2001;166:1308-13.
85. Roberts JL, Buckley RH, Luo B, et al. CD45-deficient severe combined immunodeficiency caused by uniparental disomy. Proc Natl Acad Sci U S A 2012;109:10456-61.
86. Dadi HK, Simon AJ, Roifman CM. Effect of CD3delta deficiency on maturation of alpha/beta and gamma/delta T-cell lineages in severe combined immunodeficiency. N Engl J Med 2003;349:1821-8.
87. de Saint Basile G, Geissmann F, Flori E, et al. Severe combined immunodeficiency caused by deficiency in either the delta or the epsilon subunit of CD3. J Clin Invest 2004;114:1512-7.
88. Roberts JL, Lauritsen JH, Cooney M, et al. T−B+NK+ severe combined immunodeficiency caused by complete deficiency of the CD3 zeta subunit of the T cell antigen receptor complex. Blood 2007;109:3198-206.
89. Soudais C, De Villartay JP, Le Deist F, Fischer A, Lisowska-Grospierre B. Independent mutations of the human CD3-epsilon gene resulting in a T cell receptor/CD3 complex immunodeficiency. Nat Genet 1993;3:77-81.
90. Arnaiz-Villena A, Timon M, Rodriguez-Gallego C, et al. T lymphocyte signalling defects and immunodeficiency due to the lack of CD3 gamma. Immunodeficiency 1993;4:121-9.
91. Pannicke U, Honig M, Hess I, et al. Reticular dysgenesis (aleukocytosis) is caused by mutations in the gene encoding mitochondrial adenylate kinase 2. Nat Genet 2009;41:101-5.
92. Lagresle-Peyrou C, Six EM, Picard C, et al. Human adenylate kinase 2 deficiency causes a profound hematopoietic defect associated with sensorineural deafness. Nat Genet 2009;41:106-11.
93. Markert ML. Purine nucleoside phosphorylase deficiency. Immunodef Rev 1991;3:45-81.
94. Broome CB, Graham ML, Saulsbury FT, Hershfield MS, Buckley RH. Correction of purine nucleoside phosphorylase deficiency by transplantation of allogeneic bone marrow from a sibling. J Pediatr 1996;128:373-6.
95. Myers LA, Hershfield MS, Neale WT, Escolar M, Kurtzberg J. Purine nucleoside phosphorylase deficiency (PNP-def) presenting with lymphopenia and developmental delay: successful correction with umbilical cord blood transplantation. J Pediatr 2004;145:710-2.
96. Lavin MF, Shiloh Y. Ataxia-telangiectasia. In: Ochs HD, Smith CI, Puck JM, editors. Primary immunodeficiency diseases: a molecular and genetic approach. 2nd ed. New York: Oxford University Press; 2007. p. 402-26.
97. Savitsky K, Bar-Shira A, Gilad S, et al. A single ataxia telangiectasia gene with a product similar to PI-3 kinase. Science 1995;268:1749-53.
98. Derry JMJ, Ochs HD, Francke U. Isolation of a novel gene mutated in Wiskott-Aldrich syndrome. Cell 1994;78:635-44 [erratum in Cell 1994;79:922a].
99. Orange JS, Stone KD, Turvey SE, Krzewski K. The Wiskott-Aldrich syndrome. Cell Mol Life Sci 2004;61:2361-85.
100. Jin Y, Mazza C, Christie JR, et al. Mutations of the Wiskott-Aldrich syndrome protein (WASP): hotspots, effect on transcription, and translation and phenotype/genotype correlation. Blood 2004;104:4010-9.
101. Ancliff PJ, Blundell MP, Cory GO, et al. Two novel activating mutations in the Wiskott-Aldrich syndrome protein result in congenital neutropenia. Blood 2006;108:2182-9.

102. Parolini O, Ressmann G, Haas OA, et al. X-linked Wiskott-Aldrich syndrome in a girl. N Engl J Med 1998;338:291-5.
103. Ochs HD, Thrasher AJ. The Wiskott-Aldrich syndrome. J Allergy Clin Immunol 2006;117:725-38.
104. Orange JS, Ramesh N, Remold-O'Donnell E, et al. Wiskott-Aldrich syndrome protein is required for NK cell cytotoxicity and colocalizes with actin to NK cell-activating immunologic synapses. Proc Natl Acad Sci U S A 2002;99:11351-6.
105. Gismondi A, Cifaldi L, Mazza C, et al. Impaired natural and CD16-mediated NK cell cytotoxicity in patients with WAS and XLT: ability of IL-2 to correct NK cell functional defect. Blood 2004;104:436-43.
106. Filipovich AH, Stone JV, Tomany SC, et al. Impact of donor type on outcome of bone marrow transplantation for Wiskott-Aldrich syndrome: collaborative study of the International Bone Marrow Transplant Registry and the National Marrow Donor Program. Blood 2001;97:1598-603.
107. Dewey RA, Avedillo Díez I, Ballmaier M, et al. Retroviral WASP gene transfer into human hematopoietic stem cells reconstitutes the actin cytoskeleton in myeloid progeny cells differentiated in vitro. Exp Hematol 2006;34:1161-9.
108. Boztug K, Schmidt M, Schwarzer A, et al. Stem-cell gene therapy for the Wiskott-Aldrich syndrome. N Engl J Med 2010;363:1918-27.
109. Pessach IM, Notarangelo LD. Gene therapy for primary immunodeficiencies: looking ahead, toward gene correction. J Allergy Clin Immunol 2011;127:1344-50.
110. Orange JS, Roy-Ghanta S, Mace EM, et al. IL-2 induces a WAVE2-dependent pathway for actin reorganization that enables WASp-independent human NK cell function. J Clin Invest 2011;121:1535-48.
111. Elder ME. Severe combined immunodeficiency due to defects in T cell receptor-associated protein tyrosine kinases. In: Ochs HD, Smith CI, Puck JM, editors. Primary immunodeficiency diseases: a molecular and genetic approach. 2nd ed. New York: Oxford University Press; 2007. p. 203-11.
112. Feske S, Muller JM, Graf D, et al. Severe combined immunodeficiency due to defective binding of the nuclear factor of activated T cells in T lymphocytes of two male siblings. Eur J Immunol 1996;26:2119-26.
113. Feske S, Gwack Y, Prakriya M, et al. A mutation in Orai1 causes immune deficiency by abrogating CRAC channel function. Nature 2006;441:179-85.
114. Elder ME. Severe combined immunodeficiency due to a defect in the tyrosine kinase ZAP-70. Pediatr Res 1996;39:743-8.
115. de la Salle H, Donato L, Hanau D. Peptide transporter defects in human leukocyte antigen class I deficiency. In: Ochs HD, Smith CI, Puck JM, editors. Primary immunodeficiency diseases: a molecular and genetic approach. 2nd ed. New York: Oxford University Press; 2007. p. 242-50.
116. de la Salle H, Zimmer J, Fricker D, et al. HLA class I deficiencies due to mutations in subunit 1 of the peptide transporter TAP1. J Clin Invest 1999;103:R9-13.
117. Donato L, de la Salle H, Hanau D, et al. Association of HLA class I antigen deficiency related to a TAP2 gene mutation with familial bronchiectasis. J Pediatr 1995;127:895-900.
118. Reith W, Lisowska-Grospierre B, Fischer A. Molecular basis of major histocompatibility complex class II deficiency. In: Ochs HD, Smith CI, Puck JM, editors. Primary immunodeficiency diseases: a molecular and genetic approach. 2nd ed. New York: Oxford University Press; 2007. p. 227-41.
119. Steimle V, Durand B, Barras E, et al. A novel DNA-binding regulatory factor is mutated in primary MHC class II deficiency (bare lymphocyte syndrome). Genes Dev 1995;9:1021-32.
120. Durand B, Sperisen P, Emery P, et al. RFXAP, a novel subunit of the RFX DNA binding complex is mutated in MHC class II deficiency. EMBO J 1997;16:1045-55.
121. Masternak K, Barras E, Zufferey M, et al. A gene encoding a novel RFX-associated transactivator is mutated in the majority of MHC class II deficiency patients. Nat Genet 1998;20:273-7.
122. Zhou H, Glimcher LH. Human MHC class II gene transcription directed by the carboxyl terminus of CIITA, one of the defective genes in type II MHC combined immune deficiency. Immunity 1995;2:545-53.
123. Doffinger R, Smahi A, Bessia C, et al. X-linked anhidrotic ectodermal dysplasia with immunodeficiency is caused by impaired NF-kappaB signaling. Nat Genet 2001;27:277-85.
124. Courtois G, Smahi A, Reichenbach J, et al. A hypermorphic IkappaBalpha mutation is associated with autosomal dominant anhidrotic ectodermal dysplasia and T cell immunodeficiency. J Clin Invest 2003;112:1108-15.
125. Dai YS, Liang MG, Gellis SE, et al. Characteristics of mycobacterial infection in patients with immunodeficiency and nuclear factor-kappaB essential modulator mutation, with or without ectodermal dysplasia. J Am Acad Dermatol 2004;51:718-22.
126. Orange JS, Brodeur SR, Jain A, et al. Deficient natural killer cell cytotoxicity in patients with IKK-gamma/NEMO mutations. J Clin Invest 2002;109:1501-9.
127. Fish JD, Duerst RE, Gelfand EW, Orange JS, Bunin N. Challenges in the use of allogeneic hematopoietic SCT for ectodermal dysplasia with immune deficiency. Bone Marrow Transplant 2009;43:217-21.
128. Calle-Martin O, Hernandez M, Ordi J, et al. Familial CD8 deficiency due to a mutation in the CD8 alpha gene. J Clin Invest 2001;108:117-23.
129. Regueiro JR, Espanol T. CD3 and CD8 deficiencies. In: Ochs HD, Smith CI, Puck JM, editors. Primary immunodeficiency diseases: a molecular and genetic approach. 2nd ed. New York: Oxford University Press; 2007. p. 216-26.
130. Ridanpaa M, Sistonen P, Rockas S, et al. Worldwide mutation spectrum in cartilage-hair hypoplasia: ancient founder origin of the major70A→G mutation of the untranslated RMRP. Eur J Hum Genet 2002;10:439-47.
131. Buckley RH, Wray BB, Belmaker EZ. Extreme hyperimmunoglobulinemia E and undue susceptibility to infection. Pediatrics 1972;49:59-70.
132. Buckley RH. The hyper-IgE syndrome. Clin Rev Allergy Immunol 2001;20:139-54.
133. Grimbacher B, Holland SM, Gallin JI, et al. Hyper-IgE syndrome with recurrent infections—an autosomal dominant multisystem disorder. N Engl J Med 1999;340:692-702.
134. Minegishi Y, Saito M, Tsuchiya S, et al. Dominant-negative mutations in the DNA-binding domain of STAT3 cause hyper-IgE syndrome. Nature 2007;448:1058-62.
135. Holland SM, Deleo FR, Elloumi HZ, et al. STAT3 mutations in the hyper-IgE syndrome. N Engl J Med 2007;357:1608-19.
136. Milner JD, Brenchley JM, Laurence A, et al. Impaired T(H)17 cell differentiation in subjects with autosomal dominant hyper-IgE syndrome. Nature 2008;452:773-6.
137. Claassen JL, Levine AD, Schiff SE, Buckley RH. Mononuclear cells from patients with the hyper IgE syndrome produce little IgE when stimulated with recombinant interleukin 4 in vitro. J Allergy Clin Immunol 1991;88:713-21.
138. Renner ED, Puck JM, Holland SM, et al. Autosomal recessive hyperimmunoglobulin E syndrome: a distinct disease entity. J Pediatr 2004;144:93-9.
139. Zhang Q, Davis JC, Lamborn IT, et al. Combined immunodeficiency associated with DOCK8 mutations. N Engl J Med 2009;361:2046-55.
140. Engelhardt KR, McGhee S, Winkler S, et al. Large deletions and point mutations involving the dedicator of cytokinesis 8 (DOCK8) in the autosomal-recessive form of hyper-IgE syndrome. J Allergy Clin Immunol 2009;124:1289-302.
141. Minegishi Y, Karasuyama H. Hyperimmunoglobulin E syndrome and tyrosine kinase 2 deficiency. Curr Opin Allergy Clin Immunol 2007;7:506-9.
142. Driscoll DA, Sullivan KE. DiGeorge syndrome: a chromosome 22q11.2 deletion syndrome. In: Ochs HD, Smith CI, Puck JM, editors. Primary immunodeficiency diseases: a molecular and genetic approach. 2nd ed. New York: Oxford University Press; 2007. p. 485-95.
143. Zweier C, Sticht H, Aydin-Yaylagul I, Campbell CE, Rauch A. Human TBX1 missense mutations cause gain of function resulting in the same phenotype as 22q11.2 deletions. Am J Hum Genet 2007;80:510-7.
144. Daw SC, Taylor C, Kraman M, et al. A common region of 10p deleted in DiGeorge and velocardiofacial syndromes. Nat Genet 1996;13:458-60.
145. McDonald-McGinn DM, Sullivan KE. Chromosome 22q11.2 deletion syndrome (DiGeorge syndrome/velocardiofacial syndrome). Medicine (Baltimore) 2011;90:1-18.
146. Markert ML, Devlin BH, Alexieff MJ, et al. Review of 54 patients with complete DiGeorge anomaly enrolled in protocols for thymus transplantation: outcome of 44 consecutive transplants. Blood 2007;109:4539-47.

Diseases of Immune Dysregulation

147. Schuster V, Terhorst C. X-linked lymphoproliferative disease due to defects of SH2D1A. In: Ochs HD, Smith CI, Puck JM, editors. Primary immunodeficiency diseases: a molecular and genetic approach. 2nd ed. New York: Oxford University Press; 2007. p. 470-84.
148. Nichols KE, Harkin DP, Levitz S, et al. Inactivating mutations in an SH2 domain-encoding gene in X-linked lymphoproliferative syndrome. Proc Natl Acad Sci U S A 1998;95:13765-70.
149. Sayos J, Wu C, Morra M, et al. The X-linked lymphoproliferative-disease gene product SAP regulates signals induced through the co-receptor SLAM. Nature 1998;395:462-9.

150. Tangye SG, Phillips JH, Lanier LL, Nichols KE. Functional requirement for SAP in 2B4-mediated activation of human natural killer cells as revealed by the X-linked lymphoproliferative syndrome. J Immunol 2000;165:2932-6.
151. Morra M, Silander O, Calpe-Flores S, et al. Alterations of the X-linked lymphoproliferative disease gene SH2DIA in common variable immunodeficiency syndrome. Blood 2001;98:1321-5.
152. Rigaud S, Fondaneche MC, Lambert N, et al. XIAP deficiency in humans causes an X-linked lymphoproliferative syndrome. Nature 2006;444:110-4.
153. Rigaud S, Lopez-Granados E, Siberil S, et al. Human X-linked variable immunodeficiency caused by a hypomorphic mutation in XIAP in association with a rare polymorphism in CD40LG. Blood 2011;118:252-61.
154. Huck K, Feyen O, Niehues T, et al. Girls homozygous for an IL-2-inducible T cell kinase mutation that leads to protein deficiency develop fatal EBV-associated lymphoproliferation. J Clin Invest 2009;119:1350-8.
155. Bennett CL, Christie J, Ramsdell F, et al. The immune dysregulation, polyendocrinopathy, enteropathy, X-linked syndrome (IPEX) is caused by mutations of FOXP3. Nat Genet 2001;27:20-1.
156. Bacchetta R, Passerini L, Gambineri E, et al. Defective regulatory and effector T cell functions in patients with FOXP3 mutations. J Clin Invest 2006;116:1713-22.
157. Baud O, Goulet O, Canioni D, et al. Treatment of the immune dysregulation, polyendocrinopathy, enteropathy, X-linked syndrome (IPEX) by allogeneic bone marrow transplantation. N Engl J Med 2001;344:1758-62.
158. Peltonen-Palotie L, Halonen M, Perheentupa J. Autoimmune polyendocrinopathy, candidiasis, ectodermal dystrophy. In: Ochs HD, Smith CI, Puck JM, editors. Primary immunodeficiency diseases: a molecular and genetic approach. 2nd ed. New York: Oxford University Press; 2007. p. 342-53.
159. Kisand K, Boe Wolff AS, et al. Chronic mucocutaneous candidiasis in APECED or thymoma patients correlates with autoimmunity to Th17-associated cytokines. J Exp Med 2010;207:299-308.
160. Puel A, Cypowyj S, Bustamante J, et al. Chronic mucocutaneous candidiasis in humans with inborn errors of interleukin-17 immunity. Science 2011;332:65-8.
161. Pedroza LA, Kumar V, Sanborn KB, et al. Autoimmune regulator (AIRE) contributes to Dectin-1-induced TNF-alpha production and complexes with caspase recruitment domain-containing protein 9 (CARD9), spleen tyrosine kinase (Syk), and Dectin-1. J Allergy Clin Immunol 2012;129:464-72, 472.e1-3.
162. van de Veerdonk FL, Plantinga TS, Hoischen A, et al. STAT1 mutations in autosomal dominant chronic mucocutaneous candidiasis. N Engl J Med 2011;365:54-61.
163. Glocker EO, Hennigs A, Nabavi M, et al. A homozygous CARD9 mutation in a family with susceptibility to fungal infections. N Engl J Med 2009;361:1727-35.
164. Puck JM, Rieux-Laucat F, LeDiest F, Straus SE. Autoimmune lymphoproliferative syndrome. In: Ochs HD, Smith CI, Puck JM, editors. Primary immunodeficiency diseases: a molecular and genetic approach. 2nd ed. New York: Oxford University Press; 2007. p. 326-41.

Disorders of Phagocytic Cells

165. Lekstrom-Himes JA, Gallin JI. Immunodeficiency diseases caused by defects in phagocytes. N Engl J Med 2000;343:1703-14.
166. Roos D, Kuijpers TW, Curnutte JT. Chronic granulomatous disease. In: Ochs HD, Smith CI, Puck JM, editors. Primary immunodeficiency diseases: a molecular and genetic approach. 2nd ed. New York: Oxford University Press; 2007. p. 525-49.
167. Dinauer MC, Orkin SH, Brown R. The glycoprotein encoded by the X-linked chronic granulomatous disease locus is a component of the neutrophil cytochrome *b* complex. Nature 1987;327:717.
168. Winkelstein JA, Marino MC, Johnston Jr RB, et al. Chronic granulomatous disease. Report on a national registry of 368 patients. Medicine (Baltimore) 2000;79:155-69.
169. Greenberg DE, Porcella SF, Stock F, et al. *Granulibacter bethesdensis* gen. nov., sp. nov., a distinctive pathogenic acetic acid bacterium in the family Acetobacteraceae. Int J Syst Evol Microbiol 2006;56(Pt 11):2609-16.
170. Greenberg DE, Ding L, Zelazny AM, et al. A novel bacterium associated with lymphadenitis in a patient with chronic granulomatous disease. PLoS Pathog 2006;2:e28.
171. Vowells SJ, Fleisher TA, Sekhsaria S, et al. Genotype-dependent variability in flow cytometric evaluation of reduced nicotinamide adenine dinucleotide phosphate oxidase function in patients with chronic granulomatous disease. J Pediatr 1996;128:104-7.
172. Gallin JI, Alling DW, Malech HL, et al. Itraconazole to prevent fungal infections in chronic granulomatous disease. N Engl J Med 2003;348:2416-22.
173. International Chronic Granulomatous Disease Cooperative Study Group. A controlled trial of interferon gamma to prevent infection in chronic granulomatous disease. N Engl J Med 1991;324:509-16.
174. Seger RA. Hematopoietic stem cell transplantation for chronic granulomatous disease. Immunol Allergy Clin North Am 2010;30:195-208.
175. Ott MG, Schmidt M, Schwarzwaelder K, et al. Correction of X-linked chronic granulomatous disease by gene therapy, augmented by insertional activation of MDS1-EVI1, PRDM16 or SETBP1. Nat Med 2006;12:401-9.
176. Etzioni A, Harlan JM. Cell adhesion and leukocyte adhesion defects. In: Ochs HD, Smith CI, Puck JM, editors. Primary immunodeficiency diseases: a molecular and genetic approach. 2nd ed. New York: Oxford University Press; 2007. p. 550-64.
177. Lubke T, Marquardt T, Etzioni A, et al. Complementation cloning identifies CDG-IIc, a new type of congenital disorders of glycosylation, as a GDP-fucose transporter deficiency. Nat Genet 2001;28:73-6.
178. Nagle DL, Karim MA, Woolf EA, et al. Identification and mutation analysis of the complete gene for Chédiak-Higashi syndrome. Nat Genet 1996;14:307-11.
179. Spritz RA. Chédiak-Higashi syndrome. In: Ochs HD, Smith CI, Puck JM, editors. Primary immunodeficiency diseases: a molecular and genetic approach. 2nd ed. New York: Oxford University Press; 2007. p. 570-88.

Defects of Innate Immunity

180. Jouanguy E, Altare F, Lamhamedi S, et al. Interferon-gamma-receptor deficiency in an infant with fatal bacille Calmette-Guerin infection. N Engl J Med 1996;335:1956-61.
181. Newport MJ, Holland SM, Levin M, Casanova JL. Inherited disorders of the interleukin-12/23-interferon gamma axis. In: Ochs HD, Smith CI, Puck JM, editors. Primary immunodeficiency diseases: a molecular and genetic approach. 2nd ed. New York: Oxford University Press; 2007. p. 390-401.
182. Altare F, Durandy A, Lammas D, et al. Impairment of mycobacterial immunity in human interleukin-12 receptor deficiency. Science 1998;280:1432-5.
183. de Jong R, Altare F, Haagen I, et al. Severe mycobacterial and *Salmonella* infections in interleukin-12 receptor-deficient patients. Science 1998;280:1435-8.
184. Dupuis S, Dargemont C, Fieschi C, et al. Impairment of mycobacterial but not viral immunity by a germline human STAT1 mutation. Science 2001;293:300-3.
185. Dupuis S, Jouanguy E, Al Hajjar S, et al. Impaired response to interferon-alpha/beta and lethal viral disease in human STAT1 deficiency. Nat Genet 2003;33:388-91.
186. Ku CL, Yang K, Bustamante J, et al. Inherited disorders of human Toll-like receptor signaling: immunological implications. Immunol Rev 2005;203:10-20.
187. Picard C, von Bernuth H, Ghandil P, et al. Clinical features and outcome of patients with IRAK-4 and MyD88 deficiency. Medicine (Baltimore) 2010;89:403-25.
188. Orange JS. Human natural killer cell deficiencies. Curr Opin Allergy Clin Immunol 2006;6:399-409.
189. Hsu AP, Sampaio EP, Khan J, et al. Mutations in GATA2 are associated with the autosomal dominant and sporadic monocytopenia and mycobacterial infection (MonoMAC) syndrome. Blood 2011;118:2653-5.
190. Cuellar-Rodriguez J, Gea-Banacloche J, Freeman AF, et al. Successful allogeneic hematopoietic stem cell transplantation for GATA2 deficiency. Blood 2011;118:3715-20.

Complement Component Deficiencies

191. Sullivan KE, Winkelstein JA. Genetically-determined deficiencies of the complement system. In: Ochs HD, Smith CI, Puck JM, editors. Primary immunodeficiency diseases: a molecular and genetic approach. 2nd ed. New York: Oxford University Press; 2007. p. 589-608.
192. Westberg J, Fredrikson GN, Truedsson L, Sjoholm AG, Uhlen M. Sequence-based analysis of properdin deficiency: identification of point mutations in two phenotypic forms of an X-linked immunodeficiency. Genomics 1995;29:1-8.
193. Hartmann D, Fremeaux-Bacchi V, Weiss L, et al. Combined heterozygous deficiency of the classical complement pathway proteins C2 and C4. J Clin Immunol 1997;17:176-84.

Approach to Treatment of Primary Immunodeficiency Disorders

194. Hacein-Bey-Abina S, Garrigue A, Wang GP, et al. Insertional oncogenesis in 4 patients after retrovirus-mediated gene therapy of SCID-X1. J Clin Invest 2008;118:3132-42.

73

Human Immunodeficiency Virus and Allergic Disease

SARAH K. NICHOLAS | MARY E. PAUL | WILLIAM T. SHEARER

CONTENTS

SUMMARY OF IMPORTANT CONCEPTS

» The immune dysregulation of human immunodeficiency virus (HIV) infection may lead to de novo or recrudescent atopic disease.
» Asthma and atopic dermatitis occur with increased incidence in patients receiving highly active antiretroviral therapy (HAART) for HIV infection.
» Autoimmune conditions, such as psoriatic arthritis, also occur with increased frequency among HIV-infected patients undergoing immunoreconstitution with anti-HIV drugs.
» Drug allergy in HIV infection, even with antiretroviral agents, is a common occurrence that requires careful management.

Introduction

Human immunodeficiency virus (HIV)—more specifically, HIV-1—is important to consider in the context of allergic disease because it probably is responsible for an increased incidence of atopy. Owing to the very high worldwide HIV burden, even a small increase in atopic disease represents a large change in overall incidence. The most recent estimate by the Joint United Nations Programme on HIV/AIDS (UNAIDS) puts 34 million people living with HIV infection or acquired immunodeficiency disease (AIDS) worldwide in 2010.[1] In the United States, approximately 1.2 million adolescents and adults were living with HIV infection at the end of 2008, with a steady increase of 40,000 to 50,000 new infections annually.[2]

Human Immunodeficiency Virus: Background

HIV is a retrovirus and is further classified into the lentivirus group. It is an enveloped, positive-sense RNA virus. Once it infects a host cell, it replicates its RNA genome into DNA (by means of reverse transcriptase) and inserts itself into the host genome, where it can produce viral proteins and new viruses using host machinery. The virus is transmitted by sexual contact, parenterally, and perinatally, with 70% to 80% of infections worldwide being sexually acquired.

THE VIRAL STRUCTURE

HIV has an outer coat, known as the viral envelope, and a core (Fig. 73-1). The envelope is composed of two lipid layers taken from the membrane of a human cell when a newly formed virus particle buds from the cell. Implanted in the viral envelope are envelope proteins that protrude through the surface of the viron. The envelope protein, glycoprotein (gp) 160, is formed from gp120 on the surface and a transmembrane protein, gp41. The core is composed of a capsid protein, p24, that surrounds the duplicate copies of single-stranded RNA viral genetic material. A matrix protein, p17, the nucleocapsid protein, p7, and three enzymes, reverse transcriptase, integrase, and protease, are included in the viral core.

THE VIRAL GENOME

HIV genome is 9.8 kb long and contains nine genes that are structural or regulatory and accessory in nature. The structural genes, *gag, pol,* and *env*, contain information needed to make structural proteins for new viral particles. The *env* gene codes for gp160 and the *gag* gene codes for p24. The *pol* gene encodes reverse transcriptase. Six regulatory genes, *tat, rev, nef, vif, vpr,* and *vpu*, contain information necessary for production of proteins that control cell infectivity, viral replication, and cause disease. The protein encoded by *nef*, for instance, is necessary for the virus to replicate efficiently, and the *vpu*-encoded protein influences the release of new virus particles from infected cells. The protein encoded by *vif* interacts with an antiviral defense protein in host cells causing inactivation of the antiviral effect and enhancing HIV replication. The ends of each strand of HIV RNA contain an RNA sequence called the long terminal repeat (LTR). Regions in the LTR act as switches to control production of new viruses and can be triggered by proteins from either HIV or the host cell.

ENTRY OF VIRUS INTO CELLS

HIV requires CD4 and coreceptors to infect target cells. Viral gp120 binds the CD4 molecule on the host cell surface, resulting

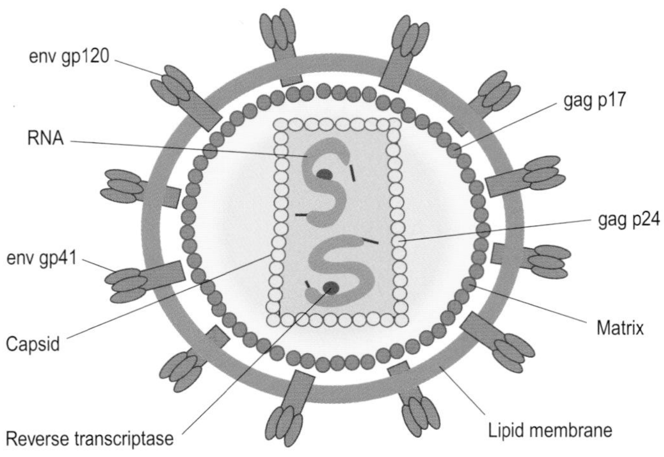

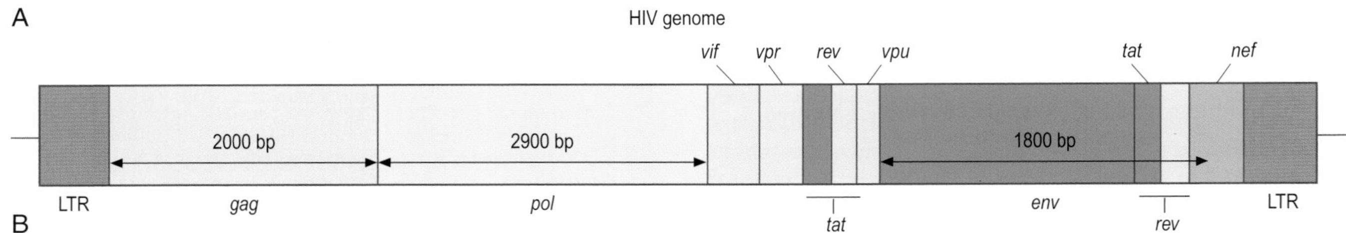

Figure 73-1 The human immunodeficiency virus, type 1 (HIV-1). **A,** HIV-1 virion, an icosahedral particle composed of an outer envelope and a central core. Outer envelope is acquired during virion budding and contains two major viral envelope glycoproteins, gp120 and gp41, in a lipid bilayer. Central core contains core proteins (capsid p24, matrix p17, p9, nucleocapsid p7), two copies of HIV-1 RNA, and viral enzymes (reverse transcriptase, integrase, protease). **B,** HIV-1 genome. The 9-kilobase genome contains three genes (*gag, env, pol*) that code for precursor proteins of the core and the envelope and for viral enzymes, respectively. Other genes with known function mediate regulatory (*tat, nef, vpr, rev*) and other functions in the life cycle of HIV-1, such as viral budding (*vpu, vif*). *bp,* Base pairs; *LTR,* long terminal repeat.

in a conformational change in gp120 to expose the binding site for the coreceptor, generally a chemokine receptor. One of two chemokine coreceptors, CCR5 and CXCR4, are used by a majority of HIV viruses; however, others have been found to be utilized by rare HIV isolates. Researchers classify the strain of HIV based on coreceptor usage, depending on whether the viral isolates exhibit tropism for T cell lines or macrophage cell lines in vitro.

CCR5 is the coreceptor for macrophage-tropic HIV strains called R5 strains. CCR5 is a G protein–coupled receptor with seven transmembrane segments. It is a receptor for RANTES (*r*egulated on *a*ctivation, *n*ormal *T* cells *e*xpressed and *s*ecreted), macrophage inflammatory protein (MIP)-1α, and MIP-1β—all chemokines that have been shown to suppress HIV-1 infection. Mutations in the CCR5 gene protect cells from HIV infection.[3]

CXCR4 acts as the coreceptor for the fusion of HIV strains adapted for growth in transformed T cell lines (T-tropic strains). T-tropic strains of HIV are called X4 strains. Antibodies to CXCR4 block cell fusion and infection with normal $CD4^+$ human target cells. The ligand for CXCR4, the α chemokine stromal cell–derived factor-1 (SDF-1α), inhibits HIV entry into the cell.

The cell first infected by HIV (R5 strains, non–syncytium-inducing phenotype) probably is the macrophage, through cooperative binding by the CD4 and CCR5 surface molecules. Later, the $CD4^+$ T cell becomes infected by HIV (X4 strains, syncytium-inducing phenotype) through cell surface CD4 and CXCR4 molecules. CXCR4 is more broadly expressed on $CD4^+$ T cells than CCR5. Dual-tropic HIV strains, designated R5X4 viral strains, and strains using additional coreceptors, also have been described.

Once gp120 has bound to CD4 and the coreceptor, gp41 of the viral envelope fuses with the cell membrane, allowing entry of the viral core components into the cell cytoplasm. The virus then uses host cell machinery, viral enzymes, and proteins to transcribe viral RNA into DNA, to integrate proviral DNA into the host genome, and to form new viral particles that bud from the host cell.

HUMAN IMMUNODEFICIENCY VIRUS DIAGNOSIS

HIV diagnosis is by serologic and virologic testing (Fig. 73-2). In children older than 18 months of age and adults, recommended screening is serologic, using enzyme immunoassays (EIAs) for antibodies against HIV-1. Newer rapid tests also pick up the p24 viral antigen, which shortens the window between initial infection and the time it can be detected.[4] Nonserologic tests must be used in children younger than 18 months of age, owing to the potential for false-positive results from lingering maternally derived anti-HIV antibodies. In these young patients, as well as in people with impaired humoral immune responses, it is imperative that polymerase chain reaction (PCR) testing for HIV DNA be used, because EIA testing is reliable only if the host can make an appropriate antibody response. Use of serologic testing in these populations is likely to yield false-negative results, with loss of opportunities for early intervention.

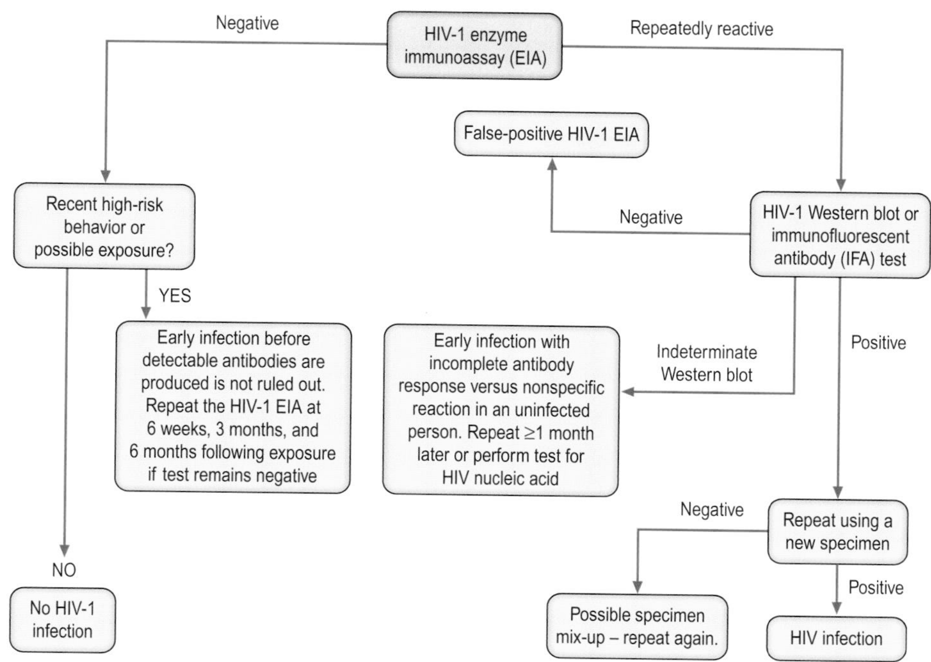

Figure 73-2 Diagnosis of human immunodeficiency virus (HIV)-1 infection in children 18 months of age and older using HIV-1 enzyme immunoassay and Western blot analysis.

HIV is divided into subtypes based on the genetic divergence in the *env* gene. The predominant HIV subtype in the United States is subtype B. The currently available HIV DNA PCR test is less sensitive in detecting non–subtype B HIV, and caution is warranted in interpreting a negative result on HIV DNA PCR testing in infants whose mothers may have been infected with a non–subtype B virus. PCR assay for HIV DNA and RNA can be used to detect HIV shortly after exposure, before antibody-based tests become positive.

The T cell receptor excision circle (TREC) analysis being developed and used for statewide severe combined immunodeficiency (SCID) newborn screening programs also may find patients with severe congenital HIV infection, although none has been detected to date.[5]

Immune Dysregulation and Human Immunodeficiency Virus

IMMUNOGLOBULIN E LEVELS: REFLECTION OF HUMAN IMMUNODEFICIENCY VIRUS DISEASE PROGRESSION

Increased immunoglobulin E (IgE) levels have been found in HIV-infected persons by many investigators. The immune mechanism for increased IgE levels in this disorder has not been well described. However, a polyclonal gammopathy and activated B cells are found in HIV-infected patients: B cells are highly and abnormally activated, and many of these patients are hypergammaglobulinemic, with increased production of immunoglobulins IgG, IgA, and IgD. Much of the immunoglobulin produced is specific for HIV; however, many HIV-infected persons have decreased production of specific antibody to other antigens and increased serum antibodies reactive with self-antigens. Also, although activated in vitro, B cells exhibit decreased in vitro proliferation after stimulation with pokeweed mitogen or antigen.

IL-4 is the cytokine that promotes the class switch to IgE production in the B cell. Increased levels of IL-4 have been reported in some stages of HIV-1 infection. Increased production of IL-4 correlated with increased IgE levels in a study of unstimulated and mitogen-stimulated peripheral blood mononuclear cells (PBMCs) from a group of vertically infected children. Also, both the increased IL-4 and IL-10 production and the higher IgE levels were found in the more symptomatic patients.

T CELLS IN HUMAN IMMUNODEFICIENCY VIRUS INFECTION: LOSS OF CD4$^+$ AND GAIN OF CD8$^+$ CELLS

Decrease in CD4$^+$ T cell number and function is the hallmark of HIV infection, although every component of immunity is affected.[6] Evidence suggests that HIV destroys CD4$^+$ T lymphocytes by a number of mechanisms. First, the virus is trophic for these lymphocytes, and destruction occurs in some infected cells owing to replication of the virus within the cell or release of virus from the cell. Cell death also can result from formation of a syncytium. Syncytium production is associated with the merging of infected cells expressing gp120 with CD4$^+$ T lymphocytes (grapelike cluster of infected CD4$^+$ T cells). Apoptosis occurs to destroy CD4$^+$ T cells as well. Fas-mediated activation–induced cell death is one such mechanism, or apoptosis may be stimulated in uninfected bystander cells by released or cell surface–expressed HIV gene products including accessory proteins and *env* proteins.[7] Specifically, autophagy has been proposed as a mechanism of CD4$^+$ T cell destruction in advanced disease, in which CXCR4 engagement in bystander CD4$^+$ T cells by the HIV glycoprotein activates a lysosomal degradation (autophagy) pathway.[8] Another mechanism of CD4+ destruction is stimulation of activation-induced cell death by HIV gp120/V3-derived epitopes of superantigen-activated CD4+ memory T cells.[9] CD4+ T lymphocyte depletion also may result from abnormal production of lymphocytes. One indication of the role of the thymus in the pathogenesis of HIV infection is the measure of T cell receptor rearrangement excision circles (i.e., TRECs found in naive T cells).[10] HIV infection leads to a decrease in the levels of TRECs in peripheral blood T cells. Th17 helper T cells are lost in subjects who are rapid HIV progressors and are preserved in slow HIV progressors, and in some instances a small Th17 component (especially in the infected mucosa) can predict loss of immune control of HIV replication.[11]

Hersperger and colleagues[12] reported that the expression of the T-bet transcription factor increases the levels of perforin and granzyme B in cytotoxic CD8+ T cells. This augmentation causes them to be powerful cytolytic agents against HIV-infected target CD4+ T cells, allowing some patients, so-called elite controllers, to survive well without antiretroviral drugs and with extremely low HIV viral burden.

Major histocompatibility complex (MHC)-restricted CD8+ T cells have been shown to exhibit a variety of effector functions important in HIV-1 disease progression, in addition to cytolytic activity. CD8+ memory and effector T cells suppress HIV replication by producing cytokines such as gamma interferon (IFN-γ), which induces cellular proteins that suppress HIV replication, and tumor necrosis factor α (TNF-α), which induces apoptosis of HIV-infected cells. CD8+ T cells also produce chemokines such as RANTES and MIP-1β, both of which can suppress viral replication by inhibiting viral entry via CCR5.[13] In addition, IFN-γ increases the surface expression of human leukocyte antigen (HLA) molecules and can activate macrophages that predominantly synthesize MIP-1β.

B CELLS IN HUMAN IMMUNODEFICIENCY VIRUS INFECTION: LOSS OF MEMORY CELLS

B cell dysfunction in HIV-1 disease may be caused by decreased contribution of CD4+ helper cells and decreased regulation of antibody production.[14] A study of children with vertical HIV-1 infection showed a smaller rise in CD40 ligand expression in infected children than in control subjects, suggesting a defect in T and B cell cooperation in the infected children. Likewise, the proportion of CD4+ T cells with the CD45RO isoform failed to increase in HIV-infected patients compared with control subjects, suggesting a disturbance in the generation of memory to T cell–dependent antigens. In vitro, the gp120-CD4 interaction has been shown to interfere with signal transduction through the CD3 antigen-receptor complex.

HIV-infected persons who have experienced a recent infection mount a vigorous antibody response against autologous HIV. HIV rapidly evolves in response to the neutralizing antibody after recent infection, and antibody escape emerges. During early HIV disease, antibody responses are more likely to recognize earlier autologous viruses than evolved current autologous virus species in the patient.[15]

INNATE IMMUNITY IN HUMAN IMMUNODEFICIENCY VIRUS INFECTION

The role of innate immunity in HIV infection has not been sufficiently explored. Newer studies are uncovering a substantial role for components of innate immunity: epithelial cells, complement proteins, dendritic cells, phagocytes, and natural killer (NK) cells.[16] NK cell activity in response to IL-2 is decreased in HIV infection as is antibody-dependent cell–mediated cytotoxicity. Inheritance of certain NK cell *KIR* (killer inhibitor receptor) alleles has been shown to be associated with decreased rapid progression of HIV infection.[17]

CYTOKINES IN HUMAN IMMUNODEFICIENCY VIRUS INFECTION: PROINFLAMMATORY MILIEU

The cytokine milieu is altered in HIV-infected patients, and the alterations are associated with level of immune activation, HIV viremia, chemokine production, chemokine receptor expression, and disease progression (Table 73-1). For example, whereas the production of IFN-γ is reduced in patients with AIDS, and persons at risk for AIDS-related opportunistic infections (OIs) have impaired IFN-γ production, symptomatic patients with primary infection show elevations of IFN-γ.[18] In chronically infected patients with high viral load, CD8+ cells consistently produce IFN-γ.[19] Interleukin (IL)-2, a cytokine secreted by T lymphocytes, regulates the proliferation and differentiation of both T and B lymphocytes. IL-2 production is decreased in both acute and chronic HIV infection and HIV-specific IL-2 production in CD4+ T cells has been correlated inversely with viremia.[19] Infusions of IL-2 result in substantial increases in CD4+ T cell count in HIV-infected patients with CD4+ counts greater than 200 cells/μL. Other cytokines that can restore some cellular immune functions in HIV-infected patients include IL-13, IL-16, and IL-12. TNF-α is a proinflammatory, monocyte-derived cytokine that has been implicated in HIV disease progression partly because of its ability to stimulate HIV expression in vitro. Mononuclear phagocytes from HIV patients produce elevated levels of TNF-α, and serum levels of TNF-α may increase as infection progresses. Other cytokines that can upregulate HIV expression on cells of chronically infected monocyte and T cell lines include IL-1β, IL-6, and granulocyte-macrophage colony-stimulating factor (GM-CSF).

IL-10 is an antiinflammatory cytokine that is produced primarily by Th0 and Th2 cells, CD8+ T cells, regulatory T cells, monocytes, and B cells.[20] IL-10 inhibits the antigen-driven activity of both Th1 and Th2 cells and has potent inhibitory action on macrophages. IL-10 production is increased during HIV infection and antiretroviral treatment results in the reduction of IL-10 production. IL-10 inhibits the expression of CCR5 on T cells and inhibits HIV replication.[21] In addition, IL-10 has been shown to increase CXCR4 expression on dendritic cells. Because monocytes act as viral reservoirs for HIV, IL-10 production may enhance the virus's ability to escape from immune surveillance and promote disease progression. IL-12 production may be altered in HIV-infected patients as well. Both reduced IL-12 secretion in response to stimulation of PBMCs of HIV-infected subjects with *Staphylococcus aureus* in vitro and reduced constitutive messenger RNA (mRNA) expression in PBMCs from HIV-infected persons have been reported.

Constitutive expression of cytokines in lymph nodes of adults with early, intermediate, and advanced stages of HIV-1 infection has included overexpression of IL-6, TNF-α, IFN-γ, and IL-10, relative to expression from lymph nodes of patients with other diseases.

Certain chemokines including RANTES, MIP-1α, MIP-1β, and SDF-1α can block HIV-1 entry into the cell by binding

TABLE 73-1 Modulation of Cytokines in HIV Disease Progression and Subsequent Effects on Chemokine Receptors in Affected Cell Types

Cytokine	Cytokine Level with HIV Disease Progression	Cytokine Effect on Chemokine Receptor	Cytokine Effect on CCR5 Chemokine
IL-2	Decreased	CCR5 ↑ CCR5 ↓	CCR5 ↑
IL-4	Unchanged to increased	CCR5 ↓, CXCR4 ↑ CCR5 ↓ CXCR4 ↑	CCR5 ↓
IL-10	Increased	CCR5 ↓, CXCR4 ↓ CCR5 ↑ CXCR4 ↑	CCR5 ↓
IFN-γ	Increased	CCR5 ↑, CXCR4 ↓ CCR5 ↑ CXCR4 ↓	CCR5 ↑ CCR5 ↑
TNF-α	Increased	CCR5 ↑↓ CCR5 ↓	CCR5 ↑ CCR5 ↓

Adapted from Kinter A, Arthos J, Cicala C, Fauci AS. Chemokines, cytokines and HIV: a complex network of interactions that influence HIV pathogenesis. Immunol Rev 2000;177:88-98; and from Norris PJ, Pappalardo BL, Custer B, et al. Elevations in IL-10, TNF alpha, and IFN gamma from the earliest point of HIV type 1 infection. AIDS Res Hum Retroviruses 2006;22:757-62.

DC, Dendritic cell; *IFN*, interferon; *IL*, interleukin; *M/M*, monocyte-macrophage; *NK*, natural killer [cell]; *TNF*, tumor necrosis factor.

respective chemokine coreceptors CCR5 and CXCR4. IL-4 upregulates CXCR4 and favors entry of lymphocytotrophic HIV-1 strains in CD4$^+$ T cells.

Clinical Phenotypes of Allergic Disease in Human Immunodeficiency Virus Infection

The most common clinical entities suggesting allergy in HIV-infected persons are drug hypersensitivity reactions and pruritic cutaneous disorders. Because IgE-mediated allergy is sometimes associated with these symptoms, investigators have postulated an increased incidence of atopy in HIV-infected patients. Few studies have detailed the pattern of atopic disease in such patients, and efforts to better define its occurrence have been hampered by the presence of confounders such as infection or other illness, the concurrent administration of multiple medications, and immunologic alterations in patients with HIV infection.

IMMUNE RECONSTITUTION INFLAMMATORY SYNDROME AND HYPERALLERGENIC STATE ASSOCIATED WITH IMMUNORECONSTITUTION IN HUMAN IMMUNODEFICIENCY VIRUS INFECTION

Immune reconstitution inflammatory syndrome (IRIS) is seen in HIV-infected patients who start on HAART, typically manifested as paradoxical worsening of HIV-related OIs or other pathologic conditions.[22] Such exacerbations may occur both with concurrently treated OIs and with previously unrecognized OIs. The syndrome is thought to represent an overactivation of the immune system in response to the OI pathogen. Based on a recent meta-analysis of data on 13,102 patients, the incidence of IRIS is thought to be 13% to16% in patients starting HAART, with significant variation based on the type of previously diagnosed OI or other HIV-associated condition. The incidence with previously diagnosed AIDS-related illnesses was 6.4% for Kaposi sarcoma, 12.2% for herpes zoster, 15.7% for tuberculosis, 16.7% for progressive multifocal leukoencephalopathy, 19.5% for cryptococcal meningitis, and 37.7% for cytomegalovirus retinitis. Low CD4$^+$ T cell count (particularly less than 50 cells/μL) at initiation of HAART also was a significant risk factor for development of IRIS, independent of preexisting OIs. The overall mortality rate for IRIS is 4.5%; disease-specific rates will vary, however, ranging from 2.5% in patients with tuberculosis to 20.8% in those with cryptococcal meningitis.

IRIS also is potentially associated with the increased rate of asthma and other allergic disease in patients with HIV infection who are on HAART. We postulate that this atopy is mediated by CD4$^+$ T cell activation, Th2 cytokine alterations as described previously, and loss of regulatory T cells and tolerance.

DRUG HYPERSENSITIVITY IN HUMAN IMMUNODEFICIENCY VIRUS INFECTION

Drug hypersensitivity is relatively common in HIV-infected patients and greatly affects clinical care. It is important to recognize that patients with AIDS have up to a 1000 times greater chance of developing Stevens-Johnson syndrome or toxic epidermal necrosis and other severe cutaneous drug reactions compared with the general population. The mortality rate with these reactions is the same as for the general population, but at 5% to 30%, this is an important cause of death.[23]

The most common clinical manifestations of adverse drug reactions are dermatologic reactions, fever, hepatotoxicity, nephrotoxicity, anaphylactic reactions, and hematologic toxicity, although lungs, pancreas, and other organs also can be involved. Reactions indicating IgE-mediated hypersensitivity include urticaria and anaphylactic reactions. The number of skin condition diagnoses increases with increasing severity of HIV disease. A morbilliform rash is the most common type of drug-related eruption in HIV-infected patients, followed by urticaria. Photodermatitis also has been reported.

Less frequent reactions that are potentially life-threatening include erythema multiforme, Stevens-Johnson syndrome, toxic epidermal necrolysis, rash occurring with abacavir (ABC)-associated systemic hypersensitivity reaction, and the syndrome of drug rash with eosinophilia and systemic symptoms (DRESS).

Trimethoprim-sulfamethoxazole (TMP-SMX), which is the mainstay of prophylaxis and treatment for *Pneumocystis jirovecii* pneumonia, is associated with a remarkably high rate of reactions, which include rash, fever, hematologic disturbances, transaminase disturbances, anaphylaxis, and Stevens-Johnson syndrome–toxic epidermal necrolysis. Reactions are reported in 44% to 83% of HIV-infected persons, compared with less than 10% of the general population.[23] Many other drugs are important causes of drug hypersensitivity reactions in HIV infection, particularly HIV treatment medications. Currently, more than 20 drugs are available that are used in combination in accordance with consensus guidelines. In general, highly active antiretroviral therapy (HAART) regimens consist of at least three drugs that target at least two stages in the viral life cycle. The currently available medications are briefly summarized in Table 73-2. The most up-to-date information can be found at the National Institutes of Health (NIH)–sponsored AIDSinfo website.[24] Table 73-3 summarizes the hypersensitivity reactions to these medications.[25] The hypersensitivity reactions with HAART that are of greatest concern are those associated with ABC and nevirapine (NVP). ABC causes a potentially fatal systemic illness in up to 8% of patients,[26] characterized by high fever, diffuse rash (in 70%), malaise, nausea, headache, myalgia, diarrhea, vomiting, flank or abdominal pain, and arthralgia. Less common manifestations include respiratory problems, adenopathy, mucositis, myocarditis, hepatitis, rhabdomyolysis, and nephritis. Pretreatment with prednisone fails to prevent this reaction.

ABC hypersensitivity reactions generally occur in the first 9 to 11 days of treatment. They are more frequent in white, treatment-naïve patients who have higher $CD8^+$ T cell counts at treatment initiation and are HLA B5701-positive. HLA B5701 allele is the dominant risk factor for ABC hypersensitivity, with greater than 70% positive predictive value and 95% to 98% negative predictive value.[23] Prescreening for this allele before initiation of an ABC–containing regimen is now recommended. If a reaction occurs, ABC must be discontinued, because symptoms worsen with continued use; the drug should never be reintroduced, because fatal hypersensitivity has occurred with rechallenge.

TABLE 73-2 Antiretroviral Agents Approved for the Treatment of Human Immunodeficiency Virus (HIV) Infection

Generic Drug	Trade Name	Other Names/Designations
ENTRY AND FUSION INHIBITORS		
Enfuvirtide	Fuzeon	DP 178, DP178, pentafuside, T 20, T-20, T20
Maraviroc	Selzentry	Celsentri, MVC, UK-427,857
INTEGRASE INHIBITORS		
Raltegravir	Isentress	MK-0518, MK0158, RAL
NON-NUCLEOSIDE REVERSE TRANSCRIPTASE INHIBITORS		
Delavirdine	Rescriptor	136817-59-9, DLV, delavirdine mesylate, U-90152S
Efavirenz	Sustiva	DMP-266, EFV, L 743726, Stocrin
Etravirine	Intelence	ETR, ETV, TMC 125, TMC-125, TMC125
Nevirapine	Viramune XR, Viramune	BI-RG-587, extended-release nevirapine, NVP
Rilpivirine	Edurant	R278474, RPV, rilpivirine hydrochloride, TMC278
NUCLEOSIDE REVERSE TRANSCRIPTASE INHIBITORS		
Abacavir	Ziagen	ABC, ABC sulfate, abacavir sulfate
Abacavir-lamivudine	Epzicom	Abacavir sulfate–lamivudine, ABC/3TC
Abacavir-lamivudine-zidovudine	Trizivir	Abacavir sulfate–lamivudine–zidovudine, ABC/3TC/ZDV
Didanosine	Videx EC, Videx	BMY 40900, BRN 3619529, CCRIS 805, dideoxyinosine (ddI), HSDB 6548
Emtricitabine	Emtriva	524W91, FTC
Emtricitabine–tenofovir disoproxil fumarate	Truvada	FTC/TDF
Lamivudine	Epivir	3TC, Epivir-HBV
Lamivudine-zidovudine	Combivir	ZDV/3TC
Stavudine	Zerit	BMY-27857, d4T
Tenofovir disoproxil fumarate	Viread	GS-4331-05, PMPA Prodrug, TDF, tenofovir DF
Zidovudine	Retrovir	Azidothymidine (AZT), ZDV
PROTEASE INHIBITORS		
Amprenavir	Agenerase	APV, VX-478, Vertex VX478
Atazanavir	Reyataz	ATV, BMS 232632 (atazanavir), BMS-232632-05 (atazanavir sulfate)
Darunavir	Prezista	DRV, TMC 114, TMC114
Fosamprenavir	Lexiva	FPV, fosamprenavir calcium, GW 433908, GW433908, Telzir, VX 175
Indinavir	Crixivan	IDV, indinavir sulfate, L-735,524, MK-639
Lopinavir/ritonavir	Kaletra	Aluvia, LPV/RTV, LPV/r
Nelfinavir	Viracept	NFV, nelfinavir mesylate
Ritonavir	Norvir	RTV
Saquinavir mesylate	Invirase	Ro 31-8959/003 (saquinavir mesylate), saquinavir (SQV)
Tipranavir	Aptivus	TPV

TABLE 73-3 Human Immunodeficiency Virus (HIV) Drugs Associated with Drug Hypersensitivity

Drug	Reaction(s)	Hepatotoxicity	Frequency
NUCLEOSIDE REVERSE TRANSCRIPTASE INHIBITORS			
Zidovudine	Exanthema	Not reported	Rare
Abacavir	Exanthema, DiHS	Elevated LFTs, hepatitis, liver failure	2.3%-9%
Emtricitabine	Rash	Elevated LFTs	17%
NON-NUCLEOSIDE REVERSE TRANSCRIPTASE INHIBITORS			
Efavirenz	SJS, TEN, exanthema	Elevated LFTs	0.1% 4.6-20%
Nevirapine	Exanthema, TEN, SJS, DiHS	Elevated LFTs, immune-mediated hepatitis, liver failure	17%-32% 0.3%-2% 2%-10% discontinuation
Etravirine	Rash, SJS, TEN	Elevated LFTs	16% 2% discontinuation
PROTEASE INHIBITORS			
Tipranavir	Rash, dyslipidemia	Elevated LFTs, toxic hepatitis	2%-14% 2%-6.4%
Atazanavir	Rash	Hyperbilirubinemia	6%
Fosamprenavir	Rash, DiHS	Elevated LFTs	1%-19% Discontinuation <1%
Lopinavir	Rash	Elevated LFTs	2%-4%
Darunavir	Rash, DiHS	Elevated LFTs	6.7% Rare
ENTRY INHIBITORS			
Enfuvirtide	Injection-site reactions, DiHS	Not reported	Rare
Maraviroc	Rash, cough	Elevated LFTs	Rash

From Davis CM, Shearer WT. Diagnosis and management of HIV drug hypersensitivity. J Allergy Clin Immunol 2008;121:826-32, e825.
DiHS, Drug-induced hypersensitivity syndrome; *LFTs,* liver function tests; *SJS,* Stevens-Johnson syndrome; *TEN,* toxic epidermal necrolysis.

A rash develops in approximately 15% of NVP recipients, and 1.5% are severe.[27] Stevens-Johnson syndrome occurs in 0.3% to 1%. NVP-associated hypersensitivity syndrome may occur without rash and includes systemic symptoms such as fever, myalgia, arthralgia, hepatitis, and eosinophilia. Severe, life-threatening, and, in rare cases, fatal hepatotoxicity, manifesting as fulminant and cholestatic hepatitis, hepatic necrosis, or hepatic failure, has occurred sometimes in association with rash or other signs or symptoms of hypersensitivity reaction. The hypersensitivity reaction most commonly occurs early in therapy; it is unusual after 12 weeks of treatment. Risk factors include female gender, Chinese ethnicity, and higher $CD4^+$ T cell counts and lower HIV RNA levels at initiation of therapy. HLA-DRB1*0101 also has been associated with NVP hypersensitivity.[27] The erythematous, maculopapular rash usually appears on the trunk and arms within the first 2 to 4 weeks of treatment. Patients with mild to moderate rash only can continue NVP therapy with close monitoring.

Other NNRTIs, including efavirenz (EFV), commonly cause hypersensitivity. A mild rash occurred in 4 of 10 children receiving this drug as the most common adverse effect.[23] In adults, rash occurs in up to 10% of subjects (1% severe). In general, these reactions are less severe than those with NVP, and resolution of the rash during treatment continuation is common. Two other NNRTIs, zidovudine and lamivudine, have rarely been associated with anaphylactic or anaphylactoid reactions.

The protease inhibitors, especially amprenavir, fosamprenavir, darunavir, and tipranavir/ritonavir, also commonly cause rash. These drugs are sulfonamides and have the potential for cross-reactivity with other sulfa drugs; they should be used with caution in patients with a prior history of sulfa hypersensitivity.

Enfuvirtide (T-20), an HIV-1 fusion inhibitor, is administered by subcutaneous injection. Injection site reactions occur in nearly all patients who receive T-20 (up to 98% in published clinical trials). The injection site reactions include tenderness, induration, erythema, and formation of subcutaneous nodules. On histopathologic analysis, the lesions are interstitial granulomatous drug reactions.

The pathophysiology of drug-related reactions in HIV-infected patients is not well understood. Possible pathogenetic mechanisms include allergic or immune-mediated reactions, formation of toxic metabolites, metabolic disturbances, and genetic factors. In addition, chronic immune activation may enhance the formation of an immune reaction to the medication. HLA associations other than those mentioned previously may yet be identified. This sensitization may be an example of metabolites undergoing haptenization to endogenous proteins during metabolism to achieve antigenicity or binding directly to MHC molecules, resulting in T cell activation.

Studies have shown that $CD4^+$ T cell clones derived from allergic patients proliferate in response to SMX and its metabolites. The metabolism of sulfonamides occurs primarily through *N*-acetylation. Risk of cutaneous hypersensitivity to TMP-SMX increases for those patients who are slow acetylators, possibly because of the slow metabolism of the sulfonamide component. However, polymorphisms in genes that encode the drug-metabolizing enzymes were not associated with hypersensitivity to TMP-SMX.[28]

It is unlikely that any one mechanism accounts for all adverse drug reactions in HIV-infected individuals. As with drug reactions in non–HIV-infected persons, dose and duration of therapy will have an impact on the development of hypersensitivity, with higher dose and longer duration of therapy increasing the frequency of hypersensitivity for many drugs.

In general, most cutaneous adverse events that follow the use of antiretroviral agents are mild or moderate, occur within the first few weeks of therapy, and resolve spontaneously following drug discontinuation. For some patients, medications may be continued or reintroduced safely despite the presence or history of a rash, because spontaneous resolution of the rash may occur despite continued use. Discontinuation is mandatory, however, and rechallenge is contradicated if a life-threatening reaction occurs, the offending drug is abacavir, or the rash is accompanied by systemic symptoms.

Oral and intravenous desensitization protocols have been successful for some HIV-infected patients whose reactions to TMP-SMX were non–life-threatening, nonblistering cutaneous reactions. Enfuvirtide desensitization protocols have been devised for patients with generalized rash only. They should not be implemented in patients who have systemic symptoms.

ALLERGIC RHINITIS/SINUSITIS: PROMINENCE IN HUMAN IMMUNODEFICIENCY VIRUS INFECTION

Rhinitis and sinusitis are common chronic problems in HIV-infected individuals. Rhinosinusitis is reported in up to 68% of the HIV-infected population. Early in HIV disease, patients may develop obstructive nasal symptoms secondary to polyclonal B cell activation leading to lymphoid hyperplasia. This obstructive component contributes to the burden of rhinosinusitis in these patients.[29]

The immunodeficiency resulting from HIV infection probably predisposes the patient to the development of sinus infections. In the HIV-infected population, sinusitis is most common among patients with AIDS, and sinus severity is correlated with stage of HIV infection. Additionally, an increase in IgE levels was significantly associated with sinusitis in HIV infection. No correlation has been found between sinusitis and a history of allergy; however, skin test positivity to allergens frequently is observed.

The causative organisms also vary by stage of infection. In patients with $CD4^+$ counts greater than 50 cells/μL, acute sinusitis most often is caused by *Streptococcus pneumoniae, Haemophilus influenzae, Moraxella catarrhalis,* and *Streptococcus viridans.* Chronic sinusitis in this population most often is caused by *S. aureus, Staphylococcus epidermidis,* gram-negative bacilli (including *Pseudomonas aeroginosa*), and anaerobic organisms. In patients with $CD4^+$ counts less than 50 cells/μL, the most common causative bacteria include *Pseudomonas aeruginosa, Legionella pneumophila, Klebsiella pneumoniae,* and *Listeria monocytogenes.* At this advanced stage of disease, fungal, viral, protozoal, and atypical mycobacterial organisms also must be considered. *Mycobacterium avium, Aspergillus* spp., members of Mucoraceae, *Candida albicans, P. jirovecii, Microsporidium, Acanthamoeba,* and cytomegalovirus all have been reported. Owing to the wide range of pathogens at this stage of HIV infecction, cultures are recommended to guide treatment.[30]

A relationship between increased allergy and chronic rhinitis in HIV infection is controversial. As detailed earlier, an increase in IgE levels has been well documented in HIV-infected patients; the significance of this increase, however, is less clear. The incidence of allergic rhinitis and conjunctivitis is increased after HIV seroconversion in symptomatic HIV-infected men with cancer or secondary infections. These men have a higher percentage of radioallergosorbent tests (RASTs) detecting specific IgE antibody to aeroallergens than control subjects or less symptomatic patients.[31] A study of 43 HIV-infected children showed 28% with positive immediate hypersensitivity to common aeroallergens as measured by prick test, but IgE levels did not correlate with allergic disease or with $CD4^+$ T cell counts.[32] The paucity of more current data on rhinitis and HIV infection complicates the issue, because changes may emerge with studies beginning in the HAART era, as discussed further on.

PULMONARY HYPERREACTIVITY AND ASTHMA: NEW DISCOVERIES IN HUMAN IMMUNODEFICIENCY VIRUS INFECTION

HIV-infected patients may have many pulmonary manifestations of disease, including bronchitis, pneumonia, and lymphoid infiltrates such as lymphoid interstitial pneumonitis. In keeping with the increased incidence of viral upper respiratory tract infection and sinusitis in HIV-infected persons, both of which are associated with asthma, asthma could be increased in HIV-infected patients as well, although few studies have examined asthma in HIV-seropositive persons. Older studies in the pre-HAART era showed mixed results regarding pulmonary hypersensitivity in HIV infection. For example, O'Donnell and colleagues[33] showed a frequent occurrence of abnormal airway function, as defined by low forced expiratory flow rates without evidence for a restrictive pattern of disease, among persons with AIDS in a retrospective analysis of pulmonary function tests of 105 patients with AIDS. Schnipper and associates[34] evaluated for the presence of reversible airway dysfunction in acute *Pneumocystis* pneumonia and found evidence for both reversible airway obstruction and airway hyperreactivity (AHR) in HIV-infected patients with acute *Pneumocystis* pneumonia. In a survey of HIV outpatients, 17% reported asthma, and asthma occurred in greater proportion in those with $CD4^+$ T cell counts greater than 200/μL.[35] Other studies of HIV-infected persons failed to show an increase in airway hyperresponsiveness.

The impact of HAART has not yet been fully established; some studies, however, show that $CD4^+$ T cell reconstitution resulting from HAART results in an increased rate of asthma. In one study examining airway hyperresponsiveness in the HAART era, Poirier and colleagues reported that HIV-infected men have increased rates of wheezing and bronchial hyperresponsiveness and higher serum IgE levels compared with uninfected control subjects.[36]

An analysis of asthma medication usage in 193 HIV-infected children and 2464 HIV-exposed uninfected children in the Women and Infants Transmission Study (WITS) showed that HIV-infected children on HAART were more likely to use asthma medications than their HIV-infected counterparts who were not receiving HAART.[37] The study further showed that HIV-infected patients who experienced immune reconstitution after initiation of HAART were at increased risk for asthma development.

In a cross-sectional systematic analysis of adult HIV-infected patients, Gingo and coworkers[38] collected data on symptoms and diagnosis, pulmonary function, sputum cell counts, and asthma-related cytokines and chemokines in 223 HIV-infected adults recruited at a Veterans Affairs Hospital affiliated with the University of Pittsburgh. These workers found a 20.6% prevalence of asthma (diagnosed by a physician) that was associated with female gender, body mass index (BMI) greater than 29.6, prior history of bacterial or *Pneumocystis* pneumonia, lack of ART, and elevated levels of IL-4 and RANTES in the sputum.

Bronchodilator responsiveness was found in 9% of this cohort and was associated with increased levels of plasma MIP-1α and sputum MIP-1β. Both asthma and bronchodilator responsiveness were associated with increased sputum eosinophil percentages.

Increased incidence of asthma diagnosed by physicians, medication use, or both in pediatric patients was reported in a study from the Pediatric HIV/AIDS Cohort Study (PHACS)[39] comparing 451 HIV-infected and 227 HIV-exposed but uninfected (HEU) children aged 7 to 16 years. The prevalence of asthma was significantly increased in the HIV-infected group (34%) versus the HEU group. By the age of 15 years, the cumulative incidence of asthma was 37% for the HIV-infected group and 29% for the HEU group. The risk of asthma was 1.37 times greater for the HIV-infected group (Fig. 73-3).

In this study, atopic dermatitis also was significantly increased in HIV-infected children (20%) compared with HEU children (12%). Among the HIV-infected children, the prevalence of asthma was significantly greater in those with atopic dermatitis (41%) than in those without atopic dermatitis (29%) (Table 73-4). Children with atopic dermatitis were more likely to have asthma in either population. In addition, the median age at onset of atopic dermatitis was 2.89 years for the HIV-infected children and 5.03 for the HEU children. The overall increased burden of atopic disease in the HIV infected population is significant, with a 30% increased risk of asthma and atopic dermatitis found in the PHACS study.

Of the HIV-infected cohort, 86% were receiving HAART, and most had $CD4^+$ T cells greater than 25% of the total lymphocyte population, with RNA plasma viral load of less than 400 copies. The immune data are consistent with the hypothesis that increased $CD4^+$ counts in patients on HAART contribute to the development of atopic disease in this population (Fig. 73-4).

In a study of 85 pediatric HIV-seropositive patients treated at an urban medical center, 28% were found to have persistent asthma. All patients in the persistent asthma group had $CD4^+$ T cell counts within the normal range for age at the time of asthma diagnosis. Two patients in this group had transient decreases in their $CD4^+$ T cell counts, with resolution of asthma symptoms during this period. Four of the patients had $CD4^+$ T cell numbers in the *P. jirovecii* prophylaxis range (i.e., <200 cells/μL for age 6 years and above) before diagnosis of persistent asthma, but all were reconstituted to normal for age range by the time of asthma diagnosis due to HAART initiation. In the same center, no patients in a series 148 had asthma diagnosed in the pre-HAART era (prior to mid-1990s).[40]

TABLE 73-4 Prevalence of Asthma History among Persons with and without a History of Atopic Dermatitis*

Method of Asthma Classification	Atopic Dermatitis (*N* = 117)	No Atopic Dermatitis (*N* = 561)	*P* Value†
Diagnosis	36 (31%)	124 (22%)	.045
Medication use	45 (38%)	146 (26%)	.007
Diagnosis and/or medication use	48 (41%)	162 (29%)	.010

*The diagnosis of atopic dermatitis may have occurred before, at the same time as, or after the first occurrence of asthma.
†Chi-square test.

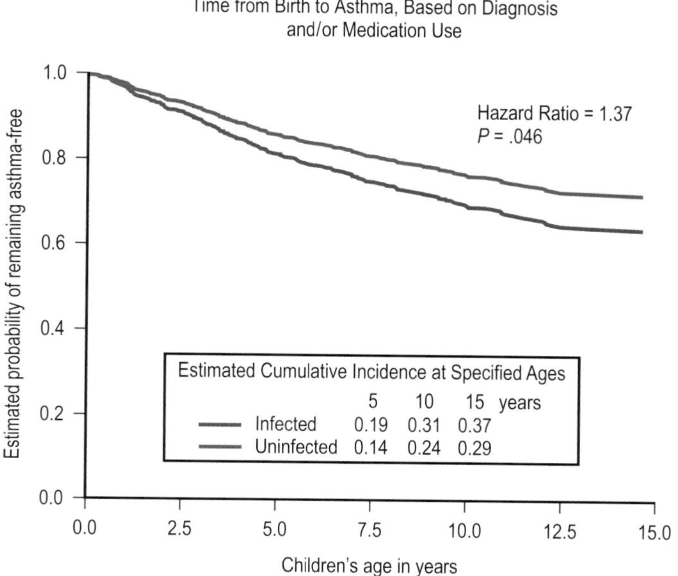

Figure 73.3 Probability of remaining asthma-free in human immunodeficiency virus (HIV) infection.

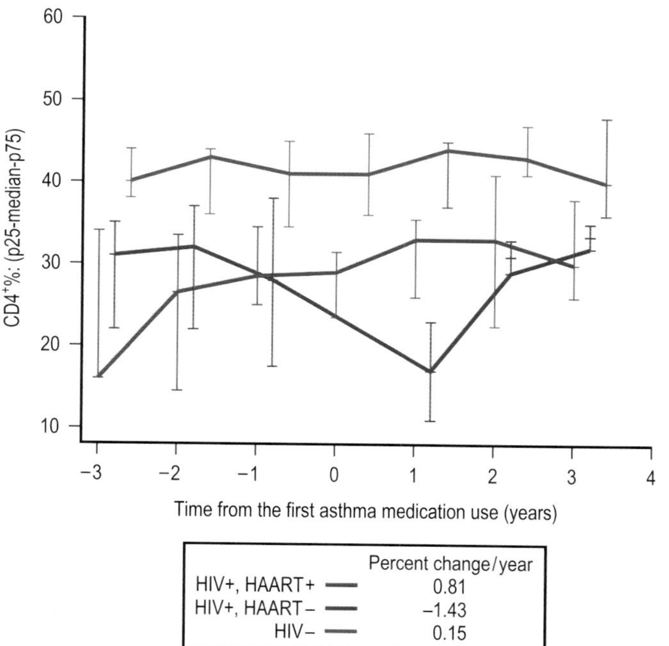

Figure 73-4 Increase in $CD4^+$ T cell percentage in asthmatic patients receiving highly active antiretroviral therapy (*HAART*) drugs. The results are expressed as the median and interquartile range.

Foster and coworkers[41] found that certain HLA alleles were linked to either increased risk for or protection from asthma development. HLA-A68 was associated with increased likelihood of medication use (33% of patients with at least one allele versus 9% without had used asthma medications), whereas HLA-Cw6 was protective (none of the patients with at least one allele versus 18% without had used asthma medications). These investigators also noted that patients who use asthma medications were more likely to have received HAART than their counterparts who do not require asthma medications.

No other large systematic studies of asthma in HIV-infected adults have been performed since the introduction of HAART in the mid-1990s, and no large studies have examined the prevalence of asthma in children with HIV infection. A pilot study of HIV-infected children suggests that the prevalence of asthma has increased in this pediatric population in the HAART era in that 28 of 83 (34%) of such children had asthma, as confirmed by an International Classification of Diseases, Ninth Revision (ICD-9) code for asthma in the medical record.[42]

This prevalence is much higher than the 6% rate reported by the Centers for Disease Control and Prevention (CDC) for children in the United States and also exceeds the prevalence of physician-diagnosed asthma in inner-city youth (predominantly African-American and Hispanic children), which ranges from 11% to 17%.[43] The CDC investigators hypothesized that this increase is due in part to maintenance or reconstitution of the immune system in the HAART era. Rationale for this hypothesis is provided by the observation that annual models with asthma lose their asthma when $CD4^+$ T cells are depleted and regain asthma when $CD4^+$ T cells are restored.[44] Porter and colleagues[45,46] have shown that common fungi in the airway of immune-dysregulated animals in asthma models produce a powerful bronchospastic response, consistent with what appears to happen in humans with a return of $CD4^+$ T cells after initiation of HAART. Figure 73-5 is a summary of the flow of concepts contained in the hypothesis. The central theme is depicted by the arrows descending from immunologic activation events resulting from the preservation or restoration of $CD4^+$ T cell–mediated immunity in HIV-seropositive children treated with HAART/ART with release of inflammatory (Th2) cytokines and a loss of Tregs and tolerance.

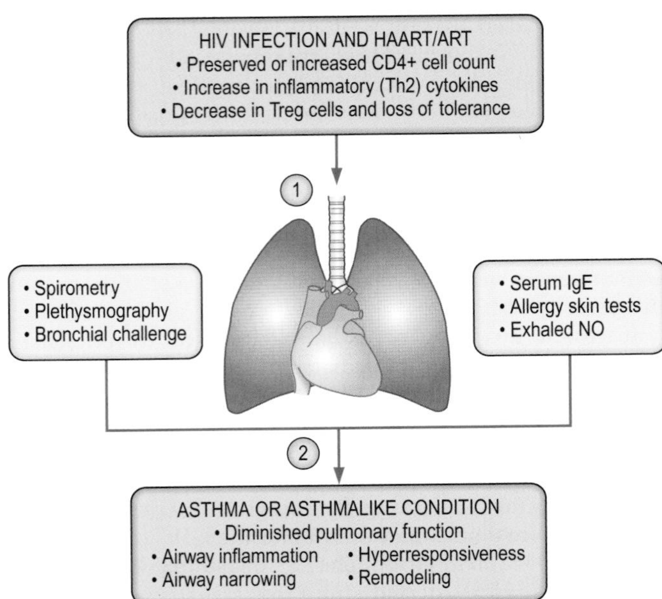

Figure 73-5 Human immunodeficiency virus (HIV) infection and highly active antiretroviral therapy (HAART)/antiretroviral therapy (ART). Immune factors (*arrow 1*) produce an effect upon the pulmonary tissues that produces asthma or an asthmalike condition with airway inflammation, narrowing, hyperresponsiveness, and possible remodeling. To distinguish asthma from an asthmalike condition, pulmonary function tests and tests for pulmonary factors that may contribute to asthma may be used (*arrow 2*). *ART*, Antiretroviral therapy; *IgE*, immunoglobulin E; *NO*, nitric oxide; *Treg*, regulatory T [cell].

ATOPIC DERMATITIS

A possible increase in the incidence of atopic dermatitis in HIV-infected individuals is important to recognize and address, because it is associated with decreased quality of life in all populations and may pose a particular burden in the HIV-seropositive population by decreasing the skin barrier protective function in patients who already have depressed immune function.

The available data are inconclusive regarding the prevalence of atopic dermatitis in HIV-infected patients. Studies have reported increased rates, decreased rates, and similar rates relative to those in the general population. In a 2002 review of these findings to characterize the relationship between atopic dermatitis and HIV infection, Rudikoff[47] suggested that the inconclusive nature of the data reflects in part the use of poorly defined criteria for diagnosis of atopic dermatitis, the fact that many conditions mimic atopic dermatitis in HIV-infected patients (including seborrheic dermatitis, pruritic papular eruption of HIV infection, eosinophilic folliculitis, and papular urticaria), and a lack of specific studies. Patients with HIV infection have excessively dry skin compared with HIV-seronegative persons, which this investigator suggested may lead to decreased skin barrier function and skewing toward a Th2 cytokine milieu. Increased CD30 expression on T cells may be associated with development of atopic dermatitis in HIV-infected patients, but this correlation has not been definitively established. Elevated IgE levels have been documented in patients with HIV infection. The exact role that this pattern plays in the development of atopic dermatitis is not yet established. Staphylococcal superantigens may contribute to the development of atopic dermatitis in HIV-seropositive patients, with a 30% to 50% colonization rate and 57% of *S. aureus* strains isolated from patients with atopic dermatitis secreting superantigens.

Ball and Harper[48] first reported an association between atopic dermatitis and HIV in 1987. They noted that three of nine HIV-infected pediatric hemophiliac patients either had atopic dermatitis for the first time or experienced a recurrence of previously resolved atopic dermatitis soon after acquiring HIV infection.

FOOD ALLERGY

Solid evidence for or against an altered rate of food allergy in HIV-infected patients is lacking. Two older studies[32,49] actually show decreased rate of food allergy in this population. No more recent publications are available to help determine whether this remains true in the HAART era or if, as in other atopic conditions, an increase in food allergy occurs with immune reconstitution.

Treatment of Atopic Disease in Human Immunodeficiency Virus–Infected Patients

The asthma and other atopic manifestations in HIV disease are likely to constitute the same entity as the atopic disease seen in non–HIV-infected patients. PHACS data suggest that asthma is commonly linked to atopic dermatitis, as is the case in the HIV–noninfected population. The presence of Th2 inflammatory cells, cytokines, and chemokines in appropriate studies further supports this hypothesis. Based on these findings and the lack of alternative therapeutic options, treatment of atopic disease is essentially the same regardless of HIV status.

One important caveat oncerns the potentially harmful interaction between fluticasone and ritonavir-boosted protease inhibitors. Concurrent use of these medications has resulted in increased serum levels of fluticasone, which can result in Cushing syndrome and adrenal suppression.

Success in treatment of atopic dermatitis may be augmented by oral antibiotics active against *S. aureus,* because a high rate of staphylococcal skin colonization in the HIV-infected population is well documented. In refractory cases, early initiation of phototherapy should be considered, to spare the use of systemic corticosteroids and avoid further immunosuppression.[47]

As mentioned, drug desensitization protocols can be used for TMP-SMX and enfuvirtide in appropriate settings.[23] The mainstays of treatment in most cases, however, are withdrawal of the offending agent and appropriate use of diphenhydramine, epinephrine, and corticosteroids. As more HIV drugs become combined into single-pill regimens, determination and elimination of the offending agents may become more complicated. The goal of eliminating only the offending agent instead of all contained in combination pills is difficult to achieve, because no skin testing protocols have been established for nonirritating concentrations of HAART drugs. Stevens-Johnson syndrome–toxic epidermal necrolysis, abacavir hypersensitivity reactions, and hepatotoxicity from nevirapine are absolute contraindications to reintroduction, because they carry a high risk of irreversible organ damage and mortality.

Summary

Immunologic changes that occur as HIV infection progresses and is treated may directly or indirectly contribute to the development or recrudescence of allergic disease. Patients with HIV infection have increased symptomatology suggesting allergy. The perturbations of the immune system in HIV-infected persons—in particular, altered cytokine production patterns—may be predisposing factors for development of allergic disease. The relationship of HIV infection and antiretroviral agents to specific allergic diseases such as asthma, allergic rhinitis, and atopic dermatitis has not yet been fully established. Additional study into the immunopathogenesis of HIV infection is likely, to further clarify the links between allergy and HIV disease progression. In fact, study of the human with HIV infection may serve as a model system to elucidate the immune mechanisms of allergic disease, such as the epidemic of asthma in developed countries.

Acknowledgments

Work on which this chapter is based was supported by NIH grants HD079533, HL052102, AI027551, AI036211, AI009441, HD41983, and RR0188; by the Pediatric Research and Education Fund, Baylor College of Medicine, and the Pediatric AIDS Fund; and by the Immunology Research Fund, Texas Children's Hospital. Janelle Allen assisted in the preparation of the manuscript.

REFERENCES

Introduction

1. Joint United Nations Programme on HIV/AIDS (UNAIDS). Global report: UNAIDS report on the global AIDS epidemic 2010. Available at: http://www.unaids.org/globalreport/; accessed May 5, 2013.
2. Centers for Disease Control and Prevention. HIV Surveillance—United States 1981-2008. Morbid Mortal Wkly Rep 2011;60:689-93.

Human Immunodeficiency Virus: Background

3. Gorry PR, Ancuta P. Coreceptors and HIV-1 pathogenesis. Curr HIV/AIDS Rep 2011;8: 45-53.
4. Branson BM. The future of HIV testing. J Acquir Immune Def Syndr 2010;55:S102-5.
5. Hanson IC, Shearer WT. Ruling out HIV when testing for severe combined immunodeficiency and other T cell disorders. J Allergy Clin Immunol 2012;129:875-6.e5.

Immune Dysregulation and Human Immunodeficiency Virus

6. McMichael AJ, Borrow P, Tamaras GD, Goonetilleke N, Haynes BF. The immune response during acute HIV-1 infection: clues for vaccine development. Nat Rev Immunol 2010; 10:11-23.
7. Gougeon ML. Apoptosis as an HIV strategy to escape immune attack. Nat Rev Immunol 2003; 3:392-404.
8. Espert L, Denizot M, Grimaldi M, et al. Autophagy is involved in T cell death after binding of HIV-1 envelope proteins to CXCR4. J Clin Invest 2006;116:2161.
9. Porichis F, Vlata Z, Hatzidakis G, et al. HIV-1 gp120/V3-derived epitopes promote activation-induced cell death to superantigen-stimulated CD4(+)/CD45RO(+) T cells. Immunol Lett 2007;108:97.
10. Douek DC, Betts MR, Hill BJ, et al. Evidence for increased T cell turnover and decreased thymic output in HIV infection. J Immunol 2001;167: 6663.
11. Hersperger AR, Martin JN, Shin LY, et al. Increased HIV-specific CD8 T-cell cytotoxic potential in HIV elite controllers. Blood 2011; 117:3799-808.
12. Hartigen-O'Conner J, Hirau LA, McCune JM, et al. Th17 cells and regulatory T cells in elite control over HIV and SIV. Curr Opin HIV AIDS 2011;6:221-7.
13. Fujiwara M, Takata H, Oka S, et al. Patterns of cytokine production in human immunodeficiency virus type 1 (HIV-1)-specific human $CD8^+$ T cells after stimulation with HIV-1-infected $CD4^+$ T cells. J Virol 2005;79:12536.
14. Moir S, Fauci AS. Pathogenic mechanisms of B cell dysfunction in HIV disease. J Allergy Clin Immunol 2008;122:12-9.
15. Deeks SG, Schweighardt B, Wrin T, et al. Neutralizing antibody responses against autologous and heterologous viruses in acute versus chronic human immunodeficiency virus (HIV) infection: evidence for a constraint on the ability of HIV to completely evade neutralizing antibody responses. J Virol 2006;80: 6155.
16. Tomescu C, Abdulhaqq S, Montaner LJ. Evidence for the innate immune response as a correlate of protection in human immunodeficiency virus (HIV)-1 highly exposed seronegative subjects (HESN). Clin Exp Immunol 2011; 164:158-69.
17. Vieillard V, Fausther-Bovendo H, Samri A, et al. Specific phenotypic and functional features of natural killer cells from HIV-infected long-term nonprogressors and HIV controllers. J Acquir Immune Defic Syndr 2010;53:564-73.
18. Norris PJ, Pappalardo BL, Custer B, et al. Elevations in IL-10, TNF alpha, and IFN gamma from the earliest point of HIV type 1 infection. AIDS Res Hum Retroviruses 2006; 22:757.
19. Kapogiannis BG, Henderson SL, Nigam P, et al. Defective IL-2 production by HIV-1-specific

CD4 and CD8 T cells in an adolescent/young adult cohort. AIDS Res Hum Retroviruses 2006;22:272.
20. Gee K, Angel JB, Mishra S, et al. IL-10 regulation by HIV-Tat in primary human monocytic cells: involvement of calmodulin/calmodulin-dependent protein kinase-activated p38 MAPK and SP-1 and CREB-1 transcription factors. J Immunol 2007;178:798.
21. Managlia EZ, Landay A, Al-Harthi L. Interleukin-7 induces HIV replication in primary naive T cell through a nuclear factor of activated T cell (NFAT)-dependent pathway. Virology 2006;350:443.

Clinical Phenotypes of Allergic Disease in Human Immunodeficiency Virus Infection

22. Müller M, Wandel S, Colebunders R, et al; IeDEA Southern and Central Africa. Immune reconstitution inflammatory syndrome in patients starting antiretroviral therapy for HIV infection: a systematic review and meta-analysis. Lancet Infect Dis 2010;10:251-61.
23. Davis CM, Shearer WT. Diagnosis and management of HIV drug hypersensitivity. J Allergy Clin Immunol 2008;121:826-32.e825.
24. AIDSinfo website: http://aidsinfo.nih.gov/drugs; accessed 5/11/13.
25. Chaponda M, Pirmohamed M. Hypersensitivity reactions to HIV therapy. Br J Clin Pharmacol 2011;71:659-71.
26. Violari A, Cotton M, Gibb D, et al. Early antiretroviral therapy and mortality among HIV-infected infants. N Engl J Med 2008;359:2233-44.
27. Martin AM, Nolan D, James I, et al. Predisposition to nevirapine hypersensitivity associated with HLA-DRB1*0101 and abrogated by low CD4 T-cell counts. AIDS 2005;1997-9.
28. Lin D, Tucker MJ, Rieder MJ. Increased adverse drug reactions to antimicrobials and anticonvulsants in patients with HIV infection. Ann Pharmacother 2006;40:1594.
29. Gurney TA, Lee KC, Murr AH. Contempoary issues in rhinosinusitis and HIV infection. Curr Opin Otolaryngol Head Neck Surg 2003;11:45-8.
30. Shah AR, Hairston JA, Tami TA. Sinusitis in HIV: microbiology and therapy. Curr Allergy Asthma Rep 2005;5:495-9.
31. Gurney TA, Murr AH. Otolaryngologic manifestations of human immunodeficiency virus infection. Otolaryngol Clin North Am 2003;36:607-24.
32. Bacot BK, Paul ME, Navarro M, et al. Objective measures of allergic disease in children with human immunodeficiency virus infection. J Allergy Clin Immunol 1997;100:707.
33. O'Donnell CR, Bader MB, Zibrak JD, et al. Abnormal airway function in individuals with the acquired immunodeficiency syndrome. Chest 1988;94:945.
34. Schnipper S, Small CB, Lehach J, et al. *Pneumocystis carinii* pneumonia presenting as asthma: increased bronchial hyperresponsiveness in *Pneumocystis carinii* pneumonia. Ann Allergy 1993;70:141.
35. Lin RY, Lazarus TS. Asthma and related atopic disorders in outpatients attending an urban HIV clinic. Ann Allergy 1995;74:510.
36. Poirier CD, Inhaber N, Lalonde RG, et al. Prevalence of bronchial hyperresponsiveness among HIV-infected men. Am J Respir Crit Care Med 2001;164:542.
37. Foster SB, McIntosh K, Thompson B, et al. Increased incidence of asthma in HIV-infected children treated with antiretroviral therapy in the National Institutes of Health Women and Infants Transmission Study. J Allergy Clin Immunol 2008;122:159-65.
38. Gingo MR, Wenzel SE, Steele C, et al. Asthma diagnosis and airway bronchodilator response in HIV infected individuals. J Allergy Clin Immunol 2012;129:708-14.e8.
39. Siberry GK, Leister E, Jacobson DL, et al. Increased risk of asthma and atopic dermatitis in perinatally HIV-infected children and adolescents. Clin Immunol 2012;142:201-8.
40. Gutin F, Butt A, Alame W, Thomas R, Secord E. Asthma in immune-competent children with human immunodeficiency virus. Ann Allergy Asthma Immunol 2009;102:438.
41. Foster SB, Lu M, Thompson B, et al. Association between HLA inheritance and asthma medication use in HIV positive children. AIDS 2010;24:2133-5.
42. Foster SB, Paul ME, Kozinetz CA, et al. Prevalence of asthma in children and young adults with HIV infection. J Allergy Clin Immunol 2007;119:750.
43. Health, United States, 2005. Hyattsville, Md.: National Center for Health Statistics; 2005. Online. Available at: http://www.cdc.gov/nchs/data/hus/hus05.pdf; accessed November 30, 2006.
44. Gavett SH, Chen X, Finkelman F, et al. Depletion of murine $CD4^+$ T lymphocytes prevents antigen-induced airway hyperreactivity and pulmonary eosinophilia. Am J Respir Cell Mol Biol 1994;10:587.
45. Porter P, Susarla SC, Polikepahad S, et al. Link between allergic asthma and airway mucosal infection suggested by proteinase-secreting household fungi. Mucosal Immunol 2009;2:504-17.
46. Porter PC, Yang T, Luong A, et al. Proteinases as molecular adjuvants in allergic airway disease. Biochim Biophys Acta 2011;1810:1059-65.
47. Rudikoff D. The relationship between HIV infection and atopic dermatitis. Curr Allergy Asthma Rep 2002;2:275-81.
48. Ball LM, Harper JI. Atopic eczema in HIV-seropositive haemophiliacs. Lancet 1987;2:627-8.
49. Tubiolo VC, Vazzo LA, Beall GN. Food allergy in human immunodeficiency virus (HIV) infection. Ann Allergy Asthma Immunol 1997;78:209-12.

74

Laboratory Tests for Allergic and Immunodeficiency Diseases

ROBERT G. HAMILTON

CONTENTS

The clinical immunology laboratory performs a broad spectrum of analytic measurements that aid in the diagnosis and management of human allergic and immunodeficiency diseases.[1,2] These assays can be subdivided into immunologic tests that measure the humoral and cellular components of the immune system and those that measure the antigenic proteins (allergens) and infectious agents in the environment that drive the allergic and infectious disease processes. This chapter focuses on methods used in the diagnostic immunology laboratory that have particular relevance for assessing humoral immune responses (immunoglobulins with a focus on IgE antibodies and serologic markers of anaphylaxis) and cellular immune responses (including cell-derived mediators of inflammation and lymphocyte subsets and function). Laboratory methods for assessing deficiencies in complement (total hemolytic complement) and phagocytosis (neutrophil-related tests) are discussed elsewhere.[3,4]

SUMMARY OF IMPORTANT CONCEPTS

» The assessment of immunodeficiency disease involves a combination of laboratory methods to assess cellular (cell type distribution and function) and humoral immunoglobulin, complement) components of the immune system.
» Allergen-specific immunoglobulin E (IgE) antibody measurements by serologic or skin testing are confirmatory tests that are not sufficient in themselves for the diagnosis of human allergic disease but are used to support the clinical history in this setting.
» Allergen-specific IgG antibody measurements by serologic testing can be useful in evaluating patients for chronic antigen exposure (e.g., before immunotherapy); however, their levels generally are not predictive of protection.
» Quantification of environmental allergen levels in surface (reservoir) dust promotes avoidance therapy by providing benchmarks for identifying potentially injurious environments and documenting successful remediation efforts to reduce allergen exposure.

Humoral Immune Responses Important in Allergic and Immunodeficiency Disease

Of the five human immunoglobulin isotypes, IgE, IgG, and IgA are the antibodies that are measured principally to assess humoral immune responses to allergens in individuals who manifest immediate-type hypersensitivity reactions, and to protein and carbohydrate antigens administered as vaccines to persons suspected of having immunodeficiency disease. There has been minimal interest in IgM and IgD immune responses in persons suspected of having either allergic or immunodeficiency diseases.

IMMUNOGLOBULIN E

Human IgE was identified in 1967 as a unique immunoglobulin of 190 kD that mediates the immediate-type hypersensitivity response.[5-7] IgE's variable regions possess an estimated 10^6 to 10^8 allergen-binding specificities, whereas its Fc region mediates biologic effector functions, such as mast cell and basophil Fcε receptor binding. By 1968, assays were available for the quantification of total IgE and allergen-specific IgE antibody.[8,9] With these assays, serum concentrations of IgE were shown to be highly age-dependent. Cord serum IgE levels are low, usually less than 2 kIU/L, because IgE does not pass the placental barrier in significant amounts.[10,11] Mean serum IgE levels progressively increase up to the age of 10 to 15 years at a rate slower than for IgG but comparable with that for IgA. An age-dependent decline in total serum IgE then occurs from the second to eighth decades of life.[12,13] IgE does not appear to be necessary for maintaining health in countries where parasites are absent, because adults may remain healthy for years with no detectable serum IgE.[14] The state of atopy has been defined as a genetic predisposition toward the development of immediate hypersensitivity reactions against common environmental antigens, manifested most commonly as allergic rhinitis but also as asthma, atopic dermatitis, or food allergy. Although atopic infants exhibit an apparent earlier and steeper rise in serum IgE levels during their early years compared with nonatopic control subjects,[11] high infant IgE levels are not always predictive for atopy in adult life.

In clinical practice, total serum IgE levels are reported in comparison with IgE levels measured in an age-adjusted control group of healthy, nonatopic persons. After age 14, serum IgE levels greater than 333 kU/L (800 μg/L) may be considered abnormally elevated and strongly associated with atopic disorders such as allergic rhinitis, atopic asthma, and atopic dermatitis.[10-12] Owing to the wide overlap in total serum IgE levels among nonatopic and atopic populations, however, total serum IgE is rarely measured today in the diagnosis of human allergic disease. With the licensing of omalizumab (Xolair) in 2003 for the treatment of IgE-dependent asthma, there has been a minor resurgence in the clinical measurement of total serum IgE, which is required to properly determine the dose of therapeutically administered anti-IgE. Moreover, some clinicians have begun ordering total serum IgE levels to evaluate a patient's IgE "specific activity," or the allergen-specific IgE–to–total IgE ratio, to aid in their interpretation of the clinical significance of the patient's allergen-specific IgE levels. This is a useful strategy because the IgE-specific activity, together with the patient's IgE antibody concentration, affinity, and clonality, has been shown to influence the translation of IgE responses into clinically evident allergic symptoms after allergen exposure.[15-17]

In contrast with total serum IgE, the presence of allergen-specific IgE antibodies to environmental allergens has been more strongly associated with allergic symptoms and the risk of systemic allergic reactions in patients who have a positive history of prior adverse reactions. The clinical utility of IgE antibody measurements in the diagnosis of human allergic disease is thus limited to diseases in which the role of IgE has been documented (e.g., allergic rhinitis, atopic asthma, urticaria, and anaphylaxis to insect venoms, drugs, or foods). However, IgE antibody can be detected in the skin or blood of a person who manifests no apparent allergy symptoms after allergen exposure. Thus, an allergen-specific IgE antibody response is necessary but not sufficient for the manifestation of allergic symptoms. IgE antibody presence and levels must be interpreted within the context of the individual's clinical history.

IgE plays an important role in transfusion reactions consequent to blood product administration.[18] Although the biologic mechanisms for allergic transfusion reactions remain largely unknown, recipient atopic predisposition as defined by IgE sensitization is one risk factor associated with these reactions. High serum levels of IgE antibodies to various allergens have been detected in the blood of donors.[19] The question of whether allergy screening of blood donors is necessary to minimize the risk of cross-transfusion sensitization[20] continues to be debated.

In contrast with its role in allergic disease, the measurement of IgE has demonstrated minimal value in the diagnosis or management of immunodeficiency. Early studies have examined the significance of total serum IgE levels after allogeneic bone marrow transplantation in patients with aplastic anemia, leukemia, Wiskott-Aldrich syndrome and infantile agranulocytosis.[21-23] Total serum IgE levels were shown to increase from 7- to 2000-fold in 10 of 12 individuals as early as 14 days after allogeneic bone marrow transplantation.[21] However, IgE levels returned to baseline levels by 60 days. In more than half of these subjects, the increase in IgE was associated with clinical and biochemical evidence for graft-versus-host disease (GVHD). In another study of 135 bone marrow transplant recipients,[22] statistically significant increases in IgE levels coincided in time with engraftment and acute GVHD, but not with herpes simplex virus or cytomegalovirus infections or chronic GVHD. In some of the nonatopic bone marrow recipients, persistently raised total serum IgE levels developed after transplantation, with specific IgE to the same allergen specificities as for their atopic donors.[23] Immunologic mechanisms inducing transient changes in plasma IgE have been investigated in 100 patients admitted to the intensive care unit for trauma. Substantial but transient increases in serum IgE concentrations were observed in association with the degree of sepsis after trauma. The time course of the IgE increase in these individuals correlated with the magnitude of infection and level of plasma IL-4, rather than with the actual traumatic event.[24,25]

IMMUNOGLOBULIN G

IgG antibody responses are considered by some to be a useful marker of antigen exposure, especially in allergic individuals receiving allergen immunotherapy or individuals receiving gamma globulins or protein and polysaccharide vaccines to diagnose immunodeficiency. In healthy adults, the four-polypeptide chain IgG monomer (150 kD) constitutes approximately 75% of total serum immunoglobulins.[26] IgG is equally distributed between intravascular and extravascular serum pools, and it thus affords protection to the fetus and newborn because of its ability to cross the placental barrier. Human IgG can be divided into four subclasses on the basis of unique antigenic determinants on their heavy chain constant-region domains and associated biologic functions.[27] Any two IgG subclasses show greater than 95% amino acid sequence homology. The greatest differences are found in the number of amino acids in the hinge region (IgG1: 15; IgG2: 12; IgG3: 62; IgG4: 21) and the number of cysteine residues probably involved in inter–heavy chain disulfide bridges (IgG1: 2; IgG2: 4; IgG3: 11; IgG4: 2). The IgG subclasses circulate in blood in the following relative percentages: 60% to 70% IgG1, 14% to 20% IgG2, 4% to 8% IgG3, and 2% to 6% IgG4.[26-28]

Structural differences among the four human IgG subclasses translate into different biologic effector functions involving complement activation and cell Fc receptor binding.[27,29] IgG3 and IgG1 activate complement efficiently, whereas IgG2 is less efficient, and IgG4 does not appear to bind C1 or activate complement. Of the four IgG subclasses, IgG4 antibody has been of particular interest to investigators of allergic disease disorders because of its observed potential for blocking allergen-induced basophil histamine release in vitro[30] and its increases after chronic antigen exposure during immunotherapy. Some IgG4 antibodies have been shown to function as monovalent antibodies as a result of asymmetry caused by unstable inter–heavy chain disulfide bonds of IgG4 that are in equilibrium with intrachain disulfide bonds. As a result, some IgG4 molecules possess two different antigen-binding sites and functional bispecificity.[31,32] The clinical importance of these bispecific IgG4 antibodies has yet to be elucidated; however, IgG4's apparent functional monovalency is an attractive feature that may produce allergen blocking activity in vivo.

The diagnosis of primary or secondary immunodeficiency in a patient 2 years of age or older begins with a detailed history concentrating on past infections and a physical examination. If the clinical picture is suggestive of immunodeficiency, preliminary screening with quantitative serum immunoglobulins and isohemagglutinins should be performed, and the diagnosis is confirmed if the total serum IgG concentration is less than 30% of the patient's age-adjusted normal range. In this patient population, confirmation of immunodeficiency by further testing of IgG antibody responses after intentional vaccination generally is considered unnecessary.[33] Lesser reductions in circulating IgG levels should, however, be confirmed by an impaired ability to produce antigen-specific IgG antibody responses to both protein (e.g., tetanus toxoid) and polysaccharide (e.g., pneumococcal) antigens after active immunization. For children younger than 2 years of age it is not always possible to distinguish between a permanent antibody deficiency and a developmental delay in IgG production, especially because IgG antibody responses to carbohydrate antigens often are deficient at this age. Although absolute standards for determining an adequate IgG antibody response after vaccination are lacking, some reference laboratories provide useful "protective" IgG antipneumococcal serotypes ranges for children and adults. Some clinicians use the criteria of a fourfold or greater rise in IgG antibodies specific for tetanus toxoid and presence of two or more pneumococcal polysaccharide serotypes as confirmatory evidence of a successful IgG antibody response.[33]

IMMUNOGLOBULIN A

IgA is the predominant immunoglobulin detected in human colostrum, saliva, tears, bronchial secretions, nasal mucosa, vaginal secretions, prostatic fluid, and mucous secretions of the small intestine.[34] In serum, IgA circulates primarily in a monomeric form (160 kD), accounting for 90%; however, 10% is polymeric, with two four-chain basic units (400 kD) combined by a J chain. Two subclasses of IgA, IgA1 and IgA2 have been identified, along with two allotypic forms of IgA2—IgA2m(1) and IgA2m(2).[35]

Total IgA and antigen-specific IgA immune responses have been measured in fluids lavaged from the nasal passages, bronchi, and alveoli of allergic individuals with rhinitis after antigen challenge.[36] In one study,[37] ragweed-specific IgA in bronchoalveolar lavage fluid that was collected after a segmental lung challenge correlated significantly with the release of eosinophil cationic protein (ECP), a marker of eosinophil degranulation. Ragweed-specific IgE in serum from the same subjects also correlated with ECP release, indicating a role for IgA antibodies in allergic pulmonary inflammation and a potential role for antigen-specific IgA in eosinophil degranulation in the lung after antigen challenge. More recent evidence seems to indicate that ragweed-specific IgE and IgA antibodies are independently involved in the pathogenesis of the late phase reaction induced in the lung by an antigen insult.[38] In addition, dust mite–specific IgE, IgA, and IgG4 antibodies have been measured in serum and saliva from 72 allergic and 14 nonallergic healthy children.[39] Serum IgE and serum and salivary IgG4 levels specific for dust mite, Der p 1, and Der p 2 allergens were higher in allergic children, whereas serum and salivary dust mite–specific IgA levels were higher in nonallergic children. The presence of allergen-specific IgA appears to have a key role in the healthy immune response to mucosal allergens.[39] Finally, successful allergen immunotherapy is reported to be accompanied by the suppression of T helper 2 (Th2) effector cells and the induction of IL-10 and/or TGF-β^+ T regulatory cells, which induce an increase in "protective" noninflammatory blocking antibodies, particularly IgG4 and IgA2 subclasses.[40,41]

Immunologic Methods for Quantifying Antigens and Antibodies

LAW OF MASS ACTION–BASED ASSAY KINETICS

A group of immunologic assays are used by clinical and research laboratories to detect and quantify multivalent antigens and antibodies in biologic fluids. Their chemistries are all governed by the law of mass action, which states that free antigen (Ag) and free antibody (Ab) reversibly interact to form antigen-antibody complexes (Ag-Ab). The relationship between free and antibody-bound antigen concentrations—that is, [Ag] and [Ab -Ag]—is determined by the equilibrium or affinity constant K_a, which is the ratio of the association (k_1) and dissociation (k_2) constants.

$$[\text{Ag}]+[\text{Ab}] \underset{k_2}{\overset{k_1}{\rightleftharpoons}} [\text{Ag-Ab}]$$

$$K_a = (k_1/k_2) = [\text{Ag-Ab}]/[\text{Ag}][\text{Ab}]$$

The addition of increasing amounts of antigen to a fixed quantity of antibody leads to the formation of increasing amounts of Ag-Ab complexes. At a certain concentration of antigen, half of the antibody binding sites become saturated, and [Ag-Ab] = [Ab]. This results in an affinity constant equal to the reciprocal of the free antigen concentration at half maximum saturation binding, or K_a = 1/[Ag]. As the concentration of antigen increases further, molar excess quantities of antigen drive the binding reaction toward complete saturation of the antibody-binding sites. At that point, the molar ratio of bound antigen to total antibody approximates 2, which is the valence of monomeric antibody (Fig. 74-1).

Scatchard analysis[42] is performed by plotting the bound to free molar ratio of antigen that is unitless versus the molar concentration of bound antigen. The affinity constant or strength of binding of the antibody is defined numerically as the negative inverse of the slope of the curve. Figure 74-1 displays a representative Scatchard analysis plot for a human insulin–specific antibody. Because most antigens are complex mixtures of proteins with multiple antigen binding epitopes, Scatchard plots of polyclonal antisera and complex antigens are usually not linear. Each antigen possesses several binding sites and thus binds to a spectrum of antibodies of different isotypes, each with a slightly different affinity. With polyclonal antisera, high-affinity antibodies define the slope of the Scatchard plot at low antigen concentrations. Low-affinity antibodies contribute more to the slope of the Scatchard plot when the antigen concentrations are high.

The interaction of multivalent antigens with polyclonal antisera is not as easily described mathematically with Scatchard

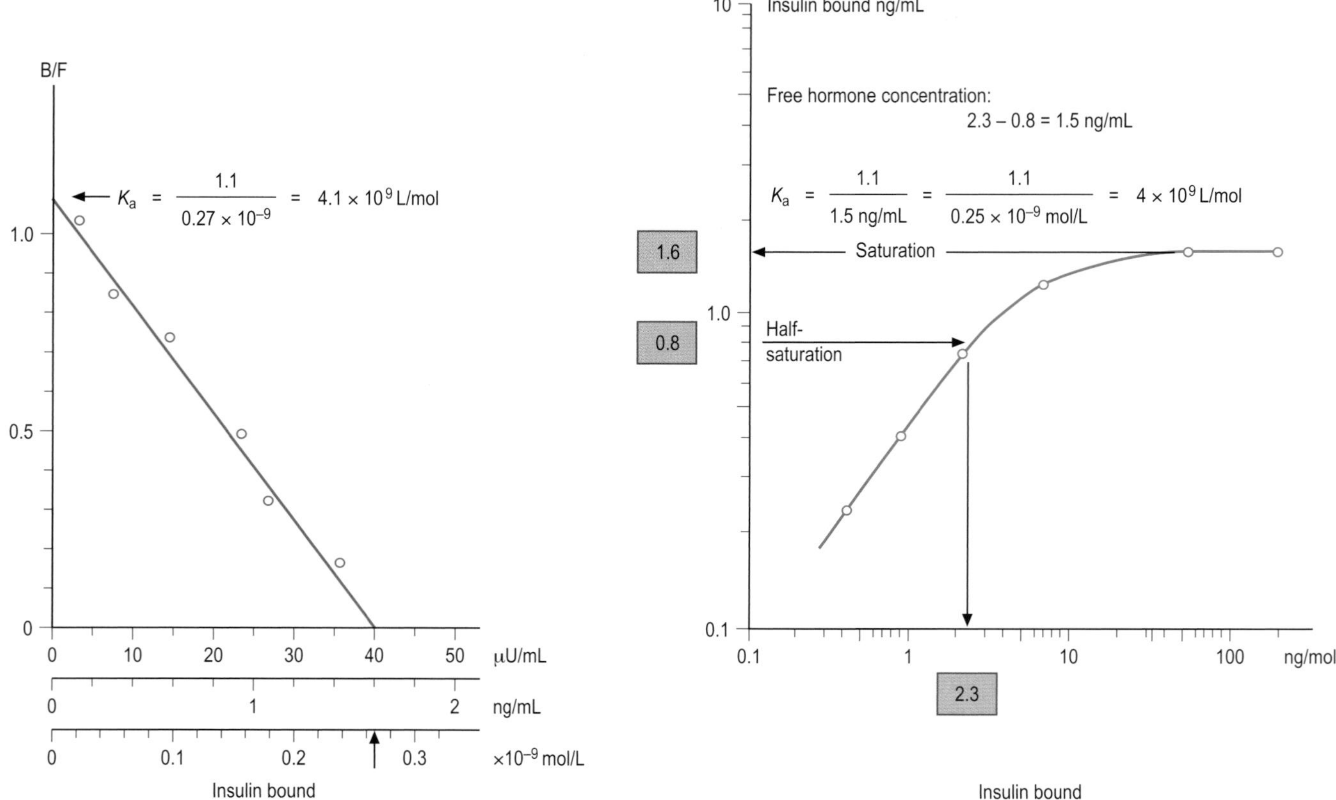

Figure 74-1 Calculation of the affinity constant (K_a) of the antigen (human insulin in units of µU/mL or ng/mL) and antibody (polyclonal antihuman insulin)-binding reaction (see law of mass action in text) by means of Scatchard analysis (*left panel*) and from the concentration of unbound ligand at half-saturation of antibody (*right panel*). In the Scatchard plot, K_a is derived from the slope of the line (y intercept/x intercept) in which the concentration of bound insulin (abscissa) is plotted against the molar ratio of bound insulin to free insulin ([AgB]/[Ab] [AgF]). In the saturation plot on the right, K_a is calculated as the inverse of the free hormone concentration at half-saturation of the antibody. *(Reproduced with permission from Thorell JI, Larson SM. Radioimmunoassay and related techniques: methodology and clinical applications. St. Louis: Mosby; 1978. p. 29.)*

analysis. The term *avidity* is used to describe the strength of binding of complex multivalent interactions. Binding at one site or epitope on an antigen may affect the rate of binding to other antigen-binding epitopes on the same antigen. When the binding of antibody to one antigenic epitope facilitates the binding of a different antibody at a second epitope on the same antigen, positive cooperativity occurs in which the final observed avidity appears to be greater than the sum of the affinities for the individual antigen-antibody interactions. This results in generally lower affinities for monoclonal antibodies (e.g., less than 10^8 L/mol) than are observed for polyclonal antisera (as much as 10^{11} L/mol).

ALLERGEN COMPONENTS IN DIAGNOSTIC IMMUNOGLOBULIN E ANTIBODY ASSAYS

Humans are exposed to a broad spectrum of biologic substances through inhalation, ingestion, and injection, many of which are recognized as foreign and immunogenic. In addition to eliciting IgG, IgA, and IgM antibody responses, several hundred of these elicit IgE antibody responses in genetically predisposed individuals and thus are classified as allergens. Allergens are most broadly categorized according to their origin grouping (e.g., weed pollens, grass pollens, tree pollens, mites, molds, epidermals and animal proteins, foods, venoms, insects, drugs, occupational/miscellaneous allergens). They are then subcategorized by their common name (e.g., dust mite), by taxonomic (genus, species) descriptors (e.g., *Dermatophagoides farinae*), and most recently by known individual allergenic components from extracted mixtures that have defined molecular weights, structures, and biologic functions (e.g., Der f 1, Der f 2). A comprehensive listing of known allergens used in diagnostic assays is provided in the Appendix to the Clinical Laboratory Standard Institute's guideline on IgE antibody assays.[43]

Subsequent to the discovery of IgE in 1968,[5-8] the first IgE antibody assay, called the radioallergosorbent test (RAST),[9] was developed that employed a radiolabeled anti-IgE to detect IgE antibodies that were bound to allergen extracts immobilized on a cellulose solid phase. Until recently, the allergen reagents have been principally crude extracts of homogeneous biologic substances, most of which contain mixtures of allergenic proteins. Protein chemistry and chromatography and molecular biology methods have been more recently used to identify individual allergenic components from these mixtures and produce recombinant forms in high purity that accurately reflect the native allergenic molecules. These are increasingly used as diagnostic reagents in serologic assays for "dissecting" the specificity of human IgE antibody responses and investigating allergenic cross-reactivity of IgE antibodies, which sometimes can induce clinically evident symptoms after relevant allergenic exposures. The exceptions to the complex nature of extracted allergens have been a number of pure allergenic drugs, such as insulin and penicillin, and industrial chemicals, such as trimethyl anhydride, used in paints.

The allergen is the key component of the IgE antibody assay that contributes to interlot variation.[43] There are multiple causes for observed variability in quality of allergen extracts used as diagnostic reagents. The allergen source may be misidentified or contaminated during collection, or there may be an inherent biologic variation in the source material. Allergen extraction conditions (time, buffer, agitation, temperature) from the biologic material often vary widely, which leads to the extraction of different compositions of allergenic proteins between batches and manufacturers. For instance, cat hair–dander extracts are prepared using variable ratios of cat hair and dander in a physiologic buffer. Alternatively, once extracted, they are precipitated with acetone and then resolubilized with saline containing glycerin. Stability of allergenic molecules may also vary over time, depending on the conditions of storage. Quality control programs for allergens used in antibody assays include extensive documentation of their identity and relative quantity and immunoreactivity or potency using nonimmunologic assays (e.g., total protein, isoelectric focusing, polyacrylamide gel electrophoresis), antibody-based immunochemical methods (e.g., Western blot analysis, specific IgE antibody assay inhibition, immunodiffusion; see further on), and cellular or in vivo assays (e.g., basophil histamine release, skin test titration) (Table 74-1).

TABLE 74-1 Performance Documentation for Allergosorbent Reagents: Illustrative Example Using Natural Rubber Latex Allergen

Parameter	Method or Source Information
Allergen extract designation: genus, species, common name, code	*Hevea brasiliensis,* natural rubber latex, K82 (occupational allergen)
Allergen extract source	Clone 600, *Hevea brasiliensis,* rubber tree sap, Malaysia (nonammoniated); identity test confirmed by supplier; (analytic and in vitro/in vivo safety tests[62])
Binding capacity	10 ng of IgE antibody per tube based on plateau of dilution recovery analysis
Parallelism	<15% interdilutional coefficient of variation based on dilution recovery analysis with 10 human sera
Specificity	<1% cross-reactivity based on inhibition with heterologous pollen, food, and mold allergens; comparison of regression slopes of dose-response curve
Interlot reproducibility	IgE-binding capacity range: 5-15 ng of IgE antibody per tube based on testing of quality control serum pool with three lots of latex allergosorbent (lot 2009, lot 2010, lot 2011)
Stability (document expiration date)	1 year based on real-time repetitive testing of quality control serum
Nonspecific binding (NSB) analysis	Evaluation with two or more sera containing >10 ng/mL levels of IgE antibody to pollens and negative for history of latex allergy
Known purified allergens (identified, cloned, and sequenced)	Hev b 1, 2, 3, 4, 5, 6, 7, 8, 9, 10, 11, 12, 13
Source of human antisera used to qualify allergosorbent reagent	CBER-FDA IgE antilatex serum pool S2 (not available for many allergen specificities)
Reference allergen used for validation studies	E8—nonammoniated latex from CBER-FDA (not available for many allergen specificities)

Adapted from Matsson P, Hamilton RG, and the CSLI Task Force.[43]
CBER, Center for Biological Evaluation and Research; *FDA,* U.S. Food and Drug Administration; *IgE,* immunoglobulin E.

ASSAYS FOR ANTIGENS AND ANTIBODIES

Immunoprecipitin-Based Assays

Research and clinical laboratories use a variety of assays to quantify both antigens and antibodies in biologic specimens. The earliest immunoassays that were used to quantify the concentration of antibody or antigen in a biologic specimen involved the use of visually detectable precipitating immune complexes in a gel or solution.[44,45] When antigen is being measured, a precipitate composed of antigen-antibody complexes is formed by adding increasing quantities of antigen to a fixed quantity of specific polyclonal antibody. The amount of precipitating antigen-antibody complexes increases to a maximum at equivalence (optimal lattice formation) and then declines. As the antigen concentration increases from zero to low levels, antigen-antibody immune complexes are formed, but they remain small and in solution, in a so-called antibody excess zone (Fig. 74-2, *C*). As the amount of antigen added increases, the reaction passes into the equivalence zone (see Fig. 74-2, *A*), characterized by optimal cross-linking of antigens and antibodies and maximal precipitate formation. As antigen concentrations become even higher, the complexes again become progressively smaller on moving into an antigen excess zone (see Fig. 74-2, *B*). Figure 74-2, *D*, illustrates the small soluble complexes that are formed when antigen is added to a monoclonal antibody that binds to a single antigen epitope and thus prevents cross-linking. The earliest quantitative precipitin-based assays used the measurement of total nitrogen or total protein precipitated as the objective end point for assessing the amount of immune complexes that had formed. As antigen increased from zero through a maximal peak at equivalence or maximal lattice formation, a progressive rise in protein was detected in the precipitate. It then declined with greater antigen addition as the immune complexes became small. The dose-response relationship—the amount of antigen or analyte relative to the amount of immune complexes formed—is defined using a reference or calibration preparation from which unknown analyte concentrations can be determined.

Radial Immunodiffusion Assay

The precipitin reaction can be performed in a variety of media, such as agar, that permit the migration of the initial reactants (antigens and antibodies) by diffusion or electrophoresis. Agar is useful because it traps large insoluble antigen-antibody

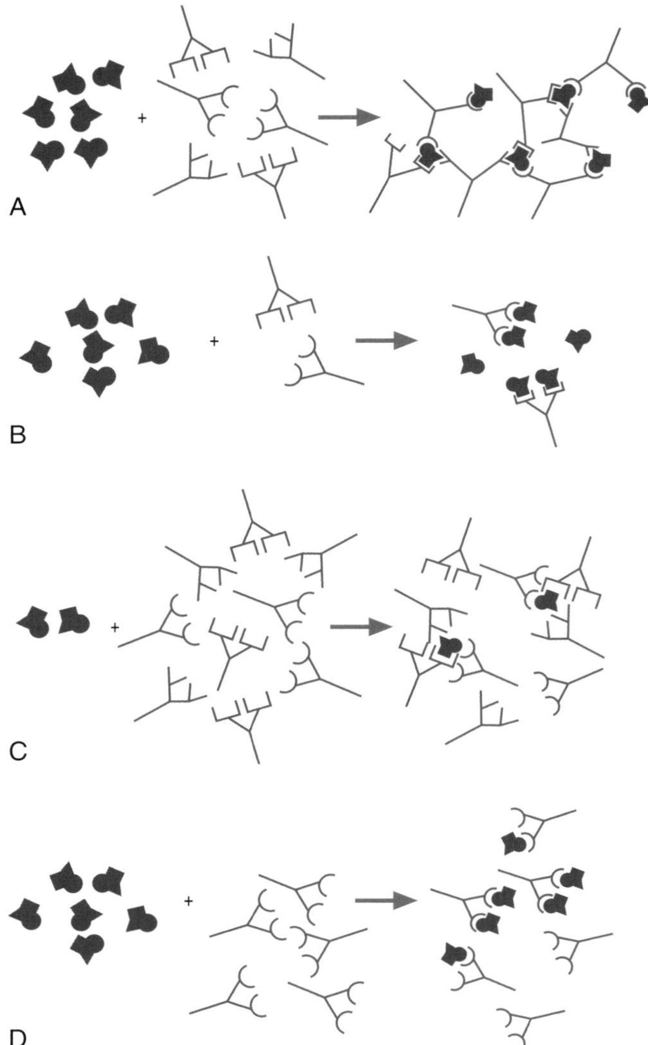

Figure 74-2 Schematic of precipitin reactions on moving from molar antigen excess **(B)**, through equivalence **(A)** to molar antibody excess **(D)**. Antigenic proteins that elicit antibody responses are depicted as having three different antibody binding sites on their surface. Polyclonal antibodies with three different specificities (*box, triangle, circle*) also are depicted. **A**, Equivalence zone. Maximum lattice formation (cross-linking) near equivalence at which a visible precipitin is formed. **B**, Antigen excess zone. The presence of molar excess quantities of antigen cause the formation of small immune complexes that are soluble and do not form a visible precipitate. **C**, Antibody excess zone. The presence of molar excess quantities of antibody cause small immune complexes that are soluble to form. This leads to insufficient lattice formation and no visible precipitate. **D**, The presence of monoclonal antibodies causes each antigen to bind at a single site. Such binding prevents cross-linking, with the result that small soluble immune complexes produce no precipitate.

complexes so they can be visually detected. In the quantitative radial immunodiffusion (RID) reported by Mancini and co-workers,[46] a gel containing polyclonal antibody specific for the analyte of interest (e.g., immunoglobulin, complement) is dissolved and layered onto a glass slide. Unknown, standard, and control serum specimens are pipetted into wells punched into the gel. After a 24- to 72-hour incubation, precipitin ring diameters are visually measured and interpolated from a standard curve. The RID is an attractive assay for low-volume tests that are performed in small clinical laboratories, because it requires no sophisticated instrumentation. Its primary limitation is its inability to accurately measure analytes with total serum protein concentrations, such as IgE, below 10 μg/mL.

Nephelometry and Turbidimetry

The precipitin reaction has also been performed in solution by adding variable concentrations of antigen to a fixed amount of antibody in a spectrophotometric reaction cell. As the immune complexes increase in size, they scatter increasingly greater amounts of incident light on the reaction cell. This antigen-antibody binding reaction occurs rapidly and is monitored by an instrument called a nephelometer that is designed to measure the extent of the incident light that is scattered. A photo detector at 31 degrees (for nephelometry) or in line (for turbidimetry) with the incident light beam collects the light-scattering signals on a recorder. As the antigen concentration in the specimen increases, it binds a constant amount of antibody, producing larger immune complexes and more scatter of light. Equilibrium (end point) and rate nephelometric and turbidimetric assays work from the antibody excess zone up to the zone of equivalence. In this region a stoichiometric relationship exists between the number of immune complexes formed and concentration of antigen in test sample. Equilibrium nephelometry involves incubating variable amounts of antigen for 30 minutes to 2 hours in separate tubes with a single concentration of antibody specific for the analyte of interest. After equilibrium has been achieved, the extent of light scatter is measured and compared with an antigen concentration–versus–light scatter standard.

Nephelometry is more sensitive than RID, measuring from 1 to 10 μg/mL of protein. Moreover, it is a homogeneous assay that does not require a physical separation of the free and antibody-bound analytes. Use of immobilized antibody on the microparticles has permitted nephelometric measurement of analytes in low concentrations in serum, such as IgE, which normally circulates at ng/mL levels, well below its routine analytic sensitivity threshold. Finally, nephelometry is attractive because it can be automated and is highly reproducible, and results can be obtained in minutes, in contrast with the required 1 to 2 days for RID measurements.

Immunoassay

In 1960, Berson and Yalow[47] made the observation that radioiodinated insulin exhibited a longer biologic half-life when injected into adult subjects with insulin-dependent diabetes than when injected into healthy normal control subjects. This observation led to the discovery that small molecules such as insulin can induce antibody formation in humans, and that insulin in the serum of individuals with diabetes exhibits a longer biologic half-life because a portion of it circulates bound to antibody. Antibody-bound insulin is therefore cleared more slowly from the circulation than is unbound insulin. The quantity of insulin bound to antibody is influenced by the equilibrium constants of the binding reaction (in accordance with the law of mass action) and, ultimately, the avidity of the antibody.

Since these investigators' original description of radioimmunoassay, many alternative immunoassay formats have been reported. These vary in their requirements for separation of free (unbound) antigen from antibody-bound antigen, their binding chemistry (solution or solid phase), the type of labeled reagent used, type of label (radioactive or nonisotopic [enzyme,

TABLE 74-2 Immunoassay Descriptors Used in the Diagnostic Immunology Laboratory

Criterion	Descriptor
1. Separation step	Heterogeneous = separation step Homogeneous = no separation
2. Method of separation	Solution or liquid phase Solid phase
3. Binding chemistry	Competitive Simultaneous reagent addition Sequential addition of reagents Noncompetitive
4. Labeled reagent	Labeled antigen Labeled antibody or immunometric
5. Type of label used	Isotopic (radionuclide: ^{3}H, ^{14}C, ^{125}I) Enzyme Horseradish peroxidase Alkaline phosphatase β-Galactosidase Fluorophor
6. Mode of calibration	Homologous standard curve (antigens) Heterologous reference curve (antibodies)

fluorophor, colloidal gold, or latex nanoparticles]), and the mode of calibration (Table 74-2). The most widely used clinical and research assays are the competitive binding liquid phase (labeled-antigen) immunoassay and the noncompetitive solid phase immunometric (labeled-antibody) assay. These assays typically display an analytic sensitivity of 1 to 10 ng of protein per mL.

Liquid Phase Immunoassay. Using unlabeled and radiolabeled insulin and insulin-specific polyclonal antibody as reagents, Yalow and Berson[47] configured the first competitive binding radioimmunoassay (Fig. 74-3, *A1*). Ekins[48] concurrently reported on a competitive binding, liquid phase equilibrium dialysis assay for thyroxine. These liquid phase competitive binding assays were called heterogeneous assays because they required the separation of free and antibody-bound antigen. Early separation techniques exploited differences in charge (electrophoresis), size (gel filtration), solubility (ammonium sulfate, trichloroacetic acid, polyethylene glycol treatment), surface configuration (immunologic epitopes, second antibody–immune precipitation), and adsorption properties (activated charcoal) to separate the free and receptor-bound labeled reagents. Moreover, by limiting the antibody concentration, these assays could achieve remarkable analytic sensitivity. These assays initially were used to quantify antigens in biologic fluids such as serum; however, they also were successfully used to detect antibodies such as the IgG-blocking antibody specific for radiolabeled pollen and venom allergens in serum.[49] A variety of radioiodination methods were employed to prepare radiolabeled antigens required for the radioimmunoprecipitation assay for allergen-specific IgG antibody.[50,51]

For labeling immunoassay reagents, radioiodine (first ^{131}I and then ^{125}I), used in early studies, has been largely replaced by enzymes (horseradish peroxidase, alkaline phosphatase, β-galactosidase), which in combination with defined substrates produce either a colorimetric, fluorescent, or chemiluminescent response. Most recently, nanoparticle labels (e.g., colored latex or colloidal gold) have permitted the development of rapid point-of-care lateral flow assays for antigen and antibody detection for which results are displayed on a visual readout. The magnitude of these final responses is proportional to the amount of label (enzyme or nanoparticle) present in the final reaction mixture.

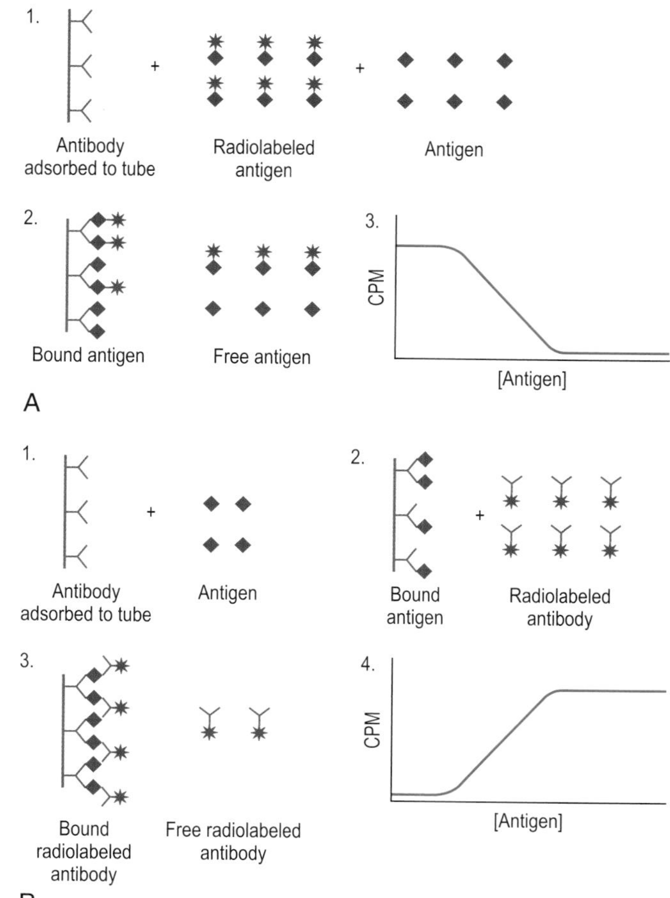

Figure 74-3 **A,** Competitive binding radioimmunoassay. *A1,* Antibody is adsorbed on a plastic surface (tube, microtiter plate well) or covalently coupled to a solid phase matrix (*not shown*). A variable amount of standard or unknown amount of unlabeled antigen (*diamond*) is added in the presence of a fixed amount of radiolabeled antigen into their respective tubes. *A2,* Radiolabeled and unlabeled antigens can both bind to the solid phase antibody. If unlabeled antigen is present, it competes with radiolabeled antigen for a limited number of antibody binding sites. Solution phase antigens (both radiolabeled and unlabeled) are washed away or decanted and bound radioactivity is measured in a gamma counter. In the absence of competing antigen, a maximal amount of radioactivity is bound. *A3,* With increasing amounts of competing unlabeled antigen, decreasing amounts of radiolabeled antigen are bound. **B,** Noncompetitive (two-site) immunoradiometric assay (IRMA). *B1,* Antibody bound to the surfaces of plastic tubes or microtiter plate wells bind unlabeled antigen from either standards with defined amounts of antigen or unknowns with variable amounts of antigen. After the binding reaction, unbound antigen is removed by decanting during buffer washes. *B2,* Radiolabeled antibody is added to all tubes and binds to bound antigen. *B3,* Unbound (residual) radiolabeled antibody is then removed with buffer washes, and bound radioactivity is measured. If no antigen is present in the standard or unknown, then no radioactivity is bound to the insolubilized antibody. *B4,* The amount of bound radiolabeled detection antibody increases in proportion to the amount of antigen that is bound from the standard or unknown specimens. *CPM,* Counts per minute.

Solid Phase Immunoassay. Although the solution phase chemistry of the liquid phase immunoassays rapidly achieves equilibrium, it suffers from the need to separate free from bound antigen. Direct adsorption of antibody onto a solid surface (glass and plastic test tubes, beads or microparticles, and 96 well microtiter plates) using noncovalent binding chemistry techniques became an attractive and inexpensive alternative (see Fig. 74-3, *B1*).[52] Adsorption of receptors or ligands onto microtiter plates was a useful alternative because fluids could be more easily manipulated. Antibodies could be covalently bound through primary amide linkages to cyanogen bromide (CNBr)-activated carbohydrate particles.[53] This method of covalent coupling of proteins to microparticles permitted complex protein mixtures to be insolubilized, thereby allowing simultaneous antibody measurements of multiple isotypes (e.g., IgG, IgE) to the many proteins in biologic extracts of pollen, mold, pet epidermal, and food allergens. Second, it allowed the concentration of solid phase allergen to be manipulated in a manner to optimize specific binding while minimizing nonspecific binding. Third, it maximized the stability of the proteins and increased the shelf life of biologic reagents in clinical assays for antibody. The use of a solid phase permitted the separation of bound and free labeled antibody or antigen in both competitive and noncompetitive binding immunoassays (see Fig. 74-3).

Immunometric Assay. Immunoassays that use a labeled antibody are classified as immunometric (see Fig. 74-3, *B*). Because antibodies are inherently stable proteins, they are readily labeled with radionuclides, enzymes, fluorophors or nanoparticles. Transition from the use of radioisotopes as labels to enzymes such as alkaline phosphatase and horseradish peroxidase and nanoparticles such as colloidal gold has been one of the single most important enhancements of immunoassays. When non–isotopically labeled detection antibody is used together with a solid phase (capture) antibody with specificity to the same antigen(s), the assay is called a two-site immunoenzymetric assay. In immunometric assays, both the solid phase (capture) antibody and the labeled (detection) antibody are added either sequentially or simultaneously to the reaction vessel (tube, microtiter plate well) in molar excess to the amount of antigen being detected (see Fig. 74-3, *B1-3*). With this assay configuration, the amount of the unlabeled antigen (ligand) becomes the rate-limiting component of the binding reaction. A noncompetitive binding reaction occurs when the immobilized capture antibody and solution phase labeled-detection antibody are added to the antigen (unknown, standard, or control) in different incubation periods. The more antigen present, the higher the amount of labeled-detection antibody bound (see Fig. 74-3, *B4*). The noncompetitive two-site immunoenzymetric assay is a robust assay configuration that minimizes nonspecific binding after buffer washes and maximizes specificity by using both a capture and a detection antibody specific for the analyte of interest.

Immunochemical Methods for Measurement of Immunoglobulin E Protein

Of the assay methods discussed in this chapter, immunodiffusion and the early nephelometric assays possessed insufficient analytic sensitivity to detect the ng/mL levels of IgE in human serum, secretions, and cell culture supernatants. The initial assay used to quantify total human serum IgE was the radioimmunosorbent test (RIST)[54] (see Fig. 74-3, *B*). One useful version of the RIST employed a polyclonal anti-human IgE Fc that was covalently attached to CNBr-activated paper disks to bind IgE from test, control, and calibrated reference sera. ^{125}I-labeled polyclonal anti human IgE Fc was added to detect bound IgE. The quantity of bound radioactivity (radioiodinated anti-human IgE) was directly related to the IgE content in the original serum. Cited advantages of this assay have been its analytic sensitivity (as low as 1 ng of IgE per mL) and precision, expressed as the absolute value of the coefficient of variation (CV)—more specifically, the relative standard deviation (intraassay CV values less than 5%). Total serum IgE assays in clinical use today are standardized with a reference serum that has been cross-calibrated against an international reference standard for human IgE.[55,56] A nonisotopic, monoclonal antibody, microtiter plate–based two-site immunoenzymetric assay (IEMA) is used by researchers.[57] The use of two monoclonal antibody clones that bind to different epitopes on the Fc region of the ε chain of the human IgE molecule ensures specificity while maximizing sensitivity (1 ng/mL), precision (intraassay CV values less than 10%), reproducibility (interassay CV values less than 15%), and parallelism (interdilutional CV values less than 20%).

Total serum IgE is routinely measured in clinical laboratories by nephelometric or non-competitive immunoassays that are cleared by the U.S. Food and Drug Administration (FDA).[58] The intermethod agreement among these different commercial IgE assays is excellent (inter-method CV values typically are less than 10% for serum IgE levels greater than 30 kU/L [1 U of IgE = 2.44 ng]).[59] This good agreement has been attributed to cross-calibration using well-characterized IgE reference preparations such as the World Health Organization (WHO) 75/502. Because total serum IgE is an analyte regulated by the federal Clinical Laboratory Improvement Act of 1988 (CLIA-88) statute, laboratories that perform total serum IgE measurements for clinical application must successfully participate in an external proficiency survey such as the one conducted by the College of American Pathologists (CAP).[58]

Immunochemical Methods for Measurement of Immunoglobulin E Antibodies of Defined Allergen Specificity

In 1967, Wide and colleagues[9] described the RAST for detection of human IgE antibodies of defined allergen specificities. This assay employed allergen covalently coupled to CNBr-activated paper disks to make an allergosorbent (solid phase allergen reagent) (Fig. 74-4). Incubation of human serum with the allergosorbent in a test tube permitted allergen-specific antibodies of any isotype to bind. Unbound serum proteins were then removed with a physiologic buffer wash, and bound IgE was detected with radioiodinated anti-human IgE Fc. The quantity of radioactivity bound to the allergosorbent was proportional to the amount of allergen-specific IgE antibody in the test serum. Assay response data (bound counts per minute) were interpolated from a calibration curve constructed with multiple dilutions of a birch-specific human IgE

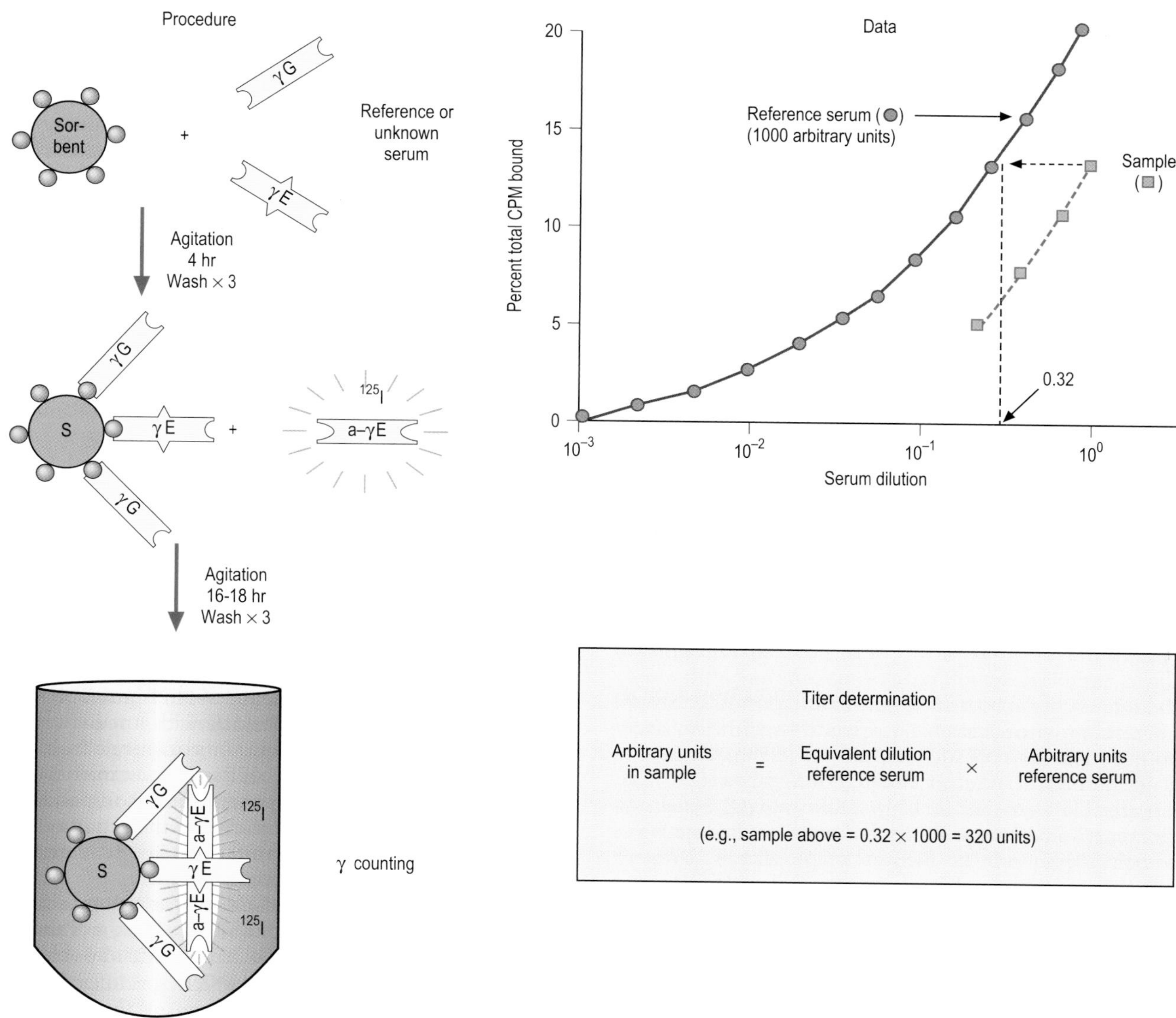

Figure 74-4 Schematic diagram of the original radioallergosorbent test reported in 1967. In the first assay incubation, human antibody of different isotypes (e.g., immunoglobulins IgG and IgE) in the reference and unknown sera bind to antigens coupled to the sorbent (*S*) (i.e., allergosorbent). Following isotonic buffer washes to remove unbound serum proteins, bound IgE antibody is detected with a ^{125}I-labeled rabbit anti-human IgE detection antibody. The percentage of the total radioactivity in counts per minute (CPM) bound to the allergosorbent was then measured in a gamma counter and plotted against the serum dilution analyzed. The amount of specific IgE in the reference and original sera was proportional to the amount of radioactivity bound. Interpolated units of antibody were corrected for sample dilution and reported as the number of arbitrary units of allergen-specific IgE in the original serum. Newer technology has allowed the use of more potent and quality-controlled allergosorbents, safer and more stable nonisotopic labels, more rapid assay kinetics, and a standardized reference serum dilution curve calibrated in kIU/L of IgE based on the World Health Organization (WHO) IgE standard. However, the general design of the assay and the data processing and computation strategies have remained unchanged. *(Reproduced with permission from Adkinson NF Jr. Measurement of total serum immunoglobulin E and allergen specific IgE antibody. In: Rose NR, Friedman H, editors. Manual of clinical laboratory immunology. Washington, D.C.: American Society for Microbiology; 1976. p. 590-602.)*

antibody and a birch allergosorbent. Results were reported in semiquantitative class groupings (0 = undetectable to 5 = very high IgE antibody) or in arbitrary Phadebas RAST Units (PRU/mL). These classifications are now obsolete as results are reported in kUa/L after interpolation from a total IgE calibration curve. A consensus guideline is available that presents an overview of the analytic performance and clinical utility of immunologic assays for human IgE antibodies of defined allergen specificity.[43]

ALLERGOSORBENT

Of the reagents used in allergen-specific IgE antibody assays, the allergosorbent is the principal component that defines its specificity. In some research applications, CNBr-activated carbohydrate particles are still used as an allergosorbent matrix. Alternatively, adsorption of allergens onto plastic microtiter plate wells has been used by researchers because of its simplicity, ease of preparation, and low cost.[60] However, complex mixtures of allergenic proteins bind differentially to plastic surfaces, and this specificity limits the protein-binding capacity of the allergosorbent for any single allergen component. Thus, some allergens may be poorly represented or absent from microtiter plate–based allergosorbents. High μg/mL levels of IgG antibody that occur in the serum of immunized allergic patients also can interfere by blocking the binding of ng/mL levels of IgE antibody to a more limited number of allergen-binding sites.[43] Thus, commercially available allergosorbents or liquid phase labeled-allergen reagents have tended to be as allergen-rich as possible to ensure that all of the allergen-specific IgE antibody specificities can bind to the allergosorbent.[58,61,62]

In one currently used clinical assay (ImmunoCAP System, ThermoFisher Scientific, Kalamazoo, Michigan), an activated cellulose sponge is used to bind large amounts of allergens. In a second clinical assay (Immulite System, Siemens Healthcare Diagnostics, Tarrytown, New York), allergen is conjugated with biotin; once added to the reaction mixture in a solution phase chemistry, biotin-allergen–IgE antibody complexes are bound to a solid phase by means of an avidin-biotin bridge. A third clinically used assay employs the activated paper disk to which allergen is coupled (HYTEC-288 System, Hycor Biomedical, Indianapolis). Because clinical assays no longer use radioisotopes, the designation "RAST" for specific IgE assays is outdated; the terms *allergen-specific IgE assays* and *IgE antibody serologic testing* are preferred.

Although not yet approved by some regulatory agencies for clinical use, chip-based microarrays[63-65] and paper-based lateral flow point-of-care assays[66] are now used to measure IgE antibodies in human serum. In one version called the ISAC (Immuno Solid-Phase Allergen Chip) assay (ThermoFisher Scientific), an activated chip is imprinted with purified native or recombinant allergenic components from more than 100 specificities in triplicate dots in a defined matrix pattern.[63,64] Human serum (30 μL) is layered over the allergen coated chip area and specific antibodies of any isotype bind. Fluorescence-labeled anti-IgE is layered over the same surface to detect bound IgE. The ISAC is able to provide a highly sophisticated assessment of IgE antibody cross-reactivity, especially between pollen and food allergens. Its analytic sensitivity also approaches that of the single-plex assays, even though its data are presented as semiquantitative. Its limitations reside in its fixed repertoire of allergen specificities that must be analyzed and the potential for interference by non-IgE antibodies due to the use of allergen-limiting microdots. Another reported version of this chip-based microarray for IgE antibody detection uses allergen extracts.[65]

In contrast with the chip-based assay, the FDA-cleared lateral flow point-of-care IgE antibody assay (e.g., ImmunoCAP Rapid, ThermoFisher Scientific) uses paper immunochromatography to qualitatively detect the presence of IgE antibodies to a panel of aeroallergens from a drop of blood.[66] For this assay, a sophisticated handheld device uses colloidal gold–conjugated anti-IgE to provide a visual confirmation of IgE antibody binding to paper impregnated with lines of 10 allergen extracts. It utilizes the simplicity and rapidity of lateral flow assay technology combined with a qualitative readout from an optical scanner.

CALIBRATION SCHEMES

IgE antibody assays have been classified as qualitative, semiquantitative, or quantitative in nature, depending on the degree to which their results accurately reflect the quantity of IgE antibody in serum (Table 74-3). In *qualitative* IgE antibody assays, a preassigned positive threshold level is used to determine whether a result is positive (reactive) or negative (nonreactive). An example is the multiallergen IgE antibody screening test discussed later on. The positive threshold is assigned by analyzing sera from nonatopic individuals with low total serum IgE levels who are known to be clinically not allergic by history and skin testing. *Semiquantitative* IgE antibody assays provide a relative magnitude of the response measured in addition to a positive or negative result. The level of the response is related in terms of rank order to, but not always directly proportional to, the quantity of IgE antibody in serum.

Quantitative IgE antibody assays use the most advanced assay calibration methods. A homologous (same allergen specificity) calibration curve would be desirable because it promotes assay parallelism (agreement between specimen results analyzed at different dilutions) and maximizes the assay's working range. However, difficulty in obtaining sufficient quantities

TABLE 74-3 Classification of Immunoglobulin E (IgE) Antibody Assays

Classification	Results	Method of Standardization	Calibrators and Controls
Qualitative	Reactive or nonreactive Positive or negative Indeterminate (equivocal) zone may be present Based on preassigned positive threshold	Single or dual calibrators used to normalize assay No calibration curve	One reference sample Negative and positive control
Semiquantitative	Arbitrary units or classes Single-point calibration curve: modified or alternative scoring system Multipoint calibration curve (class 0, I, II, III, IV, V, IV; PRU/mL)	Single or dual calibrators to normalize assay	Negative and bilevel positive control sera References unique for test system; made from pooled patient sera
Quantitative	Units (kIU/L or ng/mL) related to a recognized reference preparation (e.g., WHO IgE standard 75/702)	Multipoint homologous or heterologous standard curve used for interpolation of response data into dose results	Trilevel positive quality control sera Reference calibrated by comparison with a widely available, international reference preparation

Adapted from Matsson P, Hamilton RG, and the CSLI Task Force.[43]
WHO, World Health Organization.

of serum from IgE antibody–positive individuals for all of the clinically used allergen specificities has forced adoption of a heterologous (different allergen specificity) calibration approach. The most widely used heterologous calibration system in commercial IgE antibody assays is a total serum IgE reference curve that is traceable to the WHO 75/502 total serum IgE primary standard.[55] For clinicians who use international units, allergen-specific IgE antibody response data are interpolated from the total serum IgE calibration curve in kUa/L levels of allergen-specific IgE antibody. As in the total serum IgE assay, 1 U is roughly equivalent to 2.44 ng of IgE antibody. Clinically used IgE antibody assays have undergone a transition in their reported minimum detectable concentration from a "clinically defined" positive threshold of 0.35 kUa/L to their true analytic sensitivity of 0.1 kUa/L (0.244 ng/mL). Although these assays can analytically detect IgE antibody levels as low as 0.1 kUa/L, the clinical significance of low levels between 0.1 and 0.35 kUa/L is unknown. There is also evidence that in at least one such assay, 1 kUa/L of allergen-specific IgE antibody may be equivalent to 1 kU/L of total serum IgE.[67]

ALLERGEN COMPONENTS

Allergens can be grouped according to their route of exposure or based on their source. Extensive structural similarity or cross-reactivity of allergenic molecules has been reported within particular pollen groups, such as the grasses (June, brome, timothy, perennial rye, fescue, orchard, red top, salt, sweet vernal, velvet). Cross-reactivity also has been shown at the allergen component level using native and recombinant proteins. The best illustration is that of the PR10 family of allergens, which share extensive structural similarity (e.g., Bet v 1–birch, Cor a 1–hazelnut, Mal d 1–apple, Pru p 1–peach, Gly m 4–soybean, Ara h 8–peanut, Aln g 1–alder, Act d 8–kiwi, Api g 1–celery, and Dau c 1–carrot). Other clinically monitored component-based cross-reactivity groups include the tropomyosins (Pen a 1–shrimp, Der p 10–house dust mite, Bla g 7–cockroach, Ani s 3–*Anisakis*), serum albumins (Fel d 2–cat, Can f 3–dog, Bos d 6–cow, Equ c 3–horse, Gal d 5–chicken), parvalbumins (Gad c 1–Cod, Cyp c 1–carp), profilins (Bet v 2–birch, Phl p 12–timothy grass, Ole e 2–olive, Hev b 8–latex), calcium-binding proteins (Bet v 4–birch, Phl p 7–timothy grass), and lipid transfer proteins (Pru p 3–peach, Per j 2–wall pellitory, Art v 3–mugwort, Cor a 8–hazelnut). The component-based chip assay allows detection of IgE antibody to these clinically important component allergens.[63,64]

MULTIALLERGEN IMMUNOGLOBULIN E SCREENING ASSAY

The multiallergen screen is a single qualitative assay that simultaneously detects IgE antibody to any or all of a group of allergens either within or across allergen groups (e.g., inhaled indoor and outdoor aeroallergens or ingested food allergens). It differs from a "panel" of specific IgE antibody measurements in that it is a single analysis involving one allergosorbent that contains 5 to 15 different allergen specificities, whereas the panel involves a number of individually run specific IgE antibody measurements for different allergen specificities, all run at the same time. The specificities of aeroallergens immobilized on the multiscreen allergosorbent (e.g., a cross section of weed, grass, and tree pollens; mold, pet epidermal; dust mites) are intentionally not specified by manufacturer or the laboratory because the precise allergen specificities can vary among different commercial reagent sources. The allergen specificities are selected on the basis of knowledge of those allergens that induce allergic disease in a majority of adults in a particular region or country.[43] In analyzing sera from children younger than 6 years of age, a food allergen mix antibody to key foods (e.g., milk, egg, peanut, wheat, soybean, fish) often is tested as a second analysis with the aeroallergen screen to detect IgE. Manufacturers intentionally do not disclose which allergen specificities are on their multiaeroallergen screen, to discourage formulation of a treatment plan based on a qualitative IgE antibody result. Rather, with a positive multiallergen screen result that is consistent with a positive atopic history, the clinician should evaluate the patient further for sensitization to individual allergen specificities using an extended clinical history and individualized skin testing and/or IgE antibody serologic testing. A negative multiallergen screen result reduces the probability that IgE-mediated allergic disease is involved in the patient's clinical problem. Caution in interpretation is warranted, however: Inappropriate use of this screening test in unselected populations may produce positive results in asymptomatic patients, because IgE antibody responses are more frequent than symptomatic disease.

QUALITY ASSURANCE

IgE assays are highly complex immunologic tests that require multiple levels of quality assurance. Quality assurance testing begins at the time of manufacturing immediately after the assembly of the assay's components. Sera from clinically documented nonallergic (IgE antibody negative) and allergic (IgE antibody–positive) individuals are used in quality control of the allergen-containing reagent and to confirm the assay's analytic performance (minimum detectable concentration, precision and reproducibility, parallelism, nonspecific binding properties). The manufacturer assesses the diagnostic sensitivity and specificity of the test in clinically characterized allergic and nonallergic populations. Reproducibility of the assay is documented with a precision profile (CV_{dose} versus dose plot), and the limits of detection, linearity, and parallelism of the assay are confirmed with dilution recovery analyses.[43]

Once in the laboratory, semiquantitative and quantitative assays are quality controlled with each run by analyzing a minimum of three quality control sera with IgE antibody, which cover two to three times the assay detection limit and the assay's range midpoint and within 10% of the upper extreme plateau level. Clinical laboratories that perform total and allergen-specific IgE antibody measurements are required by the CLIA-88 legislation to perform interlaboratory proficiency testing. A well-subscribed external proficiency survey is the Diagnostic Allergy (SE) Survey, conducted by the College of American Pathologists (CAP).[58,59] In this survey, five challenge sera and two wildcard test sera are sent at 17-week intervals over the year and tested for five allergen specificities of IgE antibody, a multiallergen screen, and a total serum IgE. The total serum IgE and quantitative allergen-specific IgE antibody assay results are compared with peer group means and ranges; reported values that exceed the 99% confidence limit for a laboratory's peer group represent outlier results. IgE antibody assay results are reported in quantitative kUa/L units. Qualitative grade or class results that reflect the presence and relative levels of IgE antibodies in the test sera are now discouraged and will eventually be phased out. In specific Laboratory reports, the detection of allergen-specific IgE antibody in a serum specimen from a nonatopic person (clinical history–negative, puncture skin test–negative) constitutes gross outlier data, with relevant implications for the reporting laboratory. Moreover, a negative IgE antibody assay result that is reported for an IgE antibody–containing serum sample from an atopic individual (with a positive clinical history and positive result on puncture skin test) is considered an outlier. The CAP survey operates on the basis of peer group consensus. Thus, if more than 90% of laboratories performing an allergen-specific IgE antibody assay method do not agree with the result, then that measurement is not graded in that cycle of the survey for that particular assay. Such an undesirable result indicates a highly variable assay format. Each diagnostic allergy survey participant receives a summary of the SE survey data for each cycle with a commentary that critiques general performance trends and problem areas.

Immunochemical Methods for Measurement of Allergen-Specific Immunoglobulin G Antibody

Since the 1930s, the presence of allergen-specific IgG antibodies has been considered a hallmark of an immunized allergic person. Subsequently, these antibodies were shown to block the release of histamine from IgE sensitized basophils in the presence of allergen.[68] Nonimmunized persons who are minimally exposed to clinically important environmental aeroallergens, such as weed, grass, and tree pollens, mold, and animal epidermal antigens, generally produce serum levels of specific IgG antibody that are low (in the ng/mL range) or undetectable. Increases in serum IgG antibody to μg/mL levels are observed after the injection of antigen, either intentionally or by accidental exposure (e.g., drug injection, insect sting, or occupational chemical exposure) or by active allergen immunotherapy. Quantitative immunoassays for allergen-specific IgG antibody have been developed to assess an allergic patient's relative allergen exposure by measuring the magnitude of the humoral immune response to parenterally administered allergen injections given during immunotherapy. For *Hymenoptera* venom–allergic patients, clinically successful immunotherapy is accompanied by high serum levels (in μg/mL) of allergen-specific IgG antibody,[69] even though the precise role of IgG "blocking" antibodies in conferring protection against allergic reactions remains unclear.

Knowledge of the presence or absolute levels of IgG antibodies in human serum has not always been clinically useful. Serum levels of IgG antibodies specific for food antigens, for instance, have shown no correlation with the frequency of reactions observed during double-blind, placebo-controlled food challenges. The clinical application for IgG antibody measurements in the field of allergy has been their use in the evaluation of *Hymenoptera* venom–allergic patients who have been receiving maintenance immunotherapy injections.[69] In such cases, *Hymenoptera* venom–specific IgG antibody levels are reportedly useful in individualizing venom immunotherapy doses. Although the clinical utility of IgG antibody measurements appears to be restricted to less than 4 years of venom therapy, the IgG antivenom level can be valuable for individualizing the dose and frequency of venom injections in an effort to maximize the protective effects of immunotherapy.

The first quantitative immunoassay used to measure venom-specific IgG antibody was the radioimmunoprecipitation or double-antibody assay.[49] Both the isotopic and nonisotopic versions of this assay have remained useful analytic tools for quantification of IgG antibody specific for purified protein antigens. Because the radioimmunoprecipitation assay performs best under labeled-antigen–limiting conditions, this tends to accentuate nonparallelism and differential plateauing when polyclonal sera with heterogeneous IgG antibody populations are being evaluated.[70]

To address these concerns, a noncompetitive binding solid phase immunoassay was developed in which complex antigen mixtures were covalently insolubilized onto a solid phase.[71] The limitation of this assay resides in its detection of IgE antibodies to all of the components on the sorbent, whether they are allergens or simply antigens that do not elicit IgE antibodies. More recently, IgG antibodies against purified allergenic components have been measured using a microtiter plate–based noncompetitive enzyme immunoassay and the ISAC.

Immunglobulin G Subclass Protein and Antibodies

IgG has achieved special importance in immune protection of the neonate because it is the sole immunoglobulin that is transported across the placenta in any significant quantities. The levels of total serum IgG1, IgG2, IgG3, and IgG4 protein have been quantified by a number of immunologic methods, including radial immunodiffusion, nephelometry, and immunometric assays.[72] The concentrations of IgG subclass proteins are known to increase throughout childhood, reaching adult levels by the age of 12 years.[73,74]

Reduced levels of all four IgG subclasses have been observed in common variable hypogammaglobulinemia, severe combined immunodeficiency (SCID), and the Wiskott-Aldrich syndrome. Selective deficiencies of IgG2 and IgG4 proteins are seen in some individuals with IgA deficiency. In the assessment of allergic patients, IgG4 antibodies in particular have received special attention. IgG subclass protein measurements were extensively performed in the latter decades of the twentieth century,[75] and the abundance of data has led to extensive focus on IgG subclass deficiencies.[76] Most clinicians and researchers, however, no longer view IgG subclass protein or antibody measurements as useful in a clinical workup for immunodeficiency. Total IgG, IgA, and IgM levels in serum are most useful in the evaluation of a patient for humoral immunodeficiency.

IgG4 constitutes approximately 4% of the total IgG in serum of adults. It is often produced as a result of chronic antigenic challenge, such as occurs during high-dose allergen immunotherapy. Accordingly, there has been particular research interest in IgG4 antibodies in patients with type I hypersensitivity who receive immunotherapy or who are subject to chronic natural allergen exposures. Allergen-specific IgG4 antibody has been measured by one of several immunoassay configurations. Historically, the solid phase radioimmunoassay (SPRIA)-type of assay uses allergen that is insolubilized on an allergosorbent (microtiter plate or particle) to bind specific antibodies from serum. More recently, specific IgG and IgG4 antibodies have been detected using several automated platforms provided by (e.g., ImmunoCAP System, ThermoFisher Scientific; Immulite System, Siemens Healthcare). However, the analytic performance characteristics (sensitivity, linearity, reproducibility) and the clinical utility of the IgG and IgG4 antibody results from these assays have yet to be defined.

Allergen-specific IgG4 measurements continue to be of interest in research studies involving immunotherapy because of their in vivo blocking potential. They can act as functionally monovalent antibodies that reduce IgE–allergen complex formation as a result of their tendency to undergo light chain switching.[77,78] Immunotherapy also is known to induce regulatory B cells that produce cytokines such as IL-10, which promotes IgG4 production. A newer assay involving inhibition of CD23-dependent IgE-facilitated allergen binding (IgE-FAB) reportedly correlates more closely with clinical outcomes of immunotherapy than direct measurement of allergen-specific IgG or IgG4 antibodies.[79]

Currently, IgG4 antibody and IgE-FAB inhibition measurements remain research biomarkers and have limited use in the clinical management of patients with allergic disease.

Other Analytes of Interest in Allergic Disorders and Asthma

A number of other analytes are infrequently measured in human serum to support the differential diagnosis of allergy, asthma, or hypersensitivity pneumonitis, and to aid in the management of asthmatic patients. These include cotinine, ECP, and precipitating human IgG antibody for antigens in organic dusts.

COTININE

Nicotine in the blood of smokers or individuals passively exposed to smoke is directly excreted in the urine or converted by P-450 enzymes to 5 hydroxynicotine, which is then converted by aldehyde oxidase to cotinine. As the major metabolite of nicotine, cotinine has been shown to have a longer biologic half-life than nicotine in the blood. The rate of clearance of cotinine from the urine of smokers (15.4 ± 1.2 hours) is significantly shorter than that for nonsmokers (27.3 ± 1.9 hours). Cotinine has therefore become the serum marker of choice for monitoring asthmatics for passive smoke exposure.[80] In one study, the use of preset positive threshold levels of 13.7, 14.2, and 49.7 ng/mL for cotinine in plasma, saliva, and urine specimens, respectively, produced a diagnostic sensitivity of 97% to 99% and a diagnostic specificity of 81% to 83% for passive exposure to smoke.[81]

EOSINOPHIL CATIONIC PROTEIN

Eosinophilia is associated with a variety of inflammatory disorders, such as asthma, in which primed and activated eosinophils are detectable in high numbers. Tissue destruction, such as the shedding of epithelial cells in airways, may be caused by products released from eosinophil granules. A solid phase noncompetitive immunoassay method (ImmunoCAP, ThermoFisher Scientific) is available for quantification of ECP, which is an 18.5- to 22-kD basic protein.[82] Sera from 100 healthy subjects contained ECP at levels from 2.3 to 16 ng/mL (95% confidence interval), with a geometric mean of 6 ng/mL. Results correlate strongly with total blood eosinophil counts. At present, ECP measurements have demonstrated limited clinical utility in the monitoring of patients with atopic asthma and other allergic diseases in which eosinophils are thought to induce tissue damage.

PRECIPITATING IMMUNOGLOBULIN G ANTIBODIES (PRECIPITINS)

Precipitating IgG antibodies are used as a biomarker for individuals with suspected extrinsic allergic alveolitis or hypersensitivity pneumonitis that involves the lung interstitium and terminal bronchioles.[83] Serum can be analyzed by the double diffusion method (Ouchterlony) for precipitating antibodies. More specifically, a crude antigen extract and antibody (control or patient's serum) are pipetted into closely spaced wells in a porous agarose gel. Precipitating antibodies in visible white precipitin lines are confirmed by lines of identity with known human antibody controls. Precipitin assays are clinically available with specificities for pigeon serum, *Aureobasidium pullulans* (a yeastlike fungus), fecal particles from parakeets and a variety of exotic household birds (Amazon, cockatiel, blue front parrot), thermophilic actinomycetes, and *Aspergillus fumigatus*.

Quantification of Environmental Allergens

OUTDOOR AEROALLERGENS

Daily pollen and mold spore levels in the outdoor air are evaluated in most major cities across the United States by aerobiology stations. The American Academy of Allergy, Asthma and Immunology (AAAAI) Aerobiology Committee has established an aerobiology network that certifies participating laboratories, monitors their performance, and collates longitudinal pollen and mold spore data. Fungal spores are relatively small in comparison with pollen grains. Mold spore sizes range from 1 to greater than 100 mm in diameter, with most in the 7- to 12-mm range. Pollen grains are larger, with diameters ranging from 20 to 70 mm. Until recently, the rotorod has been the primary collection device used by most aerobiology stations.[84] To address the poor efficiency of the rotorod in collecting mold spores and bacteria, aerobiology stations have been replacing their rotorod samplers with a suction impactor, which pulls particles from the air and embeds them on a moving paper tape. These devices have the advantage of being able to collect longitudinal samples over a 24-hour or a 5-day period. Clinically, the usefulness of the pollen and mold count resides in its diagnostic value, in that it defines the type of pollen and mold that can be found in the air in different regions of the country and at times when patients are experiencing allergic symptoms. Because the pollen and mold spore count measured in an air sample covers the previous 24 hours, one limitation is that the reported levels do not always accurately reflect the aeroallergen levels in the air at the time the patient reads the information.

INDOOR AEROALLERGEN

Children with asthma, in particular, have a high prevalence of IgE antibodies specific for environmental allergens found in indoor environments that are produced by dust mites, dogs, cats, cockroaches, mice, rats and molds.[85] For dust mite allergens, a dose-response relationship has been shown between increasing exposure and the likelihood of a positive skin test response to mite allergens. Exposure to even low levels of mite allergen (0.02 to 2 μg/g) has been shown to be a significant risk factor for sensitization. The level of cockroach allergen exposure also was an important determinant for sensitization to cockroach allergens. The indoor environment has therefore become an important target for control of these allergens to facilitate avoidance therapy.

A number of clinical laboratories perform house dust analyses. A "gross" surface sample, or so-called reservoir dust specimen, is collected from carpeted and upholstered areas of the home, workplace, or school using one of several inexpensive dust collectors attached to a standard household vacuum cleaner. A dust extract is prepared and its allergen content is determined by a noncompetitive (two-site) monoclonal antibody–based immunoenzymetric assay. A fluorescence-based multiplex array assay (i.e., Multiplex Assay for Indoor Allergens [MARIA])[86] using a universal allergen standard is gradually replacing the plate-based immunoenzymetric assay for measuring the following indoor aeroallergens: Der p 1, Der f 1 (*Dermatophagoides pteronyssinus* and *D. farinae*, respectively), Fel d 1 *(Felis domesticus)*, Can f 1 *(Canis familiaris)*, Bla g 1/Bla g 2 *(Blatella germanica)*, Mus m 1 *(Mus musculus)*, and Rat n 1 *(Rattus norvegicus)*. The assays are quality-controlled to ensure reproducibility using internal positive controls.

MOLD/FUNGUS EVALUATION OF INDOOR ENVIRONMENTS

Accurate assessment of the mold content in an indoor environment is problematic, because mold spores are ever present in outdoor air. Fungal spores can be viable or nonviable, and laboratory methods for evaluating each form of mold spore are different. Viable mold spores have been considered more clinically important by some allergists, because they can colonize indoor environments and mass-produce spores for release into the air. A qualitative viable mold spore analysis can be performed on small quantities (5 mg) of fine reservoir.[85] The number of mold colonies growing at 24 and 48 hours is determined by visual inspection, and the results are reported as a colony count. The species of the predominant molds growing also can be determined by repetitive subculture and morphologic identification.

Immunoassays for indicator mold allergens such as Alt a 1 *(Alternaria alternata)* and Asp f 1 *(Aspergillus fumigatus)* have not always been clinically useful. This limitation arises from the fact that molds found in indoor environments do not always produce the same repertoire of proteins, because growth depends on the specific environmental conditions present on any given day (e.g., nutrients, temperature, humidity). Other clinically important molds found indoors are *Cladosporium herbarum (Hormodendrum)* and *Penicillium notatum.*

INTERPRETATION OF INDOOR AEROALLERGEN MEASUREMENTS

Levels of Der p 1 and/or Der f 1 allergen greater than 2000 ng/g of fine dust have been associated with an increased risk of allergic symptoms in sensitized persons, whereas levels greater than 10,000 ng/g of fine dust have been associated with an increased risk of sensitization. For cat allergen, levels of Fel d 1 greater than 8000 ng/g of fine dust have been suggested as the threshold for sensitization. Because cat allergen can be transported on clothing, the Fel d 1 content in the localized airspace of an individual patient may be clinically important and not effectively assessed by environmental testing. Comparable risk targets also have been used for dog (Can f 1) allergen levels in indoor environments. Any detectable cockroach allergen in an indoor environment (more than 0.5 unit per gram of fine dust) places a cockroach-allergic individual at risk for symptoms and further sensitization.

Regarding fungal contamination, no specific mold spore levels have been established that identify an environment as posing a risk to a mold-allergic person. This is due to the multiple variables associated with heterogeneity of the mold spores, differential growth of the mold, aerosolization of the spores, and variable quantity and heterogeneous IgE antibody specificity in the patient. Variations in these parameters minimize the use of mold spore levels in predicting a clinical outcome from any tested environmental exposure. In one study, mold spore levels above 25,000 colonies per gram of fine dust place a home environment in the 75th percentile for homes monitored across the United States.[85] Increased fungal exposure has been associated with an increased risk for development of asthma symptoms and exacerbations, especially for children living in inner city environments.[87] When any of these proposed threshold levels are exceeded, the allergic individual is encouraged to remediate the living environment. A detailed discussion of strategies for remediation of indoor environments is beyond the scope of this chapter, but descriptions of such measures can be found elsewhere.[85]

Laboratory Methods in Cellular Immunology

Lymphocytes serve to eliminate foreign antigens from the host and modulate cellular responses through the release of cytokines. The peripheral blood contains several subpopulations of mature lymphocytes: T cells, B cells, and natural killer (NK) cells. Each of these subpopulations can be broadly defined by the presence of one or more glycoproteins on their cell membranes. Human leukocyte subsets are both enumerated and evaluated for function to identify abnormal cellular immune responsiveness and as part of a workup for immunodeficiency.

ENUMERATION OF LYMPHOCYTE SUBPOPULATIONS

Specific cell surface glycoprotein antigens are used to immunophenotype peripheral blood cells. In its most basic form, the technique involves incubating cells with a fluorochrome-labeled antibody specific for defined cell surface antigens and detecting the number of fluorescence-positive cells. Initially, a fluorescence microscope was used to detect fluorescent cells; however, flow cytometry has assumed this primary role because of its capacity to analyze thousands of cells in less than a minute and its greater sensitivity for fluorescence than the human eye. By the mid-1970s, the availability of monoclonal antibodies had permitted the development of highly specific reagents to cell surface antigens. In the early 1980s, this led to the first important lymphocyte immunophenotyping clinical test, which was used to identify human immunodeficiency virus (HIV)-infected patients who were deficient in $CD4^+$ T cells in peripheral blood.

The flow cytometer is an instrument with optical, fluidic, and electronic systems (Fig. 74-5). The basic optical system consists of an argon laser that emits light of a single wavelength at 488 nm (blue region). Cells are labeled with one of several

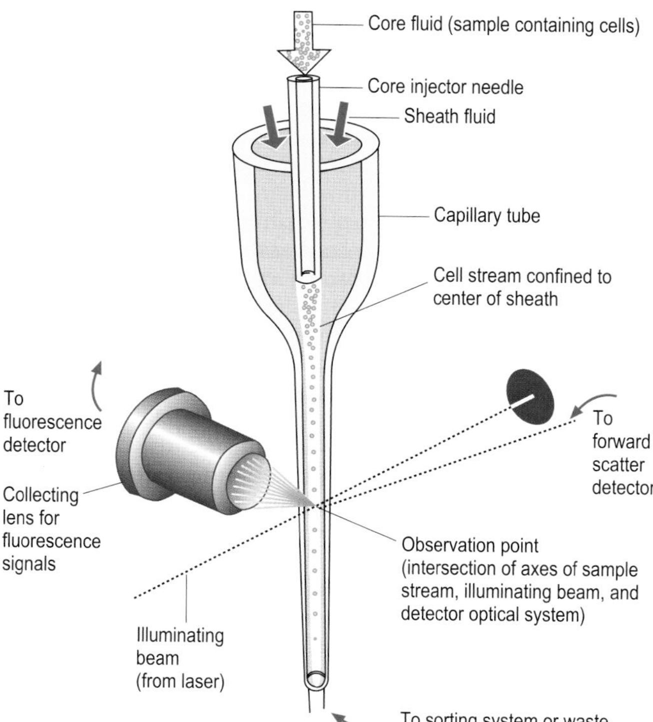

Figure 74-5 Schematic diagram of a flow cytometer. Optical, fluid, and electronic components of the flow cytometer work together to determine whether any given cell in a stream of cells has fluorophor-labeled antibody attached to its surface. Cells are sorted according to the degree of their forward scatter and by the magnitude of their fluorescence. *(Reproduced with permission from Homburger HA, Katzmann JA. Methods in laboratory immunology: principles and interpretation of laboratory tests for allergy. In: Middleton E Jr, Reed CE, Ellis EF, et al, editors. Allergy: principles and practice. 3rd ed. St. Louis: Mosby; 1998.)*

TABLE 74-4 Antibody Specificities Commonly Used in Flow Cytometry for Immunodeficiency Assessment

Antibody Designation	Detection on Normal Cells
CD2	Pan–T cell, NK cells (80-95% of T lymphocytes)
CD3	Mature pan–T cell (95% of T lymphocytes)
CD4	Helper/inducer T cells (65% of T lymphocytes) and monocytes
CD8	Cytotoxic/suppressor T cells (35% of T lymphocytes)
CD14	Maturing monocytes
CD16	Granulocytes, NK cells
CD19	Pan–B cell lymphocyte
CD20	Maturing B cells (surface immunoglobulin–positive B lymphocytes)
CD34	Immature hematopoietic cells, stem cells
CD41	Platelets and megakaryocytes
CD45	Leukocyte common antigen
CD56	NK cells, some stem cell disorders
HLA-DR	Myeloid blasts, B cells, activated T cells (90% of B lymphocytes and monocytes)
COMMON MONOCLONAL ANTIBODY PANEL SPECIFICITIES	
To evaluate lymphocyte purity and recovery	CD45, CD14 (two-color)
To evaluate helper/inducer T cell population	CD3, CD4 (two-color) CD3, CD4, CD45 (three-color) CD3, CD4, CD45, CD8 (four-color)
To evaluate cytotoxic/ suppressor T cell population	CD3, CD8 (two-color) CD3, CD8, CD45 (three-color)
To evaluate B cell lymphocyte population	CD3, CD19 (two-color) CD3, CD19, CD45 (three-color) CD3, CD19, CD45, CD16 (four-color)
To evaluate NK cell population	CD3, CD16 and/or CD56 (two-color)

HLA, Human leukocyte antigen; *NK*, natural killer.

fluorochromes, such as fluorescein (as the isothiocyanate, FITC), phycoerythrin (PE), or peridin chlorophyll protein (PerCP), as a result of monoclonal antibody fluorochrome conjugate binding to specific cell surface epitopes. The fluorochromes are excited by the laser and emit green (FITC), orange (PE), or red (PerCP) light that is measured through optical filters designed to capture its specific wavelength. Most flow cytometers measure five parameters on each cell: two nonfluorescence measures (the magnitude of forward and side scatter) and three fluorescence measures (green, orange, and red light intensity). The fluid system introduces cells in suspension into a pressurized sheath of fluid that travels through a clear cuvette. The laser light intersects a stream of cells that pass single file through the cuvette. The electronic system measures electric current signals from the detectors that provide measures of the magnitude of fluorescence intensity and the extent of light scatter associated with each cell as it passes through the laser. Particle or cell size is correlated with the degree of forward light scatter, and the cell granularity is correlated with the extent of right-angle scatter. Flow cytometers in clinical use generally have three photomultiplier tubes that permit the detection of three fluorochromes simultaneously with one argon laser. This capability allows simultaneous use of multiple markers to identify different cell populations.

Although specimen collection and processing protocols vary, whole blood collected in EDTA (ethylenediaminetetraacetic acid) tubes is preferred for flow cytometer analyses. The anticoagulated whole blood is first mixed well with fluorochrome-labeled monoclonal antibody specific for the desired cell surface marker. Table 74-4 lists the principal monoclonal antibody specificities that are used in immunophenotyping lymphocytes of patients suspected of HIV infection. The presence of sodium azide in the conjugated antibody preparations prevents any undesired capping or localization of cell receptors at discrete locations on the cell surface. Red blood cells are then lysed; the specimen is centrifuged and decanted; and remaining intact cells are resuspended in a fixative buffer such as formaldehyde (0.5% to 2% v/v) in phosphate-buffered saline.

The daily instrumentation quality control process consists of ensuring that the flow cytometer is aligned and that reproducible results are obtained with a stable fluorescent microbead standard. The mean channel numbers for maximal scatter and fluorescent peaks are plotted on a quality control chart. Moreover, the analysis of a mixture of microbeads with different fluorescence intensities from zero to very bright allows linearity to be assessed. If the investigator analyzes two or more fluorochromes at one time, spectral compensation is performed by the instrumentation with beads containing multiple fluorochromes (e.g., unlabeled, PE-labeled, and FITC-labeled microbeads) to ensure that the photomultiplier tube gains are adjusted to minimize overlapping detection of the different fluorochrome spectra. Finally, for the monoclonal antibody labeling step, an isotype-matched antibody with no specificity for lymphocyte surface antigens and matched for protein concentration and specific activity of the fluorescence is run as a negative control. A fluorescence-labeled monoclonal antibody specific for CD34, an antigen found on the surface of all immature hematopoietic cells and stem cells, is analyzed as a positive control sample. Finally, a processing control sample is run each time a patient's test specimen is prepared to ensure that immunoreactive fluorescent monoclonal antibody reagent and an effective lysing procedure have been employed.

Immunophenotyping of specific subsets of leukocytes and other cells has been invaluable in defining the cell origin of certain neoplasms (e.g., acute leukemia or non-Hodgkin lymphoma). It also has provided critical information for staging of HIV disease in patients infected with the virus (i.e., HIV-1) and other immune deficiency syndromes and for guiding therapeutic decisions. Other important applications of immunophenotyping include the quantification of hematopoietic stem cells and reticulocytes, the diagnosis of acquired or congenital immune deficiency syndrome, and detection of minimal residual leukemia after therapy.

FUNCTIONAL EVALUATION OF LYMPHOCYTES

Human lymphocyte function is evaluated by in vitro stimulation with antigen or polyclonal activators. The activation stimulus determines whether T cells, B cells, or both proliferate.[88] In clinical testing, in vitro proliferation of lymphocytes is viewed as a laboratory correlate of skin testing for delayed-type hypersensitivity to recall antigens. Abnormal lymphocyte proliferation has been associated with congenital immunodeficiencies but also with infectious diseases, malnutrition, cancer, surgery, shock, and autoimmune disease. In severe combined immunodeficiencies, both B cell and T cell functions are impaired. Using density-gradient centrifugation, mononuclear cells can be isolated from peripheral blood and exposed to various stimulants. Phytohemagglutinin, pokeweed mitogen, or concanavalin A in the role of mitogen and *Candida albicans* or tetanus toxoid in the role of recall antigen frequently are used to assess appropriate proliferative responses. After incubation in microtiter wells, cultures are pulsed with tritiated thymidine for 6 hours before harvesting. At the end of the incubation period, cultures are cooled to 4° C, harvested onto glass filter paper disks, and placed into vials containing scintillation fluid, and counted on a β scintillation counter. Mean net counts per minute (CPM) are calculated, and the quantity of ^{3}H-thymidine incorporated into the cell's DNA after antigen or mitogen stimulation is compared with the level observed with the control cells in medium alone.[89] The precise definition of a positive proliferation test result (e.g., a three- to fivefold increase in radioactivity, measured as CPM, incorporated in the cell over the buffer condition) varies among different reported studies.

Immunodeficiency disease occurs from the absence and/or functional failure of immune system components. This manifests as an increased susceptibility to infection. Functional defects in B cells increase the risk of pyrogenic infections such as pneumonia, otitis media, and sinusitis. Functional defects in the T cell compartment lead to an increase in opportunistic infections and humoral immunodeficiencies, because B cell function is largely T cell–dependent. Thus, both quantitative and functional lymphocyte studies are vital to an effective workup for evaluation of a patient with recurrent infections.

Conclusion

Various immunologic methods used to measure analytes in human blood allow assessment of the immunologic status of patients suspected of having allergic disease or an immunodeficiency. Of the analytes measured for an allergy workup, the presence and level of IgE antibody specific for a defined allergen specificity have the highest predictive value in supporting a clinical history of allergic disease. Total immunoglobulins and lymphocyte enumeration and functional assays are the most useful laboratory assays for the diagnosis of an immunodeficiency. An important but often-overlooked issue is that the assays for these analytes are considered complex tests. It is ultimately the physician ordering the test who is responsible for ensuring that the blood sample is sent to a clinical laboratory that performs accurate measurements with the least amount of variability and that reports immunologic test results in the most quantitative manner.[90] Selection of the laboratory should be based on the technical ability and diligence of the personnel performing the assays and on the quality of the assay protocols and reagent sources used. The laboratory should be certified under the statutes of CLIA-88, or its equivalent in other parts of the world, and should participate successfully in external proficiency surveys such as the diagnostic allergy, immunology, and flow cytometry surveys conducted by the CAP.

REFERENCES

Introduction

1. Hamilton RG. Immunological methods in the diagnostic allergy clinical and research laboratory. In: Detrick GB, Hamilton RG, Folds JD, editors. Manual of molecular and clinical laboratory immunology. Washington, D.C.: American Society for Microbiology; 2006. p. 955.
2. Roifman CM. Approach to the diagnosis of severe combined immunodeficiency. In: Detrick GB, Hamilton RG, Folds JD, editors. Manual of molecular and clinical laboratory immunology. Washington, D.C.: American Society for Microbiology; 2006. p. 895.
3. Giclas PC. Hereditary and acquired complement deficiencies. In: Detrick GB, Hamilton RG, Folds JD, editors. Manual of molecular and clinical laboratory immunology. Washington, D.C.: American Society for Microbiology; 2006. p. 914.
4. Holland SM. Neutropenia and neutrophil defects. In: Detrick GB, Hamilton RG, Folds JD, editors. Manual of molecular and clinical laboratory immunology. Washington, D.C.: American Society for Microbiology; 2006. p. 924.

Humoral Immune Responses Important in Allergic and Immunodeficiency Disease

5. Ishizaka K, Ishizaka T. Physicochemical properties of reaginic antibody. I. Association of reaginic activity with an immunoglobulin other than gamma A or gamma G globulin. J Allergy 1966;37:169-85.

6. Johansson SG. Raised levels of a new immunoglobulin class (IgND) in asthma. Lancet 1967;2: 951-3.
7. Bennich HH, Ishizaka K, Johansson SG, et al. Immunoglobulin E: a new class of human immunoglobulin. Immunology 1968;3:323-4.
8. Hamilton RG. The science behind the discovery of IgE. J Allergy Clin Immunol 2005;115: 648-52.
9. Wide L, Bennich H, Johansson SG. Diagnosis of allergy by an in-vitro test for allergen antibodies. Lancet 1967;2:1105-7.
10. Dati F, Ringel KP. Reference values for serum IgE in healthy non-atopic children and adults. Clin Chem 1982;28:1556.
11. Saarinen UM, Juntunen K, Kajosarri J, Bjorksten F. Serum immunoglobulin E in atopic and non-atopic children aged 5 months to 5 years. Acta Paediatr Scand 1982;71:489-94.
12. Barbee RA, Halomen M, Lebowitz M, Burrows B. Distribution of IgE in a community population sample: correlations with age, sex and allergen skin test reactivity. J Allergy Clin Immunol 1981;68:106-11.
13. Wittig HJ, Belloit J, DeFilippi I, Royal G. Age related serum IgE levels in healthy subjects and in patients with allergic disease. J Allergy Clin Immunol 1980;66:305-13.
14. Levy DA, Chen J. Healthy IgE-deficient person. N Engl J Med 1970;283:541-2.
15. Christensen LH, Holm J, Lund G, Riise E, Lund K. Several distinct properties of the IgE repertoire determine effector cell degranulation in response to allergen challenge. J Allergy Clin Immunol 2008;122:298-304.
16. Johansson SG, Nopp A, Oman H, et al. The size of the disease relevant IgE antibody fraction in relation to 'total-IgE' predicts the efficacy of anti-IgE (Xolair) treatment. Allergy 2009;64:1472-7.
17. Hamilton RG, MacGlashan Jr DW, Saini SS. IgE antibody specific activity in human allergic disease. Immunol Res 2010;47:273-84.
18. Savage WJ, Tobian AA, Savage JH, Hamilton RG, Ness PM. Atopic predisposition of recipients in allergic transfusion reactions to aphoresis platelets. Transfusion 2011;51:2337-42.
19. Johansson SG, Nopp A, Florvaag E, et al. High prevalence of IgE antibodies among blood donors in Sweden and Norway. Allergy 2005;60: 1312-5.
20. Stern A, Hage-Hamsten MV, Sondell K, Johansson SG. Is allergy screening of blood donors necessary? A comparison between questionnaire answers and the presence of circulating IgE antibodies. Vox Sang 1995;69:114-9.
21. Geha RS, Rappaport JM, Twarog FJ, et al. Increased serum immunoglobulin E levels following allogeneic bone marrow transplantation. J Allergy Clin Immunol 1980;66:78-81.
22. Abedi MR, Backman L, Persson U, Ringden O. Serum IgE levels after bone marrow transplantation. Bone Marrow Transplant 1989;4:255-60.
23. Walker SA, Riches PG, Wild G, et al. Total and allergen specific IgE in relation to allergic response patterns following bone marrow transplantation. Clin Exp Immunol 1986;66:633-9.
24. Dipiro JT, Howdieshell TR, Hamilton RG, et al. Increased plasma IgE levels in patients with sepsis after traumatic injury. J Allergy Clin Immunol 1996;97:135-6.
25. Dipiro JT, Howdieshell TR, Goddard JK, et al. Association of interleukin 4 levels with traumatic injury and clinical course. Arch Surg 1995;130:1159-62.
26. Hamilton RG. Human immunoglobulins. In: O'Gorman MR, Donnenberg AD, editors. Handbook of human immunology. Boca Raton, Fla.: CRC Press; 2008. p. 63.
27. Jefferis R. Structure-function relationships of IgG subclasses. In: Shakib F, editor. The human IgG subclasses: molecular analysis of structure, function and regulation. New York: Pergamon Press; 1990. p. 93.
28. Burton DR, Gregory L, Jefferis R. Aspects of molecular structure of IgG subclasses. Monogr Allergy 1986;19:7-35.
29. Spiegelberg HL. Biological activities of the immunoglobulins of different classes and subclasses. Adv Immunol 1974;19:259-94.
30. Van der Zee JS, Aalberse RC. The role of IgG in immediate-type hypersensitivity. Eur Respir J 1991;13(Suppl):91S-96S.
31. Schuurman J, Van Ree R, Perdok GJ, et al. Normal human immunoglobulin G4 is bispecific: it has two different antigen combining sites. Immunology 1999;97:693-8.
32. Schuurman J, Perdok GJ, Gorter AD, Aalberse RC. The inter-heavy chain disulfide bonds of IgG4 are in equilibrium with intra-chain disulfide bonds. Mol Immunol 2001;38:1-8.
33. Conley ME. Primary antibody deficiencies. In: Detrick GB, Hamilton RG, Folds JD, editors. Manual of molecular and clinical laboratory immunology. Washington, D.C.: American Society for Microbiology; 2006. p. 906.
34. Tomasi Jr TB. The gamma A globulins: first line of defense. In: Good RA, Fisher DW, editors. Immunology: current knowledge of basic concepts in immunology and their clinical applications. Stanford, Conn.: Sinauer Associates; 1971. p. 76.
35. Mestecky J, Russell MW. IgA subclasses. Monogr Allergy 1986;19:277-301.
36. Peebles Jr RS, Liu MC, Lichtenstein LM, Hamilton RG. IgA, IgG and IgM quantification in bronchoalveolar lavage fluids from allergic rhinitics, allergic asthmatics and normal subjects by monoclonal antibody based immunoenzymetric assays. J Immunol Methods 1995; 13:77-86.
37. Peebles Jr RS, Liu MC, Adkinson Jr NF, et al. Ragweed specific antibodies in bronchoalveolar lavage fluids and serum before and after segmental lung challenge: IgE and IgA associated with eosinophil degranulation. J Allergy Clin Immunol 1998;101:265-73.
38. Peebles Jr RS, Hamilton RG, Lichtenstein LM, et al. Antigen specific IgE and IgA antibodies in bronchoalveolar lavage fluid are associated with strong antigen induced late phase reactions. Clin Exp Allergy 2001;31:239-48.
39. Miranda DO, Silva DA, Fernandes JF, et al. Serum and salivary IgE, IgA, and IgG4 antibodies to *Dermatophagoides pteronyssinus* and its major allergens, Der p1 and Der p2, in allergic and nonallergic children. Clin Dev Immunol 2011;2011:302739.
40. Shamji MH, Durham SR. Mechanisms of immunotherapy to aeroallergens. Clin Exp Allergy 2011;41:1235-46.
41. Till S. Mechanisms of immunotherapy and surrogate markers. Allergy 2011;66(Suppl. 95): 25-7.

Immunologic Methods for Quantifying Antigens and Antibodies

42. Scatchard G. The attraction of proteins for small molecules and ions. Ann N Y Acad Sci 1949; 51:660-72.
43. Matsson P, Hamilton RG, and the CLSI Task Force. Analytical performance characteristics and clinical utility of immunological assays for human immunoglobulin E (IgE) antibodies of defined allergen specificities. 2nd ed. Wayne, Pa.: Clinical and Laboratory Standards Institute; 2007. I/LA20/A2.
44. Heidelberger M, Kendall FE. A quantitative study of the precipitin reaction between type III pneumococcus polysaccharide and purified homologous antibody. J Exp Med 1929;50: 809-23.
45. Ouchterlony O. In vitro method for testing the toxin producing capacity of diphtheria bacteria. Acta Pathol Microbiol Scand 1948;25:186.
46. Mancini G, Carbonara AO, Heremans JF. Immunochemical quantitation of antigens by single radial immunodiffusion. Immunochemistry 1965;2:235-54.
47. Yalow RS, Berson SA. Immunoassay of endogenous plasma insulin in man. J Clin Invest 1960;39:1157-75.
48. Ekins RP. The estimation of thyroxine in human plasma by an electrophoretic technique. Clin Chim Acta 1960;5:453-9.
49. Sobotka AK, Valentine MD, Ishizaka K, Lichtenstein LM. Measurement of IgG blocking antibodies: development and application of a radioimmunoassay. J Immunol 1976;117: 84-90.
50. Greenwood FC, Hunter WM, Glover JS. The preparation of ^{131}I labeled human growth hormone of high specific activity. Biochem J 1963;89:114-23.
51. Marchalonis JJ. An enzymatic method for the trace iodination of immunoglobulins and other proteins. Biochem J 1969;113:299-305.
52. Catt K, Tregear GW. Solid phase radioimmunoassay in antibody coated tubes. Science 1967; 158:1570-2.
53. Axen R, Porath J, Ernback S. Chemical coupling of peptides and proteins to polysaccharides by cyanogen halides. Nature 1967;214: 1302-4.

Immunochemical Methods for Measurement of Immunoglobulin E Protein

54. Zetterstrom O, Johannsson SG. IgE concentrations measured by PRIST in serum of healthy adults and in patients with respiratory allergy. Allergy 1976;35:51.
55. Seagroatt V, Anderson SG. The second international reference preparation for human serum immunoglobulin E and the first British standard for human serum immunoglobulin E. J Biol Standards 1981;9:431-7.
56. Evans R. A US reference for human immunoglobulin E. J Allergy Clin Immunol 1981;68: 79-82.
57. Hamilton RG. Immunological methods in the diagnostic allergy clinical and research laboratory. In: Detrick B, Hamilton RG, Folds JD, editors. Manual of molecular and clinical laboratory immunology. 7th ed. Washington, D.C.: American Society for Microbiology; 2006. p. 995.
58. Diagnostic Allergy Survey (Cycle A-2012). Northfield, Ill.: College of American Pathologists; 2012. p. 1-5.
59. Hamilton RG. Proficiency survey based-evaluation of clinical total and allergen-specific IgE assay performance. Arch Pathol Lab Med 2010;134:975-82.

Immunochemical Methods for Measurement of Immunoglobulin E Antibodies of Defined Allergen Specificity

60. Engvall E, Perlmann P. Enzyme linked immunosorbent assay (ELISA): quantification of specific

antibodies by enzyme linked anti immunoglobulin in antigen coated tubes. J Immunol 1972; 109:129-35.
61. Hamilton RG. Accuracy of Food and Drug Administration cleared IgE antibody assays in the presence of anti IgE (omalizumab). J Allergy Clin Immunol 2006;117:759-66.
62. Biagini RE, MacKenzie BA, Sammons DL, et al. Latex specific IgE: performance characteristics of the IMMULITE 2000 3gAllergy assay compared with skin testing. Ann Allergy Asthma Immunol 2006;97:196-202.
63. Jahn-Schmid B, Harwanegg C, Hiller R, et al. Allergen microarray: comparison to microarray using recombinant allergens with conventional diagnostic methods to detect allergen-specific serum immunoglobulin E. Clin Exp Allergy 2003;33:1443-9.
64. Scala E, Alessandri C, Palazzo P, et al. IgE recognition patterns of profilin, PR-10, and tropomyosin panallergens tested in 3,113 allergic patients by allergen microarray-based technology. PLoS One 2011;6:e24912.
65. Dottorini T, Sole G, Nunziangeli L, et al. Serum IgE reactivity profiling in an asthma affected cohort. PLoS One 2011;6:e22319.
66. Sarratud T, Donnanno S, Terracciano L, et al. Accuracy of a point-of-care testing device in children with suspected respiratory allergy. Allergy Asthma Proc 2010;31:11-7.
67. Kober A, Perborn H. Quantitation of mouse-human chimeric allergen-specific IgE antibodies with ImmunoCAP technology. J Allergy Clin Immunol 2006;117:S219 [Abstract 845].

Immunochemical Methods for Measurement of Allergen-Specific Immunoglobulin G Antibody

68. Lichtenstein LM, Norman PS, Winkenwerder WL. A single year of immunotherapy of ragweed hay fever: immunologic and clinical studies. Ann Intern Med 1971;75:663-71.
69. Golden DBK, Lawrence ID, Hamilton RG, et al. Clinical correlation of the venom specific IgG antibody level during maintenance venom immunotherapy. J Allergy Clin Immunol 1992; 90:386-93.
70. Hamilton RG, Adkinson Jr NF. Quantitation of antigen-specific IgG in human serum. II. Comparison of radioimmunoprecipitation and solid phase radioimmunoassay techniques for the measurement of IgG specific for a complex allergen mixture (yellow jacket venom). J Allergy Clin Immunol 1981;67:14-21.
71. Hamilton RG, Adkinson Jr NF. Solid phase radioimmunoassay for quantitation of antigen specific IgG in human serum with I 125 protein A from *Staphylococcus aureus*. J Immunol 1979;122:1073-9.

Immunoglobulin G Subclass Protein and Antibodies

72. Hamilton RG. Human immunoglobulins. In: Donnenberg AD, O'Gorman M, editors. Handbook of human immunology. 2nd ed. Boca Raton, Fla.: CRC Press; 2007. p. 100.
73. Morell A, Skvaril F, Hitzig WH, Barandum S. IgG subclasses: development of the serum concentrations in normal adults and children. J Pediatr 1972;80:960-4.
74. Oxelius V. IgG subclass levels in infancy and childhood. Acta Pediatr Scand 1979;68: 23-7.
75. Shaikib F. Basic and clinical aspects of IgG subclasses. In: Shaikib F, editor. Monographs in allergy, vol. 19. Basel: Karger; 1986. p. 1.
76. Hanson LA, Soderstrom T, Oxelius VA. Immunoglobulin subclass deficiencies. In: Skvaril F, Morell A, Perret B, editors. Monographs in allergy. Clinical aspects of IgG subclasses and therapeutic implications, vol. 23. Basel: Karger; 1988. p. 20.
77. Aalberse R. The role of IgG antibodies in allergy and immunotherapy. Allergy 2011;66(Suppl. 95):28-30.
78. Matsui EC, Diette GB, Krop EJ, et al. Mouse allergen specific immunoglobulin G4 and risk of mouse skin test sensitivity. Clin Exp Allergy 2006;8:1097-103.
79. Shamji MH, Ljørring C, Francis JN, et al. Functional rather than immunoreactive levels of IgG4 correlate closely with clinical response to grass pollen immunotherapy. Allergy 2012;67: 217-26.

Other Analytes of Interest in Allergic Disorders and Asthma

80. Haley NJ, Sepkovic DW, Hoffmann D. Elimination of cotinine from body fluids: disposition of smokers and non smokers. Am J Public Health 1989;79:1046-8.
81. Jarvis MJ, Tunstall Pedoe H, Feyerabend C, et al. Comparisons of tests used to distinguish smokers from non smokers. Am J Public Health 1987;77:1435-8.
82. Hallgren R, Bigelle A, Venge P. Eosinophil cationic protein in inflammatory effusions as evidence of eosinophil involvement. Ann Rheum Dis 1984;43:556-62.
83. Fink JN, Zacharisen MC. Hypersensitivity pneumonitis. In: Adkinson NF Jr, Yunginger JW, Busse WW, et al, editors. Middleton's allergy: principles and practice. 6th ed. Philadelphia: Mosby; 1988. p. 1373.

Quantification of Environmental Allergens

84. Edmonds RL. Collection efficiency of rotorod samplers for sampling fungus spores in the atmosphere. Plant Dis Rep 1972;56:704-8.
85. Hamilton RG. Assessment of indoor allergen exposure. Curr Allergy Asthma Rep 2005;5: 394-401.
86. Earle CD, King EM, Tsay A, et al. High-throughput fluorescent multiplex array for indoor allergen exposure assessment. J Allergy Clin Immunol 2007;119:428-33.
87. Pongracic JA, O'Connor GT, Muilenberg ML, et al. Differential effects of outdoor versus indoor fungal spores on asthma morbidity in inner-city children. J Allergy Clin Immunol 2010;125:593-9.

Laboratory Methods in Cellular Immunology

88. Currier JR. T-lymphocyte activation and cell signaling. In: Detrick GB, Hamilton RG, Folds JD, editors. Manual of molecular and clinical laboratory immunology. Washington, D.C.: American Society for Microbiology; 2006. p. 315.
89. Waldmann TA, Broder S. Polyclonal B cell activators in the study of the regulation of immunoglobulin synthesis in the human system. Adv Immunol 1982;32:1-63.

Conclusion

90. Hamilton RG. Responsibility for quality IgE antibody results rests ultimately with the referring physician. Ann Allergy Asthma Immunol 2001;86:353-4.

75

Eosinophilia and Eosinophil-Related Disorders

AMY D. KLION | PETER F. WELLER

CONTENTS

SUMMARY OF IMPORTANT CONCEPTS

» Mild eosinophilia (<1500 cells/μL of blood) often accompanies atopic diseases.
» Eosinophilia may indicate various types of adverse reactions to medication that may also involve specific organs.
» Many helminth parasites cause eosinophilia, and strongyloidiasis, the most important helminth infection, should be excluded with a blood antibody assay, because it can become a disseminated, fatal disease in patients treated with corticosteroids.
» Sustained blood eosinophilia (>1500/μL for months) without an apparent cause should prompt consideration of several types of hypereosinophilic syndromes.

Introduction

Many allergic, infectious, neoplastic, and idiopathic disease processes are associated with increased eosinophil numbers in the blood and tissues. Eosinophils are bone marrow–derived leukocytes, and eosinophilia develops when specific stimuli enhance eosinophilopoiesis. Among the three eosinophil growth factor cytokines—granulocyte-macrophage colony-stimulating factor (GM-CSF), interleukin-3 (IL-3), and interleukin-5 (IL-5)—IL-5 is principally responsible for increased eosinophilopoiesis. In humans, experience with hydroxyurea, an inhibitor of early eosinophilopoiesis, suggests that enhanced eosinophilopoiesis within the marrow requires several days to more than a week to increase the level of eosinophilia in blood. However, IL-5 may rapidly increase blood eosinophilia by mobilizing a marginated pool of mature eosinophils resident within the marrow.

Based on published determinations of the upper limits of normal eosinophil numbers, blood eosinophilia is defined as the presence of more than 450 cells per microliter of blood. Quantitation need not require absolute eosinophil counts and can be calculated from differential cell counts of Wright-stained blood smears. Blood eosinophil numbers exhibit a mild diurnal variation, with peak values occurring late at night and trough values occurring in the morning, which is the reciprocal of the diurnal fluctuation of circulating adrenocorticosteroid levels. Stress, fever, most bacterial and viral infections, and increased exogenous or endogenous corticosteroid levels suppress blood eosinophil levels. Increased percentages, but not absolute numbers, of blood eosinophils (i.e., pseudoeosinophilia) due to leukopenia in another white blood cell line can be misleading.

Although the intravascular compartment of eosinophils is available for enumeration, blood eosinophil numbers do not necessarily indicate the extent of eosinophil involvement in affected tissues. Eosinophils are primarily organ-dwelling leukocytes that are richly distributed within some tissues.[1] Eosinophils are several hundred-fold more abundant in tissues than in blood, and they are most abundant in tissues with a mucosal-epithelial interface with the environment, including the respiratory, gastrointestinal, and lower genitourinary tracts.[1] The life span of eosinophils is longer than that of neutrophils. Despite ambiguities in establishing their longevity in vivo, eosinophils probably survive for weeks within tissues. In some pathologic situations, tissue eosinophilia is prominent but peripheral blood eosinophilia is minimal or absent.

Conventional staining with eosin lacks sensitivity to detect eosinophils in tissues, and several techniques that use the cationic protein content of eosinophil secondary granules prove more sensitive in this regard. Specific staining techniques, such as Congo red or those based on granule autofluorescence after staining with Giemsa or fluorescein isothiocyanate, help to detect tissue eosinophilia. In tissues, loss of morphologically intact eosinophils due to degranulation, apoptosis, or necrosis leads to underestimation of the role of eosinophils, whose prior presence can be detected by immunofluorescent identification of released eosinophil granule cationic proteins, including major basic protein (MBP), eosinophil cationic protein (ECP), and eosinophil peroxidase.

In patients with eosinophilia of various origins, blood eosinophils can exhibit morphologic and functional alterations resulting from activation in vivo. These changes include increased metabolic activity, diminished density (i.e., hypodense), enhanced antibody-mediated cytotoxicity, and enhanced leukotriene C_4 formation. Morphologic changes include cytoplasmic vacuolization, alterations in granule numbers and size,

BOX 75-1 EOSINOPHIL-ASSOCIATED DISEASES AND DISORDERS

I. Allergic diseases
  A. Atopic and related diseases
  B. Medication-related eosinophilias
II. Infectious diseases
  A. Parasitic infections (mostly helminths)
  B. Specific fungal infections
  C. Other infections (infrequent)
III. Hematologic and neoplastic disorders
  A. Hypereosinophilic syndromes
  B. Leukemia
  C. Lymphomas
  D. Tumor-associated disorders
  E. Mastocytosis
IV. Diseases with specific organ involvement
  A. Skin and subcutaneous diseases
  B. Pulmonary diseases
  C. Gastrointestinal diseases
  D. Neurologic diseases
  E. Rheumatologic diseases
  F. Cardiac diseases
  G. Renal diseases
V. Immunologic reactions
  A. Specific immunodeficiency diseases
  B. Transplant rejection
VI. Endocrine disorders
  A. Hypoadrenalism
VII. Other diseases and disorders
  A. Atheroembolic disease
  B. Serosal irritation
  C. Hereditary disorders

and increased lipid body formation, all of which are visible by light microscopy, and losses within specific granules of the matrix and eosinophil MBP-containing cores (i.e., piecemeal degranulation), which are visible only by electron microscopy.[2]

Because IL-5 is a cytokine predominantly produced by $CD4^+$ helper T cell type 2 (Th2) lymphocytes, eosinophilia is common in the setting of immune responses characterized by Th2 cell activation, including allergic diseases and immune responses to helminth parasite infections. Although enhanced immunoglobulin E (IgE) production is common in these disorders, eosinophilia also develops without increased IgE levels and occurs in diverse diseases with uncertain immunopathogeneses (Box 75-1).

Evaluation of the patient with eosinophilia requires a staged approach that considers the history, the nature and types of associated clinical findings and organ involvement, and information from laboratory and imaging studies. Eosinophilia frequently is associated with common allergic diseases, which should be considered in patients with mild to moderate eosinophilia (<1500 cells/microliter of blood). Drug hypersensitivity can occur in response to a wide range of prescription and nonprescription agents and is another common cause of eosinophilia that should be excluded in the initial evaluation. Drug hypersensitivity reactions can be asymptomatic or life-threatening (e.g., drug reaction with eosinophilia and systemic symptoms [DRESS]), and the accompanying eosinophilia can range from mild to severe.

Because eosinophilia is common in the setting of helminth infection, a pertinent travel and exposure history is essential for all patients with eosinophilia. Special attention must be given to strongyloidiasis because this infection may manifest with asymptomatic eosinophilia,[3] occurs worldwide (including the southeastern United States), can persist for decades after acquisition, and may progress to fatal dissemination when immunosuppressive corticosteroids are administered.[4] A serologic test for anti-*Strongyloides* antibody has value in ascertaining that occult infection with this parasite is neither the cause of eosinophilia nor likely to disseminate with subsequent glucocorticosteroid administration.[3] Other eosinophil-associated syndromes are considered based on specific organs involved (e.g., eosinophilic pneumonia, eosinophilic gastroenteritis) or other clinical and pathologic features associated with eosinophilia.

Allergic Disorders

Eosinophilic diseases in the group of allergic disorders include atopic and related diseases and drug-induced eosinophilias, which are two of the most common causes of eosinophilia. The mechanism of drug-induced eosinophilia is unknown in most cases but typically does not involve IgE.

ATOPIC AND RELATED DISEASES

Allergic Rhinitis

Blood eosinophilia may be associated with allergic rhinitis but is less sensitive than nasal eosinophilia as an indicator of nasal allergy. Nasal eosinophilia is defined by a nasal smear showing an eosinophil count of more than 4% for children and 10% to 25% for adults.[5] Nasal secretion eosinophil numbers increase in persons with seasonal allergic rhinitis during the pollen season, and nasal eosinophilia correlates significantly with the signs and symptoms of allergic rhinitis. Nasal eosinophilia helps to differentiate allergic rhinitis from viral infections and vasomotor rhinitis, and it is an indicator of clinical responsiveness to topical steroids.[5]

Other Causes of Nasal and Upper Respiratory Tract Eosinophilia

Nasal eosinophilia may occur in asthmatic patients without symptoms of nasal allergy, and it is associated with sputum eosinophilia in asthmatic patients.[6] Nasal eosinophilia and sometimes blood eosinophilia are characteristic of the nonallergic rhinitis with eosinophilia syndrome (NARES). These patients have marked nasal eosinophilia and a propensity for nasal polyps but have negative allergic histories, negative skin test results, normal IgE levels, normal bronchial responsiveness, and no aspirin sensitivity.[7] Patients with nasal polyposis also have lesional and nasal secretion eosinophilia, and some have the triad of asthma, aspirin sensitivity, and nasal polyposis.

Eosinophilia of involved tissues is common in persons with chronic sinusitis. In children, especially those with asthma, tissue eosinophilia is a histologic feature of chronic sinusitis, but the presence of allergy does not predict tissue eosinophilia, nor does the degree of tissue eosinophilia correlate with the severity of mucosal thickening seen on computed tomography (CT).[8] In adults, chronic sinusitis correlates with blood eosinophilia, and blood eosinophilia indicates a high likelihood of extensive disease. In patients with chronic rhinosinusitis, eosinophilic inflammation and basement membrane thickening develop within the sinuses, features also found in the airways of asthmatics.[9] Allergic fungal sinusitis is associated with lesional and nasal eosinophilia.[10] When nasal polyposis or sinusitis is accompanied by marked systemic eosinophilia, Churg-Strauss syndrome (CSS) should be considered.

Asthma and Other Causes of Lower Respiratory Tract Eosinophilia

Blood eosinophilia is common in asthma, especially in allergic asthma, but it rarely exceeds a level of 1500 cells/μL of blood.[11] In allergic and nonallergic forms of asthma, eosinophil numbers are increased in airway tissues.[11] Although sputum eosinophilia is characteristic of asthma but not of chronic obstructive pulmonary disease, sputum eosinophilia may be found in some patients with chronic obstructive pulmonary disease,[12] is prominent in the syndrome of chronic cough with eosinophilic bronchitis without asthma and in the CSS, and may be present in some patients with interstitial pulmonary fibrosis.[13]

MEDICATION-RELATED EOSINOPHILIAS

Administration of diverse therapeutic agents, including clinician-prescribed medications and alternative herbal or natural therapies, can elicit eosinophilia. In evaluating a patient for the cause of eosinophilia, a detailed history of current or past medication use should be obtained. Despite the prevalent use of herbal supplements or natural therapeutics, patients may be hesitant to volunteer to physicians their use of these agents, and these specific histories must be sought. There is no official compendium of the frequency with which eosinophilia develops with various medications. Rather, the association of eosinophilia with specific therapeutic agents is recognized based on plausible mechanistic considerations (e.g., cytokine therapies), on distinct types of clinical presentations (e.g., drug-induced eosinophilic hepatitis, eosinophilic interstitial nephritis), and on resolution of eosinophilia with discontinuation of the offending agent. The mechanisms underlying most drug-associated blood or specific tissue eosinophilias have not been defined, and the expected time course for resolution of eosinophilia after cessation of a candidate medication, especially if drug derivatives become haptenated to long-lived host serum proteins, is unknown.

Tissue eosinophilia with or without blood eosinophilia can occur in a variety of drug reactions. Drug reactions can be completely asymptomatic or associated with life-threatening clinical manifestations (Table 75-1). Conversely, adverse drug reactions may occur without sentinel blood or tissue eosinophilia.[14] In the absence of organ involvement, blood eosinophilia by itself need not necessitate cessation of drug therapy if it is warranted, but drug-induced blood eosinophilia should prompt evaluation with an emphasis on organs likely to be involved in eosinophil-associated drug reactions, including the skin, lungs, liver, kidneys, and heart. When organ dysfunction develops, cessation of drug administration is indicated.

Cytokine-Mediated Eosinophilias

Some cytokine therapies may cause of eosinophilia. Administration of GM-CSF can cause prominent blood and tissue eosinophilia and less commonly associated eosinophilic diseases, including eosinophilic pneumonia and eosinophilic endomyocardial fibrosis. Administration of IL-2 or IL-2–stimulated lymphocytes frequently is followed by development of eosinophilia, most likely due to IL-2–stimulated production of IL-5. Eosinophilic myocarditis and biventricular thrombosis are possible complications of high-dose IL-2 therapy.[15]

TABLE 75-1 Eosinophilia and Drug Reactions

Drug Reaction	Examples
Cytokine-mediated response	Granulocyte-macrophage colony-stimulating factor, interleukin-2
Pulmonary infiltrates	Nonsteroidal antiinflammatory drugs
Pleuropulmonary response	Valproic acid, dantrolene
Interstitial nephritis	Semisynthetic penicillins, cephalosporins, linezolid
Necrotizing myocarditis	Ranitidine, carbamazepine
Hepatitis	Semisynthetic penicillins, tetracyclines, herbal products
Hypersensitivity vasculitis	Allopurinol, phenytoin
Gastroenterocolitis	Nonsteroidal antiinflammatory drugs
Asthma, nasal polyps	Aspirin
Eosinophilia-myalgia syndrome	L-Tryptophan contaminant
Asymptomatic	Ampicillin, penicillins, cephalosporins
Drug rash with eosinophilia and systemic symptoms (DRESS)	Anticonvulsants, minocycline, nevirapine

Drug-Induced Pulmonary Eosinophilia

Diverse agents can stimulate pulmonary eosinophilia.[16,17] The Groupes d'Études de la Pathologie Pulmonaire Iatrogène maintains a web site listing drugs that have been associated with pulmonary infiltrates and eosinophilia with literature citations (http://www.pneumotox.com).[18] Notable among these drugs are many antimicrobial agents, common cardiac medications, and nonsteroidal antiinflammatory drugs (NSAIDs). Even antiasthmatic agents, including inhaled beclomethasone and disodium cromoglycate, have been associated with pulmonary eosinophilia; but whether these reactions represent unmasking of the CSS remains conjectural.

The clinical presentation of drug-induced pulmonary eosinophilia varies and includes acute and chronic eosinophilic pneumonia and eosinophilic pleural effusion. Blood eosinophilia is usually present, and if blood eosinophilia is absent, sputum, bronchoalveolar lavage (BAL) fluid, or pleural fluid eosinophilia is necessary to help make the diagnosis. Symptoms, including dyspnea, weight loss, cough, chest pain, and fever, may appear acutely or insidiously after years of ingestion of the medication and are not specific for drug-induced pulmonary disease. Physical findings are also nonspecific and can include wheezing, rales, rhonchi, and evidence of consolidation. The erythrocyte sedimentation rate (ESR) is frequently increased. IgE levels may or may not be elevated. Arterial blood gas determinations are normal in mild cases but often indicate hypoxia with an increased alveolar-arterial gradient. Obstructive, restrictive, and normal spirometric findings have been reported. Sputum and BAL fluid usually contain eosinophils. Chest radiographic and CT patterns include peripheral subpleural infiltrations and diffuse or bibasilar alveolar and interstitial infiltration that is occasionally accompanied by pleural effusions.[19]

Clinical manifestations and eosinophilia may resolve without the use of systemic corticosteroids after discontinuation of the offending medication, but they often require several weeks to resolve completely. Corticosteroids are effective in accelerating this process, often within a matter of days. When rechallenged, pulmonary symptoms frequently recur within 48 hours, and infiltrates may develop radiographically in the same locations as the original infiltrates.

Pleuropulmonary Reactions

Drugs, especially valproic acid[20] and dantrolene, may elicit isolated pleural effusions with pleural and blood eosinophilia.[21]

Interstitial Nephritis

Although the pathogenesis of drug-induced acute interstitial nephritis remains to be elucidated, eosinophilia often is identified in the involved kidneys, urine, and the blood. Causative agents include methicillin and other penicillin congeners, NSAIDs, cimetidine, sulfonamides, captopril, allopurinol, diphenylhydantoin, rifampin, ciprofloxacin, aztreonam, triazolam, and warfarin.

Interstitial nephritis is a heterogeneous disease. Not all renal biopsies show tissue eosinophilia, and the presence of an eosinophilic renal infiltrate is not sufficient to infer a drug-induced origin. Eosinophiluria does not uniformly occur in the setting of renal tissue eosinophilia, and there are other causes of eosinophiluria. The sensitivity of eosinophiluria for acute interstitial nephritis is 25% to 40% with a positive predictive value of 3% to 38%.[22] Eosinophiluria is neither sensitive nor specific for drug-induced interstitial nephritis.

Eosinophilic Myocarditis

Acute necrotizing eosinophilic myocarditis is a serious but uncommon complication of drug hypersensitivity that has been associated with several agents, including ranitidine, carbamazepine, and clozapine.[23] Necrotizing eosinophilic myocarditis has been reported after imatinib (Gleevec) treatment in patients with platelet-derived growth factor receptor-α (PDGFRA)–associated myeloproliferative neoplasms and preexisting eosinophilic cardiac involvement, although the mechanism of drug toxicity in this setting remains unclear.

Hepatitis

Hepatitis with eosinophilia can be a manifestation of drug reactions to a wide variety of prescription and nonprescription agents, including minocycline, choline magnesium trisalicylate, halothane, methoxyflurane, salicylazosulfapyridine, ranitidine, carbamazepine, phenytoin, and sulfa antibiotics. Various herbal preparations, such as red yeast rice extract, have also been implicated.[24] Clinical manifestations range from asymptomatic transaminase elevations to fulminant hepatitis.

Other Medication-Related Eosinophilic Responses

Multisystem involvement frequently occurs in cases of drug hypersensitivity. A syndrome of drug-induced rash, eosinophilia, and systemic symptoms (DRESS) can develop several weeks after the initiation of several drugs, including aromatic anticonvulsants, sulfonamides, allopurinol, and nevirapine.[25] This syndrome typically includes a diffuse maculopapular rash, fever, eosinophilia, lymphadenopathy, and liver abnormalities, although a variety of other organs can be involved, including the heart, lungs, central nervous system, and kidneys. DRESS can be fatal in as many as 12% of cases despite discontinuation of therapy and administration of systemic glucocorticosteroids.[26] Eosinophilia can accompany drug-induced cutaneous small-vessel vasculitis.[27] Drug-induced gastroenterocolitis with eosinophilia can develop as an adverse effect of medications, including clozapine and NSAIDs. Patients with the syndrome of asthma, nasal polyps, and aspirin sensitivity exhibit eosinophilia. Adverse reactions to contaminated L-tryptophan in herbal or natural medications have caused the eosinophilia-myalgia syndrome.

Infectious Diseases

Acute bacterial or viral infections characteristically produce eosinopenia and can suppress peripheral blood eosinophilia. Suppression results from heightened endogenous corticosteroid production and release of inflammatory mediators, and it can lead to an unexpected absence of eosinophilia in the setting of allergic disease or helminth infection, including hyperinfection strongyloidiasis.[28] Increased or even normal blood eosinophil counts in a febrile patient should prompt considerations of helminthic infections and noninfectious causes, such as an eosinophilic syndrome–related illness or adrenal insufficiency.

PARASITIC INFECTIONS

Helminth parasites are multicellular, metazoan organisms that are commonly associated with eosinophilia[29] driven primarily by Th2 lymphocyte production of IL-5. Eosinophilia may provide a hematologic clue to the presence of a helminth infection, but the absence of blood eosinophilia does not exclude these infections. The eosinophilic response to helminths is determined by the host's immune response to the parasite and by the parasite itself, including its distribution, migration, and development within the infected host. The level of eosinophilia typically parallels the magnitude and extent of tissue invasion by helminth larvae or adults. For several helminth infections, migration of infecting larvae through the tissues is greatest early in infection, and the magnitude of the elicited eosinophilia is greatest during these early phases (Table 75-2). In established infections, tissue eosinophilia around helminths may not be accompanied by blood eosinophilia, especially when the organism is antigenically sequestered within tissues (e.g., intact echinococcal cysts) or is limited to the intestinal lumen (e.g., adult *Ascaris*, tapeworms). Intermittent leakage of fluids from echinococcal cysts can transiently stimulate increases in blood eosinophilia and cause allergic (e.g., urticaria, bronchospasm) or anaphylactic reactions.

The likelihood that helminth infection is the cause of eosinophilia in a given patient depends on the exposure history, degree and duration of eosinophilia, and clinical manifestations.[30] Although a wide range of helminths are associated with eosinophilia at some time during their life cycle, relatively few helminth infections cause long-lasting eosinophilia.[29] Many are tissue- or blood-dwelling helminths that require tissue biopsy or serologic tests for diagnosis. Examples include visceral larva migrans caused by *Toxocara canis*, which occurs primarily in children with a propensity for geophagous pica and ingestion of dirt contaminated by dog ascarid eggs, and trichinellosis. *Strongyloides* infection is particularly important to exclude because it can persist for decades without apparent symptoms and can develop into disseminated, often fatal disease (i.e., hyperinfection syndrome) in patients unsuspectingly given immunosuppressive corticosteroids.[4] Enzyme-linked immunosorbent assay

TABLE 75-2 Helminth Parasitic Diseases Causing Marked Eosinophilia*

Parasitic Disease	Comments
Angiostrongyliasis (*Angiostrongylus costaricensis*)	
Ascariasis	Early transpulmonary larval migration, often absent when mature
Hookworm infection	Early transpulmonary larval migration, often mild when mature
Strongyloidiasis	
Trichinellosis	
Visceral larva migrans	Primarily pediatric
Gnathostomiasis	
Filariases:	
Tropical pulmonary eosinophilia	
Loiasis	Especially in expatriates
Onchocerciasis	
Flukes:	
Schistosomiasis	During early infection in nonimmune persons (Katayama fever)
Fascioliasis	During early infection
Clonorchiasis	During early infection
Paragonimiasis	During early infection
Fasciolopsiasis	During early infection

Modified from Wilson ME, Weller PF. Eosinophilia. In: Guerrant RL, Walker DH, Weller PF, editors. Tropical infectious diseases: principles, pathogens and practice, 3rd ed. Philadelphia: Churchill Livingstone; 2011. p. 939-48.
*Marked eosinophilia: >3000 cells/μL.

(ELISA) serology is useful in detecting strongyloidiasis even when fecal examinations are unrevealing.[3]

Ectoparasite infestation, especially scabies, can cause marked eosinophilia. Myiasis, a subcutaneous infestation with the larval stages of species in the Diptera order, has been reported as a rare cause of hypereosinophilic syndrome.[31]

In contrast to infections with multicellular helminths and ectoparasite infestations, infections with single-celled protozoan parasites do not characteristically elicit blood eosinophilia. This is true of all intestinal-, blood-, and tissue-infecting protozoa with three exceptions, *Dientamoeba fragilis*, *Isospora belli*, and *Sarcocystis* species. In patients with symptoms of enteric infection and eosinophilia, diagnostic trophozoites of *D. fragilis* or oocysts of *I. belli* should be sought in stool examinations. These infections are treatable causes of diarrhea and eosinophilia. *Sarcocystis* infection is acquired by eating cysts in raw or undercooked meat. The intestinal phase of infection is often asymptomatic, and patients typically present with fever, myositis, and peripheral eosinophilia.[32] Outbreaks have been described. Other enteric protozoa, such as *Giardia lamblia*, do not elicit blood eosinophilia, and if detected in stool, they should not be accepted as causes of eosinophilia.

FUNGAL INFECTIONS

Two fungal diseases are commonly associated with eosinophilia: aspergillosis (i.e., allergic bronchopulmonary aspergillosis) and coccidioidomycosis. Eosinophilia has also been reported in cases of basidiobolomycosis, pulmonary paracoccidiomycosis, disseminated histoplasmosis, and cryptococcosis. Blood eosinophilia, which peaks during the second or third week of illness, occurs with primary coccidioidal infection. Coccidioidal infection should be included in the differential diagnosis of eosinophilic pneumonia because organisms may be absent from cultures and open lung biopsy specimens. Eosinophilia, which is sometimes prominent, may develop with disseminated coccidioidomycosis.

RETROVIRAL INFECTIONS

Eosinophilia is more common in patients infected with human immunodeficiency virus type 1 (HIV-1) than in the general population. The many reasons for this disparity include adverse reactions to medications, adrenal insufficiency due to cytomegalovirus and other infections, and concomitant fungal and parasitic infections. The prevalence of eosinophilia increases with decreasing CD4 counts, suggesting that HIV infection itself can contribute to eosinophilia, likely through the disruption of the balance between Th1 and Th2 lymphocytes.[33] Eosinophilia also accompanies eosinophilic folliculitis in HIV infection. Marked hypereosinophilia has developed in a few patients with HIV infection, including some with the hyperimmunoglobulin E syndrome and some with exfoliative dermatitis.

Eosinophil counts typically are normal or decreased in patients with human T lymphotropic virus type 1 (HTLV-1) infection. Eosinophilia in the setting of HTLV-1 infection is associated with progression to adult T cell leukemia/lymphoma and should prompt testing for concomitant strongyloidiasis.

Hematologic and Neoplastic Disorders

HYPEREOSINOPHILIC SYNDROMES

A syndrome previously called the *idiopathic hypereosinophilic syndrome* is not a single entity but rather a constellation of leukoproliferative disorders characterized by sustained overproduction of eosinophils. The three original diagnostic criteria for this syndrome were eosinophilia in excess of 1500/μL of blood persisting for longer than 6 months; lack of an identifiable parasitic, allergic, or other cause for the eosinophilia; and signs and symptoms of organ involvement attributable to eosinophilia.[34] In contemporary practice, it is no longer considered safe to wait for 6 months before diagnostic and therapeutic interventions are implemented for a hypereosinophilic patient with organ involvement. The time period in the first diagnostic criterion has been updated to require only "persisting or sustained eosinophilia."[35]

Spectrum and Causes

Hypereosinophilic syndromes (HES) encompass a spectrum of disorders, and notable progress has been made in identifying pathogenetic defects in some of these disorders.[35,36] The spectrum of HES is presented in Figure 75-1.[36] Although the precise prevalence of HES is unknown, it has been estimated from data collected in the Surveillance, Epidemiology, and End Results (SEER) database that the prevalence of HES or chronic eosinophilic leukemia in the United States is between 0.3 and 6.3 cases per 100,000 person-years.[37] Most series suggest that approximately 10% to 15% of patients with HES have

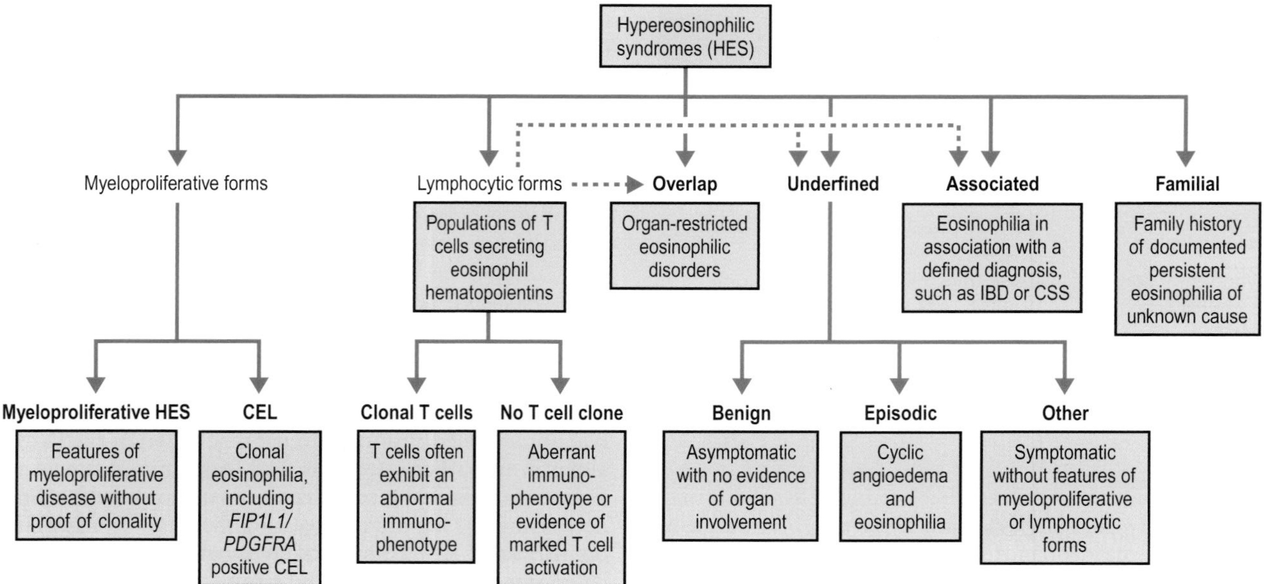

Figure 75-1. Classification of hypereosinophilic syndromes (HES). *Dashed arrows* identify HES forms for which some patients have T cell–derived disease. *CEL*, Chronic eosinophilic leukemia; *CSS*, Churg-Strauss syndrome; *IBD*, inflammatory bowel disease. *(From Simon HU, Rothenberg ME, Bochner BS, et al. Refining the definition of hypereosinophilic syndrome. J Allergy Clin Immunol 2010;126:45-9.)*

myeloproliferative disorders and an equal number have lymphocytic variants of HES.[38]

Some patients presenting with clinical features compatible with HES also have features common to myeloproliferative disorders, including elevated vitamin B_{12} levels, splenomegaly, cytogenetic abnormalities, myelofibrosis, anemia, and myeloid dysplasia without cytogenetic abnormalities or increased blasts.[39] Molecular abnormalities involving PDGFRA can be identified in 15% to 20% of these mostly male patients and are consistent with the diagnosis of a myeloproliferative neoplasm. The most common of these mutations is an interstitial deletion in chromosome 4 that yields a fusion gene encoding a FIP1L1/PDGFRA (F/P) protein that constitutively expresses receptor kinase activity.[40] This fusion gene can be diagnostically evaluated by reverse-transcription polymerase chain reaction (RT-PCR) or fluorescence in situ hybridization (FISH).[40] Serum tryptase and B_{12} levels should be measured if F/P is suspected, because levels are elevated in most patients.[38,39] Importantly, almost all patients with F/P respond dramatically to therapy with imatinib, typically used at low doses.[39-41]

X-linked clonal abnormalities in the eosinophil lineage have been reported in a few female HES patients.[42] Some patients with HES exhibit myeloproliferative features without detectable *PDGFRA* mutations (see Fig. 75-1). These patients occasionally respond to imatinib, suggesting that there may be other receptor tyrosine kinase mutations underlying the myeloproliferative forms of HES.

Another variant HES is a lymphoproliferative form due to clonal expansion of aberrant lymphocytes elaborating IL-5.[43] These aberrant T cells are most often $CD3^-CD4^+$ or $CD3^+CD4^-CD8^-$, but other phenotypes have been described. Patients with lymphocytic variant HES typically present with dermatologic manifestations and have elevated serum IgE and TARC (CCL17) levels. Flow cytometry and T cell receptor rearrangement studies are useful in confirming the diagnosis. Progression to T cell lymphomas occurs in fewer than 3% of these patients.[43]

In addition to these recognized variants of HES, there are a substantial number of HES patients for whom the cause of the eosinophilia remains unknown (see Fig. 75-1). These forms include familial hypereosinophilia, episodic angioedema with eosinophilia, overlap syndromes with other organ-targeted eosinophilic disorders, and associated disorders (discussed later). Some patients with unexplained (idiopathic) eosinophilia of 1500 cells/mm^3 are completely asymptomatic, whereas others have life-threatening end-organ manifestations. Why this occurs remains unknown.

Manifestations

The clinical manifestations of HES are extremely varied, ranging from nonspecific constitutional symptoms to life-threatening endomyocardial fibrosis and thromboembolic disease. Eosinophilic involvement in the setting of HES has been reported in all major organ systems (Table 75-3),[38,44] although the prevalence of a particular organ system involvement depends to some degree on the HES variant involved. For example, patients with the lymphocytic variant appear to be more prone to dermatologic manifestations, whereas patients with myeloproliferative HES may be more likely to develop cardiac complications. This has complicated interpretation of data from patient series compiled before the availability of molecular and immunologic testing to identify disease variants. Demographic characteristics also vary for different HES variants. The male predominance reported in early studies of HES likely reflects the overwhelming male predominance of PDGFRA-positive myeloproliferative neoplasms, which might have been overrepresented in these studies. When these patients are excluded, HES appears to occur equally frequently in men and women. Most patients with HES, regardless of the variant, are diagnosed between 20 and 50 years of age, although HES does occur in the elderly and in children.

TABLE 75-3 Frequency of Organ Involvement in Hypereosinophilic Syndromes

Organ System Involvement	Frequency at Presentation (%; *N* = 188)	Eventual Frequency (%; *N* = 188)
Dermatologic	37	70
Pulmonary	25	45
Gastrointestinal	14	38
Rheumatologic	7	NA
Constitutional	5	NA
Cardiac	5	20
Neurologic	5	21

Modified from Ogbogu PU, Bochner BS, Butterfield JH, et al. Hypereosinophilic syndrome: a multicenter, retrospective analysis of clinical characteristics and response to therapy. J Allergy Clin Immunol 2009;124:1319-25.
NA, Not available.

HES onset is often insidious, eosinophilia may be detected incidentally, or initial manifestations may result from sudden cardiac or neurologic complications.

HES is defined by the presence of more than1500 eosinophils/μL of peripheral blood.[34-36] Extremely high leukocyte counts (>90,000/μL), anemia, and thrombocytopenia are associated with a poor prognosis, perhaps indicative of underlying myeloproliferative variant disease.[34] IgE levels vary but are more likely to be elevated in the lymphocytic variant of HES. Bone marrow findings demonstrate increased levels of eosinophils and eosinophil precursors. Markedly increased cellularity, dysplastic eosinophils, myelofibrosis, and atypical mast cells are highly suggestive of PDGFRA-positive disease. Chromosomal findings are normal for most HES patients. The F/P deletion in the myeloproliferative variant of HES is not detectable by conventional chromosomal studies.

Cardiac disease is a major cause of morbidity and mortality.[34,44] The damage to the heart, ranging from early necrosis to subsequent thrombosis and fibrosis, occurs identically whether eosinophilia results from HES or other causes, including eosinophilia with carcinomas or lymphomas, GM-CSF administration or drug-reactions, or parasitic infections.[45] Some patients with sustained eosinophilia never develop cardiac disease. The pathogenesis of eosinophil-mediated cardiac damage involves increased numbers of eosinophils and other ill-defined stimuli for recruitment or activation of eosinophils.

Eosinophil-mediated heart damage evolves through three stages.[44] The acute, necrotic stage occurs in the early weeks of illness and is marked by endocardial damage, myocardial infiltration with eosinophils and lymphocytes, myocardial necrosis, and eosinophil degranulation and microabscesses. In the acute stage, patients may have normal cardiac findings, although some have prominent subungual and conjunctival splinter hemorrhages. Echocardiographic findings may be normal. Elevations of serum troponin levels can detect early myocardial involvement and should be evaluated, especially before initiating imatinib therapy for the myeloproliferative variant of HES because this is a marker for development of myocardial necrosis.[46]

The second stage of heart disease involves thrombus formation along the damaged ventricular endocardium. In the third, fibrotic stage, progressive scarring causes entrapment of

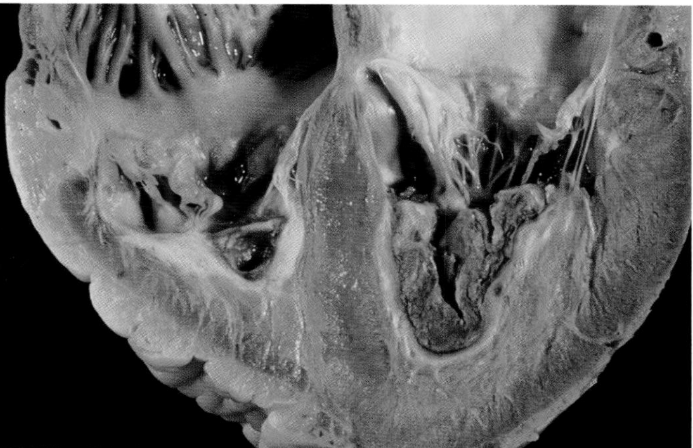

Figure 75-2 End-stage endomyocardial disease can result from hypereosinophilia. Apical ventricular thrombi form in damaged endocardium, and progressive endomyocardial fibrosis entraps the chordae tendineae, leading to mitral and sometimes tricuspid valvular incompetence. *(Courtesy Murray Resnick, MD, PhD, Brown University, Providence, RI.)*

chordae tendineae, with development of mitral or tricuspid valve regurgitation, and endomyocardial fibrosis, producing a restrictive cardiomyopathy (Fig. 75-2). HES patients often present at these later thrombotic and fibrotic stages. Common manifestations include dyspnea, chest pain, signs of left or right ventricular congestive heart failure, murmurs of atrioventricular valve regurgitation, and cardiomegaly. Echocardiography and magnetic resonance imaging (MRI) can detect and evaluate intracardiac thrombi and manifestations of endomyocardial fibrosis.[47,48] Patients with late-stage eosinophilic heart disease benefit from medical therapies for congestive heart failure and from valve replacement (with bioprosthetic but not mechanical valves[49]) when hemodynamically necessary.

Three types of neurologic complications occur in HES.[50] In the first, patients experience embolic strokes or transient ischemic episodes arising from cerebral thromboemboli that formed in the heart. Thromboembolic episodes may be the first sign of HES, and despite anticoagulation with Coumadin and antiplatelet agents, emboli can recur in HES patients.[50] The second type of HES-associated neuropathy is an encephalopathy resulting in behavioral changes, confusion, ataxia, and memory loss. This may be accompanied by upper motor neuron signs with increased muscle tone and deep tendon reflexes and a positive Babinski sign.[50] The third neurologic complication is peripheral neuropathy, which accounts for one half of the neurologic manifestations of HES.[50] Symmetric or asymmetric sensory or mixed sensory and motor forms of polyneuropathy are common. Mononeuritis multiplex (which also develops with Churg-Strauss vasculitis) and radiculopathies occur with denervation muscle atrophy. Biopsies of affected nerves usually show an axonal neuropathy with various degrees of axonal loss and no evidence of vasculitis or eosinophil infiltration. The pathogeneses of the central encephalopathic and peripheral neuropathies of HES remain unknown.

Two types of skin manifestations are common: angioedematous or urticarial lesions and erythematous, pruritic papules or nodules.[44] Patients with angioedema and urticaria are likely to have benign courses without cardiac or neurologic complications. They do not require corticosteroid therapy, or they respond to prednisone alone. Biopsies of papular or nodular lesions show perivascular infiltration with eosinophils and mild or moderate perivascular neutrophilic and mononuclear infiltrates without vasculitis. Some patients with HES experience cutaneous microthrombi or digital arteritis. Less commonly, mucosal ulcers, which often are refractory to therapy, may develop in the mouth, nose, pharynx, penis, esophagus, stomach, and anus.[51] Lymphomatoid papulosis has been reported.[52] Mucosal ulceration and lymphomatoid papulosis in the setting of HES appear to be markers of PDGFRA-positive disease.

The most common respiratory symptom is a chronic, persistent, nonproductive cough in those with usually clear chest radiographs. Asthma is not necessarily more prevalent among HES patients. Other causes of respiratory symptoms are congestive heart failure, pulmonary emboli, and eosinophilic lung infiltrates. Infiltrates occur in fewer than 25% of HES patients and may be diffuse or focal and have no predilection for any region of the lungs, unlike chronic eosinophilic pneumonia. Pulmonary fibrosis may develop over time, especially in those with cardiac fibrosis.

Eosinophilic gastritis, enterocolitis, and colitis may occur with HES.[44] Hepatic involvement may include chronic active hepatitis, focal hepatic lesions, eosinophilic cholangitis, and the Budd-Chiari syndrome from hepatic vein obstruction.[44]

Associated immunologic abnormalities indicate that HES constitute a spectrum of disorders. HES patients with elevated IgE levels constitute a subgroup with a better prognosis and likely include lymphoproliferative or episodic angioedema variants of HES. Conversely, HES patients with features common to myeloproliferative disorders, including elevated vitamin B_{12} levels, abnormal leukocyte alkaline phosphatase scores, splenomegaly, cytogenetic abnormalities, myelofibrosis, myeloid dysplasia, and basophilia, are less likely to respond to prednisone and more likely to require cytotoxic therapy. Often, in retrospect, they were found to have the myeloproliferative variant of HES.

Early reports of HES emphasized its poor prognosis; a mean survival was 9 months, and the 3-year survival rate was 12%.[34] For most HES patients who presented with advanced disease and significant cardiovascular compromise, death resulted from congestive heart failure or other complications of endomyocardial damage.[34] Earlier diagnosis, clinical and echocardiographic monitoring of heart disease, and medical and surgical management of cardiac complications have improved the longevity of HES patients. The 1989 report of 40 HES patients from France, including 17 with the myeloproliferative variant of HES, found an 80% survival rate at 5 years and a 42% survival rate at 10 and 15 years.[53]

Treatment

Patients with eosinophilia without organ involvement may have a benign course and require no therapy. However, because cardiac involvement may develop insidiously and is not correlated with specific levels of blood eosinophilia, these patients warrant careful clinical follow-up, monitoring of serum troponin levels, and echocardiographic assessments at 6-month intervals. Early in the evaluation of F/P-negative eosinophilic patients, a trial course of prednisone (60 mg/day or 1 mg/kg/day) is given to ascertain whether blood eosinophilia can be suppressed by corticosteroids. This information becomes pertinent if the patient rapidly develops organ involvement necessitating therapy.

In patients with myeloproliferative variants of HES, especially those with documented *PDGFRA* mutations, imatinib should be initiated at 100 to 400 mg/day.[33] Clinical and hematologic response usually occurs within 2 to 4 weeks. Repeat bone marrow evaluation should be performed to document the response in PDGFRA-negative patients, because partial imatinib responses have been reported for patients with underlying lymphocytic leukemia. Newer tyrosine kinase inhibitors, including nilotinib, sorafenib, and dasatinib, may be useful if imatinib is not tolerated or ineffective.

In patients with other variants of HES with organ involvement, initial therapy is prednisone (1 mg/kg/day or 60 mg/day in adults).[35] If blood eosinophilia is suppressed, daily doses are slowly tapered to an alternate-day schedule. Hydroxyurea and interferon-α (IFN-α) are effective second-line agents in up to 30% of patients with PDGFRA-negative HES,[38] although IFN-α is not advised for monotherapy for lymphoproliferative variants.[43] Neutralizing anti-IL-5 monoclonal antibodies have shown benefit in initial studies of PDGFRA-negative HES patients,[54] and ongoing studies may establish the efficacies of anti-IL-5 monoclonal antibody treatments of HESs. Bone marrow transplantation has been used successfully in the treatment of HES, but it should be reserved for aggressive disease that is unresponsive to standard therapies.[55,56]

For those with marked valvular compromise or endomyocardial thrombosis or fibrosis, cardiac surgery can provide substantial benefits.[44] Endomyocardectomy or thrombectomy has been beneficial. In patients with HES, valvular bioprostheses should be used because of difficulties in preventing thromboemboli despite adequate anticoagulation and the heightened susceptibility of mechanical valves to thrombus formation.[49]

MYELOPROLIFERATIVE DISORDERS AND MYELOID LEUKEMIAS

Marked eosinophilia is characteristic of several myeloproliferative neoplasms, including those associated with mutations in *PDGFRA*, *PDGFRB*, and fibroblast growth factor receptor 1 (*FGFR1*); acute myeloid leukemia of the M4Eo subtype; and other forms of eosinophilic leukemia, which often have specific cytogenetic and molecular genetic abnormalities.[57] Eosinophilia may occur in chronic myelogenous leukemia (often with basophilia) and in cases of *KIT* D816V mutation-positive systemic mastocytosis.[58]

LYMPHOMAS AND LYMPHOCYTIC LEUKEMIAS

As many as 15% of patients with Hodgkin disease and 5% of those with non-Hodgkin lymphoma have modest levels of peripheral blood eosinophilia. Lesional eosinophilia is most common with nodular sclerosing Hodgkin disease, and heavy eosinophilic infiltration is a significant indicator of a poorer prognosis.[59] Eosinophilia in Hodgkin disease has been correlated with the expression of IL-5 mRNA by Reed-Sternberg cells. In the Sézary syndrome, dysregulated cytokine production from Th2-like lymphocytes is associated with increased levels of IgE and eosinophilia.[60] T cell lymphoblastic lymphoma and adult T cell leukemia/lymphoma are associated with eosinophilia and IL-5 production.[61] Eosinophilia may be the presenting sign of acute lymphoblastic leukemia, particularly in children.[62] Eosinophilia and eczema typically accompany cutaneous T cell lymphomas.[63]

SOLID TUMORS

Solid tumors occasionally are associated with blood eosinophilia and more frequently with lesional eosinophil infiltration. Associated eosinophilia has been reported for a wide variety of solid tumors, including large cell nonkeratinizing cervical tumors; large cell undifferentiated lung carcinomas; squamous carcinomas of the vagina, penis, skin, and nasopharynx; adenocarcinomas of the stomach, large bowel, and uterine body; and transitional bladder cell carcinoma. Studies correlating eosinophil infiltration with prognosis have yielded various findings.

Diseases with Specific Organ Involvement

SKIN AND SUBCUTANEOUS TISSUES

Eosinophils participate in the inflammatory infiltrate in numerous dermatologic conditions. Blood and tissue eosinophilia are common in atopic dermatitis. Tissue eosinophils are seen in blistering diseases, such as bullous pemphigoid, pemphigus vulgaris, dermatitis herpetiformis, and herpes gestationis, and they can be prominent in drug-induced lesions. Eosinophils or deposited eosinophil granule proteins are found in skin sites of chronic urticaria, solar urticaria, and delayed pressure urticaria.[64] Eosinophils are prominent around migrating intradermal (e.g., cutaneous larva migrans) and subcutaneous helminths (e.g., gnathostomiasis). Eosinophils occur in pregnancy-related dermatosis, in the pruritic urticarial papules and plaques syndrome (PUPPS), and in orbital pseudotumors. An uncommon disorder, characterized by the association of nodules, eosinophilia, rheumatism, dermatitis, and swelling (NERDS), includes prominent paraarticular nodules, recurrent urticaria with angioedema, and tissue and blood eosinophilia. Blood and tissue eosinophilia can occur with Sézary syndrome and cutaneous T cell lymphomas. Eosinophilic tissue infiltration is the hallmark of IgG4-related disease.[65]

Eosinophilic Panniculitis

Eosinophilic panniculitis is characterized by prominent eosinophil infiltration of subcutaneous fat. Lesions often are nodular and less frequently manifest as plaques or vesicles. Eosinophilic panniculitis is commonly associated with leukocytoclastic vasculitis and erythema nodosum. Other disorders associated with eosinophilic panniculitis include atopic and contact dermatitis, eosinophilic cellulitis, arthropod bites, gnathostomiasis, toxocariasis, polyarteritis nodosa, injection granuloma, lupus panniculitis, malignancy, diabetes, and chronic recurrent parotitis.

Angioedema with Eosinophilia

Angioedema is a common clinical manifestation of the lymphocytic variant of HES. Two distinct clinical syndromes of angioedema with eosinophilia have been recognized. Episodic angioedema with eosinophilia is a cyclic disorder characterized by recurrent episodes of angioedema, urticaria, pruritus, fever, weight gain, elevated serum IgM, and leukocytosis with marked blood eosinophilia.[66] The level of blood eosinophilia parallels disease activity. Skin biopsies show dermal edema, perivascular $CD4^+$ T lymphocytic infiltration, and diffuse dermal eosinophilic infiltration and degranulation. The cause of this syndrome is unknown, although clonal T lymphocytes overproducing IL-5 have been described.[67] The syndrome has an excellent long-term prognosis and is responsive to glucocorticosteroids.

A syndrome of nonepisodic angioedema with eosinophilia (NEAE) also has been recognized.[68] NEAE appears to occur almost exclusively in young women of Asian descent, is limited to a single episode that may last for months, and typically involves only the extremities.

Kimura Disease and Angiolymphoid Hyperplasia with Eosinophilia

Kimura disease typically manifests as large, subcutaneous masses on the head or neck of Asian males,[69] whereas angiolymphoid hyperplasia with eosinophilia occurs in all races and is characterized by smaller and more superficial lesions. Eosinophilia is common to both, but the relationship of these two conditions to each other and to related angiomatous tumors remains unclear. Angiolymphoid hyperplasia may represent a T cell lymphoproliferative disorder with a benign or low-grade malignant nature.[70]

Shulman Syndrome

Shulman syndrome (i.e., eosinophilic fasciitis) manifests acutely with erythema, swelling, and induration of the extremities, and patients often have a history of antecedent exercise. Skin lesions are usually accompanied by elevated blood eosinophil counts. Histologically, unlike scleroderma, the epidermis and dermis are normal, and most pathology is located in the subcutaneous tissue, fascia, and muscle. Fibrous septa of the subcutaneous fat are sclerotic, and there is a perivascular inflammatory infiltration of lymphocytes, plasma cells, histiocytes, and eosinophils. In only one half to two thirds of patients are the numbers of tissue eosinophils increased. MRI findings, which include abnormal fascial signal intensity and enhancement, can be helpful diagnostically and in monitoring therapy.[71] Eosinophilic fasciitis has been reported as a paraneoplastic syndrome occurring after radiation therapy and in association with connective tissue disorders.

Wells Syndrome

Wells syndrome (i.e., eosinophilic cellulitis) is characterized by recurrent swellings on the extremities.[72] Although involved skin appears cellulitic, minimal tenderness, absence of warmth, and failure to respond to antibiotics distinguish it from bacterial cellulitis. It resolves spontaneously, leaving a granulomatous infiltration. Blood eosinophilia occurs in 50% of patients. Histologically, the edematous dermis is infiltrated by eosinophils in a perivascular pattern in the acute stage. Distinctive *flame figures*, which are masses of collagen and intact and degranulated eosinophils, occur in older lesions. Flame figures are not specific for Wells syndrome and occur in bullous pemphigoid and other eosinophil-rich skin diseases. Wells syndrome is often a manifestation of an underlying systemic disorder, such as CSS, HES, or leukemia/lymphoma.

Eosinophilic Ulcer of the Oral Mucosa

Eosinophilic ulcers often involve the tongue. They are usually tender and multiple, and trauma is often the only potential cause. Eosinophilic infiltration is prominent. Lesions usually heal spontaneously over a month. Uncommonly, these oral lesions may be manifestations of $CD30^+$ lymphoproliferative disorders.[73]

Eosinophilic Pustular Folliculitis

In eosinophilic pustular folliculitis (i.e., Ofuji disease), mixed eosinophilic and neutrophilic infiltrates are found in affected follicles, and blood eosinophilia may occur. Although described in healthy individuals, it has been increasingly recognized in those infected with HIV[74] and less commonly in HIV-negative patients being treated for hematologic malignancies or after bone marrow transplantation. The cause is not clear, but in those with HIV, similar dermal lesions develop in response to bacterial and fungal infections, mite and scabies infestations, and arthropod bites.

Recurrent Cutaneous Necrotizing Eosinophilic Vasculitis

Recurrent cutaneous necrotizing eosinophilic vasculitis affects small dermal vessels. Skin biopsies show necrotizing vasculitis with minimal or absent leukocytoclasis and an almost exclusive eosinophil infiltration in the lumen and vessel walls. Patients respond to systemic glucocorticoid treatment and have a benign, chronic course. Eosinophil-associated vasculitis is also seen in patients with connective tissue diseases with cutaneous necrotizing vasculitis, hypocomplementemia, and peripheral eosinophilia.

PULMONARY DISEASES

Eosinophilic lung diseases are a heterogeneous group of disorders unified by the presence of large numbers of eosinophils in the inflammatory cellular infiltrates in the airways and parenchyma of the lungs.[75,76] Although pulmonary eosinophilia usually manifests with symptoms referable to the respiratory system accompanied by an abnormal chest radiograph and blood or sputum eosinophilia, blood eosinophilia may be absent[77] and chest radiographs unrevealing. Pulmonary eosinophilias are classified based on recognized eliciting etiologic agents and distinct clinical and pathologic patterns (Box 75-2). Thin-section CT can be helpful in narrowing the differential diagnosis but must be correlated with clinical findings.[78]

Drug- and Toxin-Induced Eosinophilic Lung Diseases

Diverse medications and other drugs are capable of eliciting pulmonary eosinophilia. Toxic agents, including occupational exposures (e.g., rubber manufacturing, aluminum silicate, particulate metals, sulfite in vineyards) or other exposures (e.g., Scotchguard inhalation), can cause pulmonary eosinophilia. Although the pathogenesis may be different, the clinical presentation of drug- and toxin-elicited eosinophilic lung disease can resemble other forms of pulmonary eosinophilia, including acute and chronic forms of eosinophilic pneumonia. For instance, the Löffler migratory eosinophil infiltrates typical of *Ascaris* have been seen after use of crack cocaine.

BOX 75-2 TYPES AND CAUSES OF PULMONARY EOSINOPHILIA

1. Drug- and toxin-induced eosinophilic lung diseases
2. Helminth and fungal infection-related eosinophilic lung diseases
    a. Transpulmonary passage of larvae (i.e., Löffler syndrome): *Ascaris*, hookworm, *Strongyloides*
    b. Pulmonary parenchymal invasion: mostly helminths, paragonimiasis
    c. Heavy hematogenous seeding with helminths: trichinellosis, disseminated strongyloidiasis, cutaneous and visceral larva migrans, schistosomiasis
    d. Tropical pulmonary eosinophilia: filaria
    e. Allergic bronchopulmonary aspergillosis
3. Chronic eosinophilic pneumonia
4. Acute eosinophilic pneumonia
5. Churg-Strauss syndrome (vasculitis)
6. Other: neoplasia, idiopathic hypereosinophilic syndrome, bronchocentric granulomatosis

Helminth and Fungal Infection–Related Eosinophilic Lung Diseases

Helminth and fungal infections elicit distinct forms of pulmonary eosinophilia based on the behavior of the organisms in the lung and the associated immune responses.

Transpulmonary Passage of Helminth Larvae: Löffler Syndrome. Löffler originally described the syndrome of transient pulmonary infiltrates and blood eosinophilia in Swiss patients infected with *Ascaris* from the use of contaminated human night soil as fertilizer. The syndrome occurs approximately 9 to 12 days after ingestion of *Ascaris* eggs, when infecting larvae pass through the lungs by entering through the bloodstream, penetrating into alveoli, and ascending the airway to transit down the esophagus into the small bowel.[29] Although helminth larvae other than *Ascaris*, including *Strongyloides* and hookworm, transit through the lungs, pulmonary symptoms are uncommon in these infections.

Common complaints of symptomatic patients are an irritating, nonproductive cough and burning substernal discomfort. More than one half of patients have rales and wheezing. Acute symptoms usually subside within 5 to 10 days. Chest radiographs show transient, migratory, unilateral or bilateral, nonsegmental densities with indefinite borders ranging in size from several millimeters to several centimeters. Blood eosinophilia can be absent in the early symptomatic period, but it increases in magnitude after several days of symptoms and resolves over many weeks. Because at least 40 days must elapse before the larvae responsible for pulmonary infiltrates have matured sufficiently to produce eggs detectable in feces, stool examinations during the acute syndrome are not helpful in establishing the diagnosis. Conversely, finding that stools are free of eggs during the pneumonic involvement and contain *Ascaris* eggs 2 to 3 months later supports *Ascaris* as the etiologic agent of the pneumonitis.

Pulmonary Parenchymal Invasion with Helminths. In contrast to the parasites previously described that transit through the lungs, *Paragonimus* lung flukes characteristically localize within the pulmonary parenchyma and elicit eosinophil-enriched inflammatory reactions.

Heavy Hematogenous Seeding with Helminths. Eosinophilic pulmonary responses usually are elicited by helminth larvae or eggs that are carried into the lungs hematogenously in an aberrant fashion. In this category, etiologic helminths include abnormal numbers of nonhuman hookworms or ascarids causing cutaneous or visceral larva migrans (e.g., toxocariasis with an acute eosinophilic pneumonia), abnormal numbers of hematogenous larvae in heavy trichinellosis infections, acute pulmonary schistosomiasis, and disseminated strongyloidiasis.

Strongyloides has a unique autoinfection life cycle enabling it to cause chronic infection that can persist for decades. Disseminated infection develops when the autoinfection cycle becomes unbridled, most commonly due to corticosteroid administration. Large numbers of larvae traverse the lungs, eliciting pulmonary findings, and massive larval invasion of the bowel wall can lead to gram-negative bacillary bacteremia.[4] In disseminated strongyloidiasis, filariform larvae can be found in many sites, including the stool, sputum, skin, and bronchoalveolar washings. Adult parasites can develop in the bronchial tree, causing bronchospasm that can mimic asthma. The usual eosinophilia of strongyloidiasis can be suppressed in disseminated disease because of concomitant pyogenic infection or corticosteroid administration.

Acute pulmonary schistosomiasis manifests with fever, cough, and eosinophilia in a traveler with a recent history of fresh water exposure in an area endemic for schistosomiasis.[79] Diffuse pulmonary infiltrates are typically seen. Disease onset appears to coincide with schistosomule migration through the lungs and the onset egg deposition. Stool examination and serologic results may be negative at the time of clinical presentation, but they become positive within 3 to 4 weeks, confirming the diagnosis. Because praziquantel therapy is ineffective for acute schistosomiasis and can exacerbate clinical symptoms, treatment should be delayed until eggs are detected in the urine or stool.

Tropical Pulmonary Eosinophilia

Tropical eosinophilic pneumonia results from a rare hypersensitivity response to the normally bloodborne microfilarial stages of the lymphatic filariae of *Wuchereria bancrofti* and less commonly to *Brugia malayi*. Lymphatic filariasis is endemic in Asia, especially the Indian subcontinent, and specific regions in Africa, South America, and the Caribbean, and residents of or immigrants from these regions are at risk for tropical pulmonary eosinophilia.[80] Symptoms are nonspecific and include fatigue, low-grade fevers, night sweats, and weight loss. Respiratory complaints are prominent and include dyspnea, nocturnal cough, and wheezing. Laboratory findings include marked blood eosinophilia, high IgG and IgE antifilarial antibody titers, and polyclonal elevations of IgG and IgE. Microfilariae are almost never found in the blood, BAL fluid, or tissues. Examination of BAL fluid shows a predominance of eosinophils. Abnormalities on chest radiographs may be subtle and include diffuse miliary lesions 1 to 3 mm in diameter, patchy consolidations, cavitation, reticulonodular infiltrates of the lower lung zones, and an interstitial nodular pattern. Pulmonary function testing reveals diminished vital capacity, total lung capacity, residual volumes, and diffusing capacity of the lung for carbon monoxide (DLCO), with a superimposed obstructive pattern in a fourth of patients. Lung biopsies show histiocytic and eosinophilic infiltrates in the interstitial, peribronchial, and alveolar spaces during the early phases, with progression to massive eosinophilic pneumonias and later to chronic nodular interstitial disease with mixed cell infiltrates, granulomatous reactions, and marked fibrosis. Diethylcarbamazine citrate is the treatment of choice.

Allergic Bronchopulmonary Aspergillosis

Immunologic responses elicited by *Aspergillus* species in often altered airways are responsible for this syndrome (see Chapter 61). Characteristic features include a history of asthma, pulmonary infiltrates, mucoid impaction, peripheral eosinophilia, central cylindrical bronchiectasis, and elevated IgE and anti-*Aspergillus* antigen–specific IgG and IgE antibodies. Histologically, the four major lesions of allergic bronchopulmonary aspergillosis are asthmatic bronchiolitis, eosinophilic pneumonia, bronchocentric granulomatosis, and mucoid impaction of bronchi.

Chronic Eosinophilic Pneumonia

Chronic eosinophilic pneumonia has a 2-to-1 female predominance, and the cause is unknown.[77,81] Most patients are older than 30 years of age, and one half have a history of atopic disease, with asthma being the most common. Some patients developed new adult-onset asthma within the antecedent 5 years. Symptoms are usually present for more than 2 weeks, and the average time to diagnosis from symptom onset is 7.7 months. Common presenting symptoms are cough, fever, dyspnea, and significant weight loss.[77] Less than one third of patients experience sputum production, malaise, wheezing, and night sweats. Less frequently, patients have hemoptysis, fatigue, and chills and may rarely present with respiratory failure.

Although most patients with chronic eosinophilic pneumonia have blood eosinophilia,[77] the absence of blood eosinophilia does not preclude this diagnosis. Eosinophils and lymphocytes are seen in sputum and BAL fluid. ESRs and IgE levels are elevated in most patients. Pulmonary function test results may be normal but often show diminished static lung volumes, expiratory flow rates, and diffusing capacity. Hypoxia with decreased arterial oxygen tension and elevated alveolar-arterial gradient largely results from increased shunting or ventilation-perfusion mismatch.[82]

Chronic eosinophilic pneumonia, as originally observed by Carrington and coworkers,[82] is characterized radiographically by "progressive, dense, peripheral infiltrates; rapid resolution with corticosteroid medication; and the recurrence of lesions in the same unusual locations during relapse." About one fourth of patients exhibit a "photographic negative of pulmonary edema" in which peripheral infiltrates without segmental or lobar restrictions occur in the outer lung zone with central sparing in the inner and middle lung zones.[77] Peripherally located infiltration is observed in two thirds, and peripheral upper lobe involvement is seen in one third. Radiographic findings include the appearance of nodular infiltration, bilateral consolidation, atelectasis, unilateral involvement, cavitation, and pleural effusion. Chest radiographs, however, are not sensitive, and more sensitive CT scans detect peripheral infiltrates even when radiographs do not.[78] Mediastinal lymphadenopathy may be observed.

Histopathologic evaluation shows moderate to extensive consolidation, alveoli flooded with a proteinaceous exudate, and a predominantly eosinophilic infiltrate in the alveoli and interstitium.[77,82] Multinucleated histiocytic giant cells, lymphocytes, and plasma cells may be found in the alveoli. A noncaseating granulomatous reaction and a mild perivascular cuffing of venules with lymphocytes and eosinophils may be observed. True necrosis of vessel walls is not observed.

Response to corticosteroid administration is dramatic, occurring within 24 hours.[77] Blood eosinophilia declines within 12 to 24 hours, and complete resolution of symptoms for two thirds of patients occurs within 2 weeks.[77] Radiographic improvement may be observed in 60 to 72 hours, and clearance can be expected to occur within 2 weeks for half of patients.[77]

The impaired diffusing capacity and volume restriction appear to be completely reversible after treatment.[82] Most patients require more than 6 months of systemic glucocorticosteroid therapy.[77] Mean duration of initial corticosteroid therapy was 19 months. Recurrences of clinical and radiographic changes were seen in 58% of patients after discontinuation of corticosteroids, and 21% relapsed during corticosteroid taper.[77] Recurrent attacks occurred in 34%, especially those with a prior diagnosis of asthma, and about 75% of patients require long-term, low-dose corticosteroid therapy.[77]

Deaths have occurred. The long-term prognosis for most patients with chronic eosinophilic pneumonia is excellent nonetheless. Chronic eosinophilic pneumonia has sometimes been premonitory of or complicated by subsequent development of the CSS, raising questions about potential overlaps between these diseases.[81,83]

Acute Eosinophilic Pneumonia

Acute eosinophilic pneumonia is a clinical entity distinct from other eosinophilic pneumonias. There is a male predominance, and patients present with acute onset of cough, dyspnea, and fever. Diagnostic criteria for acute eosinophilic pneumonia are given in Box 75-3.[84] Because patients with clinical and histopathologic features of acute eosinophilic pneumonia have been described with up to a month of symptoms before presentation[85] and with tissue eosinophilia without BAL studies performed or without more than 25% BAL eosinophilia, defining criteria for acute eosinophilic pneumonia are not necessarily limited to less than a week.[84]

Although acute eosinophilic pneumonia may be caused by medications, hypersensitivity reactions to allergens, or adverse reactions to chemicals or metals, the cause and pathogenesis of typical acute eosinophilic pneumonia remain unknown. Acute eosinophilic pneumonia has been increasingly associated with inhalational dust exposures and especially with new-onset cigarette smoking.[86,87] Among 18 U.S. soldiers serving in Iraq who developed acute eosinophilic pneumonia, all used tobacco, and 14 (78%) had recently initiated smoking.[88]

The diagnosis of acute eosinophilic pneumonia requires exclusion of fungal, parasitic, drug-induced, and hypersensitivity causes for eosinophilic pneumonia. Originally, asthma and atopic diseases were considered to be exclusion criteria, but patients with acute eosinophilic pneumonia who had atopic histories were subsequently reported.

Physical examination is remarkable for fever, respiratory distress, crackles on auscultation, and a transient wheeze or rhonchi on forced expiratory maneuvers.[89] Laboratory examination early in the course is significant for leukocytosis without blood eosinophilia.[89] Blood eosinophilia usually peaks at 7 to 9 days after presentation. By definition, patients are hypoxic on room air. Chest radiographs show bilateral, diffuse, mixed interstitial and alveolar infiltrates, commonly with Kerley B lines and often accompanied by pleural effusions.[90] CT scans show diffuse parenchymal alveolar infiltrates, pleural effusions, pronounced septal markings, and normal lymph nodes.[89,90]

Pulmonary function shows diminished total lung and diffusing capacities and preserved forced expiratory volume in 1 second to forced vital capacity (FEV_1/FVC) ratios but with small airways dysfunction. BAL reveals lymphocytosis (20% ± 11%) and eosinophilia (45% ± 11%).[89] Histopathology shows diffuse acute and organizing alveolar damage with marked interstitial eosinophil infiltration, along with infiltration in the bronchial epithelium.[84] Vasculitis and granulomas have not been reported. Airways may show mucous plugging, but specific features of asthma are missing. Acute eosinophilic pneumonia is differentiated from the acute respiratory distress syndrome by the absence of tissue eosinophils in the latter and by the uniformly prompt response to steroid therapy and good prognosis for the former. Acute eosinophilic pneumonia is differentiated from chronic eosinophilic pneumonia by its acute presentation, rapid progression to respiratory failure, and histologic absence of the alveolar proteinaceous exudate seen in chronic eosinophilic pneumonia.

Patients respond within 24 to 48 hours to high doses of glucocorticoids.[90] Given the potential progression to respiratory failure and the dramatic response to treatment, steroids should be administered as soon as the diagnosis is ascertained. Corticosteroids are often tapered quickly over 8 weeks. Those on mechanical ventilatory support are usually weaned off in a few days. Deaths due to acute eosinophilic pneumonia occur.[88] Patients have not experienced recurrences of acute eosinophilic pneumonia,[89] and some have recovered spontaneously without corticosteroids.[85]

BOX 75-3 DIAGNOSTIC CRITERIA FOR ACUTE EOSINOPHILIC PNEUMONIA

Acute febrile illness; duration often less than 5 days but may be weeks
Hypoxemic respiratory failure
Diffuse alveolar or mixed alveolar-interstitial infiltrates seen on the radiograph
Eosinophils >25% of BAL fluid (or biopsy confirmation of lung tissue eosinophilia)
Absence of parasitic, fungal, or other infection
Prompt and complete response to corticosteroids
Failure to relapse after discontinuation of corticosteroids

Data from Allen JN, Davis WB. Eosinophilic lung diseases. Am Respir Crit Care Med 1994;150:1423-38; Tazelaar HD, Linz LJ, Colby TV, et al. Acute eosinophilic pneumonia: a study of 22 patients. Am J Respir Crit Care Med 1997;155:296-302.
BAL, Bronchoalveolar lavage.

Churg-Strauss Syndrome

CSS is characterized by allergic angiitis and granulomatosis. Antecedent asthma and pulmonary eosinophilia are typical features of this eosinophil-associated vasculitis (discussed later).

Other Forms of Pulmonary Eosinophilia

Pulmonary involvement is common in HES.[44] Peripheral blood and pulmonary eosinophilia can also be seen in pulmonary sarcoidosis. Rarely, pulmonary eosinophilia has been reported in the setting of primary or metastatic pulmonary neoplasms, lung transplantation, and autoimmune diseases, including rheumatoid arthritis. One of the two forms of bronchocentric granulomatosis, which develops in patients with asthma, peripheral eosinophilia, and *Aspergillus* in sputum and airway biopsies, is associated with pulmonary eosinophilia, and it may be related to allergic bronchopulmonary aspergillosis.

Eosinophilic Granuloma. Eosinophilic granuloma of the lung (i.e., pulmonary Langerhans cell histiocytosis or pulmonary Langerhans cell granulomatosis; formerly called histiocytosis

X) is associated with pulmonary interstitial fibrosis. The most common symptom is a nonproductive cough, which is accompanied by complaints of dyspnea, pleuritic chest pain, fever, weight loss, and hemoptysis. Occasionally, the diagnosis is made by lung biopsy in asymptomatic patients presenting with an abnormal chest radiograph. Chest radiographs show reticulonodular infiltrates, honeycombing, cystic changes, and nodules. High-resolution CT showing cysts and nodules is almost pathognomonic. Eosinophilic granuloma of the lung is usually not accompanied by blood eosinophilia. Stellate lesions with atypical histiocytes, sometimes accompanied by modest interstitial accumulation of eosinophils, are seen in pathologic specimens.

Lesions are extended by clonal expansion of Langerhans cells, which are abnormal cells of the monocyte-macrophage line that are positive for CD1 and HLA-DR markers. Various numbers of eosinophils may occur within lesions, and they may be observed in interstitial areas. Eosinophils, however, are not typically recovered from the airways as in other forms of eosinophilic lung disease.

Pleural Eosinophilia. Pleural fluid eosinophilia of more than10% of the differential cell count is a striking, albeit often nonspecific finding.[91] Pleural fluid eosinophilia can be associated with a wide variety of conditions, including malignancy, infection, drug hypersensitivity, and trauma (surgical and other). In most series, 15% to 25% of cases are idiopathic and carry a benign prognosis.[92,93] Most eosinophilic effusions are unilateral and biochemically are exudates. Blood eosinophilia usually does not accompany idiopathic pleural fluid eosinophilia.

Bronchoalveolar Lavage Eosinophilia. In addition to eosinophilic disorders involving the lung (e.g., CSS, HES), BAL fluid eosinophilia (>5% of differential cell count) is seen in 4.5% of bronchoscopies with BAL[94] and is not often accompanied by blood eosinophilia. Diseases associated with BAL eosinophilia include interstitial lung disease (40%), acquired immunodeficiency syndrome (AIDS)–related pneumonia (17%), idiopathic eosinophilic pneumonia (15%), and drug-induced lung disease (12%). Among patients with interstitial lung disease, increased numbers of eosinophils in BAL specimens have been identified in those with idiopathic pulmonary fibrosis, sarcoidosis, systemic lupus erythematosus, and hypersensitivity pneumonitis. The finding of eosinophilia in BAL fluid may indicate progressive lung disease in cases of idiopathic pulmonary fibrosis and pulmonary fibrosis associated with collagen vascular disorders.[95] Other nonallergic diseases with BAL eosinophilia include bronchiolitis obliterans organizing pneumonia, Hodgkin disease, rheumatoid arthritis, malignancy, eosinophilic granuloma, postradiation therapy, pulmonary involvement in Sjögren syndrome, graft-versus-host disease, and systemic sclerosis.

GASTROINTESTINAL DISEASES

Tissue and blood eosinophilia develop in a number of gastrointestinal and hepatobiliary disorders. Eosinophilic esophagitis is increasingly recognized in children and occurs in adults (see Chapter 68).[96,97] In the stomach, *Helicobacter pylori* infection can be associated with eosinophilia in involved tissues but not in blood. In ulcerative colitis and Crohn disease, tissue eosinophils are components of the inflammatory infiltrates, and eosinophil numbers tend to become more prominent with more extensive inflammation.[98] In celiac disease, a gluten-sensitive enteropathy, eosinophils are present in the gut and increase after gluten challenge. Tissue eosinophilia is characteristic of collagenous colitis.[99] Eosinophil enterocolitis can result from a hypersensitivity reaction to medications. Gastrointestinal eosinophilia elicited by intestinal parasites must be excluded in patients with these eosinophilic diseases. Eosinophilic gastroenteritides are considered in Chapter 68.

Hepatic eosinophilia develops in response to some medications and to helminth parasites, including schistosomes, whose eggs embolize in the portal system and generate eosinophil-enriched granulomas and fibrosis, migrating larvae (e.g., visceral larva migrans), and hepatobiliary flukes (e.g., *Clonorchis*). Eosinophilia in the liver can occur with primary biliary cirrhosis, HESs, sclerosing cholangitis, eosinophilic cholangitis, eosinophilic cholecystitis, and focal eosinophilic abscesses.[100]

NEUROLOGIC DISEASES

Tissue eosinophilia occurs within the membranes of organized chronic subdural hematomas.[101] Other eosinophil-associated neurologic diseases are uncommon and include the disorders that cause eosinophilic meningitis.[102] Cerebrospinal fluid eosinophilia can be a significant clue to central nervous system infections with *Coccidioides* species (especially in the southwestern United States) or *Angiostrongylus cantonensis* (especially in the Pacific Basin) and to adverse drug reactions to NSAIDs or antibiotics.

RHEUMATOLOGIC DISEASES

Eosinophilia is not common in connective tissue diseases.[103,104] Eosinophilia may sometimes accompany dermatomyositis, rheumatoid arthritis, progressive systemic sclerosis, and Sjögren syndrome complicated by polymyopathy and vasculitis. When eosinophilia occurs in rheumatoid arthritis, the differential diagnosis includes development of concomitant vasculitis or hypersensitivity reactions to therapeutic agents (e.g., NSAIDs, tetracyclines). Eosinophilia is unusual in systemic scleroderma, and its presence may indicate eosinophilic fasciitis. A syndrome of acute polyarthritis with hypereosinophilia was observed in a few patients in Singapore.[105] Eosinophilic infiltration into muscle is uncommon, but it accompanies trichinellosis and *Sarcocystis* infection and has been reported in cases of HES.[32] A genetic form of eosinophilic myositis has been described that is most commonly associated with mutations in calpain 3 (*CAPN3*).[106] Rare cases of idiopathic eosinophilic myositis have been reported.[107]

Synovial Fluid Eosinophilia and Idiopathic Eosinophilic Synovitis

Synovial fluid eosinophilia is uncommonly (0.1%) identified by cytologic examination, but about 0.5% of synovial fluid samples are positive for Charcot-Leyden crystals.[108] A level of synovial eosinophilia of more than 10% is seen uncommonly in tuberculous and filarial infections and in metastatic carcinoma, after arthrography and irradiation, and with urticaria, idiopathic eosinophilic synovitis, and Lyme disease. Idiopathic eosinophilic synovitis is an acute, painless monoarthritis that develops after minor trauma.[109] The knee and metatarsophalangeal joints are most frequently involved, with swelling developing rapidly over 12 to 24 hours and lasting 1 to 2 weeks. Effusions are large but not usually accompanied by other signs of arthritis such as warmth, erythema, or pain.

Eosinophilia-Myalgia Syndrome and Toxic Oil Syndrome

The features and causes of eosinophilia-myalgia syndrome and toxic oil syndrome have been compared.[110] Eosinophilia-myalgia syndrome arises from ingestion of contaminated L-tryptophan, whereas the toxic oil syndrome is caused by ingestion of edible oil adulterated with denatured rapeseed oil. Both are chronic, persistent, multisystem diseases in which eosinophilia develops, although the pathogenic roles of eosinophils have been difficult to define.

Vasculitis

Churg-Strauss Syndrome. Among the major forms of vasculitis, CSS (i.e., allergic angiitis and granulomatosis) is notable for its distinct association with blood and lesional eosinophilia and its frequent association with allergic rhinoconjunctivitis, sinusitis, and asthma.[111] CSS may develop in patients with asthma may be associated with specific asthma treatments, as reviewed by a National Institutes of Health workshop panel.[83] CSS has developed in asthmatic patients receiving several cysteinyl leukotriene receptor 1 antagonists, a 5-lipoxygenase inhibitor, inhaled corticosteroids, or salmeterol.[83] It is likely that these structurally and mechanistically distinct agents did not cause CSS. Instead, by controlling symptoms, these agents may have unmasked the incipient vasculitis in those with asthma, including those receiving oral steroids for their asthma, or may have been used as contemporary antiasthmatic medications in those otherwise destined to develop CSS. Tapering of corticosteroids might have revealed evolving CSS or variant formes frustes.[112-114]

Several published criteria may be applied to the diagnosis of CSS (Table 75-4). Churg and Strauss presented three pathologic criteria—vasculitis of small- and medium-sized arteries and veins, eosinophil infiltration around vessels and in tissues, and extravascular granuloma—that established CSS as a distinct form of vasculitis.[115] In practice, knowledgeable pathologists recognize that early lesions in evolution and those amenable for diagnostic biopsy may reveal only eosinophil infiltration around vessels without the need to demonstrate the full-blown triad.[83] To overcome the restraints of using only pathologic criteria, Lanham and colleagues at the Hammersmith Hospital defined CSS to include a history of asthma, eosinophilia of more than 1500 cells/μL, and vasculitis in two or more extrapulmonary organs.[11]

The American College of Rheumatology (ACR) published criteria (see Table 75-4) that were designed and validated to diagnose CSS in patients already known to have vasculitis.[117] The ACR principles were developed as research standards and were not meant to serve as robust criteria for the routine clinical diagnosis and management of patients.

In practice, CSS remains primarily a clinical diagnosis that largely depends on the evaluation and judgment of clinicians. In its common presentation, CSS is often a triphasic illness.[116] In the prodromal phase, patients experience allergic rhinitis, sinusitis, and asthma of variable severity that often develops in adulthood. Asthma may exist for several years at this level. The second phase is characterized by blood eosinophilia and eosinophilic tissue infiltrates. The third phase involves potentially life-threatening vasculitis that may involve multiple organs but often includes the lung, heart, gastrointestinal tract, and nervous system. Although this triphasic pattern may be common, it is by no means uniform, and published reports are replete with patients who present initially with acute vasculitic complications without antecedent asthma. Lacking a history of asthma, delayed diagnosis and treatment may contribute to death from vasculitic complications involving the heart, gastrointestinal tract, or other organs.[118]

Asthma, eosinophilia, and transient pulmonary infiltrates antedate the development of systemic vasculitis in about half of cases. Pulmonary involvement is seen in almost all patients, and pulmonary infiltrates, which are best detected by high-resolution CT, occur in three fourths of patients.[119] High-resolution CT findings include air-space consolidation or ground-glass opacities, septal lines, and bronchial wall thickenings.[120]

Nasal and sinus involvement is common, and one series reported nasal symptoms in 69% and radiologic evidence of pansinusitis in 88% of cases.[121] Cutaneous involvement occurs in 70% of patients. Typical lesions include macular or papular erythematous rashes; hemorrhagic, often-palpable lesions

TABLE 75-4 Definitions of Churg-Strauss Syndrome

Study	Criteria	Purpose and Limitations
Churg and Strauss, 1951[115]	Necrotizing vasculitis of small- and medium-sized arteries and veins, eosinophil infiltration around involved vessels and in tissues, and extravascular granulomas	Identified CSS as a pathologically distinct form of vasculitis but was based on autopsy examination of multiple organs of those with end-stage disease
Lanham et al (Hammersmith Hospital), 1984[116]	History of asthma, peak blood eosinophilia >1500 cells/μL, and systemic vasculitis involving two or more extrapulmonary organs	Expanded the defining features of CSS beyond pathologic criteria by including clinical criteria, notably a history of asthma; would not identify those with CSS without asthma
Masi et al (American College of Rheumatology), 1990[117]	*At least four of six criteria*: asthma, >10% blood eosinophilia, mononeuropathy (including multiplex) or polyneuropathy, nonfixed pulmonary infiltrates on chest radiograph, paranasal sinus abnormalities, extravascular eosinophils	Designed and validated solely to distinguish and classify forms of vasculitis in patients with documented vasculitis; intended for studies of vasculitis, not for clinical diagnosis

Modified from Weller PF, Plaut M, Taggart V, et al. The relationship of asthma therapy and Churg-Strauss syndrome: NIH workshop summary report. J Allergy Clin Immunol 2001;108:175-83.
CSS, Churg-Strauss syndrome.

ranging from petechiae to purpura to extensive ecchymoses; and cutaneous and subcutaneous nodules. Subcutaneous nodules are tender and tend to occur on the scalp and symmetrically on the extremities. The nervous system is frequently involved with peripheral neuropathies, including mononeuritis multiplex.[122] Cerebral infarctions occur and can be a cause of death in this syndrome. Gastrointestinal involvement is seen in 40% of patients. Cardiac involvement is observed clinically in one third, although as many as 62% of autopsied cases show cardiac involvement. Cardiac disease accounts for 50% of deaths due to CSS. Renal involvement occurs less frequently in CSS than in polyarteritis nodosa or Wegener granulomatosis.

Laboratory findings include a leukocytosis with blood eosinophilia, an elevated ESR, and sometimes, increases in serum IgE. Antineutrophil cytoplasmic antibodies (ANCAs) are detected in one half of the patients with CSS. Biopsies of involved tissues may show only eosinophilic perivascular and tissue infiltration or the more specific necrotizing vasculitis of small arteries and veins, tissue eosinophilia, and extravascular necrotizing granulomas.[123] Biopsies of nodular skin lesions may or may not reveal the characteristic extravascular granulomas with eosinophilic infiltrates that differentiate CSS from polyarteritis nodosa.[124] In lung biopsy specimens, there can be massive infiltration by eosinophils in the air spaces and interstitium and around blood vessels, which is histologically similar to acute or chronic eosinophilic pneumonia.[83] Extravascular necrotizing granulomas and nonnecrotizing sarcoid-like granulomas occasionally involving the vessel walls can be found. The angiitis may vary from eosinophilic infiltration of vessel walls to full necrotizing fibrinoid vasculitis of small- to medium-sized vessels. Histologic features of asthma may be seen in the bronchial tree.

A principal diagnostic dilemma is recognizing the evolution of CSS in patients who have preexisting asthma. The level of eosinophilia in asthma is usually less than 1500 cells/μL of blood,[11] but it is greater in CSS.[83] In asthma, the ESR is usually not elevated, and the ANCA test results are not positive. In patients with asthma, the development of pulmonary infiltrates or cutaneous, neurologic, gastrointestinal, cardiac, or systemic manifestations of CSS vasculitis need to be recognized as likely signs of CSS. The differential diagnosis includes Wegener granulomatosis (in which eosinophilia and asthma are rare), forms of HES (in which asthma and vasculitis are uncommon), and chronic eosinophilic pneumonia (which may antedate the development of CSS[81,83]). Deaths often occur from extrapulmonary vasculitis, and treatment includes principally corticosteroids, possibly interferon-α, and sometimes cyclophosphamide.[111,125]

Other Forms of Vasculitis. Cutaneous necrotizing eosinophilic vasculitis with hypocomplementemia and eosinophilia occurs in patients with connective tissue diseases.[126] Thromboangiitis obliterans with eosinophilia of the temporal arteries has been described.[127] Although classic Wegener granulomatosis is not commonly associated with blood or lesional eosinophilia, it has been reported.[128] Cases of likely HES- or CSS-eosinophil–associated vasculitis leading to digital necrosis also have been recognized.

CARDIAC DISEASES

Eosinophilic coronary arteritis, often a manifestation of CSS, can develop.[129,130] The principal cardiac sequela of eosinophilic diseases is damage to the endomyocardium. This can occur rarely with drug- or immunization-induced hypersensitivity myocarditis[23] and with eosinophilias associated with HESs, eosinophilic leukemia, sarcomas, carcinomas, and lymphomas, GM-CSF or IL-2[15] administration, prolonged drug-induced eosinophilia, and parasitic infections. The cardiac damage evolves to endomyocardial fibrosis and intraventricular thrombosis as discussed for HESs.[34] Rarely, eosinophilic endomyocardial diseases manifest without recognized antecedent eosinophilia.[131] Elevations of serum troponins are sensitive measures in the early stages of endomyocardial damage,[46] and echocardiography and MRI[48] are effective for evaluating later stages of endomyocardial thrombosis and fibrosis.

RENAL DISEASES

In addition to drug-induced interstitial nephritis and CSS, eosinophils may be associated with other urinary tract and renal diseases.

Eosinophiluria

Eosinophiluria is best detected in fresh urine using Hansel stain, which is more sensitive than Wright stain.[132] The clinical importance of eosinophiluria was first seen in patients with drug-induced acute interstitial nephritis in which eosinophils constituted 10% to 60% of urine leukocytes. Various degrees of eosinophiluria have since been found in other conditions, including urinary tract infections (typically <5% of total white blood cells[133]), rapidly progressive and acute poststreptococcal glomerulonephritis, eosinophilic prostatitis, eosinophilic cystitis, transplant rejection, bladder cancer, cholesterol embolization, and schistosomiasis with bladder involvement caused by *Schistosoma haematobium.*

Eosinophilic Cystitis

Eosinophilic cystitis can manifest with hematuria, urinary frequency, dysuria, and suprapubic pain. It occurs more often in children than in adults, and the cause is unknown.[134,135] Cystoscopy reveals diffusely hyperemic mucosa with areas of elevation or nodularities that extends to the urinary tract in some cases. Biopsies obtained during acute presentations show prominent eosinophilic infiltration, numerous IgA or IgE plasma cells, mucosal edema, and muscle necrosis. Subsequently, chronic inflammation and fibrosis of the mucosa and muscularis develop. The diagnosis can be suggested by CT and is usually made histologically. Bladder carcinoma is the principal differential diagnosis. Although most patients have a benign course with spontaneous resolution, some chronic cases progress to bladder destruction and renal failure.

Other Renal Conditions

Patients on hemodialysis may have mild eosinophilia, and initiation of peritoneal dialysis usually leads to self-limited episodes of peritoneal eosinophilia, with more than half of cases accompanied by blood eosinophilia.[136,137] Isolated renal hydatid disease has been reported.

Immunologic Reactions

IMMUNODEFICIENCY DISEASES

Several primary immunodeficiency syndromes are associated with eosinophilia. Hyper-IgE syndromes, including Job syndrome and dedicator of cytokinesis 8 (DOCK8) expression deficiency, are characterized by recurrent staphylococcal abscesses of the skin, lungs, and other sites; pruritic dermatitis; very high serum IgE levels; and eosinophilia of the blood, sputum, and tissues.[138] Eosinophilia is also characteristic of Omenn syndrome, a form of severe combined immunodeficiency.[139] Other immunodeficiency syndromes, including immune dysregulation, polyendocrinopathy, enteropathy, X-linked (IPEX) syndrome; autoimmune lymphoproliferative syndrome (ALPS); and X-linked ectodermal dysplasia with immunodeficiency, are associated with eosinophilia in a subset of patients.

TRANSPLANT REJECTION

Infiltration of eosinophils accompanies rejection of lung,[140] kidney,[141] and liver[142] allografts. In contrast, eosinophils in cardiac allografts may not be indicative of rejection.[143] Blood and urinary eosinophilias have been monitored as signs of acute rejection in kidney transplant allografts. Tissue eosinophilia and extracellular deposition of MBP and ECP, eosinophiluria, and urinary levels of MBP were elevated in acute renal allograft rejection but not in cyclosporine nephrotoxicity. The eosinophilia seen in renal allograft biopsies may be associated with drug-induced interstitial nephritis rather than rejection.[144] In lung allograft recipients, eosinophil infiltration has correlated with acute cellular rejection episodes.[145] Tissue and blood eosinophilia occur early in hepatic allograft rejection processes, and eosinophil counts and granule protein levels have correlated with prognosis, severity, and response to rejection therapy.[146] Eosinophils are also associated with chronic renal allograft rejections.[147] The absolute blood eosinophil count, biliary tract eosinophilia, and tissue deposition of extracellular ECP and MBP were significantly increased in patients with allogeneic liver rejection compared with recipients who had dysfunction from other causes.[142,148] Tissue eosinophils may be present in cutaneous graft-versus-host disease, but the histopathology alone cannot distinguish between drug hypersensitivity reactions and graft-versus-host reactions.[149]

Eosinophils in Other Disorders

Hypoadrenalism is an endocrine disorder. Glucocorticosteroids exert eosinopenic effects in part by stimulating apoptosis of eosinophils but not neutrophils. The loss of endogenous adrenoglucocorticosteroids in Addison disease, adrenal hemorrhage, or hypopituitarism causes increased blood eosinophilia, and eosinophilia may be a clue to adrenal insufficiency in at-risk patients with serious infections or other illnesses requiring intensive care.[150]

Cholesterol embolization occurring spontaneously or after vascular or intravascular procedures can lead to an increased ESR, hypocomplementemia, thrombocytopenia, eosinophilia, and eosinophiluria. Additional organ involvement may be evidenced by renal insufficiency, livedo reticularis, and purple toes.[151] Sometimes, blood eosinophilia is the sole clinical clue.

Irritation of serosal surfaces is associated with eosinophilia. Examples include the Dressler syndrome, eosinophilic pleural effusions, and eosinophilic peritoneal effusions that develop during chronic peritoneal dialysis. A kindred with hereditary eosinophilia has been identified.[152]

Summary

Studies have recognized roles for eosinophils in normal homeostatic responses, but many disorders are marked by enhanced involvement of eosinophils. There is a need to develop therapeutic agents that can mitigate their deleterious effects by suppressing eosinophil development, recruitment, and activation.

REFERENCES

Introduction

1. Rothenberg ME, Hogan SP. The eosinophil. Annu Rev Immunol 2006;24:147-74.
2. Dvorak AM, Weller PF. Ultrastructural analysis of human eosinophils. Chem Immunol 2000;76:1-28.
3. Loutfy MR, Wilson M, Keystone JS, Kain KC. Serology and eosinophil count in the diagnosis and management of strongyloidiasis in a non-endemic area. Am J Trop Med Hyg 2002;66: 749-52.
4. Newberry AM, Williams DN, Stauffer WM, et al. Strongyloides hyperinfection presenting as acute respiratory failure and gram-negative sepsis. Chest 2005;128:3681-4.

Allergic Disorders

5. Mullarkey MF. Eosinophilic nonallergic rhinitis. J Allergy Clin Immunol 1988;82:941-9.
6. Amorim MM, Araruna A, Caetano LB, et al. Nasal eosinophilia: an indicator of eosinophilic inflammation in asthma. Clin Exp Allergy 2010;40:867-74.
7. Ellis AK, Keith PK. Nonallergic rhinitis with eosinophilia syndrome and related disorders. Clin Allergy Immunol 2007;19:87-100.
8. Baroody FM, Hughes CA, McDowell P, et al. Eosinophilia in chronic childhood sinusitis. Arch Otolaryngol Head Neck Surg 1995;121: 1396-402.
9. Ponikau JU, Sherris DA, Kephart GM, et al. Features of airway remodeling and eosinophilic inflammation in chronic rhinosinusitis: is the histopathology similar to asthma? J Allergy Clin Immunol 2003;112:877-82.
10. Ryan MW. Allergic fungal rhinosinusitis. Otolaryngol Clin North Am 2011;44: 697-710.
11. Bousquet J, Chanez P, Lacoste JY, et al. Eosinophilic inflammation in asthma. N Engl J Med 1990;323:1033-9.
12. Brightling CE, Monteiro W, Ward R, et al. Sputum eosinophilia and short-term response to prednisolone in chronic obstructive pulmonary disease: a randomised controlled trial. Lancet 2000;356:1480-5.
13. Birring SS, Parker D, McKenna S, et al. Sputum eosinophilia in idiopathic pulmonary fibrosis. Inflamm Res 2005;54:51-6.
14. Romagosa R, Kapoor S, Sanders J, Berman B. Inpatient adverse cutaneous drug eruptions and eosinophilia. Arch Dermatol 2001;137: 511-2.
15. Junghans RP, Manning W, Safar M, Quist W. Biventricular cardiac thrombosis during interleukin-2 infusion. N Engl J Med 2001; 344:859-60.
16. Allen JN. Drug-induced eosinophilic lung disease. Clin Chest Med 2004;25:77-88.
17. Camus P, Fanton A, Bonniaud P, et al. Interstitial lung disease induced by drugs and radiation. Respiration 2004;71:301-26.
18. Foucher P, Camus P. Pneumotox on line: the drug-induced respiratory disease website. Available at http://www.pneumotox.com (accessed February 14, 2013).
19. Souza CA, Muller NL, Johkoh T, Akira M. Drug-induced eosinophilic pneumonia: high-resolution CT findings in 14 patients. AJR Am J Roentgenol 2006;186:368-73.
20. Bullington W, Sahn SA, Judson MA. Valproic acid-induced eosinophilic pleural effusion: a case report and review of the literature. Am J Med Sci 2007;333:290-2.
21. Huggins JT, Sahn SA. Drug-induced pleural disease. Clin Chest Med 2004;25:141-53.
22. Fletcher A. Eosinophiluria and acute interstitial nephritis. N Engl J Med 2008;358: 1760-1.
23. Barton M, Finkelstein Y, Opavsky MA, et al. Eosinophilic myocarditis temporally associated with conjugate meningococcal C and hepatitis B vaccines in children. Pediatr Infect Dis J 2008;27:831-5.
24. Schoepfer AM, Engel A, Fattinger K, et al. Herbal does not mean innocuous: ten cases of

severe hepatotoxicity associated with dietary supplements from Herbalife products. J Hepatol 2007;47:521-6.
25. Cacoub P, Musette P, Descamps V, et al. The DRESS syndrome: a literature review. Am J Med 2011;124:588-97.
26. Wolf R, Orion E, Marcos B, Matz H. Life-threatening acute adverse cutaneous drug reactions. Clin Dermatol 2005;23:171-81.
27. Bahrami S, Malone JC, Webb KG, Callen JP. Tissue eosinophilia as an indicator of drug-induced cutaneous small-vessel vasculitis. Arch Dermatol 2006;142:155-61.

Infectious Diseases

28. Gil H, Magy N, Mauny F, Dupond JL. Valeur de l'eosinopenie dans le diagnostic des syndromes inflammatoires disorders: un "vieux" marquer revisite. Rev Med Interne 2003;24:431-5.
29. Wilson ME, Weller PF. Eosinophilia. In: Guerrant RL, Walker DH, Weller PF, editors. Tropical infectious diseases: principles, pathogens and practice. 3rd ed. Philadelphia: Churchill Livingstone; 2011. p. 939-49.
30. Kim YJ, Nutman TB. Eosinophilia: causes and pathobiology in persons with prior exposures in tropical areas with an emphasis on parasitic infections. Curr Infect Dis Rep 2006;8:43-50.
31. Starr J, Pruett JH, Yunginger JW, Gleich GJ. Myiasis due to *Hypoderma lineatum* infection mimicking the hypereosinophilic syndrome. Mayo Clin Proc 2000;75:755-9.
32. Centers for Disease Control and Prevention. Notes from the field: acute muscular sarcocystosis among returning travelers—Tioman Island, Malaysia. MMWR Morb Mortal Wkly Rep 2012;61:37-8.
33. Cohen AJ, Steigbigel RT. Eosinophilia in patients infected with human immunodeficiency virus. J Infect Dis 1996;174:615-8.

Hematologic and Neoplastic Disorders

34. Chusid MJ, Dale DC, West BC, Wolff SM. The hypereosinophilic syndrome: analysis of fourteen cases with review of the literature. Medicine (Baltimore) 1975;54:1-27.
35. Klion AD, Bochner BS, Gleich GJ, et al. Approaches to the treatment of hypereosinophilic syndromes: a workshop summary report. J Allergy Clin Immunol 2006;117:1292-302.
36. Simon HU, Rothenberg ME, Bochner BS, et al. Refining the definition of hypereosinophilic syndrome. J Allergy Clin Immunol 2010;126:45-9.
37. Crane MM, Chang CM, Kobayashi MG, Weller PF. Incidence of myeloproliferative hypereosinophilic syndrome in the United States and an estimate of all hypereosinophilic syndrome incidence. J Allergy Clin Immunol 2010;126:179-81.
38. Ogbogu PU, Bochner BS, Butterfield JH, et al. Hypereosinophilic syndrome: a multicenter, retrospective analysis of clinical characteristics and response to therapy. J Allergy Clin Immunol 2009;124:1319-25.
39. Klion AD, Noel P, Akin C, et al. Elevated serum tryptase levels identify a subset of patients with a myeloproliferative variant of idiopathic hypereosinophilic syndrome associated with tissue fibrosis, poor prognosis, and imatinib responsiveness. Blood 2003;101:4660-6.
40. Cools J, DeAngelo DJ, Gotlib J, et al. A tyrosine kinase created by fusion of PDGFRA and FIP1L1 genes as a therapeutic target of imatinib in idiopathic hypereosinophilic syndrome. N Engl J Med 2003;348:1201-14.
41. Metzgeroth G, Walz C, Erben P, et al. Safety and efficacy of imatinib in chronic eosinophilic leukemia and hypereosinophilic syndrome: a phase-II study. Br J Haematol 2008;143:707-15.
42. Chang HW, Leong KH, Koh DR, et al. Clonality of isolated eosinophils in the hypereosinophilic syndrome. Blood 1999;93:1651-7.
43. Roufosse F, Cogan E, Goldman M. Lymphocytic variant hypereosinophilic syndromes. Immunol Allergy Clin North Am 2007;27:389-413.
44. Weller PF, Bubley GJ. The idiopathic hypereosinophilic syndrome. Blood 1994;83:2759-79.
45. Tai PC, Ackerman SJ, Spry CJ. Deposits of eosinophil granule proteins in cardiac tissues of patients with eosinophilic endomyocardial disease. Lancet 1987;1:643-7.
46. Pitini V, Arrigo C, Azzarello D, et al. Serum concentration of cardiac troponin T in patients with hypereosinophilic syndrome treated with imatinib is predictive of adverse outcomes. Blood 2003;102:3456-7; author reply, 3457.
47. Ogbogu PU, Rosing DR, Horne MK 3rd. Cardiovascular manifestations of hypereosinophilic syndromes. Immunol Allergy Clin North Am 2007;27:457-75.
48. Plastiras SC, Economopoulos N, Kelekis NL, Tzelepis GE. Magnetic resonance imaging of the heart in a patient with hypereosinophilic syndrome. Am J Med 2006;119:130-2.
49. Fuzellier JF, Chapoutot L, Torossian PF. Mitral valve repair in idiopathic hypereosinophilic syndrome. J Heart Valve Dis 2004;13:529-31.
50. Moore PM, Harley JB, Fauci AS. Neurologic dysfunction in the idiopathic hypereosinophilic syndrome. Ann Intern Med 1985;102:109-14.
51. Barouky R, Bencharif L, Badet F, et al. Mucosal ulcerations revealing primitive hypereosinophilic syndrome. Eur J Dermatol 2003;13:207-8.
52. McPherson T, Cowen EW, McBurney E, Klion AD. Platelet-derived growth factor receptor-alpha-associated hypereosinophilic syndrome and lymphomatoid papulosis. Br J Dermatol 2006;155:824-6.
53. Lefebvre C, Bletry O, Degoulet P, et al. Facteurs pronostiques du syndrome hyperéosinophilique. Étude de 40 observations. Ann Med Interne (Paris) 1989;140:253-7.
54. Rothenberg ME, Klion AD, Roufosse FE, et al. Treatment of patients with the hypereosinophilic syndrome with mepolizumab. N Engl J Med 2008;358:1215-28.
55. Cooper MA, Akard LP, Thompson JM, Dugan MJ, Jansen J. Hypereosinophilic syndrome: long-term remission following allogeneic stem cell transplant in spite of transient eosinophilia post-transplant. Am J Hematol 2005;78:33-6.
56. Ueno NT, Anagnostopoulos A, Rondon G, et al. Successful non-myeloablative allogeneic transplantation for treatment of idiopathic hypereosinophilic syndrome. Br J Haematol 2002;119:131-4.
57. Bain B. The idiopathic hypereosinophilic syndrome and eosinophilic leukemias. Haematologica 2004;89:133-7.
58. Pardanani A, Reeder T, Li CY, Tefferi A. Eosinophils are derived from the neoplastic clone in patients with systemic mastocytosis and eosinophilia. Leuk Res 2003;27:883-85.
59. Enblad G, Sundstrom C, Glimelius B. Infiltration of eosinophils in Hodgkin's disease involved lymph nodes predicts prognosis. Hematol Oncol 1993;11:187-93.
60. Borish L, Dishuk J, Cox L, et al. Sézary syndrome with elevated serum IgE and hypereosinophilia: role of dysregulated cytokine production. J Allergy Clin Immunol 1993;92:123-31.
61. Samoszuk M, Ramzi E, Cooper DL. Interleukin-5 mRNA in three T-cell lymphomas with eosinophilia. Am J Hematol 1993;42:402-4.
62. Wilson F, Tefferi A. Acute lymphocytic leukemia with eosinophilia: two case reports and a review of the literature. Leuk Lymphoma 2005;46:1045-50.
63. Tancrede-Bohin E, Ionescu MA, de La Salmoniere P, et al. Prognostic value of blood eosinophilia in primary cutaneous T-cell lymphomas. Arch Dermatol 2004;140:1057-61.

Diseases with Specific Organ Involvement

64. Staumont-Salle D, Dombrowicz D, Capron M, et al. Eosinophils and urticaria. Clin Rev Allergy Immunol 2006;30:13-8.
65. Stone JH, Zen Y, Deshpande V. IgG4-related disease. N Engl J Med 2012;366:539-51.
66. Gleich GJ, Schroeter AL, Marcoux JP, et al. Episodic angioedema associated with eosinophilia. N Engl J Med 1984;310:1621-6.
67. Morgan SJ, Prince HM, Westerman DA, McCormack C, Glapole I. Clonal T-helper lymphocytes and elevated IL-5 levels in episodic angioedema and eosinophilia (Gleich's syndrome). Leuk Lymphoma 2003;44:1623-5.
68. Matsuda M, Fushimi T, Nakamura A, Ikeda S. Nonepisodic angioedema with eosinophilia: a report of two cases and a review of the literature. Clin Rheumatol 2006;25:422-5.
69. Yuen HW, Goh YH, Low WK, Lim-Tan SK. Kimura's disease: a diagnostic and therapeutic challenge. Singapore Med J 2005;46:179-83.
70. Kempf W, Haeffner AC, Zepter K, et al. Angiolymphoid hyperplasia with eosinophilia: evidence for a T-cell lymphoproliferative origin. Hum Pathol 2002;33:1023-9.
71. Moulton SJ, Kransdorf MJ, Ginsburg WW, Abril A, Persellin S. Eosinophilic fasciitis: spectrum of MRI findings. AJR Am J Roentgenol 2005;184:975-78.
72. Moossavi M, Mehregan DR. Wells' syndrome: a clinical and histopathologic review of seven cases. Int J Dermatol 2003;42:62-7.
73. Alobeid B, Pan LX, Milligan L, Frizzera G. Eosinophil-rich $CD30^+$ lymphoproliferative disorder of the oral mucosa: a form of "traumatic eosinophilic granuloma" Am J Clin Pathol 2004;121:43-50.
74. Rajendran PM, Dolev JC, Heaphy MR Jr, Mauerer T. Eosinophilic folliculitis: before and after the introduction of antiretroviral therapy. Arch Dermatol 2005;141:1227-31.
75. Fernandez Perez ER, Olson AL, Frankel SK. Eosinophilic lung diseases. Med Clin North Am 2011;95:1163-87.
76. Allen JN, Davis WB. Eosinophilic lung diseases. Am J Respir Crit Care Med 1994;150:1423-38.
77. Jederlinic PJ, Sicilian L, Gaensler EA. Chronic eosinophilic pneumonia: a report of 19 cases and a review of the literature. Medicine (Baltimore) 1988;67:154-62.
78. Johkoh T, Muller NL, Akira M, et al. Eosinophilic lung diseases: diagnostic accuracy of

thin-section CT in 111 patients. Radiology 2000;216:773-80.
79. Ross AG, Vickers D, Olds GR, Shah SM, McManus DP. Katayama syndrome. Lancet Infect Dis 2007;7:218-24.
80. Boggild AK, Keystone JS, Kain KC. Tropical pulmonary eosinophilia: a case series in a setting of nonendemicity. Clin Infect Dis 2004;39:1123-8.
81. Marchand E, Reynaud-Gaubert M, Lauque D, et al. Idiopathic chronic eosinophilic pneumonia: a clinical and follow-up study of 62 cases. The Groupe d'Etudes et de Recherche sur les Maladies "Orphelines" Pulmonaires (GERM"O"P). Medicine (Baltimore) 1998;77: 299-312.
82. Carrington CB, Addington WW, Goff AM, et al. Chronic eosinophilic pneumonia. N Engl J Med 1969;280:787-98.
83. Weller PF, Plaut M, Taggart V, Trontell A. The relationship of asthma therapy and Churg-Strauss syndrome: NIH workshop summary report. J Allergy Clin Immunol 2001;108: 175-83.
84. Tazelaar HD, Linz LJ, Colby TV, Myers JL, Limper AH. Acute eosinophilic pneumonia: histopathologic findings in nine patients. Am J Respir Crit Care Med 1997;155:296-302.
85. Philit F, Etienne-Mastroianni B, Parrot A, et al. Idiopathic acute eosinophilic pneumonia: a study of 22 patients. Am J Respir Crit Care Med 2002;166:1235-9.
86. Rom WN, Weiden M, Garcia R, et al. Acute eosinophilic pneumonia in a New York City firefighter exposed to World Trade Center dust. Am J Respir Crit Care Med 2002;166:797-800.
87. Watanabe K, Fujimura M, Kasahara K, et al. Acute eosinophilic pneumonia following cigarette smoking: a case report including cigarette-smoking challenge test. Intern Med 2002;41: 1016-20.
88. Shorr AF, Scoville SL, Cersovsky SB, et al. Acute eosinophilic pneumonia among US military personnel deployed in or near Iraq. JAMA 2004;292:2997-3005.
89. Pope-Harman AL, Davis WB, Allen ED, Christoforidis AJ, Allen JN. Acute eosinophilic pneumonia: a summary of 15 cases and review of the literature. Medicine (Baltimore) 1996; 75:334-42.
90. King MA, Pope-Harman AL, Allen JN, Christoforidis GA, Christoforidis AJ. Acute eosinophilic pneumonia: radiologic and clinical features. Radiology 1997;203:715-9.
91. Kalomenidis I, Light RW. Pathogenesis of the eosinophilic pleural effusions. Curr Opin Pulm Med 2004;10:289-93.
92. Krenke R, Nasilowski J, Korczynski P, et al. Incidence and aetiology of eosinophilic pleural effusion. Eur Respir J 2009;34:1111-7.
93. Rubins JB, Rubins HB. Etiology and prognostic significance of eosinophilic pleural effusions: a prospective study. Chest 1996;110:1271-4.
94. Allen JN, Davis WB, Pacht ER. Diagnostic significance of increased bronchoalveolar lavage fluid eosinophils. Am Rev Respir Dis 1990; 142:642-7.
95. Boomars KA, Wagenaar SS, Mulder PG, van Vetzen-Blad H, van den Bosch JM. Relationship between cells obtained by bronchoalveolar lavage and survival in idiopathic pulmonary fibrosis. Thorax 1995;50:1087-92.
96. Straumann A, Spichtin HP, Grize L, et al. Natural history of primary eosinophilic esophagitis: a follow-up of 30 adult patients for up to 11.5 years. Gastroenterology 2003;125: 1660-9.
97. Teitelbaum JE, Fox VL, Twarog FJ, et al. Eosinophilic esophagitis in children: immunopathological analysis and response to fluticasone propionate. Gastroenterology 2002;122: 1216-25.
98. Bischoff SC, Wedemeyer J, Herrmann A, et al. Quantitative assessment of intestinal eosinophils and mast cells in inflammatory bowel disease. Histopathology 1996;28:1-13.
99. Levy AM, Yamazaki K, Van Keulen VP, et al. Increased eosinophil infiltration and degranulation in colonic tissue from patients with collagenous colitis. Am J Gastroenterol 2001;96: 1522-8.
100. Kim YK, Kim CS, Moon WS, et al. MRI findings of focal eosinophilic liver diseases. AJR Am J Roentgenol 2005;184:1541-8.
101. Golden J, Frim DM, Chapman PH, Vonsettel JP. Marked tissue eosinophilia within organizing chronic subdural hematoma membranes. Clin Neuropathol 1994;13:12-6.
102. Lo Re V 3rd, Gluckman SJ. Eosinophilic meningitis. Am J Med 2003;114:217-23.
103. Kargili A, Bavbek N, Kaya A, Kosar A, Karaaslan Y. Eosinophilia in rheumatologic diseases: a prospective study of 1000 cases. Rheumatol Int 2004;24:321-4.
104. Bavbek N, Kargili A, Cipil H, Kosar A, Karaaslan Y. Rheumatologic disease with peripheral eosinophilia. Rheumatol Int 2004;24:317-20.
105. Tay C. Eosinophilic arthritis. Rheumatology (Oxford) 1999;38:1188-94.
106. Krahn M, Lopez de Munain A, Streichenberger N, et al. CAPN3 mutations in patients with idiopathic eosinophilic myositis. Ann Neurol 2006;59:905-11.
107. Kaufman LD, Kephart GM, Seidman RJ, et al. The spectrum of eosinophilic myositis: clinical and immunopathogenic studies of three patients, and review of the literature. Arthritis Rheum 1993;36:1014-24.
108. Brown JP, Rola-Pleszczynski M, Menard H-A. Eosinophilic synovitis: clinical observations on a newly recognized subset of patients with dermatographism. Arthritis Rheum 1986;29: 1147-51.
109. Atanes A, Fernandez V, Nunez R, et al. Idiopathic eosinophilic synovitis: case report and review of the literature. Scand J Rheumatol 1996;25:183-5.
110. Kaufman LD, Krupp LB. Eosinophilia-myalgia syndrome, toxic-oil syndrome, and diffuse fasciitis with eosinophilia. Curr Opin Rheumatol 1995;7:560-7.
111. Guillevin L, Cohen P, Gayraud M, et al. Churg-Strauss syndrome: clinical study and long-term follow-up of 96 patients. Medicine (Baltimore) 1999;78:26-37.
112. Churg A, Brallas M, Cronin SR, Churg J. Formes frustes of Churg-Strauss syndrome. Chest 1995;108:320-3.
113. Bili A, Condemi JJ, Bottone SM, Ryan CK. Seven cases of complete and incomplete forms of Churg-Strauss syndrome not related to leukotriene receptor antagonists. J Allergy Clin Immunol 1999;104:1060-5.
114. Priori R, Tomassini M, Magrini L, Conti F, Valesini G. Churg-Strauss syndrome during pregnancy after steroid withdrawal. Lancet 1998;352:1599-600.
115. Churg J, Strauss L. Allergic granulomatosis, allergic angiitis, and periarteritis nodosa. Am J Pathol 1951;27:277-301.
116. Lanham JG, Elkon KB, Pusey CD, Hughes GR. Systemic vasculitis with asthma and eosinophilia: a clinical approach to the Churg-Strauss syndrome. Medicine (Baltimore) 1984;63: 65-81.
117. Masi AT, Hunder GG, Lie JT, et al. The American College of Rheumatology 1990 criteria for the classification of Churg-Strauss syndrome (allergic granulomatosis and angiitis). Arthritis Rheum 1990;33:1094-100.
118. Chen KR, Ohata Y, Sakurai M, Nakayama H. Churg-Strauss syndrome: report of a case without preexisting asthma. J Dermatol 1992; 19:40-7.
119. Choi YH, Im JG, Han BK, et al. Thoracic manifestation of Churg-Strauss syndrome: radiologic and clinical findings. Chest 2000;117: 117-24.
120. Silva CI, Müller NL, Fujimoto K, et al. Churg-Strauss syndrome: high resolution CT and pathologic findings. J Thorac Imaging 2005; 20:74-80.
121. Olsen K, Neel H, DeRemee R, Weiland LH. Nasal manifestations of allergic granulomatosis and angiitis (Churg-Strauss). Otolaryngol Head Neck Surg 1980;88:85-9.
122. Sehgal M, Swanson JW, DeRemee RA, Colby TV. Neurologic manifestations of Churg-Strauss syndrome. Mayo Clin Proc 1995;70: 337-41.
123. Lie JT. Histopathologic specificity of systemic vasculitis. Rheum Dis Clin North Am 1995;21: 883-909.
124. Schwartz RA, Churg J. Churg-Strauss syndrome. Br J Dermatol 1992;127:199-204.
125. Tatsis E, Schnabel A, Gross WL. Interferon-alpha treatment of four patients with the Churg-Strauss syndrome. Ann Intern Med 1998;129:370-4.
126. Chen KR, Su WP, Pittelkow MR, et al. Eosinophilic vasculitis in connective tissue disease. J Am Acad Dermatol 1996;35:173-82.
127. Lie JT, Michet CJ Jr. Thromboangiitis obliterans with eosinophilia (Buerger's disease) of the temporal arteries. Hum Pathol 1988;19: 598-602.
128. Lane SE, Watts RA, Barker TH, Scott DG. Evaluation of the Sørensen diagnostic criteria in the classification of systemic vasculitis. Rheumatology (Oxford) 2002;41:1138-41.
129. Hunsaker JC 3rd, O'Connor WN, Lie JT. Is spontaneous dissection of the coronary artery with eosinophilia a limited form of Churg-Strauss syndrome? Arch Pathol Lab Med 1994;118:863-4.
130. Huang CY, Lu TM, Hsu CP, et al. Eosinophilia presenting as acute coronary syndrome. Am J Hematol 2004;76:94-5.
131. Blauwet LA, Breen JF, Edwards WD, Klarich KW. Atypical presentation of eosinophilic endomyocardial disease. Mayo Clin Proc 2005; 80:1078-84.
132. Nolan CRI, Anger MS, Kelleher SP. Eosinophiluria: a new method of detection and definition of the clinical spectrum. N Engl J Med 1986;315:1516-9.
133. Corwin HL, Korbet SM, Schwartz MM. Clinical correlates of eosinophiluria. Arch Intern Med 1985;145:1097-9.
134. Verhagen PC, Nikkels PG, de Jong TP. Eosinophilic cystitis. Arch Dis Child 2001;84:344-6.
135. Kilic S, Erguvan R, Ipek D, et al. Eosinophilic cystitis: a rare inflammatory pathology mimicking bladder neoplasms. Urol Int 2003;71: 285-9.

136. Chan MK, Chow L, Lam SS, Jones B. Peritoneal eosinophilia in patients on continuous ambulatory peritoneal dialysis: a prospective study. Am J Kidney Dis 1988;11:180-3.
137. Fontan MP, Rodriguez-Carmona A, Galed I, et al. Incidence and significance of peritoneal eosinophilia during peritoneal dialysis-related peritonitis. Perit Dial Int 2003;23:460-4.

Immunologic Reactions

138. Sowerwine KJ, Holland SM, Freeman AF. Hyper-IgE syndrome update. Ann N Y Acad Sci 2012;1250:25-32.
139. Wada T, Toma T, Okamoto H, et al. Oligoclonal expansion of T lymphocytes with multiple second-site mutations leads to Omenn syndrome in a patient with RAG1-deficient severe combined immunodeficiency. Blood 2005; 106:2099-101.
140. Mogayzel PJ Jr, Yang SC, Wise BV, Colombani PM. Eosinophilic infiltrates in a pulmonary allograft: a case and review of the literature. J Heart Lung Transplant 2001;20:692-5.
141. Saisu K, Morozumi K, Suzuki K, Fujita K. Significance of interstitial lesions as the early indicator for acute vascular rejection in human renal allografts. Clin Transplant 1999;13: 17-23.
142. Nagral A, Quaglia A, Sabin CA, et al. Blood and graft eosinophils in acute cellular rejection of liver allografts. Transplant Proc 2001;33: 2588-93.
143. Gollub SB, Huntrakoon M, Dunn MI. The significance of eosinophils in mild and moderate acute cardiac allograft rejection. Am J Cardiovasc Pathol 1990;3:21-6.
144. Emovon OE, King JA, Smith SR, et al. Clinical significance of eosinophils in suspicious or borderline renal allograft biopsies. Clin Nephrol 2003;59:367-72.
145. Yousem SA. Significance of clinically silent untreated mild acute cellular rejection in lung allograft recipients. Hum Pathol 1996;27: 269-73.
146. Ben-Ari Z, Dhillon AP, Garwood L, et al. Prognostic value of eosinophils for therapeutic response in severe acute hepatic allograft rejection. Transplant Proc 1996;28:3624-8.
147. Nolan CR, Saenz KP, Thomas CA III, Murph KD. Role of the eosinophil in chronic vascular rejection of renal allografts. Am J Kidney Dis 1995;26:634-42.
148. de Groen PC, Kephart GM, Gleich GJ, Ludwig J. The eosinophil as an effector cell of the immune response during hepatic allograft rejection. Hepatology 1994;20:654-62.
149. Marra DE, McKee PH, Nghiem P. Tissue eosinophils and the perils of using skin biopsy specimens to distinguish between drug hypersensitivity and cutaneous graft-versus-host disease. J Am Acad Dermatol 2004;51:543-6.

Eosinophils in Other Disorders

150. Beishuizen A, Vermes I, Hylkema BS, Haanen C. Relative eosinophilia and functional adrenal insufficiency in critically ill patients. Lancet 1999;353:1675-6.
151. Fukumoto Y, Tsutsui H, Tsuchihashi M, et al. The incidence and risk factors of cholesterol embolization syndrome, a complication of cardiac catheterization: a prospective study. J Am Coll Cardiol 2003;42:211-6.
152. Klion AD, Law MA, Riemenschneider W, et al. Familial eosinophilia: a benign disorder? Blood 2004;103:4050-5.

76 Mastocytosis

DEAN D. METCALFE

CONTENTS

SUMMARY OF IMPORTANT CONCEPTS

» Mast cells arise from pluripotential stem cells.
» The one obligatory growth factor for human mast cell proliferation and survival is stem cell factor, which acts through the receptor KIT.
» Most adult patients with mastocytosis have an activating mutation in KIT.
» The signs and symptoms in mastocytosis are caused by the release of mast cell mediators, the increase in mast cell burden, and in some patients an associated hematologic disorder.
» The treatment of mastocytosis is largely symptomatic, with specific treatment of any associated hematologic disorder.
» Newer tyrosine kinase inhibitors show promise for the treatment of some specific variants of mastocytosis.

Introduction

Mastocytosis is a disease with clinical features that include pruritus, flushing, nausea, vomiting, diarrhea, abdominal pain, and vascular instability. The most remarkable pathologic features of mastocytosis are mast cell hyperplasia in the skin, gastrointestinal (GI) tract, bone marrow, liver, spleen, and lymph nodes, as well as the frequent association of mast cell hyperplasia with hematologic disorders.

Mastocytosis is further classified into disease variants based on clinical presentation, pathologic findings, and prognosis. The diagnostic criteria and classification of variants of systemic mastocytosis are shown in Boxes 76-1 and 76-2.[1] Patients with cutaneous mastocytosis (CM) who do not meet the criteria for systemic disease have the best prognosis, followed by those with indolent systemic mastocytosis (ISM). Patients with systemic mastocytosis with an associated clonal, hematologic non–mast cell lineage disease (SM-AHNMD), aggressive systemic mastocytosis (ASM), or mast cell leukemia (MCL) experience a more rapid and complex disease course. Patients with CM or ISM may experience progressive difficulties, but their condition may be managed for decades with medications that offer largely symptomatic therapy. In patients with SM-AHNMD, examination of the peripheral blood and bone marrow leads to the diagnosis of one of several hematologic disorders. Survival of these patients is determined by the course of the hematologic disorder.

Patients with ASM or MCL have a poor prognosis, as do those with mast cell sarcoma (MCS). Patients with ASM experience a rapid increase in the number of mast cells. Medical management may be difficult, and prognosis is less favorable. MCL is rare, with the most fulminant behavior and where numerous immature mast cells are found in peripheral blood smears. MCL is distinguished from the other disease types by its clinicopathologic picture. MCS is exceedingly rare, and a leukemia phase may occur.

Historical Perspective

Mast cells are easily identified because their cytoplasm is filled with dense, metachromatic granules that stain red or violet when treated with basic aniline dyes. Using this "metachromasia," Ehrlich[2] first described mast cells, or "mastzellen," in 1878 and speculated that these granules were the product of overfeeding. He also noted that mast cells tend to be associated with blood vessels, nerves, and glandular ducts. In 1894, Unna[3] reported that the cutaneous lesions termed *urticaria pigmentosa* (UP) were associated with increased mast cells below each lesion. Following reports that mast cells could "explosively" release their granules on contact with irritants, Webb[4] reported in 1931 that the peritoneal cells of the rat undergo degranulation after irritation by such agents as egg white, known to cause a peculiar, urticaria-like reaction when injected intraperitoneally into the rat. Within a few years, mast cells had been identified as carriers of heparin[5] and histamine.[6] These observations, as well as knowledge that histamine and heparin were released simultaneously from dog liver in anaphylactic shock, led to the conclusion by the 1950s that mast cells played an important function in allergic diseases.

Over time, researchers observed that significant mast cell hyperplasia occurred in association with pathologic conditions (e.g., parasitosis) and in diseases that would later be classified as variants of mastocytosis. The first description of a disease that was apparently UP is attributed to Nettleship and Tay[7] in 1869, later termed UP by Sangster[8] in 1878. In 1949, Ellis[9]

BOX 76-1 WHO DIAGNOSTIC CRITERIA FOR CUTANEOUS AND SYSTEMIC MASTOCYTOSIS

CUTANEOUS MASTOCYTOSIS

Typical clinical findings of urticaria pigmentosa/maculopapular cutaneous mastocytosis (UP/MPCM), diffuse cutaneous mastocytosis (DCM), or solitary mastocytoma, with typical infiltrates of mast cells in a multifocal or diffuse pattern on skin biopsy.

SYSTEMIC MASTOCYTOSIS

Diagnosis is made if one major and one minor criterion are present, or if three minor criteria are met.

Major Criterion

Multifocal, dense infiltrates of mast cells (≥15 in aggregates) detected in sections of bone marrow and/or another extracutaneous organ and confirmed by tryptase immunohistochemistry or other special stains.

Minor Criteria

a. In biopsy sections of bone marrow or other extracutaneous organs, more than 25% of the mast cells in the infiltrate are spindle shaped or have atypical morphology, or of all mast cells in bone marrow aspirates smears, more than 25% are immature or atypical mast cells.
b. Detection of an activating point mutation at codon 816 of KIT in bone marrow, blood, or another extracutaneous organ.
c. Mast cells in bone marrow, blood, or another extracutaneous organ express CD117 with CD2 and/or CD25.
d. Serum total tryptase persistently greater than 20 ng/mL in the absence of an associated clonal myeloid disorder.

Modified from Horny H-P, et al. Mastocytosis. In: Swerdlow SH, et al, editors. WHO classification of tumors of haematopoietic and lymphoid tissues. Lyon: IARC Press; 2008.
WHO, World Health Organization.

described an autopsy report of a fatal case of UP in a 1-year-old child, documenting mast cell infiltrations in the skin, liver, spleen, lymph nodes and bone marrow. The many descriptions of variants of mastocytosis that followed were organized into classification schemes, most recently by the World Health Organization (WHO).[1]

Epidemiology

Mastocytosis is a rare disease, with a reported male/female ratio of 1 : 1 to 1 : 3. Although its prevalence is unknown, an estimated 20,000 to 30,000 individuals are affected in the United States. Patients from all ethnic backgrounds have the disease, but mastocytosis is more frequently reported in Caucasians.[10] Mastocytosis may occur at any age, including infancy, and may be present at birth; familial occurrence is unusual. Variants of disease are now believed to depend in part on specific inherited genetic polymorphisms and acquired somatic mutations.

Pathogenesis and Etiology

Clonal mast cell disorders arise from mutations in critical receptors and intracellular signaling pathways that control mast cell proliferation and survival. As human mast cells develop from a bone marrow–derived hematopoietic pluripotential precursor cell (CD34$^+$, KIT [CD117]$^+$), systemic mast cell disorders may be accompanied by disturbances in number and function of other hematopoietically derived cells.[11] Human mast cells then complete maturation in vascularized tissues. During this maturation, the cells downregulate CD34 but remain CD117$^+$. Mature mast cells have prominent cytoplasmic granules that contain histamine, other chemical mediators, and surface receptors that bind the Fc portion of immunoglobulin E (IgE) with high affinity. Mast cells within tissues are often found adjacent to blood vessels and under epithelial surfaces. They are prominent in the GI and respiratory tracts, lymphoid tissues, and skin. Mature mast cells normally do not circulate, are long-lived, and appear to retain a limited capacity to proliferate.

When CD34$^+$ cells from human bone marrow are cultured with stem cell factor (SCF), mast cells are generated.[12] Correspondingly, stromal cells within tissues produce SCF, which then interacts with KIT and promotes mast cell differentiation and survival. When factors that support mast cell growth are withdrawn, mast cells undergo apoptosis.[13]

The protooncogene *c-kit* encodes KIT, the transmembrane tyrosine kinase receptor for SCF. KIT is expressed on mast cells, hematopoietic stem cells, melanocytes, and germ cell lineages. Loss-of-function mutations in KIT are involved in the hereditary disease *piebaldism,* which is characterized by loss of pigmentation. Gain-of-function point mutations have been identified in patients with systemic mast cell proliferative disorders. The most common mutation consists of a substitution of valine for aspartic acid (ASP 816 VAL).[14] An activating point mutation at codon 816 in KIT is present in most adults with various forms of mastocytosis. However, the mutation cannot be identified in many children with CM. These latter observations support the concept that mastocytosis is partly the result of "overactive" KIT in most patients with mastocytosis, with other, secondary or coexisting events giving rise to the mastocytosis disease variants. One such example is the identification of a mutation in NRAS in addition to an activating mutation in KIT in some patients with aggressive mastocytosis.[15] There is yet no convincing evidence that the ASP 816 VAL (D816V) mutation is passed from generation to generation.

Additional *c-kit* mutations have since been identified that may play a role in the etiology of mastocytosis in some patients. These mutations consist of V560G within the juxtamembrane domain of KIT and detected in the human MCL cell line HMC-1; D816Y, D816F, and D816H; the E839K-dominant inactivating mutation in several reported cases of pediatric mastocytosis; and the rare germline mutation F522C. Exceedingly rare *c-kit* mutations, reported in less than 1% of patients with mastocytosis, include R815K, D820G, V533D, V559A, del419, K509I, and A533D. KIT-dependent downstream signaling events, including the JAK-STAT pathway, may also magnify the consequences of mutations in KIT.[16]

In addition to KIT-dependent pathways, inhibition of mast cell apoptosis through other biologic pathways may also contribute to the pathogenesis of mast cell–related disorders. A subset of patients with increased mast cells and peripheral eosinophilia and an increase in serum tryptase levels has been described that carry the Fip1-like-1-platelet-derived growth factor receptor (FIP1L1-PDGFRA) fusion oncogene in pluripotential hematopoietic progenitor cells, which results from an approximately 800-kb interstitial deletion of chromosome 4q12.[17] Similarly, a rare case of systemic mastocytosis and chronic basophilic leukemia was found secondary to a PRKG2-PDGFRB fusion.[18] Disease associated with mutations in *c-kit* may be modified by the patient's genetic composition. For example, a polymorphism in the gene for the interleukin-4

BOX 76-2 WHO CRITERIA FOR VARIANTS OF SYSTEMIC MASTOCYTOSIS

Indolent Systemic Mastocytosis (ISM)*

Meets criteria for systemic mastocytosis (SM; see Box 76-1).
No "C" findings (see below).
No evidence of an associated clonal, hematologic non–mast cell lineage disease (AHNMD).
In this variant the mast cell burden is low, and skin lesions are usually present.
Bone marrow mastocytosis
As above for ISM with bone marrow involvement, but no skin lesions.
Smoldering systemic mastocytosis
As above for ISM, but with two or more "B" findings* and no "C" findings.†

Systemic Mastocytosis with Associated Clonal, Hematologic Non–Mast Cell Lineage Disease (SM-AHNMD)

Meets criteria for SM and criteria for AHNMD (MDS, MPN, AML, lymphoma, or other hematologic neoplasm that meets criteria for distinct entity in WHO classification).

Aggressive Systemic Mastocytosis (ASM)

Meets criteria for SM with one or more "C" findings.†
No evidence of mast cell leukemia.
Usually without skin lesions.
Lymphadenopathic mastocytosis with eosinophilia
Progressive lymphadenopathy with peripheral blood eosinophilia, often with extensive bone involvement, and hepatosplenomegaly, but usually without skin lesions.
Cases with rearrangement of PDGFRA are excluded.

Mast Cell Leukemia (MCL)

Meets criteria for SM.
Bone marrow biopsy shows a diffuse infiltration by atypical, immature mast cells.
Bone marrow aspirate smears show 20% or more mast cells; mast cells account for 10% or more of peripheral blood white cells.
Variant: Leukemic mast cell leukemia as above, but less than 10% of white blood cells are mast cells; usually without skin lesions.

Mast Cell Sarcoma (MCS)

Unifocal mast cell tumor.
No evidence of SM.
Destructive growth pattern; high-grade cytology.

Extracutaneous Mastocytoma

Unifocal mast cell tumor.
No evidence of SM.
No skin lesions; nondestructive growth pattern; low-grade cytology.

Modified from Horny H-P, et al. Mastocytosis. In: Swerdlow SH, et al, editors. WHO classification of tumors of haematopoietic and lymphoid tissues. Lyon: IARC Press; 2008.

AML, Acute myeloid leukemia; *ANC,* absolute neutrophil count; *Hb,* hemoglobin; *MDS,* myelodysplasia; *MPN,* myeloproliferative neoplasm.

*"B" findings
1. Bone marrow biopsy showing greater than 30% infiltration by mast cells (focal, dense aggregates) and/or serum total tryptase level greater than 200 ng/mL.
2. Signs of dysplasia or myeloproliferation in non–mast cell lineages, but insufficient criteria for definitive diagnosis of a hematopoietic neoplasm with normal or slightly abnormal blood counts.
3. Hepatomegaly without impairment of liver function, and/or palpable splenomegaly without hypersplenism, and/or lymphadenopathy.

†"C" findings
1. Bone marrow dysfunction manifested by one or more cytopenia (ANC <1.0 × 10^9/L, Hb <10 g/dL, or platelets <100 × 10^9/L), but no obvious non–mast cell hematopoietic malignancy.
2. Palpable hepatomegaly with impairment of liver function, ascites, and/or portal hypertension.
3. Skeletal involvement with large osteolytic lesions and/or pathologic fractures.
4. Palpable splenomegaly with hypersplenism.
5. Malabsorption with weight loss caused by gastrointestinal mast cell infiltrates.

(IL-4) receptor α chain is associated with less extensive mast cell involvement. In addition, the bone marrow cells of patients with mastocytosis constitutively express the antiapoptotic proteins Bcl-XL and Bcl-2.

PATHOLOGIC EFFECTS OF INCREASED MAST CELLS

Mast cells secrete chemicals that initiate inflammation. The pathologic changes observed in mastocytosis are the result of the increased number of mast cells within tissues and the local release of mast cell mediators. These mediators also circulate through the bloodstream and lymphatic system to produce biologic effects at sites distant from the site of their release (Table 76-1). These effects appear similar regardless of the specific defect underlying the pathologic increase in mast cells or the category of disease.

The biologic effects of *histamine* result from the activation of H_1 through H_4 cell surface receptors and are prominent in mastocytosis. The H_1 receptors are blocked by antihistamines such as hydroxyzine and fexofenadine and are involved in the histamine-induced contraction of bronchial and GI smooth muscle. The H_2 receptors play a major role in the increased secretion of gastric acid by parietal cells and are blocked by drugs such as famotidine and ranitidine. Histamine enhances vascular permeability by acting on the endothelial cells in the postcapillary venules. The protease *tryptase* is a major component of the mast cell secretory granule, and the mature form (measured as the major component of total tryptase in commercial assays) is released after mast cell stimulation. Histamine and tryptase levels are usually found to be elevated in the serum of mastocytosis patients.[1] Human mast cells make prostaglandin D_2 (PGD_2) and leukotriene C_4 (LTC_4). These lipid-derived molecules have a wide spectrum of biologic activities (see Box 76-1). Mast cells also produce a variety of proinflammatory and growth factor cytokines, including tumor necrosis factor-α (TNF-α), interleukin-3 (IL-3), IL-16, and IL-33.

Clinical Features

All variants of mastocytosis present similar clinical features, although some aspects of disease may predominate in a specific

TABLE 76-1 Major Human Mast Cell–Derived Mediators*

Class	Mediators	Physiologic Effects
Preformed mediators	Histamine, heparin, neutral proteases (tryptase and chymase, carboxypeptidase, cathepsin G), major basic protein, acid hydrolases, peroxidase, phospholipases	Vasodilation Vasoconstriction Angiogenesis Mitogenesis Pain Arachidonic acid generation Tissue damage and repair Inflammation
Lipid mediators	LTB_4, LTC_4, PGE_2, PGD_2, PAF	Leukocyte chemotaxis Vasoconstriction Bronchoconstriction Platelet activation Vasodilation
Cytokines	TNF-α, TGF-β, IFN-α, IFN-β, IL-1α, IL-1β, IL-5, IL-6, IL-13, IL-16, IL-18, IL-33	Inflammation Leukocyte migration and proliferation
Chemokines	IL-8 (CXCL8), I-309 (CCL1), MCP-1 (CCL2), MIP-1αS (CCL3), MIP-1β (CCL4), MCP-3 (CCL7), RANTES (CCL5), eotaxin (CCL11), MCAF (MCP-1)	Chemoattraction and tissue infiltration of leukocytes
Growth factors	SCF, M-CSF, GM-CSF, bFGF, VEGF, NGF, PDGF	Growth of various cell types Vasodilation Neovascularization Angiogenesis

CSF, Colony-stimulating factor; *IFN*, interferon; *IL*, interleukin; *LT*, leukotriene; *PAF*, platelet-activating factor; *PG*, prostaglandin; *SCF*, stem cell factor.

*Examples only; those listed may have been identified only in human mast cell lines or primary cultures of human mast cells.

category (see Box 76-2). The skin, GI tract, lymph nodes, liver, spleen, bone marrow, and skeletal system contribute the most significant management problems. The respiratory tract and endocrine and renal systems are seldom, if ever, primarily involved. Patients in every category of mastocytosis sometimes experience flushing and episodic hypotension. Occasionally, hypotension may be provoked by alcohol, aspirin, insect stings, infection, or exposure to iodinated contrast materials. Patients with mastocytosis do not experience an increase in bacterial, fungal, or viral infections.

CHARACTERISTIC PATTERNS OF SKIN INVOLVEMENT

The most common skin manifestation of mastocytosis in both children (Fig. 76-1, *A* and *B*) and adults (Fig. 76-2) is urticaria pigmentosa (UP)/maculopapular cutaneous mastocytosis (MPCM) (see Box 76-2). It is the most common pattern of skin involvement. UP is also observed in more than 90% of patients with ISM and about 50% of patients with SM-AHNMD or those with ASM. UP lesions appear as small, yellowish tan to reddish brown macules or slightly raised papules (Fig. 76-3) and occasionally as raised nodules or plaquelike lesions (see Fig. 76-1, *C* and *D*). The palms, soles, face, and scalp tend to remain free of lesions. Rubbing of the lesions usually leads to urtication and erythema over and around the macules, known as Darier sign.[19,20] UP may be associated with pruritus that is exacerbated by changes in temperature, local friction, ingestion of hot beverages or spicy foods, ethanol, and certain drugs. Histologically, UP lesions are composed of a collection of mast cells within the papillary dermis, with variable extension throughout the reticular dermis and into the subcutaneous fat. An increase in dermal mast cells approximately 10 times that of normal skin, in the absence of other pathology, is generally diagnostic of UP.[19] Petechiae, ecchymoses, or telangiectasias may be present in or adjacent to UP lesions.

Diffuse cutaneous mastocytosis (DCM) results from diffuse mast cell infiltration into the dermis and has no discrete lesions (Fig. 76-4). It usually has its onset before age 3 years. The entire cutaneous integument is involved. The skin is normal to yellowish brown, thickened, and may exhibit discoloration with a peau d'orange appearance. A generalized erythroderma may be present, in which severe edema gives the skin a doughy appearance. Additionally, yellow and cream-colored papules have been described that resemble xanthomas and pseudoxanthoma elasticum. The diagnosis is confirmed by the demonstration of diffuse mast cell infiltrates in the skin (Fig. 76-5).

Young children with UP or DCM may have bullous eruptions with hemorrhage (Fig. 76-6). Blisters may erupt spontaneously or in association with infection or immunization. Blisters may also occur at birth. CM is thus included in the differential diagnosis of neonatal disorders with blisters.

Solitary mastocytomas of the skin are a fairly common cutaneous variant of CM. They may be present at birth but more often appear before age 3 months. Cases usually spontaneously involute during childhood. Solitary extracutaneous mastocytomas of the lung have been reported in adults. As stated earlier, MCS is exceedingly rare and is characterized by a tumor consisting of highly atypical immature mast cells. Distant spread is possible, and a leukemia phase may occur.

Telangiectasia macularis eruptiva perstans (TMEP) is observed in less than 1% of patients with mastocytosis and has been reported only in adults.[20] The characteristic skin lesion in TMEP is a telangiectatic, red macule on a tan-brown background. Individual lesions are 2 to 6 mm in diameter and are without sharply defined borders. Pruritus, purpura, and blister formation are not generally associated with TMEP. Lesions may become edematous when rubbed. TMEP may occasionally coexist with UP.

GASTROINTESTINAL SYMPTOMS

In patients with mastocytosis, GI symptoms are almost as common as pruritus or flushing.[21-23] One typical study examined 16 consecutive patients referred with biopsy-proven mastocytosis, all of whom had fasting hyperhistaminemia and evidence of internal organ involvement.[22] Approximately 80% of patients had significant GI symptoms, second only to pruritus and almost twice as common as flushing.

Abdominal pain is the most common GI symptom, followed by diarrhea, nausea, and vomiting. GI bleeding is uncommon. Peptic ulcer disease is relatively infrequent despite hyperhistaminemia, occurring in 4% to 44% of all patients with systemic mastocytosis. In patients with positive endoscopic findings, most had abdominal pain classified as dyspeptic because it was

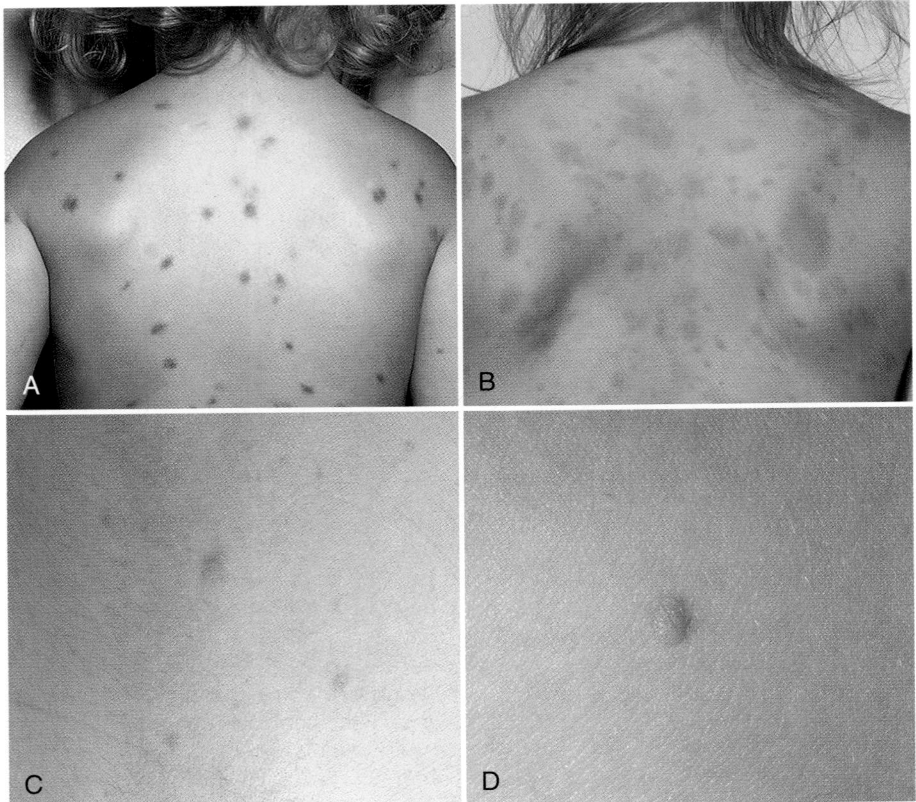

Figure 76-1 Urticaria pigmentosa in childhood. Lesions in **A** are smaller and more discrete than lesions in **B. C,** Example of nodular lesions of urticaria pigmentosa, with close-up view in **D.**

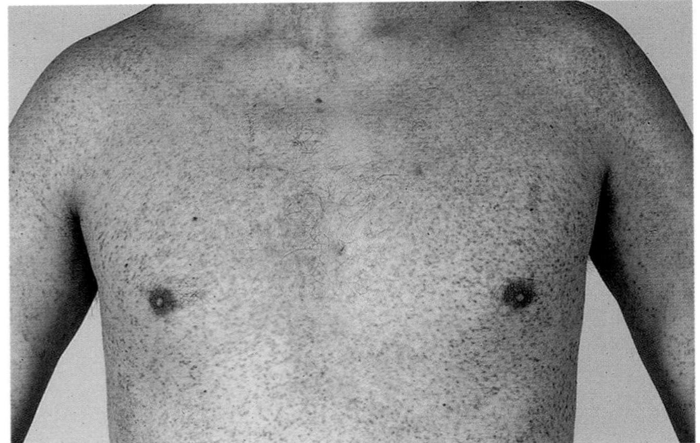

Figure 76-2 Urticaria pigmentosa in adult. Patient has indolent systemic mastocytosis.

Figure 76-3 Close-up of urticaria pigmentosa. This adult patient has indolent systemic mastocytosis.

relieved by antacids or H_2-receptor antagonists. Approximately 70% of patients with dyspeptic types of abdominal pain had evidence of gastric acid hypersecretion. Furthermore, the plasma concentration of histamine correlated with basal acid output.

The pathogenesis of abdominal symptoms in patients with systemic mastocytosis appears multifactorial. Abdominal pain thus has been reported secondary to peptic ulcer disease, edema or urticarial lesions of the GI tract, or a motility disorder.[22,23] Diarrhea is rarely secondary to gastric hypersecretion or malabsorption; studies suggest that it is secondary to altered intestinal secretion, structural disease of the small intestinal mucosa, or a hypermotility or transit disorder. In one study, most pain was described as peptic; in the remaining 30% of patients with abdominal pain, the pain was nonpeptic, was located in the lower abdomen, was not relieved by antacids or

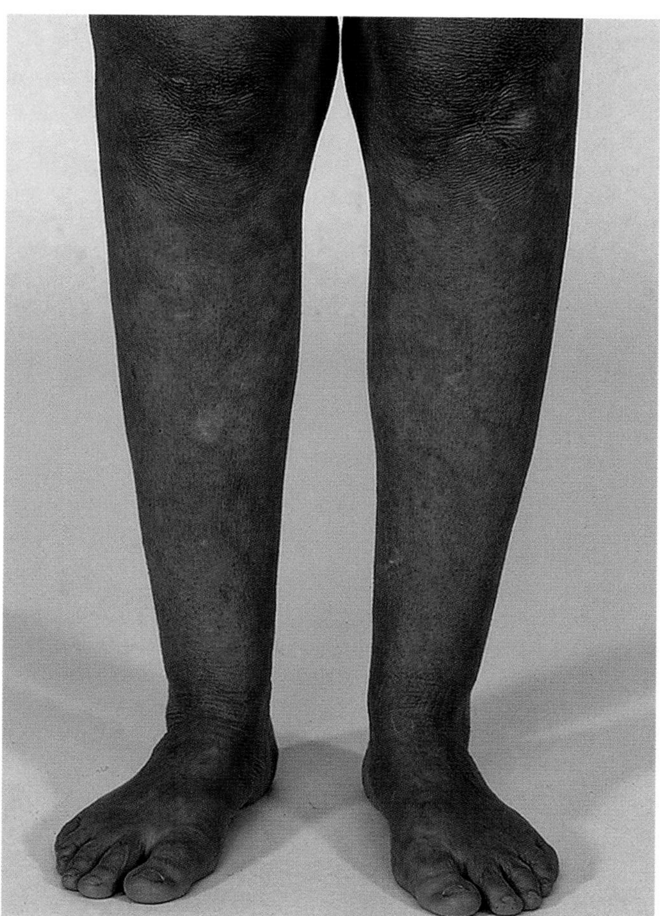

Figure 76-4 Diffuse cutaneous mastocytosis in adult.

H_2-receptor antagonists, and was not associated with abnormal endoscopy or gastrin hypersecretion.[22] Half the patients with diarrhea had an increased frequency of bowel movements and an increased fecal output (>200 g/day); the remaining half with diarrhea had an increased frequency of bowel movements but a normal fecal output. In patients with elevated fecal output, two thirds had an increased basal acid output, suggesting that gastric hypersecretion may be a contributing factor to the diarrhea. Some evidence of malabsorption was found in 31% of patients with systemic mastocytosis.[22] It was usually not severe and was manifested primarily as mild steatorrhea with impaired

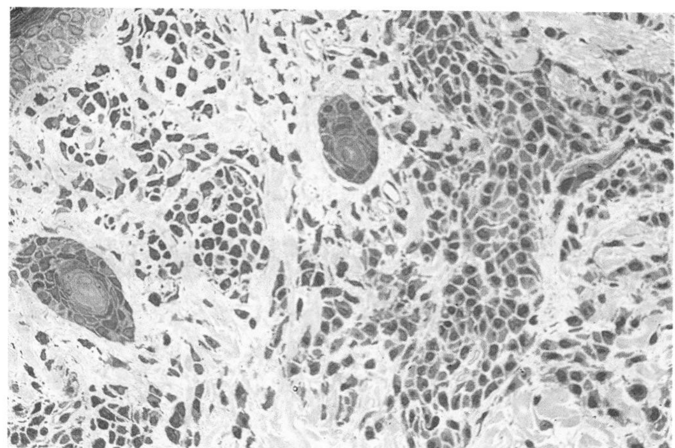

Figure 76-5 Diffuse cutaneous mastocytosis in child. Skin biopsy shows extensive mast cell infiltration. (Toluidine blue; ×250.)

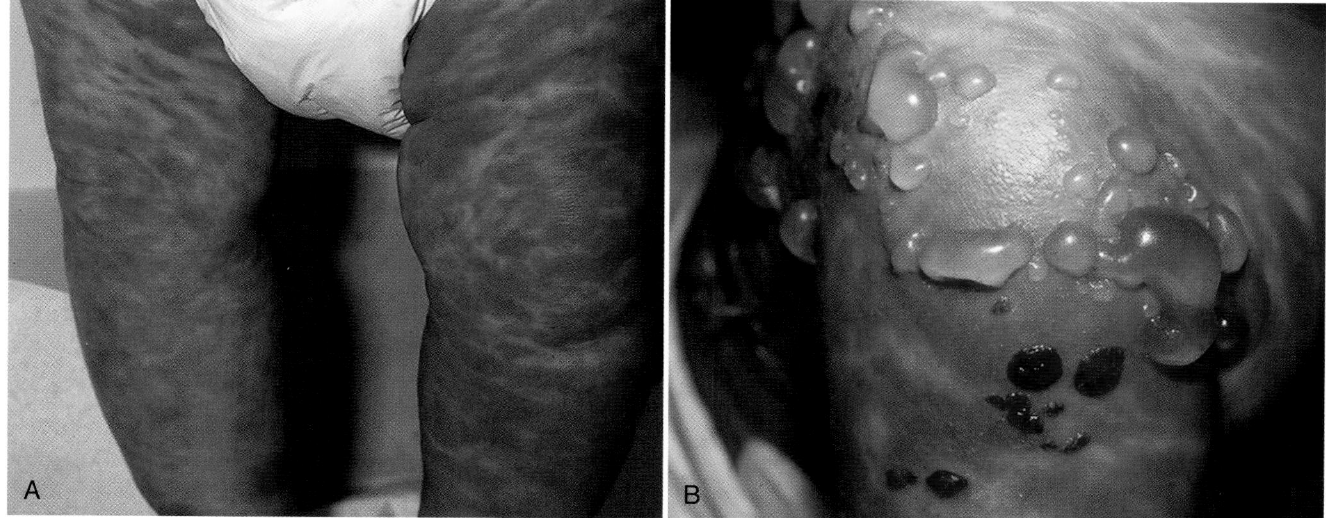

Figure 76-6 Diffuse cutaneous mastocytosis in child. Also called confluent urticaria pigmentosa. A, Extensive diffuse skin involvement. B, Bullous eruption.

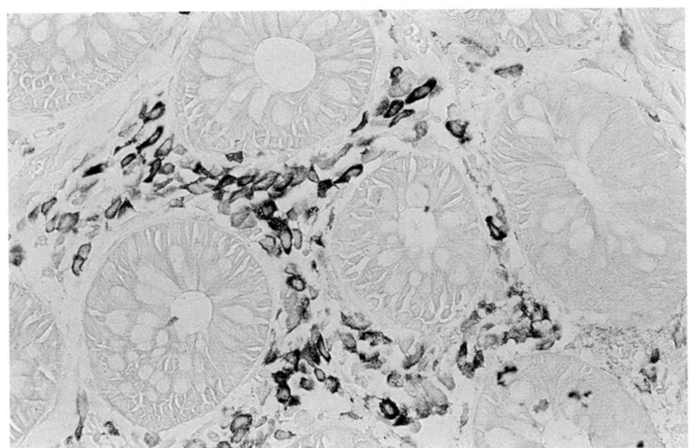

Figure 76-7 Indolent systemic mastocytosis. Colon biopsy shows increased mast cell numbers in mucosa of patient. (Toluidine blue; ×400.)

absorption of D-xylose or vitamin B_{12}. Diffuse, small intestinal mucosal dysfunction has been proposed as the basis of this malabsorption.[24,25] A structural basis for this intestinal mucosal dysfunction has been suggested by the finding of blunted villi associated with an increased number of mast cells in the mucosa[22,24] (Fig. 76-7).

MUSCULOSKELETAL PAIN

Musculoskeletal pain in patients with mastocytosis is well documented, although of uncertain etiology unless associated with osteopenia or osteoporosis, with more aggravated cases of osteoporosis leading to pathologic fractures. In some unusual cases, osteoporosis or pathologic fractures, or both, may be the initial manifestation of mastocytosis, with back pain secondary to osteoporosis and vertebral compression fractures as one presentation of systemic mast cell disease.

Bone marrow infiltration with mast cells is associated with radiographically detectable lesions in up to 70% of patients. The proximal long bones are most often affected, followed by the pelvis, ribs, and skull. Skeletal scintigraphy is more sensitive than radiographic surveys in detecting and locating active lesions and may aid in evaluating the extent of disease and disease progression.[26]

HEPATIC AND SPLENIC INVOLVEMENT

Mastocytosis frequently involves the liver and the spleen. In one study of 41 patients with mastocytosis, 61% of patients had evidence of liver disease.[27] Hepatomegaly was detected in 24%, and elevated levels of serum alkaline phosphatase (ALP), serum aminotransaminases, 5'-nucleotidase, or γ-glutamyl transpeptidase (GGTP) was detected in 54% of patients. ALP levels correlated with GGTP levels, hepatomegaly, splenomegaly, and liver mast cell infiltration and fibrosis. Elevated ALP levels were observed more frequently in patients with SM-AHNMD or ASM. Five patients with SM-AHNMD or ASM developed ascites or portal hypertension. Severe liver disease, however, is uncommon except in patients with aggressive disease, in which it may contribute to both morbidity and mortality.[27]

NEUROPSYCHIATRIC ABNORMALITIES

Neuropsychiatric difficulties reported in adults with mastocytosis include decreased attention span, memory impairment, and irritability.[28,29] Medicines administered to patients with mastocytosis as well as circulating mediators may contribute to these findings. However, an assessment of behavioral problems in children with mastocytosis found no clear excess pathology.[29] Rather, children treated with antihistamines appeared to have a nonspecific increase in behavioral difficulties at rates similar to those in other medically ill groups. No specific behavioral pattern implicating histamine overproduction was identified.

Patient Evaluation, Diagnosis, and Differential Diagnosis

Characteristics for the diagnosis of systemic mastocytosis are presented in Box 76-1. One major and one minor or three minor criteria are required for the diagnosis of SM.[1] The classic lesions of mastocytosis consist of multifocal dense mast cell aggregates and represent the sole major criteria. Minor criteria include atypical mast cell morphology, detection of codon 816 mutations in KIT, expression of CD2 and/or CD25 by bone marrow mast cells, and a total serum tryptase level greater than 20 ng/mL.

The majority of patients with mastocytosis have cutaneous disease. The diagnosis of CM should be confirmed by skin biopsy.[1,19] Mastocytosis should be suspected and the diagnostic criteria applied in patients without skin lesions if one or more of these features is present: unexplained ulcer disease or malabsorption, radiographic or technetium-99 bone scan abnormalities, hepatomegaly, splenomegaly, lymphadenopathy, peripheral blood abnormalities, and unexplained flushing or anaphylaxis. Elevated levels of plasma[30] or urinary histamine or of histamine metabolites,[31] urine PGD_2 metabolites,[32] or plasma (total) mast cell tryptase[1] are not definitive diagnostic findings but are consistent with the diagnosis of mastocytosis.

Serum mast cell tryptase is the most frequently used surrogate marker for mastocytosis and is quantified using a commercial enzyme-linked immunosorbent assay. A total tryptase level greater than 20 ng/mL suggests mastocytosis and is a minor criterion in the diagnosis of SM.[1] Tryptase levels less than 20 ng/mL have been detected in patients with CM and in those with limited SM. In general, higher tryptase values increase the likelihood of multiorgan involvement.

Other mast cell mediators that are surrogate disease markers for mastocytosis are serum histamine and 24-hour urine sampling for the urinary histamine metabolites, *N*-methylhistamine, and methylimidazoleacetic acid. These tests are less often used now with the availability of a commercial tryptase assay. Disadvantages of using blood and urinary histamine levels for diagnosis and prognosis in patients with mastocytosis include the variability of histamine levels among healthy individuals and patients, difficulty in assay standardization, and false-positive results caused by presumed synthesis of histamine by bacteria in the urinary tract and sample. Other variables that alter results of histamine assays are prior ingestion of histamine-rich foods and improper storage of the urine sample. Because basophils also contain histamine, hematologic disorders presenting with basophilia or allergic events that lead to basophil and mast cell activation also result in elevated histamine levels.

Metabolites of arachidonic acid may be elevated in patients with mastocytosis. These include urinary PGD-M or 9α,11β-dihydroxy-15-oxo-2,2,18,19-tetranorprost-5-ene-1,20-dioxic acid, as well as plasma thromboxane B_2 and its metabolites. Because the source of prostaglandins and thromboxanes in mastocytosis is not exclusively limited to mast cells, reliance on assays that measure these metabolites is unlikely to be sufficiently specific for diagnostic purposes. However, elevations in one or more mast cell mediators raise the suspicion of mastocytosis and warrant further diagnostic evaluation. A 24-hour urinary study of 5-hydroxyindoleacetic acid and urinary metanephrines will help eliminate the possibility of a carcinoid tumor or pheochromocytoma.

Plasma levels of soluble KIT and soluble IL-2 receptor α chain (CD25), which are elevated in some patients with hematologic malignancy, are also elevated in patients with mastocytosis, and correlate to severity of disease, total tryptase, and bone marrow pathology.[33] Reliable tests for these substances may not be generally available except in research laboratories.

In patients with suspected mastocytosis in the absence of skin lesions, a bone marrow biopsy and aspiration should be performed to confirm the diagnosis and to determine the disease category. The presence of mast cell aggregates is the major diagnostic criterion for the diagnosis of mastocytosis.[1] Note that patients with UP or DCM should also undergo this procedure, particularly if peripheral blood abnormalities, hepatomegaly, splenomegaly, or lymphadenopathy is present, to determine whether they have an associated hematologic disorder. Examination of other tissue specimens, such as those from the lymph nodes, spleen, liver, and GI mucosa, can help define the extent of mast cell involvement. Such studies are performed only when necessary. For example, a GI workup is dictated by symptoms of GI involvement, and lymph nodes are biopsied if lymphoma is suspected.

Identification of genetic markers of mastocytosis, such as point mutations of *c-kit*, help support the diagnosis. The identification of the D816V mutation fulfills a minor diagnostic criterion in the diagnosis of mastocytosis.[1] Such mutations are more easily identified in patients with more severe disease because of the relative clonal expansion of cells derived from the neoplastic progenitor. Such mutations may be helpful in following disease progression by assessing the relative intensity of the reverse-transcriptase polymerase chain reaction (RT-PCR) complementary DNA bands over the patient's course. Analysis for *c-kit* mutations are best performed on bone marrow and specifically on sorted malignant mast cells so as to increase sensitivity. Inability to identify the presence of a point mutation at codon 816 in *c-kit* does not eliminate the possibility that cells bearing this mutation are present; the malignant clone may not have expanded to sufficient cell number to allow for detection of the mutation in *c-kit*. In patients with coexisting eosinophilia, peripheral blood should be examined for the presence of the FIP1L1/PDGFRA fusion gene. Several techniques to detect *c-kit* mutations have been reported, but current recommendations for the most sensitive assays comprise either: RT-PCR plus restriction fragment length polymorphism (RFLP) testing, PNA-mediated PCR, or allele-specific PCR. When employing *c-kit* mutations as a diagnostic criterion for systemic mastocytosis, it is important to be aware that such mutations (e.g., D816V) are also detectable in a few patients with germ cell tumors or other non–mast cell tumors with or without coexisting systemic mastocytosis.

Additional diagnostic studies that may be helpful in evaluating extent of systemic disease include bone scans or skeletal surveys, ultrasound or computed tomography scan of the abdomen, upper GI series, small bowel radiography, and when indicated, endoscopy to rule out peptic ulcer disease or esophageal reflux. A dual-energy x-ray absorptiometry (DEXA) scan should be done to monitor osteoporosis; sites usually measured are the lumbar spine and hip.

MONOCLONAL MAST CELL ACTIVATION SYNDROME

As adopted by a consensus conference, monoclonal mast cell activation syndrome (MMAS) is applied to patients who are found on bone marrow examination to have met one or two minor diagnostic criteria for mastocytosis but lack the full diagnostic criteria for systemic mastocytosis (three minor or one major and one minor criteria).[34] Patients with such findings have been identified within groups diagnosed with idiopathic anaphylaxis and with anaphylaxis to stinging insects.[35-37] Most of these patients have tryptase levels below 20 ng/mL. It has been suggested that these findings may be identifying patients with a progressive clonal mast cell disorder that in the future may meet the diagnostic criteria for systemic mastocytosis.

For now, such patients are treated under guidelines for the treatment of anaphylaxis. Follow-up should occur yearly and include a physical examination to rule out evolving organomegaly or lymphadenopathy, serum tryptase level to determine if there is indirect evidence of an expanding mast cell compartment, and complete blood count (CBC) with differential and platelet count to help rule out an evolving hematologic disorder.

MAST CELL ACTIVATION DISORDER/SYNDROME

The term *mast cell activation syndrome* (MCAS) is sometimes applied as a diagnosis for patients who present with episodic allergy-like signs and symptoms (e.g., flushing, urticaria, diarrhea, wheezing) involving two or more organ systems and in whom an extensive medical evaluation has failed to identify an etiology. The assumption is that this diagnosis is applied to those who are having episodes caused by release of mediators associated with hyperreactivity of mast cells, which then activate spontaneously.

Diagnostic criteria have been proposed to separate possible MCAS from other causes of such clinical findings. These additional criteria include response to antimediator therapy and an increase in a validated urinary or serum marker of mast cell activation (e.g., tryptase) with an episode.[38,39] Primary (clonal) and other clinical disorders associated with mast cell activation, as well as other conditions associated with vasoactive mediator release, must be eliminated as possible causes of the clinical findings. Clonal disorders to be considered include mastocytosis and MMAS. Other disorders associated with mast cell activation, including allergic diseases, mast cell activation associated with chronic inflammatory or neoplastic disorders, and chronic autoimmune urticaria, must be eliminated as diagnostic possibilities. Conditions such as carcinoid syndrome must also be sought and rejected.[40] Once the diagnostic criteria are met, therapy is symptomatic. Vigilance must be maintained so that one of the diagnoses eliminated during the initial evaluation does not reach the level of diagnosis.

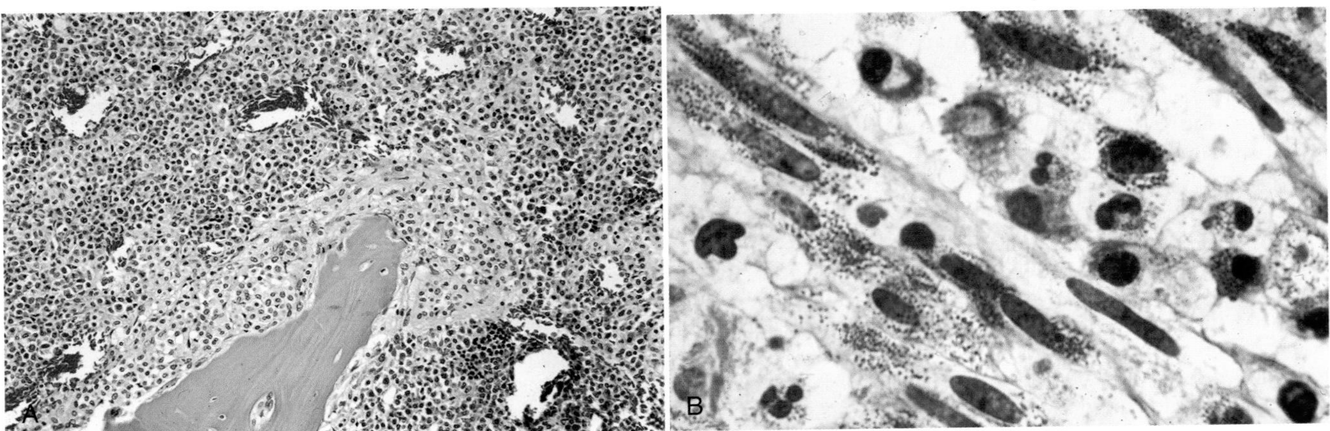

Figure 76-8 Morphologic appearance of mastocytosis-related bone marrow infiltrates. **A,** Paratrabecular aggregate of spindle-shaped mast cells. Hematopoietic marrow is hypercellular, and bone trabeculae are slightly thickened. This patient has an aggressive form of systemic mastocytosis. (Hematoxylin-eosin stain; ×20.) **B,** Higher magnification demonstrates spindle shape of the mast cells and faint granularity of the cytoplasm. (Giemsa stain; plastic imbedded; ×250.)

Pathology

DERMIS

In urticaria pigmentosa, there is an increase in the number of mast cells beneath UP macules and papules, where there is often a tenfold to twentyfold increase in mast cell numbers.[19] Occasionally, only a twofold to fourfold increase is found beneath these lesions. Because similar increases have been noted in patients with recurrent anaphylaxis, scleroderma, chronic urticaria, and prolonged antigenic contact, the diagnosis of UP cannot be made solely on the basis of small increases in the number of dermal mast cells. Gross skin examination must be correlated with the number of mast cells in the skin. In DCM, prominent bandlike infiltrates are observed that may be indistinguishable from some lesions of UP or from mastocytomas. In TMEP, cutaneous mast cell hyperplasia is observed around the capillary venules of the superficial plexus.

BONE MARROW

The bone marrow is the most common site of pathologic mast cell infiltrates in mastocytosis, followed by the spleen, liver, and lymph nodes.[41,42] The frequency of pathologic involvement at sites other than the bone marrow is not known because these are not routinely biopsied in every patient. However, palpable splenomegaly, hepatomegaly, and lymphadenopathy have been reported at initial diagnosis in 48%, 41%, and 26% of mastocytosis patients, respectively.[41] The bone marrow is the most useful biopsy site for establishing the pathologic diagnosis of systemic mastocytosis and includes inspection of the aspirate. Examination of the bone marrow both reveals diagnostic infiltrates and allows study of the hematopoietic marrow, which provides important prognostic information. Immunohistochemical (IHC) staining of the bone marrow biopsy with antitryptase is the method of choice to visualize mast cells in paraffin-imbedded decalcified specimens.

The morphologic appearance of mastocytosis-related bone marrow infiltrates in trephine core biopsy sections is distinctive. The majority of infiltrates in the bone marrow are focal, although they may be diffuse in some cases. Focal mastocytosis lesions are most often situated paratrabecularly and consist of nodular aggregates of spindle-shaped mast cells, which may be accompanied by lymphocytes and eosinophils (Fig. 76-8). Perivascular and parafollicular distributions are the next most common. In patients with tryptase-positive round cell infiltrates where the infiltrates comprise greater than 95% round cells and greater than 5% spindle-shaped cells, application of additional IHC markers to confirm the diagnosis of SM should be applied as possible (e.g., 2D7 or BB1) because basophils and sometimes blast cells also express tryptase.

Mastocytosis infiltrates have been confused with a variety of lesions, including granulomas, myelofibrosis, Hodgkin disease, metastatic carcinoma, Kaposi sarcoma, and histiocytosis X, because these cells resemble fibroblasts and histiocytes. The bone marrow lesions are cellular in the early stages of mastocytosis. As the disease progresses, the number of mast cells may decrease and the lesions may become fibrotic. Mastocytosis infiltrates in the bone marrow may be associated with osteosclerotic or osteolytic changes in the bone trabeculae.

The coexpression of CD2 and CD25 in CD117 (KIT)–positive mast cells by flow cytometry of bone marrow aspirates or by IHC analysis of bone marrow biopsies is generally accepted as the most sensitive and specific method to support the diagnosis of SM in bone marrow.[1] The cellular composition of lymphoid collections is evaluated using lineage-specific antibodies against CD3 and CD20. Other stains used to detect mast cell infiltrates include Wright-Giemsa and toluidine blue, along with reticulin staining to detect fibrosis and Masson trichrome staining to evaluate the extent of collagen deposition. Mast cells also stain positively for chloroacetate esterase and aminocaproate esterase.

Prognostic features of the bone marrow in mastocytosis patients have been reported. In one review of 58 cases of systemic mast cell disease, a hypercellular marrow with a decreased percentage of fat cells emerged as a significant predictor of poor prognosis.[41] In most cases the hypercellular marrow was caused by an increase in hematopoietic elements or, less often, extensive mast cell infiltration. Most mastocytosis patients with hypercellular hematopoietic marrow had an associated hematologic disorder. Approximately one third of patients had associated hematologic disorders defined by traditional criteria, including dysmyelopoietic syndromes, myeloproliferative disorders, de novo acute leukemia, malignant lymphoma, and chronic neutropenia.[34,41,42] Mastocytosis patients with hematologic disorders had significantly reduced 5-year survival rates. Although systemic mast cell lesions in patients with hematologic disorders may be discovered incidentally during examination of bone marrow biopsy specimens, most patients have manifestations of mastocytosis, and the hematologic disorder is detected after mastocytosis is diagnosed.

Mast cell leukemia is a separate clinical entity. The bone marrow shows a diffuse infiltration by atypical, immature mast cells.[1,43] Mast cells account for 10% or more of the peripheral white blood cells (see Box 76-2). MCL differs from the rare case of aggressive mastocytosis with a terminal leukemic phase, in which circulating mast cells appear late in the disease course and the percentage of circulating mast cells is relatively low.

Cytologic abnormalities in hematopoietic cells, as well as mast cells, may be detected in bone marrow aspirates. In most cases, evidence of dysplastic or neoplastic hematopoietic cells forms the basis for the classification of the associated hematologic disorders. Atypical or poorly differentiated mast cells may be identified in the bone marrow aspirates of patients with MCL and with aggressive forms of mastocytosis. The cytoplasmic granules of atypical mast cells are often very fine and smaller in number compared with the coarsely granular mast cells from patients with the indolent form of mastocytosis. Nuclear mast cell atypia may take the form of lobated nuclei and have binucleation or multinucleation and mitotic figures. Mitoses are rarely seen in mast cells, even in aggressive forms of mastocytosis, except in patients with MCL. In one study the presence of lobated mast cell nuclei in bone marrow aspirates was associated with a significantly reduced 5-year survival rate.[41]

The relative number of mast cells in the bone marrow aspirate versus the number in the bone marrow biopsy is not always a useful measure of pathologic mastocytosis infiltrates. In some cases, few mast cells are found in the bone marrow aspirate despite evidence of mastocytosis in trephine core biopsy sections because of the increased reticulin associated with the infiltrates in the marrow itself. Mast cell hyperplasia in bone marrow is also found in uremia, osteoporosis, and hematologic conditions (lymphomas, preleukemias, leukemias).

The most common finding in spleens affected by mastocytosis is trabecular fibrotic thickening. Splenic mast cell lesions have been found in a paratrabecular, parafollicular, follicular, or diffuse red pulp distribution. The most common location in the lymph node for a mastocytosis infiltrate is the paracortical region. Parafollicular and follicular replacement, as well as medullary cord and sinus infiltration, are less frequent. Mastocytosis infiltrates in the spleen and lymph nodes may resemble follicular and T cell lymphomas, monocytoid B cell hyperplasia and lymphoma, Kaposi sarcoma, hairy cell leukemia, and histiocytosis X.

Mast cell infiltration is observed in liver biopsy specimens, is more severe in patients with SM-AHNMD or ASM, and correlates with hepatomegaly, splenomegaly, ALP levels, and GGTP levels. Portal fibrosis correlates with mast cell infiltration and portal inflammation. Nodular regenerative hyperplasia, portal venopathy, and venoocclusive disease are reported and may contribute to portal hypertension.

Treatment

MAST CELL–MEDIATED SYMPTOMS

A principal objective of treatment in all categories of mastocytosis is the control of mast cell mediator–induced signs and symptoms, especially systemic hypotension, gastric hypersecretion, GI cramping, and pruritus. H_1-receptor antagonists such as the classic antihistamine hydroxyzine or the nonsedating antihistamines loratadine or fexofenadine are instituted to reduce pruritus and flushing. If this is insufficient, the addition of an H_2 antagonist such as ranitidine, cimetidine or famotidine may be beneficial. One approach is to administer a nonsedating antihistamine during the day and a potent sedating antihistamine at bedtime. Even with these medications, many patients continue to complain of musculoskeletal pain, headaches, and flushing; thus adding a leukotriene-modifying agent may be beneficial.

Disodium cromoglycate (cromolyn sodium) inhibits degranulation of mast cells and has some efficacy in mastocytosis, particularly in the relief of GI complaints, but does not reduce plasma or urinary histamine levels in patients with mastocytosis.[44] Ketotifen, an antihistamine with mast cell–stabilizing properties, helps relieve the pruritus and whealing associated with mastocytosis but appears to offer no advantage over hydroxyzine.

Epinephrine is used to treat episodes of systemic hypotension. Patients should be taught to administer this medication themselves. If intramuscular epinephrine is inadequate, intensive therapy for systemic hypotension, as for anaphylaxis, should be instituted. Patients with recurrent episodes of hypotension may be given H_1 or H_2 antihistamines to reduce the severity of attacks. Episodes of profound hypotension may be spontaneous but have also been observed after insect stings and administration of contrast media.

The oral administration of 8-methoxypsoralen with long-wave ultraviolet photochemotherapy (PUVA) has been used to relieve pruritus and whealing in adult patients after 1 to 2 months of treatment.[20] Improvement is associated with a transient decrease in the number of dermal mast cells. Relapse of pruritus occurs within 3 to 6 months after discontinuation of therapy. Photochemotherapy should be used only in patients with extensive cutaneous disease unresponsive to other forms of therapy. Some patients report a diminution in the number or intensity of cutaneous lesions after repeated exposure to natural sunlight.

Topical steroids, such as 0.05% betamethasone dipropionate ointment applied under plastic wrap occlusion for 8 hours a day over 8 to 12 weeks, may be used to treat UP or DCM. The number of mast cells decreases as lesions resolve. Lesions eventually recur after discontinuation of therapy, although the treatment may lead to improvement in cutaneous lesions for up to 1 year.

GASTROINTESTINAL SYMPTOMS

The treatment of GI disease is dictated by the degree of peptic symptoms, diarrhea, and malabsorption. Gastric acid hypersecretion leading to peptic symptoms and ulcerations is controlled with H_2 antagonists and proton pump inhibitors such as omeprazole. Diarrhea is difficult to manage, and H_2 agonists are generally not effective for this symptom. Anticholinergics may give partial relief. In patients with severe malabsorption, oral steroids may be effective. Ascites is also difficult to control, and a portacaval shunt may be considered.

OSTEOPOROSIS

Osteoporosis in patients with mastocytosis may go unrecognized, especially in patients with milder forms such as ISM. It is thus important to use DEXA scanning in their evaluation. Recommended approaches to the treatment of osteoporosis include calcium supplementation, consideration of estrogen replacement in postmenopausal women, and use of bisphosphonates.[45] Narcotic analgesics may potentiate mast cell degranulation and thus should be used with care, particularly at high doses. Radiotherapy may have a palliative role in decreasing bone pain in localized areas in patients with aggressive forms of disease. Interferon-α2b may have some efficacy in decreasing musculoskeletal pain and improving bone mineralization in patients with extensive bony involvement.

HEMATOLOGIC ABNORMALITIES

Patients with mastocytosis and an associated hematologic disorder are managed as dictated by the specific hematologic abnormality.[34,45-47] For patients with aggressive forms of mastocytosis, interferon alpha-2b (IFN-α2b) and 2-chloro-2-deoxyadenosine (cladribine, 2-CdA) are potential first-line therapeutic options.[46] The decision to initiate therapy with IFN-α2b should consider potentially debilitating side effects such as fever, malaise, nausea, and hypothyroidism.

Cladribine, a nucleoside analog, does not appear to require cells in active cell cycle to exert its cytotoxic activity, and thus appears beneficial in slowly progressing neoplastic processes.

Bone marrow transplantation has been investigated as a treatment option for patients with advanced categories of mastocytosis associated with poor survival in only a few reported instances. Although these studies reported favorable responses of the associated hematologic disorders, the overall effect on mast cell hyperplasia has to date been poor.

Imatinib mesylate (Gleevec; Novartis, Basel, Switzerland) is approved by the U.S. Food and Drug Administration for treatment of chronic myelogenous leukemia, KIT-positive gastrointestinal stromal tumors, and aggressive forms of mastocytosis when the patient does not have the D816V mutation. This is because in vitro studies investigating the ability of imatinib to inhibit various mutant forms of *c-kit* revealed that, although the drug effectively inhibited wild-type KIT and KIT-bearing juxtamembrane activating mutations, it failed to inhibit KIT-bearing codon 816 mutations associated with most common forms of SM. Consistent with these observations, imatinib showed a strong in vitro cytotoxic effect on mast cells bearing wild-type KIT, whereas mast cells bearing a codon 816 mutation isolated from bone marrow aspirates of patients with mastocytosis were relatively resistant to the drug. Imatinib mesylate has been shown to be of value in unusual clinical presentations of mastocytosis, which are associated with novel mutations in *c-kit*. Patients with increased mast cells and peripheral eosinophilia that carry the FIP1L1-PDGFRA fusion oncogene also respond to imatinib.[17] A careful mutational analysis of a sample enriched for lesional mast cells thus appears essential before contemplating imatinib therapy. In vitro studies found that other tyrosine kinase inhibitors such as midostaurin (PKC412) were able to inhibit KIT with the D816V mutation, and clinical trials report encouraging initial results.[47] Treatment response criteria for mastocytosis are available.[48]

Chemotherapy has not been shown to produce remission or prolong survival in MCL and has no place in the treatment of indolent mastocytosis. Chemotherapy, including cladribine, may be considered for advanced disease, but data thus far are not compelling for most regimens with regard to long-term outcome. Splenectomy may somewhat improve survival times in patients with forms of mastocytosis associated with poor prognosis. Radiotherapy has been used in the management of refractory bone pain in patients with aggressive disease. Bone marrow transplantation may be considered for extremely ill patients, although such procedures may yield a better prognosis if mast cell suppression is attempted before the transplantation.[49]

Prognosis

The prognosis differs for each category of mastocytosis. Variables strongly associated with poor survival include advanced age, weight loss, anemia, thrombocytopenia, hypoalbuminemia, and excess bone marrow blasts.[50]

Patients with CM only have the best prognosis, followed by those with ISM.[51] For children with isolated UP, at least 50% of cases are reported to resolve by adulthood. UP in adulthood may evolve into systemic disease. Occasionally, ISM converts to SM-AHNMD, and the course in these patients depends largely on the prognosis of the specific hematologic disorder and response to aggressive therapy.[51] The mean survival time for patients with MCL is usually less than 12 months. The survival time with ASM is 2 to 4 years with aggressive symptomatic management.

Conclusion

The understanding of mast cell disorders over the past decade has expanded to include not only the classification of variants of mastocytosis, but also the adaptation of available therapeutic approaches based on disease severity. Most promising are trials of tyrosine kinase inhibitors that target KIT with activating mutations and the recognition that patients with aggressive forms of mastocytosis may have additional mutations that contribute to pathogenesis and offer additional targets for a combined therapeutic approach. The most surprising and insightful clinical research has documented mutations in KIT within populations of patients with idiopathic anaphylaxis and with anaphylaxis to stinging insects. These patients have unrecognized mastocytosis by standard diagnostic criteria, and others have mutations in KIT but do not meet the diagnostic criteria for systemic mastocytosis, now with the diagnosis of mononuclear mast cell activation syndrome. Identification of hyperreactive mast cell responses in such patients has shown that mast cell reactivity is altered by mutations in critical receptors and signal transduction molecules, the basis of ongoing studies to assess mast cell variability in responsiveness in allergic diseases in general. Unfortunately, targeted therapy specific to the mast cell compartment remains elusive, suggesting the need to revisit nonablative bone marrow transplantation for patients with aggressive mastocytosis.

Acknowledgment

This work was supported by the Division of Intramural Research, NIAID/NIH.

REFERENCES

Introduction

1. Horny H-P, Metcalfe DD, Bennett JM, et al. Mastocytosis. In: Swerdlow SH, Campo E, Harris NL, et al, editors. WHO classification of tumors of haematopoietic and lymphoid tissues. Lyon: IARC Press; 2008. p. 54-63.

Historical Perspective

2. Ehrlich P. Beitrage zur theorie und praxis der histologischen färbung. University of Leipzig; 1878.
3. Unna PG. Die spezifische färbung der mastzellenkörnung. Monatsh Prakt Dermatol 1894;19: 367.
4. Webb RL. Peritoneal reactions in the white rat, with especial reference to the mast cells. Am J Anat 1931;49:283-334.
5. Jorpes JE. The site of formation of heparin. In: Heparin: its chemistry, physiology, and application in medicine. London: Humphrey Milford (Oxford University Press); 1939. p. 30.
6. Riley JF. Histamine in tissue mast cells. Science 1953;118(3064):332.
7. Nettleship E, Tay W. Rare forms of urticaria. BMJ 1869;2:323-30.
8. Sangster A. An anomalous mottled rash, accompanied by pruritus, factitious urticaria and pigmentation, "urticaria pigmentosa?" Trans Clin Soc Lond 1878;11:161-3.
9. Ellis JM. Urticaria pigmentosa: a report of a case with autopsy. AMA Arch Pathol 1949;48: 426-35.

Epidemiology

10. Robyn J, Metcalfe DD. Systemic mastocytosis. Adv Immunol 2006;89:169-243.

Pathogenesis and Etiology

11. Kirshenbaum AS, Goff JP, Semere T, et al. Demonstration that human mast cells arise from a progenitor cell population that is CD34(+), *c-kit*(+), and expresses aminopeptidase N (CD13). Blood 1999;94:2333-42.
12. Kirshenbaum AS, Goff JP, Kessler SW, et al. Effect of IL-3 and stem cell factor on the appearance of human basophils and mast cells from CD34+ pluripotent progenitor cells. J Immunol 1992;148:772-7.
13. Akin C, Brockow K, D'Ambrosio C, et al. Effects of tyrosine kinase inhibitor STI571 on human mast cells bearing wild-type or mutated *c-kit*. Exp Hematol 2003;31:686-92.
14. Nagata H, Worobec AS, Oh CK, et al. Identification of a point mutation in the catalytic domain of the protooncogene *c-kit* in peripheral blood mononuclear cells of patients who have mastocytosis with an associated hematologic disorder. Proc Natl Acad Sci USA 1995;92: 10560-4.
15. Wilson TM, Maric I, Simakova O, et al. Clonal analysis of NRAS activating mutations in KIT-D816V systemic mastocytosis. Haematologica 2011;96:459-63.
16. Lasho T, Tefferi A, Pardanani A. Inhibition of JAK-STAT signaling by TG101348: a novel mechanism for inhibition of KITD816V-dependent growth in mast cell leukemia cells. Leukemia 2010;24:1378-80.
17. Maric I, Robyn J, Metcalfe DD, et al. KIT D816V-associated systemic mastocytosis with eosinophilia and FIP1L1/PDGFRA-associated chronic eosinophilic leukemia are distinct entities. J Allergy Clin Immunol 2007;120:680-7.
18. Lahortiga I, Akin C, Cools J, et al. Activity of imatinib in systemic mastocytosis with chronic basophilic leukemia and a PRKG2-PDGFRB fusion. Haematologica 2008;93:49-56.

Clinical Features

19. Garriga MM, Friedman MM, Metcalfe DD. A survey of the number and distribution of mast cells in the skin of patients with mast cell disorders. J Allergy Clin Immunol 1988;82: 425-32.
20. Soter NA. Mastocytosis and the skin. Hematol Oncol Clin North Am 2000;14:537-55, vi.
21. Parwaresch MR, Horny HP, Lennert K. Tissue mast cells in health and disease. Pathol Res Pract 1985;179:439-61.
22. Cherner JA, Jensen RT, Dubois A, et al. Gastrointestinal dysfunction in systemic mastocytosis: a prospective study. Gastroenterology 1988;95: 657-67.
23. Ammann RW, Vetter D, Deyhle P, et al. Gastrointestinal involvement in systemic mastocytosis. Gut 1976;17:107-12. [Comparative study.]
24. Bredfeldt JE, O'Laughlin JC, Durham JB, Blessing LD. Malabsorption and gastric hyperacidity in systemic mastocytosis: results of cimetidine therapy. Am J Gastroenterol 1980; 74:133-7.
25. Broitman SA, McCray RS, May JC, et al. Mastocytosis and intestinal malabsorption. Am J Med 1970;48:382-9.
26. Chen CC, Andrich MP, Mican JM, Metcalfe DD. A retrospective analysis of bone scan abnormalities in mastocytosis: correlation with disease category and prognosis. J Nucl Med 1994;35:1471-5.
27. Mican JM, Di Bisceglie AM, Fong TL, et al. Hepatic involvement in mastocytosis: clinicopathologic correlations in 41 cases. Hepatology 1995;22:1163-70.
28. Rogers MP, Bloomingdale K, Murawski BJ, et al. Mixed organic brain syndrome as a manifestation of systemic mastocytosis. Psychosom Med 1986;48:437-47.
29. McFarlin KE, Kruesi MJ, Metcalfe DD. A preliminary assessment of behavioral problems in children with mastocytosis. Int J Psychiatry Med 1991;21:281-9.

Patient Evaluation, Diagnosis, and Differential Diagnosis

30. Friedman BS, Steinberg SC, Meggs WJ, et al. Analysis of plasma histamine levels in patients with mast cell disorders. Am J Med 1989;87: 649-54.
31. Keyzer JJ, de Monchy JG, van Doormaal JJ, van Voorst Vader PC. Improved diagnosis of mastocytosis by measurement of urinary histamine metabolites. N Engl J Med 1983;309: 1603-5.
32. Roberts LJ 2nd, Sweetman BJ, Lewis RA, Austen KF, Oates JA. Increased production of prostaglandin D_2 in patients with systemic mastocytosis. N Engl J Med 1980;303:1400-4.
33. Akin C, Schwartz LB, Kitoh T, et al. Soluble stem cell factor receptor (CD117) and IL-2 receptor alpha chain (CD25) levels in the plasma of patients with mastocytosis: relationships to disease severity and bone marrow pathology. Blood 2000;96:1267-73.
34. Valent P, Akin C, Escribano L, et al. Standards and standardization in mastocytosis: consensus statements on diagnostics, treatment recommendations and response criteria. Eur J Clin Invest 2007;37:435-53.
35. Akin C, Scott LM, Kocabas CN, et al. Demonstration of an aberrant mast-cell population with clonal markers in a subset of patients with "idiopathic" anaphylaxis. Blood 2007;110: 2331-3.
36. Ludolph-Hauser D, Rueff F, Fries C, Schopf P, Przybilla B. Constitutively raised serum concentrations of mast-cell tryptase and severe anaphylactic reactions to Hymenoptera stings. Lancet 2001;357(9253):361-2.
37. Bonadonna P, Perbellini O, Passalacqua G, et al. Clonal mast cell disorders in patients with systemic reactions to Hymenoptera stings and increased serum tryptase levels. J Allergy Clin Immunol 2009;123:680-6.
38. Akin C, Valent P, Metcalfe DD. Mast cell activation syndrome: proposed diagnostic criteria. J Allergy Clin Immunol 2010;126:1099-104, e4.
39. Valent P, Akin C, Arock M, et al. Definitions, criteria and global classification of mast cell disorders with special reference to mast cell activation syndromes: a consensus proposal. Int Arch Allergy Immunol 2011;157:215-25.
40. Metcalfe DD. Differential diagnosis of the patient with unexplained flushing/anaphylaxis. Allergy Asthma Proc 2000;21:21-4.

Pathology

41. Travis WD, Li CY, Bergstralh EJ, Yam LT, Swee RG. Systemic mast cell disease: analysis of 58 cases and literature review. Medicine (Baltimore) 1988;67:345-68.
42. Lawrence JB, Friedman BS, Travis WD, et al. Hematologic manifestations of systemic mast cell disease: a prospective study of laboratory and morphologic features and their relation to prognosis. Am J Med 1991;91:612-24.
43. Travis WD, Li CY, Hoagland HC, Travis LB, Banks PM. Mast cell leukemia: report of a case and review of the literature. Mayo Clin Proc 1986;61:957-66.

Treatment

44. Frieri M, Alling DW, Metcalfe DD. Comparison of the therapeutic efficacy of cromolyn sodium with that of combined chlorpheniramine and cimetidine in systemic mastocytosis: results of a double-blind clinical trial. Am J Med 1985;78: 9-14.
45. Worobec AS. Treatment of systemic mast cell disorders. Hematol Oncol Clin North Am 2000;14:659-87, vii.
46. Lim KH, Pardanani A, Butterfield JH, Li CY, Tefferi A. Cytoreductive therapy in 108 adults with systemic mastocytosis: outcome analysis and response prediction during treatment with interferon-alpha, hydroxyurea, imatinib mesylate or 2-chlorodeoxyadenosine. Am J Hematol 2009;84:790-4.
47. Pardanani A. Systemic mastocytosis in adults: 2012 update on diagnosis, risk stratification, and management. Am J Hematol 2012;87: 401-11.
48. Pardanani A, Tefferi A. A critical reappraisal of treatment response criteria in systemic mastocytosis and a proposal for revisions. Eur J Haematol 2010;84:371-8.

49. Nakamura R, Chakrabarti S, Akin C, et al. A pilot study of nonmyeloablative allogeneic hematopoietic stem cell transplant for advanced systemic mastocytosis. Bone Marrow Transplant 2006;37:353-8.

Prognosis

50. Lim KH, Tefferi A, Lasho TL, et al. Systemic mastocytosis in 342 consecutive adults: survival studies and prognostic factors. Blood 2009;113: 5727-36.
51. Pardanani A, Lim KH, Lasho TL, et al. Prognostically relevant breakdown of 123 patients with systemic mastocytosis associated with other myeloid malignancies. Blood 2009;114: 3769-72.

Anaphylaxis

SIMON G.A. BROWN | STEPHEN F. KEMP | PHILLIP L. LIEBERMAN

CONTENTS

SUMMARY OF IMPORTANT CONCEPTS

» The incidence of anaphylaxis is increasing.
» Anaphylaxis is underdiagnosed and underreported.
» Epinephrine autoinjectors are often underprescribed.
» Mortality risk from anaphylaxis is increased in asthmatic patients, teenagers, and elderly patients with comorbidities.
» Patients with recurrent anaphylactic episodes should avoid drugs that complicate therapy or that may increase the severity of a reaction.

Terminology

Traditionally, the term *anaphylaxis* has referred to a systemic, immediate hypersensitivity reaction caused by IgE-mediated immunologic release of mediators from mast cells and basophils. In the past, "anaphylactoid reaction" referred to a clinically similar event not mediated by immunoglobulin E.[1,2] The World Allergy Organization proposed a change in terminology that *anaphylaxis* refer to a "severe, life-threatening, generalized or systemic hypersensitivity reaction."[3] Further, the term *allergic anaphylaxis* should be used when this reaction "is mediated by an immunologic mechanism, e.g., IgE, IgG, and immune-complex-complement related," and anaphylaxis from a nonimmunologic reaction called "nonallergic anaphylaxis." Therefore this terminology eliminated "anaphylactoid." (Fig. 77-1).[4]

The difficulty in defining anaphylaxis was highlighted in symposia jointly sponsored by the U.S. National Institutes of Health (Allergy and Infectious Disease) and the Food Allergy and Anaphylaxis Network.[5,6] Panels of experts from different organizations and government bodies with representatives from North America, Europe, and Australia convened to define anaphylaxis and establish criteria for treatment. Although no true definition of anaphylaxis in the classic sense resulted, they established a clear-cut constellation of signs and symptoms defining the necessity for treatment with epinephrine (Box 77-1).[1,5,6]

Incidence and Causative Agents

The exact incidence of anaphylaxis is unknown[7-15] (Table 77-1). An expert panel concluded that the incidence is 50 to 2000 episodes per 100,000 person-years, with a possible "lifetime" prevalence of 0.05% to 2%, and that the best estimate of incidence to date is probably from real-time data obtained from prescriptions dispensed for outpatient use of injectable epinephrine.[14] Such data indicate that approximately 1% of the population is dispensed outpatient epinephrine.[7] Regardless of overall estimates, the incidence of anaphylaxis clearly is increasing and a worldwide phenomenon, at least in industrialized populations.[8,9,16-18] In addition, the incidence of anaphylaxis is probably underestimated in part because episodes are underreported.[2,14,19-22]

INCIDENCE FOR SPECIFIC AGENTS

Drugs and foods are the most frequent causes of anaphylaxis (Table 77-2).[2,23-37] Drug reactions account for perhaps as many as 230,000 hospital admissions in the United States annually,[29] although such reactions are probably underreported.[2] As many as 6% of children and 3% to 4% of adults suffer from food allergy.[28] Evidence shows that the incidence of anaphylaxis to foods is increasing (Box 77-2).[31,38,39] Anaphylactic reactions during anesthesia[40] and frequency of reactions to biologic agents[41,42] seem to be increasing as well.

FACTORS AFFECTING INCIDENCE

Geographic location, economic status, race, age, gender, route of administration of antigen, constancy of administration of antigen, chronobiologic factors, and atopy have been evaluated for their effects on the incidence of anaphylaxis (Table 77-3).[2,19,43-54] Race exerts no known effect. Data for geographic location show that, at least in the United Kingdom, incidence may be higher for those living in rural versus urban areas.[44] In the United States, epinephrine autoinjector prescriptions were fewer in states with warmer climates and more year-round sunlight.[45] These findings could not be accounted for based on access to allergists, number of pharmaceutical salesmen, or other factors. In Australia, epinephrine prescription rates and

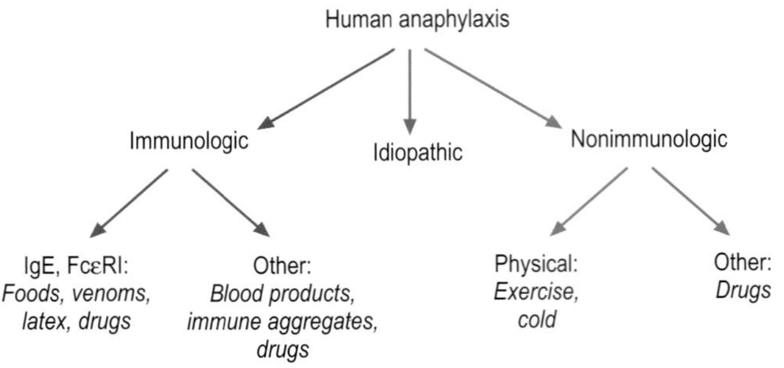

Figure 77-1 Visual schema of change in anaphylaxis terminology. *(From Simons FER. Anaphylaxis, killer allergy: long-term management in the community. J Allergy Clin Immunol 2006;117:367-77.)*

BOX 77-1 CRITICAL CRITERIA FOR DIAGNOSING ANAPHYLAXIS

Anaphylaxis is highly likely when any *one* of the following three criteria is fulfilled:

1. Acute onset of an illness (minutes to several hours) with involvement of the skin, mucosal tissues, or both (e.g., generalized hives, pruritus or flushing, swollen lips-tongue-uvula)
   And at least one of the following:
   a. Respiratory compromise (e.g., dyspnea, wheeze-bronchospasm, stridor, reduced PEF, hypoxemia)
   b. Reduced BP or associated symptoms of end-organ dysfunction (e.g., hypotonia [collapse], syncope, incontinence)
2. Two or more of the following that occur rapidly after exposure *to a likely allergen for that patient* (minutes to several hours):
   a. Involvement of skin-mucosal tissue (e.g., generalized hives, itch-flush, swollen lips-tongue-uvula)
   b. Respiratory compromise (e.g., dyspnea, wheeze-bronchospasm, stridor, reduced PEF, hypoxemia)
   c. Reduced BP or associated symptoms of end-organ dysfunction (e.g., hypotonia [collapse], syncope, incontinence)
   d. Persistent gastrointestinal symptoms (e.g., crampy abdominal pain, vomiting)
3. Reduced BP after exposure *to known allergen for that patient* (minutes to several hours):
   a. Infants and children: low systolic BP (age specific) or greater than 30% decrease in systolic BP*
   b. Adults: systolic BP less than 90 mm Hg or greater than 30% decrease from their baseline

From Sampson HA et al. Second symposium on the definition and management of anaphylaxis. J Allergy Clin Immunol 2006;117:391-7.

PEF, Peak expiratory flow; *BP,* blood pressure.

*Low systolic BP for children is defined as less than 70 mm Hg from 1 month to 1 year, less than (70 mm Hg + [2 × age]) from 1 to 10 years, and less than 90 mm Hg from 11 to 17 years.

TABLE 77-1 Summary of Studies Assessing Overall Incidence of Anaphylaxis

Study (Year)	Description/Findings
Simons et al.[7] (2002)	Real-time data from administrative claims pharmaceutical database; generalized dispensing data for all epinephrine formulations over 5 consecutive fiscal years. In population base of 1.15 million persons in Manitoba, Canada, approximately 1% of this defined general population had injectable epinephrine dispensed for out-of-hospital treatment.
Gupta et al.[8] (2003)	Identified admissions for anaphylaxis to hospital; used 11-year study period. Anaphylaxis rates rose from 6 to 41 per million between 1990–1 and 2000–1.
Peng, Jick[9] (2004)	Used observational follow-up study encompassing approximately 8 million person-years based on UK General Practice Research Database from Jan. 1, 1994, to Dec. 31, 1999. Based on 675 cases of anaphylaxis, estimated incidence of 8.4 per 100,000 person-years. Approximately 10% had hypotension and shock. Common causes were insect stings and oral drugs.
Helbling et al.[10] (2004)	Investigated incidence and cause of severe anaphylactic episodes with circulatory signs in the Canton Bern, Switzerland. Capture area was approximately 240,000 inhabitants; 3-year study period. Incidence of severe life-threatening anaphylaxis was 7.9 to 9.6 per 100,000 inhabitants per year.
Bohlke et al.[11] (2004)	Study population of children and adolescents enrolled in health maintenance organization; 6-year study period. Results from automated database and medical records review. Incidence of 10.5 episodes per 100,000 person-years. Did not observe increasing incidence; 11% resulted in hospitalization.
Mehl et al.[12] (2005)	Retrospective study between October 2002 and December 2003. Pediatricians throughout Germany were asked to identify anaphylactic reactions over 12-month period; 103 cases evaluated.
Moneret-Vautrin et al.[13] (2005)	Review; severe anaphylactic episodes affect 1-3 per 10,000 people. Highest results in U.S. and Australia. Anaphylaxis will cause death in estimated 0.65%-2% of patients (1-3 per million people); concluded incidence is increasing.
Lieberman et al.[14] (2006)	Panel review of incidence studies led to frequency estimate of 50-2000 episodes per 100,000 person-years, or lifetime prevalence of 0.05%-2%. Largest number of incident cases occurs in children and adolescents. Noted possible underdiagnosis as well as undertreatment of anaphylaxis.

anaphylaxis admissions to hospitals are higher in the southern versus northern part of the country. These factors imply that the incidence of anaphylaxis is increased with lower exposure to sunlight, and that lower vitamin D levels might predispose to anaphylactic events.[46]

Economic status may play a role in the incidence of anaphylactic episodes. Simons and colleagues[47] found that epinephrine was dispensed more frequently for individuals in higher-income groups in an urban Canadian population; this could not be attributed to access to specialist care. Sheikh and Alves[44] noted a similar effect of income in the United Kingdom.[44]

TABLE 77-2 Summary of Incidence for Common Triggers of Anaphylaxis

Agent	Comment/Findings
Antibiotics[27]	Arguably most common cause of drug-induced anaphylaxis, most frequently β-lactams, accounting for as many as 22% of all drug-related episodes. Nonfatal drug-induced anaphylaxis to penicillin may affect 1.9-27.2 million Americans.
Latex[32]	Populations at risk experience multiple mucosal exposures to latex, e.g., health care workers, patients with multiple catheterizations/surgeries. Overall incidence of latex allergy in U.S. is 2.7-16 million. Although incidence of latex allergy has risen greatly over last 15 years, with reduced use of powdered gloves and substitution of nonlatex gloves in hospitals, incidence appears to have stabilized.
Perioperative anaphylaxis[33,40]	Depending on the country, perioperative anaphylactic reactions represent 9%-19% of complications of anesthesia. Fatality rate approximates 5%-7%. Muscle relaxants account for 62% and latex 16%; remainder of reactions result from hypnotics, antibiotics, plasma substitutes, and opioids. Serial data collected in France showed increased incidence of perioperative anaphylactic events. Muscle relaxants still remain most common cause.
Radiocontrast media[34]	Adverse reactions to ionic contrast media (hyperosmolar agents) occur with a frequency of 4%-12% and to nonionic (lower osmolar agents) of 1%-3%. Severe adverse reactions occur in 0.16% of ionic media administration and 0.03% with nonionic media. Paradoxically, mortality rate (1-3 per 100,000 contrast administrations) appears similar for both ionic and nonionic media.
Hymenoptera stings[35]	Potentially life-threatening systemic reactions to insect stings occur in and estimated 0.4%-0.8% of children and 3% of adults.
Food[25,28]	As many as 6% of children and 3%-4% of adults have food allergy. Based on incidence in Colorado, approximately 0.0004% of the U.S. population, or 1080 Americans, have anaphylactic reactions to food each year. Shellfish is probably most common source in adults and peanuts in children. Also, 1.1% of U.S. population may be allergic to tree nuts or peanuts.
Nonsteroidal antiinflammatory drugs[24]	Incidence varies depending on whether or not asthmatic patients are included. NSAIDs are probably second most common medication offender after antibiotics.
Antisera	Once the most important cause of anaphylaxis, antisera now have greatly diminished in importance with their decreased use as therapeutic agents, but antiserum is still used for snakebites and immunosuppression. Incidence in patients receiving antilymphocyte globulin may be as high as 2%, and incidence to antivenom 4.6%-10%. Incidence may decline further with recent release of Crotalidae Polyvalent ImmunFab, a purified preparation of Fab fragment obtained from sheep immunized with venom. Although urticaria reported, no anaphylactic episodes have occurred with this agent.
Reactions associated with hemodialysis[36]	Incidence appears to be increasing. Drug administration data show 3.5 severe hypersensitivity reactions per 100,000 hollow-fiber dialyzers sold. In 260,000 dialysis treatments, 21 severe reactions occurred, including one fatality.
Idiopathic anaphylaxis[37]	Cause remains unidentified in as many as two thirds of adults presenting to allergist/immunologist for evaluation of anaphylaxis. Survey of 75 U.S. allergists found 633 cases encountered. The authors extrapolated data to U.S. population and estimated as many as 20,592 to 47,024 cases.
Biologic agents[41,42]	With increased use of biologic agents, anaphylactic reactions to these products have also increased, including omalizumab, tumor necrosis factor antagonists, cetuximab, tocilizumab, and natalizumab.

BOX 77-2 SEVEN CONCLUSIONS REGARDING INCIDENCE OF ANAPHYLAXIS

1. No exact incidence of anaphylaxis can be established based on available data.
2. Most studies indicate a significant underreporting, and therefore the true incidence of anaphylaxis is probably significantly higher than formally reported.
3. In adults, based on series of episodes evaluated by allergy or immunology specialists, events of unknown cause (idiopathic) account for as many as 60% of cases. In childhood, idiopathic anaphylaxis events are rare.
4. Foods are probably the most frequent triggers, followed by drugs. The incidence of food allergy, especially to peanuts, appears to be increasing.
5. The agents most frequently causing anaphylaxis are nonsteroidal antiinflammatory drugs and antibiotics. Reactions to radiocontrast media appear to be diminishing in frequency.
6. Perioperative episodes of anaphylaxis may be increasing, with muscle relaxants being the most common offenders in this setting.
7. The overall incidence of anaphylactic reactions to latex greatly increased in the 1990s, but with the institution of nonpowdered gloves and nonlatex gloves in hospitals, the incidence may have stabilized.

Gender plays a role in the incidence of anaphylaxis. Simons and associates[47] demonstrated an age-related gender effect, where episodes are more common in males until age 15 years and in females older than 15 years. A similarly increased incidence in women has been reported.[2,37,49,51] The reason for this increased susceptibility in women is unclear; in animal models, however, mast cells have enhanced releasability and higher cell counts during the estrus phase of the menstrual cycle, and progesterone enhances sensitivity to anaphylaxis.[2] Anaphylaxis to insect sting is predominant in men, probably by virtue of increased exposure.[53]

Route of administration can affect both frequency of occurrence and severity of anaphylaxis caused by a provocative agent. Although anaphylaxis can occur with any route of administration—oral, subcutaneous, intramuscular, intravenous, intranasal, intraocular, cutaneous, intravaginal, intrarectal, and endotracheal—attacks appear to be more frequent and more severe with injection versus ingestion.[2]

The constancy of administration of antigen affects occurrence of anaphylaxis. For example, in most patients with insulin allergy, an anaphylactic reaction will not occur as long as drug administration is uninterrupted. Interruption in therapy, as

TABLE 77-3 Factors Affecting Incidence and Severity of Anaphylaxis

Factor	Effect
Age	More frequent in adults than children for some agents (radiocontrast media, plasma expanders, anesthetics); may be function of exposure frequency.
Socioeconomic status	Higher socioeconomic status associated with increased frequency of anaphylaxis based on outpatient epinephrine-dispensing rates.
Gender	Reportedly more common in women for latex, aspirin, and muscle relaxants. Random surveys show more frequent in females. May be more frequent in males for Hymenoptera stings, perhaps a function of exposure. Age-related effect shown, with males affected more frequently under age 15 years, and females affected more frequently after age 15.
Route of administration	Oral less likely to produce reaction, and reaction usually less severe.
Constancy of administration	Gaps in administration may predispose to reactions.
Time since last reaction	The longer the interval, the less likely the recurrence for many allergens.
Atopy	Risk factor for anaphylaxis as a result of ingested antigens, exercise anaphylaxis, idiopathic anaphylaxis, radiocontrast media reactions, latex reactions; probably not a risk factor for insulin, penicillin, and Hymenoptera reactions.
Geographic location	In most cases, no known effect documented; however, geographic location as well as rural environment affected incidence in one study. Investigations have now shown a clear north-south gradient in the Northern Hemisphere, with reactions more frequent in northern climes; the explanation remains unclear.
Race	No known effect
Chronobiology	No known effect of time of day or lunar cycle
Asthma	UK and U.S. studies have shown that asthma is a risk factor for anaphylactic events and that the more severe the asthma, the higher the risk.

occurs between pregnancies in women with gestational diabetes, increases the frequency of insulin anaphylaxis.[2]

Boleman and colleagues[48] examined the effect of chronobiologic factors on the incidence of anaphylaxis in patients receiving immunotherapy and retrospectively reviewed 210 anaphylactic reactions after immunotherapy from 1996 to 2000. They found no relationship between time of day or lunar cycle and the incidence of anaphylactic episodes. The lack of effect of the circadian cycle on the incidence has also been reported.[37]

Whether atopy is a risk factor for anaphylaxis appears to depend on several variables, including the antigen involved and the route of administration. Early investigations found that anaphylaxis to penicillin was more common in atopic individuals, but later reviews have not confirmed this observation. A multicenter cooperative study of penicillin allergy by the American Academy of Allergy found no correlation between penicillin reactivity and a personal or family history of atopy.[2] Similar observations have been made regarding anaphylactic reactions to insulin, Hymenoptera stings, and muscle relaxants. On the other hand, the incidence of anaphylaxis to latex is clearly increased in atopic individuals.[43] This probably relates to the nature of the antigen, its cross-reactivity with foods, and the route of sensitization (inhalation of latex-coated powder from gloves). These observations are in keeping with experimental data showing that atopic individuals appear to be more prone to producing IgE antibody when antigen is administered topically than when given by injection.[2]

Atopic individuals account for an inordinate percentage of anaphylaxis cases in random series,[37] as well as in series of idiopathic anaphylaxis,[37] exercise-induced anaphylaxis,[2] and anaphylactic reactions to radiocontrast media.[2,34] It is unclear why atopic persons exhibit such heightened predisposition. An increased level of IgE alone is insufficient to account for this phenomenon, and only a minority of atopic individuals are prone to anaphylaxis. For example, most tolerate large amounts of allergen administered during immunotherapy. Also, many people have elevated amounts of IgE to insect venom, latex, or food, but fail to develop systemic reactions on exposure. Thus additional factors account for the idiosyncrasy of anaphylactic events. Possible abnormalities include autonomic nervous system dysfunction (e.g., β-blockade) and the phenomenon of basophil hyperreleasability, seen in many atopic states, including food allergy, atopic dermatitis, asthma, and bronchopulmonary aspergillosis.[2] This in vitro phenomenon could reflect increased in vivo sensitivity to agents capable of causing mast cell and basophil degranulation. In atopic patients the time of year the antigen is administered may also play a role, because anaphylactic reactions to allergen immunotherapy are increased during pollen season.

Frequency of exposure is an important factor in terms of incidence. This is self-evident in most cases but can be cryptic in others. For example, diabetic patients treated with protamine-containing insulin are 40 to 50 times more likely to have reactions to protamine when this agent is administered to reverse heparin anticoagulation. Also, previous administration of protamine for heparin neutralization can sensitize a patient to insulin preparations containing protamine. Reactions to these preparations can be confused with anaphylactic reactions to insulin, and the previous sensitization experience to protamine can be missed, resulting in delayed recognition of protamine as the responsible agent.[2]

Asthmatic individuals experience anaphylaxis more often than those without asthma. Data from the UK Health Improvement Network database also suggest that people with asthma have a greater risk of anaphylaxis, and that the more severe the asthma, the greater the risk, with women at higher risk than men, especially those with severe asthma.[49] A managed care organization in northern California also noted increased risk for anaphylaxis in patients with asthma.[54]

Pathology

Despite an overall lack of autopsied cases, several series describe the pathology of anaphylactic deaths.[55-58] Pumphrey and Roberts[55] reported the largest series, 56 cases, with histology performed in only 20 necropsies. Mosbech[57] reviewed the findings in 26 deaths caused solely by insect stings, and Delage and Irey[56] evaluated 43 anaphylactic deaths. The remaining pathologic findings are described in case reports, small series, and reviews of previously published data.[59-69] An important finding from these reports is that anaphylactic deaths may have no significant macroscopic pathology. In 23 of 56 cases, nothing was indicative of anaphylaxis on macroscopic examination, possibly because death can occur rapidly, in this series within 1 hour after onset of symptoms in 39 patients.[55]

Macroscopically identifiable pathologic findings most often involve the respiratory tract. In one series the most common macroscopic findings were pharyngeal or laryngeal edema (23 of 56 cases) and mucus plugging or hyperinflated lungs (15 cases).[55] In another series, upper airway edema was found in about 60% of deaths, and bronchial obstruction with hyperinflation occurred in about 50% of cases.[56] Bronchial obstruction was caused by a combination of bronchospasm, submucosal edema, and secretions. Upper airway edema was the result of the accumulation of transudate in the submucosa.

Mosbech[57] reported that preexisting atherosclerotic heart disease contributed to cardiovascular collapse in 5 of the 26 cases, consistent with myocardial damage reported in the majority of cases on extensive histologic review.[68] Other findings included dilatation of the right ventricle; diffuse eosinophilic infiltration of the pulmonary vessels, lamina propria of gastrointestinal (GI) tract, and sinusoids of spleen; and congestion of abdominal viscera.[55-57] Greenberger and associates[58] reported 25 pathology results in documented fatal anaphylactic events. The reactions began within 30 minutes of exposure in 21 of the 25 cases, with death within 60 minutes in 13 of 25. Urticaria occurred in only one of these 25 cases. Anatomic findings consistent with anaphylaxis were present in 18 of the 23 subjects undergoing autopsy. At least one significant comorbid disease was identified in 22 of the 25 subjects. Fifteen of the 18 subjects had upper airway edema. This series consisted of elderly patients with a number of comorbidities.[58]

In view of the lack of significant findings in a large number of these cases, anaphylactic deaths presumably are underreported.[55] Also, death from anaphylaxis is usually the result of respiratory obstruction involving the upper or lower airway (or both) or cardiovascular collapse. When death is caused by cardiovascular collapse, especially if it occurs rapidly after onset of symptoms, pathologic findings can be sparse.

Over the last 2 decades, postmortem measurements of serum tryptase and antigen-specific IgE levels have suggested the incidence of anaphylactic death may be underestimated, and that a significant portion of unexplained sudden deaths may be caused by anaphylaxis.[70-78] Initial studies of postmortem antigen-specific IgE and serum tryptase found that a number of deaths of unknown cause in the spring and summer months might have been the result of undetected insect sting–induced anaphylaxis.[70,71] Also, serum tryptase levels were higher in patients experiencing anaphylactic deaths from venom injection versus ingested allergen. Connective tissue mast cells are preferentially degranulated when antigen is injected, whereas mucosal mast cells are preferentially degranulated when antigen is ingested. Connective tissue mast cells contain more tryptase than do mucosal mast cells.[70,71] These results suggested that measurement of antigen-specific IgE, and especially serum tryptase, might be used to determine whether death of unknown cause resulted from an anaphylactic episode.[72,74]

However, other evaluations have shown that serum tryptase levels may be less specific than previously proposed.[75,78] Deaths caused by trauma, sudden infant death syndrome, and heroin injection could also result in elevated postmortem tryptase. The presence of heterophilic antibodies could also lead to false-positive tryptase levels.[79] Thus, although useful for confirmation of anaphylaxis, elevated tryptase level postmortem does not conclusively establish anaphylaxis as the cause of death.

Pathophysiology

Anaphylaxis can result from several pathways of inflammation (Box 77-3). Mouse models demonstrate two distinct mechanisms that probably also apply to humans. The first, the classic IgE-dependent mechanism, depends on both interleukin-4 and IL-4 receptors and is characterized by allergen cross-linking of FcεRI receptors (high-affinity IgE receptors) on mast cells and basophils, from which subsequent release and fulminant propagation of inflammatory mediators and cytokines cause the smooth muscle contraction and increased vascular contractility associated with clinical anaphylaxis.[80,81] The second mechanism is IgE independent; is mediated by IgG, FcγRIII receptors, and either macrophages or basophils (depending on the experimental system); and requires proportionately more antigen and antibody than the IgE-dependent pathway.[80,82-85] Both mechanisms release platelet-activating factor (PAF), whereas only the IgE-dependent mechanism releases histamine.[80,82]

IgG-dependent anaphylaxis has not been proved in humans. However, human IgG receptors are capable of activating macrophages to release PAF,[80] which can activate mast cells in vitro.[86] Therefore PAF may contribute to human anaphylaxis.[87,88]

BOX 77-3 PATHOPHYSIOLOGIC CLASSIFICATION OF ANAPHYLAXIS

IgE DEPENDENT, IMMUNOLOGIC

- Foods
- Drugs
- Insect stings and bites
- Exercise (food dependent)
- Other causes

IgE INDEPENDENT, IMMUNOLOGIC

- Immune aggregates
- IgG anti-IgA
- Cytotoxic
- Disturbance of arachidonic acid metabolism
  - Aspirin
  - Other nonsteroidal antiinflammatory drugs
- Activation of kallikrein-kinin contact system
  - Dialysis membranes
  - Radiocontrast media
- Multimediator recruitment
  - Complement
  - Clotting
  - Clot lysis
  - Kallikrein-kinin contact system
- Other causes

NONIMMUNOLOGIC

- Direct mediator release from mast cells and basophils
  - Drugs, e.g., opiates
  - Physical factors, e.g., cold and sunlight
- Exercise
- *c-kit* Mutation (D816V)
- Other causes

IDIOPATHIC

Some agents can cause degranulation of mast cells and basophils without help from immunoglobulins, and this can lead to nonimmunologic anaphylaxis. Examples include physical factors, such as heat or cold, and opioids and vancomycin, which directly degranulate mast cells.[2]

IDIOPATHIC ANAPHYLAXIS

By definition, the cause of idiopathic anaphylaxis is unknown and its pathogenesis unclear. Grammer and colleagues[89] compared flow cytometric patterns in patients with recent idiopathic anaphylactic episodes, patients serving as normal controls, and patients with previous idiopathic episodes in remission. Patients with idiopathic anaphylaxis who had experienced a recent event had a significantly higher percentage of $CD3^+HLA\text{-}DR^+$ cells. The control group had a significantly lower percentage of $CD3^+HLA\text{-}DR^+$ cells than the other groups. The authors concluded that patients experiencing acute episodes had more activated T cells and postulated a role for these cells in the pathogenesis of idiopathic episodes.[60] These investigators also found that the chemokine MCP-1 was not responsible for histamine release in idiopathic events.[90,91]

Tejedor and associates[92] evaluated mast cell releasability in patients with idiopathic anaphylaxis. These patients showed a higher cutaneous response to codeine than atopic patients without anaphylaxis. The authors concluded that an increase in mast cell releasability might contribute to idiopathic anaphylaxis.

Reed and coworkers,[93] however, could not confirm an increased cutaneous sensitivity to codeine in 18 subjects with idiopathic anaphylaxis and 18 controls. The control group consisted of atopic and nonatopic individuals without episodes of anaphylaxis. No difference was found between the patient and control groups when skin was tested to serial dilutions of codeine or histamine, or in basophil sensitivity (CD63 activation) to formyl-Met-Leu-Phe (fMLP). In addition, baseline serum levels of IL-4, IL-5, and IL-13 were the same in all groups. In contrast, peripheral blood monocyte production of IL-4, IL-5, and IL-13 after anti-CD3 stimulation followed by 24-hour incubation revealed that subjects with idiopathic anaphylaxis, independent of atopic disease, had higher levels of IL-4 and trended toward higher levels of IL-5 and IL-13. The authors postulated that this helper T cell type 2 (Th2) cytokine milieu might have a role in the pathogenesis of idiopathic episodes.[93]

Basophil and Mast Cell Degranulation Syndromes

The majority of anaphylactic events involve basophil and mast cell degranulation with the release of biochemical mediators and chemotactic substances. Table 77-4 briefly summarizes the activities of these mediators and pathophysiologic consequences and clinical correlates. Anaphylaxis also depends on cellular responsiveness to these mediators. IL-4 and IL-13 are cytokines important in the initial responses to anaphylaxis. No comparable human studies have been conducted, but anaphylactic effects in the mouse depend on IL-4Rα–dependent IL-4/IL-13 activation of the transcription factor signal transducer and activator of transcription 6 (STAT6).[80]

The major pathophysiologic events caused by the release of these mediators include smooth muscle spasm (especially of bronchi, coronary arteries, and GI tract), increased vascular permeability, vasodilation, stimulation of sensory nerve endings with reflex activation of vagal effector pathways and antidromic pathways, and myocardial depression. These effects result in the classic symptoms of flush; urticaria and angioedema; wheeze; fall in blood pressure with potential features of both distributive and hypovolemic shock; GI smooth muscle contraction with

TABLE 77-4 Mast Cell and Basophil Mediators and Roles in Producing Anaphylactic Events

Mediators	Pathophysiologic Activity	Clinical Correlates
Histamine and products of arachidonic acid metabolism (leukotrienes, thromboxane, prostaglandins, platelet-activating factor)	Smooth muscle spasm, mucus secretion, vasodilation, increased vascular permeability, activation of nociceptive neurons, platelet adherence, eosinophil activation, eosinophil chemotaxis	Wheeze, urticaria, angioedema, flush, itch, diarrhea, abdominal pain, hypotension, rhinorrhea, bronchorrhea
Neutral proteases: tryptase, chymase, carboxypeptidase, cathepsin G	Cleavage of complement components, chemoattractants for eosinophils and neutrophils, further activation and degranulation of mast cells, cleavage of neuropeptides, conversion of angiotensin I to angiotensin II	May recruit complement by cleaving C3; may ameliorate symptoms by invoking hypertensive response through angiotensin I-II conversion and by inactivating neuropeptides, although angiotensin II also may cause deleterious coronary artery vasoconstriction. Also, proteases can magnify response because of further mast cell activation.
Proteoglycans: heparin, chondroitin sulfate	Anticoagulation, inhibition of complement, phospholipase A_2 binding, chemoattractant for eosinophils, cytokine inhibition, kinin pathway activation	Can prevent intravascular coagulation and recruitment of complement. Can recruit kinins, increasing severity of reaction.
Chemoattractants: chemokines, eosinophil chemotactic factors	Summons cells to site	May be partly responsible for recrudescence of symptoms in late phase reaction or extension and protraction of reaction
Tumor necrosis factor α activates nuclear factor-κB	Produces platelet-activating factor (PAF)	Vascular permeability and vasodilation; PAF synthesized and released late, involved in late phase reactions

nausea, vomiting, and diarrhea; and myocardial ischemia. Data also suggest splenic involvement might be more important than previously thought.[94]

In addition, many of these mediators are capable of activating other inflammatory pathways. Mast cell kininogenase and basophil kallikrein can activate the kinin system. Tryptase also has kallikrein activity and can activate the complement cascade and cleave fibrinogen with potential clinical consequences of angioedema, hypotension, and disseminated intravascular coagulation (DIC).[2,95] Platelet-activating factor induces clotting and DIC. In a prospective controlled study of 41 subjects (age 15 to 74 years) and 23 nonallergic adult controls, serum PAF levels correlated directly and PAF acetylhydrolase levels correlated indirectly with severity of anaphylaxis.[87] In a companion retrospective analysis, PAF acetylhydrolase activity was significantly lower in subjects experiencing fatal peanut-induced anaphylaxis than in five control groups.

In addition, chemotactic agents have the capacity to prolong and intensify reactions by activating eosinophils and other cells. Other agents may modify the pathophysiologic events. Heparin opposes complement activation, modulates tryptase activity, and inhibits clotting, plasmin, and kallikrein. Chymase is capable of converting angiotensin I to angiotensin II, independent of angiotensin-converting enzyme, and therefore theoretically could enhance the compensatory response to hypotension.[96] However, these effects may also cause deleterious coronary artery vasoconstriction. Cells, especially eosinophils, activated by chemotactic substances originally released from mast cells and basophils can be responsible for protracted episodes of anaphylaxis and for clinical recurrence after an initial improvement (late phase or biphasic response). For example, eosinophil-derived substances can activate mast cells, resulting in a secondary release of mediators. Eosinophil cationic protein levels were elevated in a 6-year-old boy with protracted anaphylaxis caused by either thiopental or cisatracurium.[97] Tumor necrosis factor-α (TNF-α), as observed in a murine model of penicillin-induced anaphylaxis, can also factor in protracted or recurrent anaphylaxis by initiating PAF production. Prolonged mast cell degranulation also could cause such events.[98]

A mouse model indicates that IL-33 can induce antigen-independent anaphylaxis and can directly induce degranulation and eicosanoid and cytokine production in IgE-sensitized mast cells.[99] Its role in human anaphylaxis has not been determined, but five atopic patients who sustained perioperative anaphylaxis had pronounced elevations in IL-33 compared with both atopic and nonatopic controls. IL-25 produced by Th17 lymphocytes induces eosinophilia and also upregulates tissue expression of IL-4, IL-5, and IL-13.[100] Conversely, regulatory T lymphocytes can suppress mast cell release of histamine, thus inhibiting anaphylaxis.[101,102]

HISTAMINE

Infusions of histamine experimentally produce the majority of the signs and symptoms of anaphylaxis,[2] and histamine has been the most intensively studied mediator. The actions relevant to anaphylaxis occur through activation of three histamine receptors (H_1, H_2, and H_3) and possibly a fourth (H_4) as well. The overall vascular effect of histamine is vasodilation. This produces flushing and decreased peripheral resistance, with a subsequent fall in systolic blood pressure. Vascular permeability increases because of the exposure of the permeable basement membrane secondary to separation of endothelial cells at the level of the postcapillary venule. Vasodilation is mediated by both H_1 and H_2 receptors. H_2 receptors exert their effect directly on the vascular smooth muscle. H_1 receptors also exert some direct effect, but their major activity is indirect via the stimulation of endothelial cells to manufacture nitric oxide.[2] The H_3 receptor can be found on presynaptic sites of histaminergic nerve terminals and tend to be inhibitory receptors. H_3 receptors are also found on peripheral afferent neurons, reducing nerve repolarization when stimulated, and in vascular beds. H_4 receptors are found principally on peripheral blood cells.

Cardiac effects of histamine are mediated primarily through the H_2 receptor, but the H_1 receptor also plays a role. H_2 receptor stimulation increases both rate and force of atrial and ventricular contraction, probably by enhancing calcium influx. This increases myocardial oxygen demand. H_1 receptor activity increases the heart rate by hastening diastolic depolarization at the sinoatrial node. H_1 receptor stimulation also produces coronary artery vasospasm.[2]

Histamine produces varying effects on extravascular smooth muscle. It causes smooth muscle contraction in the bronchial tree, which is mediated entirely via the H_1 receptor. H_1 receptor stimulation also causes modest contraction of the human uterus, whereas H_2 receptor stimulation can produce uterine relaxation. The dominant effect of histamine on GI smooth muscle is H_1 receptor–mediated contraction.

Glandular secretion is mediated by both H_1 and H_2 receptors. Stimulation of H_2 enhances glycoprotein secretion from goblet cells and bronchial glands, whereas stimulation of H_1 increases mucus viscosity. Infusion of histamine into humans produces symptoms similar to those observed during anaphylaxis. A combination of H_1 and H_2 receptor blockade is required for maximal inhibition of flushing, headaches, hypotension, and tachycardia.[2] This observation is clinically important. The H_3 receptor may have a role in anaphylaxis because its stimulation of presynaptic terminals of sympathetic effector nerves innervating the heart and systemic vasculature results in inhibition of norepinephrine release. Since norepinephrine is involved in the correction of hypotension in shock, blockade of H_3 stimulation may be beneficial in reversing hypotension, as demonstrated in a dog model of anaphylaxis.[103]

Murine models suggest H_4 receptors might be involved in chemotaxis and mast cell cytokine release and might also help to mediate pruritus.[104,105] However, potential human implications have not been studied.

RECRUITMENT OF OTHER INFLAMMATORY PATHWAYS

Mast cell and basophil contents can activate a number of inflammatory pathways, including the kallikrein-kinin and complement systems, as well as clotting and clot lysis. In addition, platelets are also activated during anaphlaxis (Box 77-4).[106] Strong in vivo evidence indicates that these recruitment pathways play an important role in the clinical events of anaphylaxis.

In three patients experiencing shock during controlled insect sting challenges,[107] peak histamine levels rose dramatically and correlated with the severity of hypotension. In addition, two of the three patients had decreased factor V, factor VIII, fibrinogen, and high-molecular-weight kininogen. One patient had decreased C4 and C3 levels. Later evaluation of eight patients

BOX 77-4 MULTIMEDIATOR RECRUITMENT DURING ANAPHYLAXIS

Coagulation pathway
- Decreased factor V
- Decreased factor VIII
- Decreased fibrinogen

Complement cascade
- Decreased C4
- Decreased C3
- Formation of C3a

Kallikrein-kinin contact system (kinin formation)
- Decreased high-molecular-weight kininogen
- Formation of kallikrein-C1-inhibitor complexes and factor XIIa-C1-inhibitor complexes

Platelet activation

showed C3a levels correlated with severity of anaphylaxis in sting challenge.[108]

Other investigations have demonstrated activation of the kallikrein-kinin system.[109] Kallikrein–C1 inhibitor complexes, factor XIIa–C1 inhibitor complexes, antigenic prekallikrein, and antigenic factor XII were measured in serial blood samples obtained from 16 subjects with a history of insect sting anaphylaxis immediately after insect sting challenge. Peak levels of kallikrein–C1 inhibitor complexes and factor XIIa–C1 inhibitor complexes were observed 5 minutes after the onset of symptoms. By 15 minutes, antigenic prekallikrein levels had decreased in patients with angioedema as a component of the anaphylactic event. These findings occurred only in subjects experiencing reactions. Therefore activation of the kallikrein-kinin contact system was strongly related to development of angioedema after sting challenge.

Mast cells secrete a number of cytokines during the degranulation process. Lin and Trivino[110] examined 85 patients admitted to the emergency department with acute allergic reactions, including anaphylaxis and measured levels of histamine, C-reactive protein (CRP), and IL-6. The levels of IL-6 and CRP were highly correlated. IL-6 and histamine levels were both significantly correlated with the extent of erythema. However, histamine was not positively correlated with IL-6 or CRP. Histamine levels correlated with the extent of urticaria, but IL-6 and CRP did not. A negative correlation was demonstrated between IL-6 concentration and the mean arterial blood pressure. The authors concluded that CRP and IL-6 were not surrogate markers for histamine release in mast cells and basophils. However, IL-6 levels did correlate with erythema and lower arterial blood pressure. IL-6 levels might correspond to a decrease in peripheral vascular resistance, and CRP and IL-6 increases might be markers of a late phase response, which might also explain the inverse correlation between CRP and histamine levels. As histamine from the acute phase response declines, the levels of CRP and IL-6 from macrophages and monocytes increase.

As previously noted, recruitment of other inflammatory pathways could be caused by tryptase, mast cell kininogenase, and basophil kallikrein. The additional cellular and biochemical events (e.g., hypoxia, endothelial damage) that occur during shock could activate the kallikrein-kinin contact system, coagulation pathway, and complement system. Activation of these systems has been noted in severe hypotension of other etiologies (e.g., cardiovascular shock, endotoxic shock). Hypotension can be correlated with elevations of histamine, tryptase, and C3a, but levels of these mediators may not correlate with the presence of flushing, urticaria, or bronchospasm.[2] Angioedema may be related to the appearance of activation products of the contact (kallikrein-kinin) system[111] or to angiotensin-converting enzyme (ACE) levels, which also influence kinin levels.[112]

Levels of two enzymes involved in bradykinin metabolism, serum ACE and aminopeptidase P (APP), were measured in 122 patients with peanut and tree nut allergy who presented with acute allergic reactions after ingestion of these agents.[112] Of these, 46 had moderate to severe pharyngeal edema, 36 had moderate to severe bronchospasm, and 40 lacked these findings. Patients clinically judged to have severe pharyngeal edema had significantly lower serum ACE levels than those with no pharyngeal edema. Multivariate analysis indicated that patients with serum ACE concentrations in the lowest quartile were almost 10 times more likely to have severe pharyngeal edema than those with higher ACE concentrations. However, patients with serum ACE levels in the lowest quartile were no more likely than others to have urticaria, bronchospasm, or reduced consciousness. Serum APP levels did not correlate with clinical severity and had no statistical trends. More studies are needed, but these findings suggest a clinical scenario in which some patients who experience angioedema during anaphylaxis might be more resistant to treatment with epinephrine and other therapeutic agents recommended for use after epinephrine.

INDUCTION OF NITRIC OXIDE SYNTHESIS

Nitric oxide (NO) is a potent autocoid vasodilator that participates in the homeostatic control of vascular tone and regional blood pressure.[113,114] The L-arginine is converted to NO as histamine binds to H_1 receptors during phospholipase C–dependent calcium mobilization through the activity of nitric oxide synthase (NOS). There are three isoforms of NOS. The constitutively expressed isoforms endothelial NOS (eNOS) and neuronal NOS (nNOS) presumably produce low amounts of NO for physiologic and antiinflammatory functions. Conversely, inflammation-associated expression of the isoform inducible NOS (iNOS) and subsequent overproduction of NO and activation of guanylate cyclase have been implicated in the adverse cardiovascular effects associated with septic shock. Many have presumed that iNOS has a similar role in anaphylaxis.[115] However, subsequent studies in knockout mice suggest that eNOS, rather than iNOS, is a critical mediator of PAF-mediated anaphylactic shock.[116] Human data are unavailable, but these findings suggest NOS involvement in anaphylaxis is more complex than previously thought.

Nitric oxide has the potential to be both beneficial and detrimental in anaphylaxis (Box 77-5). NO relaxes bronchial smooth muscle while dilating vascular smooth muscle. In addition to inducing peripheral vasodilatation, NO can enhance vascular permeability. Its effect on smooth muscle thus can improve bronchospasm while worsening hypotension. NO can also inhibit mediator release from mast cells. However, the total effects appear to be adversarial, resulting in hypotension, loss of intravascular volume, and hemoconcentration. At least in animal models of anaphylaxis, an NO synthesis inhibitor exerts a beneficial effect in shock,[2] and similar effects have been seen in humans with hypotension caused by cardiogenic shock.[2]

Nitric oxide is increased in exhaled air during anaphylaxis.[117] However, the role of NO in the production of anaphylactic

BOX 77-5 NITRIC OXIDE EFFECTS RELATIVE TO ANAPHYLAXIS

POTENTIALLY DETRIMENTAL

Vasodilatation (peripheral vascular bed)
Increased vascular permeability

POTENTIALLY BENEFICIAL

Bronchodilatation
Vasodilatation (coronary arteries)
Decreased mast cell degranulation

reactions has been questioned. In a study of 77 patients with acute allergic reactions, NO levels were assayed in stored serum. Histamine, tryptase, IL-6, and CRP were also measured. No correlation was found between NO levels and plasma histamine or serum tryptase levels. NO levels also were not correlated with urticaria or erythema and were no higher in patients with hypotension or bronchospasm.[118]

Mechanisms in Anaphylactic Shock

Many of the pathophysiologic events that occur during anaphylactic shock are easily explained by the actions of mediators cited earlier, all of which have overlapping actions of similar clinical importance. However, the mechanism producing hypotension and shock is more complicated and deserves special mention.

The balance of evidence from human observations and animal studies suggests that the main pathophysiologic features of anaphylactic shock are a profound reduction in venous tone and fluid extravasation. The resulting mixed hypovolemic-distributive shock involves reduction in blood volume (hypovolemia) from extravasation and distribution of blood to the wrong areas. Both combine to cause reduced venous return to the heart and an empty ventricle. Animal models and a few human case reports also suggest that depressed myocardial function can be a factor in some cases, introducing a component of temporary cardiogenic shock as well.[119] Electrocardiographic (ECG) changes are seen in some cases, but it is not known if this represents a mediator effect on myocardium, a reduction in coronary perfusion caused by low diastolic blood pressure (blood flow through coronary arteries occurs during diastole when heart relaxes), or a coronary spasm or sometimes plaque rupture. Box 77-6 summarizes likely key pathologic mechanisms of human anaphylactic shock.[119]

Arguably the most important human study to date is a series of 205 episodes of anaphylactic shock occurring under anesthesia, where the treating anesthesiologist was asked to provide detailed clinical and laboratory information immediately after the event.[120,121] Increases in hematocrit signaled extravasation of up to 35% of circulating blood volume within 10 minutes. Forty-six patients with central or pulmonary artery catheters placed before or soon after onset of anaphylaxis had a significant fall in filling pressures, except in 9 of 11 patients with cardiac disease, who had elevated pressures. Even so, these patients appeared to need volume expansion to achieve a stable blood pressure. In all six patients with balloon pulmonary artery catheters, pulmonary pressure rose initially and then fell over the next 10 minutes.

A report of eight closely observed hypotensive anaphylactic reactions found that hypotension was preceded by a fall in diastolic blood pressure (suggesting reduced systemic vascular resistance) with tachycardia. Following this, in every case the onset of hypotension was accompanied by a *relative* bradycardia. That is, rather than the heart rate further increasing to compensate for falling blood pressure, it fell as the blood pressure fell.[122] This may have been caused by a neurocardiogenic reflex, triggered by cardiac mechanoreceptors, and enhanced by increased levels of various mediators known to potentiate this reflex that are also elevated during anaphylaxis. However, bradycardia may also be a nonspecific feature of severe hypovolemic-distributive shock in awake animals. Paradoxic bradycardia has been reported as a common feature of traumatic hypotension in humans. Physiologic studies of awake mammals have identified two phases of response to hypovolemia, an initial phase of blood pressure maintenance by tachycardia and peripheral arteriolar constriction, followed by a second phase with more severe hypovolemia, characterized by bradycardia, reduced peripheral arteriolar tone, and a profound fall in blood pressure. However, bradycardia has *not* been reported as a feature of anaphylaxis under anesthesia, where tachycardia is the norm except when the patient had prior β-adrenergic blockade or severe hypoxia. This may be explained by the blunting of central reflexes that occurs under anesthesia and with different allergen routes and dosage.

Upright or semirecumbent (sitting upright) posture has been associated with fatal anaphylaxis. Movement from a supine

BOX 77-6 KEY PATHOPHYSIOLOGIC MECHANISMS OF HUMAN ANAPHYLACTIC SHOCK

COMMON/CLEARLY DEMONSTRATED*

Fluid extravasation causing hemoconcentration, hypovolemia, and reduced venous return to the heart manifested as low filling pressures and reduction in cardiac output.

LIKELY†

Venodilation and blood pooling, contributing to reduced venous return.
Impaired myocardial contractility contributing, along with reduced venous return, to reduced cardiac output.
Relative bradycardia (neurally mediated) in awake patients, contributing to reduced cardiac output.
Early transient increase in pulmonary vascular resistance, contributing to reduced cardiac output by obstructing venous return to left side of heart.
Early arteriolar dilation, manifested as a widened pulse pressure and contributing to hypotension. (However, an *increase* in systemic vascular resistance caused by increased arteriolar tone may predominate after this early phase.)

UNCOMMON/POSTULATED‡

Severe global depression of myocardial contractility, with nonspecific ST-segment electrocardiographic changes (unresponsive to adrenaline) possibly more likely in those with underlying cardiac disease or taking β-blockers.
Severe arteriolar dilation as well as venous dilation.
Coronary ischemia caused by coronary vasospasm and plaque ulceration.

Modified from Brown SGA. The pathophysiology of shock in anaphylaxis. Immunol Allergy Clin North Am 2007;27:165-75.
*Supported by unambiguous observations of human anaphylaxis.
†Unproven but supported by animal studies, studies of histamine infusion in volunteers, known mediator actions, or indirect physiologic observations during human anaphylaxis.
‡Based on case reports, speculation, and plausible mechanisms.

to an upright or semi-upright position reduces venous return to the heart and is likely to exacerbate all the pathophysiologic processes involved in anaphylaxis (reduced venous return, profound bradycaria with further reduction in cardiac output myocardial ischemia). Thus keeping a patient flat to maximize venous return to the heart is a key component of first aid for anaphylaxis.[123]

A fall in blood pressure and reduced tissue perfusion lead to compensatory mechanisms that involve secretion of catecholamines (norepinephrine, epinephrine),[124,125] activation of the angiotensin system (with angiotensin I and II production),[126] and production of endothelin-1, a potent vasoconstrictor peptide increased in patients with heart failure, stroke, or hypotension.[127] Failure to mobilize these compensatory mechanisms may predispose patients to anaphylaxis.[128,129]

Anaphylactic episodes are dynamic, and cardiovascular status can change during different stages of the event (Table 77-5). The changes can also be quite variable. For example, during the initial phase, at the onset of shock, systemic vascular resistance (SVR) can be reduced with a drop in diastolic blood pressure (but normal systolic blood pressure) and a compensatory tachycardia, whereas SVR can rise later, presumably through the compensatory vasoconstrictor response, administration of endogenous vasoconstrictors, or both. In other patients it is thought that a profound loss of vascular tone can occur despite standard doses of epinephrine. Cardiac output, which can initially be increased, characteristically declines as the event progresses. Central venous pressure may be normal during the early phases of anaphylaxis and then should consistently fall with progression of the reaction. The same occurs with pulmonary capillary wedge pressure.

These changes are important to therapy. The one consistent and most important finding in regard to the production of hypotension is the mixed hypovolemic-distributive shock and modestly reduced cardiac output. In most patients a combination of epinephrine and fluid resuscitation will overcome these effects. When patients fail to respond to these first-line measures, fluid resuscitation is adequate; often it has not because up to 5 L of fluid may be required in the first 20 minutes.[120,121] An intravenous infusion of epinephrine may be required because intramuscular doses may not be well absorbed when blood pressure is low. Intravenous atropine may be required to treat profound bradycardia, but this will be of little use if fluid status is not corrected.[122] Then, recognizing that some patients may have profound vasodilation, a trial of selective vasoconstrictor (e.g., metaraminol, vasopressin) may be warranted if blood pressure remains low. Also, because some patients have profound but reversible myocardial depression, urgent bedside echocardiographic assessment, phosphodiesterase inhibitor inotropes (particularly if patient taking β-blockers), and mechanical circulatory support may be required.

TABLE 77-5 Dynamics of Cardiovascular Abnormalities in Anaphylactic Shock

	At Onset of Reaction	Early Stage (Minutes) with No Treatment	Prolonged Shock
Blood pressure	↓	↓↓	↓↓↓
Pulse	↑	↑	↑↑
Cardiac output	↑	↓	↓↓
PVR	↓	→↓(*)	→↑↓(*)
Intravascular volume	→↓	↓	↓↓↓

(*)Peripheral vascular resistance (PVR) can vary, likely depending on internal compensation response.

Signs and Symptoms

The clinical manifestations of anaphylaxis can best be ascertained by a review of published series (Table 77-6).[2,52,122,130-137] This summary includes series of patients with exercise-induced anaphylaxis or idiopathic anaphylaxis; series limited to pediatric patients; and series of randomly selected patients of all ages. Overall, the clinical similarities shared by patients in these series are striking. The most common manifestations are cutaneous, followed by respiratory, cardiovascular, and gastrointestinal.

However, there are exceptions to these prototypical clinical manifestations. For example, cardiovascular collapse with shock can occur immediately without any cutaneous or respiratory symptoms.[2] In fact, in a series of 27 severe episodes[130] only 70% of patients with circulatory and/or cardiovascular collapse had cutaneous manifestations. About 30% of these had GI symptoms, and 85% had neurologic symptoms (seizures, impaired consciousness, muscle spasms). The lack of cutaneous symptoms, specifically urticaria, in severe events was also noted in a series of fatal reactions.[58] In these severe episodes, incidence of cutaneous manifestations was also extremely low. Thus, in severe episodes, cutaneous features do not seem to occur. The relative paucity of cutaneous symptoms may be the result of symptom data recorded after emergency personnel arrival. Alternately, the lack of cutaneous symptoms may have been caused by an inability to manifest them because of profound hypotension with loss of blood volume into the third space. The postmortem series of deaths was reported in older patients,[58] who more often have cardiovascular involvement than younger persons.[131]

TABLE 77-6 Signs and Symptoms of Anaphylaxis: Frequency of Occurrence*

Signs/Symptoms	Percentage of Cases†
CUTANEOUS	>90
Urticaria and angioedema	85-90
Flush	45-55
Pruritus without rash	2-5
RESPIRATORY	40-60
Dyspnea, wheeze	45-50
Upper airway angioedema	50-60
Rhinitis	15-20
DIZZINESS, SYNCOPE, HYPOTENSION	30-35
ABDOMINAL	
Nausea, vomiting, diarrhea, cramping pain	25-30
MISCELLANEOUS	
Headache	5-8
Substernal pain	4-6
Seizure	1-2

*Based on a compilation of 1784 patients reviewed in Lieberman P. Anaphylaxis and anaphylactoid reactions. In: Middleton E et al, editors. Allergy: principles and practice, 5th ed. St Louis: Mosby–Year Book; 1998. p. 1079-92.

†Percentages are approximations (see text).

In addition, although common manifestations of food allergy[2] in double-blind placebo-controlled food challenges, cutaneous symptoms may occur less frequently during anaphylaxis. For example, in 100 children evaluated for food allergy by oral food challenge, skin symptoms were the most frequent manifestations, overall approximately 84%, slightly lower than in random series.[132] In 57 children presenting to the emergency department (ED) with anaphylaxis, cutaneous symptoms were much less common, with pruritus in 40%, history of generalized erythema in 26% and found on examination in 25%, urticaria in 54%, and angioedema in 32%. The overall percentage with cutaneous features was 82%. However, the incidence of cutaneous features may have been reduced because of the time between the onset of symptoms and ED presentation.[133] In contrast, in a larger series of anaphylaxis in children, cutaneous symptoms were clearly predominant.[134]

The signs and symptoms of anaphylaxis that occur during anesthesia may be different from those noted in episodes occurring outside the operating room (OR). Significant differences also may exist between operative IgE-mediated events and non-IgE-mediated events.[2] The incidence of cutaneous manifestations is approximately 75% for IgE-mediated events and slightly higher for non-IgE-mediated episodes. Cardiovascular collapse appears to occur more often in operative events than those occurring outside the OR. During operative events, cardiovascular collapse is significantly more common during IgE-mediated events than those nonallergic in nature. The same holds true for wheezing and bronchospasm. Overall, surgical IgE-mediated events are more severe than those caused by non-IgE-mediated mechanisms. There are no clear explanations for these observations.

Also, the signs and symptoms in infants can clearly differ from those in older children and adults. Infants may exhibit nonspecific behavioral changes such as crying, fussing, irritability, and fright. Infants may flush, feel hot, and cry. Hoarseness and dysphonia with drooling and increased secretions can occur, as well as nasal congestion and GI symptoms (e.g., regurgitation, spitting up, loose stools, colicky pain). Infants may exhibit drowsiness and somnolence. This stage can be followed by unresponsiveness and lethargy. Seizures can occur. Examination may show a weak pulse, pallor, and diaphoresis. Coughing and choking with stridor can occur as well.[135] In toddlers and infants who present with anaphylactic episodes, the major manifestation may mimic foreign body aspiration.[2] Vomiting without aspiration minutes after the ingestion of an allergenic food is also a common presentation in this age group.

When antigen has been administered by injection, symptoms usually begin within 5 to 30 minutes; however, the onset of symptoms can be 1 hour or more after injection. When antigen has been ingested, symptoms usually occur within the first 2 hours but can be delayed for several hours. However, onset of symptoms can occur immediately after ingestion, which can be fatal. The immediacy of symptom onset is thought to correlate directly with the severity of a given attack; the more rapid the onset, the more severe the episode.

An anaphylactic episode can abate and then exhibit a recrudescence several hours after symptoms have disappeared, termed *biphasic anaphylaxis.* In addition, attacks can be protracted, persisting for several days, and characterized by multiple recurrences interrupted by hours-long asymptomatic periods. Protracted shock and adult respiratory distress syndrome can occur despite appropriate therapy. The exact incidence of biphasic reactions is unknown, but reports range from 1% to 20% of episodes.[70] The severity of the second response is highly variable. Events range from mild to severe, with fatalities reported. Delayed administration and underdosing of epinephrine predispose to a late phase response. No clear evidence shows that the recurrent response can be suppressed by corticosteroids. Most biphasic reactions occur within the first 8 hours after resolution of the primary phase, although recurrent events have been described as late as 72 hours. Such events are more common when antigen has been ingested rather than injected. The mechanism of production of biphasic anaphylaxis is not known.

The cardiac manifestations of anaphylaxis can be varied and profound.[2] Characteristically, anaphylaxis is associated with a compensatory tachycardia that occurs in response to a decreased effective vascular volume. This has often been used as a sign to differentiate an anaphylactic episode from a vasodepressor reaction. However, bradycardia, presumably caused by increased vagal reactivity, can also occur in anaphylaxis. This is probably due to the Bezold-Jarisch reflex, a cardioinhibitory reflex that has its origin in sensory receptors in the inferoposterior wall of the left ventricle. Unmyelinated vagal C fibers transmit the reflex, which is activated by ischemia. The most extensive study of bradycardia in anaphylaxis in humans involved 21 healthy adults with systemic allergic reactions to insect venom with provocative stings in a controlled setting; 18 required intervention.[122] Hypotension was always accompanied by an initial relative bradycardia severe enough to require atropine therapy in two patients.

Myocardial depression with decreased cardiac output as a result of contractile depression can occur and persist for several days, thought to result from hypoxemia.[2] Coronary artery vasospasm has been documented with coronary angiography and can be severe enough to result in myocardial infarction (Kounis syndrome).[136] ECG abnormalities include ST-segment elevation, flattened T waves, inverted T waves, and arrhythmias (e.g., from heart block). Cardiac enzyme elevations also occur. Arterial blood gas abnormalities usually involve a fall in oxygen (Po_2) and carbon dioxide (Pco_2) partial pressure early in the course. If severe respiratory difficulty supervenes, the hypoxia worsens and Pco_2 may increase, along with a decrease in pH likely caused by a combination of CO_2 retention and metabolic acidosis.

Anaphylaxis can present with unusual manifestations that make diagnosis difficult. Syncope without other manifestations can occur and has been reported in episodes caused by fire ant sting and mastocytosis.[2] Individuals experiencing syncope alone can present with a seizure or simply spontaneous loss of consciousness. With this form of presentation, unnecessary cardiovascular and neurologic evaluations are often done before establishing the diagnosis of anaphylaxis.

Rarely, anaphylaxis can cause adrenal hemorrhage. Hypotension is prolonged in these patients. It is important to consider adrenal hemorrhage in patients with resolution of all manifestations except hypotension.[2] Profound anaphylactic episodes with hypotension can also result in fibrinolysis and DIC. Four patients who experienced hypotensive reactions (three with elevated plasma tryptase) had abnormal thromboelastograms and clear-cut evidence of DIC. The events occurred through both IgE-mediated and non–IgE-mediated mechanisms. Tranexamic acid rapidly reversed the coagulopathy in all patients.[137]

BOX 77-7 DIFFERENTIAL DIAGNOSIS OF ANAPHYLAXIS

Anaphylaxis
- Anaphylaxis to exogenously administered agents
- Physical factors
  - Exercise
  - Cold, heat, sunlight
- Idiopathic

Vasodepressor Reactions
- Flush syndromes
  - Carcinoid
  - Menopause
  - Chlorpropamide, alcohol
- Medullary carcinoma thyroid
- Autonomic epilepsy

Restaurant Syndromes
- Monosodium glutamate (MSG)
- Sulfites
- Scrombroidosis

Other forms of shock
- Hemorrhagic
- Cardiogenic
- Endotoxic

Excess Endogenous Production of Histamine Syndromes
- Systemic mastocytosis
- Urticaria pigmentosa
- Basophilic leukemia
- Acute promyelocytic leukemia (tretinoin)
- Hydatid cyst

Nonorganic Disease
- Panic attacks
- Munchausen stridor
- Vocal cord dysfunction syndrome
- Globus hystericus
- Undifferentiated somatoform anaphylaxis

Miscellaneous
- Hereditary angioedema
- Progesterone anaphylaxis
- Urticarial vasculitis
- Pheochromocytoma
- Hyper-IgE, urticaria syndrome
- Neurologic (seizure, stroke)
- Pseudoanaphylaxis
- Red man syndrome (vancomycin)
- Capillary leak syndrome

Differential Diagnosis

The differential diagnosis of anaphylaxis is presented in Box 77-7. This classification includes conditions that should be considered by the physician who sees the patient during the acute event, as well as those conditions that should be considered when the patient is seen after the episode for determining the cause of the event.

Perhaps the most common condition mimicking anaphylaxis is the vasodepressor reaction. The mechanisms underlying the vasodepressor response have not been clarified, but such reactions may be caused by the activation of the Bezold-Jarisch reflex. This reflex is initiated by excessive venous pooling, with a resulting decrease in ventricular volume and an increase in ventricular inotropy. These events activate sensory receptors that respond to wall tension in the inferoposterior portions of the left ventricle, paradoxically increasing neural response through the vagus nerve. The result is vasodilatation, bradycardia, hypotension, and loss of consciousness. Characteristic features of vasodepressor reactions are therefore hypotension, pallor, weakness, nausea, vomiting, and diaphoresis. Patients with severe reactions lose consciousness.[2] These reactions often result from a threatening event or emotional trauma. The characteristic bradycardia is used to distinguish these episodes from anaphylaxis. However, as previously noted, the Bezold-Jarisch reflex can be elicited in anaphylactic events characterized by hypotension, and therefore bradycardia can also be a feature of anaphylaxis.[122] Another important differential diagnostic factor is that vasodepressor reactions are not accompanied by cutaneous manifestations such as urticaria, angioedema, or flush.

FLUSHING SYNDROMES

Entities that produce flush should also be considered in the differential diagnosis of anaphylaxis. Flushing is a common phenomenon and can result from a variety of agents, including niacin, nicotine, catecholamines, ACE inhibitors, and alcohol (with and without associated drugs). Flush is also seen in association with carcinoid syndrome, pancreatic tumors, medullary carcinoma of the thyroid, hypoglycemia, rosacea, pheochromocytoma, menopause, autonomic epilepsy, panic attacks, and systemic mastocytosis.[2]

Flush occurs in wet and dry forms. The *wet* form is associated with sweating and mediated by sympathetic cholinergic nerves that supply sweat glands in the skin. This type of flush is characteristic in menopausal women. It also occurs after the ingestion of spicy foods containing capsaicin. Direct vasodilation without stimulation of the sweat glands produces a *dry* flush, as is seen in the carcinoid syndrome. Not surprisingly, carcinoid syndrome produces symptoms similar to anaphylaxis because carcinoid tumors secrete histamine, kallikrein, neuropeptides, and prostaglandins, in addition to 5-hydroxytryptamine (5-HT, serotonin).[2] A similar mechanism underlies the flush caused by pancreatic tumors and thyroid medullary carcinoma. These tumors also can secrete prostaglandins, histamine, substance P, and 5-HT. Patients with medullary carcinoma of the thyroid have telangiectasia, a positive family history for the disease, and mucosal neuromas.

Menopausal flush lasts approximately 3 to 5 minutes, can occur several times a day, is associated with sweating, and may occur intermittently. Episodes usually occur over 5 months to 5 years. Menopausal flush is often aggravated by alcohol and stress. There are no respiratory tract symptoms or decreases in blood pressure.

Autonomic epilepsy is a rare condition thought to be caused by paroxysmal autonomic discharges. Blood pressure may fall or rise, and tachycardia, flush, and syncope can occur.

In alcohol-induced flush, a nonelevated intense erythema, mainly over the face and trunk, occurs within minutes after the person drinks even small amounts of alcohol. Symptoms usually peak 30 to 40 minutes after ingestion and subside within 2 hours. There are two forms of alcohol-induced flushing: (1) the event is associated with the intake of drugs, and (2) alcohol alone is sufficient stimulus to produce the episode. The second form, occurring independent of drug ingestion, is extremely common in Asians (47% to 85%)[2] but also occurs in non-Asians (3% to 29%).[2] Symptoms are worse in the drug-independent form. Both types can be associated with nausea, anxiety, lightheadedness, headache, and vomiting. In the drug-independent form, wheezing and conjunctivitis can be seen as well. Drugs linked to alcohol-induced flushing include disulfiram, griseofulvin, and cephalosporins. Alcohol-induced flush has also been described in patients with Hodgkin disease or other malignancy, hypereosinophilic syndrome, mastocytosis, or splenectomy. In the drug-independent form in Asians, the reaction may be caused by abnormal alcohol metabolism, occurring in those with homozygous or heterozygous null alleles for the mitochondrial enzyme aldehyde dehydrogenase-2. Without the action of this enzyme, aldehyde accumulates after alcohol ingestion. In patients with this disorder the increased aldehyde levels have caused mast cell degranulation.[2]

In many cases the cause of flushing cannot be determined, and the patient is said to have an "idiopathic" flush reaction.

This occurs more frequently in women than men and may be associated with palpitations, diarrhea, syncope, and hypotension. There is no wheezing or abdominal pain.[2]

RESTAURANT SYNDROMES AND SCOMBROIDOSIS

A group of postprandial syndromes (restaurant syndromes) resembling anaphylaxis have been attributed to the ingestion of monosodium glutamate (MSG), sulfites, or histamine. Ingestion of MSG can produce chest pain, facial burning, flushing, paresthesias, sweating, dizziness, headaches, palpitations, nausea, and vomiting. Children can experience shivering and chills, irritability, screaming, and delirium. The occurrence of these symptoms has been termed the *Chinese restaurant syndrome.* The mechanism is unknown, but MSG is thought to cause a transient acetylcholinosis. About 15% to 20% of the general population appears to be sensitive to small doses of MSG, but reactions can occur in any individual if the dose is large enough. Symptoms usually begin no later than 1 hour after ingestion, but can be delayed in onset up to 14 hours. There may be a familial tendency to develop these reactions.[2]

Scombroidosis, histamine poisoning caused by the ingestion of histamine in spoiled fish, appears to be increasing in frequency. Histamine is the major chemical involved in symptoms, but symptoms are not caused by the uncomplicated ingestion of histamine alone. For unclear reasons, the ingestion of histamine-contaminated spoiled fish is more toxic than the ingestion of equal amounts of pure histamine administered by mouth. However, *cis*-urocanic acid, an imidazole compound similar to histamine derived from histidine in spoiled fish, could account for this phenomenon. urocanic acid can degranulate mast cells, thus perhaps augmenting the response to endogenous histamine.[2] Histamine itself is produced by histidine decarboxylase from bacteria that cleave histamine from histidine in the spoiled fish. When caught, fish are not contaminated. The increase in histamine content occurs after death on board the fishing vessel, at the processing plant, in the distribution system, or in the restaurant or home. Fish with elevated histamine levels can look and smell normal. Cooking neither destroys the histamine nor alters the activity of urocanic acid.

The production of histamine and urocanic acid is increased when fish are stored at elevated temperatures. These agents are formed by bacteria such as *Morganella morganii, Klebsiella pneumoniae*, and *Hafniae alvei.* The optimal temperature for amine production is about 30° C (86° F). However, once the bacterial population is enlarged, ongoing histamine production can occur even during refrigeration at temperatures ranging from 0° to 5° C (32° to 41° F). Scombroidosis is the most prevalent form of seafood-borne disease in the United States.[2] It is probably underreported, because most episodes are mild. In addition, many episodes are reported as allergic reactions. It is most often produced by scombroid fish belonging to the family Scombroidae (e.g., tuna, mackerel) or Scomberesocidae (e.g., saury), but nonscombroid species (e.g., mahi-mahi, anchovies, herring), can also cause the problem.

As expected, the features of scombroidosis are very similar to those of anaphylaxis and can include cardiovascular, GI, cutaneous, and neurologic manifestations. Episodes can occur in outbreaks, with morbidity as high as 100%. However, individual susceptibility appears to vary greatly; episodes can occur from a few minutes to several hours after fish ingestion. The symptoms usually last for a few hours but occasionally persist for several days. The typical signs and symptoms, similar to histamine toxicity, include urticaria, flush, angioedema, nausea, vomiting, diarrhea, and hypotension. Neurologic findings are also common, with occasional wheezing. The most common symptom is flushing of the face and neck, accompanied by a sensation of heat and discomfort. The rash most frequently takes the appearance of a sunburn rather than urticaria. These cutaneous manifestations are the most common symptoms, with GI symptoms being second in frequency. Serious complications can occur in patients with preexisting cardiovascular or respiratory tract disease.

Although similar, several features distinguish histamine fish poisoning from food-induced anaphylaxis. First, many people dining at the same table can be affected—everyone who ingests significant quantities of the fish. Second, the cutaneous symptoms, as noted, are usually somewhat different, consisting of a prolonged flush without urticaria. This is also true of anaphylaxis triggered by foods, including fish. Patients taking isoniazid appear to have enhanced susceptibility to episodes of scombroidosis.[2]

Syndromes characterized by excessive endogenous production of histamine include systemic mastocytosis and leukemias with overproduction of histamine-containing cells (acute promyelocytic, basophilic). Anaphylaxis can occur in such patients after relevant stimuli. For example, episodes can be precipitated in patients with systemic mastocytosis on the ingestion of opiates and in patients with promyelocytic leukemia on treatment with tretinoin.[2]

NONORGANIC CONDITIONS

Nonorganic disease also can mimic anaphylaxis. Such episodes can be involuntary, such as in panic attacks, undifferentiated somatoform anaphylaxis, and vocal cord dysfunction syndrome, or they can be consciously self-induced, as in Munchausen stridor. Panic attacks are accompanied by tachycardia, flushing, GI symptoms, and shortness of breath. Vocal cord dysfunction syndrome is caused by an involuntary adduction of the vocal cords that occludes the glottal opening. A bunching together of the false vocal cords produces obstruction in both inspiration and expiration; the patient is unaware of the process. The term *Munchausen stridor* was coined to describe patients who intentionally adduct their vocal cords and present to the ED with self-induced manifestations of laryngeal edema. This entity occurs in psychologically disturbed individuals and can be distinguished from vocal cord dysfunction syndrome by laryngoscopy during the acute episode. Also, patients with Munchausen stridor can be distracted from their vocal cord adduction by asking them to perform maneuvers such as coughing.[2]

Undifferentiated somatoform anaphylaxis is a term used to describe patients who present with manifestations that mimic idiopathic anaphylaxis but who lack objective confirmatory findings, do not respond to therapy, and exhibit psychologic signs of an undifferentiated somatoform disorder.

OTHER DIFFERENTIAL DIAGNOSES

Other entities traditionally listed in the differential diagnosis of anaphylaxis include hereditary angioedema, progesterone anaphylaxis, anaphylaxis associated with recurrent and chronic urticaria, pheochromocytoma, neurologic disorders, tracheal foreign body, pseudoanaphylactic syndrome occurring after administration of procaine penicillin, and red man syndrome, often occurring after administration of vancomycin. Hereditary angioedema can cause laryngeal edema, abdominal pain, and an erythematous rash that can be confused with urticaria, although these two entities can usually be differentiated without difficulty.

Some patients diagnosed with "idiopathic anaphylaxis" were found to have progesterone-related anaphylactic episodes.[2] Patients with this disorder experience anaphylactoid reactions to the infusion of luteinizing hormone–releasing hormone (LHRH) and the intradermal injection of medroxyprogesterone. LHRH analog therapy is beneficial. The mechanism of this disorder is unknown, but the increased level of progesterone associated with menses may predispose patients to the anaphylactic event. This entity should be considered in women, usually over age 35, who present with recurrent episodes of anaphylaxis exhibiting a temporal relationship with the menstrual cycle. Some women with this disorder demonstrate an IgE antiprogesterone antibody, but others do not.

The vast majority of patients with chronic idiopathic urticaria or recurrent episodes of urticaria are not considered to be at risk for the development of anaphylaxis episodes. However, anaphylaxis can occur in patients who previously had only recurrent episodes of acute or chronic urticaria. Case reports include a patient with recurrent episodes of acute urticaria resulting in anaphylaxis who also had hyper-IgE and another with episodes of chronic urticaria who had urticarial vasculitis associated with an episode of shock, leukopenia, and thrombocytopenia, thought to be caused by activation of the complement cascade.[2] Occasionally, patients with pheochromocytoma can have symptoms suggestive of an anaphylactic reaction.

Pseudoanaphylaxis is a term used to describe the reaction in patients who develop syncope and neurologic symptoms after administration of procaine penicillin. These reactions are caused by procaine and not penicillin. Similar episodes have resulted from lidocaine administration. Lastly, capillary leak syndrome can present as anaphylaxis. This rare, often fatal disorder characterized by angioedema, GI symptoms, and shock with hemoconcentration is usually associated with a monoclonal gammopathy. Recurrent episodes can mimic idiopathic anaphylaxis.

Laboratory Findings

In some patients, laboratory evaluations can help establish a diagnosis of anaphylaxis or exclude other conditions. For example, plasma, serum, or urinary levels of serotonin, 5-hydroxyindoleacetic acid, catecholamines or catecholamine metabolites, substance P, vasointestinal polypeptide (VIP) hormones, urokinase A, and pancreastatin can be measured if a VIP-secreting tumor, carcinoid, or paradoxic pheochromocytoma is being considered.

Traditionally, serum tryptase, plasma histamine, and 24-hour urinary histamine metabolites (e.g., *N*-methylhistamine) have been used clinically to confirm the diagnosis of anaphylaxis. Tryptases are a subgroup of trypsin-family serine peptidases. Almost all human mast cells contain tryptases, and small amounts are also found in human basophils. Serum tryptase is specific to these cells, and elevated tryptase levels are a useful marker in the diagnosis of anaphylaxis. Tryptase is secreted constitutively in small amounts. Although α-tryptase was once thought to make up the majority of this tryptase, subjects with null alleles for α-tryptase exhibit normal levels of constitutively secreted tryptase, a mixture of α- and β-protryptase (mostly β). Also, the marked increases in tryptase levels seen during an anaphylactic event consist of mature β-tryptase.[138]

If a patient is seen shortly after onset of anaphylaxis, plasma and urinary histamine (or histamine metabolites) and serum tryptase determinations may be helpful. Plasma histamine levels begin to rise within 5 to 10 minutes and remain elevated for 30 to 60 minutes and therefore are of little help if the patient is seen even 1 hour after event onset. However, urinary histamine metabolites are elevated for a longer period and thus may be useful. Serum tryptase levels peak 60 to 90 minutes after onset of anaphylaxis and persist longer than plasma histamine levels do. Elevated tryptase concentrations are sometimes seen up to 5 hours after symptom onset and in rare cases can persist several hours longer.[2]

Disparities between histamine and tryptase levels occur. One patient exhibited a hypotensive reaction to thiopental in which plasma histamine was elevated 10 minutes after onset of hypotension without concomitant elevation in β-tryptase at 45 minutes, interpreted as activation of basophils without mast cell degranulation.[139] In a study of allergic reactions in the ED, plasma histamine concentration was elevated in 42 of 97 adult patients, but serum trypase was elevated in only 20.[140] Histamine levels correlated better with clinical signs than tryptase. Patients with elevated histamine were more likely to have urticaria, more extensive erythema, abnormal abdominal findings, and wheezing.

Other markers of mast cell and basophil degranulation evaluated for their ability to confirm a diagnosis of anaphylaxis include CD63 and CD203c, prostaglandin D_2, and carboxypeptidase. CD63 and CD203c are surface markers on basophils. The expression of CD63 and CD203c is upregulated and can be detected by flow cytometry,[93,141,142] shown to be reliable in assisting allergy diagnosis for reactions induced by food, latex, Hymenoptera venom, and drugs.[143] Prostaglandin D_2 levels have been used to confirm the diagnosis of anaphylaxis in patients with mastocytosis.[2] In mastocytosis patients, mast cell carboxypeptidase A levels in serum or plasma collected within 8 hours of the onset of allergic reactions were significantly greater than in control groups. Carboxypeptidase concentration was elevated in 83% of cases of elevated tryptase, as well as in 77 of 110 cases (70%) of suspected anaphylaxis that were tryptase negative.[144]

It might also be beneficial to obtain serum for the analysis of specific IgE against suspected antigens. Leftover or vomited food may be a useful source of antigen for the creation of a customized specific IgE test to identify the source in patients with possible anaphylaxis to food. The specific agent causing anaphylaxis may not be identifiable in many cases, especially in adults. The search for such an agent should include, when appropriate, tests for foods. Such tests can sometimes determine the offending agent in cases previously designated idiopathic. Tests should include not only foods but also spices and vegetable gum products. A detailed history is always the most important evaluation and should be repeated after each episode, occasionally, revealing a previously undetermined cause.

Prevention and Management

Anaphylactic reactions are an unavoidable aspect of the practice of medicine. Some episodes are so severe that treatment is

BOX 77-8 MEASURES TO REDUCE ANAPHYLAXIS AND ANAPHYLACTIC DEATHS

GENERAL INTERVENTIONS

Obtain thorough history for drug allergy.
Avoid drugs that have immunologic or biochemical cross-reactivity with any agents to which patient is sensitive.
Administer drugs orally rather than parenterally, when possible.
Check all drugs for proper labeling.
Keep patients in the office 20 to 30 minutes after injections.
Because of the potential for delayed anaphylaxis after monoclonal antibody therapy (e.g., omalizumab), observation periods of 2 hours for the first three injections and 30 minutes for subsequent injections are recommended.

MEASURES FOR PATIENTS AT RISK

Have patient wear and carry warning identification tags.
Teach self-injection of epinephrine, and advise patients to carry an epinephrine autoinjector.
Discontinue β-adrenergic blockers, angiotensin-converting enzyme inhibitors, angiotensin receptor blockers, monoamine oxidase inhibitors, and certain tricyclic antidepressants, when possible.
Use preventive techniques when patients undergo a procedure or take an agent that places them at risk, including pretreatment, provocative dose challenge, and desensitization.

unsuccessful. This underscores the critical importance of education, avoidance, and prevention, which together can decrease the incidence and severity of such reactions (Box 77-8).

Agents that cause anaphylaxis must be identified whenever possible, and patients should be instructed how to minimize future exposure to those agents. A thorough history for drug allergy should be taken for every patient. Proper interpretation of this history requires knowledge of the immunologic and biochemical cross-reactivities among drugs. When a history of an allergic reaction to a drug is present, a non–cross-reactive drug should be substituted whenever possible. Parenteral administration of medication usually produces more severe reactions than oral administration. Therefore drugs should be administered orally whenever possible. If the parenteral route is required, the patient should remain under medical observation for 20 to 30 minutes after administration. Anaphylaxis resulting from drug mislabeling is rare but occurs. Therefore proper labeling of drugs is essential, and whenever a drug is suspected as the cause of an episode, the contents of the container should be checked against the label.

Patients subject to anaphylaxis should wear a MedicAlert bracelet or neck chain and should carry an identification card.[4] They should also carry epinephrine autoinjectors at all times and know how to administer. β-Adrenergic blockers, ACE inhibitors, angiotensin receptor blockers (ARBs), monoamine oxidase inhibitors (MAOIs), and some tricyclic antidepressants (TCAs) should not be taken by patients who are at risk for anaphylaxis if other agents will suffice. These drugs decrease the effectiveness of epinephrine (β-blockers), interfere with endogenous compensatory responses to hypotension (ACE inhibitors, ARBs),[2] or affect use of epinephrine through side effects (MAOIs, some TCAs).

If patients are required to take medications or diagnostic agents or to undergo procedures that are known to place them at risk for an anaphylactic episode, specific preventive measures, such as pretreatment, provocative challenges, or desensitization, should be instituted when appropriate. Published preventive regimens are helpful in specific situations.

BOX 77-9 THERAPY FOR ANAPHYLAXIS

IMMEDIATE ACTION

Perform assessment.
Check airway and secure if needed.
Rapidly assess level of consciousness.
Vital signs

TREATMENT

Epinephrine
Supine position, legs elevated
Oxygen
Tourniquet proximal to injection site

DEPENDENT ON EVALUATION

Start peripheral intravenous fluids
H_1 and H_2 antihistamines
Vasopressors
Corticosteroids
Aminophylline
Glucagon
Atropine
Electrocardiographic monitoring
Transfer to hospital

HOSPITAL MANAGEMENT

Medical antishock trousers
Continued therapy with listed agents and management of complications

MANAGEMENT OF THE ACUTE EVENT

Boxes 77-9 and 77-10 outline the basic therapeutic approach, medications, and equipment in the emergency management of anaphylaxis. It is important to stress that these are subject to the discretion of the physician managing the care of the patient, and variations in their sequence and performance depend on clinical judgment and facilities at hand. In addition, the determination of when a patient should be transferred to an emergency department or intensive care unit also depends on the skill, experience, and assessment of the individual physician. Position statements on office equipment for management of anaphylaxis and other common emergencies include those from the American Academy of Pediatrics Committee on Drugs; American Academy of Allergy, Asthma, and Immunology;(Joint Task Force on Practice Parameters, Board of Directors); American College of Allergy, Asthma, and Immunology; and World Health Organization.

The emergency management of anaphylaxis is notable for the lack of guidance from high-level clinical trials. Current knowledge relies on observational human studies of likely mechanisms (from which appropriate treatment is inferred), nonrandomized assessments of therapeutic protocols, and controlled trials in animals. Nevertheless, more recent consensus guidelines are broadly consistent.[6,145,146] The following three guidelines direct the current approach to anaphylaxis management:

1. Giving epinephrine as soon as possible by the intramuscular (IM) route before shock intervenes is safe (even if diagnosis wrong) and likely effective in most cases. Injection into a large muscle (lateral thigh) probably results in more reliable absorption.[147]
2. When shock (hypotension) occurs, absorption from IM route may be poor. Intravenous bolus injections may cause dangerous blood pressure surges and may have only

BOX 77-10 EQUIPMENT AND MEDICATIONS FOR OFFICE THERAPY OF ANAPHYLAXIS

PRIMARY

- Tourniquet
- 1-mL and 5-mL disposable syringes
- Oxygen tank and mask/nasal prongs
- Epinephrine solution (aqueous) 1 : 1000 (1-mL ampules and multidose vials)
- Epinephrine solution (aqueous) 1 : 10,000 (preloaded syringe)
- Diphenhydramine injectable
- Ranitidine or cimetidine injectable
- Injectable corticosteroids
- Ambu-bag, oral airway, laryngoscope, endotracheal tube, No. 12 needle
- Intravenous setup with large-bore catheter
- Intravenous fluids: 2000 mL crystalloid, 1000 mL hydroxyethyl starch
- Aerosol β_2-bronchodilator and compressor nebulizer
- Glucagon
- Electrocardiogram
- Normal saline (10-mL vial for epinephrine dilution)

SUPPORTING

- Suction apparatus
- Dopamine
- Sodium bicarbonate
- Aminophylline
- Atropine
- Intravenous setup with needles, tape, and tubing
- Nonlatex gloves

OPTIONAL

- Defibrillator
- Calcium gluconate
- Medications for seizures
- Lidocaine

a transient therapeutic effect, whereas a controlled infusion of epinephrine is more likely to be efficacious.[148]

3. Severe reductions in venous return to the heart are a prominent feature of anaphylaxis because of a combination of vascular dilation and fluid extravasation. A supine posture is therefore a key part of basic life support, and aggressive fluid resuscitation is recommended for hypotensive anaphylaxis.[121,123,149]

Standard life support procedures should also be followed: airway, oxygen, and interventions for arrhythmias, including atropine for severe bradycardia, defibrillation for ventricular fibrillation, and external cardiac massage and bolus IV adrenaline, 1 mg every 2 to 3 minutes, for cardiac arrest. Treatments with steroids and antihistamines are unproven,[150,151] and animal data suggest potential for harm with antihistamines.[152] Therefore steroids and antihistamines are considered to be second-line therapies.

The initial step in managing anaphylaxis is a rapid assessment of the patient's status, with emphasis on evaluation of the airway, circulation, and state of consciousness and giving IM dose of adrenaline (lateral thigh) as soon as possible based on a quick estimate of patient weight. The patient should be placed in the supine position. Elevation of the legs may help with improving venous return if a few pillows are available, but the patient should not be placed head-down on a trolley, because this may actually impair ventilation by increasing pressure on the diaphragm. Modification of this position may be necessary if the patient has extreme respiratory distress (and then may insist on sitting) or vomiting (left lateral position used to keep upper airway clear of vomit). If the airway is compromised, it should be supported with such measures as ventilatory assistance. Invasive airway maneuvers may be needed and applied according to operator skill.

A rapid assessment of heart rate and blood pressure is essential, to document severity and guide management, but the assessment can be delayed until after the first IM dose of epinephrine is given. To do this, in quick succession, take a pulse (radial or brachial), inflate the manual cuff to determine systolic blood pressure (point at which pulse disappears, then reappears as cuff is deflated slightly), and then deflate the cuff further, thus using it as a venous tourniquet to facilitate IV insertion. It is a common mistake to rely on automatic machines that can give unreliable readings in an emergency, or to waste time trying to auscultate a blood pressure that may be too low. The approach with finger (pulse) and a manual cuff is quick, reliable, and comprehensive and doubles as the first step for IV line insertion.

EPINEPHRINE

Prescription for Outpatient Use

Over the past several years a number of studies have uncovered problems regarding the use of epinephrine by outpatients.[153-156] Physicians, especially in hospital emergency departments, often underprescribe epinephrine and fail to demonstrate the use of epinephrine autoinjectors to patients given prescriptions. Physicians themselves are often unaware of proper epinephrine autoinjector technique. In addition, patients may neglect to carry the autoinjector or fail to administer the drug at all or in a timely manner. The lack of an adequate dosage range for children prescribed epinephrine autoinjectors increases the chances for underdosing or overdosing. On the other hand, careful instruction on the importance of outpatient epinephrine can help patients adhere to keeping epinephrine on their person and administering it appropriately.[37] Administration of epinephrine in the lateral thigh (vastus lateralis muscle) results in a faster rate of rise of blood concentrations than IM administration in the deltoid or subcutaneous administration in the arm. In addition, outdated epinephrine autoinjectors still contain some epinephrine, although the concentration and thus the dose are reduced. Therefore an outdated epinephrine autoinjector should be employed if it is the only therapy available.[7,47,155,156]

Administered by Physician

Epinephrine should be administered simultaneously while the patient is being assessed. The dose and route depend on the severity of the reaction. In almost all office management situations, the vastus lateralis muscle is the site of choice. The dose in adults is 0.3 to 0.5 mL of 1 : 1000 solution (0.3 to 0.5 mg) and in children, 0.01 mg/kg up to the maximal adult dose. This dose can be repeated two or three times as needed, at intervals of 5 to 15 minutes.

If severe hypotension is present, especially with cardiovascular collapse, and no response is obtained to IM administration, epinephrine can be administered intravenously. Animal models[148] and human studies[157] show that continuous infusion is superior to IV bolus injection. Numerous IV regimens are available. Regardless of the dose and regimen used, special care should be taken and the patient monitored for arrhythmias. We

TABLE 77-7 Drugs and Other Agents Used in Anaphylaxis Therapy

Drug	Dose/Route of Administration	Comment
EPINEPHRINE	Adult: 0.3-0.5 mL of 1:1000 dilution IM lateral thigh Child: 0.01 mg/kg or 0.1-0.3 mL of 1:1000 solution IM lateral thigh	Initial drug of choice for all anaphylactic episodes; should be given immediately; may repeat every 5-15 minutes
	0.1-1.0 mL (0.1-1.0 mg) of 1:1000 aqueous epinephrine diluted in 10 mL normal saline IV Alternatively, epinephrine infusion prepared: 1 mg (1 mL) of 1:1000 dilution added to 250 mL D5W to yield concentration of 4.0 μg/mL. Solution infused at 1-4 μg/min (15-60 drops/min with microdrip) [60 drops/min = 1 mL = 60 mL/h], increasing to maximum 10 μg/min	If no response to IM administration and patient in shock with cardiovascular collapse
ANTIHISTAMINES		
Diphenhydramine	Adult: 25-50 mg IM or IV Child: 12.5-25 mg PO, IM, or IV	Route depends on episode severity
Cimetidine	Adult: 4 mg/kg IV	Cimetidine given slowly; rapid rate associated with hypotension
Ranitidine	Adult: 1 mg/kg IV	Child doses not well established
CORTICOSTEROIDS		
Hydrocortisone	Adult: 100 mg to 1 g IV or IM Child: 10-100 mg IV	Exact dose not established Methylprednisolone and other corticosteroids also used Prednisone, 30-60 mg, used for milder episodes
DRUGS FOR RESISTANT BRONCHOSPASM		
Aerosolized β-agonist: albuterol, metaproterenol	Dose as for asthma: 0.25-0.5 mL in 1.5-2 mL saline every 4 hours as needed	Useful for bronchospasm not responding to epinephrine
Aminophylline	Dose as for asthma	Rarely used for recalcitrant bronchospasm; β-agonist preferred
VOLUME EXPANDERS		
Crystalloids: normal saline, Ringer's lactate	Adult: 1000-2000 mL rapidly Child: 30 mL/kg in first hour	Rate titrated to BP response for IV volume expander After initial infusion, further administration requires tertiary care monitoring; larger amounts may be needed in β-blocked patients
Colloids (hydroxyethyl starch)	Adult: 500 mL rapidly, followed by slow infusion	
VASOPRESSORS		
Dopamine	400 mg in 500 mL D5W as IV infusion; 2-20 μg/kg/min	Dopamine probably drug of choice; rate titrated to BP response; continued infusion requires intensive care monitoring
DRUGS IN β-BLOCKED PATIENTS		
Atropine sulfate	Adult: 0.3-0.5 mg IV; may repeat every 10 minutes to maximum 2 mg	
Glucagon	Initial dose of 1-5 mg IV, followed by infusion of 5-15 μg/min titrated to BP response	Glucagon probably drug of choice, with atropine useful only for bradycardia
Ipratropium		As alternative or added to inhaled β-blockers for wheezing

BP, Blood pressure; *D5W*, dextrose 5% in water; *IM*, intramuscularly; *IV*, intravenously; *PO*, orally.

counsel strongly *against* the use of IV bolus injections, unless the patient is in cardiac arrest. Bolus injections can be dangerous, however carefully given. An infusion is safer and can be quickly prepared and administered even if a mechanical infusion pump is not available. Table 77-7 presents one approach widely approved by specialist bodies (e.g., emergency physicians, general practitioners) for use in Australiasia.[146] A dilute infusion (epinephrine 1 mg in saline 1000 mL) is unlikely to do harm and is thus acceptable to use outside a critical care environment without a mechanical infusion pump. Furthermore, if a high infusion rate is required, adequate volume is given at the same time to push the drug centrally. It is important to emphasize that patients who die from anaphylaxis generally do so before they reach a hospital. If a patient is hypotensive, the potential benefits of this infusion outweigh potential risks.

Alternative Routes of Administration

The rich vascularity of the sublingual area also may offer an improved route of administration of epinephrine for outpatient use.[158] In a rabbit model, a 40-mg tablet of epinephrine that dissolves sublingually within seconds had a roughly equivalent area under the plasma concentration versus time curve as 0.3 mg injected intramuscularly. Availability of a sublingual epinephrine tablet for outpatient management would eliminate difficulties related to injection and therefore would likely improve adherence rates.

Aerosolized epinephrine for inhalation has previously been used, but the aerosol devices are no longer available because of issues with shelf life.[159]

Nebulized epinephrine, 5 mL of 1:1000 dilution (5 mg in 5 mL) has been recommended for the treatment of upper airway compromise in anaphylaxis and should be given in addition to parenteral (IM or IV) epinephrine.[160] Anecdotal reports suggest supplemental nebulized epinephrine works well, but no randomized controlled trial (RCT) data are available.

Protracted Reactions and Repeat Doses

As mentioned, anaphylaxis can occur in both a protracted and a biphasic pattern. Patients must be equipped to deal with such episodes and should understand that more than one epinephrine autoinjector may be needed per episode in the outpatient setting. Studies have shown that 16% to 36% of anaphylactic episodes require two epinephrine injections.[161-163] The studies did not address whether the two doses were needed because of prolonged symptoms during protracted episodes or a biphasic response.

FLUIDS AND SELECTIVE VASOCONSTRICTORS

Perhaps the most difficult-to-treat manifestation of anaphylaxis and the most threatening, except for acute upper airway obstruction, is profound, protracted hypotension and shock. Hypotension can be severe and resistant to therapy and is caused by a shift of fluid from the intravascular to the extravascular space. Up to 30% of blood volume may shift in the first 10 minutes of a reaction because of extravasation of fluid; combined with the effects of vasodilation, this means that up to 50 mL/kg of crystalloid (normal saline or Ringer's lactate) may be required during initial resuscitation.[121] Alternatives such as hydroxyethyl starch, gelofusine, or albumin may be used, but a large multicenter study of critically ill patients found that colloids provide no benefit over crystalloids for volume expansion.[164] Colloids are also more expensive and can precipitate anaphylaxis.

Evidence for the use of vasoconstrictors other than epinephrine in cardiovascular collapse from anaphylaxis includes metaraminol,[165] methoxamine,[166] and vasopressin.[167] For cardiopulmonary resuscitation, vasopressin was similar to epinephrine in managing ventricular fibrillation and pulseless electrical activity but was superior in patients with asystole. Vasopressin followed by epinephrine was postulated to be more effective than epinephrine alone in treating refractory cardiac arrest.[168] However, other trials have not found vasopressin to improve survival in cardiac arrest.[169] At this time, data are insufficient to make a conclusive statement on the usefulness of alternative vasopressors in treating cardiovascular collapse caused by anaphylaxis. Nevertheless, when faced by the rare patient with anaphylactic shock in whom both epinephrine by infusion and fluid resuscitation have failed to restore blood pressure, it is reasonable to try one of these agents in an attempt to maintain coronary and cerebral perfusion while considering further investigations (urgent bedside echocardiography) and other interventions (mechanical support such as intraaortic balloon pump or left ventricular assist device).

ATROPINE

Patients with anaphylaxis may experience bradycardia, which can be absolute or relative; heart rate is not as fast as might otherwise be expected given the degree of hypotension. Atropine has been used to treat episodes of bradycardia, but because the trigger is probably poor venous return, it is unlikely to be effective on its own. If used, atropine should only be as an adjunct to adequate volume resuscitation and adrenaline.

GLUCAGON

Patients taking β-adrenergic blockers may present a special problem in anaphylaxis treatment: resistance to standard therapeutic regimens.[170] These patients can experience refractory hypotension, bradycardia, and relapsing manifestations. Both inotropic and chronotropic functions of the heart are suppressed, resulting in marked hypotension with bradycardia. Glucagon, a polypeptide hormone produced by the α cells of the pancreas, has both positive inotropic and chronotropic effects on the heart. The inotropic effect does not depend on catecholamines or their receptors and is therefore unaltered by β-adrenergic blockade. For this reason, glucagon is probably the drug of choice for β-blocked patients. The dose of glucagon is 1 to 5 mg intravenously as a bolus, followed by an infusion of 5 to 15 μg/min titrated against the clinical response. The cardiotonic effects of glucagon are not associated with increased myocardial irritability. Cardiotonic effects are seen within 1 to 5 minutes and are maximal at 5 to 15 minutes after a single 5-mg bolus. Nausea and vomiting are the major limiting factors of glucagon therapy.

INHALED β-ADRENERGIC AGONISTS

If wheezing unresponsive to epinephrine occurs, aerosolized β-adrenergic agonists are the drug of choice. The doses are the same as those used in treating asthma. It is now usual practice to use 10 to 12 puffs through a spacer, which is as effective as a nebulizer and easier to administer. For intubated patients, puffers may also be given directly into a ventilator circuit using a special connector.

CORTICOSTEROIDS

The role of corticosteroids in managing anaphylaxis has not been established. However, based on an extrapolation of the effects in other allergic diseases, corticosteroid administration is reasonable. Given the proven value of steroids for treating acute exacerbations of asthma, which has pathophysiologic similarities to anaphylaxis, corticosteroid treatment is most reasonable for severe or persistent bronchospasm. Because anaphylaxis can be biphasic, a role for corticosteroids in preventing such a recurrence has been postulated.[98] However, a review of available studies showed no clear-cut benefit of corticosteroids in anaphylaxis recurrence. Although there is no established dose or drug of choice, suggested corticosteroid doses are listed in Table 77-7.

ANTIHISTAMINES

Although antihistamines are not life-saving, they can offer dramatic relief of itching and urticaria. One clinical study found a combination H_1 and H_2 antagonists to be superior to an H_1 antagonist alone.[171] However, this study was confined to relatively mild reactions (only 2 of 91 were hypotensive) and was probably confounded by a higher rate of epinephrine administration in the combined $H_1 + H_2$ group. Antihistamines have a vasodilating (α-blocking) effect and can trigger hypotension, particularly if given without epinephrine. One animal study clearly demonstrated increased mortality when antihistamines were given.[152] In the absence of adequate human clinical trials or a known risk/benefit ratio, it is difficult to recommend these

BOX 77-11 INDICATIONS FOR PROLONGED OBSERVATION OF ANAPHYLACTIC PATIENT*

Moderate to severe reaction
Episode in asthmatic patient with wheezing
Ingested antigen with possibility of continued absorption
Previous history of biphasic response

*8 to 24 hours after resolution of symptoms.

agents.[150] It is, however, reasonable to use antihistamines for relief of skin symptoms that persist despite adequate treatment with epinephrine. Current consensus guidelines either restrict use of antihistamines to this scenario[146] or list antihistamines as second-line agents after treatment with epinephrine and fluids.[6,145]

OBSERVATION PERIOD

No consensus or RCT indicates the ideal observation period after resolution of symptoms of anaphylaxis. The recognition of the frequency of biphasic episodes has altered the perception of an adequate observation time. Resuscitation guidelines list indications for prolonged observation of 8 to 24 hours after resolution of symptoms[172] (Box 77-11).

One of the risk factors for prolonged or recurrent reactions is antigen exposure through ingestion. This might be caused by prolonged absorption as antigen is retained in the gut. Substances that prolong absorption in the bowel can produce delayed and protracted reactions. One example is *Bacillus natto*–fermented soybeans (natto). The viscous substance of natto has poly–γ-glutamic acid produced by *B. natto* during fermentation. Polyglutamic acid has been used in drug delivery applications to facilitate controlled, sustained release. Delayed and prolonged release of natto allergens in food bound to polyglutamic acid (which degrades slowly in GI tract) can cause late-onset and protracted anaphylactic reactions.[173]

PROGNOSIS FOR RECURRENCE

The prognosis for patients with recurrent anaphylactic episodes is reasonably good. Although prognosis is better when the allergen is known versus unknown, even in idiopathic cases, frequency of episodes usually diminishes over time, and resolution is the rule.[37] Prognosis is based on not only natural history but also the amount of allergen necessary to produce a reaction and the ability to avoid exposures to triggering agents. In one study, approximately one of every 12 patients who experienced an episode of anaphylaxis had recurrent symptoms each year of follow-up evaluation.[174] One quarter of these reactions were classified as serious, and the other 75% were less severe than the original episode. Neither the presence of asthma nor atopy was a risk factor for recurrence. The best predictor of a serious recurrence was the presence of serious symptoms during the initial event. Peanuts and tree nuts were the most common original causes and the most common triggers for recurrence of anaphylaxis.

Fatalities

Anaphylactic deaths are relatively rare, but many are preventable and a significant percentage iatrogenic. Therefore it is important to consider the characteristics that place a patient at risk for death and learn what might be done to prevent fatal episodes. In a series of 25 retrospectively reviewed fatalities from anaphylaxis, Greenberger and colleagues[58] found seven reactions due to medication, six to radiocontrast media, six to Hymenoptera stings, four to foods, and a final case that may have been caused by insect repellent in a hair-coloring product. The mean age of the individuals in this series was 59 years. Death occurred within 60 minutes of the onset of symptoms in 13 of the 25 cases and in 1 to 6 hours in six. At least one comorbid disease was identified in 22 cases. The authors concluded that elderly patients with comorbid diseases are at mortality risk from anaphylaxis, and that a rapid onset after exposure might also be a risk factor. In one case, death ensued despite appropriate use of epinephrine.

Pumphrey[95] collected the largest series of anaphylaxis fatalities in 2004. In 212 cases in the UK, there was a very low rate of fatality outside the hospital, even for untreated reactions. However, avoidance, self-treatment, and medical management still failed to prevent anaphylactic death in many cases. The most common causes of reactions were insect sting, foods, and drugs; however, anesthetic agents and radiocontrast media also produced a significant number of fatalities. Airway obstruction and cardiovascular collapse were the most common causes of death. Disseminated intravascular coagulation was the cause in several instances. Because many patients who died had only minor previous reactions, mild severity of initial reaction did not indicate future reactions would be mild, as also noted by Simons.[156] The most common foods to cause fatalities were nuts, which included peanuts and true nuts. Asthma was a risk factor. The median time from onset to cardiac arrest was faster for injected than for ingested antigen: 30 minutes for foods, 15 minutes for venom, and 5 minutes for iatrogenic reactions caused by injections. Many patients were not carrying their epinephrine autoinjector, and others had epinephrine but failed to use it. In a few cases, even when epinephrine was administered appropriately, death ensued.

In the UK series, four deaths occurred when patients assumed the upright or sitting posture during treatment. Pumphrey[95] postulated that these patients died because of cardiac electromechanical dissociation, with empty heart syndrome and pulseless electrical activity predisposing to arrhythmias.[123] This observation has prompted recommendations to maintain hypotensive patients in the recumbent (preferably Trendelenburg) position until the anaphylactic event has completely resolved.

REFERENCES

Terminology

1. Lieberman P, Kemp S, Oppenheimer J, et al. The diagnosis and management of anaphylaxis: an updated practice parameter. Joint Task Force on Practice Parameters, American Academy of Allergy, Asthma, and Immunology, American College of Allergy, Asthma, and Immunology, and Joint Council of Allergy, Asthma, and Immunology. J Allergy Clin Immunol 2005;115:S483-523.
2. Lieberman P. Anaphylaxis. In: Adkinson N, Bochner, B, Busse W, et al, editors. Middleton's

allergy: principles and practice. 7th ed. St Louis: Mosby-Elsevier; 2009. p. 1027-49; also Anaphylaxis and anaphylactoid reactions. In: Middleton E et al, editors. Allergy: principles and practice, 5th ed. St Louis: Mosby–Year Book; 1998. p. 1079-92.
3. Johansson SGO, Bieber T, Dahl R, et al. Revised nomenclature for allergy for global use: report of the Nomenclature Review Committee of the World Allergy Organization, October 2003. J Allergy Clin Immunol 2004; 113:832-6.
4. Simons FER. Anaphylaxis, killer allergy: long-term management in the community. J Allergy Clin Immunol 2006;117:367-77.
5. Sampson HA, Munoz-Furlong A, Bousquet J, et al. Symposium on the definition and management of anaphylaxis: summary report. J Allergy Clin Immunol 2005;115:584-92.
6. Sampson HA, Munoz-Furlong A, Bock SA, et al. Second symposium on the definition and management of anaphylaxis: summary report. Second National Institute of Allergy and Infectious Disease/Food Allergy and Anaphylaxis Network Symposium. J Allergy Clin Immunol 2006;117:391-7.

Incidence and Causative Agents

7. Simons FER, Peterson S, Black CD. Epinephrine dispensing patterns for an out-of-hospital population: a novel approach to studying the epidemiology of anaphylaxis. J Allergy Clin Immunol 2002;110:647-51.
8. Gupta R, Sheikh A, Strachan D, et al. Increasing hospital admissions for systemic allergic disorders in England: analysis of national admission data. BMJ 2003;327:1142-3.
9. Peng M, Jick H. A population-based study of the incidence, cause, and severity of anaphylaxis in the United Kingdom. Arch Intern Med 2004;164:317-9.
10. Helbling A, Hurni T, Mueller UR, et al. Incidence of anaphylaxis with circulatory symptoms: a study over a three-year period comprising 940,000 inhabitants of the Swiss Canton Bern. Clin Exp Allergy 2004;34: 285-90.
11. Bohlke K, Davis R, DeStefano F, et al. Epidemiology of anaphylaxis among children and adolescents enrolled in a health maintenance organization. J Allergy Clin Immunol 2004; 113:536-42.
12. Mehl A, Wahn U, Niggemann B. Anaphylactic reactions in children: a questionnaire-based survey in Germany. Allergy 2005;60:1440-5.
13. Moneret-Vautrin DA, Morisset M, Flabbee J, et al. Epidemiology of life-threatening and lethal anaphylaxis: a review. Allergy 2005;60: 443-51.
14. Lieberman P, Camargo CA, Bohlke K, et al. Epidemiology of anaphylaxis: findings of American College of Allergy, Asthma, and Immunology Epidemiology of Anaphylaxis Working Group. Ann Allergy Asthma Immunol 2006;97:596-602.
15. Walker S, Sheikh A. Managing anaphylaxis: effective emergency and long-term care are necessary. Clin Exp Allergy 2003;33:1015-8.
16. Liew W, Williamson E, Tang M. Anaphylaxis fatalities and admissions in Australia. J Allergy Clin Immunol 2009;123:434-42.
17. Decker W et al. The etiology and incidence of anaphylaxis in Rochester, Minnesota: a report from the Rochester Epidemiology Project. J Allergy Clin Immunol 2008;122:1161-5.
18. Anderson AS, Lin R, Shah S. Increase in hospitalizations for anaphylaxis in the first two decades of life. J Allergy Clin Immunol 2008;121:S27.
19. Harduar-Morano ML, Simon M, Watkins S, Blackmore C. Algorithm for the diagnosis of anaphylaxis and its validation using population-based data on emergency department visits for anaphylaxis in Florida. J Allergy Clin Immunol 2010;126:98-104.
20. Ross M, Ferguson M, Street D, Clontz K, et al. Analysis of food-allergic and anaphylactic events in the National Electronic Injury Surveillance System. J Allergy Clin Immunol 2008;121:166-71.
21. Simons FER, Sampson H. Anaphylaxis epidemic: fact or fiction? J Allergy Clin Immunol 2008;122:1166-8.
22. Lin RY, Anderson A, Shah S, Naurruzzaman F. Increasing anaphylaxis hospitalizations in the first two decades of life: New York state, 1990-2006. Ann Allergy Asthma Immunol 2008;101: 387-93.
23. Pereira B, Benter C, Grundy J, et al. Prevalence of sensitization to food allergens, reported adverse reactions to foods, food avoidance, and food hypersensitivity among teenagers. J Allergy Clin Immunol 2005;116:884-92.
24. Moneret-Vautrin DA, Kanny G, Morisset M, et al. The food anaphylaxis vigilance network in France. Allergy Clin Immunol Int 2003;15: 155-9.
25. Palmer K, Burks W. Current developments in peanut allergy. Curr Opin Allergy Clin Immunol 2006;6:202-6.
26. MacDougall CF, Cant AJ, Colver AF. How dangerous is food allergy in childhood? The incidence of severe and fatal allergic reactions across the UK and Ireland. Arch Dis Child 2002;86:236-9.
27. Leone R, Conforti A, Venegoni M, et al. Drug-induced anaphylaxis: case/non-case study based on Italian pharmacovigilance database. Drug Safety J 2005;28:547-56.
28. Sicherer SH, Sampson HA. Food allergy. J Allergy Clin Immunol 2006;117:S470-5.
29. Sicherer SH, Leung D. Advances in allergic skin disease, anaphylaxis, and hypersensitivity reactions to foods, drugs, and insect stings. J Allergy Clin Immunol 2004;114:118-24.
30. Adkinson NF, Essiayan D, Gruchalla R, et al. Task force report: future research needs for prevention and management of immune-mediated drug hypersensitivity reactions. J Allergy Clin Immunol 2002;109:S461-78.
31. Gupta R, Sheikh A, Strachand P, et al. Burden of allergic disease in the UK: secondary analysis of national databases. Clin Exp Allergy 2004;34:520-6.
32. Hetner D, Casdell SM. Latex allergy: an update. Anesth Analg 2003;96:1219-29.
33. Mertes P, Laxenaire M, Lienhart A, et al. Reducing the risk of anaphylaxis during anesthesia: guidelines for clinical practice. J Invest Allergol Clin Immunol 2005;15:91-101.
34. Cochran ST. Anaphylactoid reactions to radiocontrast media. Curr Allergy Asthma Rep 2005;5:28-31.
35. Moffitt JE, Golden D, Reisman R, et al. Stinging insect hypersensitivity: a practice parameter update. J Allergy Clin Immunol 2004;114: 869-86.
36. Ebo D, Bosmans J, Couttenye M, et al. Hemodialysis-associated anaphylaxis and anaphylactoid reactions. Allergy 2006;61:211-20.
37. Webb L, Lieberman P. Anaphylaxis: a review of 601 cases. Ann Allergy Asthma Immunol 2006;97:39-43.
38. Koplin JJ, Martin PE, Allen KJ. An update on epidemiology of anaphylaxis in children and adults. Curr Opin Allergy Clin Immunol 2011;11:492-6.
39. Gupta RS, Springston EE, Warrier MR, Smith B, et al. The prevalence, severity, and distribution of childhood food allergy in the United States. Pediatrics 2011:e9-17.
40. Mertes PM, Alla F, Trechot P, Auroy Y, et al. Anaphylaxis during anesthesia in France: an 8-year national survey. J Allergy Clin Immunol 2011;128:366-73.
41. Pichler WJ. Adverse side effects to biological agents. Allergy 2006;61:912-20.
42. Paoloa C, Mauriziob B, Mariangelec M, et al. Hypersensitivity reactions to biological agents with special emphasis on tumor necrosis factor alpha antagonists. Curr Opin Allergy Clin Immunol 2007;7:393-403.
43. Hamann CP. Natural rubber latex protein sensitivity in review. Am J Contact Dermat 1993; 4:4-21.
44. Sheikh A, Alves B. Age, sex, geographical and socioeconomic variations in admissions for anaphylaxis: analysis of four years of English hospital data. Clin Exp Allergy 2001;31: 1571-6.
45. Camargo CA Jr, Clark S, Kaplan MS, et al. Regional differences in EpiPen prescriptions in the United States. J Allergy Clin Immunol 2006;117:S139.
46. Mullins RJ, Clark S, Camargo CA. Regional variation in epinephrine autoinjector prescriptions in Australia: more evidence for the vitamin D–anaphylaxis hypothesis. Ann Allergy Asthma Immunol 2009;103:488-95.
47. Simons FER, Peterson S, Black C. Epinephrine dispensing for out-of-hospital treatment of anaphylaxis in infants and children: a population-based study. Ann Allergy Asthma Immunol 2001;86:622-6.
48. Boleman W, Harper D, Hagan L, et al. Chronobiology of immunotherapy reactions. J Allergy Clin Immunol 2001;105:S310.
49. Gonzalez-Perez A, Aponte Z, Vidaurre C, Rodriguez L. Anaphylaxis epidemiology in patients with and patients without asthma: a United Kingdom database review. J Allergy Clin Immunol 2010;125:1098-104.
50. Sheehan W, Graham D, Phipatanakul L. Higher incidence of pediatric anaphylaxis in southern areas of the United States. J Allergy Clin Immunol 2009;123:S185.
51. Tejedor MA, Moro M, Mugica M, Bila C, et al. Incidence of different causes of anaphylaxis in an emergency room of a Spanish hospital. J Allergy Clin Immunol 2008;121:S26.
52. Campbell RL, Hagan JB, Li JTC, Vukov SC, et al. Anaphylaxis in emergency department patients 50 or 65 years or older. Ann Allergy Asthma Immunol 2011;106:401-6.
53. Harduar-Morano ML, Simon ML, Watkins S, Blackmore C. A population-based epidemiologic study of emergency department visits for anaphylaxis in Florida. J Allergy Clin Immunol 2011;128:594-600.
54. Iribarren C, Tolstykh I, Miller M, Eisner M. Asthma and the perspective risk of anaphylactic shock and other allergy diagnoses in a large integrated healthcare delivery system. Ann Allergy Asthma Immunol 2010;104: 371-7.

Pathology

55. Pumphrey RSH, Roberts ISD. Postmortem findings after fatal anaphylactic reactions. J Clin Pathol 2000;53:273-6.
56. Delage C, Irey NS. Anaphylactic deaths: a clinical pathologic study of 43 cases. J Forensic Sci 1972;17:525.
57. Mosbech H. Death caused by wasp and bee stings in Denmark 1960-1980. Allergy 1983;38:195-200.
58. Greenberger PA, Rotskoff BD, Lifschultz B. Fatal anaphylaxis: postmortem findings and associated comorbid diseases. Ann Allergy Asthma Immunol 2007;98:252-7.
59. Patel F. Seafood-induced fatal anaphylaxis. Med Sci Law 1998;38:354-7.
60. Ansari M, Zamora J, Lipscomb M. Postmortem diagnosis of acute anaphylaxis by serum tryptase analysis: a case report. Am J Clin Pathol 1993;99:101-3.
61. Ciesielski-Carlucci C, Leong P, Jacobs C. Case report of anaphylaxis from cisplatin/paclitaxel and a review of their hypersensitivity reaction profiles. Am J Clin Oncol 1997;20:373-5.
62. Belton AL, Chira T. Fatal anaphylactic reaction to hair dye. Am J Forensic Med Pathol 1997;18:290-2.
63. Prahlow JA, Barnard JJ. Fatal anaphylaxis due to fire ant stings. Am J Forensic Med Pathol 1998;19:137-42.
64. Vaughn STA, Jones GN. Systemic mastocytosis presenting as profound cardiovascular collapse during anesthesia. Anaesthesia 1998;53:804-9.
65. Hunt EL. Death from allergic shock. N Engl J Med 1993;228:502-4.
66. Lamson RW. So-called fatal anaphylaxis in man with a special reference to diagnosis and treatment of clinical allergies. JAMA 1929; 93:1775-8.
67. Sheppe WM. Fatal anaphylaxis in man. J Lab Clin Med 1980;16:372.
68. Delage C, Mullick FG, Irey NS. Myocardial lesions in anaphylaxis. Arch Pathol Lab Med 1973;95:1985.
69. James LP, Jr., Austen KF. Fatal and systemic anaphylaxis in man. N Engl J Med 1964;270: 597.
70. Yunginger JW, Nelson DR, Squillace DL, et al. Laboratory investigation of deaths due to anaphylaxis. J Forensic Sci 1991;36:857-65.
71. Schwartz HJ, Sutheimer C, Gauerke M, et al. Hymenoptera venom-specfic IgE antibodies in post-mortem sera from victims of sudden, unexpected death. Clin Allergy 1988;18:461-8.
72. Schwartz HJ, Yunginger J, Schwartz LB. Unrecognized anaphylaxis may be a cause of sudden unexpected death. J Allergy Clin Immunol 1993;91:S154.
73. Schwartz LB, Irani AMA, Roller K, et al. Quantitation of histamine, tryptase, and chymase in dispersed human T and TC mast cells. J Immunol 1987;138:2611-5.
74. Schwartz LB, Irani AM. Serum tryptase and the laboratory diagnosis of systemic mastocytosis. Hematol Oncol Clin North Am 2000;14: 641-57.
75. Randall B, Butts J, Halsey J. Elevated postmortem tryptase in the absence of anaphylaxis. J Forensic Sci 1995;40:208-11.
76. Edston E, Gidlund E, Wickman M, et al. Increased mast cell tryptase in sudden infant death - anaphylaxis, hypoxia, or artifact? Clin Exp Allergy 1999;29:1648-54.
77. Edston E, van Hagge-Hamsten M. Beta-tryptase measurements postmortem in anaphylactic deaths and in controls. Forensic Sci Int 1998;93:135-42.
78. Edston E, Eriksson O, van Hage M. Mast cell tryptase in postmortem serum: reference values and confounders. Int J Legal Med 2007; 121:275-80.
79. Sargur R, Cowley D, Murng S, et al. Raised tryptse without anaphylaxis or mastocytosis: heterophilic antibody interference in the serum tryptase assay. Clin Exp Allergy 2011; 163:339-45.

Pathophysiology

80. Finkelman FD. Anaphylaxis lessons from mouse models. J Allergy Clin Immunol 2007; 120:506-15.
81. Kalesnikoff J, Galli SJ. Anaphylaxis: mechanisms of mast cell activation. Chem Immunol Allergy 2010;95:45-66.
82. Strait RT, Morris SC, Finkelman FD. IgG-blocking antibodies inhibit IgE-mediated anaphylaxis in vivo through both antigen interception and FcγRIIb cross-linking. J Clin Invest 2006;116:833-41.
83. Tsujimura Y, Obata K, Mukai K, et al. Basophils play a pivotal role in immunoglobulin-G-mediated but not immunoglobulin-E-mediated systemic anaphylaxis. Immunity 2008;28:581-9.
84. Karasuyama H, Tsujimura Y, Obata K, et al. Role for basophils in systemic anaphylaxis. Chem Immunol Allergy 2010;95:85-97.
85. Arias K, Chu DK, Flader K, et al. Distinct immune effector pathways conribute to the full expression of peanut-induced anaphylactic reactions in mice. J Allergy Clin Immunol 2011;127:1552-61.
86. Kajiwara N, Sasaki T, Bradding P, et al. Activation of human mast cells through the platelet-activating factor receptor. J Allergy Clin Immunol 2010;125:1137-45.
87. Vadas P, Gold M, Perelman B, et al. Platelet-activating gactor, PAF acetylhydrolase, and severe anaphylaxis. N Engl J Med 2008;358: 28-35.
88. Yost CC, Weyrich AS, Zimmerman GA. The platelet activating factor (PAF) signaling cascade in systemic inflammatory responses. Biochimie 2010;92:692-7.
89. Grammer L, Shaughnessy M, Harris K, et al. Lymphocyte subsets and activation markers in patients with acute episodes of idiopathic anaphylaxis. Ann Allergy Asthma Immunol 2000;85:368-71.
90. Hogan MB. Progress toward an understanding of idiopathic anaphylaxis. Ann Allergy Asthma Immunol 2000;85:332-3.
91. Mozelsio N, Grammer L. Quantitation of monocyte chemoattractant protein-1 in patients with idiopathic anaphylaxis. J Allergy Clin Immunol 2001;107:S80.
92. Tejedor M, Perez C, Sastre, et al. Mast cell releasability in idiopathic anaphylaxis subtypes. J Allergy Clin Immunol 2000;105:S348.
93. Reed J, Yedulapuram M, Lieberman P, et al. Differences in cytokine production between idiopathic anaphylaxis (IA) subjects and controls. J Allergy Clin Immunol 2006;117: S305.

Basophil and Mast Cell Degranulation Syndromes

94. Trani N, Bonetti LR, Gualandri G, Barbolini G. Immediate anaphylactic death following antibiotics injection: splenic eosinophilia easily revealed by pagoda red stain. Forensic Sci Int 2008;181:21-5.
95. Pumphrey RSH. Fatal anaphylaxis in the UK, 1992-2001. Anaphylaxis 2004;257:116-32.
96. Richard V, Hurel-Merle S, Scalbert E, et al. Functional evidence for a role of vascular chymase in the production of angiotensin II in isolated human arteries. Circulation 2001;104: 750-2.
97. Briassoulis G, Hatzis T, Mammi P, et al. Persistent anaphylactic reaction after induction with thiopentone and cisatracurium. Paediatr Anaesth 2000;10:429-34.
98. Lieberman P. Biphasic anaphylactic reactions. Ann Allergy Asthma Immunol 2005;95: 217-28.
99. Pushparaj PN, Tay HK, H'ng SC, et al. The cytokine inerleukin-33 mediates anaphylactic shock. Proc Natl Acad Sci USA 2009;106: 9773-8.
100. Dong C. Regulation and pro-inflammatory function of interleukin-17 family cytokines. Immunol Rev 2008;226:80-6.
101. Gri G, Piconese S, Frossi B, et al. $CD4^+CD25^+$ regulatory T cells suppress mast cell degranulation and allergic responses through OX40-OX40L interaction. Immunity 2008;29:771-81.
102. Akdis CA, Akdis M. Mechanisms and treatment of allergic disease in the big picture of regulatory T cell. J Allergy Clin Immunol 2009;123:735-48.
103. Chrusch C, Sharma S, Unruh H, et al. Histamine H_3 receptor blockade improves cardiac function in anaphylaxis. Am J Respir Crit Care Med 1999;160:1142-9.
104. Godot V, Arock M, Garcia G, et al. H_4 histamine receptor mediates optimal migration of mast cell precursors to CXCL12. J Allergy Clin Immunol 2007;120:827-34.
105. Dunford PJ, Williams KN, Desai PJ, et al. Histamine H_4 receptor antagonists are superior to traditional antihistamines in the attenuation of experimental pruritus. J Allergy Clin Immunol 2007;119:176-83.
106. Kasperska-Zajac A, Rogala B. Platelet function in anaphylaxis. J Invest Allergol Clin Immunol 2006;16:1-4.
107. Kaplan AP, Hunt KJ, Sobotka AK, et al. Human anaphylaxis: a study of mediator systems. Clin Rev 1977;25:361.
108. Van der Linden PW, Hack CE, Kerckhaert J, et al. Preliminary report: complement activation in wasp-sting anaphylaxis. Lancet 1990; 336:904-6.
109. Van Hagge-Hamsten M, Hack CE, Eerenberg AJ, et al. Contact system activation and angioedema in insect-sting anaphylaxis. J Allergy Clin Immunol 1993;91:283.
110. Lin R, Trivino M. C-reactive protein and interleukin-6 levels relate to key clinical manifestations and laboratory parameters in acute allergic reactions. J Allergy Clin Immunol 2001;107:S269.
111. Van der Linden PW, Struyvenberg A, Kraaijenhagen RJ, et al. Anaphylactic shock after insect-sting challenge in 138 persons with a previous insect-sting reaction. Ann Intern Med 1993; 118:161-8.
112. Summers CW, Pumphrey RS, Woods WN, et al. Factors predicting anaphylaxis to peanuts and tree nuts in patients referred to a specialist center. J Allergy Clin Immunol 2008;121: 632-8.
113. Palmer RM, Ferrige AG, Moncada S. Nitric oxide release accounts for the biological

activity of endothelium-derived relaxing factor. Nature 1987;327:524-6.
114. Marsden PA, Brenner BM. Nitric oxide and endothelins: novel autocrine/paracrine regulators of the circulation. Semin Nephrol 1991; 11:169-85.
115. Lowenstein CJ, Michel T. What's in a name? eNOS and anaphylactic shock. J Clin Invest 2006;116:2075-8.
116. Cauwels A, Janssen B, Buys E, et al. Anaphylactic shock depends on PI3K and eNOS-derived NO. J Clin Invest 2006;116:2244-51.
117. Rolla G, Nebiolo F, Guida G, et al. Level of exhaled nitric oxide during anaphylaxis. Ann Allergy Asthma Immunol 2006;97:264-5.
118. Lin RY, Gupta A. Nitric oxide levels in patients with acute allergic reactions. J Allergy Clin Immunol 2003;111:S100.

Mechanisms in Anaphylactic Shock

119. Brown SGA. The pathophysiology of shock in anaphylaxis. Immunol Allergy Clin North Am 2007;27:165-75.
120. Fisher M. Clinical observations on the pathophysiology and implications for treatment. New York: Springer-Verlag; 1989.
121. Fisher MM. Clinical observations on the pathophysiology and treatment of anaphylactic cardiovascular collapse. Anaesth Intensive Care 1986;14:17-21.
122. Brown SGA, Blackman KE, Stenlake V, Heddle RJ. Insect sting anaphylaxis; prospective evaluation of treatment with intravenous adrenaline and volume resuscitation. Emerg Med J 2004; 21:149-54.
123. Pumphrey R. Fatal posture in anaphylactic shock. J Allergy Clin Immunol 2003;112: 451-2.
124. Fahmy NR. Hemodynamics, plasma histamine and catecholamine concentrations during an anaphylactoid reaction to morphine. Anesthesiology 1981;55:329-31.
125. Moss J, Fahmy NR, Sunder N, et al. Hormonal and hemodynamic profile of an anaphylactic reaction in man. Circulation 1981;63:210-3.
126. Rittweger R, Hermann K, Ring J. Increased urinary excretion of angiotensin during anaphylactic reactions. Int Arch Allergy Immunol 1994;104:255-61.
127. Gawlik R, Rogala E, Jawor B. Endothelin-1 in plasma of patients with Hymenoptera venom anaphylaxis. J Allergy Clin Immunol 1998; 101:S160.
128. Hermann K, von Tschirschnitz M, von Eschenbach C, et al. Histamine, tryptase, norepinephrine, angiotensinogen, angiotensin-converting enzyme, angiotensin I and II in plasma of patients with Hymenoptera venom anaphylaxis. Int Arch Allergy Immunol 1994;104: 379-84.
129. Hermann K, Donhauser S, Ring J. Angiotensin in human leukocytes in patients with insect sting venom anaphylaxis and healthy volunteers. Int Arch Allergy Immunol 1995;107: 385-6.

Signs and Symptoms

130. Soreide E, Busrod T, Harber S. Severe anaphylactic reactions outside hospital; etiology, symptoms, and treatment. Acta Anaesthesiol Scand 1988;32:339-44.
131. Moro M, Tejedor M, Esteban J, et al. Severity of anaphylaxis according to causes and demographic characteristics. J Allergy Clin Immunol 2008;121:S24.
132. Sampson HA. Utility of food-specific IgE concentrations in predicting symptomatic food allergy. J Allergy Clin Immunol 2001;107: 891-6.
133. Braganza SC, Acworth JP, McKinnon DR, et al. Pediatric emergency department anaphylaxis: different patterns from adults. Arch Dis Child 2006;91:159-63.
134. Simons FER, Chad ZH, Gold M. Anaphylaxis in children. Allergy Clin Immunol Int 2004; 1:S242-4.
135. Simons FER. Anaphylaxis in infants: can recognition and management be improved? J Allergy Clin Immunol 2007;2007;120:3.
136. Kounis NG. Kounis syndrome (allergic angina and allergic myocardial infarction): a natural paradigm. Int J Cardiol 2006;110:7-14.
137. DeSouza RL, Short T, Warman GR, et al. Anaphylaxis associated with fibrinolysis, reversed with tranexamic acid and demonstrated by thromboelastography. Anaesth Intensive Care 2004;32:580-7.

Laboratory Findings

138. Caughey GH. Tryptase genetics and anaphylaxis. J Allergy Clin Immunol 2006;117: 1411-4.
139. Sprung J, Schoenwald PK, Schwartz LB. Cardiovascular collapse resulting from thiopental-induced histamine release. Anesthesiology 1997;86:1006-7.
140. Lin RY, Schwartz LB, Curry A, et al. Histamine and tryptase levels in patients with acute allergic reactions: an emergency department-based study. J Allergy Clin Immunol 2000;106: 65-71.
141. Da Broi U, Moreschi C. Post-mortem diagnosis of anaphylaxis: a difficult task in forensic medicine. Forensic Sci Int 2010;204:1-5.
142. Gernez Y, Tirouvanziam R, Yu G, et al. Basophil CD203c levels are increased at baseline and can be used to monitor omalizumab treatment in subjects with nut allergy. Int Arch Allergy Immunol 2011;154:318-27.
143. Ebo DG, Hagendorens MM, Bridts CH, et al. In vitro allergy diagnosis: should we follow the flow? Clin Exp Allergy 2004;34:332-9.
144. Zhou X, Buckley MG, Lau LC, et al. Mast cell carboxypeptidase as a new clinical marker for anaphylaxis. J Allergy Clin Immunol 2006; 117:S85.

Prevention and Management

145. Simons FER, Ardusso LRF, Bilo MB, et al. World Allergy Organization guidelines for the assessment and management of anaphylaxis. World Allergy Org J 2011;4:13-37.
146. Anaphylaxis wall chart. Australian Prescriber 2011.
147. Simons FE, Gu X, Simons KJ. Epinephrine absorption in adults: intramuscular versus subcutaneous injection. J Allergy Clin Immunol 2001;108:871-3.
148. Mink SN, Simons FE, Simons KJ, Becker AB, Duke K. Constant infusion of epinephrine, but not bolus treatment, improves haemodynamic recovery in anaphylactic shock in dogs. Clin Exp Allergy 2004;34:1776-83.
149. Fisher M. Blood volume replacement in acute anaphylactic cardiovascular collapse related to anaethesia. Br J Anaesth 1977;49:1023-6.
150. Sheikh A, Ten Broek V, Brown SGA, Simons FE. H_1-antihistamines for the treatment of anaphylaxis: Cochrane systematic review. Allergy 2007;62:830-7.
151. Choo KJ, Simons E, Sheikh A. Glucocorticoids for the treatment of anaphylaxis: Cochrane systematic review. Allergy 2010;65: 1205-11.
152. Bellou A, Lambert H, Gillois P, et al. Constitutive nitric oxide synthase inhibition combined with histamine and serotonin receptor blockade improves the initial ovalbumin-induced arterial hypotension but decreases the survival time in brown Norway rats' anaphylactic shock. Shock 2003;19:71-8.
153. Lieberman P. Use of epinephrine in the treatment of anaphylaxis. Curr Opin Allergy Clin Immunol 2003;3:313-8.
154. Pouessel G, Deschildre A, Castelain C, et al. Parental knowledge and use of epinephrine autoinjector for children with food allergy. Pediatr Allergy Immunol 2006;17:221-6.
155. Sicherer S, Simons FER. Quandaries in prescribing emergency action plan and self-injectable epinephrine for first-aid management of anaphylaxis in the community. J Allergy Clin Immunol 2005;115:575-83.
156. Simons FER. First-aid treatment of anaphylaxis to food: focus on epinephrine. J Allergy Clin Immunol 2004;113:837-44.
157. Gei A, Pacheco L, van Hook J, et al. The use of a continuous infusion of epinephrine for anaphylactic shock during labor. Obstet Gynecol 2003;102:1332-5.
158. Rawas-Qualaji MM, Simons FER, Simons KJ. Sublingual epinephrine tablets versus intramuscular injection of epinephrine: dose equivalents for potential treatment of anaphylaxis. J Allergy Clin Immunol 2006;117: 398-403.
159. Muller UR, Bonifazi F, Przybilla B, et al. Withdrawal of the Medihaler-Epi/Adrenaline Medihaler: comments of the Subcommittee on Insect Venom Allergy of the EAACI. Allergy 1998;53:619-20.
160. Brown SGA, Mullins RJ, Gold MS. Anaphylaxis: diagnosis and management. Med J Aust 2006;185:283-9.
161. Korenblatt P, Lundie MJ, Dankner RF, et al. A retrospective study of epinephrine administration for anaphylaxis: how many doses are needed? Allergy Asthma Proc 1999;20: 383-6.
162. Uguz A, Lack G, Pumphrey R, et al. Allergic reactions in the community: a questionnaire survey of members of the anaphylaxis campaign. Clin Exp Allergy 2005;35:746-50.
163. Kelso JM. A second dose of epinephrine for anaphylaxis: how often needed and how to carry. J Allergy Clin Immunol 2006;117: 464-5.
164. Finfer S, Bellomo R, Boyce N, et al. A comparison of albumin and saline for fluid resuscitation in the intensive care unit. N Engl J Med 2004;350:2247-56.
165. Heytman M, Rainbird A. Useof alpha-agonists for management of anaphylaxis occurring under anesthesia: case studies and review. Anaesthesiology 2004;59:1210-5.
166. McBrien ME, Breslin DS, Atkinson S, et al. Use of methoxamine in the resuscitation of epinephrine-resistant electromechanical dissociation. Anaesthesiology 2001;56:1085-9.
167. Schummer W, Schummer C, Wippermann J, et al. Anaphylactic shock: is vasopressin the drug of choice? Anaesthesiology 2004;101: 1025-7.
168. Wenzel V, Krismer AC, Arntz HR, et al. A comparison of vasopressin and epinephrine for

out-of-hospital cardiopulmonary resuscitation. N Engl J Med 2004;350:105-13.
169. Stiell IG, Hebert PC, Wells GA, et al. Vasopressin versus epinephrine for in-hospital cardiac arrest: a randomized controlled trial. Lancet 2001;358:105-9.
170. Lieberman P, Kemp SF. Beta-blockers and anaphylaxis: are the risks overstated? J Allergy Clin Immunol 2005;116:933-5.
171. Lin RY, Curry A, Pesola G, et al. Improved outcomes in patients with acute allergic syndromes who are treated with combined H_1 and H_2 antihistamines. Ann Emerg Med 2000;36: 462-8.
172. Soar J, Deakin C, Nolen J, et al. European Resuscitation Council guidelines for resuscitation 2005. Section 7. Cardiac arrest in special circumstances. Resuscitation 2005;6751:S135-70.
173. Inomata N, Osuna H, Ikezawa Z. Late-onset anaphylaxis to *Bacillus natto*–fermented soybeans (natto). J Allergy Clin Immunol 2004;113:998-1000.
174. Mullins RJ. Anaphylaxis: risk factors for recurrence. Clin Exp Allergy 2003;33:1033-40.

78

Insect Allergy

DAVID B.K. GOLDEN

CONTENTS

SUMMARY OF IMPORTANT CONCEPTS

» Anaphylaxis to insect stings occurs in 3% of adults and 1% of children, and even the first reaction can be fatal.
» Cutaneous-systemic reactions are most common in children, hypotensive shock is most common in adults, and respiratory complaints occur equally in all age groups.
» The chance of a systemic reaction to a sting is low in those with large local reactions and in children with mild (cutaneous) systemic reactions; the rate varies from 25% to 70% among adults, depending on the severity of previous systemic sting reactions.
» Venom skin tests are most accurate for diagnosis, but the serum specific immunoglobulin E (IgE) test is an important complementary test. The degree of sensitivity on skin or serum tests does not predict the severity of a sting reaction. The history is important because venom sensitization can be detected in up to 25% of adults.
» Patients discharged from emergency care for anaphylaxis should be well educated on how to use an epinephrine kit and should understand that using the kit is not a substitute for emergency medical attention. Allergy consultation and preventative treatment should be arranged.
» Venom immunotherapy is 75% to 98% effective in preventing sting anaphylaxis, and it is as safe as inhalant allergen immunotherapy. Most patients can discontinue treatment after 5 years with a low residual risk of a severe sting reaction.
» Better tests are needed for markers of susceptibility (e.g., determining who are at high risk for sting anaphylaxis) and markers of tolerance (e.g., determining who can safely discontinue venom immunotherapy).

Stinging Insect Allergy

Insect stings are a common cause of allergic reactions, but they also have been the subject of myth and a source of misunderstanding. Physicians and nonphysicians have offered counsel ranging from dire predictions ("The next one will kill you.") to dismissive advice ("Don't worry; you will outgrow it."). Most affected patients think that the reaction was a fluke and that it will never happen again. Most primary care physicians are unaware that venom immunotherapy (VIT) is available, is rapidly protective, and is virtually curative. Decades of epidemiologic, clinical, and laboratory research have revealed the natural history, risk factors, mechanisms, and optimal treatment for insect sting allergy. This improved understanding of the condition provides a framework for the evaluation, management, and guidance of affected individuals. Prevention of severe reactions to stings requires continued research and public and professional educational efforts to dispel misunderstandings and to disseminate the knowledge we have gained.

HISTORICAL PERSPECTIVE

The potential for life-threatening allergic reactions to insect stings has been understood for a long time. The recognition of anaphylaxis in 1902 and the description of immunotherapy in 1911 provided the framework for the first report of immunotherapy for insect sting allergy in 1930.[1] That study used a whole-body extract of the insects, with the reasoning that the relevant allergen was an "intrinsic bee protein" that was present in the bodies and the venom. The fact that this treatment was erroneously recognized as effective for 50 years and endorsed by the American Academy of Allergy provides important lessons in the need for robust knowledge of the natural history of the disease and for controlled clinical trials. Although venom was suspected to be superior to the whole-body extract in case reports by Mary Loveless, the first controlled trial conducted in 1976 showed no difference between whole-body extract and placebo, whereas venom was 95% protective.[2] Only subsequent studies of the epidemiology and natural history revealed the variability and complexity of sting reactions and enabled a stratification of risk that has become the basis for current therapy. VIT has become a unique model for advancing our understanding of the mechanisms of immunotherapy and for the development of improved diagnostic and therapeutic modalities.[3]

EPIDEMIOLOGY

Insect sting allergy can occur at any age, often after a number of uneventful stings, and is more common than once thought. In the United States, systemic allergic reactions are reported by up to 3% of adults, and almost 1% of children have a medical history of severe sting reactions.[4] In some Mediterranean studies, the prevalence of systemic reactions to stings was about 5% among adults and children.[5] The frequency of large local reactions is less certain, but estimates range from 5% to 25% for adults and children.[5]

At least 40 fatal stings occur each year in the United States and 16 to 38 occur in France, but many other sting fatalities may be unrecognized.[4,5] Although the number of deaths in recent years declined in one report from Australia, there was no change in the United States over a 30-year period.[6] Most fatal sting reactions occur in adults older than 45 years of age, but some have occurred in very young children. Approximately one half of the fatal reactions occur in persons with no prior history of allergic reactions to stings. In postmortem blood samples, it has proved possible to document the presence of venom-specific immunoglobulin E (IgE) antibodies and elevated serum tryptase, suggesting a possible mechanism for some cases of unexplained sudden death.[7] However, the presence of IgE antibodies to Hymenoptera venom is common. More than 30% of adults who were stung in the previous few months showed venom-specific IgE antibodies by skin testing or immunoassay, and 10% to 20% of all adults demonstrate positive skin test or blood test results for yellow jacket or honeybee venom.[4,5,8]

Allergic sensitization to insect venoms requires at least one previous sting, but it may be remote and forgotten. Cross-sensitization from pollen or food allergens may occur. Positive serum IgE test results of uncertain clinical significance may result from sensitization to cross-reacting carbohydrate determinants present in a variety of foods.[9-11] Although insect sting allergy is sometimes familial, it is not statistically more likely in those with a family history of sting reactions, and there is only a weak correlation with other allergic conditions.[4,5,8] The frequency of venom sensitization (regardless of history) is higher among individuals with sensitization to inhalant allergens (with or without symptoms).

ETIOLOGY

Stinging insects belong to the order Hymenoptera. The sting apparatus is a modified ovipositor; therefore, only the female insects can sting. Although some species sting offensively as a method of disabling and capturing prey, most sting primarily in defense of themselves and their nest. The Hymenoptera of importance in allergy are from three families: Apidae, Vespidae, and Formicidae (Table 78-1). Selected representatives of these families are depicted in Figure 78-1. Yellow jackets are the most frequent culprits in northern North America and Europe, whereas the *Polistes* species are more commonly implicated in the Gulf coast areas of the United States and the Mediterranean coast of Europe.[12] Common names in general usage can be misleading: the term *bee* can refer to honeybees only or to all stinging insects. Similarly, *wasps* may refer to any of the social wasps or vespids or only to the *Polistes* species. The stinging ants are an increasingly prevalent cause of anaphylaxis in the United States, Asia, and Australia.[12,13]

TABLE 78-1 Taxonomy of the Hymenoptera Insect Order

Family and Subfamily	Scientific Name	Common Name
Apidae	*Apis mellifera*	Honeybee
	Bombus spp.	Bumblebee
	Megabombus spp.	
	Halictus spp.	Sweatbee
	Dialictus spp.	
Vespidae		
Vespinae	*Vespula* spp.	Yellow jacket
	Dolichovespula arenaria	Yellow hornet
	Dolichovespula maculata	White-faced hornet
Polistinae	*Polistes* spp.	Paper wasp
Formicidae	*Solenopsis invicta*	Fire ant
	Myrmecia spp.	Jack jumper ant
	Pogonomyrmex spp.	Harvester ant
	Pachycondyla spp.	

Apids

Feral honeybees often nest in natural hollows such as in trees, although in recent years, natural pests have decimated most of these colonies. Domestic honeybees are relatively docile and rarely sting or swarm without considerable provocation, mostly in defense of their nest and their queen. The sting apparatus of the honeybee is barbed and breaks away from the insect body when it remains in the skin after a sting (i.e., sting autotomy). This eviscerates the insect and leads to its death. Most honeybee stings (other than in beekeepers) occur in children and others who run outdoors without shoes or who handle flowering plants without gloves.

African-European hybrid bees escaped into the wild in Brazil in 1957, migrated over many decades through Central America, and entered the southern United States in 1990.[12] Although an individual Africanized honeybee appears no different from a domestic honeybee and delivers the same venom when it stings, groups of Africanized bees have an unusual tendency to swarm with little provocation and to sting in large numbers. Delivery of large numbers of stings at one time can cause toxic reactions that have been fatal to livestock and humans; this has earned these insects the common name of *killer bees*.

Bumblebees, like honeybees, usually are not aggressive and do not usually sting. Systemic reactions to bumblebee stings (*Bombus* species) occur especially in areas of higher exposure (e.g., greenhouse workers) and show very limited cross-reactivity with honeybee sting reactions.[14] There are very few reports of allergic reactions to sweat bee stings (*Halictus* species), which are unrelated to honeybee allergy.[4]

Vespids

Vespids use a wood pulp to construct nests that contain one or more layers of comb, each of which contain a large number of cells. These comb layers are attached in a vertical arrangement and usually are enclosed in papier mâché outer layers. New queens mate, survive the winter, and initiate new nests the next spring. The other members of the hive, including the existing queen, die in the fall. The vespid sting apparatus usually has finer barbs than in the apids and does not commonly autotomize, and vespids are able to sting repeatedly. Some yellow jacket species often leave the sting apparatus in the skin, so sting autotomy is not unique to the honeybee.[15]

Yellow jackets (genus *Vespula*) are scavengers; they seek their food at picnics and in orchards, trashcans, and dumpsters. Yellow jackets are highly aggressive and sting for no apparent reason, particularly in the autumn, when larger populations compete for limited food supplies. Yellow jacket nests are located in the ground or in cracks in buildings or residential landscape materials.

Yellow hornets and white-faced (bald-faced) hornets (genus *Dolichovespula*) are aerial nesting yellow jackets that are present in North America but not in Europe. They often build their nests in shrubs and trees, and their sensitivity to vibration can initiate their defensive sting behavior. The true hornets (genus *Vespa*) include the European hornet (*Vespa crabro*) and the Asian hornet (*Vespa orientalis*); the former exists in significant numbers in eastern North America.

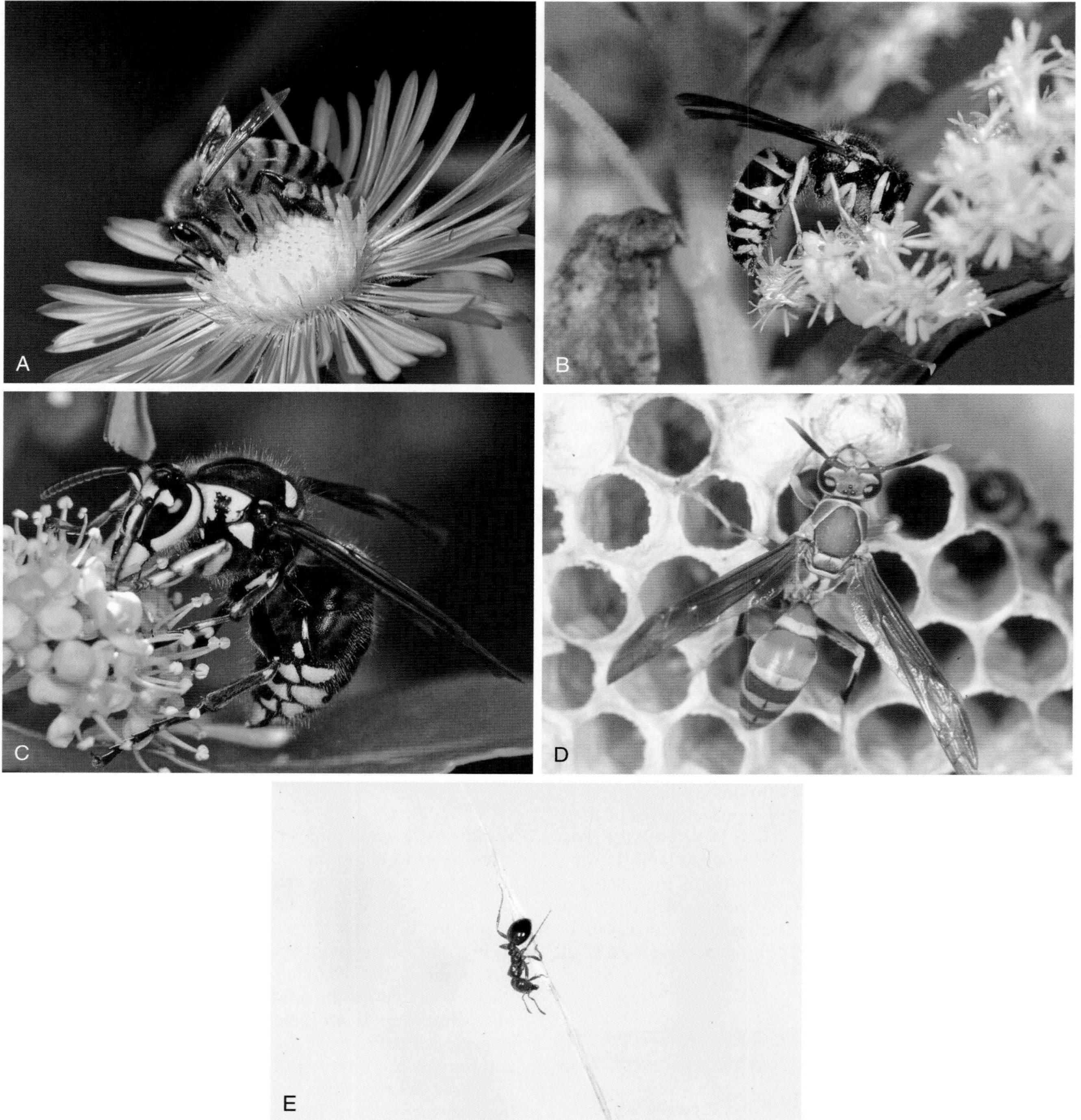

Figure 78-1 Stinging insects of the order Hymenoptera. **A,** Honeybee (*Apis mellifera*). **B,** Yellow jacket (*Vespula maculifroms*). **C,** White-faced hornet (*Dolichovespula maculata*). **D,** Paper wasp (*Polistes exclamans*). **E,** Imported fire ant (*Solenopsis invicta*). *(Reproduced by permission of ALK-Abelló A/S, Hørsholm, Denmark © 2012 ALK.)*

Paper wasps are primarily of the genus *Polistes*. Most build a nest similar to those of other vespids but usually are limited to a single layer of open cells (i.e., comb) with minimal outer covering. These nests are often found on the eaves or windowsills of a home and on the railings of wood decks. Some solitary species do not construct large nests and may differ in some ways from other wasps. Wasps are recognizable by the narrow wasp waist and their characteristic dangling legs when in flight. The coloring of wasps varies greatly, and they can be black, brown, red, or striped. A European species, the Mediterranean wasp (*Polistes dominulus*), has an increasing presence in the United States and is often mistaken for a yellow jacket due to the bright yellow and black stripes on its body. *Polistes* wasps are less aggressive than yellow jackets and hornets, but they sting readily when disturbed and can sting repeatedly without losing their sting apparatus.

Formicids

The ants of the Formicidae family have a true sting apparatus. When they bite, they anchor by their mandibles and pivot to administer multiple stings. Ants of the genus *Solenopsis* are widespread in the southeastern United States, and stings occur so frequently that in many areas, as much as 50% of the population is stung each year.[13,16] These imported fire ants arrived in Mobile, Alabama, in 1940 and have spread slowly through the surrounding states and Gulf coast. Although they were not expected to infest the northern part of North America, nests have been found in Maryland, suggesting that they are capable of adapting to cooler climates. In most cases, multiple ants each administer multiple stings, although they are not painful. The unique lesions form sterile pustules that can become infected if excoriated or opened.

Other genera of the formicid ants include the harvester ants (*Pogonomyrmex* spp.) found in western areas of the United States, Canada, and Mexico; the Australian jack jumper ants (*Myrmecia* spp.); and Asian ants (*Pachycondyla* spp.), which have been reported to cause allergic reactions.[17,18]

INSECT VENOMS

Insect whole-body extracts contain little or no venom protein. Compared with Hymenoptera venoms, whole-body extracts are inaccurate for diagnosis by skin testing and serologic IgE testing and are ineffective for immunotherapy.[4] Although imported fire ant venom is superior, their whole-body extracts contain sufficient quantities of venom allergens to be clinically useful.[13,19]

The biochemical, physicochemical, and immunologic characteristics of the venoms of most of the clinically relevant species have been elucidated and reviewed.[12] Most of the venoms contain vasoactive amines (e.g., histamine, dopamine, norepinephrine), acetylcholine, and kinins, which account for the burning, pain, and itching normally experienced from a sting. Some venom components can cause toxic reactions, including neurologic complications.[4] When a very large number of stings are sustained by the patient, renal failure can occur as a result of rhabdomyolysis. The major allergenic components of Hymenoptera venoms are described in Chapter 26. Most are protein enzymes with molecular weights in the range of 13 to 50 kD. Phospholipase A is the major allergen in honeybee venom; antigen 5 is the common name for the major allergen in the vespid venoms (e.g., Ves v 5). Fire ant venoms are quite different; they contain very little protein in an unusual suspension of alkaloid toxins, which cause the characteristic vesicular eruption.[12] The allergenic proteins are unique except for one that shows limited cross-reactivity with vespid antigen 5.

Within the vespid family, there is extensive cross-allergenicity of the venoms of different genera. This is not the case in the apid and formicid families. There is limited cross-reactivity of honeybee and bumblebee venoms, but there are reports of patients with bumblebee allergy who did not cross-react to honeybee venom.[14] There is significant cross-reactivity among the various fire ant (*Solenopsis*) species and among the harvester ant (*Pogonomyrmex*) species, but the two genera do not cross-react with each other.[4] Vespid venoms have been extensively analyzed, and the primary allergens have been identified and sequenced.[4] Within each genus, there are some species that show only limited cross-reactivity with the other species (e.g., *Vespa squamosa*, *P. dominulus*). A few individuals react only to a single species. The commercial yellow jacket venom is a mix of species (including *V. squamosa* in the United States). The commercial *Polistes* venom is also a species mix, but it does not include *P. dominulus* or some of the solitary wasp species.[4]

The venoms of different insect families have almost no cross-reactivity. There is no cross-allergenicity between honeybee phospholipase A (i.e., the major honey bee venom allergen) and the vespid phospholipase A (i.e., a minor vespid venom allergen). There is limited and infrequent cross-reactivity between honeybee and vespid venom hyaluronidases, some of which may be related to cross-reacting carbohydrate determinants of uncertain clinical significance.[10] When a patient has detectable IgE antibodies against the venoms of different families or genera, it is possible to distinguish cross-reactivity from multiple sensitization by testing the serum in an inhibition immunoassay.[20,21] However, in clinical practice, it is more common to recommend immunotherapy with each of the venoms to which the patient demonstrates sensitivity. Newer in vitro methods using recombinant allergens may more accurately distinguish between clinically relevant (specific) and irrelevant (cross-reactive) venom sensitivities.[11,22]

Commercial Hymenoptera venom products are available in many countries as lyophilized protein extracts for honeybee, yellow jacket, and *Polistes* wasp venoms. In the United States, similar preparations are available for the two *Dolichovespula* venoms (i.e., yellow hornet and white-faced hornet), and an additional mixed vespid product containing equal parts of the three *Vespula* venoms is available. Filtered and delayed-release venom extracts are available in Europe. Honeybee venoms are standardized for their content of phospholipase A, whereas *Vespula* venoms are standardized for their content of hyaluronidase. Lyophilized products are reconstituted and diluted with buffered saline diluent containing 0.03% human serum albumin. This method stabilizes the very small amounts of protein allergens in the solutions and prevents adsorption to the walls of the vials. Technical developments in allergen materials have improved diagnosis and treatment with recombinant venom allergens and venom peptides.[11,12,22]

CLINICAL FEATURES

Classification of Reactions

Insect stings cause reactions that are classified as local or systemic in distribution, and they can have an immediate or delayed time course. Local reactions are limited to the area contiguous with the sting site. Most large local reactions represent a late-phase, IgE-dependent reaction that is mild initially but that develops after 12 to 24 hours to a diameter often exceeding 20 cm and occasionally involving an entire limb. These reactions may manifest with a lymphangitic streak toward the axilla or the inguinal region. This pattern represents the drainage of inflammatory mediators rather than an infectious process. A large local reaction subsides after 5 to 10 days and is not dangerous except for potential local anatomic compression, especially on the head, neck, tongue, or throat.

A systemic reaction causes symptoms and signs in one or more anatomic systems distant from the site of the sting. Almost all systemic reactions are IgE mediated and cause anaphylaxis.[23] Patients may exhibit cutaneous signs (e.g., generalized urticaria, angioedema, flushing, pruritus), respiratory changes (e.g., throat tightness, dysphagia, dyspnea, stridor or dysphonia, chest tightness, wheezing), or a circulatory component (e.g., dizziness, hypotension, unconsciousness, shock).[24] Less frequently, gastrointestinal complaints (e.g., cramps, diarrhea, nausea, vomiting) or uterine cramping occur. Cardiac anaphylaxis after insect stings can cause coronary vasospasm, tachyarrhythmias, or bradycardia, even with no underlying coronary or cardiac abnormality. The diagnosis of the acute reaction can be difficult when hypotension or cardiac manifestations occur with no other signs or symptoms. The absence of urticaria or angioedema is associated with more severe reactions to stings.[25] Protracted anaphylaxis occurs much less often with insect stings than with food allergy.[4] Of 2602 subjects in a registry of sting-allergic patients, 16% reported only cutaneous symptoms, and 24% had life-threatening reactions, including 15% with loss of consciousness; 44% had moderate systemic reactions.[26] Cutaneous signs and symptoms are the sole manifestation in 15% of adults, but children have a higher frequency (60%) of these isolated cutaneous reactions and a lower frequency of vascular symptoms or anaphylactic shock compared with adults.[4] Patients with repeated systemic reactions typically report an individual pattern of reaction that is consistent from one episode to another.[4] Another delayed manifestation of unclear mechanism that has been reported in some individuals with demonstrable venom-specific IgE antibodies is the occurrence of cold urticaria beginning in the weeks after the sting and persisting for months, usually without any immediate allergic reaction to the sting.[12]

Systemic reactions may be caused by underlying mast cell disorders in 1% to 2% of cases.[27,28] Up to 25% of patients with severe anaphylactic reactions to venom have elevated baseline serum tryptase.[29] Systemic reactions may occasionally be caused by toxic effects from the vasoactive substances in a large number of stings. Massive envenomation from large numbers of stings can cause life-threatening reactions with renal failure, rhabdomyolysis, hemolysis, and acute respiratory distress syndrome or diffuse intravascular coagulation. Seizures have occurred, particularly after multiple fire ant stings.[12] Unusual reactions of unknown mechanisms are usually delayed and include serum sickness-like reactions, encephalitis, peripheral and cranial neuropathies, glomerulonephritis, myocarditis, and Guillain-Barré syndrome.[4] If there is a question about whether the observed reaction was truly anaphylactic, the detection of elevated serum tryptase level in blood samples drawn within 1 to 3 hours after the onset of the reaction may provide confirmation. Even if the tryptase level is not clearly elevated, comparison with a baseline level may demonstrate a significant change that confirms anaphylaxis.[30]

PATIENT EVALUATION AND DIAGNOSIS

Clinical History

The diagnosis of insect sting allergy rests on the history as the primary evidence of allergic reactivity because, as with all types of allergens, venom-specific IgE antibodies are present in a large number of clinically nonreactive individuals. Physicians should inquire about severe reactions to insect stings when obtaining a complete medical history, because most affected individuals fail to mention the event during routine interrogation. The history should be reviewed in detail with respect to the nature and timing of stings in the past, the time course of the reaction, and all associated symptoms and treatments. The identity of the culprit is a notoriously unreliable part of the history, but the location and timing of the sting or the location of the nest may suggest the type of insect. The number of stings and the location on the body may also help to differentiate systemic or local reactions. Concurrent medications, such as β-adrenergic blocking agents and angiotensin-converting enzyme inhibitors (ACEIs), can contribute significantly to the severity of the anaphylactic reaction. In some cases, medications used for treatment of the reaction may account for some of the delayed symptoms. Antihistamines may cause somnolence that can be confused with a reduced level of consciousness. Epinephrine causes tachycardia and nausea, which can also be related to the anaphylactic reaction.

Skin Tests

The standard method of skin testing employs an intradermal technique that uses the five Hymenoptera venom protein extracts. Fire ant sensitivity can be tested with reasonable diagnostic sensitivity and specificity using whole-body extracts of imported fire ants. Preliminary studies suggest the superiority of fire ant venom extract, but commercial preparations are not available.[4] For Hymenoptera venom testing, intradermal tests are performed with venom concentrations in the range of 0.001 to 1.0 μg/mL to find the minimum concentration that gives a positive result. Epicutaneous tests at concentrations of 1 to 100 μg/mL may be used initially for patients with a history of very severe reactions, but if results are negative, they should be followed by intradermal skin tests. Sensitization may have occurred to multiple venoms even when there has only been a reaction to only a single insect. Skin testing should be performed with a complete set of the five Hymenoptera venoms available in the United States and with a negative diluent control (i.e., human serum albumin-saline) and a positive histamine control.[31,32]

Skin test results are clearly positive for most patients with a convincing history, but they often can be negative. In the days or weeks after a sting reaction, some patients have negative skin test results attributed to a refractory period of anergy; for them, skin tests should be repeated after 4 to 6 weeks.[33] Negative skin test results for a history-positive patient may represent the loss of sensitivity in a person with a remote history of sting reaction. Some cases of sting anaphylaxis may be non–IgE mediated or be attributable to subclinical (indolent) mastocytosis.[27,28] Some persons with negative venom skin test results have systemic reactions to subsequent stings.[4,34] Skin test results for individual venoms can vary over a short period, and identification of all sensitivities requiring treatment may require skin testing on two separate occasions.[35] Venom skin tests are limited in their diagnostic range because of their nonallergenic ingredients, which may cause false-positive reactions at concentrations higher than 1.0 μg/mL. Most insect-allergic patients with negative venom skin test results have detectable venom-specific IgE antibodies in the serum, but some are detected only by skin testing with a higher concentration of a dialyzed venom extract.[36] Commercial venom extracts available in other countries are purified (i.e., filtered or dialyzed), as are the venom products used in most venom-specific IgE assays.[37] The serum-specific IgE test is positive in 10% of patients with negative skin test results, and venom skin test results can be negative on one occasion and positive on another. For these reasons, patients with negative skin test results and a convincing history of anaphylaxis should be further investigated with serologic testing, and if results remain negative, the skin tests should be repeated after 3 to 6 months.[38]

Venom skin test sensitivities have different patterns. Because of cross-reactivity, almost all patients who have a positive skin test result in response to yellow jacket venom will also have positive results for skin tests for one or both of the hornet venoms, and approximately one half will have positive results for challenge to *Polistes* wasp venom. The degree of skin test sensitivity does not correlate reliably with the degree of sting reaction.[12,39] The most reactive skin tests may occur in patients who have had only large local reactions and have a very low risk of anaphylaxis, whereas some patients who have had near-fatal anaphylactic shock show only weak skin test reactivity. Approximately 25% of patients evaluated for systemic allergic reactions to stings have positive skin test reactions only at the 1.0 μg/mL concentration, demonstrating the importance of skin testing with the full diagnostic range of concentrations.[4,31,32]

In Vitro Tests

The diagnosis of insect sting allergy by detection of allergen-specific IgE antibodies in serum is a method with great potential, but performance varies.[21,40] Improved methods have led to improved diagnostic accuracy, but they are not used by all commercial laboratories in the United States. A high level of venom-specific IgE is usually diagnostic, but low levels are more difficult to detect with reliability. Venom skin tests and venom-specific IgE assays correlate imperfectly.[4] The latter produce negative results in up to 20% of skin test–positive subjects, and venom skin test results are negative for approximately 10% of persons with elevated IgE antibodies. Neither test alone can detect all cases of insect sting allergy, and each test is useful as a supplement to the other. The clinical significance of a positive IgE antibody assay result with a negative skin test result is not known in all cases, but it is clearly associated with a risk of systemic reaction to a sting.[4,34,41]

Alternate diagnostic methods that measure basophil activation or basophil sensitivity may be useful in difficult cases, but their methodology and diagnostic accuracy have been inconsistent compared with the combination of venom skin tests and measurement of specific serum IgE.[21,42,43] There may be specific applications for basophil activation tests in patients with negative skin test and serologic test results and to predict VIT failure, systemic reactions to VIT, relapse after stopping VIT, and outcomes for children.[42,44,45]

Venom skin test sensitivity may be improved with the use of recombinant venom allergens.[12] Component-resolved diagnosis with recombinant allergens can improve the specificity and prognostic value of serologic testing.[11,22] These materials are expressed without the carbohydrate components that are present in the natural allergens (i.e., cross-reacting carbohydrate determinants), which are thought to be responsible for a double-positivity reaction to honeybee and yellow jacket venoms in patients who are only clinically reactive to one of the insects. However, the activity of these recombinant component allergens is often less than the native allergens, and multiple allergen components should be included in the test to detect all patients with clinical sting allergy.[9,46]

Sting Challenge Test

It has been assumed that the ultimate test of whether an individual will have a systemic reaction to a sting is to observe the outcome of a supervised live sting challenge.[2,47] This procedure has been used as the gold standard in research studies of the efficacy of VIT and to determine the relapse rate after discontinuation of VIT. Sting challenge of untreated patients with a history of previous systemic reactions to stings and with positive venom skin test results has resulted in systemic reaction rates ranging between 21% and 73%. This variability in part reflects the variability of the culprit insect. The quantity of venom protein injected during a sting is relatively consistent for honeybees but varies greatly for vespids. The species of vespid used may also affect the outcome.[4,39] The routine use of a live sting challenge as a diagnostic procedure for selection of patients for immunotherapy has been proposed, but there have been many objections.[4] Moreover, the lack of reaction to a single challenge sting has limited clinical significance, because a subsequent sting can still cause a systemic reaction in up to 20% of cases.[39,48] The use of sting challenge in research has been considered unethical in many European centers, making it more difficult to evaluate the diagnostic accuracy of new methods such as recombinant allergens and the basophil activation test.

TREATMENT OF ACUTE REACTIONS

Large local reactions, especially those involving the head and neck, are best treated with a brief burst of an oral corticosteroid (e.g., initial dose of 40 to 60 mg of prednisone, tapering to 0 in 5 days). For best results, steroids should be started within a few hours of the sting in patients with a known history of large local reactions to stings. Large local reactions can be mistaken for cellulitis, especially on the extremities, where intense inflammation can cause an apparent lymphangitis directed toward the axillary or inguinal nodes. When such a reaction presents 24 to 48 hours after the sting, infection is unlikely, and treatment should include ice and moderate-dose oral steroids, but antibiotics are not necessary.

Systemic reactions require more urgent intervention and close monitoring. Urticaria may respond to antihistamines alone, but anaphylactic reactions require epinephrine injection. Any sign of hypotension or respiratory obstruction should be treated promptly with aqueous epinephrine intramuscularly and should have full emergency medical attention and observation for 3 to 6 hours (see Chapter 77).[23,32] The recommended dose of epinephrine is 0.3 to 0.5 mg (0.3 to 0.5 mL of 1 : 1000 weight/volume solution) for adults and 0.01 mg/kg for children to a maximum of 0.3 mg. After use of self-injectable epinephrine, the individual should be taken to an emergency department for observation and further treatment, if necessary. Some patients who have a history of rapid-onset or very severe systemic reactions may warrant treatment immediately after the sting. Delay in the use of epinephrine has contributed to fatal reactions, and some individuals with anaphylactic shock are resistant to epinephrine. Patients taking β-blocker medications may be resistant to the effects of epinephrine. Glucagon injection can be beneficial in these cases. For some patients, anaphylaxis is prolonged or recurrent for 6 to 24 hours, and it may require intensive medical care.[23,49] The patient with hypotension should be kept supine with legs raised because upright posture has been associated with sudden death due to lack of venous return (i.e., empty ventricle syndrome).[50]

Emergency treatment of anaphylaxis requires patient education before discharge. The risk of recurrence should be clearly described, and the use of self-injectable epinephrine requires consistent instruction and follow-up. Many patients are not specifically instructed about the need for self-injectable epinephrine, and they are not referred for an allergy consultation and preventive treatment.[49] This is important because affected individuals may think the reaction was a chance occurrence and fail to inform their personal physicians about it.[8]

PREVENTION OF ACUTE REACTIONS

Patients allergic to insect stings seem to have a higher frequency of being stung, although this tendency disappears during VIT.[4] Patients should avoid high-risk exposures such as yard and garden work, trash containers, and outdoor areas where food and drink are exposed. Food and flavored drinks in cans, bottles, and straws can be an unsuspected source of a sting to the tongue or throat. Avoidance of wearing brightly colored clothes is of uncertain benefit, and insect repellants have little or no effect.[51]

Epinephrine Kits

Epinephrine autoinjectors (0.3-mg EpiPen and 0.15-mg EpiPen Jr, Dey Labs, Napa, Calif.; 0.3-mg Twinject and 0.15-mg Adrenaclick, Shionogi Pharma, Atlanta, Ga.; 0.3-mg and 0.15-mg Auvi-Q, Sanofi, Bridgewater, N.J.) should be prescribed and explained to all patients at risk for anaphylaxis. The age at which to prescribe an adult-dose instead of pediatric-dose autoinjector is uncertain, but the question may be considered when the child reaches a weight of 25 kg.[52] Even when epinephrine kits are prescribed, patients often fail to carry the injector with them and delay or defer using them when they have a reaction.[49] Patients, caretakers in homes and schools, and physicians need initial and follow-up education about the correct use of the device and how to recognize the expiration date on the unit and replace outdated units promptly.[12,32]

PREDICTORS OF RISK FOR STING ANAPHYLAXIS

Natural History

The prognosis for affected patients is based on the understanding of the natural history of the condition (Table 78-2), including clinical factors and biologic markers (Table 78-3). The chance that a future sting will cause an allergic reaction depends on the history and immunologic status of the patient.[4,39] The ability to predict the occurrence of systemic reactions is especially desirable, because many fatal reactions to stings occur in individuals who did not know they had been sensitized. Because one of five healthy adults has detectable venom-specific IgE antibodies, testing of asymptomatic individuals is not recommended. In one study, the normal adults with positive venom skin test results had a 17% incidence of systemic reactions to subsequent stings, although the results became negative in 30% to 50% of these individuals after 2 to 5 years.[53]

In a patient who had previous systemic reactions, the outcome of the next sting is unpredictable because systemic reactions may occur on some occasions but not on others.[4] This inconsistency may reflect variations in the insect species and delivery of allergen as much as variations in the patient's physiology or immune status.[39] Additional factors favoring a systemic reaction include older age, male gender, multiple stings, and repeated stings occurring in temporal proximity (e.g., only weeks apart).

In studies of challenge stings or field stings in patients with positive venom skin test results and previous systemic reactions, the average frequency of systemic reaction has been 45%. However, a subsequent sting caused a systemic reaction in 20% of patients who had no reaction to the first sting.[39,48] The risk of recurrence in patients with a history of systemic reactions to stings is higher for those who are allergic to honeybee stings than for those with vespid allergies, higher for adults than for children, and higher for patients who had more severe systemic reactions previously than for those with milder systemic reactions.[4] Patients who previously had severe reactions have a higher chance that any future reaction will be severe. Most patients exhibit a characteristic and individual pattern of reaction; contrary to popular belief, it is uncommon for patients to have more severe reactions with each subsequent sting.[39,41] There appears to be a gradual decline in the chance of systemic reaction over time, decreasing from almost 50% after a recent reaction to 25% 7 to 10 years later.[54] However, the risk never disappears, and some patients have had severe reactions to stings after decades without an intervening sting.

Large local reactions are not usually a precursor of systemic reactions. The risk of eventual anaphylaxis in those with large local reactions is only 5% to 10%.[4] In one study, the frequency of systemic sting reactions among high school children was greater for those with previous large local reactions.[55] Most large local reactors consistently have similar reactions with repeated stings, even some whose family members have had systemic reactions. The level of sensitivity shown by a venom skin test or specific IgE level does not predict future occurrences, and no known clinical or laboratory characteristics differentiate patients who will progress to systemic reactions from those who will continue to have only large local sting reactions.

The natural history of insect sting allergy in children is not as well studied as in adults. The results of skin tests or specific

TABLE 78-2 Risk of Systemic Reaction in Untreated Patients with History of Sting Anaphylaxis and Positive Venom Skin Test Results

Original Sting Reaction		Risk of Systemic Reaction (%)	
Severity	Age	1-9 Years	10-20 Years
No reaction	Adult	17	
Large local	All	10	10
Cutaneous-systemic	Child	10	5
	Adult	20	10
Anaphylaxis	Child	40	30
	Adult	60	40

TABLE 78-3 Predictors of Risk of Systemic Reaction to Insect Stings

Natural History	Screening Tests and Markers
Severity of previous reaction	Venom skin test
Insect species	Venom-specific IgE
Age, gender	Basophil activation test
No urticaria or angioedema	Baseline serum tryptase value
Medications	Platelet-activating factor (PAF) acetylhydrolase
Multiple or sequential stings	Angiotensin-converting enzyme (ACE)

IgE level became negative in 25% to 50% of untreated children after an average of 10 years of follow-up.[4] The outcome of subsequent stings into adulthood is not as benign as once thought. During 10 to 20 years of follow-up, children who had had strictly cutaneous reactions had only a 10% to 15% chance of subsequent systemic reactions (mostly milder than the previous reaction) and only about a 3% chance of more severe reactions with respiratory or circulatory symptoms.[56] Those who had moderate or severe reactions in childhood had a significantly higher risk of reaction in adulthood, estimated to be 30%.

The chance of progression from a mild reaction to a severe reaction is a central issue in determining whether many patients require VIT. Although this possibility has been studied in children, it has not been conclusively determined in adults. Some retrospective studies showed more frequent progression,[26,57] but prospective sting challenge studies found a very low risk of progression (<5%).[39,41]

Markers of Risk for Sting Anaphylaxis

The history (i.e., severity of previous sting reactions) has been the most reliable predictor of the severity of subsequent sting reactions. Absence of urticaria or angioedema during anaphylaxis was associated with a higher frequency of severe reaction.[25] Measurable markers that predict the risk of systemic reaction to a sting are summarized in Table 78-3. Results of skin tests and specific IgE tests correlate better with the frequency of sting reactions than with the severity of reactions. The baseline serum tryptase level correlates closely with the risk of severe anaphylaxis from a sting, and together with other variables, it has been used to develop a mathematical model of the risk of severe sting anapahylaxis.[58] It is likely that abnormal measurements of other mast cell mediators will be found to reflect an increased risk of severe anaphylaxis. This is true for platelet-activating factor (PAF). The level of PAF correlates with the serum activity of PAF acetylhydrolase.[59] This finding reveals that abnormal metabolism of mast cell mediators can increase the risk of severe anaphylaxis.

Another growing concern has been the effect of medications on the risk of reaction. β-Blockers can increase the risk of anaphylaxis primarily by interfering with the effects of epinephrine.[23] However, it has not been determined whether the risk is similar for β_1-selective agents as it is for β_2-blockers. β-Blockers should be avoided in all patients who are at risk for anaphylaxis, including those with insect sting allergy and those receiving allergen immunotherapy. However, risk analysis has suggested that in many patients with cardiovascular disease, stopping β-blockers can create greater risk than not stopping the drug during VIT.[60] It is therefore acceptable, when necessary, to proceed with VIT in patients receiving β-blockers. Another concern has been the risk of anaphylaxis in patients taking ACEIs. Some case reports have suggested a significant risk; one study showed no increased risk for VIT, and one large, multicenter study found a significant correlation of ACEI with severe anaphylaxis.[58,61] In another report, ACEIs were not associated with increased frequency of severe systemic reactions to stings.[25] It is unknown whether angiotensin receptor blockers (ARBs) carry the same risk, but their mechanism of action is not expected to influence the kinin pathways that are affected by ACEIs.

Baseline serum tryptase activity can predict severe sting anaphylaxis, and it has been useful as a predictor of systemic reactions during VIT, failure of VIT, and relapse of sting anaphylaxis after discontinuing VIT.[27,29,58,62] Elevated baseline tryptase levels often indicate underlying mastocytosis, which occurs in approximately 1% to 2% of patients with sting anaphylaxis. Sting anaphylaxis is the most common cause of anaphylaxis in patients with indolent mastocytosis, and it can be the presenting sign of the disease.[28]

VENOM IMMUNOTHERAPY

Indications

VIT is the treatment of choice for prevention of systemic allergic reactions to insect stings, but it requires careful selection of patients.[4,32,63] Since its introduction, the indication for VIT includes only patients with a history of previous systemic allergic reaction to a sting and evidence of venom-specific IgE antibodies with a positive venom skin test result or elevated specific IgE level. Some patients with positive skin test results do not require VIT because they are judged to be at relatively low risk for anaphylaxis. Those with recent and severe anaphylaxis are at highest risk (40% to 70%); a low risk (<10%) has been found for children and adults with a history of large local reactions[4,56] and for children with reactions limited to cutaneous signs and symptoms but with no respiratory or vascular manifestations.[4,56,64]

Some low-risk patients request treatment because of their fear of reaction and its impact on their lifestyle. The quality of life is impaired in patients with a history of systemic reactions and is improved by VIT but not by prescription of self-injectable epinephrine.[65,66] Adults with a history of mild systemic reactions have a low risk of severe reaction to a later sting, but there are known cases of progression from cutaneous-only reactions to life-threatening anaphylaxis on subsequent stings. For this reason, adults with cutaneous-systemic reactions are advised to undergo VIT. There is no test for large local or cutaneous reactions that predicts which patients will progress to more severe reactions, although elevated levels of mast cell mediators predict the severity of reactions in patients with sting anaphylaxis.[58,59] There is increasing evidence that VIT can inhibit large local reactions to stings, which may benefit patients with frequent and severe local reactions.[67,68]

Safety

Adverse reactions to VIT are no more common than reactions during inhalant allergen immunotherapy.[63,69,70] Systemic symptoms occur in 5% to 15% of patients during the initial weeks of treatment, regardless of which standard schedule is used. Adverse reactions to VIT may be associated with greater basophil sensitivity to venom allergen.[71] There is also an association between severe or repeated systemic reactions to injections and underlying mast cell disease (e.g., mastocytosis, urticaria pigmentosa, elevated baseline serum tryptase levels).[27,28,72,73]

Systemic reactions to venom injections occur more frequently in patients treated with honeybee venom than in those treated with yellow jacket venom.[4] Systemic reactions during initial immunotherapy with Jack Jumper ant (*Myrmecia pilosula*) venom were much more frequent (34%) than for other venoms.[74] Most systemic reactions are mild, and less than 5% of patients receiving VIT ever require epinephrine treatment for a reaction to an injection.

Pretreatment with antihistamines appears to reduce the local and systemic reactions to injections, and it may reduce the frequency of systemic reactions to subsequent stings.[75,76]

Pretreatment with a leukotriene modifier can significantly reduce the occurrence of large local reactions to VIT injections.[77] In the unusual case of recurrent systemic reactions to injections, therapy may be streamlined to a single venom and given in divided doses 30 minutes apart. Rarely, therapy has to be suspended for 6 to 12 months and then restarted, often without producing severe reactions. In patients with recurrent systemic reactions to VIT, rush VIT, or omalizumab treatment have been successful.[78-81] Large local reactions to venom injections occur in up to 50% of patients, especially in the dose range of 20 to 50 µg. Unlike standard inhalant immunotherapy, there is a uniform target dose in VIT, and it is occasionally necessary to advance the dose in the face of moderately severe local reactions. Although large local reactions to venom injections have not predicted systemic reactions to subsequent doses, an association has been reported for fire ant immunotherapy.[82] Like inhalant immunotherapy, maintenance VIT is considered acceptable during pregnancy, even though limited data are available.[4]

Efficacy

VIT can be 95% to 100% effective in preventing systemic reactions to stings. These results were reported in U.S. clinical trials in which the most common treatment employed a maintenance dose of 300 µg of mixed vespid venoms.[4] Studies of immunotherapy with a 100-µg dose of individual venoms (i.e., honeybee, yellow jacket, or *Polistes* wasp) have been associated with 75% to 95% efficacy.[4,83] In a controlled trial of immunotherapy with Jack Jumper ant venom, a maintenance dose of 100 µg was associated with complete protection from sting challenge in more than 95% of patients.[74] Even in cases considered to be treatment failures, the repeat sting reactions usually are milder than pretreatment reactions.[83] Although the serum level of venom-specific IgG antibodies has been proposed as a marker of the efficacy of VIT, it has shown good positive predictive value but poor negative predictive value.[4] No marker has been able to reliably predict the reaction to a sting in an individual patient. Treatment failure can often be overcome with higher treatment doses (e.g., 200 µg).[4,83] Failure of VIT has been associated with abnormal basophil activation test responses[84] and with underlying mastocytosis in some cases.[27,28]

The mechanism of protection induced by VIT, like inhalant allergen immunotherapy, has been elucidated only in part. Early observations centered on the apparent therapeutic increase in levels of venom-specific IgG antibodies, particularly the role of IgG4 subclass antibodies in long-term protection.[4] In some cases, passive immunization with hyperimmune globulin from beekeepers has been effective.[4] Evidence supports the role of IgG in intercepting allergen and in facilitating lymphocyte responses.[12,85] Immunotherapy induces suppression of venom skin test and specific IgE antibodies,[4] and it reduces basophil release of histamine or leukotrienes.[12]

Altered antibody responses are related to the effects of VIT on T lymphocyte activities. As with inhalant allergen immunotherapy, VIT causes a shift in the T lymphocyte responses from a helper T cell type 2 (Th2) pattern to a helper T cell type 1 (Th1) pattern, which is more pronounced with more rapid treatment regimens.[12] Further studies have elucidated an important role for interleukin 10 (IL-10) in the suppression of the Th2 cytokines during VIT for systemic or late-phase local reactions to stings and suggest a role for regulatory T cells and osteopontin in the protective effects of VIT.[12,86] Additional investigation has identified more specific pathways of T cell regulation and identified a role for dendritic cells.[87,88] Another novel pathway involves the role of IgG4 antibodies in facilitated antigen presentation to T cells and B cells that regulate the allergic response to venom.[85] Newer approaches to VIT using T cell epitope peptides, recombinant allergens, and DNA sequences may expand our understanding of the immune mechanisms involved.[9,11,12,22]

Venom Species and Dose

The selection of venom extracts to be used for immunotherapy depends on the venom skin test reaction or venom-specific IgE antibody level to those venoms. Therapy should include all that elicit a positive response, because a guarantee of not reacting to the next sting is not possible without therapy, and anaphylaxis to one venom may predispose to anaphylaxis to another venom. For this reason, the most common therapy for vespid sensitivities in the United States is with the mixed vespid venoms preparation: 100 µg each of yellow jacket, yellow hornet, and white-faced hornet venoms. Although therapy with yellow jacket venom alone can protect against hornet stings because of the marked cross-reactivity of the *Vespula* venoms, there are reports that therapy with any single venom gives 15% to 20% less immune response and less reliable clinical protection than mixed vespid venoms.[4,83] The skin test result is also positive to *Polistes* wasp venoms in at least 50% of vespid allergic patients, and treatment is usually given as a separate injection. Therapy with yellow jacket or mixed vespid venoms can protect against wasp stings, but this has been established only for patients whose wasp IgE showed complete cross-reactivity with yellow jacket venom as assessed by inhibition immunoassays.[4]

The standard recommended dose of 100 µg of each venom was originally selected to be equivalent to the estimated venom protein content of two to four stings. The amount of venom protein injected by a honeybee sting is consistently in the range of 50 µg, but there is considerable variability in the amount of venom injected by the vespids, with estimates of 2 to 20 µg per sting.[4] The efficacy of the 100-µg dose has contributed to its widespread acceptance. Data on the use of lower doses are limited, with various degrees of efficacy reported for adults.[4] Patients who are not adequately protected with the 100-µg dose usually can be protected with higher doses.[83] The treatment recommendations for children 3 years old or older are the same as for adults. However, some studies have shown similar efficacy and long-term outcomes using a 50-µg maintenance dose in children.[89,90]

Schedules

Initial VIT follows a schedule that can vary according to the recommendations of the source laboratory that prepared the allergen extract and the level of caution preferred by the clinician. Table 78-4 shows the recommended schedules for the two products available in the United States. The modified rush regimen (ALK-Abelló, Round Rock, Tex.) is more rapid than the traditional regimen (Hollister-Stier Laboratories, Spokane, Wash.), achieving maintenance dose in eight weekly injections instead of 15 weeks, respectively. These regimens are equally effective, and the frequency of systemic reactions was the same with both.[4] Treatment often requires multiple venoms, which can be administered on the same day. Although the *Vespula* venoms are mixed for the commercial preparation of mixed vespid venom, it has been recommended not to mix other

TABLE 78-4 Examples of Conventional Dosing Schedules for Venom Immunotherapy

Schedule 1*

Week No.	Concentration (μg/mL)	Volume (mL)
1	1.0	0.05
2	1.0	0.1
3	1.0	0.2
4	1.0	0.4
5	10	0.05
6	10	0.1
7	10	0.2
8	10	0.4
9	100	0.05
10	100	0.1
11	100	0.2
12	100	0.4
13	100	0.6
14	100	0.8
15	100	1.0
16	100	1.0
18	100	1.0
21	100	1.0
Monthly	100	1.0

Schedule 2*

Week No.	Concentration (μg/mL)	Volume (mL)
1a	0.01	0.1
1b	0.1	0.1
1c	1.0	0.1
2a	1.0	0.1
2b	1.0	0.5
2c	10	0.1
3a	10	0.1
3b	10	0.5
3c	10	1.0
4a	100	0.1
4b	100	0.2
5a	100	0.2
5b	100	0.3
6a	100	0.3
6b	100	0.3
7a	100	0.4
7b	100	0.4
8a	100	0.5
8b	100	0.5
9	100	1.0
Monthly	100	1.0

*Injections usually are given weekly. Schedule 2 prescribes two or three doses, at 30-minute intervals for the first 8 weeks. When the maintenance dose is achieved, the interval may be advanced from weekly to monthly. Schedule 1 is based on the package insert for Hollister-Stier venom extracts (Spokane, Wash.). Schedule 2 is based on the package insert for ALK-Abelló venom extracts (Round Rock, Tex.).

venoms because of the potential proteolytic effects of enzyme allergens. When the full dose is achieved, it is usually repeated in 1 week, again after another 2 weeks, and then after 3 weeks before beginning maintenance treatment every 4 weeks.

Rush regimens refer to a variety of build-up schedules that vary from semirush cluster regimens given over 3 to 4 weeks, to 2- to 3-day rush regimens, and to ultrarush regimens given over just a few hours. Rush VIT regimens administered over 2 to 3 days have been highly effective and generally safe, with adverse reactions occurring no more often than with traditional regimens.[4,12] Ultra-rush regimens are associated with an increased risk of severe reactions.[91] Rush VIT has been used successfully in patients unable to achieve maintenance doses due to repeated systemic reactions using standard schedules.[79,80] Use of rush regimens has become routine in Europe due to the regional availability of specialized treatment and in the U.S. military to hasten return to duty.

Maintenance

Based on early clinical trials and the regulatory approval for Hymenoptera venoms in the United States, maintenance therapy is administered every 4 weeks for at least 1 year. There are few studies on longer maintenance intervals, but clinical experience supports the practice of extending the maintenance interval to every 6 to 8 weeks over several years in most cases.[32,63] A few patients require maintenance doses every 2 to 3 weeks to avoid systemic reactions. VIT with a 12-week interval may be effective for extended maintenance treatment after 4 years of routine therapy.[92,93] Maintenance evaluation should include a review of the dose and frequency of injections, all adverse reactions, any intervening stings, and all current medications. Repeat skin tests or immunoassays may be performed every 2 to 3 years. Bousquet and colleagues[94] reported negative skin test results for honeybee treatment in 19% of patients after 1 year and in 30% after 3 years of treatment.[94] In that study, skin test results became negative during yellow jacket treatment in 35% of patients after 1 year and in 54% after 3 years. Golden and associates[95,96] reported that 20% of patients have negative skin test results after 5 years but that 50% to 60% had negative results after 7 to 10 years. Venom-specific IgE antibody levels before immunotherapy average 10 ng/mL (4.2 kU/L) in adults and 20 ng/mL (8.4 kU/L) in children; the level rises during the first months of therapy, returns to baseline after 12 months, and then declines steadily during maintenance treatment (even after therapy is stopped and after a sting).[4]

The level of venom-specific IgG antibodies can be measured during maintenance VIT as a marker of clinical efficacy.[4,97] Some argue that this is unnecessary because of the high degree of overall efficacy of the treatment. The test can be used to confirm protective levels after initial therapy (especially with honeybee or other single venoms) and then to determine whether the venom IgG level is adequately maintained at longer maintenance intervals. In the assay clinically validated by one laboratory, the venom IgG level was considered protective when it was more than 3 μg/mL during the first 4 years of maintenance therapy.[97]

Discontinuation

The duration of VIT is described in the U.S. product package inserts as indefinite, but finite options have been studied. The question is no longer whether VIT can be discontinued, but when and in which patients. It was initially suggested that treatment could be stopped when venom skin test results or specific IgE antibody levels become negative.[4] This has been successful for the small number of patients who do achieve negative results in the first 5 years of therapy. It does not apply to the majority of treated patients who continue to have positive reactions; if they prematurely discontinue therapy after just 1 to 2 years, these patients still have a substantial risk of systemic reaction to a sting.[4]

Early studies focusing on the duration of VIT recommended 3 years of treatment, but the results included patients with up to 10 years of treatment, and patients were excluded if they did not have an uneventful sting during treatment.[4] Subsequent studies found that compared with 3 years, 5 years of treatment was associated with better suppression of allergic sensitivity and lower risk of relapse.[96,98-100] After stopping venom treatment, the venom IgE level continues to decline steadily with time, even after challenge stings.[99,100] Although there is usually no reaction to a sting 1 to 2 years after stopping treatment, the chance of relapse increases in years 3 to 5 after discontinuation and does not disappear for up to 13 years after stopping.[95,96]

As in untreated patients, systemic reactions can be unpredictable, occurring on one occasion and not on another. There is an approximately 10% chance of systemic reaction with each sting after stopping treatment, with a cumulative risk of relapse of 15% to 20% after 10 years off treatment (repeat stings increase the chance of reaction). Fortunately, most reactions are mild and less severe than the pretreatment reaction, but patients who had very severe reactions before VIT can have severe reactions again if they do relapse after stopping treatment. Reactions have occurred even in patients who developed negative venom skin test or specific serum IgE test results.[100,101] A higher chance of relapse has been observed for patients with honeybee allergy and for those who had a systemic reaction during VIT for an injection or a sting.[96,100,102]

Basophil activation test results may predict the outcome of stopping VIT.[44] Elevated baseline serum tryptase increases the risk of relapse after stopping VIT, and mastocytosis has been associated with fatal reactions to stings after a course of immunotherapy.[12,27,28] In these cases, as in those with near-fatal reactions before treatment, VIT may be continued indefinitely. There have been few reports of the outcomes for these high-risk patients if VIT is discontinued after 10 to 15 years.[103]

Collectively, the published studies on discontinuing VIT suggest that treatment may be stopped after 5 years for most patients, with the possible exception of those treated for honeybee allergy, those who had systemic reactions to an injection or sting during VIT, those with elevated baseline serum tryptase levels, and those who had very severe sting reactions before treatment. These caveats may lead to continued treatment of more than one third of the patients on VIT. Long-term extension of treatment may also be considered for patients who are not willing to accept the 10% to 20% chance of reaction to a subsequent sting, particularly if they have frequent exposures, which increases the cumulative risk of systemic reaction. In these cases, treatment at 12-week intervals can maintain protection.

Fire Ant Immunotherapy

The natural history of fire ant allergy is not as well described as for other Hymenoptera, but there is a clear need for effective immunotherapy.[19,104,105] Although immunotherapy using whole-body extracts of imported fire ants has been reported to be effective in preventing systemic reactions to fire ant stings, there have been no placebo-controlled trials.[19] The superiority of fire ant venom for skin testing suggests that it also would be superior for immunotherapy. The suggested materials, methods, regimens, and doses for fire ant immunotherapy have been reviewed.[19,32,106] The duration of fire ant immunotherapy is still uncertain, because attempts at discontinuation led to relapse within several years in a significant minority of cases.[4]

Biting Insect Allergy

There are few credible reports of allergic reactions to biting insects. Sensitization to salivary proteins may cause abnormal local swelling following insect bites, but anaphylaxis is rarely reported.[4] An attempt to collect such cases through a registry at the American Academy of Allergy and Immunology yielded a small number of cases with a convincing history of systemic reactions and detectable allergen-specific IgE antibodies in the serum.[4]

TRIATOMA (KISSING BUG, CONE-NOSE BUG)

The most common confirmed cause of systemic reactions to insect bites is the kissing bug (*Triatoma* spp.).[107] The relevant species in the United States are found throughout the arid areas of the southwest states and California. These insects feed exclusively by sucking the blood of vertebrate animals, and they may find shelter in homes at night. The bite causes an erythematous plaque, but because it is painless, the victim may be unaware of the cause of an allergic reaction. The allergens are salivary gland proteins, and they have little cross-reactivity between species.[4] Immunotherapy with a salivary gland extract was effective in preventing anaphylaxis from *Triatoma* bites in a small number of patients.[4]

CULICOIDAE (MOSQUITO)

Considering the widespread exposure to mosquitoes and the frequency of mosquito bites, which are painless, it is remarkable that so few cases of anaphylaxis have been reported.[108] There has also been increased recognition of the clinical impact of large local reactions to mosquito bites in children (i.e., skeeter syndrome).[109] Unfortunately, the mosquito extracts commercially available in the United States are of unreliable composition and activity and are not approved for therapeutic use.

Research has focused on the identification of the major allergens in mosquito extracts and their activity in clinical allergy. These efforts have led to the development and production of recombinant allergens, which may aid in diagnosis and therapy.[110] These studies demonstrated significant cross-reactivity of the major worldwide mosquito species. Although immunotherapy with whole-body extracts may be effective, further studies with improved materials are needed. In some cases, natural desensitization may occur with frequent and numerous bites.[108] Treatment with second-generation antihistamines can prevent and relieve the large local reactions to mosquito bites.[4]

TABANIDAE (HORSEFLY, DEERFLY)

The tabanid species are large flies that suck blood and inflict painful bites. They have widespread distribution in rural and suburban areas. They affect humans and animals. Allergic reactions to insect bites from horseflies and deerflies have been reported.[4] In some cases of allergic reactions to deerfly bites, a whole-body extract was able to induce marked histamine release from the patients' leukocytes and strong skin test responses. The possibility of immunotherapy has been little studied.

ALLERGIC REACTIONS TO OTHER BITING INSECTS

There have been anecdotal reports of allergic reactions to a number of other biting insects.[4,107] As with the biting insects, most have been local reactions, and very few were anaphylactic. Black flies present an annual nuisance in the early summer months in the northeastern United States and Canada. Large local reactions to black fly bites have been reported, but convincing anaphylactic reactions have not.

Fleas (order Siphonaptera) are an uncommon cause of allergy in humans, unlike dogs and cats, which have been extensively studied for flea hypersensitivity. Efforts more than 50 years ago to prevent reactions to flea bites with the use of flea antigen have not been confirmed. The most commonly encountered reaction to flea bites in humans is papular urticaria, a form of persistent papular inflammation. The reaction usually begins about the ankles and becomes generalized over a period of weeks, often persisting for months and resolving spontaneously.[4]

Inhalant Insect Allergy

Seasonal respiratory exposures to outdoor insects (e.g., caddis flies, midges, lake flies) or perennial exposure to indoor insects (e.g., cockroaches) may cause allergic respiratory symptoms. These insect allergens are discussed in Chapters 27 and 28. In other cases, airborne insect antigens produce occupational disease and are discussed in Chapter 59.

Conclusions

Stinging insects are a common cause of allergic reactions ranging from large local reactions to life-threatening anaphylaxis. Clinical and immunologic features can predict the risk of future severe reactions to stings. Skin or serum tests for venom-specific IgE antibodies are useful to confirm sensitization to venom allergens. VIT is recommended for patients at moderate to high risk for systemic reactions to future stings, but it is not required for low-risk patients despite positive venom-IgE test results. VIT can rapidly achieve complete clinical protection from systemic reactions to stings in 75% to 95% of patients. VIT can be discontinued after 5 years in most patients but may be continued indefinitely in those at high risk for relapse. An elevated baseline serum tryptase level predicts the severity of reactions to stings, systemic reactions to VIT, limited protection with VIT, and chance of relapse if VIT is stopped after 5 years. Anaphylaxis is rare from biting insects, but large local reactions can be severe, especially with mosquito bites.

REFERENCES

Stinging Insect Allergy

1. Benson R, Semenov H. Allergy in its relation to bee sting. J Allergy Clin Immunol 1930;1:105-11.
2. Hunt KJ, Valentine MD, Sobotka AK, et al. A controlled trial of immunotherapy in insect hypersensitivity. N Engl J Med 1978;299:157-61.
3. Golden DB. Insect sting allergy and venom immunotherapy: a model and a mystery. J Allergy Clin Immunol 2005;115:439-47.
4. Golden DBK. Insect allergy. In: Adkinson NF, Yunginger JW, Busse WW, et al., editors. Middleton's allergy: principles and practice. 6th ed. St. Louis: Mosby; 2003. p. 1475-86.
5. Bilo MB, Bonifazi F. The natural history and epidemiology of insect venom allergy: clinical implications. Clin Exp Allergy 2009;39:1467-76.
6. Graft DF. Insect sting allergy. Med Clin North Am 2006;90:211-32.
7. Hoffman DR. Fatal reactions to Hymenoptera stings. Allergy Asthma Proc 2003;24:123-7.
8. Golden DBK, Marsh DG, Kagey-Sobotka A, et al. Epidemiology of insect venom sensitivity. JAMA 1989;262:240-4.
9. Eberlein B, Krischan L, Darsow U, Ollert M. Double positivity to bee and wasp venom: improved diagnostic procedure by recombinant allergen-based IgE testing and basophil activation test including data about cross-reactive carbohydrate determinants. J Allergy Clin Immunol 2012;130:155-61.
10. Jappe U, Raulf-Heimsoth M, Hoffmann M, et al. In vitro Hymenoptera venom allergy diagnosis: improved by screening for cross-reacting carbohydrate determinants and reciprocal inhibition. Allergy 2006;61:1220-9.
11. Muller UR, Johansen N, Petersen AB, Fromberg-Nielsen J, Haeberli G. Hymenoptera venom allergy: analysis of double positivity to honey bee and *Vespula* venom by estimation of IgE antibodies to species-specific major allergens Api m1 and Ves v5. Allergy 2008;64:543-8.
12. Golden DBK. Insect allergy. In: Adkinson NF, Yunginger JW, Bochner BS, et al., editors. Middleton's allergy: principles and practice. 7th ed. Philadelphia: Mosby Elsevier; 2009. p. 1005-17.
13. Freeman TM. Clinical practice: hypersensitivity to Hymenoptera stings. N Engl J Med 2004;351:1978-84.
14. deGroot H. Allergy to bumblebees. Curr Opin Allergy Clin Immunol 2006;6:294-7.
15. Greene A, Breisch NL, Golden DB, Kelly D, Douglass LW. Sting embedment and avulsion in yellowjackets (Hymenoptera: Vespidae): a functional equivalent to autotomy. Am Entomologist 2012;58:50-7.
16. Kemp SF, deShazo RD, Moffitt JE, et al. Expanding habitat of the imported fire ant: a public health concern. J Allergy Clin Immunol 2000;105:683-91.
17. Brown SG, Franks RW, Baldo BA, Heddle RJ. Prevalence, severity and natural history of jack jumper ant venom allergy in Tasmania. J Allergy Clin Immunol 2003;111:187-92.
18. Kim S-S, Park H-S, Kim H-Y, Lee S-K, Nahm D-H. Anaphylaxis caused by the new ant, *Pachycondyla chinensis*: demonstration of spe-

cific IgE and IgE-binding components. J Allergy Clin Immunol 2001;107:1095-9.
19. Freeman TM, Hyghlander R, Ortiz A, Martin ME. Imported fire ant immunotherapy: effectiveness of whole body extracts. J Allergy Clin Immunol 1992;90:210-5.
20. Hamilton RH, Wisenauer JA, Golden DBK, Valentine MD, Adkinson Jr NF. Selection of Hymenoptera venoms for immunotherapy based on patients' IgE antibody cross-reactivity. J Allergy Clin Immunol 1993;92:651-9.
21. Hamilton RG. Diagnostic methods for insect sting allergy. Curr Opin Allergy Clin Immunol 2004;4:297-306.
22. Mitterman I, Zidarn M, Silar M, Markovic-Housley Z, Aberer W. Recombinant allergen based IgE testing to distinguish bee and wasp allergy. J Allergy Clin Immunol 2010;125: 1300-7.
23. Lieberman P, Nicklas RA, Oppenheimer J, Kemp SF, Lang DM. The diagnosis and management of anaphylaxis practice parameter: 2010 update. J Allergy Clin Immunol 2010; 126:477-80.
24. Brown SG. Clinical features and severity grading of anaphylaxis. J Allergy Clin Immunol 2004;114:371-6.
25. Stoevesandt J, Hain J, Kerstan A, Trautmann A. Over- and underestimated parameters in severe Hymenoptera venom-induced anaphylaxis: cardiovascular medication and absence of urticaria/angioedema. J Allergy Clin Immunol 2012;130:698-704.
26. Lockey RF, Turkeltaub PC, Baird-Warren IA, et al. The Hymenoptera venom study: I, 1979-1982. Demographic and history-sting data. J Allergy Clin Immunol 1988;82:370-81.
27. Muller UR. Elevated baseline serum tryptase, mastocytosis and anaphylaxis. Clin Exp Allergy 2009;39:620-2.
28. Niedoszytko M, deMonchy J, vanDoormaal JJ, Jassem E, Oude-Elberink JNG. Mastocytosis and insect venom allergy: diagnosis, safety and efficacy of venom immunotherapy. Allergy 2009;64:1237-45.
29. Bonadonna P, Perbellini O, Passalacqua G, et al. Clonal mast cell disorders in patients with systemic reactions to Hymenoptera stings and increased serum tryptase levels. J Allergy Clin Immunol 2009;123:680-6.
30. Borer-Reinhold B, Haeberli G, Bitzenhofer M, et al. An increase in serum tryptase even below 11.4 ng/ml may indicate a mast cell-mediated hypersensitivity reaction: a prospective study in Hymenoptera venom allergic patients. Clin Exp Allergy 2011;41:1777-83.
31. Biló BM, Rueff F, Mosbech H, Bonifazi F, Oude-Elberink JN, EAACI Interest Group on Insect Venom Hypersensitivity. Diagnosis of Hymenoptera venom allergy. Allergy 2005;60: 1339-49.
32. Golden DBK, Moffitt J, Nicklas RA, et al. Joint Task Force on Practice Parameters; American Academy of Allergy, Asthma & Immunology (AAAAI); American College of Allergy, Asthma & Immunology (ACAAI; Joint Council Of Allergy, Asthma, and Immunology. Stinging insect hypersensitivity: a practice parameter update 2011. J Allergy Clin Immunol 2011;127: 852-4.
33. Goldberg A, Confino-Cohen R. Timing of venom skin tests and IgE determinations after insect sting anaphylaxis. J Allergy Clin Immunol 1997;100:183-4.
34. Golden DBK, Kagey-Sobotka A, Hamilton RG, Norman PS, Lichtenstein LM. Insect allergy with negative venom skin tests. J Allergy Clin Immunol 2001;107:897-901.
35. Graif Y, Confino-Cohen R, Goldberg A. Reproducibility of skin testing and serum venom-specific IgE in Hymenoptera venom allergy. Ann Allergy 2006;96:24-9.
36. Golden DBK, Kelly D, Hamilton RG, Wang NY, Kagey-Sobotka A. Dialyzed venom skin tests for identifying yellow jacket-allergic patients not detected using standard venom. Ann Allergy Asthma Immunol 2009;102:7-50.
37. Biló MB, Severino M, Cilia M, et al. The VISYT trial: venom immunotherapy safety and tolerability with purified vs non-purified extracts. Ann Allergy Asthma Immunol 2009;103: 57-61.
38. Golden DBK, Tracy JM, Freeman TM, Hoffman DR, Insect CA. Negative venom skin test results in patients with histories of systemic reaction to a sting [Rostrum article]. J Allergy Clin Immunol 2003;112:495-8.
39. Golden DBK, Breisch NL, Hamilton RG, et al. Clinical and entomological factors influence the outcome of sting challenge studies. J Allergy Clin Immunol 2006;117: 670-5.
40. Hamilton RG. Clinical laboratory assessment of immediate-type hypersensitivity. J Allergy Clin Immunol 2010;125:S284-96.
41. vanderLinden PG, Hack CE, Struyvenberg A, vanderZwan JK. Insect-sting challenge in 324 subjects with a previous anaphylactic reaction: current criteria for insect-venom hypersensitivity do not predict the occurrence and the severity of anaphylaxis. J Allergy Clin Immunol 1994;94:151-9.
42. Korosec P, Erzen R, Silar M, et al. Basophil responsiveness in patients with insect sting allergies and negative venom-specific immunoglobulin E and skin prick test results. Clin Exp Allergy 2009;39:1730-7.
43. Sturm GJ, Bohm E, Trummer M, et al. The CD63 basophil activation test in Hymenoptera venom allergy: a prospective study. Allergy 2004;59:1110-7.
44. Kucera P, Cvackova M, Hulikova K, Juzova O, Pachl J. Basophil activation can predict clinical sensitivity in patients after venom immunotherapy. J Investig Allergol Immunol 2010;20: 110-16.
45. Zitnik SE, Vesel T, Avcin T, et al. Monitoring honeybee venom immunotherapy in children with the basophil activation test. Pediatr Allergy Immunol 2011;23:166-72.
46. Sturm GJ, Hemmer W, Hawranek T, et al. Detection of IgE to recombinant Api m 1 and rVes v 5 is valuable but not sufficient to distinguish bee from wasp venom allergy. J Allergy Clin Immunol 2011;128:247-8.
47. Rueff F, Przybilla B, Muller U, Mosbech H. The sting challenge test in Hymenoptera venom allergy. Allergy 1996;51:216-25.
48. Franken HH, Dubois AEJ, Minkema HJ, vanderHeide S, deMonchy JGR. Lack of reproducibility of a single negative sting challenge response in the assessment of anaphylactic risk in patients with suspected yellow jacket hypersensitivity. J Allergy Clin Immunol 1994;93: 431-6.
49. Clark S, Long AA, Gaeta TJ, Camargo CC. Multicenter study of emergency department visits for insect sting allergies. J Allergy Clin Immunol 2005;116:643-9.
50. Pumphrey RS. Fatal posture in anaphylactic shock. J Allergy Clin Immunol 2003;112: 451-2.
51. Greene A, Breisch NL. Avoidance of bee and wasp stings: an entomological perspective. Curr Opin Allergy Clin Immunol 2005;5: 337-41.
52. Simons FER, Gu X, Silver NA, Simons KJ. EpiPen Jr versus EpiPen in young children weighing 15 to 30 kg at risk for anaphylaxis. J Allergy Clin Immunol 2002;109:171-5.
53. Golden DBK, Marsh DG, Freidhoff LR, et al. Natural history of Hymenoptera venom sensitivity in adults. J Allergy Clin Immunol 1997; 100:760-6.
54. Reisman RE. Duration of venom immunotherapy: relationship to the severity of symptoms of initial insect sting anaphylaxis. J Allergy Clin Immunol 1993;92:831-6.
55. Graif Y, Romano-Zelekha O, Livne I, Green MS, Shohat T. Allergic reactions to insect stings: results from a national survey of 10,000 junior high school children in Israel. J Allergy Clin Immunol 2006;117:1435-9.
56. Golden DBK, Kagey-Sobotka A, Norman PS, Hamilton RG, Lichtenstein LM. Outcomes of allergy to insect stings in children with and without venom immunotherapy. N Engl J Med 2004;351:668-74.
57. Golden DBK, Langlois J, Valentine MD. Treatment failures with whole body extract therapy of insect sting allergy. JAMA 1981; 246:2460-63.
58. Rueff F, Przybilla B, Bilo MB, et al. Predictors of severe systemic anaphylactic reactions in patients with Hymenoptera venom allergy: importance of baseline serum tryptase. A study of the EAACI Interest Group on Insect Venom Hypersensitivity. J Allergy Clin Immunol 2009;124:1047-54.
59. Vadas P, Gold M, Perelman B, et al. Platelet-activating factor, PAF acetylhydrolase, and severe anaphylaxis. N Engl J Med 2008;358: 28-35.
60. Muller U, Haeberli G. Use of beta-blockers during immunotherapy for Hymenoptera venom allergy. J Allergy Clin Immunol 2005; 115:606-10.
61. White KM, England RW. Safety of angiotensin converting enzyme inhibitors while receiving venom immunotherapy. Ann Allergy Asthma Immunol 2008;101:426-30.
62. Haeberli G, Bronnimann M, Hunziker T, Muller U. Elevated basal serum tryptase and hymenoptera venom allergy: relation to severity of sting reactions and to safety and efficacy of venom immunotherapy. Clin Exp Allergy 2003;33:1216-20.
63. Bonifazi F, Jutel M, Biló BM, Birnbaum J, Muller U, EAACI Interest Group on Venom Hypersensitivity. Prevention and treatment of Hymenoptera venom allergy: guidelines for clinical practice. Allergy 2005;60:1459-70.
64. Reisman RE. Natural history of insect sting allergy: relationship of severity of symptoms of initial sting anaphylaxis to re-sting reactions. J Allergy Clin Immunol 1992;90: 335-9.
65. Oude-Elberink JNG, deMonchy JGR, vanderHeide S, Guyatt GH, Dubois AEJ. Venom immunotherapy improves health-related quality of life in yellow jacket allergic patients. J Allergy Clin Immunol 2002;110: 174-82.
66. Oude-Elberink JN, vanderHeide S, Guyatt GH, Dubois A. Analysis of the burden of treatment in patients receiving an Epi-Pen for yellow jacket anaphylaxis. J Allergy Clin Immunol 2006;118:699-704.

67. Golden DBK, Kelly D, Hamilton RG, Craig TJ. Venom immunotherapy reduces large local reactions to insect stings. J Allergy Clin Immunol 2009;123:1386-90.
68. Severino MG, Cortellini G, Bonadonna P, et al. Sublingual immunotherapy for large local reactions caused by honeybee sting: a double-blind placebo-controlled trial. J Allergy Clin Immunol 2008;122:44-8.
69. Lockey RF, Turkeltaub PC, Olive ES, et al. The Hymenoptera venom study III: safety of venom immunotherapy. J Allergy Clin Immunol 1990;86:775-80.
70. Mosbech H, Muller U. Side effects of insect venom immunotherapy: results from an EAACI study. Allergy 2000;55:1005-10.
71. Kosnik M, Silar M, Bajrovic N, Music E, Korosec P. High sensitivity of basophils predicts side effects in venom immunotherapy. Allergy 2005;60:1401-6.
72. Bonadonna P, Zanotti R, Caruso B, et al. Allergen specific immunotherapy is safe and effective in patients with systemic mastocytosis. J Allergy Clin Immunol 2008;121:256-7.
73. Gonzalez-de-Olano D, Alvarez-Twose I, Esteban-Lopez MI, et al. Safety and effectiveness of immunotherapy in patients with indolent systemic mastocytosis presenting with Hymenoptera venom anaphylaxis. J Allergy Clin Immunol 2008;121:519-26.
74. Brown SG, Wiese MD, Blackman KE, Heddle RJ. Ant venom immunotherapy: a double-blind placebo-controlled crossover trial. Lancet 2003;361:1001-6.
75. Brockow K, Kiehn M, Riethmuller C, Vieluf D, Berger J, Ring J. Efficacy of antihistamine pretreatment in the prevention of adverse reactions to Hymenoptera immunotherapy: a prospective, randomized, placebo-controlled trial. J Allergy Clin Immunol 1997;100:458-63.
76. Muller UR, Jutel M, Reimers A, et al. Clinical and immunologic effects of H1 antihistamine preventive medication during honeybee venom immunotherapy. J Allergy Clin Immunol 2008;122:1001-7.
77. Wohrl S, Gamper S, Hemmer W, et al. Premedication with montelukast reduces large local reactions of allergen immunotherapy. Int Arch Allergy Immunol 2007;144:137-42.
78. Galera C, Soohun N, Zankar N, et al. Severe anaphylaxis to bee venom immunotherapy: efficacy of pretreatment with omalizumab. J Investig Allergol Clin Immunol 2009;19:225-9.
79. Goldberg A, Confino-Cohen R. Rush venom immunotherapy in patients experiencing recurrent systemic reactions to conventional venom immunotherapy. Ann Allergy 2003;91:405-10.
80. Oren E, Chegini S, Hamilos DL. Ultrarush venom desensitization after systemic reactions during conventional venom immunotherapy. Ann Allergy Asthma Immunol 2006;97:606-10.
81. Tartibi HM, Majmundar AR, Khan DA. Successful use of omalizumab for prevention of fire ant anaphylaxis. J Allergy Clin Immunol 2010;126:664-5.
82. LaShell MS, Calabria CW, Quinn JM. Imported fire ant field reaction and immunotherapy safety characteristics: the IFACS study. J Allergy Clin Immunol 2010;125:1294-9.
83. Rueff F, Wenderoth A, Przybilla B. Patients still reacting to a sting challenge while receiving conventional Hymenoptera venom immunotherapy are protected by increased venom doses. J Allergy Clin Immunol 2001;108:1027-32.
84. Peternelj A, Silar M, Erzen R, Kosnik M, Korosec P. Basophil sensitivity in patients not responding to venom immunotherapy. Int Arch Allergy Immunol 2008;146:248-54.
85. Varga EM, Francis JN, Zach MS, et al. Time course of serum inhibitory activity for facilitated allergen-IgE binding during bee venom immunotherapy in children. Clin Exp Allergy 2009;39:1353-7.
86. Larche M, Akdis C, Valenta R. Immunological mechanisms of allergen-specific immunotherapy. Nat Rev Immunol 2006;6:761-71.
87. Dreschler K, Bratke K, Petermann S, et al. Impact of immunotherapy on blood dendritic cells in patients with Hymenoptera venom allergy. J Allergy Clin Immunol 2011;127:487-94.
88. Kerstan A, Albert C, Klein D, Brocker EB, Trautmann A. Wasp venom immunotherapy induces activation and homing of CD4+CD25+ forkhead box protein 3-positive regulatory T cells controlling Th1 responses. J Allergy Clin Immunol 2011;127:495-501.
89. Houliston L, Nolan R, Noble V, et al. Honeybee venom immunotherapy in children using a 50-mcg maintenance dose. J Allergy Clin Immunol 2011;127:98-9.
90. Konstantinou GN, Manoussakis E, Douladiris N, et al. A 5-year venom immunotherapy protocol with 50 mcg maintenance dose: safety and efficacy in school children. Pediatr Allergy Immunol 2011;22:393-7.
91. Brown SG, Wiese MD, van Eeden P, et al. Ultrarush versus semirush initiation of insect venom immunotherapy: a randomized controlled trial. J Allergy Clin Immunol 2012;139:162-8.
92. Cavalucci E, Ramondo S, Renzetti A, et al. Maintenance venom immunotherapy administered at a 3 month interval preserves safety and efficacy and improves adherence. J Investig Allergol Clin Immunol 2010;20:63-8.
93. Goldberg A, Confino-Cohen R. Maintenance venom immunotherapy administered at 3-month intervals is both safe and efficacious. J Allergy Clin Immunol 2001;107:902-6.
94. Bousquet J, Knani J, Velasquez G, et al. Evolution of sensitivity to Hymenoptera venom in 200 allergic patients followed for up to 3 years. J Allergy Clin Immunol 1989;84:944-50.
95. Golden DBK, Kwiterovich KA, Kagey-Sobotka A, Valentine MD, Lichtenstein LM. Discontinuing venom immunotherapy: outcome after five years. J Allergy Clin Immunol 1996;97:579-87.
96. Golden DBK, Kwiterovich KA, Addison BA, Kagey-Sobotka A, Lichtenstein LM. Discontinuing venom immunotherapy: extended observations. J Allergy Clin Immunol 1998;101:298-305.
97. Golden DBK, Lawrence ID, Kagey-Sobotka A, Valentine MD, Lichtenstein LM. Clinical correlation of the venom-specific IgG antibody level during maintenance venom immunotherapy. J Allergy Clin Immunol 1992;90:386-93.
98. Graft DF, Golden D, Reisman R, Valentine M, Yunginger J. The discontinuation of Hymenoptera venom immunotherapy: report from the Committee on Insects. J Allergy Clin Immunol 1998;101:573-5.
99. Keating MU, Kagey-Sobotka A, Hamilton RG, Yunginger JW. Clinical and immunologic follow-up of patients who stop venom immunotherapy. J Allergy Clin Immunol 1991;88:339-48.
100. Lerch E, Muller U. Long-term protection after stopping venom immunotherapy. J Allergy Clin Immunol 1998;101:606-12.
101. Golden DBK, Kagey-Sobotka A, Lichtenstein LM. Survey of patients after discontinuing venom immunotherapy. J Allergy Clin Immunol 2000;105:385-90.
102. Muller U, Helbling A, Berchtold E. Immunotherapy with honeybee venom and yellow jacket venom is different regarding efficacy and safety. J Allergy Clin Immunol 1992;89:529-35.
103. Golden DBK. Long-term outcome after venom immunotherapy. Curr Opin Allergy Clin Immunol 2010;10:337-41.
104. Kemp SF, Lockey RF, Wolf BL, Lieberman P. Anaphylaxis: a review of 266 cases. Arch Intern Med 1995;155:1749-54.
105. Tracy JM, Demain JG, Quinn JM, et al. The natural history of exposure to the imported fire ant. J Allergy Clin Immunol 1995;95:824-8.
106. Moffitt JE, Barker JR, Stafford CT. Management of imported fire ant allergy: results of a survey. Ann Allergy Asthma Immunol 1997;79:125-30.

Biting Insect Allergy

107. Hoffman DR. Allergic reactions to biting insects. In: Levine MI, Lockey RF, editors. Monograph on insect allergy. 4th ed. Milwaukee: American Academy of Asthma Allergy and Immunology; 2003. p. 161-74.
108. Peng Z, Ho MK, Li C, Simons FE. Evidence for natural desensitization to mosquito salivary allergens: mosquito saliva specific IgE and IgG levels in children. Ann Allergy Asthma Immunol 2004;93:553-6.
109. Simons FER, Peng Z. Skeeter syndrome. J Allergy Clin Immunol 1999;104:705-7.
110. Simons FER, Peng Z. Mosquito allergy: recombinant mosquito salivary antigens for new diagnostic tests. Int Arch Allergy Immunol 2001;124:403-5.

79

Drug Allergy

GÜLFEM E. ÇELIK | WERNER J. PICHLER | N. FRANKLIN ADKINSON, JR.

CONTENTS

SUMMARY OF IMPORTANT CONCEPTS

» Drug hypersensitivity reactions are restricted to a small subset of the population that is vulnerable for either immunologic or idiosyncratic reactions.
» Drug-specific immune responses depend on host factors and on the chemical structure and metabolism of the drug.
» Nonallergic hypersensitivity (pseudoallergic) reactions to drugs look like immunopathology but usually have an idiosyncratic mechanism; aspirin reactions are the best studied of these.
» Predictive skin testing after acute allergic drug reactions is available mainly for macromolecules and a few haptenic drugs, most notably β-lactam antibiotics.
» Some drugs induce severe systemic reactions in a subgroup of patients who carry a certain human leukocyte antigen (HLA) class I allele. Examples are abacavir (associated with HLA-B*5701) and carbamazepine (associated with HLA-B*1502 or A*3101). HLA testing is recommended before use in some cases.
» Using provocative testing and drug desensitization when indicated, almost all drug-sensitive patients can receive drugs associated with prior reactions. The principal exception to this claim is for patients with severe exfoliative dermatoses and hypersensitivity reactions.

Introduction

Adverse reactions to pharmaceutical and diagnostic products constitute a major hazard in the practice of medicine[1-3] and are responsible for substantial morbidity and cost.[4,5] Although different classifications have been proposed, adverse drug reactions (ADRs) are usefully organized into two subtypes: *type A* reactions, which are predictable from known pharmacologic properties, and *type B* reactions, which are unpredictable or unexpected syndromes restricted to a vulnerable subpopulation. This scheme distinguishes between reactions that can affect most patients, given sufficient therapeutic intensity, and reactions usually conceptualized as hypersensitivity, the risk for which is restricted to a small subset of treated patients (Table 79-1).

One form of hypersensitivity is seen in patients who experience the pharmacologically predictable toxicity of one or more drugs at low and sometimes subtherapeutic doses. This reaction putatively reflects altered drug metabolism or end-organ hyperacuity.

Idiosyncratic drug reactions are qualitatively distinct from the known pharmacologic toxicity profiles. The reactions may result from a defined genetic defect, as in the well-studied example of primaquine-sensitive hemolytic anemia, which depends on deficiency of the enzyme glucose-6-phosphate dehydrogenase (G6PD).[6] The mechanism of most idiosyncratic drug reactions remains obscure and often reflects a complex interaction of metabolic and constitutional factors (e.g., reactions to radiocontrast media).

Because some drug allergies are defined by human leukocyte antigen (HLA) alleles, the previously postulated unpredictability of type B reactions no longer holds. Avoidance of drug hypersensitivity is one of the early successes of personalized medicine. Drug reactions resulting from consequences of a drug-specific immune response constitute *immunologic drug reactions*, usually referred to as *drug allergies*.

The World Allergy Organization has recommended use of the adjectives *immediate* and *delayed* to refer to the onset of symptoms within or later than 1 hour after dosing, because these terms are helpful in distinguishing whether the probable immunologic mechanism is antibody mediated (e.g., immunoglobulin E [IgE]) or T lymphocyte mediated, respectively.[7] The distinction between idiosyncratic drug reactions and drug allergy can be difficult to discern clinically, but it is important because diagnosis and management are different for the two conditions.

This chapter reviews the ways in which drugs can sensitize the immune system, the factors that influence drug immunogenicity, and the cross-reactivity of drug-induced immune responses. The effector mechanisms recognizable in drug allergy syndromes are distinguished from idiosyncratic reactions that mimic drug allergy (i.e., pseudoallergic or nonallergic drug hypersensitivity). An approach to the diagnosis of drug allergy is offered, followed by a discussion of the management of drug-allergic states, with emphasis on the issues involved in readministration of a drug to previously reactive patients. Other chapters in this textbook deal with special cases of drug hypersensitivity.

TABLE 79-1 Classification of Adverse Drug Reactions

Drug Reaction	Examples
TYPE A: REACTIONS OCCURRING IN MOST NORMAL PATIENTS GIVEN SUFFICIENT DOSE AND DURATION OF THERAPY	
Overdose	Hepatic failure (acetaminophen)
Side effects	Nausea, headache (with methylxanthines)
Secondary or indirect effects	GI bacterial alteration after antibiotics
Drug interactions	Erythromycin increasing theophylline/digoxin blood levels
TYPE B: DRUG HYPERSENSITIVITY REACTIONS RESTRICTED TO A SMALL SUBSET OF THE GENERAL POPULATION	
Intolerance*	Tinnitus after a single aspirin tablet
Idiosyncrasy† (pharmacogenetics)	G6PD deficiency: anemia after antioxidant drugs
Immunologic drug reactions (allergy)	Anaphylaxis from β-lactam antibiotics

GI, Gastrointestinal; *G6PD*, glucose-6-phosphate dehydrogenase.
*Side effects at subtherapeutic doses.
†Drug effect not attributable to known pharmacologic properties of drug and not immune mediated.

The focus of this chapter is the recognition and management of immunologic drug reactions.

Epidemiology and Burden of Drug Hypersensitivity

ADRs have been reported to affect 10% to 20% of hospitalized patients and up to 25% of outpatients.[5,8,9] Most ADRs are type A reactions. Type B reactions are much less common, with an estimated frequency of 10% to 15% of all ADRs.[5] Immune-mediated drug reactions may constitute 6% to 10% of ADRs. The most common drug groups causing hypersensitivity reactions are β-lactam antibiotics and nonsteroidal antiinflammatory drugs (NSAIDs).[5] Other common causes of drug hypersensitivity reactions are radiocontrast media, neuromuscular blocking agents, and antiepileptic drugs. Increasingly, reports have been published on hypersensitivity reactions to anticancer drugs such as platins and taxanes and to biologic cytokines and anticytokines. Immediate hypersensitivity to local anesthetics is rare, despite common complaints.[10]

Epidemiologic studies indicate that cutaneous reactions, such as maculopapular eruptions and urticaria, are the most common clinical manifestations for ADRs.[5,9] Rarely, drugs induce more severe and potentially life-threatening reactions such as toxic epidermal necrolysis (TEN), Stevens-Johnson syndrome (SJS), immune hepatitis, and drug-induced hypersensitivity syndromes (DiHS), one form of which is drug reaction with eosinophilia and systemic symptoms (DRESS).[5,8,9] In the United States, about 1 of every 300 hospitalized patients dies from an ADR (amounting to 106,000 estimated deaths in 1994), and 6% to 10% of these reactions may be allergic in origin.[1] Several studies have documented drug allergy as a frequent cause of anaphylaxis, accounting for 8% to 62% of cases, depending on the inclusion of diagnostic codes.[11]

Limited data are available on the cost of drug allergy. A study of hospital practice showed that penicillin-allergic patients had higher medical costs related to the use of alternative antibiotics.[12] Alternative treatments for drug-allergic patients are commonly more expensive and often more toxic than first-line drugs.

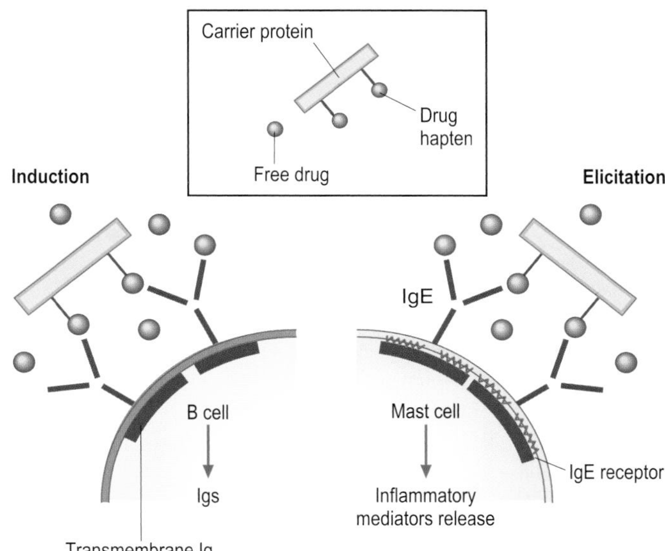

Figure 79-1 Multivalency theory of haptenic drug allergy. Multivalent presentation of drug haptens on carrier proteins is necessary both for B cell activation (induction of immunoglobulin [*Ig*] synthesis) and for mast cell activation (type I effector mechanism).

How Drugs Are Recognized by the Immune System

Karl Landsteiner first proposed an essential requirement for multivalency in the initiation of immune responses to foreign substances.[13] The current paradigm insists that with few exceptions, an antigen must be presented to the immune system in multivalent form to elicit a specific immune response (i.e., sensitization) and to activate immunopathologic mechanisms (i.e., effector functions) (Fig. 79-1). Some macromolecules used therapeutically meet this requirement intrinsically by virtue of large molecular weight with multiple repeating epitopes (Table 79-2). A few interesting small molecules have multiple recurrences of a single epitope and qualify as *complete allergens* potentially able to cross-link immune receptors. The best-studied example is quaternary ammonium epitopes, which render drugs such as succinylcholine as bivalent and related neuromuscular blockers as multivalent.[14,15]

Most pharmaceutical agents have simple structures and small molecular weights; most do not qualify as drug allergens. There are two ways in which small chemicals (<1 kD) can be recognized by the immune system: Under physiologic conditions, drugs such as penicillins can directly bind *covalently* with macromolecules on cell surfaces and in plasma to form hapten-carrier complexes. When direct haptenation results in a sufficient density of drug epitopes (multivalency), a drug-specific immune response can ensue.[16,17] In the case of β-lactam antibiotics such as penicillins, the critical chemical structure is the β-lactam ring itself, which is unstable and readily acylates lysine residues in proteins[18] (Fig. 79-2). This results in the penicilloyl epitope, which is immunodominant in penicillin-specific immune responses. Other molecular rearrangements allow β-lactams to haptenate covalently through carboxyl and thiol

TABLE 79-2 Drugs as Immunogens

Mechanism	Examples
Complete allergens	
Foreign macromolecules	Insulin and other hormones Enzymes and protamine Antisera Recombinant proteins Vaccines
Functionally multivalent chemicals	Succinylcholine Other quaternary ammonium compounds
Direct haptenation	β-Lactam antibiotics Quinidine *Cis*-platinum Penicillamine Barbiturates Antithyroid drugs Heavy metals (gold)
Metabolism to haptenic form	Sulfonamides* Acetaminophen† Phenacetin* Phenytoin‡ Procainamide* Halothane§
Monomeric stimulation of TCR or direct drug binding to HLA allele‖	Sulfamethoxazole Lidocaine, mepivacaine Carbamazepine, abacavir, allopurinol Lamotrigine

HLA, Human leukocyte antigen; *TCR*, T lymphocyte receptor.
*Postulated intermediate: hydroxylamine.
†Postulated intermediate: quinone imine.
‡Postulated intermediate: arene oxide.
§Postulated intermediates: radicals, acylhalides.
‖According to the p-i mechanism.

groups, resulting in a variety of less dominant or minor determinants. Minor determinant–specific IgE responses to β-lactams are of major clinical importance because of their association with anaphylaxis,[19] whereas penicilloyl IgE responses may be more associated clinically with urticarial reactions.

The penicillins, cephalosporins, and carbapenems share a bicyclic nucleus (Fig. 79-3), which apparently conveys an appreciable but variable immunologic cross-reactivity in immune responses to these drugs. The cross-reactivity among penicillins is virtually complete[20] if IgE-mediated reactions are considered. Cephalosporins are similar to penicillins immunochemically, but individual immune responses vary greatly.[20] Third-generation cephalosporins (e.g., ceftazidime) appear less likely to engender cross-allergic responses than first-generation cephalosporins (e.g., cephalothin).[21] Carbapenems have a similar degree of cross-reactivity by skin testing to first-generation cephalosporins,[22] but studies have consistently shown that penems are well tolerated clinically even in patients with positive penicillin skin test results. The monobactam class (prototype: aztreonam) is poorly immunogenic and very weakly cross-reactive with other β-lactams,[23,24] possibly because of the absence of a second nuclear ring structure (see Fig. 79-3).

Other simple drugs that are in their native state unreactive with macromolecules can be converted into reactive intermediates during drug metabolism.[25,26] Xenobiotic metabolism occurs largely in the liver by cytochrome P-450–associated enzymes,[27-29] which can produce protein-reactive intermediates.[30,31] Intracellular proteins may be rapidly haptenated, with the resulting multivalent complex secreted from the cell or in antigen-presenting cells (APCs) and processed for T and B lymphocyte activation.[32,33] One example of this pathway to immunogenicity is the acetylation and oxidation metabolism of sulfonamides to yield the predominant N^4-sulfonamidoyl hapten (Fig. 79-4). Aromatic sulfonamides, often with antimicrobial activity (i.e., sulfamethoxazole, sulfadiazine, sulfisoxazole, and sulfacetamide), differ from other sulfonamide-containing medications by having an aromatic amine at the N^4 position and a substituted ring at the N^1 position; these features are not found in nonantibiotic sulfonamide-containing drugs such as thiazide diuretics and sulfonylurea antiglycemic drugs. Based on chemical structure, cross-reactivity between these groups of sulfonamides is considered unlikely, and clinical studies have confirmed that cross-sensitivity is rare.[34] Other protein-reactive intermediates have been implicated for other immunogenic drugs with different metabolic pathways (see Table 79-2).[33]

Drugs may stimulate the immune system by another method. Pichler and colleagues described a direct pharmacologic interaction of drugs with immune receptors, which they called the *p-i concept* (Fig. 79-5).[35,36] According to this concept, a chemically inert drug that is unable to covalently bind to peptides or proteins may nevertheless activate the immune system by binding directly and reversibly to HLA molecules on APCs or to T cell receptors (TCRs) on certain T cells. If the drug fits with sufficient affinity into a peculiar HLA molecule (e.g., HLA-B*5701), some T cells react with the HLA-drug complex (similar to an allo-HLA allele), resulting in a strong T cell immune response. This association of a certain drug with a peculiar HLA allele explains the HLA connection of some severe drug allergies (discussed later). Alternatively, the drug may bind noncovalently to some of the approximately 10^{12} different TCRs available, resulting in stimulation of T cells with cytokine production, proliferation, and cytotoxicity. In these cases, interaction of the drug-reactive TCRs with major histocompatibility complex (MHC) molecules enhances the T cell signal. The drug-TCR interaction is akin to the interaction of drugs with other pharmacologic receptors and is therefore distinct from the recognition of processed hapten-carrier complexes by TCRs. Direct drug binding to TCRs can result in no signal, inhibitory signals, or partial or full activation. Full activation may result in a clinical picture that is indistinguishable from that of a normal, hapten-specific T cell immune response. In p-i and hapten-dependent pathways, a selective T cell population is stimulated, expands, and infiltrates the skin and other organs. The clinical manifestations of drug allergy due to the p-i mechanism are expected to be a T cell–orchestrated inflammation, such as that observed with drug exanthems and drug-induced hepatitis. Whether B cells can be similarly stimulated by monomeric drug binding to surface immunoglobulin remains unclear.

The threshold of T cell activation by drugs can be further lowered by generalized immune stimulation of T cells, such as occurs during a systemic viral infection (e.g., Epstein-Barr virus [EBV], cytomegalovirus [CMV], human herpesvirus 6 [HHV6], human immunodeficiency virus [HIV]) and during exacerbations of autoimmune diseases. These diseases, which represent risk factors for T cell–dependent drug hypersensitivity, often involve broad stimulation of T cells, high cytokine levels, and increased expression of MHC and costimulatory molecules, all of which can enhance the readiness of T cells to react.

The p-i mechanism of T cell stimulation does *not* require biotransformation of an inert drug to a chemically reactive

Figure 79-2 Fundamental immunochemistry of penicillin molecules. Acylation of lysine residues in serum or cell surface proteins results in the penicilloyl or major antigenic determinant. From its isomer penicillanic acid, other covalent linkages to macromolecules can occur to produce a variety of less common or less dominant minor epitopes. *(Reproduced with permission from Adkinson NF Jr. Tests for immunological reactions to drugs and occupational allergens. In: Rose NR, Conway de Macario E, Folds JD, et al., editors. Manual of clinical laboratory immunology. Washington, D.C.: American Society of Microbiology; 1997. p. 893.)*

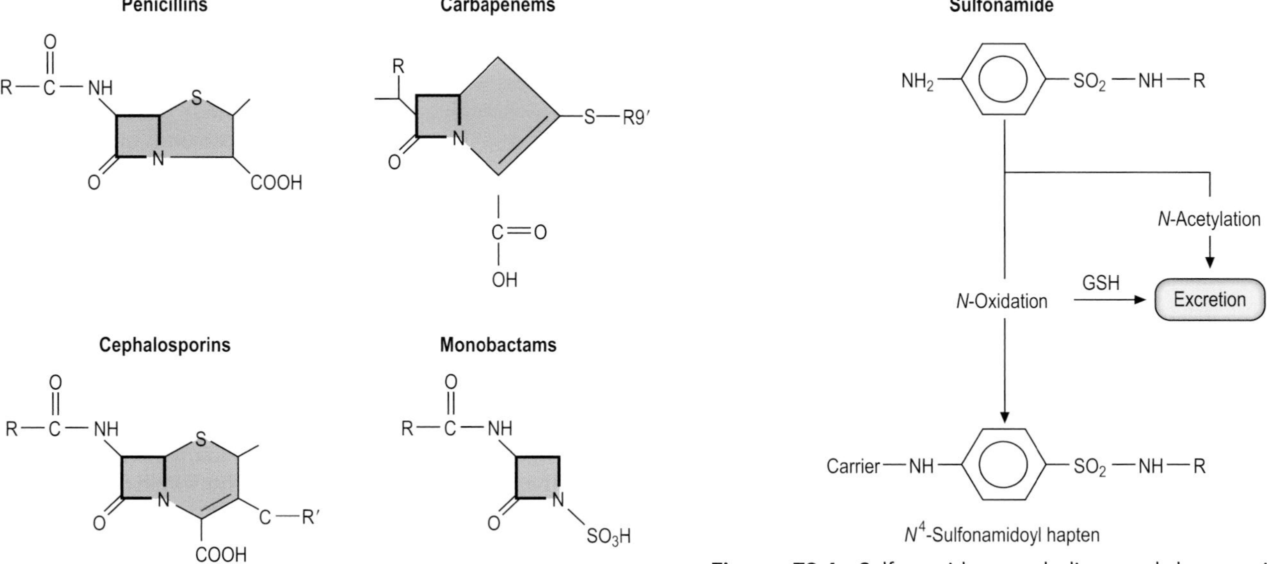

Figure 79-3 Classes of β-lactam antibiotics.

Figure 79-4 Sulfonamide metabolism and haptenation. Sulfonamides are metabolized by N^4-oxidation by cytochrome P-450 enzymes or by N^4-acetylation. *N*-acetyl sulfonamides and glutathionyl (GSH) sulfonamides are then excreted. Free sulfonamides, *N*-acetyl sulfonamides, and GSH sulfonamides can act as univalent inhibitors of antibody-mediated reactions. Carrier haptenation can occur after *N*-oxidation if the capacity for GSH conjugation is exceeded.

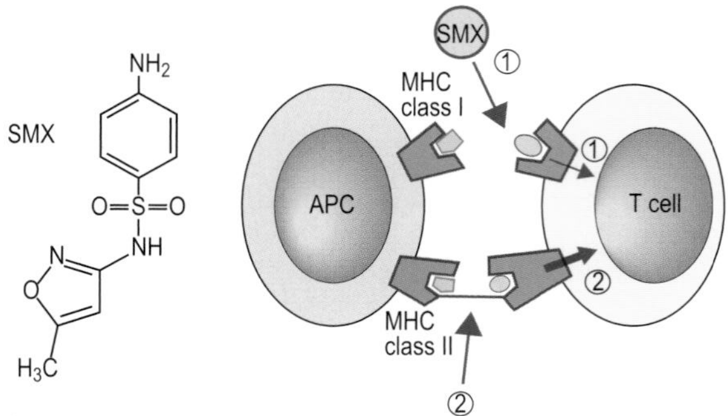

Figure 79-5 The p-i concept of T lymphocyte activation. *1,* The drug fits into some TCR with sufficient affinity to cause a signal. *2,* This drug-TCR interaction is supplemented by a MHC interaction (*2*). The T cells react and proliferate. No metabolism of drugs required. The reactive T cell is probably preactivated and has an additional peptide specificity. Alternatively, the drug binds first to the HLA molecule, and the new drug-HLA complex stimulates T cells. *APC,* Antigen-presenting cell; *HLA,* human leukocyte allergen; *MHC,* major histocompatibility complex; *SMX,* sulfamethoxazole; *TCR,* T cell receptor.

compound. Moreover, it is thought to be independent of the generation of its own hapten-specific antibody response.[36] The p-i concept is a radically different way to explain drug-induced hypersensitivity reactions, because it postulates that T cell–mediated drug allergies can occur as a result of drug-stimulated T cells.

Drug hypersensitivity due to the p-i pathway is more likely to be operative for generalized drug hypersensitivity reactions such as maculopapular, bullous, or pustular exanthems, whereas the hapten/prohapten pathway may be more relevant for contact dermatitis and antibody formation. Direct activation of T cells by drugs is well documented for carbamazepine and abacavir, two model drugs for systemic hypersensitivity reactions.[37,38] The old dogma that small chemicals are not full antigens remains valid, but drugs may have other ways to stimulate the immune system, and hapten and p-i mechanisms may occur simultaneously.[39]

The p-i concept can explain some of the so-called bizarre features of drug hypersensitivity, such as the rapid flow of symptoms at the first encounter with the drug, notably without a sensitization phase; drug hypersensitivity in generalized viral infections, which can lower the threshold for T cell reactivity; and the preferential involvement of the skin in drug allergy. The skin is a repository for an enormous number of T cells, many of which are effector memory T cells that perform sentinel functions and react rapidly if immunogenic agents penetrate the skin barrier.[40]

Factors That Influence Influencing Drug Immunogenicity

Several genetic, metabolic, and environmental factors influence the rate at which potentially sensitizing drugs elicit a specific immune response (Box 79-1). Even with recurrent high-dose exposures, highly immunogenic drugs may not induce a detectable drug-specific immune response in most patients. For penicillins, the IgG response rate for the major penicilloyl determinant is only about 50% among hospitalized patients receiving more than 20 g of drug.[41] This suggests that a clinically significant immune response is restricted by host and

BOX 79-1 FACTORS THAT INFLUENCE IMMUNOGENICITY OF DRUG HAPTENS

- Genetic factors
  - Incomplete responsiveness
  - Haptenation (MHC presentation or augmentation of response)
  - Acetylator phenotype
- Metabolic factors
  - Rate of haptenation
  - Hapten inhibition
  - Dehaptenation
  - Glutathione levels
- Preformed multivalent drug forms
- Adjuvants
- Concomitant infections
- Occult exposure to native or cross-reactive epitopes

MHC, Major histocompatibility complex.

environmental factors despite haptenation being a nominally universal event. Haptenation of soluble, cell-bound proteins or an HLA surface molecule or its presented peptides may be the mechanism of hapten presentation.[17,42,43] The immune response may be T cell mediated (i.e., CD4 and CD8) and B cell mediated (i.e., antibody mediated). Complete drug allergens and hapten-protein immunogens may be created by intracellular drug metabolism, followed by processing along MHC class II and possibly class I pathways,[44,45] although few experimental data support this concept. Only certain carriers (e.g., HLA molecules on cell surfaces) may be of immunogenic importance, and haptenation rates for these carriers may not parallel general acylation rates as determined for serum proteins in vitro. Among structural classes of simple chemicals, the story is quite different. Experimental studies of contact sensitizers show an excellent correlation between protein reactivity and sensitizing potential in vivo.[46,47]

Haptenation is by no means irreversible, and rapid dehaptenation of penicillin-protein conjugates has been observed.[48] Haptenation is facilitated by unidentified serum factors.[48,49] For penicillins, less than 0.01% of drug is covalently bound to protein in plasma. This observation suggests that serum levels of free drug may be an important determinant of the density of haptenation. For cytochrome metabolism of drugs, condensation with glutathione is a preferred pathway for elimination of certain drugs. When drug overdoses or other insults overwhelm metabolic resources and deplete glutathione, reactive intermediates of drugs such as acetaminophen and halothane can become immunogenic by conjugating instead to intracellular proteins.[50,51] Patients with a genetic limitation of the drug acetylation pathway (i.e., slow acetylation) shunt the metabolism of drugs such as sulfonamides toward more protein-reactive intermediates, enhancing immunogenicity.[28,52]

The chemical reactivity of a drug or its metabolite is important for the haptenic pathway, but the drug properties favoring p-i interactions are different. In this case, it is the steric configuration of the drug and its ability to interact with TCRs or with a peculiar HLA allele that determine its stimulatory potential. In case of HLA-restricted T cell reactions, the drug binds with high affinity to the particular HLA allele. It elicits an immune response by T cells (CD8 mostly, because the restricting HLA allele is HLA-A or HLA-B). The resulting allergy can be very severe (e.g., SJS).

TABLE 79-3 **Genetic Susceptibility to Drug Hypersensitivity Is Specific for the Drug, Clinical Phenotype, and Ethnicity**

Culprit Drug	Disease	HLA Allele (*P* Value*)	Ethnicity	PPV %†	Number to HLA Test to Prevent One Reaction
Carbamazepine[55]	SJS/TEN	HLA-B*1502 (3.1×10^{-27})	Han Chinese	3	1000
Carbamazepine[56]	SJS/TEN	HLA-B*1511	Japanese		
Carbamazepine[57]	HSS, SJS/TEN	HLA-A*3101	Caucasians		
Allopurinol[58]	SJS/TEN	HLA-B*5801 (4.7×10^{-24})	Han Chinese	3	250
Allopurinol[59]	HSS; SJS/TEN	HLA-B*5801	Caucasians		
Abacavir[60]	HSS	HLA-B*5701 (5.2×10^{-20})	Caucasians	55	13
Flucloxacillin[61]	Hepatitis	HLA-B*5701	Caucasians	0.12	13,819

DIHS, (Drug-induced) hypersensitivity syndrome; *HLA*, human leukocyte antigen; *SJS*, Stevens-Johnson syndrome; *TEN*, toxic epidermal necrolysis.
*Probability value corrected for Bonferroni's adjustment for association between drug and disease.
†Positive predictive value, or percentage of those with the designated HLA type who will display hypersensitivity if given the drug. For abacavir, the negative predictive value (i.e., percentage of those without the HLA allele do not react to the drug) is 100%.

In the case of preferential drug binding to the TCR, the reactive T cells are those that carry TCRs to which the drug can bind with a sufficient affinity. Small structural alterations of the drug may abrogate its stimulatory capacity.[53] For T cells to be stimulated by the noncovalently bound drug, a supplementing interaction of the TCR with the MHC molecule is required. Because the MHC-embedded peptides can be exchanged or removed without inhibiting TCR reactivity to the drug,[54] some drug-specific T cell clones can be stimulated independently of the MHC-presented peptide.

The prominent HLA association of some severe drug hypersensitivity reactions with certain HLA alleles in some populations is summarized in Table 79-3.[55-61] Development of SJS in response to carbamazepine in Han Chinese patients demonstrates a strong association with the HLA-B*1502 allele.[62] European Caucasians have a low frequency of this allele and do not show the association of HLA-B*1502 with SJS; however, an association with HLA-A*3101 has been established.[57] Data show that only certain HLA alleles, such as HLA-B*1502 or B*5701 (for abacavir), are able to bind the drug like a peptide and thereby augment drug-specific TCR stimulation in keeping with the p-i concept.[63]

Other pathways to immunogenicity may exist. The ability of aminopenicillins (e.g., ampicillin, amoxicillin) to polymerize may be a determinant of the high rate of late-occurring exanthems observed with these antibiotics, especially when given to patients with viral infection, acute lymphocytic leukemia, or mononucleosis or when coadministered with allopurinol.[64,65] The basis for these interactions is not known.

Repository preparations, such as benzathine penicillin and the oil-emulsified penicillins, which are no longer available, produce an adjuvant effect that enhances immunogenicity and the frequency of allergic reactions. Certain infections may create an inflammatory milieu that enhances drug allergy.[66-68] Noteworthy in this regard is the very high rate of putatively immunologic dermatologic reactions to sulfonamides and other drugs in patients infected with HIV.[69,70] A diverse set of clinical reactions is accompanied by an intense humoral immune response to drug antigens.[51,71] Whether the reduced hepatic glutathione level resulting from polypharmacy in these patients or some immunologic dysfunction associated with acquired immunodeficiency syndrome (AIDS) is a contributing factor is unknown.[72] Some drugs may sensitize more readily because of common exposures to cross-reacting epitopes. The quaternary ammonium epitope in muscle relaxant drugs is widely distributed in a variety of foods and cosmetics.[73]

DANGER HYPOTHESIS

The generation of a specific cellular and antibody response to an antigen usually requires the involvement of innate and acquired forms of immunity. Bacterial or viral products can interact with pattern recognition receptors (i.e., Toll-like receptors) on dendritic cells to initiate antigen processing. A close connection between these "danger signals" and immunogenicity has been shown for drugs that cause contact dermatitis, which are also frequently involved in toxic-irritative skin lesions. The danger effect of contact sensitizers was suggested by their ability to cause upregulation of costimulatory molecules such as CD86 or CD40 and phosphorylation of signaling molecules in dendritic cells exposed in vitro.[74,75] The data are less clear for drugs causing systemic reactions.

Specificity of Drug-Induced Immune Responses

Macromolecules contain numerous but finite epitopes, each of which can engender an immune response with various degrees of intensity. Surprisingly, even small-molecular-weight drugs such as penicillins may generate heterogeneous immune responses. The predominant epitope that is strongly cross-reactive among β-lactam antibiotics is the penicilloyl moiety. This neodeterminant is contributed to by the nuclear rings of the antibiotic, the carrier protein, and the connecting amide linkage (Fig. 79-6). Penicilloyl antibodies bind free penicillin molecules very weakly or not at all.[76] This property may be important in the pathogenicity of penicilloyl antibodies because hapten inhibition by the free drug is minimal. In contrast, immune responses specific for the side chains of β-lactams,[77,78] which are especially prevalent when the side chain is large relative to the nucleus (e.g., in third-generation cephalosporins), can be competitively inhibited by free drug.[23] This distinction may explain why side-chain–specific β-lactam drug allergy is rare relative to the frequency of side-chain–, β-lactam ring–specific immune responses.[20,79,80] Less often, drug haptens appear to function as the carrier to facilitate autoimmune responses against the native proteins they bind. The best-characterized example of this innocent bystander mechanism

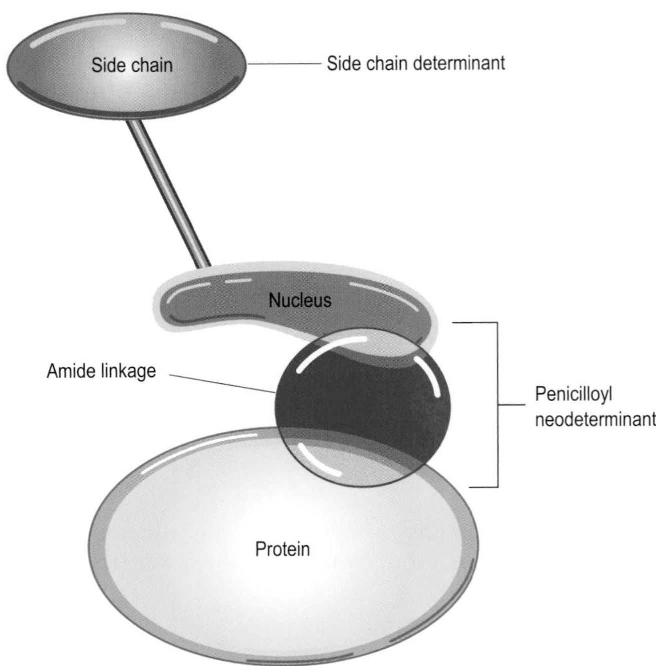

Figure 79-6 Specificities of drug hapten immune responses. The immunodominant major penicilloyl epitope contains constituents from the bicyclic nucleus, the amide linkage, and the adjacent carrier protein. Antibodies recognizing side chains of β-lactam antibiotics are produced and, as in the case of the monobactam aztreonam, may be the predominant specificity. *(Reproduced with permission from Kelkar PS, Li JT. Cephalosporin allergy. N Engl J Med 2001;345:794.)*

of drug-induced autoimmunity is methyldopa-induced hemolytic anemia. Persistent anti-Rh_o–specific antibodies mediate hemolysis and can persist for many months after discontinuation of drug.[81]

Immunopathologic Features of Drug Allergy

Allergenic drugs can induce the entire spectrum of immunopathologic reactions, which for antibody-mediated reactions are clinically indistinguishable from the reactions elicited by macromolecules. For penicillins, the range of clinical syndromes is classified by the predominant immunologic effector mechanism (Table 79-4). IgE-mediated drug reactions may involve acute anaphylaxis or urticaria, the latter of which can occur early or late in a course of therapy and persist for weeks or months after drug withdrawal. Type II cytolytic reactions usually are confined to rapidly haptenating drugs such as penicillin. Drug-specific immune complexes result from high-dose, prolonged therapy and may produce drug fever, a classic serum sickness syndrome, and various forms of cutaneous vasculitis. Contact dermatitis from topically applied drugs may occur,[82] although highly sensitizing drugs such as penicillins are no longer provided in this form.

Morbilliform eruptions are presumed to have an immunologic cause because of their increased frequency with sensitizing drugs. Although the mechanism remains obscure, most evidence implicates T lymphocyte involvement.[83,84] Severe exfoliative dermatitis syndromes, such as SJS and TEN, are often drug associated and presumed to be immune mediated.[85,86] The

TABLE 79-4 Immunopathologic Penicillin Reactions

Gell-Coombs Classification	Mechanism	Examples of Adverse Penicillin Reactions
I	Anaphylactic (IgE-mediated)	Acute anaphylaxis Urticaria
II	Complement-dependent cytolysis (IgG/IgM)	Hemolytic anemias Thrombocytopenia
III	Immune complex damage	Serum sickness Drug fever Some cutaneous eruptions and vasculitis
IV	Delayed or cellular hypersensitivity	Contact dermatitis Morbilliform eruptions SJS/TEN Hepatitis

Ig, Immunoglobulin; *SJS*, Stevens-Johnson syndrome; *TEN*, toxic epidermal necrolysis.

involvement of drug specific $CD8^+$ T cells and possibly natural killer (NK) cells has been suggested.[87]

The Gell and Coombs classification of drug hypersensitivity was established before a detailed analysis of T cell subsets and functions was available. Since then, immunologic research has revealed that the three antibody-dependent types of reactions require the involvement of helper T (Th) cells. Moreover, T cells can orchestrate different forms of inflammation. T cell–meditated immunopathology has been further subclassified as types IVa through IVd reactions (Fig. 79-7).[86] This subclassification considers the distinct cytokine production patterns by T cells and incorporates the well-accepted distinction between type 1 and type 2 (Th1/Th2) T cells. It includes the cytotoxic activity of both CD4 and CD8 T cells (type IVc), and it emphasizes the participation of effector cells such as monocytes (type IVa), eosinophils (type IVb), or neutrophils (type IVd), which are the important ancillary cell types contributing to the inflammation and tissue damage.

TYPE IVa REACTIONS

Type IVa reactions involve Th1-type immune reactions: Th1 cells activate macrophages by secreting large amounts of interferon-γ (IFN-γ), drive the production of complement-fixing antibody isotypes involved in type II and III reactions (e.g., IgG1, IgG3), and are costimulatory for proinflammatory responses (e.g., tumor necrosis factor [TNF], interleukin 12 [IL-12]) and for $CD8^+$ T cell responses. The T cells promote these reactions by secretion of cytokines (e.g., IFN-γ, TNF-α, IL-18). An in vivo correlate would be monocyte activation (e.g., in skin tests to tuberculin, granuloma formation in sarcoidosis). These Th1 cells also activate CD8 cells, which may explain the frequently observed combination of IVa and IVc reactions (e.g., in contact dermatitis).

TYPE IVb REACTIONS

Type IVb reactions follow a Th2-type immune response. Th2 cells secrete the cytokines IL-4, IL-13, and IL-5, which promote B cell production of IgE and IgG4, macrophage deactivation, and mast cell and eosinophil responses. The Th2 cytokine IL-5

Type	Type IVa	Type IVb	Type IVc	Type IVd
Cytokines	IFN-γ, TNF-α (Th1 cells)	IL-5, IL-4/IL-13 (Th2 cells)	Perforin/granzyme B (CTL)	CXCL8, GM-CSF (T cells)
Antigen	Antigen presented by cells or direct T cell stimulation	Antigen presented by cells or direct T cell stimulation	Cell-associated antigen or direct T cell stimulation	Antigen presented by cells or direct T cell stimulation
Cells	Macrophage activation	Eosinophils	T cells	Neutrophils
Pathomechanism	IFN-γ, Th1 Chemokines, cytokines, cytotoxins	Th2, IL-4, IL-5, Eotaxin, Eosinophil Cytokines, inflammatory mediators	CTL	CXCL8, GM-CSF, PMN Cytokines, inflammatory mediators
Example	Tuberculin reaction, contact dermatitis (with IVc)	Chronic asthma, chronic allergic rhinitis Maculopapular exanthema with eosinophilia	Contact dermatitis Maculopapular and bullous exanthema hepatitis	AGEP Behçet disease

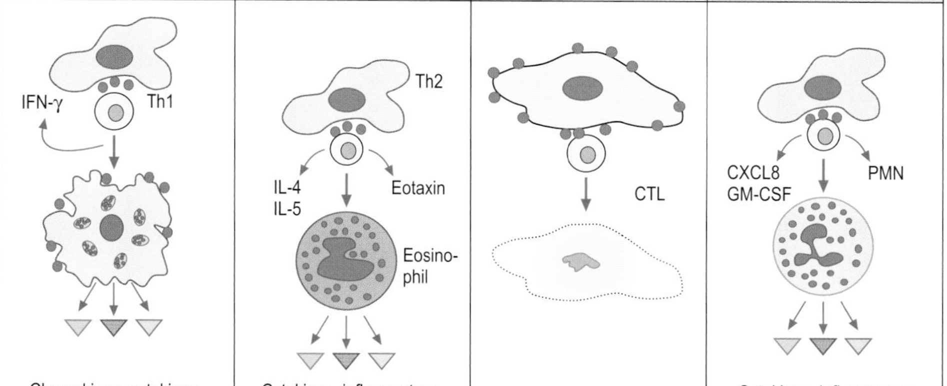

Figure 79-7 T cell–orchestrated hypersensitivity reactions (Gell and Coombs types IVa through IVd). *AGEP,* Acute generalized exanthematous pustulosis; *CTL,* cytotoxic T lylmphocyte; *CXCL8,* chemokine formerly called interleukin-8; *GM-CSF,* granulocyte-macrophage colony-stimulating factor; *IFN-γ,* interferon-γ; *IL,* interleukin; *PMN,* polymorphonuclear neutrophil; *Th1*; helper T cells type 1; *Th2,* helper T cells type 2; *TNF-α,* tumor necrosis factor-α.

leads to eosinophilic inflammation, which is the characteristic inflammatory cell type in many drug hypersensitivity reactions.[86] There also is a link to type I reactions, because Th2 cells boost IgE production by secretion of IL-4/IL-13. Type IVb reactions may be involved in late phase allergic (IgE-dependent) inflammation of the bronchi or nasal mucosa (i.e., asthma and rhinitis). Other immunopathology may include infestations with nematodes, eosinophil-rich maculopapular exanthems, or other T cell–dependent diseases with hypereosinophilia.

TYPE IVc REACTIONS

T cells themselves can act as cytotoxic effector cells. They emigrate to the tissue and can kill tissue cells such as hepatocytes or keratinocytes in a perforin/granzyme B– and FAS ligand–dependent manner.[87,88] These responses occur in most drug-induced delayed hypersensitivity reactions, usually together with other type IV reactions involving recruitment and activation of monocytes, eosinophils, or polymorphonuclear neutrophils (PMNs). Cytotoxic T cells play an important role in maculopapular and bullous skin diseases, in neutrophilic inflammation (e.g., acute generalized exanthematous pustulosis [AGEP]), and in contact dermatitis. Type IVc reactions appear to be prominent in bullous skin reactions such as SJS and TEN, in which activated CD8⁺ T cells kill keratinocytes (Fig. 79-8), but they may also be the dominant cell type in drug-induced hepatitis or nephritis.[87,88]

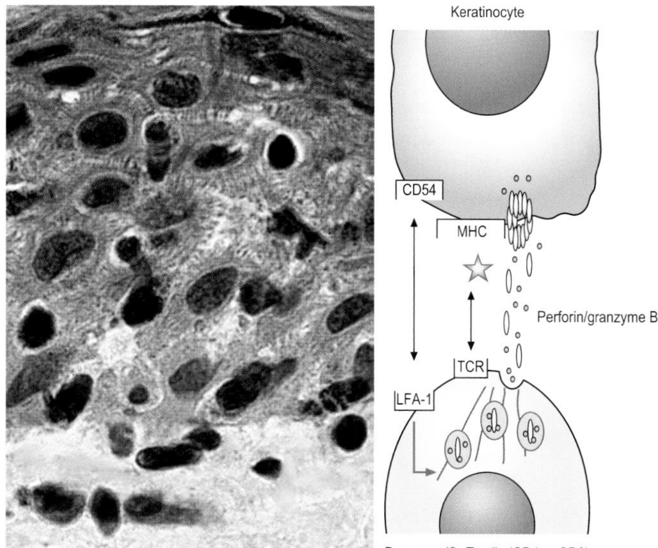

Figure 79-8 Cytotoxic T lymphocyte–mediated dermatitis (type IVc). $CD4^+$ or $CD8^+$ T cells injure keratinocytes in the dermis using the perforin/granzyme B pathways. Perforin-positive cells (*left*) are identified in the epidermis of a patient with drug-induced maculopapular exanthem. T lymphocytes and keratinocytes (*right*) interact through the TCR-MHC and CD54-LFA-1 ligand interactions. *LFA-1,* Lymphocyte function-associated antigen 1; *MHC,* major histocompatibility complex; *TCR,* T cell receptor.

TYPE IVD REACTIONS

Rather neglected by early researchers was the possibility that T cells could coordinate (sterile) neutrophilic inflammation. Typical examples include sterile neutrophilic inflammation of the skin, particularly AGEP. In this drug-induced disease, T cells that produce the chemokine CXCL8 and granulocyte-macrophage colony-stimulating factor (GM-CSF) recruit neutrophilic leukocytes through CXCL8 release and prevent their apoptosis through GM-CSF release.[89]

Drug-induced lupuslike syndrome has been reported for a variety of unrelated drugs, including procainamide, phenytoin, isoniazid, sulfasalazine, amiodarone, minocycline, and penicillamine. Despite intensive scrutiny, the mechanisms involved in these drug-induced autoimmune processes have not been elucidated.[90]

Risk Factors for Drug Hypersensitivity

Many risk factors have been shown to modify the clinical expression of immunologic drug reactions. They can be associated with the drug itself (intrinsically or by use), with the disease state in which the drug is used, or with the individual patient receiving the drug (Table 79-5). All the drug features that convey or enhance immunogenicity also promote the expression of immunopathology. This is especially true for haptenic drugs, because the requirement for multivalency applies as much to activation of immunologic mechanisms as to initiation of immune responses. Multivalent epitope presentation is required for IgE-dependent mast cell activation, antibody- or complement-mediated cytolysis, and immune complex damage, but it is less clear for T cell activation.[91] Type II and type III reactions are promoted by high-dose, long-term, and frequent drug treatment. The existence of naturally occurring cross-reacting epitopes (or, in children, earlier drug exposure in utero or in breast milk) likely explains acute drug allergy that occurs with first clinical use. Trace macromolecular contaminants[64,92] and excipients that facilitate solubility (e.g., Cremophor) are also implicated in acute drug allergy.[93]

Excess allergic reactions can be expected in patients with chronic diseases such as cystic fibrosis that require continuous or frequently repeated courses of therapy with the same drugs or cross-reactive drugs.[94] Allopurinol administered with aminopenicillins was reported to enhance the rate of exanthematous reactions.[66]Some allergic drug reactions are much more likely to occur if the drug is administered to patients with particular disease backgrounds, such as when aminopenicillins are given to patients with atypical or abnormal lymphocytes[66] or sulfonamides to patients with HIV infection.[69,70,95]

Patient factors that convey risk include any history of allergic reactions to the same drug or to cross-reactive drugs. In some patients, a history of allergic reactions to unrelated drugs also carries an increased risk for further drug allergies. Positive penicillin skin test results do not occur more frequently for atopic individuals,[41] but an atopic background is a substantial risk factor for severe and fatal penicillin anaphylaxis.[96] Penicilloyl IgE immune responses progressively decay in most individuals, but at highly variable rates.[97] Over 3 to 8 years, more than 75% of prior penicillin reactors have negative skin test results, including patients with histories of anaphylaxis and urticaria.[98,99] Patients with rapid disappearance of drug-specific immune responses are presumably at much lower risk for clinical expression of drug allergy with repeated therapy.

Evidence has demonstrated a familial propensity for immunologic drug reactions.[100] Having an antibiotic-sensitive parent carries a fifteenfold increased risk of drug sensitivity for the offspring.[101,102] A history of other drug allergies is reported more frequently among penicillin reactors.[103,104] This observation is consistent with prospective data showing a tenfold increased risk for allergic reactions to unrelated antibiotics in patients with a history of antibiotic sensitivity.[67] A wide variety of clinical reactions was observed in this study, suggesting that the risk may be attributable to enhanced immunogenicity for drugs, rather than facilitated expression of a particular pathogenic mechanism. The genetic or metabolic basis for this aggregation of multiple reactions to unrelated haptenic drugs has not been determined.[105] At least one subset of patients[13,104] carries the drug-reactive T cells in an in vivo preactivated cell fraction. A major step forward in understanding of drug hypersensitivity reactions came from the elucidation that some severe drug allergies are strongly associated with certain HLA alleles.[106]

The reverse-transcriptase inhibitor abacavir is the prototype of a drug whose T cell reactions are strongly associated with an HLA allele (B*5701).[107] This allele predisposes to a delayed rash in about 50% of individuals, most of whom have positive skin patch test results to the drug. (see Table 79-3). The same allele is associated with flucloxacillin-induced hepatitis, but with a much lower frequency.[61] Weaker HLA associations of delayed hypersensitivity reactions to nevirapine[106] and aminopenicillin-induced exanthems have been reported.

TABLE 79-5 Risk Factors for Clinical Expression of Drug Allergy

Association	Risk Factors
Drug	Polymerization or macromolecular contamination Protein reactivity Dose and duration of therapy Exposure to cross-reactive epitopes Frequency of drug treatment Impurity of the preparation (e.g., containing acetylsalicylic acid-anhydride in acetylsalicylic acid)
Disease	Need for prolonged or repeated courses of therapy (e.g., cystic fibrosis, chronic sinusitis, immunodeficiencies) Concomitant medications (e.g., allopurinol, amoxicillin) Concomitant diseases (e.g., Epstein-Barr viral infections and amoxicillin; AIDS and sulfonamides)
Individual	Prior reaction history Atopy (IgE-mediated reactions) Multiple drug allergy syndromes Persistence of drug-specific immune response Female sex in certain reactions (gemifloxacin rash) HLA class I (B and A) allele

AIDS, Acquired immunodeficiency syndrome; *HLA*, human leukocyte antigen; *IgE*, immunoglobulin E.

Nonallergic Drug Hypersensitivity Reactions

Drug reaction syndromes with manifestations that suggest or are compatible with immunopathologic mechanisms but that

TABLE 79-6 Common Examples of Drug Hypersensitivity

Immunologic (Allergic)	Nonimmunologic
Anaphylaxis from β-lactam antibiotics	Shock after radiocontrast media
Halothane hepatitis	Aspirin-induced asthma
Hypotension after protamine	Opiate-related urticaria
Dermatitis from sulfonamides	Protamine-induced pulmonary hypertension
Serum sickness from phenytoin or cefaclor	NSAID-related urticaria (most common)
Hypotension after succinylcholine	Hemolytic anemia due to choline
Quinine-induced thrombocytopenia	Syncope after local anesthetics
Phenolphthalein-induced fixed drug eruption	Acute ciprofloxacin reactions (most)
Cis-platinum–associated urticaria	Isoniazid hepatitis
	Flushing during vancomycin infusion

NSAID, Nonsteroidal antiinflammatory drug.

TABLE 79-7 Distinction between Allergic and Idiosyncratic Drug Reactions

Feature	Allergic	Idiosyncratic
Increased risk of drug reactions	Yes	No
Persistence of risk	Dissipates with time	Variable
Cross-reactivity pattern	Common structure	Common function

lack an immune basis are usefully aggregated under the term *nonallergic hypersensitivity reactions*, previously called *pseudoallergic drug reactions*.[7] These reactions constitute a subset of idiosyncratic reactions and clinically must be distinguished from immunologic (allergic) reactions (Table 79-6).

Nonallergic drug hypersensitivity responses must be distinguished from true drug allergy because counseling considerations, management options, and prognosis are fundamentally different (Table 79-7). Whereas cross-reactivity patterns depend on common structure for immunologic drug reactions, common biologic function is important for idiosyncratic and pseudoallergic reactions. In most cases of drug idiosyncrasy, the critical functional property is not known.

Most nonallergic hypersensitivity reactions that qualify as anaphylactoid (or pseudoallergic) involve the same clinical findings and often the same final common pathway as type I reactions. In these cases (e.g., radiocontrast media reactions, opiate-induced urticaria, aspirin-exacerbated respiratory disease [AERD]), basophils and mast cells are activated, and vasoactive mediators are released by nonimmune mechanisms.

For radiocontrast media, many biologic effects have been described, but none has been directly related to idiosyncratic activation of circulating basophils or tissue mast cells. Earlier literature postulated a correlation with "iodine sensitivity," which putatively manifested as urticarial reactions to seafood rich in inorganic iodine. This myth was debunked by evidence that contrast media reactors tolerate iodine-containing surgical scrubs, and vice versa.[108] Many of the adverse consequences of radiocontrast media infusion are attributable to its hypertonicity, which augments basophil and mast cell histamine release.[109]

TABLE 79-8 Premedication for Repeat Administration of Radiocontrast Media to Prior Anaphylactoid Reactors*

Time before Procedure (hr)	Drug	Dose
13	Prednisone	1 mg/kg PO
7	Prednisone	1 mg/kg PO
1	Prednisone	1 mg/kg PO
1	Diphenhydramine	1 mg/kg PO or IM
1	Cimetidine†	4 mg/kg PO or IM

IM, Intramuscularly; *PO*, orally.
*Isotonic contrast media should be used for treatment of all high-risk patients.
†Optional H_2 antihistamine therapy if desired. Some authorities have recommended inclusion of ephedrine (25 mg).

Newer nonionic contrast media, which are almost isotonic, have substantially reduced but not eliminated hypersensitivity reactions.[110] Accumulating evidence suggests that some severe reactions to some nonionic contrast agents may be IgE mediated.[111,112] Risk factors for contrast media reactions include an atopic background (relative risk: 3 to 5), female gender, underlying severe cardiovascular disease, a history of radiocontrast reactions, and, less clearly, a history of drug allergy in general.[110-112] Although several clinical trials have shown that anaphylactoid reactions to radiocontrast media can be reduced fivefold to tenfold using an empirically derived premedication regimen that at least includes corticosteroids and antihistamines (Table 79-8),[113] severe anaphylactic reactions induced by contrast media injections have occurred despite prophylactic use of these drugs. In addition to repeat treatment of prior reactors, this premedication regimen should be considered for high-risk patients, especially strongly atopic individuals and those with extensive cardiovascular disease.[113] Exactly why these regimens help remains unknown. The premedication regimens cannot dependably prevent true IgE-mediated anaphylaxis. Contrast media also can cause delayed exanthems, which are clearly T cell mediated.[114]

Aspirin and related NSAIDs may be implicated in two distinct nonallergic hypersensitivity syndromes (see Chapter 80).[115] Aspirin can induce acute bronchospasm in patients with preexisting asthma or flares of rhinosinusitis in susceptible patients; this clinical syndrome is referred to as AERD. Other NSAIDs, with the exception of cyclooxygenase 2 (COX-2) inhibitors, exhibit virtually complete cross-reactivity in this syndrome, suggesting that the common functional property of COX inhibition (especially COX-1) is somehow involved in the pathogenesis. An unrelated set of patients may develop urticarial reactions to aspirin-like drugs. Among urticarial reactions, two distinct clinical patterns can be identified. Up to 30% of the patients with chronic urticaria experience an urticarial flare in response to aspirin. In this clinical condition, a cross-reactivity among COX-1 inhibitors is very likely. However, some individuals without underlying chronic urticaria experience urticarial episodes after aspirin and other NSAIDs; in these cases, cross-reactivity with other NSAIDs is less likely. The possibility of an IgE-mediated drug reaction to a frequently administered NSAID needs to be considered when there is no NSAID cross-sensitivity. Desensitization for urticaria-angioedema is usually not as readily achievable as in AERD.[115]

Hemolytic anemia can be immunologic, as in the case of penicillins, or idiosyncratic, as in primaquine-sensitive anemia.[6] In the latter case, a genetic G6PD deficiency renders erythrocytes sensitive to the metabolic consequences of primaquine and other drugs with antioxidant properties. The clinical phenotype is similar to immune hemolysis except for the absence of drug antibodies. Future studies will undoubtedly uncover a genetic basis for other obscure idiosyncratic and pseudoallergic drug reactions.

Local anesthetic agents are relatively good sensitizers when applied topically (i.e., contact allergy).[116] In contrast, antibody-mediated allergic reactions to these agents are rare events.[10,117-119] However, nonallergic responses to local anesthetics, particularly in dentistry, often lead to allergy consultations. Most alarming for patients and dentists are episodes of vasovagal syncope, which can mimic anaphylaxis. Paresthesias and lightheadedness can be explained on the basis of the pharmacologic toxicity of the "caines," and the symptoms are more common in drug-intolerant patients. Episodes of anxiety or panic associated with a procedure contribute to some reactions and may predispose some patients to conditioned responses and anticipatory recurrences. Because rare IgE responses to local anesthetics are documented,[119] intradermal skin testing followed by a series of provocative dose challenges is the recommended approach to diagnosis and management.[117,118] Because antibody-mediated reactions to local anesthetic agents are very rare, a consideration of cross-reactivity patterns based on the presence of *para*-aminophenol side chains, as determined by contact sensitivity studies, appears moot.

Taxanes such as paclitaxel and docetaxel can lead to mast cell degranulation by nonimmune mechanisms.[120,121] Such reactions commonly occur with the first infusion. Slowing the infusion and pretreatment with corticosteroids and antihistamines can prevent hypersensitivity reactions in most cases. Successful readministration of taxanes using gradual dose escalation has been reported.[120,121]

Recombinant biological cytokines and antibodies are in frequent medical use and are the source of many infusion-related reactions.[122,123] Although antibody formation to recombinant proteins requires multiple exposures, adverse reactions at the first exposure are not uncommon and reflect a variety of mechanisms, including acute induction or release of cytokines, protein infusion reactions, and secondary toxicities of the product. Carbohydrate epitopes such as α-galactose added by bacteria during recombinant synthesis are the object of IgE-dependent reactions.[124] Skin testing can be helpful for identifying IgE-mediated reactions. Desensitization protocols involving slow dose escallations with succesful outcomes have been published for immunologic and nonimmunologic reactivity to biologicals and other injectable pharmaceuticals.[125]

Diagnosis of Drug Allergy

Acute drug allergy occurring within 2 hours after a dose of a single drug is readily diagnosed, often by patients themselves or their physicians. Unfortunately, most clinical presentations of drug allergy are much more complex in terms of timing of the reaction and use of multiple drugs at the time of the reaction. Consulting allergy specialists are often asked to render an opinion about whether a syndrome of adverse events is drug related, which of multiple drug treatments may be responsible, and what action should be taken. The paucity of immunodiagnostic tests notwithstanding, a well-informed and rehearsed consultant can often contribute substantially to patient management in such cases. One systematic approach to the evaluation of putative drug allergy in patients receiving multiple medications involves six specific steps (Box 79-2). The key elements for success are careful assembly of the chronology of all relevant events and knowledge of the relative sensitizing potential of various candidates, as found in a critical evaluation of the medical literature.

BOX 79-2 STEPS IN DRUG ALLERGY EVALUATION FOR PATIENTS RECEIVING MULTIPLE MEDICATIONS

1. Assemble clinical data set.
   a. Complete drug reaction history
   b. Atopic history
   c. List of concomitant medications, with chart of starts, stops, and dose changes
   d. Previous exposures to same or cross-reacting drugs
   e. Chronology of all drug reactions: attributable signs and symptoms, useful nonspecific laboratory tests (e.g., eosinophilia, ESR, tryptase, proteinuria)
2. Narrow candidate list by focusing on the following.
   a. Temporal association between drug starts and stops and onset
   b. Intensification and waning of signs and symptoms of reactions
3. Consider pharmacoepidemiology of the candidate list, and rank candidates by allergenic potential from published data.
4. Stop and/or substitute all candidate drugs with good temporal relationship to syndrome and known allergic potential. Observe consequences of stopping medications.
5. Consider skin testing if suspected drug is clinically imperative to assess IgE response. Disregard negative results within 28 days of acute anaphylaxis (i.e., false negative), and for all haptenic drugs without validated negative predictive value.
6. Readminister incriminated drugs as clinically indicated. Use gradual dose escalation (if skin test negative) or desensitization protocol (if reaction IgE dependent or skin test positive).

ESR, Erythrocyte sedimentation rate; *IgE*, immunoglobulin E.

Often, it is helpful to remind referring physicians that drug skin testing with invalidated reagents is uninformative if the result is negative. Because a positive wheal and flare response to nontoxic concentrations of drug has considerable inferential value, the decision to attempt skin testing with unvalidated drug allergens is influenced substantially by the likelihood of a positive result. This depends on published experience with such testing and the likelihood that the patient's drug reaction was IgE dependent. The consultant also recommends which drugs may be readministered safely and helps to supervise gradual dose escalation or desensitization as warranted (Fig. 79-9). This schema further suggests that reintroduction of a drug by serial dose escalations may be useful in the diagnosis of idiosyncratic drug reactions of limited severity. However, most authorities agree that rechallenge for diagnosis is strongly contraindicated in severe exfoliative dermatitis syndromes and even with milder dermatoses that include mucous membrane lesions (e.g., SJS-like), as well as in patients with substantial involvement of internal organs (as in DRESS or DiHS).

HISTORY

Drug allergy syndromes are recognized by the constellation of signs and symptoms identified with a particular mechanism of

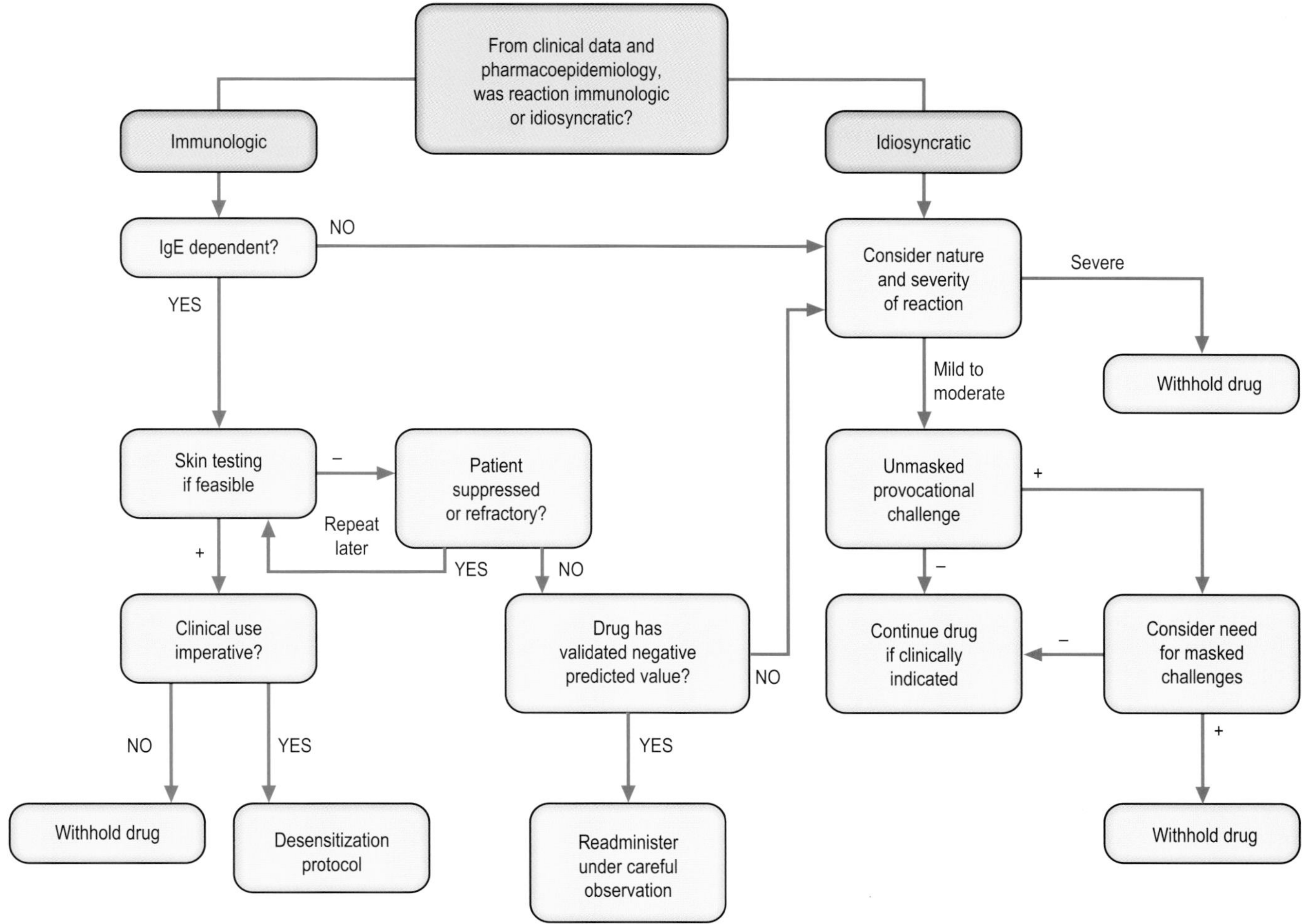

Figure 79-9 Approach to establishing current hypersensitivity status in patients with prior drug reactions to known agents. *IgE*, Immunoglobulin E.

immunopathology. The Gell and Coombs classification scheme is widely taught and conceptually useful (see Table 79-4 and Fig. 79-8). Some putative drug allergies are presumed to be immunologic in origin despite defying the Gell and Coombs classification. The most common example is morbilliform drug rashes, with or without pruritus, which typically occur late in the course of therapy or even after drug treatment has ceased. This category also includes SJS, TEN, and the usually benign fixed drug eruption.

Appropriate diagnosis of these cases depends largely on careful history taking, with attention to prior drug experience and the chronology of the reaction that is supplemented by compatible physical and laboratory findings. Use of the terms *immediate* or *delayed* reaction to qualify the onset of symptoms has been recommended because they indicate the probable responsible immune mechanism (i.e., IgE or lymphocyte mediated).[7] However, some IgE-mediated reactions may start after 1 hour, and very strong T cell–mediated immune reactions may start rapidly, within hours, defying the original definitions of these terms.

History alone is often not sufficient for establishing current drug sensitivity. Provocative drug test results from a large series of patients with a history of drug allergy have shown that less than 20% are currently allergic to the previously offending drugs.[126,127] Possible explanations include the presence of confounding factors at the time of reaction, such as infections or other comorbid situations, and waning sensitivity to the offending drug over time.[128] For a more accurate assessment of current allergy, subjects with a compatible history of drug allergy should be evaluated by further diagnostic tests for definite diagnosis. In the following sections, we suggest an approach to the patient with a history of drug allergy according to the onset of signs and symptoms.

SKIN TESTING

Immediate Reactions

Skin prick and intradermal tests can be used for the diagnosis of IgE-mediated drug reactions such as urticaria, angioedema, anaphylaxis, dyspnea, and rhinitis.[129,130] However, interpretation of these tests can be confounded by a drug-induced reaction within the past 4 to 6 weeks, use of interfering medication such as antihistamines, underlying diseases such as active urticaria or dermographism, uncontrolled asthma, or uncontrolled cardiac diseases. Prick tests usually are applied first as a safety measure, and then intradermal tests are recommended in case of negative puncture results.[129,130]

Immediate-type skin testing has been usefully applied to β-lactam antibiotics and a variety of other immunogenic drugs, but the rate of clinically false-negative test results is well

TABLE 79-9 **Predictive Value of Penicillin Skin Testing**

Prior Reaction	Penicillin Skin Tests	Immunoglobulin E–Dependent Reaction (%)	Any Immunologic Reaction (%)
Any	Positive	50-80*	—
All histories	Negative	2.6†	5.4
Anaphylaxis		3.6	7.1
Urticaria		4.7	7.1
Exanthem		2.0	6.8
Other/unknown		1.1	3.0
None	Positive	<50‡	—
	Negative	0.4†	1.0

*Limited data from inadvertent treatment or provocative challenge.[140]
†Data from large, outpatient, sexually transmitted disease clinical study.[101]
‡Data unavailable for major and minor determinant testing. Early studies with penicilloyl polylysine in history-negative subjects indicated a low reaction rate (5.5%).[140]

established only for penicillins (Table 79-9).[98,99,130-138] Application of these tests in clinical practice has demonstrated that most patients with a history of immediate reactions to β-lactams will later have negative skin test results and tolerate retreatment with penicillins and related β-lactam antibiotics. Results from one large outpatient study[137] are typical of many studies using penicilloyl polylysine (PPL) as a synthetic major determinant allergen and benzylpenicilin (with or without other hydrolyzate products) as a minor determinant reagent (see Fig. 79-9). Allergic reactions observed in retreatment of history-positive, skin test–negative patients have virtually all been mild and self-limited; no life-threatening, false-negative reactions have been reported. Because recurrent therapy can resensitize patients, although at a low rate,[135] patients with IgE-mediated reactions can be retested before subsequent courses of therapy.

Skin testing regimens for IgE-mediated penicillin allergy vary by geography. Spanish allergists have documented a high rate of IgE specific for the amino side chain of amoxicillin, which is the predominant penicillin in use there.[139] They also reported anaphylactic reactions occurring in patients with negative skin test results, which included amoxicillin.[136] As a result, European recommendations for penicillin skin testing include amoxicillin skin testing in addition to PPL and minor determinants.[136] This protocol has been adopted in North America despite a low frequency of patients with only aminopenicillin sensitivity.[138] Because of the European experience and the fact that minor determinants for skin testing constitute an orphan drug in the United States, directly observed drug challenges are increasingly being used after negative results on penicillin skin testing. Studies also suggest helpful results with the use of some cephalosporins. Concentrations of 2 to 3 mg/mL of a parental cephalosporin preparation are usually nonirritating, but each cephalosporin requires concurrent evaluation for its irritation potential in nonallergic subjects.[21,139-141] Although a positive cephalosporin skin test result implies the presence of drug-specific IgE antibodies, a negative result does not exclude immediate hypersensitivity.[139-141] Positive results for intradermal skin tests have been reported for imipenem and other β-lactams, but validated skin testing protocols are not available.[141]

Sulfonamidoyl poly-L-tyrosine, a synthetic multivalent sulfonamide antigen, has been shown to elicit positive type I skin test results in a few patients with sulfonamide allergy by history.[142,143] Other haptenic drugs have been reported to elicit positive type I skin test results in their native form and may be used as probes for drug-specific IgE responses. They include a variety of β-lactam antibiotics, trimethoprim (but not sulfonamides), carboplatin and related drugs, neuromuscular blockers, thiobarbiturates, some anticonvulsants, and local anesthetics. Specific IgE-mediated reactions to NSAIDs such pyrazolones, diclophenac, and propionic acid derivates have been reported.[115]

Enzymes and other recombinant or native proteins (e.g., heteroantisera) are complete antigens and can engender an immune response under appropriate circumstances. Exceptions include protamine, a highly charged foreign protein that does not reliably provoke wheal and flare responses in all patients who have circulating IgE antibody.[144]

Delayed-Onset Reactions

In vivo assays of delayed cutaneous responses to putative drug allergens may have diagnostic utility. Late-onset maculopapular rash is the most common form of drug allergy, and increasing evidence indicates that these rashes are likely mediated by T cells.[145] Aminopenicillins induce delayed exanthems with a frequency threefold to fivefold higher than with other penicillins, and evidence suggests that the risk of rash is related to class II MHC genes.[65] Studies suggest that patch tests and intradermal tests with delayed cutaneous readouts are useful in evaluating nonimmediate reactions to aminopenicillins and that both can reliably predict the results of rechallenge.[146-148] Patch tests with drugs are safer than intradermal tests.[146,147] The value of patch tests in DRESS or DiHS is high, but occasional mild systemic reactions may appear. The value of patch tests in SJS or TEN is much less clear, and some groups recommend avoiding them because of anecdotal reports of reactivated disease. Additional studies are required to confirm and extend these results to other drug allergies and to define more precisely the clinical correlation and predictive value for retreatment.

IN VITRO EVALUATIONS

Laboratory assessment of drug allergy patients can help diagnostically in selected cases. Most useful are biochemical or immunologic markers that confirm the activation of particular immunopathologic pathways.[149]

Immediate Reactions

Solid-phase immunoassays have been established for a wide variety of drug allergies, using sera from skin test–positive patients for standardization. These serologic tests for IgE antibody have been useful in confirming positive skin test results, in evaluating allergenic specificities and the contributions of various macromolecular carriers, in evaluating cross-reactivity with similar compounds, and in longitudinal studies of the fluxes of such antibodies over time.[150] Only with penicillin allergy have in vitro test results been systematically compared with those of skin tests.[150,151] The consistent finding has been diagnostic sensitivity for penicilloyl-IgE of 65% to 85% compared with penicilloyl-polylysine skin tests and 32% to 50% compared with a combination of skin testing and provocative challenge.[151,152] Minor determinant penicillin IgE antibodies are not reliably detected by available allergosorbent-type immunoassays. For these reasons, skin testing remains the diagnostic procedure of choice for IgE-dependent penicillin allergy.[20,136,152] Immunoassays for documenting IgE antibodies to quinolone antibiotics, rocuronium, and other drugs have been reported, but their validity is unknown.[153,154]

Flow cytometry has been increasingly studied in the diagnosis of drug allergy.[155] Assessment of drug-induced basophil activation by means of increased surface markers such as CD63 and CD203c has been investigated in the diagnosis of hypersensitivity reactions to several drugs, including penicillin, amoxicillin, quinolone antibiotics, aspirin, and neuromuscular blocking agents.[156-160] Even hypersensitivity reactions to aspirin or NSAIDs, which are not mediated by drug-specific IgE, have been associated with in vitro basophil activation, but these drugs also activate the basophils of normal subjects.[159] Determination of cysteinyl leukotrienes released from blood leukocytes after drug incubation has been suggested to increase the diagnostic value of flow cytometry alone.[160] As for unvalidated skin tests, a clearly positive result is of greater clinical value than a negative result, and these tests remain investigational.

Detectable serum mast cell β-tryptase (>1 ng/mL) or plasma histamine (>10 nmol/L) taken within 4 hours of a putative acute allergic event suggest mast cell and basophil activation.[161,162] Mild anaphylaxis without hemodynamic changes may still be falsely negative.[162]

Delayed-Onset Reactions

Drug-related T cell activity can be assessed by lymphocyte transformation tests and the flow cytometric lymphocyte activation test (LAT).[163] Results of earlier lymphocyte activation tests using drugs as stimulants were often strongly positive in drug-allergic subjects, but the response usually was not distinguishable from patients receiving equally intense and recent therapy but without reactions.[164] Studies have reported more favorable results with a variety of drugs.[164] The lymphocyte transformation test was positive in 78% of patients classified as highly likely to be drug allergic on clinical grounds. Overall specificity was 85%; however, false-positive results were observed, especially with NSAIDs.[164] This study was retrospective and did not include recently treated, nonreactive patients as controls, but the results indicate the need for reevaluation of this and the pursuit of other in vitro T cell assays, especially those involving drug-stimulated cytokines such as IL-5, IFN-γ, and IL-2.[165]

Immunoassays for IgG, IgM, or IgA responses to drug allergens have not proved to be clinically useful. IgG immune responses to the penicilloyl determinant occur in half of patients receiving high-dose therapy,[41] but the IgG response is not associated with drug allergy or risk for retreatment. IgG antidrug can attenuate the biologic activity of complete drug allergens such as antisera, enzymes, and cytokines.

Total hemolytic complement (CH_{50}) and major complement proteins (C3 and C4) are useful indicators of the presence and severity of complement activation in immune complex disorders such as serum sickness syndromes. The diagnostic utility of anaphylatoxin measurements (C3a, C4a, and C5a) remains to be defined.[166]

PROVOCATIVE DRUG TESTING

Definite diagnosis of drug allergy involves provocative drug testing, during which gradually increasing doses of the offending drug are given by various routes, including oral, parenteral, conjunctival, and mucosal challenges.[128] It may be necessary to accurately identify the responsible agent when multiple drugs are given simultaneously and a reaction occurs. Experience has shown that very few subjects with a positive history have positive drug challenge results.[126,127] Provocative drug tests should be implemented only after consideration of the risk-benefit ratio for an individual patient and should be performed only by experienced personnel in an appropriate setting. Informed consent should be obtained from the patient before the procedure. Factors to consider include the severity of the prior reaction, how recently it occurred, and the mechanism of immunopathology. Provocative drug tests should not be performed if an acute reaction occurred within the last 4 to 6 weeks, antihistamines or oral steroids are being used, or there are active signs of underlying disease such urticaria, uncontrolled asthma (i.e., forced expiratory volume in 1 second [FEV_1] value less than 70% of predicted), or uncontrolled cardiac, renal, or hepatic disease or current upper airway infection. For IgE-dependent reactions, the principal concern is anaphylaxis, and lower initial doses are warranted. Rechallenge, even with incremental dosing, is relatively contraindicated in patients with histories of TEN, SJS, DRESS, DiHS, AGEP, or severe organ-specific involvements.[128]

Readministration of the drug is usually accomplished by graded challenge. If the previous reaction occurred less than 1 hour after drug administration, the starting challenge dose should be between 1:10,000 and 1:10 of the therapeutic dose, depending on the severity of the historical reaction. Sequential doses are incremented by at least 30- to 60-minute intervals. The test challenge can usually be completed in 1 day with a maximum of four to five incremental doses for a patient with history of an immediate-type reaction. For delayed or nonimmediate types of reactions, provocative drug testing may last days or weeks. Inclusion of a placebo is strongly recommended to eliminate false-positive results for patients with largely subjective reactions.[128]

Management of Drug Allergy

ACUTE TREATMENT

Management of acute allergic drug reactions involves identification and withdrawal of the offending agent; introduction of required supportive, suppressive, or remittive therapy; and consideration of whether and how the incriminating drug should be substituted. An approach to discovering the offending drug when multiple drugs are coadministered was discussed earlier. Withdrawal of the identified drug allergen is almost always prudent and may immediately attenuate the reaction. There are some exceptions to this rule. In patients with life-threatening enterococcal endocarditis who require long-term treatment with high-dose penicillin to effect a cure, "treating through" isolated episodes of urticaria and generalized pruritus may be necessary. Experience suggests that most such episodes are self-limited and will remit with continuous therapy. H_1 antihistamines can be used to suppress symptoms while careful surveillance is established for multisystem immunopathology, such as drug fever, hepatitis, and renal damage. When treating through mild type I reactions, it is imperative to avoid lapses in treatment because restarting treatment after a lapse may invoke anaphylaxis. Late-occurring maculopapular exanthems with minimal or no pruritus is another setting for continuing treatment through relatively mild reactions, provided there is a compelling clinical need to do so. A high success rate with spontaneous resolution of ampicillin rashes despite continuation of therapy has been reported in children,[68] but anecdotal experience suggests that this is not always achievable in adults or with other drugs. Careful monitoring for fever, eosinophilia, proteinuria, arthralgia, lymphadenopathy, and hepatitis is warranted, with prompt cessation of therapy if new signs or symptoms appear. Severe exfoliative syndromes, including SJS and toxic epidermal necrolysis, and any drug rash involving mucosal surfaces warrant immediate drug withdrawal and often require hospitalization.[167]

Drug-induced allergic syndromes are pharmacologically treated similar to non–drug-induced immunopathology. Treatment of urticaria and angioedema, anaphylaxis, serum sickness, immune cytopenias, and contact sensitivity is detailed in other chapters. Severe drug-induced immunopathology of any type usually prompts the use of corticosteroids. Whether high-dose steroids constitute an effective remittive agent for exfoliative dermatitis syndromes is controversial. Studies indicate the apparent success of high-dose intravenous immune globulin (IVIG) when used early in SJS or TENS patients.[167]

When ambiguity surrounds which drug induced a severe immunologic reaction, plans should be made to pursue a definitive diagnosis after the patient's convalescence. Any type I drug skin testing should be delayed at least 4 weeks after an acute anaphylactic episode to avoid testing during a refractory period. When the drug culprit is identified, the patient should be provided instruction on avoidance, including a written list of cross-reactive drugs. The use of wallet cards, identification jewelry, and registry services (e.g., MedicAlert) should be recommended for patients with documented severe reactions.

ALTERNATIVES FOR DRUG-ALLERGIC PATIENTS

There are three approaches to providing acceptable pharmacotherapy for the underlying condition in drug-allergic patients.

Administration of an Unrelated Alternative Medication

The most common approach is administration of an unrelated alternative medication that is safe and effective for the disease requiring treatment. Careful attention should be given to the risks of second-line therapy, especially treatment failure with antibiotics, and to the toxicity and cost of alternative regimens. Studies have shown that prophylactic vancomycin use in patients with a history of penicillin or cephalosporin allergy undergoing elective orthopedic surgery was substantially reduced by a targeted allergy consultation and penicillin allergy skin testing.[168] For most common outpatient infections, alternative antibiotics provide a reasonable choice for the penicillin-allergic patient. For hospitalized patients with serious systemic infections, such as enterococcal endocarditis, bacterial meningitis, and brain abscess, the risk of treatment failure with a second-line drug is an important consideration.

Administration of a Potentially Cross-reactive Medication

The second alternative for drug-sensitive patients is to receive a medication not identical to but potentially cross-reactive with the offending drug allergen. Cross-reactivity usually is confined to the same drug class (e.g., within the quinolone or sulfa-antibiotics class), but cross-reactivity does not occur outside the class. Common clinical examples are the use of cephalosporins and penems in penicillin-allergic subjects,[20,21] drugs containing a sulfa moiety (e.g., sulfonylureas, sulfasalazine) in patients reactive to sulfamethoxazole,[169] and alternative anticonvulsants within a broadly cross-reactive group.[170] Cross-reactivity among some β-lactam antibiotics can be explained by similarities in the R1 side chain structure.[20,21,139] Cephalosporins that share a similar (e.g., cephalothin, cefamandol) or identical (e.g., cefaclor, cephalexin, cefatrizine) R1 side chain with benzylpenicillin can be cross-reactive with penicillins. Amoxicillin has cross-reactivity with cefadroxil in 38% of the patients.[21] A cross-reactivity pattern among cephalosporins was also demonstrated.[20,21,139] Use of aztreonam appears safe in penicillin-allergic patients.[171]

Although the absolute risk of cross-allergic reactions is small (<25%), when β-lactam reactions involve a type I mechanism, preliminary skin testing with the chosen alternative and slow dose escalation (e.g., usual intravenous dose at incremental rates over 4 to 6 hours) under observation can minimize the potential for life-threatening anaphylaxis. Whether gradual dose escalation is advantageous for late-occurring, non–IgE-dependent reactions is unstudied. Potentially cross-reactive drugs should not be reintroduced even in graded doses for patients who have experienced SJS or toxic epidermal necrolysis, because small doses have reactivated serious manifestations of these syndromes.[167]

Readministration of the Offending Drug

The third alternative for drug-allergic subjects is readministration of the offending drug by desensitization. If an offending drug is irreplaceable or significantly more effective than the alternatives, the drug may need to be readministrated.[152,172] Although classic desensitization is applied only to type I allergy in patients with demonstrable or presumed IgE antibody responses, the same procedure has been used to achieve drug tolerance when sensitivity is not conveyed by specific IgE antibodies, as in the case of aspirin desensitization (see Chapter 41). Desensitization is achieved by administering progressive doses of a drug every 15 to 30 minutes for IgE-mediated reactions until a full therapeutic dose is clinically tolerated. The procedure entails risk of acute allergic reactions, which occur in mild form in 30% to 80% of penicillin-allergic patients undergoing desensitization (Box 79-3).[173,174]

The mechanism by which clinical tolerance is induced during drug desensitization is complex but depends fundamentally on achieving antigen-specific basophil and mast cell desensitization.[175-179] Specific mast cell desensitization is poorly understood but may involve low-level, subthreshold antigen stimulation by hapten-carrier conjugates.[178] The consecutive

BOX 79-3 DRUG DESENSITIZATION FOR IMMUNOGLOBULIN E–DEPENDENT ALLERGY

Generic Protocol

PREPARATION

1. Obtain a skin test to determine the patient's degree of sensitivity (if available).
   a. Dilute available drug solution or suspension to 1-3 mg/mL.
   b. Prepare three tenfold dilutions.
   c. Perform prick or puncture testing with a 1:1000 dilution.
   d. If the result is negative, perform serial intradermal tests, using 0.02 mL (3- to 4-mm bleb) in duplicate, up to and including 3 mg/mL stock; discontinue testing when >8 mm wheal is observed. Test result is positive if both duplicate wheals increase significantly (>2-3 mm) 20 minutes after placement compared with diluent control.
2. Prepare sufficient quantities of drug solution or suspension for desensitization regimen in tenfold dilutions from full therapeutic dose (1/10, 1/100, and 1/1000 dilutions if necessary).

PROCEDURE

1. Establish baseline monitoring of the patient in a medical setting appropriate for his or her clinical conditions and the nature or severity of prior reaction. Start a secure intravenous infusion.
2. Starting dose: if the skin test result negative and the test is unvalidated, begin with 0.1 mL of a 1/100 dilution (start with a 1/1000 dilution in severe reactions); if the skin test result is positive, begin 100-fold below dose that produces midpoint reaction (5- to 8-mm wheal).
3. Route: oral by ingestion or nasogastric tube in 30 mL of water; parenteral by intradermal (<0.2 mL); subcutaneous (0.2-0.6 mL); or intramuscular (>0.6 mL) injection.
4. Dosing interval: 15-20 minutes for parenteral doses; 20-30 minutes for oral dosing. Repeat dose for mild to moderate systemic reactions; drop back two doses for any reaction producing hemodynamic changes.
5. Dose escalation: twofold increments (e.g., 1, 2, 4, 8, 16 μg)

FOLLOW-UP

1. If intravenous therapy follows desensitization, continuous 24-hour drug infusion is preferable if feasible. If not, avoid rapid infusion of intermittent drug doses.
2. If drug skin test result was positive, repeat after desensitization to document shift in skin sensitivity.
3. Avoid lapses in therapeutic doses.
4. Treat through selected mild to moderate reactions (e.g., urticaria) to avoid need to repeat desensitization.
5. Before subsequent courses of therapy, repeat desensitization if skin test results remain positive; desensitization therapy is dose and drug dependent.

administration of suboptimal doses of antigen before the optimal dose seems to render these cells unresponsive to the drug compound but not to other stimuli. Low-dose therapy favors oligomer formation with monovalent inhibitors, both of which may be involved in the desensitization process. Increasing subtherapeutic doses can provide a sufficient amount of antigenic determinants to bind to IgE without cross-linking.[176] Desensitization results in a reduced skin sensitivity to drug allergens in most patients.[179] Rapid desensitization protocols have been published for non–IgE-mediated reactions caused by chemotherapeutic and biologic agents, sulfonamides, and non–β-lactam antibiotics, but the mechanisms are still largely unknown, especially for T cell–mediated sensitivities.[125,172,180]

Desensitization is an active process that depends on the continuous presence of the drug. After drug discontinuation, the desensitized state dissipates over days to weeks, and repeat desensitization is usually required for subsequent treatment courses. Desensitization also depends on drug dose, and a substantial dose increase may result in breakthrough allergic symptoms. Although deaths have occurred during desensitization attempts, in the modern era, the success rate is extremely high using recommended procedures (see Box 79-3).

Oral and parenteral routes can be used to initiate desensitization therapy, and both appear equally effective in inducing clinical tolerance. The oral approach is arguably safer,[172,173] although not always feasible. Specific protocols for desensitization by parenteral and oral routes have been widely published for penicillin.[172] The use of penicillin desensitization has included pregnant patients,[173,174] indicating that the risk of this therapy in competent hands is probably lower than the risk of treatment failure with an inferior antibiotic. Nevertheless, the potential risks are serious enough to require hospitalization and informed consent.

Classic protocols for oral and intravenous desensitization to penicillin start at 1/10,000 to 1/100 of the target dose; doubled doses are administered every 15 to 20 minutes over the course of several hours until the therapeutic dose is reached. The starting dose should be determined by taking into account the severity of reaction. In patients with histories of severe anaphylaxis (e.g., hypotension with loss of consciousness, severe bronchospasm), the initial dose should be between 1/1,000,000 and 1/10,000 of the full therapeutic one. In patients with a positive skin test result for a nonirritating concentration of a drug, the starting dose can be determined on the basis of the end-point titration.

The procedure entails risk of acute allergic reactions, which occur in mild form in 30% to 80% of penicillin-allergic patients undergoing desensitization.[173,174] In a published series by Castells and colleagues,[180] during 413 rapid desensitizations to a variety of chemotherapeutic agents, about one third were adverse reactions; 27% were mild, and only 5.8% were anaphylactic reactions. Most (75%) reactions occurred in the final steps of the 12-step desensitization protocol.

Occasionally, late-occurring reactions during therapy, including urticaria or serum sickness and hemolytic anemia, can be seen if high-dose therapy is used. Levels of IgG- and IgE-specific antibodies increase after desensitization therapy. The rising IgG titer may neutralize drug epitopes and serve a blocking function for IgE-dependent reactions. As previously noted, skin test reactivity diminishes as a result of desensitization despite a large increase in drug-specific IgE, providing further evidence for cellular desensitization as a principal mechanism.

It appears possible to maintain a desensitized state chronically by daily oral administration of penicillin for selected patients in whom recurrent infections are anticipated[175,179] or occupational exposure is unavoidable and disabling.[172] Published clinical experience with chronic desensitization, however, is very limited.

Several examples of successful insulin desensitization efforts are available.[181] A variety of desensitization protocols have been derived empirically for reintroducing sulfamethoxazole-trimethoprim (SMX-TMP), dapsone, and other antimicrobials to reactive patients with AIDS[182-184] or with cystic fibrosis[185-187] and for sulfasalazine retreatment for patients with inflammatory bowel disease.[188] Imipenem[189] and cephalosporins[190] have also been used for successful reinstitution of therapy. Some of these efforts have been directed at inducing tolerance in patients whose history is one of late-onset morbilliform eruptions. Many successful cases have been reported using dose escalations over 10 days or longer in outpatient oral protocols, but it is not clear to what degree these patients were at risk for recurrent reactions. Because sulfonamide skin tests are unreliable, the presence of drug-specific IgE could not be documented by skin test or in vitro IgE testing in the reported series. The propensity for morbilliform eruptions can be desensitized by non–IgE-dependent mechanisms using gradual dose escalation, as demonstrated with lamotrigine and with clopidogrel.[191,192]

READMINISTRATION OF PREVIOUSLY OFFENDING AGENTS

Until recently, the medical culture regarded readministration of a medicinal agent to a patient who previously reacted adversely to the drug as strongly contraindicated and fraught with concerns about violation of the Hippocratic oath and medicolegal liability. Experience has taught that dismissing the possibility of re-treatment often does the patient a disservice by withholding indicated therapy that may be well tolerated the second time. There are many reasons why a previously reactive patient may tolerate re-treatment. The most common is misdiagnosis of the original reaction based on a temporal association that was not causally linked. IgE antibody responses dissipate over time, especially for haptenic drugs, and as amply demonstrated for penicillins, most patients lose sensitivity over time. Some pseudoallergic reactions result from psychologic overgeneralization of an initial frightening or life-threatening drug treatment episode. The biologic states required for reactivity may wane over time and render the patient less vulnerable. For example, aspirin-like drugs often aggravate chronic idiopathic urticaria but are well tolerated after the urticaria remits.

These factors provide opportunities for safe re-treatment of a surprisingly large number of patients with allergic and idiosyncratic adverse drug experiences. When drugs being withheld are uniquely beneficial or alternative therapy has failed, risks need to be weighed against anticipated benefits.

With a few exceptions, the possibility of readministration can be tested safely using gradual dose escalation. Factors to consider include the severity of the prior reaction, how recently it occurred, and the mechanism of immunopathology. For IgE-dependent reactions, the principal concern is anaphylaxis, and lower initial doses are warranted. For some life-threatening reactions, such as exfoliative dermatitis syndromes and dermatoses with mucous membrane lesions (SJS-like), readministration of any dose is strongly contraindicated. Otherwise, initial doses for retreatment can generally begin at 1% of the desired therapeutic dose. The oral route is preferred, especially for haptenic drugs. At appropriate intervals, as determined by the pharmacology of the drug and the patient's prior experiences with the agent, dose escalations (about threefold) are appropriate. The strategy is to use incremental doses and intervals such that a very mild clinical reaction will be elicited if the patient remains sensitive. After the full therapeutic dose has been achieved without incident, continuous therapy should start immediately with appropriate monitoring. When there is clinical suspicion of anticipatory reactions (i.e., classic conditioning) or strong emotional elements are present, the inclusion of placebos in serial challenges is advisable. A decision tree helps to outline the prerequisites for readministration (see Fig. 79-9).

PROPHYLAXIS IN DRUG ALLERGY-PRONE PATIENTS

Some individuals are vulnerable to allergic drug reactions as a result of genetic or metabolic abnormalities (e.g., multiple drug allergy syndrome), frequent and recurrent drug exposure (e.g., antibiotics in cystic fibrosis), or certain disease states related to immune dysfunction (e.g., AIDS). Such patients are likely to benefit from a thorough and proactive evaluation that documents sensitivities (Box 79-4). Ongoing reevaluation helps to keep the list of usable drugs from becoming unacceptably limited. In a drug reaction–prone population, pharmacotherapy requires special management to avoid adverse events and to prevent (as far as possible) sensitization or resensitization. Prevention of recurrent infections is a prime objective in patients with multiple antibiotic sensitivities. Aggressive management of rhinosinusitis can help to minimize recurrent otitis media and sinusitis. Up-to-date vaccination is highly desirable. Avoidance of unnecessary exposures to contagious diseases may be helpful, especially in children. Low-dose prophylactic antibiotics may paradoxically reduce drug allergy if they prevent recurrent infections. Stringent indications for antibiotics, including a requirement for positive culture results, can help to limit cumulative drug exposures. These approaches can have substantial clinical impact on antimicrobial allergy, especially in patients constitutionally predisposed to haptenic drug allergy.

Premedication with antihistamines and corticosteroids can reduce the incidence and severity of acute pseudoallergic reactions to radiocontrast media (see Table 79-8).[193] These regimens have not been systematically studied for the prevention of IgE-mediated anaphylaxis. Numerous anecdotal reports attest to the failure of steroids and antihistamines to prevent serious

BOX 79-4 EVALUATION AND MANAGEMENT OF MULTIDRUG-SENSITIVE PATIENT

EVALUATION

1. Careful drug sensitivity data with a focus on common features (e.g., groups of related drugs, similar time to reaction, commonality of syndrome elements)
2. Skin test evaluation for drugs with validated skin test (e.g., proteins, penicillin, quaternary ammonium compounds, cisplatin) or as preliminary evaluation to provocative testing
3. Provocative testing for unconvincing reports or mild symptoms, especially if the drug therapy remains clinically indicated
4. Placebo-controlled challenges when the reaction patterns are similar for unrelated drugs to demonstrate operant conditioning in suspected cases

MANAGEMENT

1. Measures to prevent infections (if antimicrobials are implicated)
2. Stringent criteria for new drug use
3. For intolerant patients, initiation of therapy at one third to one tenth of the usual dose
4. Medical observation after first dose of new or suspect drugs
5. Careful monitoring and encouragement to allow treating through selected mild or atypical reactions
6. Gradual dose escalation or desensitization as warranted
7. Monitoring and discontinuation of drug at earliest signs of severe cutaneous reactions (e.g., Stevens-Johnson syndrome, exfoliative dermatitis, toxic epidermal necrolysis)

anaphylactic episodes. Premedication may mask early symptoms and allow dosing to proceed more rapidly than advisable. Drugs reinstituted under the cover of corticosteroids may still be problematic when steroids are withdrawn. For these reasons, use of premedication before gradual dose escalation of drugs implicated in type I allergy or when undertaking drug desensitization is not recommended.

For drug-intolerant patients, new drug therapy should begin at lower doses than required for therapy. Administration under medical observation is advisable when risk is considered substantial or the patient requires reassurance. Consideration should be given to treating through mild cutaneous reactions, including urticaria, especially early in therapy when an alternative antibiotic usually is required. High-risk patients should also be advised to monitor for constitutional signs such as fever or early evidence of mucositis. Aggressive management by a knowledgeable physician can greatly expedite the long-term care of drug allergy–prone patients by preserving and protecting therapeutic options. Some drug hypersensitivity reactions can be avoided by genetic testing to exclude individuals at risk.[194,195]

Summary

Drug hypersensitivity states present an often frustrating challenge for most practicing physicians. Knowledge of the natural history and pathogenesis of many immunologic and idiosyncratic drug reactions remains superficial and incomplete. Because immunodiagnostic tests for drug allergy are limited in number and require some sophistication to interpret, many practitioners have concluded that the only reasonable option for drug-reactive patients is permanent and total avoidance of putative offenders. In the extreme, patients with multiple drug hypersensitivity syndromes are sometimes abandoned by their primary physicians, or they are told to do without all drug therapy.

Armed with an understanding of the distinction between drug allergy and idiosyncrasy, the risk factors for drug allergy, and the pharmacoepidemiology of sensitizing drugs, a medical practitioner can safely provide useful drug therapy for a surprisingly large number of drug-sensitive patients. For allergy and immunology specialists, the willingness to undertake this task is usually appreciatively obliged by other professionals, who readily refer drug-sensitive patients and are grateful for the assistance received.

Medical progress in understanding and managing drug hypersensitivity states often requires the collaborative efforts of multiple disciplines, including basic immunology, pharmacology, toxicology, genetics, biochemistry, pathology, and epidemiology. The high morbidity rates and costs associated with drug hypersensitivity make this set of disorders a high priority for future research investment.[7]

REFERENCES

Introduction

1. Lazarou J, Pomeranz BH, Corey PN. Incidence of adverse drug reactions in hospitalized patients: a meta-analysis of prospective studies. JAMA 1998;279:1200-5.
2. McDonnell PJ, Jacobs MR. Hospital admissions resulting from preventable adverse drug reactions. Ann Pharmacother 2002;36:1331-6.
3. Stern RS. Utilization of hospital and outpatient care for adverse cutaneous reactions to medications. Pharmacoepidemiol Drug Saf 2005;14:677-84.
4. Sun DC, Woodall BS, Skin SK, et al. Clinical and economic impact of adverse drug reactions in hospitalized patients. Ann Pharmacother 2000;34:1373-9.
5. Gomes ER, Demoly P. Epidemiology of hypersensitivity drug reactions. Curr Opin Allergy Clin Immunol 2005;5:309-16.
6. Dern RJ, Beutler E, Alving AS. The hemolytic effect of primaquine V: primaquine sensitivity as a manifestation of a multiple drug sensitivity. J Lab Clin Med 1981;97:750-9.
7. Johansson SG, Bieber T, Dahl R, et al. Revised nomenclature for allergy for global use: report of the Nomenclature Review Committee of the World Allergy Organization, October 2003. J Allergy Clin Immunol 2004;113:832-6.

Epidemiology and Burden of Drug Hypersensitivity

8. Impicciatore P, Choonara I, Clarkson A, et al. Incidence of adverse drug reactions in paediatric in/out-patients: a systematic review and meta-analysis of prospective studies. Br J Clin Pharmacol 2001;52:77-81.
9. Ghandhi TK, Weingart SN, Borus J, et al. Adverse drug events in ambulatory care. N Engl J Med 2003;348:1556-64.
10. Berkun Y, Ben-Zvi A, Levy Y, Galili D, Shalit M. Evaluation of adverse reactions to local anesthetics: experience with 236 patients. Ann Allergy Asthma Immunol 2003;91:342-5.
11. Moneret-Vautrin DA, Morisset M, Flabbee J, Beaudouin E, Kanny G. Epidemiology of life-threatening and lethal anaphylaxis: a review. Allergy 2005;60:443-51.
12. Sade K, Holtzer I, Levo Y, Kivity S. The economic burden of antibiotic treatment of penicillin-allergic patients in internal medicine wards of a general tertiary care hospital. Clin Exp Allergy 2003;33:501-6.

How Drugs Are Recognized by the Immune System

13. Landsteiner K. The specificity of serological reactions. New York: Dover; 1962.
14. Vervloet D, Arnaud A, Senft M, et al. Anaphylactic reactions to suxamethonium: prevention of mediator release by choline. J Allergy Clin Immunol 1985;76:222-5.
15. Gueant JL, Aimone-Gastin I, Namour F, et al. Diagnosis and pathogenesis of the anaphylactic and anaphylactoid reactions to anaesthetics. Clin Exp Allergy 1998;28:65-70.
16. Lafaye P, Lapresk C. Fixation of penicilloyl groups to albumin and appearance of anti-penicilloyl antibodies to penicillin-treated patients. J Clin Invest 1988;88:7-12.
17. Padovan E. T cell response in penicillin allergy. Clin Exp Allergy 1998;28:33-6.
18. Dewdney JM. Immunology of the antibiotics. In: Sela M, editor. The antigens, vol. 4. New York: Academic Press; 1977. p. 73.
19. Gorevic PD, Levine BB. Desensitization of anaphylactic hypersensitivity specific for the penicillate minor determinant of penicillin and carbenicillin. J Allergy Clin Immunol 1981;68:267-72.
20. Torres MJ, Blanca M. The complex clinical picture of beta-lactam hypersensitivity: penicillins, cephalosporins, monobactams, carbapenems, and clavams. Med Clin North Am 2010;94:805-20.
21. Romano A, Gaeta F, Valluzzi RL, et al. IgE-mediated hypersensitivity to cephalosporins: cross-reactivity and tolerability of penicillins, monobactams, and carbapenems. J Allergy Clin Immunol 2010;126:994-9.
22. Saxon A, Adelman DC, Patel A, Hajdu R, Calandra GB. Imipenem cross-reactivity with penicillin in humans. J Allergy Clin Immunol 1988;82:213-7.
23. Adkinson NF Jr. Immunogenicity and cross-allergenicity of aztreonam. Am J Med 1990;88:12S-15S.
24. Patriarca G, Schiavino D, Lombardo C, et al. Tolerability of aztreonam in patients with IgE-mediated hypersensitivity to beta-lactams. Int J Immunopathol Pharmacol 2008;21:375-9.
25. Riley RJ, Leeder JS. In vitro analysis of metabolic predisposition to drug hypersensitivity reactions. Clin Exp Immunol 1995;99:1-6.
26. Rieder MJ. Mechanisms of unpredictable adverse drug reactions. Drug Saf 1994;11:196-212.
27. Park BK, Pirmohamed M, Kitteringham NR. The role of cytochrome P450 enzymes in hepatic and extrahepatic human drug toxicity. Pharmacol Ther 1995;68:385-424.
28. Clark DW. Genetically determined variability in acetylation and oxidation: therapeutic implications. Drugs 1985;29:342-75.
29. Wilson RA. The liver: its role in drug biotransformation and as a target of immunologic injury. Immunol Allergy Clin North Am 1991;11:555-73.

30. Meekins CV, Sullivan TJ, Gruchalla RS. Immunochemical analysis of sulfonamide drug allergy: identification of sulfamethoxazole-substituted human serum proteins. J Allergy Clin Immunol 1994;94:1017-24.
31. Naisbitt DJ, Hough SJ, Gill HJ, et al. Cellular disposition of sulphamethoxazole and its metabolites: implications for hypersensitivity. Br J Pharmacol 1999;126:1393-407.
32. Yang Y, Sempe P, Peterson PA. Molecular mechanisms of class I major histocompatibility complex antigen processing and presentation. Immunol Res 1996;15:208-33.
33. Park BK, Kitteringham NR, Powell H, Pirmohamed M. Advances in molecular toxicology: towards understanding idiosyncratic drug toxicity. Toxicology 2000;153:39-60.
34. Hernstreet BA, Page Rl. Sulfonamide allergies and outcomes related to use of potentially cross-reactive drugs in hospitalized patients. Pharmacotherapy 2006;26:551-7.
35. Pichler WJ. Pharmacological interaction of drugs with antigen-specific immune receptors: the p-i concept. Curr Opin Allergy Clin Immunol 2002;2:301-5.
36. Pichler WJ. Direct T cell stimulations by drugs: bypassing the innate immune system. Toxicology 2005;209:95-100.
37. Ko TM, Chung WH, Wei CY, et al. Shared and restricted T-cell receptor use is crucial for carbamazepine-induced Stevens-Johnson syndrome. J Allergy Clin Immunol 2011;128: 1266-76.
38. Wei CY, Chung WH, Huang HW, Chen YT, Hung SI. Direct interaction between HLA-B and carbamazepine activates T cells in patients with Stevens-Johnson syndrome. J Allergy Clin Immunol 2012;129:1562-9.
39. Schnyder B, Burkhart C, Schnyder-Frutig K, et al. Recognition of sulfamethoxazole and its reactive metabolites by drug specific T cells from allergic individuals. J Immunol 2000; 164:6647-54.
40. Schaerli P, Ebert L, Willimann K, et al. A skin-selective homing mechanism for human immune surveillance T cells. J Exp Med 2004; 199:1265-75.

Factors That Influence Drug Immunogenicity

41. Adkinson NF Jr. Risk factors for drug allergy. J Allergy Clin Immunol 1984;74:567-72.
42. York IA, Rock KL. Antigen processing and presentation by the class I major histocompatibility complex. Annu Rev Immunol 1996;14: 369-96.
43. Bour H, Peyron E, Gaucherand M, et al. Major histocompatibility complex class I-restricted CD8+ T cells and class II-restricted CD4+ T cells, respectively, mediate and regulate contact sensitivity to dinitrofluorobenzene. Eur J Immunol 1995;25:3006-10.
44. Pieters J. MHC class II restricted antigen presentation. Curr Opin Immunol 1997;9: 89-96.
45. Romano A, De Santis A, Romito A, et al. Delayed hypersensitivity to aminopenicillins is related to major histocompatibility complex genes. Ann Allergy Asthma Immunol 1998;80: 433-7.
46. Basketter D, Dooms-Goossens A, Karlberg AT, Lepoittevin JP. The chemistry of contact allergy: why is a molecule allergenic? Contact Dermatitis 1995;32:65-73.
47. Weltzien HU, Moulon C, Martin S, et al. T cell immune responses to haptens: structural models for allergic and autoimmune reactions. Toxicology 1996;107:141-51.
48. Sullivan TJ. Dehaptenation of albumin substituted with benzylpenicillin G determinants. J Allergy Clin Immunol 1988;81:222.
49. DiPiro JT, Adkinson NF Jr, Hamilton RG. Facilitation of penicillin haptenation to serum proteins. Antimicrob Agents Chemother 1993; 37:1463-7.
50. Martin JL, Kenna JG, Martin BM, et al. Halothane hepatitis patients have serum antibodies that react with protein disulfide isomerase. Hepatology 1993;18:858-63.
51. Carr A, Swanson C, Penny R, Cooper DA. Clinical and laboratory markers of hypersensitivity to trimethoprim-sulfamethoxazole in patients with *Pneumocystis carinii* pneumonia and AIDS. J Infect Dis 1993;167:180-5.
52. Rieder MJ, Shear NH, Kanee A, Tang BK, Spielberg SP. Prominence of slow acetylator phenotype among patients with sulfonamide hypersensitivity reactions. Clin Pharmacol Ther 1991;49:13-7.
53. Schmid DA, Depta JPH, Lüthi M, Pichler WJ. Transfection of drug specific T cell receptors into hybridoma cells: tools to monitor drug binding to TCR and to evaluate cross-reactivity to related compounds. Mol Pharmacol 2006; 70:356-65.
54. Burkhard C, Britschgi M, Strasser I, et al. Noncovalent presentation of sulfamethoxazole to human CD4+ T cells is independent of distinct HLA-bound peptides. Clin Exp Allergy 2002; 32:1635-43.
55. Chung WH, Hung SI, Hong HS, et al. Medical genetics: a marker for Stevens-Johnson syndrome. Nature 2004;428:486.
56. Kaniwa N, Saito Y, Aihara M, et al. JSAR research group. HLA-B*1511 is a risk factor for carbamazepine-induced Stevens-Johnson syndrome and toxic epidermal necrolysis in Japanese patients. Epilepsia 2010;51: 2461-5.
57. McCormack M, Alfirevic A, Bourgeois S, et al. HLA-A*3101 and carbamazepine-induced hypersensitivity reactions in Europeans. N Engl J Med 2011;364:1134-43.
58. Hung SI, Chung WH, Liou LB, et al. HLA-B*5801 allele as a genetic marker for severe cutaneous adverse reactions caused by allopurinol. Proc Natl Acad Sci U S A 2005;102: 4134-9.
59. Somkrua R, Eickman EE, Saokaew S, Lohitnavy M, Chaiyakunapruk N. Association of HLA-B*5801 allele and allopurinol-induced Stevens-Johnson syndrome and toxic epidermal necrolysis: a systematic review and meta-analysis. BMC Med Genet 2011;12: 118.
60. Mallal S, Nolan D, Witt C, et al. Association between presence of HLA-B*5701, HLA-DR7, and HLA-DQ3 and hypersensitivity to HIV-1 reverse-transcriptase inhibitor abacavir. Lancet 2002;359:727-32.
61. Daly AK, Donaldson PT, Bhatnagar P, et al. DILIGEN Study; International SAE Consortium. HLA-B*5701 genotype is a major determinant of drug-induced liver injury due to flucloxacillin. Nat Genet 2009;41:816-9.
62. Lonjou C, Thomas L, Borot N, et al. RegiSCAR Group. A marker for Stevens-Johnson syndrome: ethnicity matters. Pharmacogenomics J 2006;6:265-8.
63. Yang CW, Hung SI, Juo CG, et al. HLA-B*1502-bound peptides: implications for the pathogenesis of carbamazepine-induced Stevens-Johnson syndrome. J Allergy Clin Immunol 2007;120:870-7.
64. Knudsen ET, Dewdney JM, Trafford JA. Reduction in incidence of ampicillin rash by purification of ampicillin. Br Med J 1970;169: 469-71.
65. Hoigne R, Sonntag MR, Zoppi M, et al. Occurrence of exanthema in relation to aminopenicillin preparations and allopurinol. N Engl J Med 1987;316:1217-18.
66. Kerns D, Shira JE, Go S, et al. Ampicillin rash in children: relationship to penicillin allergy and infectious mononucleosis. Am J Dis Child 1973;125:187-90.
67. Moseley EK, Sullivan TJ. Allergic reactions to antimicrobial drugs in patients with a history of prior drug allergy. J Allergy Immunol 1991;87:226.
68. Uetrecht J. New concepts in immunology relevant to idiosyncratic drug reactions: the "danger hypothesis" and innate immune system. Chem Res Toxicol 1999;12:387-95.
69. Lanctot KL, Ghajar BM, Shear NH, Naranjo CA. Improving the diagnosis of hypersensitivity reactions associated with sulfonamides. J Clin Pharmacol 1994;34:1228-33.
70. Rose EW, McCloskey WW. Glutathione in hypersensitivity to trimethoprim/sulfamethoxazole in patients with HIV infection. Ann Pharmacother 1998;32:381-3.
71. Daftarian MP, Filion LG, Cameron W, et al. Immune response to sulfamethoxazole in patients with AIDS. Clin Diagn Lab Immunol 1995;22:199-204.
72. Lee BL, Wong D, Benowitz NL, Sullam PM. Altered patterns of drug metabolism in patients with acquired immunodeficiency syndrome. Clin Pharmacol Ther 1993;53: 529-35.
73. Birnbaum J, Vervloet D. Allergy to muscle relaxants. Clin Rev Allergy 1991;9:281-93.
74. Coulter EM, Farrell J, Mathews KL, et al. Activation of human dendritic cells by *p*-phenylenediamine. J Pharmacol Exp Ther 2007;320:885-92.
75. Ashikaga T, Hoya M, Itagaki H, Katsumura Y, Aiba Si. Evaluation of CD86 expression and MHC class II molecule internalization in THP-1 human monocyte cells as predictive endpoints for contact sensitizers. Toxicol In Vitro 2002;16:711-6.

Specificity of Drug-Induced Immune Responses

76. De Weck AL, Schneider CH. Specific inhibition of allergic reactions to penicillin in man by a monovalent hapten. Int Arch Allergy 1972; 42:782-97.
77. Adkinson NF Jr. Side-chain specific β-lactam allergy. Clin Exp Allergy 1990;20:445-7.
78. Silviu-Dan F, McPhillips S, Warrington RJ. The frequency of skin test reactions to side-chain penicillin determinants. J Allergy Clin Immunol 1993;91:694-701.
79. Moss RB, Babin S, Hsu Y-P, Blessing-Moore J, Lewiston NJ. Allergy to semisynthetic penicillins in cystic fibrosis. J Pediatr 1984;104: 460-6.
80. Romano A, Torres MJ, Fernandez J, et al. Allergic reactions to ampicillin: studies on the specificity and selectivity in subjects with immediate reactions. Clin Exp Allergy 1997;27: 1425-31.
81. Worlledge SM. Immune drug-induced hemolytic anemias. Semin Hematol 1973;10: 327-44.

Immunopathologic Features of Drug Allergy

82. Storrs FJ. Contact dermatitis caused by drugs. Immunol Allergy Clin North Am 1991;11: 509-23.
83. Hertl M, Geisel J, Boecker C, Merk HF. Selective generation of CD8+ T cell clones from the peripheral blood of patients with cutaneous reactions to β-lactam antibiotics. Br J Dermatol 1993;128:619-26.
84. Mauri-Hellweg D, Bettens F, Mauri D, et al. Activation of drug-specific CD4+ and CD8+ T cells in individuals allergic to sulfonamides, phenytoin and carbamazepine. J Immunol 1995;155:462-72.
85. Roujeau JC, Kelly JP, Naldi L, et al. Medication use and the risk of Stevens-Johnson syndrome or toxic epidermal necrolysis. N Engl J Med 1995;333:1600-7.
86. Pichler WJ. Delayed drug hypersensitivity reactions. Ann Intern Med 2003;139:683-93.
87. Nassif A, Bensussan A, Dorothee G, et al. Drug specific cytotoxic T cells in the skin lesions of a patient with toxic epidermal necrolysis. J Invest Dermatol 2002;118:728-33.
88. Schnyder B, Frutig K, Mauri-Hellweg D, et al. T-cell-mediated cytotoxicity against keratinocytes in sulfamethoxazol-induced skin reaction. Clin Exp Allergy 1998;28:1412-7.
89. Britschgi M, Steiner UC, Schmid S, et al. T cell involvement in drug-induced acute generalized exanthem. J Clin Invest 2001;107:1433-41.
90. Vergne P, Bertin P, Bonnet C, Scotto C, Trèves R. Drug-induced rheumatic disorders: incidence, prevention and management. Drug Saf 2000;23:279-93.

Risk Factors for Drug Hypersensitivity

91. Christensen LH, Holm J, Lund G, Riise E, Lund K. Several distinct properties of the IgE repertoire determine effector cell degranulation in response to allergen challenge. J Allergy Clin Immunol 2008;122:298-304.
92. Smith H, Dewdney JM, Wheeler AW. A comparison of the amounts and the antigenicity of polymeric materials formed in aqueous solution by some β-lactam antibiotics. Immunology 1971;21:527-33.
93. Szebeni J, Muggia FM, Alving CR. Complement activation by Cremophor EL as a possible contributor to hypersensitivity to paclitaxel: an in vitro study. J Natl Cancer Inst 1998;90: 300-6.
94. Burrows JA, Nissen LM, Kirkpatrick CM, Bell SC. Beta-lactam allergy in adults with cystic fibrosis. J Cyst Fibros 2007;6:297-303.
95. Floris-Moore MA, Amodio-Groton MI, Catalano MT. Adverse reactions to trimethoprim/sulfamethoxazole in AIDS. Ann Pharmacother 2003;37:1810-3.
96. Idsoe O, Guthe T, Willcox RR, de Weck AL. Nature and extent of penicillin side-reactions, with particular reference to fatalities from anaphylactic shock. Bull World Health Organ 1968;38:159-88.
97. Adkinson NF Jr, Mardiney M, Wheeler B. Natural history of IgE dependent drug sensitivities. J Allergy Clin Immunol 1986;77:65-69.
98. Sogn DD, Evans R III, Shepherd GM, et al. Results of the National Institute of Allergy and Infectious Diseases Collaborative Clinical Trial to test the predictive value of skin testing with major and minor penicillin derivatives in hospitalized adults. Arch Intern Med 1992; 152:1025-32.
99. Gadde J, Spence M, Wheeler B, Adkinson NF Jr. Clinical experience with penicillin skin testing in a large inner-city STD clinic. JAMA 1993;270:2456-63.
100. Kurtz KM, Beatty TL, Adkinson NF Jr. Evidence for familial aggregation of immunologic drug reactions. J Allergy Clin Immunol 2000; 105:184-5.
101. Sullivan TJ. Management of patients allergic to antimicrobial drugs. Allergy Proc 1992;12: 361-4.
102. Attaway NJ, Jasin HM, Sullivan TJ. Familial drug allergy. J Allergy Clin Immunol 1991;87: 227.
103. Sullivan TJ, Ong R, Gilliam LK. Studies of the multiple drug allergy syndrome. J Allergy Clin Immunol 1989;83:270.
104. Kamada MM, Twarog F, Leung DY. Multiple antibiotic sensitivity in a pediatric population. Allergy Proc 1991;12:347-50.
105. Daubner B, Groux-Keller M, Hausmann OV, et al. Multiple drug hypersensitivity: normal Treg cell function but enhanced in vivo activation of drug-specific T cells. Allergy 2011;67: 58-66.
106. Phillips EJ, Chung WH, Mockenhaupt M, Roujeau JC, Mallal SA. Drug hypersensitivity: pharmacogenetics and clinical syndromes. J Allergy Clin Immunol 2011;127(Suppl): S60-6.
107. Mallal S, Phillips E, Carosi G, et al. PREDICT-1 Study Team. HLA-B*5701 screening for hypersensitivity to abacavir. N Engl J Med 2008;358: 568-79.

Nonallergic Drug Hypersensitivity Reactions

108. Schabelman E, Witting M. The relationship of radiocontrast, iodine, and seafood allergies: a medical myth exposed. J Emerg Med 2010;39: 701-7.
109. Stellato C, de Crescenzo G, Patella V, et al. Human basophil/mast cell releasability: XI. Heterogeneity of the effects of contrast media on mediator release. J Allergy Clin Immunol 1996;97:838-50.
110. Brockow K, Ring J. Classification and pathophysiology of radiocontrast media hypersensitivity. Chem Immunol Allergy 2010;95:157-69.
111. Stellato C, Adkinson NF Jr. Pathophysiology of contrast media anaphylactoid reactions: new perspectives on an old problem. Allergy 1998; 53:1111-3.
112. Brockow K, Romano A, Aberer W, et al. European Network of Drug Allergy and the EAACI interest group on drug hypersensitivity. Skin testing in patients with hypersensitivity reactions to iodinated contrast media: a European multicenter study. Allergy 2009;64:234-41.
113. Tramèr MR, von Elm E, Loubeyre P, Hauser C. Pharmacological prevention of serious anaphylactic reactions due to iodinated contrast media: systematic review. BMJ 2006;333:675.
114. Lerch M, Keller M, Britschgi M, et al. Cross-reactivity patterns of T cells specific for iodinated contrast media. J Allergy Clin Immunol 2007;119:1529-36.
115. Kowalski ML, Makowska JS, Blanca M, et al. Hypersensitivity to nonsteroidal anti-inflammatory drugs (NSAIDs)—classification, diagnosis and management: review of the EAACI/ENDA(#) and GA2LEN/HANNA*. Allergy 2011;66:818-29.
116. Orasch CE, Helbling A, Zanni MP, et al. T-cell reaction to local anaesthetics: relationship to angioedema and urticaria after subcutaneous application—patch testing and LTT in patients with adverse reaction to local anaesthetics. Clin Exp Allergy 1999;29:1549-54.
117. Ring J, Franz R, Brockow K. Anaphylactic reactions to local anesthetics. Chem Immunol Allergy 2010;95:190-200.
118. Harboe T, Guttormsen AB, Aarebrot S, et al. Suspected allergy to local anaesthetics: follow-up in 135 cases. Acta Anaesthesiol Scand 2010;54:536-42.
119. Fuzier R, Lapeyre-Mestre M, Mertes PM, et al. French Association of Regional Pharmacovigilance Centers. Immediate- and delayed-type allergic reactions to amide local anesthetics: clinical features and skin testing. Pharmacoepidemiol Drug Saf 2009;18:595-601.
120. Lee C, Gianos M, Klaustermeyer WB. Diagnosis and management of hypersensitivity reactions related to common cancer chemotherapy agents. Ann Allergy Asthma Immunol 2009; 102:179-87.
121. Syrigou E, Makrilia N, Koti I, Saif MW, Syrigos KN. Hypersensitivity reactions to antineoplastic agents: an overview. Anticancer Drugs 2009;20:1-6.
122. Hong DI, Bankova L, Cahill KN, Kyin T, Castells MC. Allergy to monoclonal antibodies: cutting-edge desensitization methods for cutting-edge therapies. Expert Rev Clin Immunol 2012;8:43-52.
123. Puxeddu I, Giori L, Rocchi V, et al. Hypersensitivity reactions during treatment with infliximab, etanercept, and adalimumab. Ann Allergy Asthma Immunol 2012;108:123-4.
124. Commins SP, Kelly LA, Rönmark E, et al. Galactose-α-1,3-galactose-specific IgE is associated with anaphylaxis but not asthma. Am J Respir Crit Care Med 2012;185:723-30.
125. Brennan PJ, Rodriguez Bouza T, et al. Hypersensitivity reactions to mAbs: 105 desensitizations in 23 patients, from evaluation to treatment. J Allergy Clin Immunol 2009;124: 1259-66.

Diagnosis of Drug Allergy

126. Lammintausta K, Kortekangas-Savolainen O. Oral challenge in patients with suspected cutaneous adverse drug reactions: findings in 784 patients during a 25-year-period. Acta Derm Venereol 2005;85:491-6.
127. Messaad D, Sahla H, Benahmed S, et al. Drug provocation tests in patients with a history suggesting an immediate drug hypersensitivity reaction. Ann Intern Med 2004;140:1001-6.
128. Aberer W, Bircher A, Romano A, et al. European Network for Drug Allergy (ENDA); EAACI interest group on drug hypersensitivity. Drug provocation testing in the diagnosis of drug hypersensitivity reactions: general considerations. Allergy 2003;58:854-63.
129. Brockow K, Romano A, Blanca M, et al. General considerations for skin test procedures in the diagnosis of drug hypersensitivity. Allergy 2002;57:45-51.
130. Kränke B, Aberer W. Skin testing for IgE-mediated drug allergy. Immunol Allergy Clin North Am 2009;29:503-16.
131. Salkind AR, Cuddy PG, Foxworth JW. The rational clinical examination: is this patient allergic to penicillin? An evidence-based analysis of the likelihood of penicillin allergy. JAMA 2001;285:2498-505.
132. Pichichero ME, Pichichero DM. Diagnosis of penicillin, amoxicillin, and cephalosporin allergy: reliability of examination assessed by skin testing and oral challenge. J Pediatr 1998;132:137-43.

133. Macy E, Richter PK, Falkoff R, Zeiger R. Skin testing with penicilloate and penilloate prepared by an improved method: amoxicillin oral challenge in patients with negative skin test responses to penicillin reagents. J Allergy Clin Immunol 1997;100:586-91.
134. Levine BB, Zolov DM. Prediction of penicillin allergy by immunological tests. J Allergy 1969; 43:231-44.
135. Parker PJ, Parrinello JT, Condemi J, Rosenfeld SI. Penicillin resensitization among hospitalized patients. J Allergy Clin Immunol 1991;88: 213-7.
136. Blanca M, Romano A, Torres MJ, et al. Update on the evaluation of hypersensitivity reactions to beta-lactams. Allergy 2009;64:183-93.
137. Torres MJ, Romano A, Mayorga C, et al. Diagnostic evaluation of a large group of patients with immediate allergy to penicillins: the role of skin testing. Allergy 2001;56:850-6.
138. Macy E. The clinical evaluation of penicillin allergy: what is necessary, sufficient and safe given the materials currently available? Clin Exp Allergy 2011;41:1498-501.
139. Antunez C, Blanca-Lopez N, Torres MJ, et al. Immediate allergic reactions to cephalosporins: evaluation of cross-reactivity with a panel of penicillins and cephalosporins. J Allergy Clin Immunol 2006;117:404-10.
140. Romano A, Gueant-Rodriguez RM, Viola M, et al. Diagnosing immediate reactions to cephalosporins. Clin Exp Allergy 2005;35: 1234-42.
141. Empedrad R, Darter AL, Earl HS, Gruchalla RS. Nonirritating intradermal skin test concentrations for commonly prescribed antibiotics. J Allergy Clin Immunol 2003;112: 629-30.
142. Macy E. Current sulfamethoxazole skin test reagents fail to predict recurrent adverse reactions. J Allergy Clin Immunol 1995;95:121.
143. Gruchalla RS, Sullivan TJ. Detection of human IgE to sulfamethoxazole by skin testing with sulfamethoxazoly poly-L-tyrosine. J Allergy Clin Immunol 1991;88:784-92.
144. Weiss ME, Chatham F, Kagey-Sobotka A, Adkinson NF Jr. Serial immunological investigations in a patient who had a life-threatening reaction to intravenous protamine. Clin Exp Allergy 1990;20:713-20.
145. Rozieres A, Vocanson M, Saïd BB, Nosbaum A, Nicolas JF. Role of T cells in nonimmediate allergic drug reactions. Curr Opin Allergy Clin Immunol 2009;9:305-10.
146. Torres MJ, Mayorga C, Blanca M. Nonimmediate allergic reactions induced by drugs: pathogenesis and diagnostic tests. J Investig Allergol Clin Immunol 2009;1:80-90.
147. Romano A, Blanca M, Torres MJ, et al. ENDA, EAACI. Diagnosis of nonimmediate reactions to beta-lactam antibiotics. Allergy 2004;59: 1153-60.
148. Waton J, Pouget-Jasson C, Loos-Ayav C, et al. Drug re-challenges in cutaneous adverse drug reactions: information and effectiveness in the long-term management of patients. Allergy 2011;66:941-7.
149. Adkinson NF Jr. Tests for immunological reactions to drugs and occupational allergens. In: Rose NR, Conway de Macario E, Folds JD, et al, editors. Manual of clinical laboratory immunology. Washington, D.C.: American Society of Microbiology; 1997. p. 893.
150. Fontaine C, Mayorga C, Bousquet PJ, et al. Relevance of the determination of serum-specific IgE antibodies in the diagnosis of immediate beta-lactam allergy. Allergy 2007; 62:47-52.
151. Blanca M, Mayorga C, Torres MJ, et al. Clinical evaluation of Pharmacia CAP System RAST FEIA amoxicilloyl and benzylpenicilloyl in patients with penicillin allergy. Allergy 2001; 56:862-70.
152. Joint Task Force on Practice Parameters; American Academy of Allergy, Asthma and Immunology; American College of Allergy, Asthma and Immunology; Joint Council of Allergy, Asthma and Immunology. Drug allergy: an updated practice parameter. Ann Allergy Asthma Immunol 2010;105:259-73.
153. Manfredi M, Severino M, Testi S, et al. Detection of specific IgE to quinolones. J Allergy Clin Immunol 2004;113:155-60.
154. Ebo DG, Venemalm L, Bridts CH, et al. Immunoglobulin E antibodies to rocuronium: a new diagnostic tool. Anesthesiology 2007;107: 253-9.
155. Leysen J, Sabato V, Verweij MM, et al. The basophil activation test in the diagnosis of immediate drug hypersensitivity. Expert Rev Clin Immunol 2011;7:349-55.
156. Kvedariene V, Kamey S, Ryckwaert Y, et al. Diagnosis of neuromuscular blocking agent hypersensitivity reactions using cytofluorimetric analysis of basophils. Allergy 2006;61: 311-5.
157. Sanz ML, Gamboa PM, Antépara I, et al. Flow cytometric basophil activation test by detection of CD63 expression in patients with immediate-type reactions to betalactam antibiotics. Clin Exp Allergy 2002;32:277-86.
158. Pinnobphun P, Buranapraditkun S, Kampitak T, Hirankarn N, Klaewsongkram J. The diagnostic value of basophil activation test in patients with an immediate hypersensitivity reaction to radiocontrast media. Ann Allergy Asthma Immunol 2011;106:387-93.
159. Celik GE, Schroeder JT, Hamilton RG, Saini SS, Adkinson NF. Effect of in vitro aspirin stimulation on basophils in patients with aspirin-exacerbated respiratory disease. Clin Exp Allergy 2009;39:1522-31.
160. Sanz ML, Gamboa P, de Weck AL. A new combined test with flow cytometric basophil activation and determination of sulfidoleukotrienes is useful for in vitro diagnosis of hypersensitivity to aspirin and other nonsteroidal anti-inflammatory drugs. Int Arch Allergy Immunol 2005;136:58-72.
161. Lin RY, Schwartz LB, Curry A, et al. Histamine and tryptase levels in patients with acute allergic reactions: an emergency department-based study. J Allergy Clin Immunol 2000;106:65-71.
162. Schwartz LB, Metcalfe DD, Miller JS, et al. Tryptase levels as an indicator of mast cell activation in systemic anaphylaxis and mastocytosis. N Engl J Med 1987;316:1622-6.
163. Porebski G, Gschwend-Zawodniak A, Pichler WJ. In vitro diagnosis of T cell-mediated drug allergy. Clin Exp Allergy 2011;41:461-70.
164. Nyfeler B, Pichler WJ. The lymphocyte transformation test for the diagnosis of drug allergy: sensitivity and specificity. Clin Exp Allergy 1997;27:175-81.
165. Sachs B, Erdmann S, Malte BJ, et al. Determination of interleukin-5 secretion from drug-specific activated ex vivo peripheral blood mononuclear cells as a test system for the in vitro detection of drug sensitization. Clin Exp Allergy 2002;32:736-44.
166. Szebeni J. Complement activation-related pseudoallergy caused by liposomes, micellar carriers of intravenous drugs, and radiocontrast agents. Crit Rev Ther Drug Carrier Syst 2001;18:567-606.

Management of Drug Allergy

167. Letko E, Papaliodis DN, Papaliodis GN, et al. Stevens-Johnson syndrome and toxic epidermal necrolysis: a review of the literature. Ann Allergy Asthma Immunol 2005;94:419-36.
168. Li JT, Markus PJ, Osmon DR, et al. Reduction of vancomycin use in orthopedic patients with a history of antibiotic allergy. Mayo Clin Proc 2000;75:902-6.
169. Knowles S, Shapiro L, Shear NH. Should celecoxib be contraindicated in patients who are allergic to sulfonamides? Revisiting the meaning of "sulfa" allergy. Drug Saf 2001;24: 239-47.
170. Schlienger RG, Shear NH. Antiepileptic drug hypersensitivity syndrome. Epilepsia 1998; 39(Suppl. 7):3-7.
171. Patriarca G, Schiavino D, Lombardo C, et al. Tolerability of aztreonam in patients with IgE-mediated hypersensitivity to beta-lactams. Int J Immunopathol Pharmacol 2008;21: 375-9.
172. Cernadas JR, Brockow K, Romano A, et al. European Network of Drug Allergy and the EAACI interest group on drug hypersensitivity. General considerations on rapid desensitization for drug hypersensitivity: a consensus statement. Allergy 2010;65:1357-66.
173. Wendel GD, Stark BJ, Jamison RB, Molina RD, Sullivan TJ. Penicillin allergy and desensitization in serious infections during pregnancy. N Engl J Med 1985;312:1229-32.
174. Macy E. Penicillin skin testing in pregnant women with a history of penicillin allergy and group B streptococcus colonization. Ann Allergy Asthma Immunol 2006;97:164-8.
175. Naclerio R, Mizrahi EA, Adkinson NF Jr. Immunologic observations during desensitization and maintenance of clinical tolerance to penicillin. J Allergy Clin Immunol 1983;71: 294-301.
176. Sobotka AK, Dembo M, Goldstein B, Lichtenstein LM, et al. Antigen-specific desensitization of human basophils. J Immunol 1979;122:511-7.
177. Sullivan TJ. Antigen-specific desensitization of patients allergic to penicillin. J Allergy Clin Immunol 1982;69:500-8.
178. MacGlashan D Jr, Lichtenstein LM. Basic characteristics of human lung mast cell desensitization. J Immunol 1987;139:501-5.
179. Stark BJ, Earl HS, Gross GN, et al. Acute and chronic desensitization of penicillin-allergic patients using oral penicillin. J Allergy Clin Immunol 1987;79:523-32.
180. Castells MC, Tennant NM, Sloane DE, et al. Hypersensitivity reactions to chemotherapy: outcomes and safety of rapid desensitization in 413 cases. J Allergy Clin Immunol 2008;122: 574-80.
181. Patterson R, Roberts M, Grammer LC. Insulin allergy: re-evaluation after two decades. Ann Allergy 1990;64:459-62.
182. Smith RM, Iwamoto GK, Richerson HB, Flaherty JP. Trimethoprim-sulfamethoxazole desensitization in the acquired immunodeficiency syndrome. Ann Intern Med 1987;106: 335.
183. Absar N, Daneshvar H, Beall G. Desensitization to trimethoprim/sulfamethoxazole in HIV-infected patients. J Allergy Clin Immunol 1994;93:1001-5.

184. Stroup JS, Stephens JR, Reust R, Miller JA. Adverse reactions associated with dapsone therapy in HIV-positive patients: a case presentation and review. AIDS Read 2006;16:47-8.
185. Turvey SE, Cronin B, Arnold AD, Dioun AF. Antibiotic desensitization for the allergic patient: 5 years of experience and practice. Ann Allergy Asthma Immunol 2004;92:426-32.
186. Burrows JA, Toon M, Bell SC. Antibiotic desensitization in adults with cystic fibrosis. Respirology 2003;8:359-64.
187. Legere HJ 3rd, Palis RI, Rodriguez Bouza T, Uluer AZ, Castells MC. A safe protocol for rapid desensitization in patients with cystic fibrosis and antibiotic hypersensitivity. J Cyst Fibros 2009;8:418-24.
188. Purdy BH, Philips DM, Summers RW. Desensitization to sulfasalazine skin rash. Ann Intern Med 1984;100:512-4.
189. Wilson DL, Owens RC Jr, Zuckerman JB. Successful meropenem desensitization in a patient with cystic fibrosis. Ann Pharmacother 2003;37:1424-8.
190. Win PH, Brown H, Zankar A, Ballas ZK, Hussain I. Rapid intravenous cephalosporin desensitization. J Allergy Clin Immunol 2005;116:225-8.
191. Wong IC, Mawer GE, Sander JW. Factors influencing the incidence of lamotrigine-related skin rash. Ann Pharmacother 1999;33:1037-42.
192. Campbell KL, Cohn JR, Fischman DL, et al. Management of clopidogrel hypersensitivity without drug interruption. Am J Cardiol 2011;107:812-6.
193. Greenberger PA, Patterson GA, Radin RC. Two pretreatment regimens for high-risk patients receiving radiographic contrast media. J Allergy Clin Immunol 1984;74:540-3.
194. Wolf E, Blankenburg M, Bogner JR, et al. Cost impact of prospective HLA-B*5701-screening prior to abacavir/lamivudine fixed dose combination use in Germany. Eur J Med Res 2010;15:145-51.
195. Nieves Calatrava D, Calle-Martín Ode L, et al. Cost-effectiveness analysis of HLA-B*5701 typing in the prevention of hypersensitivity to abacavir in HIV+ patients in Spain. Enferm Infec Microbiol Clin 2010;28:590-5.

80 Hypersensitivity to Aspirin and Other Nonsteroidal Antiinflammatory Drugs

HAE-SIM PARK | MAREK L. KOWALSKI | MARIO SANCHEZ-BORGES

CONTENTS

SUMMARY OF IMPORTANT CONCEPTS

» Nonsteroidal antiinflammatory drugs (NSAIDs) can induce various clinical manifestations of hypersensitivity reactions. A classification to distinguish these acute processes from delayed-type reactions has been proposed, in which two phenotypes, aspirin-exacerbated respiratory disease (AERD) and aspirin-exacerbated cutaneous disease (AECD), are the most common.

» The major pathogenetic mechanisms are inhibition of cyclooxygenase 1 (COX-1) with reduction of prostaglandin E_2 (PGE_2) levels, leading to overproduction of cysteinyl leukotrienes and activation of inflammatory cells.

» To confirm the diagnosis, provocation testing performed using inhalation or the oral route remains the gold standard; in vitro diagnostic methods are still not available.

» Avoidance of cross-reacting NSAIDs with use of alternative analgesics is essential. Pharmacologic treatment should follow standard asthma, rhinitis, and urticaria guidelines according to symptom severity. Aspirin desensitization can be done when indicated.

» Delayed-type reactions to NSAIDs, including fixed drug eruptions, maculopapular eruption, contact dermatitis, and severe cutaneous adverse reactions, are rare. Such reactions are mediated by the T cell response.

Introduction and Historical Note

An adverse reaction to aspirin was first reported by Hirschberg[1] in 1902. Samter and Beers[2] further characterized this association in a large group of patients, and since then, the pattern of clinical manifestations has been variously designated the acetylsalicylic acid (ASA) triad, aspirin-intolerant asthma, or Samter disease. Szczeklik and Stevenson[3] developed aspirin desensitization protocols. The pathomechanisms of aspirin-intolerant asthma were described by Szczeklik[4] in 1990, based on the cyclooxygenase theory.

Classification

Various terms, including *sensitivity, pseudoallergy, idiosyncrasy,* and *intolerance,* have been used to describe type B adverse reactions to nonsteroidal antiinflammatory drugs (NSAIDs),[3] but the designation *hypersensitivity* seems to be the most appropriate. NSAIDs can induce a wide range of hypersensitivity reactions with variable clinical course and symptomatology and driven by differing immunologic and nonimmunologic mechanisms. Szczeklik and Stevenson[3] proposed a classification system of NSAID-induced reactions based on the clinical spectrum of symptoms, presence or absence of underlying diseases, and observed cross-reactivity between various NSAIDs. More recently, this classification was modified by the EAACI/GA^{2}LEN (European Academy of Allergology and Clinical Immunology/Global Allergy and Asthma European Network) Task Force, which proposed to clearly distinguish acute from delayed-type reactions.[5] Acute hypersensitivity reactions are further divided into the cross-reactive type (manifesting as either respiratory or skin symptoms), involving nonimmunologic mechanisms, and single drug–induced reactions (manifesting as urticaria-angioedema or anaphylaxis), which are putatively immunoglobulin E (IgE)-mediated. Delayed-type reactions exhibit various organ or systemic manifestations and are predominantly T cell–mediated (Table 80-1).

Cross-Reactive Nonsteroidal Antiinflammatory Drug Hypersensitivity

ASPIRIN-EXACERBATED RESPIRATORY DISEASE

Definition

In a subpopulation of asthmatic patients, aspirin as well as other NSAIDs may induce hypersensitivity reactions manifested primarily as acute dyspnea and usually accompanied by nasal symptoms (rhinorrhea and/or nasal congestion). These patients present with a typical "ASA triad," which includes chronic rhinosinusitis complicated by polyp formation, moderate to severe bronchial asthma, and hypersensitivity reactions occurring in response to aspirin and also to other cross-reacting NSAIDs.[3,5] The most remarkable feature of these reactions is the presence of eosinophilic inflammation of unknown etiology in both the lower and upper airway mucosa, only occasionally exacerbated by NSAIDs. Several terms have been used to describe this distinct clinical syndrome: *the aspirin triad, Widal syndrome, Samter disease, aspirin-induced* or *aspirin-sensitive asthma,* and

TABLE 80-1 Classification of Nonsteroidal Antiinflammatory Drug (NSAID) Hypersensitivity Reactions

Timing of Reaction	Clinical Manifestation	Type of Reaction	Underlying Disease	Putative Mechanism
Acute (immediate to several hours after exposure)	Rhinitis/asthma (AERD)	Cross-reactive	Asthma/rhinosinusitis	COX-1 inhibition
	Urticaria/angioedema (AECD)	Cross-reactive	Chronic urticaria	COX-1 inhibition
	Urticaria/angioedema	Multiple NSAID–induced	No underlying chronic diseases	Unknown, probably COX-1 inhibition
	Urticaria/angioedema/ anaphylaxis	Single drug–induced	Atopy Food allergy Drug allergy	IgE-mediated
Delayed-type (more than 24 hours after exposure)	Various organs involved		Usually none	Type IV delayed-type Cytotoxic T cells, NK cells, other

Modified from Kowalski ML, Makowska JS, Blanca M, et al. Hypersensitivity to nonsteroidal anti-inflammatory drugs (NSAIDs)—classification, diagnosis and management: review of the EAACI/ENDA(#) and GA²LEN/HANNA. Allergy 2011;66:818-29.*

AECD, Aspirin-exacerbated cutaneous disease; *AERD*, aspirin-exacerbated respiratory disease; *COX-1*, cyclooxygenase 1; *IgE*, immunoglobulin E; *NK*, natural killer.

aspirin-sensitive rhinosinusitis/asthma syndrome. More recently, the term *aspirin-exacerbated respiratory disease* (AERD) has been used to emphasize the chronicity of the disorder and the fact that the core issue in these patients is not ASA hypersensitivity but the underlying chronic inflammatory respiratory disease. In some patients with hyperplastic rhinosinusitis and polyps (but without bronchial asthma), the hypersensitivity to NSAIDs may manifest exclusively in the upper respiratory tract (as acute rhinorrhea and nasal congestion).[6] In this subpopulation, the mechanism of the disease seems to be identical to that in the ASA triad, and in some patients, the disease may evolve over time into the full aspirin triad, including chronic bronchial asthma and a bronchial reaction to aspirin.

Epidemiology

The true prevalence of respiratory-type ASA hypersensitivity cannot be assessed accurately, because it varies depending on the diagnostic method and patient factors including gender, age, and other characteristics. It is generally believed that this syndrome remains widely underdiagnosed. The overall incidence of ASA hypersensitivity among adult asthmatics, if assessed by history alone, ranges from 4.3% to 12% in various populations.[7,8] When aspirin hypersensitivity was assessed by oral provocation, however, the incidence increased to 21.1%, as documented in a systematic review of 15 studies.[9]

The prevalence of NSAID hypersensitivity seems to increase with increasing severity of the underlying disorder. For example, in patients admitted to the ICU with a severe asthmatic attack, the prevalence of ASA hypersensitivity may be as high as 14% to 24%.[10] The prevalence of ASA hypersensitivity has been reported to be 30% to 40% in patients with chronic rhinosinusitis and/or nasal polyps.[11] In children with asthma, the prevalence of ASA hypersensitivity was lower than in adults, approximating 1% to 3% when determined by history alone and close to 5% in asthmatic children subjected to oral provocation.[9] Gender also seems to be a predisposing factor: The condition affects more women than men in most populations by a ratio of 3:2.

Pathogenesis

The pathogenesis of AERD involves two separate but probably closely related mechanisms.[12] The first is the mechanism underlying ASA-induced acute respiratory reactions, which are the hallmark of this syndrome (although they may be only an occasional event, sometimes occurring once in a lifetime); the second is the mechanism of development of chronic intractable inflammation of the lower and upper airway mucosa, which is present even in the absence of exposure to NSAIDs and underlies the chronicity of the disease.

Pathogenetic Mechanisms of Acetylsalicylic Acid/Nonsteroidal Antiinflammatory Drug–Induced Acute Respiratory Reactions. Immunologic mechanisms of ASA-triggered hypersensitivity reactions in asthmatic patients were excluded based on the lack of detectable drug-specific immunoglobulins or sensitized T cells. Subsequent to the original observation that only NSAIDs that are strong, or at least moderate, inhibitors of prostaglandin synthesis can evoke reactions in ASA-hypersensitive patients, Szczeklik and colleagues[4] attributed the mechanism to the pharmacologic properties of these drugs and proposed a *cyclooxygenase hypothesis* to explain the phenomenon.

Cyclooxygenase Hypothesis. According to the cyclooxygenase hypothesis, inhibition of cyclooxygenase type 1 (COX-1), the enzyme that metabolizes arachidonic acid to prostaglandins, thromboxane, and prostacyclins, would lead to decreased generation of protective PGE_2, activation of inflammatory cells, release of inflammatory mediators (predominantly, but not exclusively, cysteinyl leukotrienes), and finally to bronchial or nasal symptoms[3,4,13] (Fig. 80-1). This hypothesis is based on the observation that NSAIDs with strong COX-1 inhibitory activity precipitate adverse symptoms in a significant proportion of ASA-hypersensitive patients (ranging from 30% to 80%), whereas weak (e.g., salicylic acid or acetaminophen), and selective COX-2 inhibitors usually are well tolerated by these patients.[3] In support of this theory, a local deficiency in PGE_2 synthesis has been found in nasal polyp epithelial cells and bronchial fibroblasts, and less consistently in peripheral blood leukocytes, from patients with AERD, suggesting decreased PGE_2 regulatory capacity that may be exaggerated after inhibition by NSAIDs.[14,15] Furthermore, inhalation of PGE_2 or oral pretreatment with misoprostol (a synthetic PGE_2 analog) prevents ASA-induced bronchoconstriction, suggesting a protective role for PGE_2 in this reaction.[16]

Mediators Involved in Aspirin-Induced Respiratory Reactions. ASA-induced reactions are associated with the release of

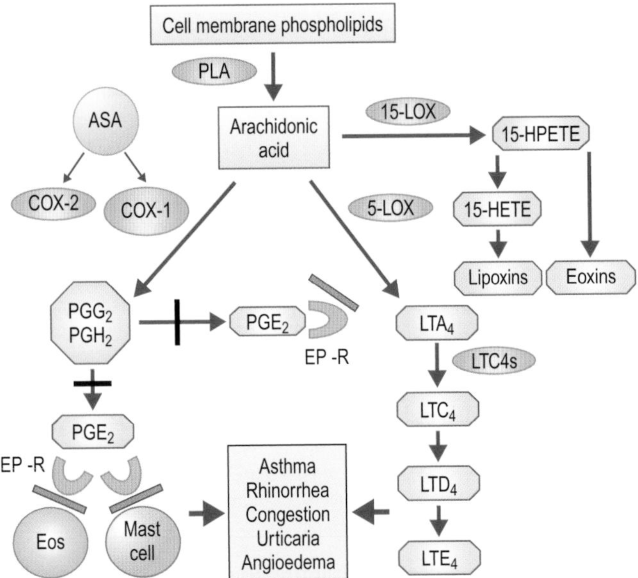

Figure 80-1 Pathomechanisms of cross-reactivity–based hypersensitivity to nonsteroidal antiinflammatory drugs (NSAIDs)—aspirin-exacerbated airway disease and aspirin-exacerbated cutaneous disease—according to the "cyclooxygenase hypothesis." In patients with NSAID hypersensitivity, PGE_2 acting via prostaglandin EP receptors (*EP-R*) is responsible for stabilization of inflammatory cells, mainly mast cells and eosinophils (*Eos*) and 5-lipoxygenase (*5-LOX*). Inhibition of cyclooxygenase (COX)-1 by aspirin/NSAIDs deprives the system of stabilizing activity of PGE_2, leading to activation of inflammatory cells and 5-LOX. Mediators released from inflammatory cells, including cysteinyl-leukotrienes, are responible for development of symptoms. The role of 15-LOX pathway activation leading to generation of 15-HETE, lipoxins, and eoxins is not clear, and the mechanism may be either proinflammatory or modulatory. *ASA,* Acetylsalicylic acid [aspirin]; *15-HETE,* 15-hydroxyeicosatetranoic acid; *15-HPETE,* hydroxyperoxyeicosatetranoic acid; *15-LOX,* 15-lipoxygenase; *LTA_4,* leukotriene A_4; *LTC_4,* leukotriene C_4; *LTD_4,* leukotriene D_4; *LTE_4,* leukotriene E_4; *PGE_2,* prostaglandin E_2; *PGG_2,* prostaglandin G_2; *PGH_2,* prostaglandin H_2; *PLA,* phospholipase. *(Reproduced and modified from Kowalski ML. Diagnosis of aspirin sensitivity in aspirin-exacerbated respiratory disease. In: Pawankar R, Holgate ST, Rosenwasser LJ, editors. Allergy frontiers: diagnosis and health economics. New York: Springer; 2009, p. 349-72.)*

both mast cell– (tryptase, histamine, PGD_2) and eosinophil-specific mediators such as eosinophil cationic protein (ECP) into nasal washes, clearly indicating activation of both types of cells.[17,18] Similarly, concentrations of PGD_2 metabolite from mast cell increase in urine after aspirin challenge.[13] Of interest, the mobilization of eosinophil progenitor cells from bone marrow has been reported for up to 20 hours after aspirin bronchial challenge.[19] The acute reaction is release of cysteinyl leukotrienes into nasal secretions[20] or induced sputum[21]; increased leukotriene metabolites also are present in the urine.[13] In vitro specific activation of the 15-LO pathway and increased generation of 15-hydroxyeicosatetranoic acid (15-HETE) from epithelial cells and leukocytes also have been demonstrated.[22]

Pathogenesis of Chronic Inflammation in the Airways

Inflammatory Cells and Cytokines. Increased severity of asthma, rhinosinusitis, and nasal polyposis in patients with AERD seems to be reflected in a characteristic airway inflammatory profile. A high degree of tissue eosinophilia and increased ECP release are prominent features of mucosal inflammation in the upper and lower airways of patients with AERD.[23,24] Tissue eosinophilia has been linked to a distinctive profile of cytokine expression, with upregulation of several cytokines related to eosinophil activation and survival (e.g., interleukin [IL]-5, granulocyte-macrophage colony-stimulating factor [GM-CSF], RANTES [regulated on activation, normal T cell expressed], eotaxins) in the airway mucosa,[25,26] in which overproduction of IL-5 might be a major factor responsible for increased eosinophil survival, resulting in increased eosinophilic inflammation in patients with AERD. Mast cells also are abundant in the upper and lower airway mucosae of these patients. In nasal polyp tissue, the density of mast cells and concentrations of presumably mast cell–derived stem cell factor (SCF) were correlated with the number of polypectomies, implicating these cells in the pathogenesis of nasal polyposis in patients with AERD.[27] A distinct T cell–derived cytokine expression profile, elevated IL-5 protein concentrations, and significantly greater numbers of $CD45RO^+$ cells (which are considered to be activated T cells with memory or effector functions) were found in nasal polyps, suggesting an important role for activated T cells in perpetuating the inflammatory response in patients with AERD.[28] Whether similarly distinct patterns of T cells and cytokines are present in the lower airways of ASA-hypersensitive subjects remains to be investigated.

Arachidonic Acid Metabolites. The most distinctive feature of the airway inflammation in patients with AERD is the presence of several baseline abnormalities of arachidonic acid metabolism (Table 80-2).

Prostaglandin E_2 Deficiency. Significantly reduced generation of PGE_2 by nasal polyps and nasal polyp epithelial cells as well as bronchial fibroblasts has been documented.[14] In view of the significant antiinflammatory activity of PGE_2, including inhibition of eosinophil chemotaxis and activation, it may be speculated that an intrinsic defect in local PGE_2 generation may contribute to the development of more severe eosinophilic inflammation in ASA-sensitive patients. Consistent with this proposal, reduced expression of COX-2 mRNA in nasal polyps of these patients was inversely correlated with PGE_2 generation and positively correlated with leukotriene production.[29] The data with regard to COX expression in the lower airways showed decreased COX-2 mRNA levels and diminished COX-1 expression in bronchial epithelial cells from patients with AERD.[30]

Overproduction of Leukotrienes. Although basal levels of leukotriene metabolites in the urine of patients with AERD are several-fold higher than in ASA-tolerant asthmatics, even in the absence of aspirin challenge,[13,31] concentrations of cysteinyl leukotrienes were found to be similar in bronchoalveolar lavage fluid from ASA-sensitive and -tolerant subjects,[32] but were significantly higher in the saliva, induced sputum, and exhaled breath air of patients with AERD.[33] A greater number of cells expressing leukotriene C_4 synthase (LTC_4S), an enzyme involved in the transformation of arachidonic acid to cysteinyl leukotrienes, were found in the bronchi of ASA-hypersensitive asthmatic patients, with significantly higher LTC_4S expression in mast cells than in eosinophils.[34] More recently, Perez-Novo and coworkers[29] found increased generation of the leukotrienes LTC_4, LTD_4, and LTE_4 and overexpression of enzymes involved in the production of leukotrienes (5-LOX and LTC_4 synthase) in nasal polyp tissue from patients with AERD, but the production of cysteinyl leukotrienes was correlated with the tissue ECP concentration in both AERD and ASA-tolerant polyps. These observations suggest that the increased basal levels of cysteinyl leukotrienes may be linked to increased tissue eosinophil (and

TABLE 80-2 Arachidonic Acid Metabolism Abnormalities in Patients with Aspirin-Exacerbated Respiratory Disease

Abnormality	PBMC	Urine	Exhaled Air	Saliva	Tissue
Decreased production of PGE_2	±	—	—	—	NPEC± BF+
Decreased expression of PGE_2 receptors	—	—	—	—	NP±
Decreased expression of COX-2	No	—	—	—	NP± BEC+
Increased generation of cysteinyl leukotrienes	±	+	±	+	NP±
Increased expression of Cys-LT1 receptors	—	—	—	—	NP+
Increased LTC_4 synthase expression	+	—	—	—	BM+ NP+
Increased 5-LO expression	—	—	—	—	NPEC+
Decreased lipoxin generation	±	—	—	—	NPEC+

BEC, Bronchial epithelial cells; *BF*, bronchial fibroblasts; *BM*, bronchial mucosa; *5-LO*, 5-lipoxygenase; *LTC_4*, leukotriene C_4; *NP*, nasal polyps; *NPEC*, nasal polyp epithelial cells; *PBMC*, peripheral blood mononuclear cells; PGE_2, prostaglandin E_2; +, documented; ±, not conclusive; —, not relevant or information not available.

possibly mast cell) numbers in patients with AERD rather than to distinct mechanisms of chronic inflammation. Along these lines, it has been suggested that increased leukotrienuria is associated with the presence and intensity of chronic hyperplastic rhinosinusitis and polyposis in both AERD and ASA-tolerant patients.[35] A significant decrease in urinary leukotrienes following nasal sinus surgery indicates that urinary leukotrienes may reflect an overall increase in the number of leukotriene-producing cells (mostly eosinophils) in different tissues, rather than real overproduction within target organs. On the other hand, in support of a special role for leukotriene pathways in patients with AERD, increased expression of type 1 cysteinyl leukotriene receptor (CysLTR1) was found in the nasal mucosa of these patients, suggesting local hyperresponsiveness to leukotrienes.[36] The role of cysteinyl leukotrienes and their receptors in the pathogenesis of chronic mucosal inflammation in ASA sensitivity needs further investigation, because chronic treatment with CysLTR1 antagonists does not more effectively relieve nasal and bronchial symptoms or reduce polyp size in ASA-hypersensitive than it does in ASA-tolerant patients.[37]

15-Lipoxygenase Pathways. Other arachidonic acid metabolites generated by the 15-LOX pathway have been associated with chronic inflammation in ASA-sensitive patients. Production of lipoxin A_4 (LXA_4), an antiinflammatory derivative of arachidonic acid generated by transcellular metabolism involving cooperation of 5-LO and 15-LO, was significantly lower in peripheral blood leukocytes from asthmatic patients with AERD.[38] In addition, decreased production of lipoxin A4 and upregulation of 15-lipoxygenase were noted in nasal polyp tissue from patients with AERD, pointing to a distinct, but not yet understood, role for 15-LO metabolites in this clinical entity.[29,38] These data suggest a role for eicosanoids in the pathogenesis of chronic eosinophilic inflammation in the lower and upper airways of patients with AERD. The specificity of these abnormalities in arachidonic acid metabolism for AERD, however, remains to be established.

Environmental Triggers. The pathogenesis of persistent eosinophilic inflammation of the airway mucosa in AERD is not related to intake of aspirin or other NSAIDs, because in most patients, the airway disease precedes, sometimes by years, the development of hypersensitivity to ASA. Moreover, in already hypersensitive patients, even complete avoidance of NSAIDs does not lead to clinical improvement. The fact that cross-reactive respiratory-type hypersensitivity reactions to ASA do not occur in healthy persons without rhinosinusitis/asthma (i.e., without underlying airway inflammation) suggests that the presence of chronic inflammation may be a prerequisite for hypersensitivity. Putative viral factors have been proposed as both primary triggers of ASA hypersensitivity and a cause of the underlying chronic inflammation in the airways of patients with AERD. This hypothesis is supported by the observation that human rhinovirus mRNA transcripts were detected in bronchial epithelial cells from 100% of patients with AERD but only 73% of ASA-tolerant patients with well-controlled asthma.[39]

A role for a specific immune response to *Staphylococcus* enterotoxin in perpetuating chronic eosinophilic inflammation in the airways of patients with AERD also has been suggested. IgE antibodies to staphylococcal enterotoxins (SEAs) were more abundant in the nasal polyp tissue of patients with AERD, and their concentration was correlated with ECP, eotaxin, and IL-5 levels.[40] However, higher levels of serum specific IgE to staphylococcal superantigen was observed in AERD patients.[41] From a clinical perspective, an important point is that a significant proportion of patients with AERD had atopy and high total IgE level: IgE-mediated mechanisms may therefore also contribute to the chronicity of inflammation in some patients with AERD.

Genetic Mechanisms

Much effort has in recent years been devoted to investigating the genetic mechanisms of AERD. A candidate gene approach was used in most studies; however, ethnic differences were found that require further clarification. The human leukocyte antigen (HLA) allele DPB1*0301 has been identified as a strong genetic marker for AERD in a Polish and a Korean population,[42] in which the prevalence of this allele was significantly higher in persons with AERD than in control groups. Patients with this allele showed typical clinical characteristics of AERD, including lower forced expiratory volume in 1 second (FEV_1) and a very high prevalence of rhinosinusitis with nasal polyps,[42] as previously noted in a Polish population.[43]

Genetic polymorphism studies of AERD have focused on two lines of inquiry[43]: (1) leukotriene- and prostanoid-related genes including the lipoxygenase (LOX) pathway and the type 1 and type 2 cysteinyl leukotriene receptors, CysLTR1 and CysLTR2, and (2) eosinophil-related genes, including *CRTH2* and *CCR3*—the latter because intense eosinophil infiltration into the upper and lower airways is a key feature of AERD. Inhibition of COX in the respiratory tract by aspirin alters arachidonic acid metabolism, leading to increased production of cysteinyl leukotrienes[4] and reduced PGE_2. AERD has also been shown to be correlated with increased cysteinyl leukotriene receptor expression; increased CysLTR1 expression was detected in the nasal mucosa.[36] It was proposed that the third cysteinyl leukotriene receptor, G protein–coupled receptor 17 (GPR17), purinergic receptor (P2Y)-like receptor, is involved in cysteinyl leukotriene–related airway inflammation and eosinophil activation.[44] Moreover, COX pathway metabolite receptors, including the E prostanoids 2 and 4 (EP2 and EP4), and thromboxane A_2 receptor (TBXA2R), may be involved in the pathogenesis of AERD. Regarding the LOX pathway, 15-lipoxygenase (15-LO), a LOX family member, is a potential candidate because it catalyzes the conversion of arachidonic acid to 15-hydroxyperoxyeicosatetranoic acid (15-HPETE) and 15-hydroxyeicosatetranoic acid (15-HETE), a more stable derivative of 15-HPETE.[15] The results of the genetic polymorphism studies published in recent years are summarized in Table 80-3.

Leukotriene- and Prostanoid-Related Genes. Initial investigations focused on genes involved in the synthetic pathway of cysteinyl leukotrienes, because the C allele of the *LTC4S* −444A>C promoter polymorphism was identified as a risk factor for AERD in a Polish population.[45] However, these findings were not replicated in Japanese, American, or Korean populations. Recently, three SNPs (−634C>T, −475A>C, and −336A>G) in the promoter region of *CysLTR1* were identified; mutant variants of these were associated with the AERD phenotype[46] and with increased expression of *CysLTR1* in peripheral mononuclear cells in a Korean population. Additionally, a study performed in a Korean population showed that the frequencies of the rare −819T>G, 2078C>T, and 2534A>G alleles of *CysLTR2* were significantly higher in the AERD group, a phenomenon also noted in white and Japanese populations. Alleles of the 5-LO gene *ALOX5* at −1708G>A, 21C>T, 270G>A, 1728G>A, and *ALOX5*-activating protein (*ALOX5AP*, 218 A>G) were studied in a Korean population. The haplotype *ALOX5* ht1 [G-C-G-A] was significantly more common in the AERD group than in control groups, suggesting a possible contribution of *ALOX5* to AERD.[43] Regarding prostanoid and COX-related genes, a COX-2 promoter polymorphism at −765G>C was identified in a Polish population[47]; this was significantly associated with sex, atopy, and increased prostaglandin production in patients with AERD.

Sixty-three candidate genes were investigated in a Japanese population.[48] The functional SNP (μS5) located in the regulatory region of the *EP2* gene, was associated with risk of AERD by reducing transcription activity, leading to reduced PGE_2-protecting mechanism of inflammation. PGE_2 receptor subtype 3 (*PTGER3*) may be an important genetic factor for aspirin hypersensitivity in Korean asthmatic patients.[43]

Eosinophil-Related Genes. Several candidate genetic polymorphisms related to eosinophil activation have been reported in a Korean population. The *CRTH2* −466T>C polymorphism of the chemoattractant receptor molecule expressed in Th2 cells could increase serum and cellular eotaxin-2 production by lowering *CRTH2* expression in patients with AERD, leading to eosinophilic infiltration.[49] The chemokine CC motif receptor (CCR3) has been described as key for eosinophil migration. The frequency of variant genotypes of *CCR3* at −520T>C was

TABLE 80-3 Genetic Mechanisms of Aspirin-Exacerbated Respiratory Disease

Gene	SNP(s)	Clinical Phenotype	Mechanism
LTC4S	−444A>C	High genotype frequency of C allele compared with A allele	C allele may be the risk allele owing to overproduction of cys-LTs
CYSLTR1	−634C>T, −475A>C, −336A>G	ht2(TCG) showed higher frequency in AERD and higher promoter activity	Higher *CysLTR1* mRNA expression may be responsible for pathogenesis
CYSLTR2	—	Frequencies of rare allele increased in AERD, with decrease in FEV_1 after aspirin provocation	Elevation of cys-LT production
CRTH2	—	−466T allele had higher frequency in AERD and increased serum and cellular eotaxin-2 production and lower mRNA expression	−466T allele may be the risk allele by activation of eosinophils
CCR3	−520T>C	Frequencies of rare genotypes were higher in AERD, and −520G allele showed higher promoter activity	Higher mRNA expression of CCR3 may cause eosinophil activation
MS4A2R	E237G	FcER1b −109T allele had higher frequency and high promoter activity	Increased mRNA expression of −109T allele may cause mast cell activation mediated by MS4A2R receptor
ACE	−262A>T, −115T>C	Frequencies of the rare alleles were higher in AERD; −262T had lower promoter activity; and reduction in FEV_1 was seen after aspirin provocation	Downregulation of ACE expression
IL4	−589T>C	The frequency of rare alleles was higher in AERD; −589C had enhanced promoter and transcriptional activity induced by aspirin	Enhanced IL-4 activity with aspirin exposure

ACE, Angiotensin-converting enzyme; *AERD*, aspirin-exacerbated respiratory disease; *cys-LT*, cysteinyl leukotriene; *FEV_1*, forced expiratory volume in 1 second; *IL-4*, interleukin-4; *mRNA*, messenger ribonucleic acid.

reported to be significantly higher in patients with AERD in whom mRNA expression was significantly increased after ASA provocation.[50] IL-13 polymorphisms at −1510A>C and −1055C>T are associated with the development of rhinosinusitis in patients with AERD. *IL-13 Arg110Gln* may be associated with an increase in the eosinophil count and eotaxin-1 level, leading to an increase in eosinophilic inflammation in the upper and lower airways of patients with AERD.[43]

Genome-wide association studies (GWASs) have recently emerged as a technology that can predict genetic variations associated with human diseases and clinical responses to drug treatment. Such studies suggested that the nonsynonymous *CEP68* rs 7572857G>A variant, which replaces glycine with serine, exhibits a greater decline in FEV_1 consequent to aspirin provocation than do other variants. This gene may thus be related to AERD susceptibility. Gly74Ser also may affect the polarity of the protein structure.[51] AERD often produces a moderate to severe disease phenotype; however, diagnosis based on molecular genetic information is challenging, and replication studies in different ethnic groups will be essential to validate the data and apply this knowledge in clinical practice.

Clinical Features

The clinical presentation in AERD is one of moderate to severe asthma with chronic persistent rhinosinusitis with nasal polyps; intense eosinophil infiltrations are found in the upper and lower airway mucosae.[52] In these patients, NSAIDs induce respiratory symptoms, which may be accompanied by ocular, cutaneous (flushing, urticaria, and/or angioedema), or gastric symptoms. AERD may develop according to a distinctive pattern characterized by a natural sequence of symptoms: first, persistent rhinosinusitis, commonly with polyposis, followed by asthma, and then aspirin hypersensitivity, as described in two large studies involving European[5] and American[53] patients. Nasal symptoms appear by middle age and then progress to a chronic rhinosinusitis, often with nasal polyposis. Asthma usually is diagnosed a few years later. The "classic" adverse reaction to aspirin consists of bronchospasm of variable severity, usually accompanied by rhinitis symptoms and ocular injection. In some patients, these are combined with chronic urticaria with or without angioedema and/or anaphylaxis. Nausea and stomach pain occur only occasionally.

NSAID hypersensitivity not only is a significant risk factor for development of severe chronic asthma but is also strongly associated with near-fatal asthma. In the TENOR study, 459 adult subjects with AERD were compared with 2824 aspirin-tolerant asthmatic patients.[54] The former had significantly lower mean postbronchodilator percent predicted FEV_1 and were more likely to have had episodes of severe asthma and tracheal intubation, to have required a steroid burst in the previous 3 months, and to be using high-dose inhaled corticosteroids.

AERD usually is accompanied by significant blood, nasal, and sputum eosinophilia. Bronchial biopsies reveal eosinophil infiltration and increased numbers of IL-5–positive cells, although serum IL-5 levels remain within the normal range. Positive reaction to at least one aeroallergen on skin-prick testing was present in 34% to 64% of patients in a European cohort.[5] Atopy in adult patients with AERD is less common.[52]

The degree of polypoid hypertrophy of the sinus mucosa and the severity of inflammation is more extensive in patients with AERD than in ASA-tolerant individuals.[23,26,53] Most patients suffer from severe nasal obstruction, postnasal drainage, and anosmia. Loss of smell usually indicates development of nasal polyposis extensive enough to alter odor detection. Chronic hyperplastic eosinophilic sinusitis with nasal polyposis is responsible for an average of five to six sinus infections per year.[5] Nasal polyps characteristically undergo rapid regrowth, resulting in an average of three sinus surgeries or polypectomies per patient.[53]

Diagnosis

The diagnosis of ASA hypersensitivity is based on a history of adverse reactions precipitated by ASA or other NSAIDs. Some patients have a definitive history of adverse reactions to ASA and NSAIDs; however, 50% do not.[52] In patients without a clear history, challenge tests are necessary to confirm or exclude hypersensitivity.[5,52]

Challenge Tests. Most patients demonstrate positive responses to methacholine bronchial challenge tests. There are four types of aspirin-provocation tests: oral, inhalation (bronchial), nasal, and intravenous.[55,56] The diagnosis of AERD can be definitively established only through aspirin-provocation challenges. Oral, inhalation, and intravenous aspirin challenges in asthmatic patients should be carried out in a hospital setting under the direct supervision of a physician experienced in the performance of such testing. Emergency resuscitative equipment should be readily available. Patients should have an open intravenous line in place, and asthma should be stable. Baseline FEV_1 should be at least 70% of the predicted value. Aspirin challenge in asthmatic patients ideally should be preceded by a placebo challenge. Before any challenges, withdrawal of several types of antiasthma drugs is indicated: short-acting β_2-agonists and ipratropium bromide, 6 hours (8 hours if possible); long-acting β_2-agonists, long-acting theophylline, and tiotropium bromide, 24 hours (48 hours if possible); short-acting antihistamines, 3 days; cromolyn sodium (sodium cromoglycate), 8 hours; nedocromil sodium, 24 hours; and leukotriene modifiers, at least 1 week.[56] Performance of oral and inhalation challenges in patients with unstable asthma or an FEV_1 lower than 70% of the predicted value or less than 1.5 L is not recommended. If regular treatment with oral corticosteroids is required, the dose should not exceed 10 mg prednisolone or equivalent. Of note, however, any therapy with oral corticosteroids must be carefully recorded, because these agents may blunt the response to aspirin. The dose of bronchial and nasal corticosteroids should be as low as possible, and levels should be kept stable throughout the challenge.

Oral Challenge Test. Controlled oral challenge with aspirin is regarded as the gold standard, a definitive means by which aspirin sensitivity can be determined. However, oral aspirin challenge, which was introduced into clinical practice in the early 1970s, is time- and labor-intensive.[55,57] The oral route mimics natural exposure, and the challenge procedure does not require special equipment, except simple spirometry (an acceptable alternative is peak expiratory flow [PEF] measurement). Various oral challenge protocols exist. In the United States, only oral aspirin challenge protocols are available (Table 80-4). In Europe, the HANNA (Hypersensitivity to Aspirin and Other NSAIDs) task force, working within the framework of the GA^{2}LEN Program, developed guidelines for standardized oral, inhalation, and nasal challenges.[56]

The oral test is carried out with increasing aspirin doses of 27, 44, 117, and 312 mg (for a cumulative dose of 500 mg),

TABLE 80-4 Single-Blind Three-Day Oral ASA Challenge for Evaluation for Aspirin-Exacerbated Respiratory Disease

Time	Day 1	Day 2	Day 3
First dose	Placebo	ASA 30 mg	ASA 100-150 mg
Second dose (after 3 hours)	Placebo	ASA 45-60 mg	ASA 150-325 mg
Third dose (after 6 hours)	Placebo	ASA 60-100 mg	ASA 325-650 mg

From Berges-Gimeno M, Simon RA, Stevenson DD. The natural history and clinical characteristics of aspirin exacerbated respiratory disease. Ann Allergy Asthma Immunol 2002;89:474-8.
ASA, Acetylsalicylic acid [aspirin].

administered at 1.5- to 2-hour intervals. If a patient with a very strong suspicion of aspirin hypersensitivity shows no reaction after the final dose (i.e., after administration of a total of 500 mg), a 500-mg aspirin dose is administered within 1.5 to 2 hours, which brings the cumulative dose to 1000 mg. If the patient has a history of a severe hypersensitivity reaction (profound dyspnea and/or anaphylactic shock), the test is commenced with 10 mg aspirin, and the next dose of 17 mg is administered 1.5 to 2 hours later—that is, the 27-mg dose is divided into two for safety reasons. The time interval between administrations of consecutive aspirin doses can be shortened to 1.5 hours without compromising patient safety. This allows most challenges to be completed in 2 days (first day, placebo challenge; second day, aspirin challenge).

After ASA exposure, FEV_1 is measured before each aspirin dose and every 30 minutes thereafter. The challenge is interrupted if FEV_1 falls to 20% of baseline or lower (a positive reaction) or if the maximum cumulative dose of aspirin (1000 mg) is reached without a fall in FEV_1 of 20% or greater and in the absence of nasoocular symptoms (a negative reaction). The test result also can be regarded as positive on appearance of unequivocal extrabronchial symptoms (e.g., severe nasal congestion, pronounced rhinorrhea). Oral challenge is preferred for investigation of extrapulmonary or systemic symptoms of aspirin hypersensitivity. The threshold dose of aspirin that provokes a 20% FEV_1 fall varies among patients and depends also on level of asthma control. In rare cases, hypersensitivity to aspirin and NSAIDs may remit over time.[57]

Bronchial Challenge Test. During inhalational (bronchial) challenge, increasing doses of lysine aspirin (soluble synthetic aspirin analog, available in Europe) are administered.[56,58] The lysine ASA bronchoprovocation test is widely used in Asia[43] and in European and other countries. A detailed standardized test protocol has been published.[56] This inhalational challenge is safer and faster to carry out than the oral test, although it is slightly less sensitive. Inhalation challenge involves administration of increasing doses of lysine aspirin using a dosimeter-controlled nebulizer every 30 minutes, with FEV_1 measurement every 10 minutes after each ASA administration (Table 80-5). The criteria for a positive response are the same as for oral aspirin challenge (greater than 20% fall of FEV_1 from the baseline value), and a dose-response curve is constructed to calculate the provocative concentration causing 20% fall in FEV1 (PC_{20}). In cases of a positive reaction, symptoms are relieved by inhalation of 2 to 4 puffs of a short-acting β_2-agonist or by nebulization of an appropriate agent (e.g., 2.5 to 5.0 mg of salbutamol) until FEV_1 returns to the baseline value. If more severe reactions occur, oral or intravenous corticosteroids are administered.

TABLE 80-5 The Lysine-ASA Bronchoprovocation Test Protocol

Conc. of L-ASA (M)	No. of Inhalations	Inhaled ASA Dose (mg)	Cumulative ASA Dose (mg)
0.1	1	0.18	0.18
0.1	2	0.36	0.54
0.1	5	0.90	1.44
0.1	13	2.34	3.78
1	4	7.20	10.98
1	9	16.2	27.18
2	11	39.60	66.78
2	32	115.20	181.98

From Nizankowska-Mogilnicka E, Bochenek G, Mastalerz L, et al. EAACI/GA^{2}LEN guideline: aspirin provocation tests for diagnosis of aspirin hypersensitivity. Allergy 2007;62:1111-8.
ASA, Acetylsalicylic acid [aspirin].

Nasal and Intravenous Aspirin Challenge. Evaluation of the response following nasal instillation of 16 mg of acetylsalicylic acid (a lysine-aspirin solution) is based on symptom scores and/or rhinomanometry and/or acoustic rhinometry or peak nasal inspiratory flow (PNIF).[56] In a newer diagnostic test, ketorolac solution (2.26 mg of ketorolac per spray) is delivered as a nasal spray in increasing doses every 30 minutes.[56a] This test offers an alternative to the lysine-aspirin nasal challenge used in Europe. Unlike the oral challenge, the nasal test is very safe and does not produce systemic reactions. It is recommended for patients with predominantly nasal symptoms and for those in whom oral or inhalation tests are contraindicated because of the severity of their asthma. Because its diagnostic sensitivity is lower than that of the other two tests, a negative result on nasal challenge should be followed, whenever possible, by an oral or inhalation test. Patients with septal perforation or important nasal blockade secondary to nasal polyposis are not suitable candidates for nasal provocation testing or rhinomanometry. Intravenous tests with lysine-aspirin, with administration of increasing doses of aspirin every 30 minutes (12.5, 25, 50, 100, 200 mg), are preferred in Japan.[59]

In Vitro Diagnostic Tests. Several in vitro tests for confirming aspirin hypersensitivity in patients with AERD have been proposed, but none is recommended at this time for routine diagnosis. Aspirin can induce LTC_4 release from the peripheral blood leukocytes (PBL) in sensitive patients, and measurement of cysteinyl leukotriene release has been used for AERD diagnosis. However, the results of these studies are inconsistent.[60]

The basophil activation test, which uses measurement of CD63 expression on in vitro challenge, has been proposed for in vitro AERD diagnosis. Its reported specificity and sensitivity vary, however, and no firm conclusions on the reliability of this test in the routine setting have been reached.[61] The measurement of aspirin-triggered 15-HETE release from PBL has been proposed; this is known as the Aspirin-Sensitive Patient Identification Test (ASPI Test),[22] but its clinical utility must first be confirmed by larger studies.

Prevention and Management

Prevention and Use of Alternative Analgesics. ASA and NSAIDs that inhibit COX-1 are popular over-the-counter drugs, so patients with asthma should be alerted by their physicians and pharmacists to the possibility of cross-reactions. Simple, standardized warnings for asthmatics on packs of aspirin and some NSAIDs should perhaps be mandated. Once diagnosed, patients with AERD should avoid aspirin and any other NSAIDs that strongly inhibit COX-1; education is therefore of utmost importance. Patients should be provided with a list of contraindicated and well-tolerated analgesics (Box 80-1). Even transdermal iontophoresis with NSAIDs can induce systemic adverse reactions, albeit rarely. Similarly, topical intraocular administration of NSAID drops may cause an asthma attack and should be avoided.

Acetaminophen, coxibs, and codeine usually are safe choices for management of acute pain in these patients. Azapropazone, choline magnesium trisalicylate, and salsalate, which are very weak inhibitors of COX-1 and COX-2, also are well tolerated by the large majority of patients with AERD. Nimesulide and meloxicam generally are well tolerated, although the small degree of residual COX-1 inhibition displayed by these compounds may be enough to trigger reactions at high doses or in highly sensitive patients (see also earlier section on cross-reactions with aspirin and NSAIDs).[5] It is prudent, therefore, to administer the first dose of these drugs in the physician's office.

BOX 80-1 NONSTEROIDAL ANTIINFLAMMATORY DRUG (NSAID) TOLERANCE IN PATIENTS WITH CROSS-REACTIVE–TYPE ASA HYPERSENSITIVITY

GROUP A: NSAIDs CROSS-REACTING IN A MAJORITY OF HYPERSENSITIVE PATIENTS (60%-100%)

Ibuprofen
Indomethacin
Sulindac
Naproxen
Fenoprofen
Meclofenamate
Ketorolac
Etololac
Diclofenac
Ketoprofen
Flurbiprofen
Piroxicam
Nabumetone
Mefenamic acid

GROUP B: NSAIDs CROSS-REACTING IN A MINORITY OF HYPERSENSITIVE PATIENTS (2%-10%)

Rhinitis/Asthma Type

Acetaminophen (at doses below 1000 mg), meloxicam, nimesulide

Urticaria/Angioedema Type

Acetaminophen, meloxicam, nimesulide
Selective COX-2 inhibitors (celecoxib, rofecoxib)

GROUP C: NSAIDs WELL TOLERATED BY MOST HYPERSENSITIVE PATIENTS

Rhinitis/Asthma Type

Selective cyclooxygenase inhibitors (celecoxib, parvocoxib, parecoxib), trisalicylate, salsalate

Urticaria/Angioedema Type

New selective COX-2 inhibitors (etoricoxib, parecoxib)

Modified from Kowalski ML, Makowska JS, Blanca M, et al. Hypersensitivity to nonsteroidal anti-inflammatory drugs (NSAIDs)—classification, diagnosis and management: review of the EAACI/ENDA(#) and GA²LEN/HANNA. Allergy 2011;66:818-29.*
ASA, Acetylsalicylic acid [aspirin]; *COX-2,* cyclooxygenase 2.

Management of Asthmatic Symptoms. In general, treatment of the asthma underlying NSAID sensitivity should follow standard asthma guidelines according to symptom severity. This type of asthma often is severe, and high doses of inhaled corticosteroids with the addition of a long-acting β_2-agonist and bursts or daily doses of oral corticosteroids often are necessary.[52]

The discovery of antileukotrienes such as zileuton (5-LO inhibitor) and montelukast, zafirlukast, pranlukast (CysLT1 receptor inhibitors) provided a new opportunity for AERD treatment, and these drugs have been widely prescribed to control upper and lower airway symptoms in this disorder. A double-blind, placebo-controlled study evaluated the clinical efficacy of 6-week treatment with zileuton in 40 patients.[62] Zileuton treatment led to improved pulmonary function, lower use of rescue bronchodilators, and a remarkable return of the patient's sense of smell. Montelukast (10 mg taken once daily for 4 weeks) in a randomized, double-blind, placebo-controlled study improved asthma control and pulmonary function (10.2% increase in FEV_1) in 80 patients.[63] In other studies, montelukast treatment attenuated nasal reactions to lysine-aspirin, improved nasal function, and diminished the requirement for oral corticosteroids.[64] Against expectations, aspirin-sensitive asthmatic patients seem not to respond better to leukotriene receptor antagonists than do aspirin-tolerant asthmatics. The success of treatment with these drugs was significantly better only in patients with AERD who were carriers of the variant C allele of LTC_4 synthase, *CYSLTR1*, and the HLA-DPB1*0301 marker.[43]

Management of Chronic Rhinosinusitis and Nasal Polyposis. Aspirin-sensitive eosinophilic rhinosinusitis is particularly difficult to treat. Standard treatment aims to reduce nasal inflammation and retard the formation of nasal polyps. It includes high doses of topical steroids, antibiotics, and occasional bursts of oral corticosteroids to control symptoms and slow down nasal polyp recurrence.[52] Most patients should use high-dose intranasal corticosteroids on a long-term basis. During acute bacterial sinus infections, extended courses of broad-spectrum antibiotics are frequently needed. Many patients require a 1- to 3-week burst of systemic corticosteroids to control their nasal symptoms ("medical polypectomy"); shrinkage of nasal polyps frequently is observed after systemic steroid treatment. Nasal and oral decongestants and antihistamines may provide additional relief. Several reports have suggested that leukotriene modifiers could improve rhinosinusitis and nasal polyps without surgery.[64] In patients with severe chronic sinusitis with multiple nasal polyps and nasal passage obstruction, surgical procedures (polypectomy, functional endoscopic sinus surgery, or ethmoidectomy) usually are needed to relieve symptoms of chronic rhinsinusitis and to remove polypoid tissue from sinuses, although patients with AERD seem to respond less well to surgical intervention.

Aspirin Desensitization. Another treatment option is chronic desensitization to aspirin.[65] Aspirin desensitization can be beneficial in some patients with AERD associated with upper and lower airway inflammation; however, it is recommended for patients with corticosteroid-dependent asthma or those requiring daily ASA/NSAID therapy for other medical conditions, including coronary artery disease or chronic arthritis. After an acute reaction (i.e., after inadvertent aspirin intake or diagnostic challenge), the refractory period develops and lasts 2 to 5 days. During this period, patients may take aspirin without any adverse symptoms. After that time, aspirin may again precipitate an adverse reaction. However, by continuing administration of aspirin each day during the refractory period and thereafter for many weeks, months, or years, this state of tolerance can be maintained. This procedure is called *desensitization.* Several desensitization protocols that allow for completing the procedure within 3 to 5 days have been proposed.[55,57]

Aspirin desensitization is induced by administering increasing doses over 2 to 3 days until a mild reaction occurs, and then slowly increasing the dose, most commonly to 650 to 1300 mg. A subsequent decrease to 325 mg twice daily after 1 to 6 months is recommended. The ASA target dose to maintain desensitization differs according to the diseases underlying the aspirin sensitivity. Recommended doses are as follows: 81 mg once per day for cardiovascular disease prevention, 325 mg once per day to maintain cross-desensitization to any dose of all NSAIDs, and 650 mg twice daily as a starting dose for desensitization of patients with AERD. Once thus desensitized, the patient can take aspirin on a daily basis indefinitely, but tolerance will disappear after 2 to 5 days without aspirin intake. The mechanism of action of aspirin desensitization has not been fully elucidated. Chronic desensitization was shown to decrease peripheral monocyte synthesis of LTB_4 to the same level as in normal control subjects. The synthesis of cysteinyl leukotrienes also was diminished, as indicated by depressed urinary LTE_4 levels. A decreased bronchial response to inhaled LTE_4 also was observed.

Stevenson's group of investigators, which has the most experience with desensitization procedures, showed a significant reduction in both upper and lower airway symptoms, improvement in the sense of smell, and reduction in purulent sinus infections, in the need for further polyp surgery, in hospitalizations, and in the requirement for systemic corticosteroids.[65] Aspirin given after desensitization may be a valuable solution for patients with AERD who require chronic treatment with aspirin for coronary heart disease or rheumatic diseases. Some patients (approximately 15% to 20%) discontinue daily ASA treatment because of side effects (usually gastritis).

In several countries, the desensitization process is used for limited indications such as coronary artery disease and rheumatologic diseases.[5,52] During the state of desensitization to aspirin, both aspirin and most strong NSAIDs are tolerated, so desensitization and NSAID maintenance could be used for treatment of rheumatic diseases or chronic pain syndrome. As a practical matter, a fraction of patients with AERD will benefit from aspirin desensitization, but at present, it is not possible to identify these patients before the procedure is implemented. Aspirin desensitization also may be useful in women suffering from antiphospholipid syndrome with a history of aspirin hypersensitivity who become pregnant or plan a new pregnancy. An oral desensitization procedure could be carried out by administering rapidly escalating aspirin doses (a starting dose of 0.1 mg increasing up to 125 mg at 15-minute intervals). Tolerance in such patients can be maintained by administration of 100 to 125 mg of ASA per day, in combination with subcutaneous low-molecular-weight heparin, throughout the pregnancy.

ASPIRIN-EXACERBATED CUTANEOUS DISEASE AND MULTIPLE NONSTEROIDAL ANTIINFLAMMATORY DRUG–INDUCED URTICARIA

Hypersensitivity reactions to ASA and NSAIDs often involve the skin and mucosal surfaces in the form of urticaria (hives) and angioedema. Three different clinical pictures can be observed, according to the type of hypersensitivity-inducing drug and a patient's individual predisposing factors. The first three types—AECD, multiple NSAID–induced urticaria, and a blended or mixed reaction—are cross-reactive, do not involve immunologic mechanisms, and manifest as urticaria and or angioedema,[5] whereas a quite distinct, fourth type seems to be IgE-mediated and manifests as acute urticaria, angioedema, and anaphylaxis induced by a single NSAID (more often associated with pyrazolones), as discussed further on.

Definition and Prevalence

Up to 35% of patients with chronic spontaneous urticaria (CSU) experience exacerbation of skin symptoms when exposed to ASA/NSAIDs. Analogous to AERD, the designation AECD has been recently proposed for this condition.[66] Acute urticaria also may develop in some patients who do not have CSU on exposure to ASA/NSAIDs. The disorder in this second group of cross-reactive patients is designated *multiple NSAID–induced urticaria.*[5]

Clinical Features

Urticaria and angioedema appear usually after 1 to 4 hours of drug ingestion, although late reactions occurring up to 24 hours after ingestion can be observed (Fig. 80-2). Either local or generalized urticaria can occur, depending on severity. When urticaria is combined with angioedema, clinical manifestations are more severe. In some serious cases, facial (periorbital) angioedema is the most common manifestation. ASA/NSAID-induced urticaria or angioedema also can develop in a second group of patients who do not have any predisposing disease. This condition is sometimes called multiple NSAID–induced urticaria or ASA-intolerant acute urticaria.[67] In some of these patients, chronic urticaria may develop subsequently; these reactions have a higher prevalence among atopic individuals.[67]

Pathogenetic Mechanisms

Inflammatory Mechanism. The mechanisms of multiple-NSAID reactions in patients without CSU are unknown at present, although it is likely that COX-1 inhibition is involved. Most patients with ASA-induced urticaria and angioedema have reactions to various NSAIDs, which have in common their

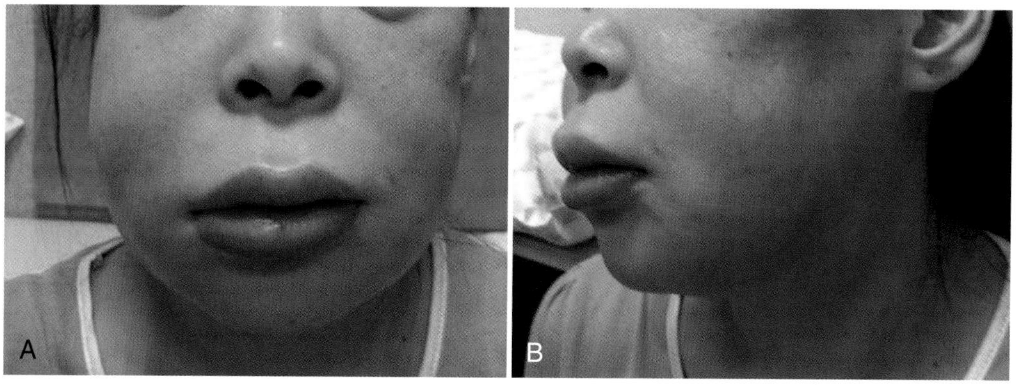

Figure 80-2 Lip angioedema induced by diclofenac in a 30-year-old woman with chronic spontaneous urticaria and angioedema.

ability to inhibit COX-1. Subjects with CSU and NSAID intolerance have increased levels of basal urinary LTE_4 when compared with patients with CSU who are tolerant to aspirin. Furthermore, increases of urinary LTE_4 occur in the first group after oral aspirin challenge.[68]

The inhibition of COX-1 by NSAIDs results in decreased prostaglandin production, enhanced inflammatory mediator release in the skin, and production of clinical symptoms. Increased cysteinyl-leukotriene production contributes to the inflammatory process, as suggested by the ability to inhibit these reactions by leukotriene receptor antagonists.[69] Patients with CSU and NSAID intolerance also exhibit, with high frequency, positive results on autologous serum and plasma skin tests, which would suggest an association among CSU, autoimmunity, and aspirin hypersensitivity. In a comparison of the clinical parameters and inflammatory markers between multiple NSAID–induced urticaria and AECD, no significant differences were found between the two phenotypes. However, the neutrophil activation marker serum myeloperoxidase was present in higher concentration in multiple NSAID–induced urticaria than in AECD, indicating that neutrophil activation may be involved in multiple NSAID–induced urticaria.[70]

Genetic Mechanisms. A few HLA alleles were suggested as potential genetic markers for multiple NSAID–induced urticaria and AECD. Most genetic polymorphism studies have focused on leukotriene synthesis or mast cell– and histamine-related genes. Neutrophil-related genes have been potential targets for multiple NSAID–induced urticaria.[67] The C allele in the LTC_4 −444A>C promoter polymorphism was reported to be a risk factor for aspirin-intolerant urticaria in a Venezuelan population,[71] a finding that has not been replicated in other populations. The frequency of the high-affinity IgE receptor FCER1A at −344T was significantly higher in patients with AECD than in the control group,[67,72] which was not replicated in a Polish population. The genetic polymorphism at *FCER1G* −237G was significantly associated with atopic status and basophil histamine releasability in patients with AECD. Although no significant associations were found between the two histamine receptor genes, *HRH1* and *HRH2,* the histamine *N*-methyl transferase (HNMT) 939A>C polymorphism was associated with the AECD phenotype by regulation of enzymatic activity and histamine release from peripheral basophils.[67] Regarding a neutrophil activation–related gene, the promoter polymorphism of *ADORA3* at −1050 G/T was found to be associated with the phenotype of aspirin-intolerant urticaria, in which the ht1 [TC] haplotype transcript was found to be associated with increased basophil histamine releasability.[67]

Diagnosis

Clinical history suggests the diagnosis of AECD and multiple NSAID–induced urticaria. Patients should be classified according to whether they have underlying CSU, which is exacerbated by aspirin or other NSAIDs, or whether they have acute urticaria, which develops only on exposure to ASA/NSAIDs. Atopy is a predisposing factor for both multiple NSAID–induced urticaria and AECD,[9] and the allergy skin-prick test or specific IgE screening to common inhalant allergens is recommended to identify atopy status and evaluate the patient for any associated allergic diseases. Reliable in vitro tests for the diagnosis of multiple NSAID–induced urticaria and AECD are not available; however, several serologic tests for the evaluation of chronic urticaria, such as thyroid autoimmunity testing and use of viral markers, are indicated for screening. The confirmative diagnosis can be established only by oral challenge tests,[73,74] and such standardized tests have recently been described.[56] Cross-reactivity with other NSAIDs should be determined. Some patients have had cross-reactivity with a wide spectrum of COX-1 inhibitors and with the highly selected COX-2 inhibitors.[5]

Prevention and Management

Patients with CSU who experience exacerbations of cutaneous symptoms after taking COX-1 inhibitors should avoid all strong inhibitors of COX-1, and it is recommended that acetaminophen or COX-2 inhibitors be prescribed for pain, fever, and inflammation. Some of these patients, however, may show wheals or angioedema from these alternative medications, especially if higher doses are taken. In patients with NSAID-induced urticaria who do not have CSU, the history of acute reactions to more than one COX-1 inhibitor is highly suggestive of NSAID cross-hypersensitivity. A confirmatory oral challenge is therefore recommended, and if the result is positive, avoidance of all COX-1 inhibitors is advisable. This step is followed by a second challenge with an alternative non–COX-1 inhibitor NSAID, as depicted in Figure 80-3.

After confirmation of sensitivity, ASA and all drugs that inhibit COX-1 or sometimes COX-2 should be avoided in patients who already have experienced AECD and multiple NSAID-induced urticaria.[7] All patients with CSU should be

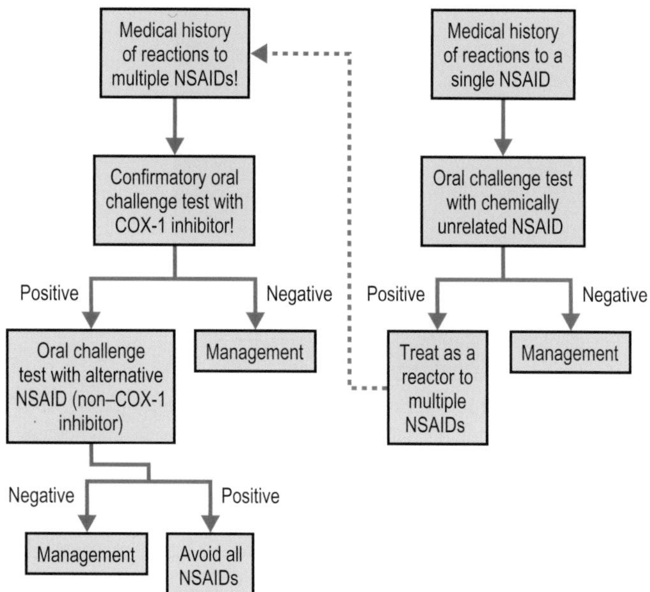

Figure 80-3 Algorithm for the management of patients with urticaria, angioedema, and anaphylaxis induced by nonsteroidal antiinflammatory drugs (NSAIDs). *COX-1,* Cyclooxygenase 1.

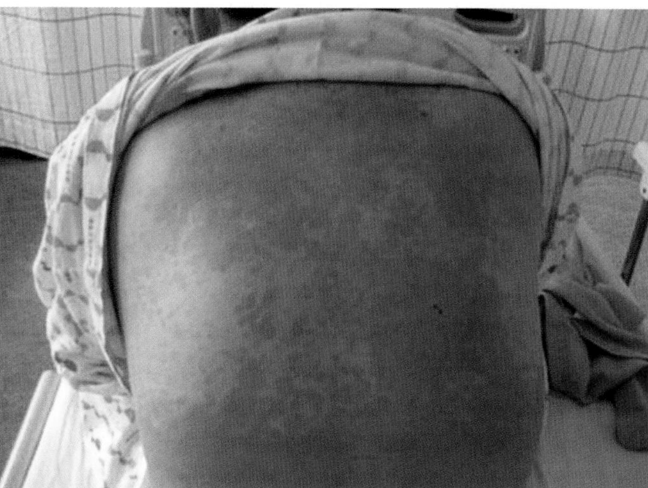

Figure 80-4 Ibuprofen-induced maculopapular exanthema, seen on the back, in a 35-year-old woman.

educated to pay attention to whether NSAIDs affect their propensity for or severity of hives. For the treatment of AECD, maintenance treatment based on stepwise doses of antihistamines should be done according to the current guidelines.[73,74] The clinical course and symptoms are more severe than in CSU without ASA hypersensitivity; in some cases, immunomodulators, leukotriene modifiers, and anti-IgE therapy may be needed. A successful desensitization to both conditions has not been reported.[74]

Allergic (or Immunologically Mediated) Types of Nonsteroidal Antiinflammatory Drug Hypersensitivity

ACUTE SINGLE NONSTEROIDAL ANTIINFLAMMATORY DRUG–INDUCED REACTION

Some patients may show hypersensitivity to a single NSAID. Serum-specific IgE antibodies specific for the drug have been detected, as has been demonstrated for pyrazolones.[75] In that study, however, specific IgE antibodies to other NSAIDs were not detected in the sera of the patient. A history of urticaria, angioedema, and anaphylaxis triggered by a single NSAID should be confirmed by means of an oral challenge with the causative NSAID and a second, chemically unrelated NSAID in the hospital, under controlled conditions and with careful medical supervision. If the reaction is positive, the patient should be managed as a "cross-reactor" (see Fig. 80-3). Strict avoidance of the culprit and potentially cross-reactive chemically similar compounds should be recommended. Use of alternative NSAIDs can be proposed but should be preceded by an oral challenge to confirm tolerance.[5] Desensitization to aspirin in patients with this type of cutaneous reaction and anaphylaxis is not recommended at present.

DELAYED HYPERSENSITIVITY REACTIONS TO NONSTEROIDAL ANTIINFLAMMATORY DRUGS

Definition

Delayed or nonimmediate reactions involving the skin and other organs develop more than 6 hours after drug administration. Symptoms usually emerge several days to weeks after initiation of a new drug; however, they may develop earlier when induced by reintroduction of the drug. The recovery period lasts from several days to weeks. The most common clinical presentations of this delayed hypersensitivity include fixed drug eruptions (FDEs), maculopapular exanthemas (MPEs), contact dermatitis, photosensitivity, and, less frequently, severe drug eruptions, such as Stevens-Johnson syndrome (SJS), toxic epidermal necrolysis (TEN), drug-induced hypersensitivity syndrome (DIHS), and acute generalized exanthematous pustulosis (AGEP). Organ-specific allergic diseases such as NSAID-induced pneumonitis, aseptic meningitis, and nephritis also may occur.[76,77]

Clinical Features

Fixed Drug Eruptions. Approximately 10% of all drug reactions are FDEs, in which lesions recur at the same anatomic location every time the drug is reintroduced, usually on the lips, hands, genitalia, and oral mucosa. NSAIDs are involved in about 30% of all cases. Pyrazolones, piroxicam, phenylbutazone, paracetamol, aspirin, mefenamic acid, diclofenac, indomethacin, ibuprofen, diflunisal, naproxen, and nimesulide have been associated with FDE.

Maculopapular Eruptions. Maculopapular or morbilliform exanthemas are among the most common drug eruptions. They are characterized by erythematous macules and infiltrated papules, mainly involving the trunk and proximal extremities (Fig. 80-4). Ibuprofen, pyrazolones, flurbiprofen, diclofenac, and celecoxib have been most frequently implicated. According to some studies, NSAIDs induce between 9% and 17% of all cases of MPE.

Contact and Photocontact Dermatitis. Localized itchy and erythematous lesions are occasionally observed with topical use

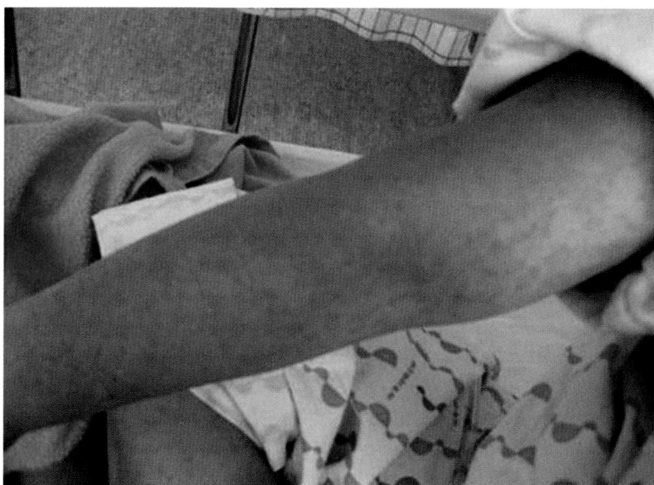

Figure 80-5 Contact dermatitis induced by etofenamate 10% gel seen on the arm of a 37-year-old woman.

of NSAIDs such as diclofenac, aceclofenac, indomethacin, flurbiprofen, bufexamac, etofenamate, flufenamic acid, ibuprofen, ketoprofen, and mefenamic acid (Fig. 80-5). Cross-reactivity among chemically related NSAIDs has been reported. Severe cutaneous reactions may develop in patients sensitized to a topical NSAID with the systemic use of the same drug, a clinical picture designated *systemic contact dermatitis.*

Severe Bullous Cutaneous Reactions. SJS and TEN are severe drug reactions characterized by fever and generalized erythematous macules or a diffuse erythema involving the trunk and extremities. These lesions evolve to necrotic bullae and epidermal detachment. SJS involves less than 10%, whereas TEN involves more than 30% of epidermal detachment. Oxicams, phenylbutazone, and oxyphenbutazone are the most common offenders. In one study, NSAIDs, including naproxen, paracetamol, aspirin, and ketoprofen, were the most common causative agents in severe cutaneous reactions.[34] More recently, an association of SJS and TEN with use of the sulfonamide COX-2 inhibitors valdecoxib and celecoxib has been described.

Drug-Induced Hypersensitivity Syndrome. DIHS is characterized by severe eruption, fever, lymphadenopathy, hepatitis, and hematologic abnormalities, along with eosinophilia and atypical lymphocytes. NSAIDs are rarely involved, but among those agents, ibuprofen is the most commonly reported.

Acute Generalized Exanthematous Granulomatosis. AGEP manifests with nonfollicular sterile pustules on a diffuse, edematous erythema predominantly involving the skin folds or the face. Fever and neutrophilia are common findings. It has been rarely reported with ibuprofen, nimesulide, celecoxib, etoricoxib, valdecoxib, metamizol, and paracetamol.

Pathogenesis

Delayed reactions to NSAIDs are mediated by type IV immunologic reactions with the participation of drug-specific cytotoxic T cells. Pichler described four subtypes of cellular reactions—IVa, IVb, IVc, and IVd—whereby different subsets of T cells and various cytokines are predominantly involved in the effector phase of the reaction.

Diagnosis

The diagnosis of delayed reactions to NSAIDs is based on compatible clinical features that include symptoms and morphology and distribution of lesions. Confirmatory tests include in vivo tests, such as intradermal and patch tests and drug provocation tests, and in vitro tests. Patch tests with the suspected drug are useful but have not been well standardized. Photopatch tests are indicated when photosensitivity is suspected. Skin biopsy is useful for differential diagnosis in some cases. The lymphocyte transformation test with drugs has been proposed for the diagnosis of nonimmediate reactions to NSAIDs but has not been validated. Oral drug provocation tests, although useful in mild cases, are contraindicated in patients who have experienced severe reactions.

Management

Patient management is based on prompt withdrawal of the culprit drug, supportive care, and symptomatic treatment with corticosteroids and antihistamines. Patients with SJS or TEN should be treated in the intensive care unit. In those diseases, the use of parenteral corticosteroids, plasmapheresis, intravenous immunoglobulins, and immunosuppressive agents is controversial. Anti-tumor necrosis factor-α therapy with infliximab has been proposed.[78] The search for an alternative NSAID belonging to a different chemical group for use under medical supervision is recommended. ASA desensitization has not been applied in cases of delayed reactions to NSAIDs.

REFERENCES

Introduction and Historical Note

1. Hirschberg [VGS]. Mitteilungübereinen Fall von Nebenwirkung des Aspirin. Dtsch Med Wochenschr 1902;28:416.
2. Samter M, Beers RF. Concerning the nature of intolerance to aspirin. J Allergy 1967;40: 281-93.
3. Szczeklik A, Stevenson DD. Aspirin-induced asthma: advances in pathogenesis, diagnosis, and management. J Allergy Clin Immunol 2003; 111:913-21.

Classification

4. Szczeklik A. The cyclooxygenase theory of aspirin-induced asthma. Eur Respir J 1990;3: 588-93.
5. Kowalski ML, Makowska JS, Blanca M, et al. Hypersensitivity to nonsteroidal antiinflammatory drugs (NSAIDs)—classification, diagnosis and management: review of the EAACI/ENDA(#) and GA^{2}LEN/HANNA*. Allergy 2011; 66:818-29.

Cross-Reactive Nonsteroidal Antiinflammatory Drug Hypersensitivity

6. Lumry WR, Curd JG, Zeiger RS. Aspirin-sensitive rhinosinusitis: the clinical syndrome and effects of aspirin administration. J Allergy Clin Immunol 1983;71:580-7.
7. Kasper L, Sladek K, Duplaga M, et al. Prevalence of asthma with aspirin hypersensitivity in the adult population of Poland. Allergy 2003;58: 1064-6.
8. Vally H, Taylor ML, Thompson PJ. The prevalence of aspirin intolerant asthma (AIA) in Australian asthmatic patients. Thorax 2002;57: 569-74.
9. Jenkins C, Costello J, Hodge L. Systematic review of prevalence of aspirin induced asthma and its implications for clinical practice. BMJ 2004;328:434.
10. Marquette CH, Saulnier F, Leroy O, et al. Long-term prognosis of near-fatal asthma. A 6-year follow-up study of 145 asthmatic patients who underwent mechanical ventilation for a near-fatal attack of asthma. Am Rev Respir Dis 1992; 146:76-81.
11. Settipane GA. Nasal polyps. Epidemiology, pathology, immunology, and treatment. Am J Rhinol 1987;1:119-26.

12. Farooque SP, Lee TH. Aspirin-sensitive respiratory disease. Annu Rev Physiol 2009;71:465-87.
13. Higashi N, Mita H, Ono E, et al. Profile of eicosanoid generation in aspirin-intolerant asthma and anaphylaxis assessed by new biomarkers. J Allergy Clin Immunol 2010;125:1084-91.
14. Kowalski ML, Pawliczak R, Woźniak J, et al. Differential metabolism of arachidonic acid in nasal polyp epithelial cells cultured from aspirin-sensitive and aspirin-tolerant patients. Am J Respir Crit Care Med 2000;161:391-8.
15. Kowalski ML, Ptasinska A, Bienkiewicz B, et al. Differential effects of aspirin and misoprostol on 15-hydroxyeicosatetraenoic acid generation by leukocytes from aspirin-sensitive asthmatic patients. J Allergy Clin Immunol 2003;112:505-12.
16. Szczeklik A, Mastalerz L, Nizankowska E, et al. Protective and bronchodilator effects of PGE_2 and salbutamol in aspirin-induced asthma. Am J Respir Crit Care Med 1996;153:567-71.
17. Fischer AR, Rosenberg MA, Lilly CM. Direct evidence for role of the mast cell in the nasal response to aspirin in aspirin-sensitive asthma. J Allergy Clin Immunol 1994;94:1046-56.
18. Nasser S, Christie PE, Pfister R, et al. Effect of endobronchial aspirin challenge on inflammatory cells in bronchial biopsy samples from aspirin-sensitive asthmatic subjects. Thorax 1996;51:64-70.
19. Makowska JS, Grzegorczyk J, Bienkiewicz B, et al. Systemic responses after bronchial aspirin challenge in sensitive patients with asthma. J Allergy Clin Immunol 2008;121:348-54.
20. Picado C, Ramis I, Rosellò J, et al. Release of peptide leukotrienes into nasal secretions after local instillation of aspirin in sensitive asthmatic patients. Am Rev Respir Dis 1992;145:65-9.
21. Obase Y, Shimoda T, Tomari SY, et al. Effects of pranlukast on chemical mediators in induced sputum on provocation tests in atopic and aspirin-intolerant asthmatic patients. Chest 2002;121:143-50.
22. Kowalski ML, Ptasinska A, Jedrzejczak M, et al. Aspirin-triggered 15-HETE generation in peripheral blood leukocytes is a specific and sensitive Aspirin-Sensitive Patient Identification Test (ASPITest). Allergy 2005;60:1139-45.
23. Adamjee J, Suh YJ, Park HS, et al. Expression of 5-lipoxygenase and cyclooxygenase pathway enzymes in nasal polyps of patients with aspirin-intolerant asthma. J Pathol 2006;209:392-9.
24. Nasser SM, Pfister R, Christie PE, et al. Inflammatory cell populations in bronchial biopsies from aspirin-sensitive asthmatic subjects. Am J Respir Crit Care Med 1996;153:90-6.
25. Sousa AR, Lams BE, Pfister R, et al. Expression of interleukin-5 and granulocyte-macrophage colony-stimulating factor in aspirin-sensitive and non-aspirin-sensitive asthmatic airways. Am J Respir Crit Care Med 1997;156:1384-9.
26. Pods R, Ross D, van Hulst S, et al. RANTES, eotaxin and eotaxin-2 expression and production in patients with aspirin triad. Allergy 2003;58:1165-70.
27. Kowalski ML, Lewandowska-Polak A, Wozniak J, et al. Association of stem cell factor expression in nasal polyp epithelial cells with aspirin sensitivity and asthma. Allergy 2005;60:631-7.
28. Hamilos DL, Leung DY, Huston DP, et al. GM-CSF, IL-5 and RANTES immunoreactivity and mRNA expression in chronic hyperplastic sinusitis with nasal polyposis. Clin Exp Allergy 1998;28:1145-52.
29. Perez-Novo CA, Watelet JB, Claeys C, et al. Prostaglandin, leukotriene, and lipoxin balance in chronic rhinosinusitis with and without nasal polyposis. J Allergy Clin Immunol 2005;115:1189-96.
30. Pierzchalska M, Soja J, Woś M, et al. Deficiency of cyclooxygenases transcripts in cultured primary bronchial epithelial cells of aspirin-sensitive asthmatics. J Physiol Pharmacol 2007;58:207-18.
31. Kumlin M, Dahlén B, Björck T, et al. Urinary excretion of leukotriene E4 and 11-dehydro-thromboxane B2 in response to bronchial provocations with allergen, aspirin, leukotriene D4, and histamine in asthmatics. Am Rev Respir Dis 1992;146:96-103.
32. Szczeklik A, Sladek K, Dworski R, et al. Bronchial aspirin challenge causes specific eicosanoid response in aspirin-sensitive asthmatics. Am J Respir Crit Care Med 1996;154:1608-14.
33. Gaber F, Daham K, Higashi A, et al. Increased levels of cysteinyl-leukotrienes in saliva, induced sputum, urine and blood from patients with aspirin-intolerant asthma. Thorax 2008;63:1076-82.
34. Cowburn AS, Sladek K, Soja J, et al. Overexpression of leukotriene C_4 synthase in bronchial biopsies from patients with aspirin-intolerant asthma. J Clin Invest 1998;15;101:834-46.
35. Higashi N, Taniguchi M, Mita H, et al. Clinical features of asthmatic patients with increased urinary leukotriene E_4 excretion (hyperleukotrienuria): involvement of chronic hyperplastic rhinosinusitis with nasal polyposis. J Allergy Clin Immunol 2004;113:277-83.
36. Corrigan C, Mallett K, Ying S, et al. Expression of the cysteinyl leukotriene receptors cysLT(1) and cysLT(2) in aspirin-sensitive and aspirin-tolerant chronic rhinosinusitis. J Allergy Clin Immunol 2005;115:316-22.
37. Ragab S, Parikh A, Darby YC, et al. An open audit of montelukast, a leukotriene receptor antagonist, in nasal polyposis associated with asthma. Clin Exp Allergy 2001;31:1385-91.
38. Sanak M, Levy BD, Clish CB, et al. Aspirin-tolerant asthmatics generate more lipoxins than aspirin-intolerant asthmatics. Eur Respir J 2000;16:44-9.
39. Wos M, Sanak M, Soja J, et al. The presence of rhinovirus in lower airways of patients with bronchial asthma. Am J Respir Crit Care Med 2008;177:1082-9.
40. Suh YJ, Yoon SH, Sampson AP, et al. Specific immunoglobulin E for staphylococcal enterotoxins in nasal polyps from patients with aspirin-intolerant asthma. Clin Exp Allergy 2004;34:1270-5.
41. Lee JY, Kim HM, Ye YM, et al. Role of staphylococcal superantigen-specific IgE antibodies in aspirin-intolerant asthma. Allergy Asthma Proc 2006;27:341-6.
42. Choi JH, Lee KW, Oh HB, et al. HLA association in aspirin-intolerant asthma: DPB1*0301 as a strong marker in a Korean population. J Allergy Clin Immunol 2004;113:562-4.
43. Shrestha Palikhe N, Kim SH, Jin HJ, et al. Genetic mechanisms in aspirin-exacerbated respiratory disease. J Allergy (Cairo) 2012;2012:794890.
44. Ciana P, Fumagalli M, Trincavelli ML, et al. The orphan receptor GPR17 identified as a new dual uracil nucleotides/cysteinyl-leukotrienes receptor. EMBO J 2006;25:4615-27.
45. Sanak M, Pierzchalska M, Bazan-Socha S, et al. Enhanced expression of the leukotriene C4 synthase due to overactive transcription of an allelic variant associated with aspirin-intolerant asthma. Am J Respir Cell Mol Biol 2000;23:290-6.
46. Kim SH, Oh JM, Kim YS, et al. Cysteinyl leukotriene receptor 1 promoter polymorphism is associated with aspirin-intolerant asthma in males. Clin Exp Allergy 2006;36:433-9.
47. Szczeklik W, Sanak M, Szczeklik A. Functional effects and gender association of COX-2 gene polymorphism G-765C in bronchial asthma. J Allergy Clin Immunol 2004;114:248-53.
48. Jinnai N, Sakagami T, Sekigawa T, et al. Polymorphisms in the prostaglandin E_2 receptor subtype 2 gene confer susceptibility to aspirin-intolerant asthma: a candidate gene approach. Hum Mol Genet 2004;13:3203-17.
49. Palikhe NS, Kim SH, Cho BY, et al. Genetic variability in CRTH2 polymorphism increases eotaxin-2 levels in patients with aspirin exacerbated respiratory disease. Allergy 2010;65:338-46.
50. Kim SH, Yang EM, Lee HN, et al. Association of the CCR3 gene polymorphism with aspirin exacerbated respiratory disease. Respir Med 2010;104:626-32.
51. Kim JH, Park BL, Cheong HS, et al. Genome-wide and follow-up studies identify CEP68 gene variants associated with risk of aspirin-intolerant asthma. PLoS One 2010;5:e13818.
52. Palikhe N, Kim JH, Park HS. Update on recent advances in the management of aspirin exacerbated respiratory disease. Yonsei Med J 2009;60:744-50.
53. Berges-Gimeno M, Simon RA, Stevenson DD. The natural history and clinical characteristics of aspirin exacerbated respiratory disease. Ann Allergy Asthma Immunol 2002;89:474-8.
54. Mascia K, Haselkorn T, Deniz YM, et al; TENOR Study Group. Aspirin sensitivity and severity of asthma: evidence for irreversible airway obstruction in patients with severe or difficult-to-treat asthma. J Allergy Clin Immunol 2005;116:970-5.
55. Dursun AB, Woessner KA, Simon RA, et al. Predicting outcomes of oral aspirin challenges in patients with asthma, nasal polyps, and chronic sinusitis. Ann Allergy Asthma Immunol 2008;100:420-5.
56. Nizankowska-Mogilnicka E, Bochenek G, Mastalerz L, et al. EAACI/GA^{2}LEN guideline: aspirin provocation tests for diagnosis of aspirin hypersensitivity. Allergy 2007;62:1111-8.
56a. Lee RU, White AA, Ding D, et al. Use of intranasal ketorolac and modified oral aspirin challenge for desensitization of aspirin-exacerbated respiratory disease. Ann Allergy Asthma immunol 2010;105:130–5.
57. Hope AP, Woessner KA, Simon RA, et al. Rational approach to aspirin dosing during oral challenges and desensitization of patients with aspirin-exacerbated respiratory disease. J Allergy Clin Immunol 2009;123:406-10.
58. Phillips GD, Foord R, Holgate ST. Inhaled lysine-aspirin as a bronchoprovocation procedure in aspirin-sensitive asthma: its repeatability, absence of a late-phase reaction, and the role of histamine. J Allergy Clin Immunol 1989;84:232-41.
59. Mita H, Higashi N, Taniguchi M, et al. Increase in urinary leukotriene B_4 glucuronide concentration in patients with aspirin-intolerant asthma after intravenous aspirin challenge. Clin Exp Allergy 2004;34:1262-9.
60. Pierzchalska M, Mastalerz L, Sanak M, et al. A moderate and unspecific release of cysteinyl leukotrienes by aspirin from peripheral blood

leucocytes precludes its value for aspirin sensitivity testing in asthma. Clin Exp Allergy 2000; 30:1785-91.
61. Sanz ML, Gamboa PM, Mayorga C. Basophil activation tests in the evaluation of immediate drug hypersensitivity. Curr Opin Allergy Clin Immunol 2009;9:298-304.
62. Dahlen B, Nizankowska E, Szczeklik A, et al. Benefits from adding the 5-lipoxygenase inhibitor zileuton to conventional therapy in aspirin-intolerant asthmatics. Am J Respir Crit Care Med 1998;157:1187-94.
63. Dahlén SE, Malmström K, Nizankowska E, et al. Improvement of aspirin-intolerant asthma by montelukast, a leukotriene antagonist: a randomized, double-blind, placebo-controlled trial. Am J Respir Crit Care Med 2002;165:9-14.
64. Berges-Gimeno MP, Simon RA, Stevenson DD. The effect of leukotriene-modifier drugs on aspirin-induced asthma and rhinitis reactions. Clin Exp Allergy 2002;32:1491-6.
65. Berges-Gimeno M, Simon RA, Stevenson DD. Long-term treatment with aspirin desensitization in asthmatic patients with aspirin-exacerbated respiratory disease. J Allergy Clin Immunol 2003;111:180-6.
66. Sánchez-Borges M, Capriles-Hulett A, Caballero-Fonseca F. The multiple faces of nonsteroidal antiinflammatory drug hypersensitivity. J Investig Allergol Clin Immunol 2004; 14:329-34.
67. Kim SH, Ye YM, Palikhe NS, et al. Genetic and ethnic risk factors associated with drug hypersensitivity. Curr Opin Allergy Clin Immunol 2010;10:280-90.
68. Mastalerz L, Setkowicz M, Sanak M, et al. Hypersensitivity to aspirin: common eicosanoid alterations in urticaria and asthma. J Allergy Clin Immunol 2004;113:771-5.
69. Pérez C, Sánchez-Borges M, Suárez-Chacón R. Pretreatment with montelukast blocks NSAID-induced urticaria and angioedema. J Allergy Clin Immunol 2001;108:1060-1.
70. Choi SJ, Ye YM, Hur GY, et al. Neutrophil activation in patients with ASA-induced urticaria. J Clin Immunol 2008;28:244-9.
71. Sánchez-Borges M, Acevedo N, Vergara C, et al. The A-444C polymorphism in the leukotriene C4 synthase gene is associated with aspirin-induced urticaria. J Investig Allergol Clin Immunol 2009;19:375-82.
72. Bae JS, Kim SH, Ye YM, et al. Significant association of FcεRIa promoter polymorphisms with aspirin-intolerant chronic urticaria. J Allergy Clin Immunol 2007;119: 449-56.
73. Marer M, Weller K, Bindslev-Jensen C, et al. Unmet clinical needs in chronic spontaneous urticaria. A GA2LEN task force report. Allergy 2011;66:317-30.
74. Zuberbier T, Asero R, Bindslev-Jensen C, et al. EAACI/GA(2)LEN/EDF/WAO guideline: management of urticaria. Allergy 2009;64: 1427-43.

Allergic (or Immunologically Mediated) Types of Nonsteroidal Antiinflammatory Drug Hypersensitivity

75. Himly M, Jahn-Schmid B, Pittertschatscher K, et al. IgE-mediated immediate type hypersensitivity to the pyrazolone drug propyphenazone. J Allergy Clin Immunol 2003;111:882-8.
76. Layton D, Marshall V, Boshiek A, et al. Serious skin reactions and selective COX-2 inhibitors: a case series from prescription-event monitoring in England. Drug Saf 2006;29:687-96.
77. Ward KE, Archambault R, Mersfelder JL. Severe adverse reactions to nonsteroidal anti-inflammatory drugs: a review of the literature. Am J Health Syst Pharm 2010;67:206-13.
78. Hunger RE, Hunziker T, Buettiker U, et al. Rapid resolution of toxic epidermal necrolysis with anti-TNF-alpha treatment. J Allergy Clin Immunol 2005;116:923-4.

81 Reactions to Foods

ANNA NOWAK-WĘGRZYN | A. WESLEY BURKS | HUGH A. SAMPSON

CONTENTS

SUMMARY OF IMPORTANT CONCEPTS

» Food allergy affects 6% of the U.S. children younger than 5 years of age and 3.5% to 4% of the general population, and the incidence of peanut allergy has tripled over the past decade in Western countries.

» Sensitization to food allergens may occur in the gastrointestinal tract (traditional or class 1 food allergy), or it may result from sensitization to cross-reacting inhalant allergens (secondary or class 2 food allergy).

» Food reactions may have immunoglobulin E (IgE)–mediated, non–IgE-mediated, or a combination of IgE- and non–IgE-mediated pathophysiologic mechanisms involving the skin, gastrointestinal tract, respiratory tract, or cardiovascular system.

» Foods are the most common triggers of anaphylaxis in children and major triggers in adults.

» Increasing levels of food-specific serum IgE antibodies or skin-prick test wheal diameters correlate with increasing probabilities of clinical reactivity, although the double-blind, placebo-controlled food challenge remains the gold standard for diagnosing food allergy.

» Strict food allergen avoidance remains the only proven therapy for treating food allergy, although several immunomodulatory approaches are in clinical trials.

Definitions and Historical Perspective

In the past 2 decades, food allergy has emerged as an important public health problem affecting people of all ages in societies with a Western lifestyle, such as the United States, Canada, United Kingdom, Australia, and Western Europe.[1,2] The overall prevalence of food allergy in American children increased by 18% from 1997 to 2007.[2] Peanut allergy tripled during a similar period in the United States, Canada, United Kingdom, and Australia.[3] In the past decade, the incidence of eosinophilic esophagitis has increased among children and adults. Food allergy is the most common cause of anaphylaxis in the outpatient setting for all ages, and it can lead to fatalities. The diagnosis of food allergy requires labor-intensive, medically supervised oral food challenges (OFCs) that carry a risk for anaphylaxis and are not readily available to all patients.[4] There is no cure for food allergy. Current management relies on food avoidance and timely treatment of acute reactions. To facilitate diagnosis and management of food allergy, the first official U.S. guidelines for food allergy were published in 2010.[5] The growing recognition of the burden of food allergies and the challenges in diagnosis and management are driving multifaceted research approaches with the ultimate goal of finding a cure.

Food allergy is defined as an adverse health effect arising from a specific immune response that occurs reproducibly on exposure to a given food. Nonallergic adverse reactions to foods may be the result of food intolerances or adverse physiologic reactions.[5]

Food intolerances are thought to comprise most adverse reactions to foods. They can be caused by factors inherent in food ingested, such as toxic contaminants (e.g., histamine in scombroid fish poisoning, toxins secreted by *Salmonella*, *Shigella*, and *Campylobacter*), pharmacologic properties of the food (e.g., caffeine in coffee, tyramine in aged cheeses), and host characteristics such as metabolic disorders (e.g., lactase deficiency) and idiosyncratic responses. *Food aversions* may mimic adverse food reactions, but they typically cannot be reproduced when the patient ingests the food in a blinded fashion.

Immunoglobulin E (IgE)–mediated food allergies, or *hypersensitivities*, occur frequently in young children and account for most well-characterized food-allergic disorders, although several non–IgE-mediated immune reactions, especially in the gastrointestinal tract, have been delineated. Food allergy must be distinguished from a variety of adverse reactions to foods that do not have an immune basis but whose clinical manifestations may resemble food allergy. Examples of adverse food reactions are presented in Table 81-1.

Hippocrates recorded the first report of an adverse food reaction (i.e., milk) more than 2000 years ago, and accounts from ancient Rome indicate that the Romans were aware that foods consumed safely by most people could occasionally provoke adverse reactions in others. It was not until 1921 that the first significant advance was made in our understanding of these disorders. Prausnitz and Kustner demonstrated that the substance responsible for Kustner's allergic reaction to fish was present in his blood serum and could be transferred to a nonsensitive individual.[6] After injecting a small amount of Kustner's serum into the skin of his forearm, Prausnitz developed a wheal and flare at the passively sensitized site after the

TABLE 81-1 Nonallergic Adverse Reactions to Consider in the Differential Diagnosis of Food Allergy

Condition	Symptoms	Mechanism and Comments
ENZYME DEFICIENCIES		
Lactose intolerance	Bloating, abdominal pain, diarrhea (dose dependent)	Lactase deficiency
Fructose intolerance	Emesis, poor feeding, jaundice, hypoglycemia, seizures	Hereditary fructose aldolase B deficiency; rare
Fructose malabsorption	Bloating, abdominal pain, diarrhea (dose dependent)	Deficiency of fructose carrier GLUT5 in the enterocytes in small intestines; 10% prevalence in Asia, up to 30% in Western Europe and Africa
Pancreatic insufficiency	Malabsorption	Deficiency of pancreatic enzymes, acquired or congenital (e.g., cystic fibrosis, Schwachman-Diamond syndrome)
Alcohol	Nasal congestion, flushing, vomiting	Polymorphism of the aldehyde dehydrogenase gene (*ALDH*), resulting in deficiency of ALDH, which metabolizes alcohol in the liver; common in Asians
Gallbladder or liver disease	Malabsorption	Deficiency of liver enzymes
GASTROINTESTINAL DISORDERS		
Gastroesophageal reflux disease	Nausea, emesis, abdominal pain, heartburn, dysphagia	Chronic symptom of mucosal damage caused by stomach acid refluxing into the esophagus
Peptic ulcer disease	Abdominal pain, bloating, loss of appetite, weight loss, melena	Ulcer of the gastrointestinal tract (commonly duodenum); 70%-90% are associated with *Helicobacter pylori* infection
ANATOMIC DEFECTS		
Hiatal hernia	Abdominal pain, shortness of breath, nausea, emesis	Protrusion (or herniation) of the upper part of the stomach into the thorax through a tear or weakness in the diaphragm
Pyloric stenosis	Severe, nonbilious, projectile vomiting in the first few months of life	Stenosis due to hypertrophy of muscle around pylorus, which spasms when stomach empties; rare case reports of eosinophilic infiltrates in pylorus and reported resolution of muscle hypertrophy with hypoallergenic formula or steroids
Hirschsprung disease	Delayed passage of meconium, constipation, ileus, emesis	Failure of neural crest cells to migrate completely during fetal development of the intestine, causing aganglіosis; usually affects short segment of the distal colon
Tracheoesophageal fistula	Copious salivation associated with choking, coughing, vomiting, and cyanosis coincident with the onset of feeding in newborns and young infants	*Congenital:* failed fusion of tracheoesophageal ridges during third week of embryologic development *Acquired:* usually sequela of surgical procedures (e.g., laryngectomy)
PHYSIOLOGIC EFFECTS OF ACTIVE SUBSTANCES		
Caffeine	Tremors, cramps, diarrhea	Xanthine alkaloid acts as stimulant drug; found in seeds, leaves, and fruit of some plants, where it acts as a natural pesticide; consumed in coffee, tea, and drinks containing kola nut, yerba mate, guarana berry, or guayusa derivatives
Theobromine	Sleeplessness, tremors, restlessness, anxiety, increased urination, loss of appetite, nausea, vomiting	Bitter alkaloid in cocoa bean and tea leaves; elderly more susceptible
Tyramine	Migraine	Naturally occurring monoamine compound derived from tyrosine; acts as a catecholamine-releasing agent; pharmacologic effects in susceptible individuals; found in pickled, aged, smoked, fermented, or marinated foods (e.g., hard cheeses, tofu, sauerkraut, fava beans)
Histamine	Flushing, headache, nausea	Naturally occurring in fermented foods and beverages (e.g., fish, sauerkraut) due to a conversion from histidine to histamine performed by fermenting bacteria or yeasts; sake contains histamine in the 20-40 mg/L range and wines in the 2-10 mg/L range
Serotonin	Flushing, diarrhea, palpitations	Monoamine neurotransmitter derived from tryptophan; found in nuts, mushrooms, fruits, and vegetables; highest values (25-400 mg/kg) in nuts of walnut and hickory genera; concentrations of 3-30 mg/kg found in plantain, pineapple, banana, kiwi, plums, and tomatoes
FOOD ADDITIVES AND CONTAMINANTS		
Sodium metabisulfite	Rare reports of bronchospasm in sensitive individuals	Antioxidant and preservative in food, also known as E223
Monosodium glutamate (MSG)	Chinese restaurant syndrome begins 15-20 min after the meal and lasts for about 2 h; symptoms include numbness at the back of the neck and gradually radiating to the arms and back, general weakness, and palpitations	Naturally occurring nonessential amino acid; flavor enhancer; in a DBPCFC study, objective reactions to MSG were observed in only 2 of 130 self-selected MSG-reactive adult volunteers[6a]
Accidental contaminants	Abdominal pain, diarrhea, nausea	Include heavy metals (e.g., mercury, copper), pesticides, antibiotics (e.g., penicillin), dust or storage mites
Infectious agents	Pain, fever, nausea, emesis, diarrhea	Include bacteria (e.g., *Salmonella, Shigella, Escherichia coli, Yersinia, Campylobacter*); parasites (e.g., *Giardia, Trichinella*); viruses (e.g., hepatitis, rotavirus, enterovirus)

Continued

TABLE 81-1 Nonallergic Adverse Reactions to Consider in the Differential Diagnosis of Food Allergy—cont'd

Condition	Symptoms	Mechanism and Comments
NEUROLOGIC DISORDERS		
Auriculotemporal syndrome (Frey syndrome)	Facial flush in trigeminal nerve distribution associated with spicy foods	Neurogenic reflex, frequently associated with birth trauma to trigeminal nerve (forceps delivery)
Gustatory rhinitis	Profuse watery rhinorrhea associated with spicy foods	Neurogenic reflex
CONDITIONS CONFUSED WITH FOOD REACTIONS		
Panic disorder	Subjective reactions, fainting on smelling or seeing the food; tachycardia, perspiration, dyspnea, shivers, uncontrollable fear (fear of dying)	Psychological; anxiety disorder affects children and adults; usually leads to extensive medical testing; controlled with medications and behavioral therapy

Modified from Nowak-Węgrzyn A, Sampson HA. Adverse reactions to foods. Med Clin North Am 2006;90:97-127.

ingestion of fish.[6] In 1950, Loveless reported the first blinded, placebo-controlled food trials and challenged the accuracy of diagnoses based on patients' historical reporting.[7,8] In one study, 8 patients were investigated for milk allergy,[7] and in another, 25 patients were evaluated for cornstarch sensitivity.[8]

About a decade later, Goldman and coworkers evaluated 89 children with suspected milk allergy.[9] The diagnosis of food allergy was established only when withdrawal of milk from the diet led to complete resolution of symptoms and each of three successive challenges with milk duplicated the presenting symptoms. In 1976, May reported on the use of double-blind, placebo-controlled oral food challenges (DBPCFCs) to diagnose food allergy,[10] ushering in the current era of scientific investigation into food allergic disorders. Recognition of the burden of food allergies and emergence of food allergy as a major public health problem worldwide prompted development of guidelines for food allergy in the past 5 years.[11] In 2010, the first clinical guidelines for the diagnosis and management of food allergy in the United States were published.[5]

Epidemiology

Food allergies are most common in the first few years of life.[1] Overall, more than 90% of food allergies in children are caused by cow's milk, hen's egg, soybean, wheat, peanut, tree nuts, fish, and shellfish. These foods have relatively high protein contents and are introduced at early stages. Local dietary habits often result in the increased presence of various food allergens in the diet. Examples include sesame in Israel, buckwheat in Japan, and mustard and lupine in France.[3] Most allergies to cow's milk, egg, soybean, and wheat are outgrown, whereas most allergies to peanut, nuts, seeds, and seafood tend to persist into adulthood.

CHILDREN

Prospective studies from several countries indicate that about 2.5% of newborn infants experience hypersensitivity reactions to cow's milk in the first year of life.[3] IgE-mediated reactions account for about 60% of these milk-allergic reactions. Chicken egg allergy is estimated to affect about 1.6% of young children in the United States and United Kingdom. A rigorous, population-based study found an 8.9% prevalence of egg allergy diagnosed by OFC to raw egg in children younger than 12 months of age in Australia, suggesting that food allergies continue to increase in the youngest age groups.[12]

Most infants with non–IgE-mediated cow's milk allergy outgrow their sensitivity by the third year of life, but about 10% to 25% of infants with IgE-mediated cow's milk and egg allergies retain their sensitivity into the second decade, and about 50% develop allergic reactions to other foods.[13,14]

Large, population-based studies have addressed the prevalence of peanut allergy (Table 81-2).[15] Three studies used random digit dialing, a standard method for selection, with administration of a survey; two studies used allergy testing and OFCs; and one was a retrospective study of a specialist referral population.[3] All of these studies determined that peanut allergy affects more than 1% of children in Canada, the United States, Australia, and the United Kingdom.

Adverse reactions to food additives affect 0.5% to 1% of children, especially those with atopic disorders,[3] who have a higher prevalence of food allergy. About 35% of children with moderate to severe atopic dermatitis have IgE-mediated food allergy, many of whom exhibit skin symptoms provoked by ingestion of the food allergen.[16] About 6% of asthmatic children attending a general pulmonary clinic reportedly had food-induced wheezing.[17] Among children with eosinophilic esophagitis, 50% have food-responsive disease (i.e., symptoms improve or resolve on elimination of the offending food).

ADULTS

Food allergy in adults appears to be less common than in children.[3] U.S. surveys indicated that peanut and tree nut allergy together affect 1.2% of American adults, and seafood allergy affects about 2.3%, giving an overall estimate of 3.5% to 4%. A survey from the United Kingdom identified 1.4% to 1.8% of adults reporting adverse food reactions, and a study in the Netherlands concluded that about 2% of the adult Dutch population was affected by adverse food reactions. The estimates of pollen-related food allergy are considerably higher. Among pollen-allergic individuals, 74% report symptoms (most had oral symptoms) to the pollen-associated foods (e.g., fruits, vegetables). Overall, 16.7% of young adults report pollen-food allergy symptoms.

Prevalence of Food Allergy

Studies of the prevalence of food allergy are hampered by the requirement of a physician-supervised OFC for the ultimate confirmation of food allergy. Food challenges are expensive,

TABLE 81-2 **Prevalence of Allergy to Specific Foods**

Food	General Population	Children (<5 years)	Adults
Cow's milk	0.4%-0.9%	0.5% (Israel) to 3.8% (US, UK)	
Hen's egg white	0.2%	≈2%-8.9% (<12 mo) (Australia)	
Soybean	0%;0.7%	1.4%	0%-0.7%
Wheat	0%-1.2%	≈0.5%	0%-1.2%
Peanut	0.75%-1.3%	0.2% (Israel) to 1.9% (US, Canada, UK)	0.7%
Tree nuts	0.6%-1.1%	1.1%-1.6%	0.5%-1%
Sesame oil or seeds	Overall: 0.1%-<1%	0.6%	
Fish	Overall: 0.3%-0.5%	0.2%; 0.5%	≈0.6%
Shellfish	0.6%-2%	0.5% 14-16 yr: 5.2% (Singapore)	1.7%-2.5%
Fruits	Up to 4.2% (SPT); up to 8.5% (symptoms)	0.4% (UK)	
Vegetables	0.1%-0.3%, up to 2.7% (SPT); up to 13.7% (symptoms)	1.2%	
Oral allergy (raw fruits or vegetables)			22 yr: 17% (Denmark)

Modified from Sicherer SH. Epidemiology of food allergy. J Allergy Clin Immunol 2011;127:594-602.
SPT, Skin-prick test; *UK*, United Kingdom; *US*, United States.

labor-intensive, and impractical in large-scale, population-based cohorts. For this reason, many studies use surrogate markers, such as evidence of specific IgE to food or self-reported food allergy to estimate prevalence figures. Several studies that applied similar methods over time showed a twofold to threefold increase in peanut allergy and peanut-IgE sensitization in children in the United States, United Kingdom, Canada, and Australia over the past 10 to 20 years. Many studies reported rates of peanut allergy of more than 1% among young children.[3]

Few data are available for the rate change of any form of food allergy over time. In one clinic in China, food allergy rates increased from 3.5% in 1999 to 7.7% in 2009 (P = .017).[18] Branum and Lukacs described several U.S. national databases that allowed information to be compared over time.[5] On the basis of diagnostic coding in U.S. national ambulatory care surveys, ambulatory care visits tripled between 1993 and 2006 (P < .01).

Food-induced anaphylaxis also appears to have increased.[19] In the United States, data from one geographic region in Minnesota from 1983 to 1987 and 1993 to 1997 show a 71% to 100% increase.[20,21] Studies focusing on pediatric food-related ambulatory and emergency department visits or food-induced anaphylaxis also suggest increases. In the United Kingdom, there was almost a doubling of anaphylaxis, from 5.6 to 10.2 cases per 100,000 hospital discharges over the 4 years from 1991 to 1995 (P < .001).[15] The proportion of cases attributed to food-induced anaphylaxis also increased over the same period.

The reasons for increased cases of food allergy are unknown. There appears to be a strong genetic contribution to peanut allergy. Monozygotic twins have 64% concordance for peanut allergy; dizygotic twins have 7% concordance.[22] However, the rapid rate of increase suggests that environmental factors play a more important role, likely by affecting the expression of genetic susceptibility.[23]

The *hygiene hypothesis* suggests that the lack of early life exposures to infectious agents (e.g., bacteria, parasites) may lead to a faulty programming of tolerogenic mechanisms, increasing the host's susceptibility to allergic diseases. A meta-analysis of six studies showed a mild effect of cesarean delivery increasing the risk of food allergy (odds ratio [OR] = 1.32; 95% confidence interval [CI], 1.12 to 0.55). The pro-allergy skewing effect of cesarean section may be explained by the abnormal bacterial colonization of a newborn's gut in the absence of exposure to the protective bacterial flora in the birth canal. Alternatively, cesarean section is associated with higher maternal age, a higher number of first-born infants, and a higher number of male births, which all have been identified as independent risk factors for atopy.

Several studies focused on dietary factors, including vitamin D, omega-3 polyunsaturated fatty acids (n-3 PUFAs), antioxidants, soluble dietary fiber, and folate during pregnancy and early childhood.[24] In animal models, maternal diet can have epigenetic effects on immune function that predispose to an allergic phenotype.[1] This suggests that pregnancy provides an important window of opportunity for disease prevention and that diet may be a noninvasive preventive strategy.

Epidemiologic findings, such as the observations that season of birth is a risk factor, that food-induced pediatric anaphylaxis is more common in northern areas of the United States (i.e., less sunlight exposure than in the southern states), and that maternal intake of vitamin D during pregnancy was associated with a decreased risk of food sensitization, support the hypothesis that relative deficiency of vitamin D may predispose offspring to development of atopy and food allergy. However, two independent studies showed that infants who received vitamin D supplementation were at increased risk of food allergy.

The typical Western diet is characterized by the reduced consumption of n-3 PUFAs (found in oily fish) and increased consumption of proinflammatory omega-6 polyunsaturated fatty acids (found in margarine and vegetable oils) led to the increased production of prostaglandin E_2 (PGE_2). This presumably results in reduced production of interferon-γ (IFN-γ) by T cells and increased production of IgE by B cells, amplifying the risk of atopy and asthma.

Timing of exposure to food allergens may be critical for the development of oral tolerance. A review of 13 studies (only one was controlled) found a consistent association between the persistence of eczema and the introduction of solid foods before 4 months of age but not with an increased risk of asthma, food allergy, allergic rhinitis, or animal allergies. Several reports suggested that early introduction of peanut, cow's milk, egg, and wheat into the infant diet was associated with decreased risk of allergy to these foods. Countries in Asia, Africa, and the Middle East have low rates of peanut allergy, and peanut consumption is unrestricted during pregnancy and early childhood. A questionnaire-based study found that the prevalence of peanut allergy in the United Kingdom was 1.85% and the prevalence in Israel was 0.17% ($P < .001$). The adjusted risk ratio for peanut allergy between countries was 9.8 (95% CI, 3.1 to 30.5) in primary English school children.[25] The only difference identified between the two populations was the timing of introduction of peanuts, which in Israel occurs during early weaning. Randomized clinical trials are underway to determine whether early introduction of peanuts and other solid foods protects against food allergy.[23]

TABLE 81-3 Gastrointestinal Barriers to Ingested Food Antigens

Barriers	Food Allergy Predisposition in Newborns and Infants
IMMUNOLOGIC BARRIERS	
Block penetration of ingested antigens Antigen-specific sIgA in gut lumen	Newborn lacks IgA and IgM in exocrine secretions. Salivary sIgA is absent at birth, and levels remain low during early months of life.
Clear antigens penetrating GI barrier Serum antigen-specific IgA and IgG Reticuloendothelial system	Immaturity of the humoral immune system, low levels of circulating antibodies
PHYSIOLOGIC BARRIERS	
Breakdown of ingested antigens Gastric acid and pepsins Pancreatic enzymes Intestinal enzymes Intestinal epithelial cell lysozyme activity	Low basal acid output during first month of life Immaturity of the intestinal proteolytic activity until about 2 years of age
Block penetration of ingested antigens Intestinal mucous coat (i.e., glycocalyx) Intestinal microvillus membrane composition Intestinal peristalsis	Intestinal microvillous membranes are immature in infants, resulting in altered antigen binding and transport through mucosal epithelial cells.

GI, Gastrointestinal; *IgM*, immunoglobulin M; *sIGA*, secretory immunoglobulin A.

Pathogenesis and Etiology

ANTIGEN HANDLING BY THE GASTROINTESTINAL MUCOSAL BARRIER

The gastrointestinal tract processes ingested food into a form that can be absorbed and used for energy and cell growth. This requires the intestinal immune system to discriminate between harmful and harmless foreign proteins.[26] As shown in Table 81-3, a variety of immunologic and nonimmunologic factors may destroy or block antigens from entering the body. However, developmental immaturity of these mechanisms in infants reduces the efficiency of their mucosal barriers and likely plays a major role in the increased prevalence of gastrointestinal infections and food allergy seen in the first few years of life. The importance of digestion was demonstrated by Michael,[27] who showed that digested bovine serum albumin (BSA) was tolerogenic when given orally or placed into the ileum, whereas undigested BSA was tolerogenic when given orally but immunogenic when placed into the ileum. The relatively low concentrations of secretory immunoglobulin A (sIgA) in the young infant's intestine and the relatively large quantities of ingested proteins place a tremendous burden on the immature gut-associated immune system.

ANTIGEN PENETRATION OF THE GASTROINTESTINAL TRACT MUCOSAL BARRIER

Despite evolution of the multilayered mucosal barrier of the gastrointestinal tract, about 2% of ingested food antigens are absorbed and transported throughout the body in an immunologically intact form, even through the mature gut. Prausnitz and Kustner[6] were the first to demonstrate how rapidly food antigens were absorbed and transported to mast cells in the skin.

In a classic series of experiments, Walzer and colleagues[28] used sera from egg- and fish-allergic patients to passively sensitize volunteers. Volunteers were given intradermal injections of food-allergic patient and control sera. Approximately 24 hours later, they were fed fish.[29] A wheal and flare reaction developed at the sensitized site within several minutes to 1 hour after ingestion of the relevant antigen in more than 90% of subjects, but no reaction occurred at the control site. Using a similar passive sensitization protocol and introducing food in specific locations along the gastrointestinal tract, it was demonstrated that food antigens were most readily absorbed from the small intestine, colon, and rectum and somewhat more slowly from the esophagus and stomach.[30] Several factors were shown to decrease antigen absorption, including increased stomach acidity and the presence of other food in the gut, whereas increased absorption resulted from decreased stomach acidity and the ingestion of alcohol.

The appearance of the gastrointestinal tract surface after ingestion of a food allergen was first investigated by passively sensitizing rectal, colonic, and ileal mucosa in normal volunteers and patients with ileostomies and colostomies. Ingestion of the responsible food allergen initially provoked pallor at the sensitized site, followed rapidly by edema, hyperemia, marked secretion of mucus, and occasionally petechiae and bleeding. Subsequent studies were carried out in food-allergic patients by instilling small amounts of food allergen in the stomach under endoscopic observation, first using a rigid endoscope and then with flexible endoscopes followed by biopsy. The physical findings described in passively sensitized patients were confirmed, and histochemical staining of biopsy samples demonstrated degranulation of mast cells after food challenge.

ORAL TOLERANCE

In normal children and adults, the intact food antigens that penetrate the gastrointestinal tract and enter the circulation do not normally cause clinical symptoms because most individuals develop tolerance to ingested antigens. In mucosal tissues, soluble antigens, such as food and inhaled antigens, are usually poor immunogens, inducing an active state of unresponsiveness known as *oral tolerance*. Oral tolerance is the specific immunologic unresponsiveness to antigens induced by their prior feeding. Unresponsiveness of T cells to ingested food proteins may result from three mechanisms: *T cell deletion*, *T cell anergy*, or *induction of regulatory T cells*. In humans, anergy and induction of the regulatory T cells appear to be more relevant than clonal deletion. The topic of oral tolerance is discussed in detail in Chapter 67.

NORMAL IMMUNE RESPONSE TO THE INGESTED FOOD ANTIGENS

Low concentrations of serum IgG, IgM, and IgA food-specific antibodies are commonly found in normal individuals. The younger an infant when a food antigen is introduced into the diet, the more pronounced the antibody response is likely to be. After introduction of cow's milk, serum levels of milk protein–specific IgG antibodies rise over the first month, achieving peak antibody levels after several months, and they then decline, even though cow's milk proteins continue to be ingested. Individuals with various inflammatory gastrointestinal disorders (e.g., celiac disease, food allergy, inflammatory bowel disease) frequently have high levels of food-specific IgG and IgM antibodies. However, these antibodies do not indicate that the patient is allergic to these foods. The increased levels of food-specific antibodies (not IgE) appear to result from increased gastrointestinal permeability to food antigens and reflect dietary intake.

Several studies have demonstrated increased lymphocyte proliferation or interleukin-2 (IL-2) production after food antigen stimulation in vitro in patients with food allergy, celiac disease, and inflammatory bowel disease. However, in vitro T cell responses are also commonly demonstrated in normal individuals.[31] Although not diagnostic, stimulation of T cells from food-allergic patients in vitro demonstrates the presence of increased numbers of type 2 helper T (Th2) cells (i.e., IL-4, IL-5, and IL-13 positive).

In animal models of food allergy, exposure to peanut and ovalbumin by the cutaneous route (i.e., tape-stripped skin) is associated with increased production of food-specific IgE, whereas oral feeding induces tolerance.[32] Genetic polymorphisms in the filaggrin gene (*FLG*) resulting in impairment of the skin barrier are found in large subsets of subjects with atopic dermatitis, especially with early onset, a more severe chronic course, and a large number of allergic sensitizations. *FLG* loss-of-function mutations are associated with peanut allergy, even after controlling for coexistent atopic dermatitis ($P = .008$).[33]

Food Allergens

Among 399 described food allergens, only 71 of 14,831 (0.5%) protein families are represented, and the top 20 (0.13%) protein families account for 80% of all described food allergens, suggesting that food allergens share common characteristics that render them allergenic.[34] (For more information, see a database of protein families [Pfam] at www.pfam.sanger.ac.uk and a database of known allergens [Allfam] at www.meduniwien.ac.at. Accessed April 28, 2013.) The allergenic potential may be linked to the stability during food processing and digestion, protein glycosylation, ability to bind lipids that protect them from degradation and enhance their absorption from the gastrointestinal tract, or the ability to stimulate innate immune responses (e.g., through the mannose receptor).[35]

About 65% of *plant food allergens* belong to one of the three classes of structurally related protein superfamilies: the prolamin superfamily (i.e., seed-storage proteins of cereals, lipid transfer proteins, α-amylase/protein inhibitors, and 2S albumins); the cupin superfamily (i.e., 7S vicilins and 11S globulins); and the PR10 protein family, of which Bet v 1 is the best known example. *Animal food allergens* belong to one of three main families: tropomyosins, EF-hand proteins, and caseins.[36] The ability to act as an allergen seems to be inversely related to the relative identity to human homologs; animal proteins with a sequence identity greater than 63% to human homologs are rarely allergenic (Table 81-4).

Functionally, based on the ability to induce allergic sensitization in the gastrointestinal tract, food proteins can be classified as class 1 (traditional) food allergens or as class 2 food allergens that do not have the capacity to sensitize in the gastrointestinal tract but become allergenic as a consequence of sensitization to inhalant allergens.[37] The major food allergens that have been identified in class 1 allergy are water-soluble glycoproteins, which have molecular masses ranging from 10 to 70 kD and are stable to treatment with heat, acid, and proteases (see Table 81-4). However, there are no obvious physicochemical properties common to the class 2 food allergens. The mostly plant-derived proteins are highly heat labile and difficult to extract intact, often making standardized extracts for diagnostic purposes unsatisfactory. Several class 1 and 2 food allergens have been identified, cloned, sequenced, and expressed as recombinant proteins (see Table 81-4). Many of the plant-related allergens are homologous to pathogenesis-related (PR) proteins, which are expressed by the plant in response to infections or other stress factors or comprise seed-storage proteins, profilins, peroxidases, or protease inhibitors common to many plants.

Cow's milk usually represents the first foreign proteins introduced into an infant's diet. It is the most common food allergy among young children (if IgE- and non–IgE-mediated hypersensitivities are considered), and it has been implicated in a variety of hypersensitivity reactions.[1] Cow's milk contains at least 20 protein components, which may lead to antibody production in humans.[38] The milk protein fractions are subdivided into casein and whey proteins. The caseins usually are found in micellar complexes, which give the liquid its milky appearance and constitute 76% to 86% of the protein in cow's milk. The casein fraction is precipitated from skim milk by acid at pH 4.6 and is composed of four basic caseins: α_{s1}, α_{s2}, β, and κ, comprising 32%, 10%, 28%, and 10% of total milk protein, respectively. The whey fraction (i.e., noncasein) consists of β-lactoglobulin, α-lactalbumin, bovine immunoglobulins, bovine serum albumin (BSA), and minute quantities of various proteins (e.g., lactoferrin, transferrin, lipases, esterases). Caseins suspended in micellar complexes are predominantly presented to the immune system by Peyer patches, whereas whey proteins (e.g., β-lactoglobulin, α-lactalbumin) are highly soluble and rapidly transported across the intestinal epithelium. As a consequence, in an animal model of milk allergy, caseins are more potent as inducers of antibody responses, including IgE. However, in animal models sensitized to casein and whey, the whey proteins induce stronger systemic allergic reactions on exposure, possibly because they are so rapidly absorbed.[39]

TABLE 81-4 Characteristics of Important Food Allergens

Protein Fraction and Nomenclature	Percent of Total Food Protein*	Molecular Mass (kD)	Protein Family and Function†
CLASS I FOOD ALLERGENS			
ANIMAL			
Cow's milk			
Caseins	76-86	19-24	Ca^{2+} binding by a cluster of phosphoserine and phosphothreonine
α_{s1}-Casein, Bos d 8	53-70	27	
α_s-Casein	45-50	23	
β-Casein	25-35	24	
κ-Casein	8-15	19	
Whey	14-24		
β-Lactoglobulin, Bos d 5	7-12	36	Lipocalins or carriers of small molecules such as lipids, steroids, and hormones
α-Lactalbumin, Bos d 4	2-5	14	α-Lactalbumin family; lactose synthesis; three-dimensional structure is superimposable with hen's egg lysozyme (C-type lysozyme)
Serum albumin, Bos d 6	0.7-1.3	69	A major component of blood plasma; binds ions (e.g., Ca^{2+}, Na^+, K^+) and hydrophobic molecules (e.g., fatty acids, hormones, drugs)
Chicken egg white			
Ovomucoid, Gal d 1	11	28	Kazal-type protease (trypsin) inhibitor
Ovalbumin, Gal d 2	54	45	Serpin serine protease inhibitor
Ovotransferrin, Gal d 3	12-13	78	Sulfur-rich glycoprotein with iron-binding function
C-type lysozyme, Gal d 4	3.4	14	C-type lysozymes secreted; bacteriolytic enzymes cleave peptidoglycan of bacterial cell walls
Chicken egg yolk			
α-Livetin, Gal d 5	50	69	Serum albumin family; a major component of blood plasma; binds ions (e.g., Ca^{2+}, Na^+, K^+) and hydrophobic molecules (e.g., fatty acids, hormones, drugs)
Fish			
Parvalbumin, Gad c 1	N/A	12	EF-hand domain, intracellular Ca^{2+} binding
Shrimp			
Tropomyosin, Pen a 1	N/A	36	Tropomyosins; regulates muscle contraction
Myosin light chain, Lit v 3.0101	N/A	19	Major allergen in adults
Sarcoplasmic calcium-binding protein	N/A	22	Major allergen in children
PLANT			
Peanut			
Vicilin, Ara h 1	N/A	63	Cupin superfamily, 7/8S globulins are trimeric seed-storage proteins
Conglutins, Ara h 2/6	N/A	17/19	Prolamin superfamily, 2S albumins, seed-storage proteins
Glycinin, Ara h 3	N/A	60	Seed storage of protein
PR10, Ara h 8	N/A	16.9	Bet v 1 homolog
Ara h 9	N/A	9.8	Nonspecific lipid transfer protein
Soybean			
Gly m 1	N/A	8	Soybean hull protein, inhalant allergen in occupational and environmental soy allergy
Profilin, Gly m 3	N/A	20	Highly homologous with Bet v 2, with an amino acid sequence homology of 73%
Gly m 4	N/A	17	PR protein with a 50% homology with Bet v 1; also called SAM 22 (starvation-associated message 22)
Gly m 5	18.5	50-71	Beta-conglycinin (vicilin, 7S globulin)
Gly m 6	51	54-63	Glycinin (legumin, 11S globulin), hexameric protein
PR Proteins Group 14		9-10	*Lipid Transfer Proteins*
Apple, Mal d 3	N/A		Trafficking of phospholipids; defense against fungal and bacterial infections
Apricot, Pru ar 3	N/A		
Peach, Pru p 3	N/A		
Plum, Pru d 1	N/A		
Corn, Zea m 14	N/A		
Peanut, Ara h 9	N/A		

TABLE 81-4 Characteristics of Important Food Allergens—cont'd

Protein Fraction and Nomenclature	Percent of Total Food Protein*	Molecular Mass (kD)	Protein Family and Function†
CLASS II FOOD ALLERGENS			
PLANT			
PR Proteins Group 2			*Involved in Fruit-Latex Syndrome*
Latex β-1,3 gluconase, Hev b 2	N/A	34-35	Catalysis of hydrolysis of β-1,3-glucosidic linkages in β-1,3-glucans in plant cell walls; implicated in protection against microbial pathogens, fertilization, pollen and seed germination, and fruit ripening
Allergens in avocado, banana, chestnut, fig, kiwi, and olive pollen	N/A		
PR Proteins Group 3			*Endochitinases; Panallergens Involved in the Fruit-Latex Syndrome*
Latex, Hev b 6.02	N/A	5	Hydrolysis of chitin in fungal cell walls and the exoskeleton of hexapods
Avocado Pers a 1	N/A	32	
Chestnut Cas s 5	N/A	31	
Grape Vit v 5	N/A	27	
PR Proteins Group 5 (Thaumatin-like)			*Rigid Structure of Antiparallel β-Sheets Stabilized by the Disulfide Bridges; Resistant to Heating and Digestion; Synthesized on Biotic and Abiotic Stress and During Fruit Ripening; Found in Pollen of Mountain Cedar (Jun a 3) and Cypress (Cup a 3)*
Apple, Mal d 2	N/A	31	
Cherry, Pru av 2	N/A	23.3	
PR Proteins Group 10			
Birch Bet v 1 homologs			Protein fold creates a large Y-shaped hydrophobic pocket that seems to bind plant steroids; some proteins have ribonuclease activity; Bet v 1 homologous proteins constitutively expressed in mature pollen, ripe fruits, roots, bulbs, and old leaves
Apple, Mal d 1	N/A	18	
Cherry, Pru av 1	N/A	18	
Apricot, Pru ar 1	N/A	17	
Pear, Pyr c 1	N/A	18	
Carrot, Dau c 1	N/A	16	
Celery, Api g 1	N/A	16	
Parsley, pcPR 1 and 2	N/A		
Hazelnut, Cor a 1	N/A	17	
Profilins birch Bet v 2 homologs			Proteins located in the cytosol that bind actin; key role in regulating intracellular transport process, cell morphogenesis, and cell division; celery-mugwort-spice syndrome
Latex, Hev b 8	N/A	14	
Celery, Api g 4	N/A	14	
Potato	N/A	14	
Cherry, Pru av 4	N/A	15	
Pear, Pyr c 4	N/A	14	
Peanut, Ara h 5	N/A	15	
Soybean, Gly m 3	N/A	14	

N/A, Not available; *PR*, pathogenesis-related protein.
*Approximate value.
†International Union of Immunological Societies (IUIS) allergen database. Information on allergen nomenclature. Available at http://www.allergen.org (accessed March 8, 2013).

Goldman and coworkers[9] investigated the relative allergenicity of milk proteins. Of 50 milk allergic children with positive skin test results, 30 were positive to two or more of the milk proteins: 34 to caseins, 22 to α-lactalbumin, 20 to β-lactoglobulin, and 21 to BSA. Of 45 children challenged with purified milk proteins, 62% reacted to β-lactoglobulin, 60% to casein, 53% to α-lactalbumin, and 52% to BSA.[40] It is likely that these proteins contained small amounts of other milk proteins, and studies with more highly purified proteins suggest that the casein proteins are more allergenic.

Immunoblotting techniques also have shown cross-reactivity among milk proteins in cows, goats, and sheep due to their high degree of homology. Oral challenge studies indicated that at least 90% of cow's milk–allergic children react to goat's milk.[41] About 10% of milk-allergic children react to beef, with a slightly higher percentage reacting to rare beef.[42]

Extensive heating (e.g., boiling at 95° C for about 20 minutes) destroys several of the whey proteins (i.e., BSA, bovine γ-globulin, and α-lactalbumin). However, routine pasteurization is not sufficient to denature these proteins, but it may increase the allergenicity of some milk proteins, such as β-lactoglobulin.[43] Sequential (linear) allergenic IgE-antibody binding epitopes have been mapped on the caseins β-lactoglobulin and α-lactalbumin, and they have been correlated with the persistence of cow's milk allergy.[44-46] About 75% of children with milk allergy tolerate extensively heated milk in baked products. Children reactive to baked milk tend to have a more severe phenotype of milk allergy with a higher likelihood of anaphylaxis and more prolonged duration of milk allergy.[47] Introduction of baked milk into the diet appears to accelerate development of tolerance to unheated milk.[48]

Chicken egg is the most common IgE-mediated food allergy in children. The white is considered more allergenic than the yolk, although IgE antibodies to chicken egg yolk immunoglobulin Y (IgY), apovitellenin I, and contaminating egg white proteins can be demonstrated.[49] The egg white contains 23 glycoproteins; ovomucoid, ovalbumin (the most abundant protein), and ovotransferrin have been identified as the major allergens. Ovomucoid is the dominant allergen when highly purified egg white proteins are used.[50] Ovomucoid (Gal d 1) is composed of 186 amino acids arranged in three tandem domains, a set tertiary structure, and six sequential (linear) IgE binding sites. Blinded OFCs with ovomucoid-depleted egg white demonstrated that ovomucoid was responsible for clinical reactivity in most egg-allergic children.[51] About 70% of egg-allergic children may be able to ingest egg protein in extensively heated (baked) products, such as breads, cakes, and cookies.[52] These children appear to lack IgE antibodies to sequential epitopes, and because the prolonged high temperature destroys the tertiary structure (discontinuous or conformational epitopes) of the egg white proteins, the children do not react.[53,54] Lack of an IgE-antibody response against ovomucoid appears to be a favorable prognostic factor for heat-denatured egg nonreactivity.[55] When baked with wheat gluten, ovomucoid polymerizes and forms high-molecular-mass complexes that are water insoluble, potentially making them less available for absorption. Another potential mechanism contributing to heat-induced decreases in allergenicity of egg white proteins is linked to decreased gastrointestinal digestibility and the inability of heated ovalbumin or ovomucoid to be absorbed in a form capable of triggering effector cells.[56]

Peanut is the most common food allergen in the population beyond the age of 4 years.[3] Peanut proteins are traditionally classified as albumins (water soluble) and globulins (saline solution soluble); the latter is further subdivided into arachin and conarachin fractions. Thirty-two protein bands have been identified on sodium dodecyl sulfate-polyacrylamide gel electrophoresis (SDS-PAGE); 12 of them have allergenic potential, and of those, three with molecular masses of 64.5 kD (Ara h 1),[57] 17.5 kD (Ara h 2),[58] and 64 kD (Ara h 3)[59] have been identified as major allergens. Ara h 5 is a profilin, whereas Ara h 4 appears to be an isoform of Ara h 3, and Ara h 6 and 7 appear to be isoforms of Ara h 2. Ara h 8 is a member of the PR10 protein family, and members are primarily involved in pollen-associated food allergy. Many peanut products, including flour and reprocessed peanuts, retain their allergenicity; however, highly refined peanut oil was found to be safe in 60 peanut-allergic individuals, whereas pressed (or extruded) oils were found to retain some of their allergenicity.[60]

Ara h 1 (64.5 kD) belongs to the vicilin family of seed-storage protein.[61] Using peanut-allergic patient sera and overlapping decapeptides representing the entire primary amino acid sequence of Ara h 1, 23 IgE-binding sequential epitopes were identified, four of which were recognized by more than 80% of peanut-allergic patient sera.[62] Mutational analysis of the immunodominant epitopes revealed that a single amino acid substitution, especially in the center of each epitope, could dramatically reduce IgE binding.[63] Expression of these mutated recombinant proteins may facilitate the development of safer vaccines for immunotherapy.[64] Ara h 1 induces activation of human dendritic cells (DCs) and enhances induction of Th2 differentiation by these DCs in naïve T cells. Ara h 1 was further shown to bind to the C-type lectin receptor (CLR) DC-SIGN. Deglycosylated Ara h 1 lacked this Th2-skewing effect, indicating that allergen-bound carbohydrate structures may act as a Th2-skewing adjuvant.[65] Incubation of DCs with Lewis-X trisaccharides suppressed production of IL-12, which suggests one mechanism for the enhanced Th2 skewing induced by these glycans.[35]

Ara h 2 (17.5 kD) is a member of the conglutin family of storage proteins, which has been fully sequenced and a full-length cDNA clone isolated.[58] Ten IgE-binding sequential epitopes have been identified, three of which are clearly immunodominant, and mutational analysis of these major allergenic epitopes demonstrated that single amino acid substitutions markedly reduced IgE binding.[63] T cell epitope mapping with peanut-specific T cell lines demonstrated four immunodominant regions on the Ara h 2 molecule, three of which mapped to locations different from the immunodominant IgE-binding epitopes.[66] Ara h 2 has been identified as an immunodominant allergen with a relative potency up to 100-fold higher than Ara h 1 and Ara h 3 in basophil activation studies and intracutaneous testing.[67] Detectable specific IgE antibodies to Ara h 2 have been associated with an increased risk of systemic reactions during OFC.[68] *Ara h 6* (15 kD) has homology with Ara h 2, especially in the middle portion and at the C-terminal end of the protein. Almost complete inhibition of the IgE-Ara h 6 interaction with Ara h 2 demonstrates that at least part of the epitopes of Ara h 6 are cross-reactive with epitopes on Ara h 2.[69] Compared with Ara h 1 and Ara h 3, Ara h 2 and Ara h 6 are significantly more resistant to pepsin digestion, even at very high concentrations of pepsin, likely due to the presence of the disulfide bridges.[70]

Ara h 3 (64 kD) is a member of the glycinin family of storage of proteins.[59] Glycinins represent a class of seed-storage proteins that are first synthesized as precursor proteins of approximately 60 kDa and then proteolytically cleaved into 40- and 20-kD proteins. A full-length cDNA of the 64-kD protein has been isolated, and four IgE-binding sequential epitopes have been identified.[59]

Ara h 8 is a Bet v 1 cross-reactive protein with low stability during roasting and no stability in gastric digestion. It has been identified as a major allergen in adults with pollen allergy and oral allergy symptoms to peanut.[71]

Soybean is a second member of the legume family that provokes a significant number of hypersensitivity reactions, predominantly in infants and young children. Because soybean is inexpensive and contains a high concentration of protein, it is used in many commercial foods.

Twenty-eight potential allergens have been identified in soy based on IgE binding from patients with soy allergy.[35] Only a few of these are recognized as major allergens by the International Union of Immunological Societies (IUIS) Allergen Nomenclature Subcommittee: Gly m 1, Gly m 2, Gly m 3, and Gly m 4. Other dominant allergens in soy include soybean Kunitz trypsin inhibitor, the thiol-protease Gly m Bd 30k, α-subunit of β-conglycinin (BC, Gly m 5), the acidic chain of the major storage protein glycinin (Gly m 6) G1 subunit, basic chain of the G2 subunit, and 2S albumin.

Gly m 1 and Gly m 2 are soybean hull proteins that are aeroallergens. These proteins in addition to Kunitz trypsin inhibitor have been implicated in development of allergic asthma. Gly m 1 (i.e., Gly m Bd30K/P34 or P34) is a soybean vacuolar protein that belongs to the group of nonspecific lipid transfer proteins. Gly m 1 shares high sequence similarity to thiol proteinases of the papain family, which includes the major allergen in dust mites, Der p 1.

Gly m 3 and Gly m 4 are related to birch pollen. With an amino acid sequence identity of 73%, Gly m 3 is highly homologous with the profilin Bet v 2. The IgE-binding epitopes of Gly m 3 are highly conformational, and fragments of Gly m 3 fail to bind IgE. Gly m 4, also called SAM 22 (starvation-associated message 22), is a PR protein with a 50% homology with Bet v 1. Serum IgE from 85% of birch pollen–allergic patients react to Gly m 4.[72] About 10% of Central European patients sensitized to birch pollen have concomitant soy allergy, mainly due to cross-reactivity with Gly m 4.[73]

Gly m 5 (β-conglycinin, 7S) and Gly m 6 (glycinin, 11S) are the seed-storage proteins from the cupin family that were found to be major allergens in a cohort of 30 patients with DBPCFC-confirmed soy allergy, suggesting that these molecules are good diagnostic markers of component-resolved in vitro testing. Gly m 5 and Gly m 6 have been associated with anaphylactic reactions in Japanese children.[74] The allergenic epitopes on the Gly m 6 acidic chain are homologous with IgE-binding epitopes on peanut Ara h 3. Similar to highly refined peanut oil, refined soy oil did not provoke allergic reactions to soy in eight patients after ingesting up to 8 mL of soy oil.[75]

Tree nut allergies affect about 0.6% of the American population.[3] In a national registry of peanut and nut allergic individuals, walnuts provoked the most allergic reactions (34%), followed by cashews (20%), almonds (15%), pecan (9%), pistachio (7%), and by hazel nut, Brazil nut, pine nut, and macadamia nut (all <5%).[76] Skin testing reveals extensive cross-reactivity among tree nuts. Although individuals allergic to one nut can tolerate other nuts, too few patients have been systematically challenged to a variety of nuts to determine the extent of clinical cross-reactivity. High immunologic and clinical cross-reactivity has been found between cashew and pistachio and between walnut and pecan.[77] Patients allergic to nuts do not necessarily need to avoid peanuts (a legume) and vice versa. However, about 30% of peanut-allergic patients also reacted to at least one tree nut.[78,79]

Fish are a common cause of food-allergic reactions in adults and in children.[80] Edible fish are found predominantly in the bony fish class (Osteichthyes), in which there are hundreds of species. The major allergen in cod, Gad c 1, is a parvalbumin that has been isolated from the myogen fraction of the white meat. A similar protein, Sal s 1, has been isolated from salmon. It is heat stable and resistant to proteolytic digestion, has a molecular mass of 12 kD and an isoelectric point of 4.75, and is composed of 113 amino acids.[81] Specific IgE-binding epitopes have been identified in Sal s 1; two of them correlate with those previously described in Gad c 1. The three-dimensional structure of Gad c 1 is arranged in three domains, two of which bind calcium. Using SDS-PAGE and immunoblot analyses, 10 common fish species were shown to have a protein that is similar to Gad c 1 and up to 29 protein fractions. Eleven patients with histories of fish allergy had multiple positive skin test results for various fish; 7 of 11 reacted to only one fish species in DBPCFCs, 1 reacted to two fish, 2 reacted to three fish, and 1 patient did not react to any fish during blinded challenges. The relative content of parvalbumin may underlie differences in allergenic potential, which is highest in white fish (e.g., swordfish, codfish, flounder), followed by salmon and tuna.[82] Unlike many other food allergens, the fish protein fractions responsible for clinical symptoms in some patients appear to be more susceptible to manipulation (e.g., heating, lyophilization) than other foods, because reactions occurred during open feedings of the fish in approximately 20% of those with negative DBPCFCs using lyophilized fish.[83] Most patients allergic to fresh, cooked salmon or tuna tolerated canned salmon or tuna, indicating that preparation led to destruction of the major allergens. Nevertheless, allergic reactions after exposure to airborne allergens emitted during the cooking of fish are not uncommon.[84] Fish has been reported as a trigger in seafood industry workers who develop occupational asthma.[85] In some patients, allergic reactions after ingestion of fish, particularly raw or marinated fish, are caused by allergy to the fish parasite *Anisakis simplex*.

Shellfish allergens are considered a major cause of food-allergic reactions in adults, affecting up to 2.3% of the U.S. adult population.[86] Shellfish allergy is also common in Asian children.[87] Shellfish include a wide variety of crustaceans (e.g., lobsters, crabs, prawns, crawfish, shrimp) and mollusks (e.g., snails, mussels, oysters, scallops, clams, squid, octopus). Shrimp allergens have been most extensively studied. Eighteen precipitating antigens have been detected by crossed immunoelectrophoresis (CRIE); seven appeared to be allergens as determined by CRIE using a pool of sera from six shrimp-allergic subjects.[88] Tropomyosin, a protein found in muscle and elsewhere, has been identified as the major allergen in shrimp.[89] Myosin light chain (MLC) has been identified as another major allergen (Lit v 3.0101 in adults with shrimp allergy), whereas sarcoplasmic calcium-binding protein (SCP) has been identified as a major allergen in children.[90,91] Considerable cross-reactivity among crustaceans has been demonstrated by skin test and in vitro IgE testing. Invertebrate tropomyosins are highly homologous and tend to be allergenic,[92] such as those from crustaceans (e.g., shrimp, crab, crawfish, lobster), arachnids (e.g., house-dust mites), insects (e.g. cockroaches), and mollusks (e.g., squid, snails), whereas vertebrate tropomyosin tends to be nonallergenic.

Wheat (e.g., spelt) and other cereal grains (e.g., rye, barley) belong to the Poaceae family and share a number of homologous proteins among themselves and with grass pollen.[93] Cereal grains are frequently implicated in food-allergic reactions in children with atopic dermatitis. On the basis of their solubility, wheat proteins can be classified as water/salt-soluble albumins and globulins and water/salt-insoluble gliadins and glutenins.[94] Among the major allergens identified in the water/salt-soluble fraction of wheat flour are the cereal α-amylase inhibitors (AAIs) and α-amylase/trypsin inhibitors (AATIs), which are capable of sensitizing by oral and inhaled routes (important allergens in baker's asthma and rhinitis). The globulin and glutenin fractions are the major allergenic fractions in IgE-mediated reactions, as are gliadins in celiac disease and in food-associated, exercise-induced anaphylaxis (ω-5 gliadin, Tri a 19).[95,96] Lipid transfer proteins have been identified as allergens in cases of reactions to beers brewed from barley and wheat. In a study of pediatric patients, 70 of 225 children were found to have at least one positive prick skin test to wheat, rye, oat, barley, rice, or corn: 28 of 70 to one grain, 16 of 70 to two grains, 12 of 70 to three grains, 6 of 70 to four grains, 6 of 70 to five grains, and 2 of 70 to six grains.[97] However, only 15 patients had at least one positive DBPCFC to a cereal grain; two children reacted to two grains, and two reacted to three grains. SDS-PAGE and immunoblot analyses with patient sera revealed 27 to 31 protein bands in the range of 7.8-66.5 kDa for each of the six cereal grains studied. Nonspecific binding to lectin fractions was seen with each grain, and extensive immunologic cross-reactivity occurred among the cereals, as was seen with skin-prick testing. Homologies to allergenic proteins in grass pollens account for a large number of clinically irrelevant positive skin tests to wheat and other cereal grains.

PR proteins comprise a large number of class 2 allergenic proteins (see Table 81-4) that are found in various vegetables and fruits.[98] These proteins are induced when pathogens, wounding, or certain environmental pressures (e.g., drought, heat) stress the plant. PR proteins have been classified as members of 14 families, although 6 PR protein families account for most cross-reactivity among plant proteins. Allergens homologous to the PR2 β-1,3-glucanase proteins are responsible for the latex-fruit cross-reactivity seen between latex (Hev b 2) and avocado, banana, chestnut, fig, and kiwi. Two families of chitinases that are similar to the latex allergen Hev b 6.02 have been identified as allergens in several vegetables. PR3-type proteins are found in chestnut and avocado (Pers a 1), and PR4-type proteins are wound-induced proteins found in tomato and potato (Win 1 and Win 2). PR5-type thaumatin-like proteins have been identified as cross-reacting proteins found in apples (Mal d 2) and cherry (Pru av 2). The PR10-type proteins are homologous with the major birch pollen allergen (Bet v 1), and they account for cross-reactivity between birch pollen and fruits of the Rosaceae species, such as apple (Mal d 1), cherry (Pru av 1), apricot (Pru ar 1), and pear (Pyr c 1); vegetables of the Apiaceae species, such as carrot (Dau c 1), celery (Api g 1), and parsley (pcPR 1 and 2); and hazel nut (Cor a 1).

Nonspecific lipid transfer proteins, or PR14-type proteins, form a family of 9-kD proteins distributed widely throughout the plant kingdom. Lipid transfer proteins have been identified as major allergenic proteins in Prunoideae family members, such as peach (Pru p 1 in peach skin and Pru p 3 in the fruit), apple (Mal d 3), apricot, plum, and cherries. Gly m 1, a major allergen in soybean, is a lipid transfer protein. Due to their low molecular mass and compact structure, nonspecific lipid transfer proteins are resistant to heating and proteases, and among plant allergens, they are considered to have a potential to induce systemic allergic reactions.

Profilins are actin-binding small proteins (12 to 15 kD) present in all eukaryotic cells. Profilin was first identified in birch pollen (Bet v 2) and is recognized as an allergenic protein in several fruits and vegetables (i.e., panallergen).[98] Plant profilins share about 75% amino acid sequence homology among themselves. Profilins have a compact globular structure with a central, seven-stranded, antiparallel β-sheet enclosed by the N- and C-terminal α-helices. Because of its conserved amino acid sequences, about 10% to 30% of all tree pollen–allergic patients react to profilin. Moreover, sensitization to profilin is considered a risk factor for developing multiple pollen-associated food allergies. Profilins are responsible for the celery-mugwort-spice syndrome and are responsible for pollen-food allergy syndrome (i.e., oral allergy syndrome) to apple, pear, carrot, celery (Api g 4), and potato in birch pollen–allergic patients. Profilins have also been identified in tomato, peanut (Ara h 5), and soybean (Gly m 3), but whether these proteins cause allergic reactions remains to be established.

CARBOHYDRATE ALLERGENS

The carbohydrate moieties present on many foods can induce IgE responses.[35] Because carbohydrate moieties share significant structural homologies beyond that of proteins, they are prone to extensive cross-reactivity and are referred to as *cross-reactive carbohydrate determinants*. Approximately 15% to 30% of allergic patients generate specific antiglycan IgE, but very few develop clinical allergy. Bromelain was identified as the first food antigen that contained an oligosaccharide with two structural features that had not been found in mammalian glycoproteins: core α1,3-fucose and xylose. Galactose-α-1,3-galactose (α-gal) has been identified as a cause of serious, even fatal, anaphylaxis.[99] In contrast to previously described cross-reactive carbohydrate determinants expressed in plants and insects, the oligosaccharide α-gal is abundantly expressed on cells and tissues of nonprimate mammals. This expression pattern makes α-gal potentially clinically relevant as a food allergen (e.g., beef, pork, lamb) or as an inhaled allergen (e.g., cat, dog).[100] IgE antibodies to α-gal are associated with an unusual form of delayed anaphylaxis, which occurs 3 to 6 hours after ingestion of mammalian meat that carries α-gal. Patients with IgE to α-gal describe generalized urticaria or frank anaphylaxis starting 3 to 6 hours after eating beef, pork, or lamb and have a consistent pattern of skin testing (likelihood of positive results is increased by testing with freshly ground meat or with intradermal testing) and serum IgE antibody results. Most patients developed anaphylaxis to red meat in adulthood; some reported receiving multiple tick bites, suggesting that tick bites, especially the lone star tick (*Amblyomma americanum*) may predispose to sensitization to α-gal.

Food additives and colorings derived from natural sources that contain proteins may induce allergic reactions. They include colors derived from turmeric, paprika, seeds (e.g., annatto), and insects (e.g., carmine, cochineal). Chemical additives are not likely to cause IgE-mediated food allergy, but some may have drug effects that cause adverse reactions, including allergy-like symptoms, or they may invoke immune responses. Tartrazine (yellow #5) is a synthetic color that has been extensively investigated because of concerns that it may trigger hives, allergic reactions, and asthma. However, well-conducted studies have not validated these concerns. Sulfites are added to foods as a preservative, an antibrowning agent, or a bleaching effect. In sensitive persons, sulfites may induce asthma.

CROSS-REACTIVITY

Structural homology among allergens underlies immunologic and clinical cross-reactivity.[101] More than 70% identity in primary sequence is considered necessary for clinical cross-reactivity. However, the expression of clinical cross-reactivity is modulated by additional factors, including: protein solubility and digestibility, concentration and affinity of the specific IgE antibody, and the dose and route of allergen exposure. High rates of clinical cross-reactivity are observed among milks from cows, goats, and sheep (>90%); melons (90%); crustacean shellfish (75%); Rosaceae fruits such as apple, pear, peach (55%); and bony fish (50%). Lower rates are observed among tree nuts (37%), grains (20%), cow's milk and beef (10%), and peanuts and other legumes (5%). The rates of pollen-fruit cross-reactivity are about 50% for birch pollen and Rosaceae fruits.

The rate of reactions to kiwi, banana, or avocado among latex-allergic individuals is about 11%. The risk of latex allergy among kiwi-, banana-, or avocado-allergic individuals is about 35%.

Pathophysiologic Mechanisms of Food Allergy

In the susceptible host, a failure to develop or a breakdown in oral tolerance, commonly as a result of heavy occupational exposure or sensitization to cross-reactive allergens, may result in allergic responses to ingested food antigens. The extended Gell and Coombs classification provides a framework for discussing hypersensitivity reactions, but food-allergic disorders usually involve more than one of the classic mechanisms described (Table 81-5).

IgE-MEDIATED FOOD ALLERGY

The best characterized food allergic reactions involve IgE antibodies that bind to high-affinity FcεRI receptors on mast cells and basophils as well as low-affinity FcεRII (CD23) receptors on macrophages, monocytes, lymphocytes, and platelets. When food allergens penetrate mucosal barriers and reach IgE antibodies bound to mast cells or basophils, mediators are released that induce vasodilatation, smooth muscle contraction, and mucus secretion, producing the symptoms of immediate hypersensitivity. The activated mast cells also release a variety of cytokines, which may contribute to the IgE-mediated late phase response. During the initial 4 to 8 hours, primarily neutrophils and eosinophils invade the site of response. These infiltrating cells are activated and release a variety of mediators, including platelet-activating factor, peroxidases, eosinophil major basic protein, and eosinophil cationic protein. In the subsequent 24 to 48 hours, lymphocytes and monocytes infiltrate the area and establish a more chronic inflammatory picture. With repeated ingestion of a food allergen, mononuclear cells are stimulated to secrete histamine-releasing factor (HRF), a cytokine that interacts with IgE molecules bound to the surface of basophils (and perhaps mast cells) and increases their releasability. The spontaneous generation of HRF by activated mononuclear cells in vitro has been associated with increased bronchial hyperreactivity in patients with asthma and increased cutaneous irritability in children with atopic dermatitis.

IgE-mediated allergic reactions are associated with a variety of symptoms: generalized (e.g., hypotension, shock), cutaneous (e.g., urticaria, angioedema, pruritic morbilliform rash), oral and gastrointestinal (e.g., lip, tongue, and palatal pruritus and swelling, laryngeal edema, vomiting, diarrhea), and upper and lower respiratory systems (e.g., ocular pruritus and tearing, nasal congestion, pharyngeal edema, wheezing). A rise in plasma histamine has been associated with the development of these symptoms after blinded food challenges. In contrast, β-tryptase levels are usually not elevated.

In one study, increased levels of serum platelet-activating factor (PAF) were reported for subjects with peanut-induced anaphylaxis who presented to the emergency department.[102] The proportion of patients with low PAF acetylhydrolase values increased with the severity of anaphylaxis. Serum PAF acetylhydrolase activity was significantly lower in patients with fatal peanut anaphylaxis than in control patients, which suggested that impaired ability to breakdown PAF might contribute to severe anaphylaxis. However, these findings require replication.

Children possessing IgE antibodies directed at more numerous epitopes on major peanut or milk allergens had histories of more severe reactions than the children with IgE antibodies directed at fewer epitopes.[103,104] Greater diversity of recognized allergenic epitopes and increased IgE antibody affinity were associated with more efficient cross-linking of the IgE receptors and degranulation of effector cells.

In IgE-mediated gastrointestinal reactions, endoscopic observation has revealed local vasodilation, edema, mucus secretion, and petechial hemorrhaging.[105] Increased stool and serum PGE_2 and PGF_2 levels have been observed after adverse food reactions leading to diarrhea.[106] Atopic dermatitis and chronic airway hyperreactivity (e.g., asthma) involve activation of other cell types (e.g., eosinophils) through IgE-mediated mechanisms.

AUGMENTATION FACTORS

Several factors have been associated with increased risk of developing food allergy and with increased severity of food-allergic reactions. Drugs lowering the gastric acidity predisposed to de novo sensitization to food allergen (i.e., hazelnut and codfish) in a mouse model and in treated humans.[107] In allergic individuals, antacids increased the severity of codfish-induced anaphylaxis.[108] Exercise and ingestion of alcohol with nonsteroidal antiinflammatory drugs are associated with increased severity of food-induced anaphylaxis. In oral milk, egg, and peanut immunotherapy trials, viral infection, febrile

TABLE 81-5 Classification of Food-Allergic Disorders Based on Pathophysiology

Disorder	IgE-Mediated Response	IgE- and Cell-Mediated Response	Non–IgE-Mediated Response
Generalized	Food-dependent, exercise-induced anaphylaxis		
Cutaneous	Urticaria, angioedema, flushing, acute morbilliform rash, acute contact urticaria	Atopic dermatitis, contact dermatitis	Contact dermatitis, dermatitis herpetiformis
Gastrointestinal	Oral allergy syndrome, gastrointestinal anaphylaxis	Allergic eosinophilic esophagitis, allergic eosinophilic gastroenteritis	Allergic proctocolitis, food protein-induced enterocolitis syndrome, celiac disease, infantile colic
Respiratory	Acute rhinoconjunctivitis, acute bronchospasm	Asthma	Pulmonary hemosiderosis (Heiner syndrome)

Modified from Nowak-Węgrzyn A, Sampson HA. Adverse reactions to foods. Med Clin North Am 2006;90:97-127.

illness, menstruation, and exercise were associated with reaction to previously tolerated maintenance doses.[109]

NON–IgE-MEDIATED FOOD ALLERGY

Type II antigen-antibody complex–dependent cytotoxic reactions occur when specific antibody binds to a surface tissue antigen or hapten associated with a cell and induces complement activation. Complement activation products promote the generation of various inflammatory mediators that lead to subsequent tissue damage. A few reports have implicated an antibody-dependent thrombocytopenia resulting from milk ingestion.[110] However, little evidence supports any significant role for type II hypersensitivity in food-allergic disorders.

Type III antigen-antibody complex–mediated hypersensitivity has been implicated in patients with a variety of complaints and elevated serum levels of food antigen-antibody complexes. However, food antigen-antibody complexes have been demonstrated in the sera of normal individuals and in patients with suspected food hypersensitivity.[111] The complexes formed by the interaction of IgG, IgA, or IgM antibodies to β-lactoglobulin are found 1 to 3 hours after ingesting milk in normal children and adults. Although IgE-food antigen complexes are more commonly found in patients with food hypersensitivity, there are a few reports of antigen-immune complex–mediated vasculitis.[112]

Type IV and delayed type IV cell-mediated hypersensitivities have been implicated in food-allergic disorders for which the onset of clinical symptoms occurred several hours after the ingestion of a suspected food allergen. Ingestion of the sensitizing antigen may provoke mucosal lesions. In humans, a few investigators have found increased lymphocyte proliferation to food antigens in food-allergic individuals, but increased proliferation also is found in many asymptomatic subjects. Cell-mediated hypersensitivity reactions contribute to several gastrointestinal disorders, such as eosinophilic esophagitis, eosinophilic gastroenteritis, atopic dermatitis, and celiac disease. In several adverse food reactions, pathogenic factors are not well defined but are believed to involve immunologic mechanisms. Antigen-antibody complexes and cell-mediated reactions in part may be responsible for these pathogenic states (see Table 81-5).

Clinical Manifestations of Food Allergy

Classification of food hypersensitivity disorders into those primarily involving IgE-mediated reactions, those not involving IgE-mediated mechanisms, and those that may involve IgE- and non–IgE-mediated mechanisms is most useful for clinical and diagnostic purposes, as depicted in Table 81-6.

GASTROINTESTINAL FOOD ALLERGY

Gastrointestinal IgE-Mediated Food Allergy

IgE–mediated gastrointestinal food allergy has been studied extensively in rodent models, which elucidated physiologic changes provoked by the ingestion of a food allergen (see Table 81-6). There is a sharp increase in gastric acid secretion in the stomach, delayed gastric emptying, and mast cell degranulation with a rise in intraluminal histamine levels. In the intestine, sodium (Na^+), chloride (Cl^-), and water absorption decrease sharply while abnormal contractility increases markedly, leading to diarrhea. Histologically, intestinal mast cells are degranulated, and although significant disruption of the basement membrane and underlying collagenous matrix is apparent by ultrastructural examination, the mucosal architecture appears largely unchanged after a reaction.[113] Cromolyn sodium, histamine H_1 antihistamines, and H_2 antihistamines do not block the allergic response.

The effect of repeated daily ingestion of allergen has been investigated using a similar model in rats sensitized with ovalbumin.[114] After the first feeding of ovalbumin in sensitized rats, serum rat mast cell protein (RMCP) II levels rose to approximately 16 times normal on the first day and ranged between two and five times normal on the subsequent 4 days. After the rats were rested for 9 days and then fed ovalbumin, serum RMCP II levels again rose, but only to five times normal concentrations. In the sensitized rats, the initial allergen challenge led to a marked mast cell activation (i.e., release of RMCP II and probably other mast cell mediators) followed by a period of partial desensitization. Subsequent exposures to allergen, even after short periods of avoidance, provoked reduced (but significant) amounts of immediate mast cell mediator release. Similar blunting of symptoms is seen in humans, which accounts for the need to have an extended period of complete food allergen avoidance to elicit a distinctive response during the OFC. The phenomenon of partial desensitization due to frequent allergen exposure also explains why food-allergic patients with primarily cutaneous symptoms (e.g., atopic dermatitis) who are placed on strict elimination diets frequently experience more severe generalized symptoms if the food allergen is accidentally ingested after prolonged avoidance.[115]

Human studies of IgE-mediated food hypersensitivity initially focused on roentgenologic changes associated with the ingestion of food allergens. In one of the first reports, a wheat-sensitive patient was studied after a deliberate feeding of wheat. Hypertonicity was seen in the transverse and pelvic colon, and hypotonicity was observed in the cecum and ascending colon.[116] In a later study, four patients were evaluated after administering barium mixtures containing specific allergens. Gastric retention, hypermotility of the intestine, and colonic spasm were observed.[117] In a third study, 12 food-allergic children underwent a single-blind food challenge and were followed fluoroscopically to compare the outcome of barium sulfate meals with and without food allergen.[118] The most prominent findings included gastric hypotonia and retention of the allergen test meal, prominent pylorospasm, and increased or decreased peristaltic activity of the intestines.

Some investigators used the rigid gastroscope in the late 1930s to observe allergic reactions in the stomach.[119] After placing a small amount of food allergen on the stomach mucosa, the mucosa of patients with gastrointestinal allergy became markedly hyperemic and edematous, with patches of thick, gray mucus and scattered petechiae, confirming the earlier discovery by Walzer and colleagues using passively sensitized intestinal mucosal sites.[28] Only mild hyperemia of the gastric mucosa was seen in patients with wheezing provoked by food ingestion. Later studies of intragastral provocation under endoscopic control (IPEC) confirmed the earlier observations.[105] Increased numbers of intestinal mast cells were observed before challenge in food-allergic patients compared with normal controls and significant decreases in stainable mast cells and tissue histamine content after a positive food challenge.

TABLE 81-6 Gastrointestinal Food-Allergic Disorders

Disorder*	Age Group	Characteristics	Diagnosis	Prognosis and Course
IgE-MEDIATED DISORDERS				
Acute gastrointestinal hypersensitivity	Any	Onset: minutes to 2 h; nausea, abdominal pain, emesis, diarrhea; typically in conjunction with cutaneous and/or respiratory symptoms	History, positive SPT and/or serum food-IgE level; confirmatory OFC	Varies, food-dependent; milk, soy, egg, and wheat typically outgrown; peanut, tree nuts, seeds, and shellfish typically persistent
Pollen-food allergy syndrome (oral allergy syndrome)	Any; most common in young adults (50% of birch pollen–allergic adults)	Immediate symptoms on contact of raw fruit with oral mucosa: pruritus, tingling, erythema, or angioedema of the lips, tongue, oropharynx; throat pruritus/tightness	History, positive SPT with raw fruits or vegetables; OFC positive with raw fruit, negative with cooked	Severity of symptoms varies with pollen season; may improve in a subset of patients with pollen immunotherapy
IgE AND NON–IgE-MEDIATED DISORDERS				
Eosinophilic esophagitis	Any, but especially infants, children, and adolescents	*Children*: chronic or intermittent symptoms of gastroesophageal reflux, emesis, dysphagia, abdominal pain, and irritability *Adults*: abdominal pain, dysphagia, and food impaction	History, positive SPT and/or food-IgE level in 50% but poor correlation with clinical symptoms; patch testing may be of value; elimination diet and OFC; endoscopy or biopsy provides conclusive diagnosis and information about treatment response	Varies, not well established; improvement with elimination diet within 6-8 wk; elemental diet may be required; often responds to swallowed topical steroids
Allergic eosinophilic gastroenteritis	Any	Chronic or intermittent abdominal pain, emesis, irritability, poor appetite, failure to thrive, weight loss, anemia, protein-losing gastroenteropathy	History, positive SPT, and/or food-IgE level in 50% but poor correlation with clinical symptoms, elimination diet, and OFC; endoscopy or biopsy provides conclusive diagnosis and information about treatment response	Varies, not well established; improvement with elimination diet within 6-8 wk; elemental diet may be required
NON–IgE-MEDIATED DISORDERS				
Allergic proctocolitis	Young infants (<6 mo), frequently breastfed	Blood-streaked or heme-positive stools; otherwise healthy appearing	History, prompt response (resolution of gross blood in 48 h) to allergen elimination; biopsy conclusive but not necessary for most	Most able to tolerate milk or soy by 1-2 yr
Food protein-induced enterocolitis syndrome	Young infants	*Chronic*: emesis, diarrhea, failure to thrive on chronic exposure *Subacute*: repetitive emesis, dehydration (15% shock), diarrhea on repeat exposure after elimination period; breastfeeding protective	History, response to dietary restriction; OFC	Most have resolution in 1-3 yr; rarely persists into late teenage years
Dietary protein-induced enteropathy	Young infants; incidence has decreased	Protracted diarrhea, (steatorrhea), emesis, failure to thrive, anemia in 40%	History, endoscopy and biopsy; response to dietary restriction	Most have resolution in 1-2 yr
Celiac disease (gluten-sensitive enteropathy)	Any	Chronic diarrhea, malabsorption, abdominal distention, flatulence, failure to thrive or weight loss; may be associated with oral ulcers and/or dermatitis herpetiformis	Biopsy diagnostic, shows villous atrophy; screening with serum IgA antitissue transglutaminase and antigliadin; resolution of symptoms with gluten elimination and relapse on oral challenge	Lifelong

Modified from Nowak-Węgrzyn A, Sampson HA. Adverse reactions to foods. Med Clin North Am 2006;90:97-127.
IgE, Immunoglobulin E; *OFC*, oral food challenge; *SPT*, skin-prick test.
*See Chapter 68 for more information on eosinophilic gastroenteropathies.

Pollen-food allergy syndrome, traditionally referred to as oral allergy syndrome, is elicited by a variety of plant proteins, especially PR proteins cross-reacting with airborne allergens. Sensitization to inhaled pollen is the primary event, with secondary reactions occurring on ingestion of the cross-reactive plant foods. Symptoms are provoked almost exclusively in the oropharynx and rarely involve other target organs. It is estimated that pollen-food allergy syndrome affects 50% to 70% of adults suffering from pollen allergy, especially to birch, ragweed, and mugwort pollens. Little is known regarding its prevalence among children. In one study, among 72 children (6 to 16 years of age) with severe rhinoconjunctivitis to birch pollen participating in a clinical trial of birch pollen immunotherapy, 93% reported symptoms after ingestion of fruits or vegetables, or both, but the prevalence rates for the general population have not been determined.[120] Local contact IgE-mediated mast cell activation provokes the rapid onset of pruritus, tingling, and angioedema of the lips, tongue, palate, and throat, and it occasionally elicits a sensation of pruritus in the ears or tightness in the throat. Symptoms are usually induced by raw fruits and vegetables, but they are short-lived due to exquisite susceptibility of the allergens to digestion. The cooked forms of these foods typically are not capable of inducing symptoms.

Ragweed-allergic patients may experience pollen-food allergy syndrome after contact with various fresh melons (e.g., watermelon, cantaloupe, honeydew) and bananas. Symptoms may vary throughout the year, as shown for birch pollen–related food allergies. Symptoms were more prominent during the birch pollen season, corresponding to the seasonal rise in birch-specific IgE levels. Birch pollen–allergic patients may develop symptoms after the ingestion of raw carrots, celery, apples, pears, hazelnuts, and kiwi. Cross-reactivity between birch pollen and various fruits and vegetables is due to homology among various PR proteins. For example, Mal d 1, the major apple allergen, is 63% homologous with the major birch pollen allergen, Bet v 1 (see Table 81-6).

Diagnosis is based on a suggestive history and positive "prick plus prick" skin tests with the implicated fresh fruits or vegetables in patients with allergic rhinitis. Skin-prick test results with commercial extracts are often negative because the responsible allergen is often destroyed in the manufacturing process. Novel platforms, such as protein microarray (ISAC chip) and ImmunoCAP with individual purified or recombinant major allergens, offer superior specificity and sensitivity compared with conventional tests. Studies report various effects on reducing or eliminating oral allergy symptoms with successful immunotherapy for pollen-induced rhinitis.[64]

Immediate gastrointestinal food allergy (i.e., gastrointestinal anaphylaxis) is a form of IgE-mediated gastrointestinal hypersensitivity that often accompanies allergic manifestations in other target organs and results in a variety of symptoms. Symptoms usually develop within minutes to 2 hours of consuming the responsible food allergen and consist of nausea, abdominal pain, cramps, vomiting, and diarrhea. In food-allergic children with atopic dermatitis, frequent ingestion of a food allergen appears to induce partial desensitization of gastrointestinal mast cells, resulting in less pronounced symptoms, such as occasional minor complaints of poor appetite and periodic abdominal pain. However, carbohydrate absorption studies, a measure of gut wall integrity, demonstrate malabsorption in such patients. A similar diminution of symptoms is seen in young infants with frequent vomiting, leading to a loss of consistent vomiting immediately after feeding.

Diagnosis is established by clinical history, determination of food-specific IgE antibodies (i.e., skin-prick tests or in vitro IgE measurement), complete elimination of the suspected food allergen for up to 2 weeks with resolution of symptoms, and OFC. OFCs usually provoke typical symptoms if the allergen has been strictly eliminated from the patient's diet for 10 to 14 days.

Mixed IgE- and Non–IgE-Mediated Gastrointestinal Food Allergy

Mixed IgE- and non–IgE-mediated disorders may involve IgE- and cell-mediated mechanisms. Allergic eosinophilic esophagitis, gastritis, and gastroenteritis are characterized by infiltration of the esophagus, stomach, and intestinal walls with eosinophils, basal zone hyperplasia, papillary elongation, absence of vasculitis, and peripheral eosinophilia in about 50% of patients. A complete discussion of these disorders is provided in Chapter 68.

Eosinophilic esophagitis (i.e., allergic eosinophilic esophagitis) is increasingly seen during infancy through adolescence, although the diagnosis appears to be occurring more frequently in adults. Eosinophilic esophagitis typically manifests with symptoms of chronic gastroesophageal reflux disease (GERD), intermittent emesis, food refusal, abdominal pain, dysphagia, irritability, sleep disturbance, and failure to respond to conventional reflux medications. In adults, abdominal discomfort, dysphagia, and food impaction are more common. Diagnosis depends on the gastrointestinal biopsy demonstrating a characteristic eosinophilic infiltration, typically more than 15 eosinophils per high-power field (×40).[121] The thymic stromal lymphopoietin (TSLP) protein is overexpressed in lesions from eosinophilic esophagitis, and mutations in the *TSLP* gene on chromosome 5q22.1 may predispose to eosinophilic esophagitis.[122]

Elimination of the responsible food allergens from the diet for up to 8 weeks may be necessary to bring about resolution of symptoms and for up to 12 weeks to bring about normalization of intestinal histology. This diet often requires the use of an amino acid–derived formula or an oligoantigenic diet. To identify the responsible foods, challenges are required that consist of reintroducing the suspect food allergen (often for 3 to 5 days) and demonstrating recurrence of symptoms and a significant eosinophilic infiltrate on biopsy.

Dietary intervention is often effective, and about 50% of children respond favorably to dietary modifications. However, institution of an elemental diet (e.g., amino acid–based formulas) is often necessary to identify the food allergens that provoke symptoms. A six-food elimination diet was effective in eliminating symptoms and esophageal pathology in more than 70% of patients treated.[123] An alternative approach is to use inhaled or oral corticosteroids, which usually bring about rapid symptomatic relief.[124] Early trials of anti-IL-5 therapy have provided mixed results.[64]

Infantile colic is an ill-defined syndrome of paroxysmal fussiness characterized by inconsolable agonized crying, drawing up of the legs, abdominal distention, and excessive gas. It usually develops in the first 2 to 4 weeks of life and persists through the third or fourth month. Although a variety of psychosocial and dietary factors have been implicated, it is difficult to establish the cause of infantile colic. However, double-blind, crossover trials of bottle-fed and breast-fed infants suggest that IgE-mediated hypersensitivity may be a pathogenic factor in some infants. Allergic mechanisms probably account for only 10% to 15% of colicky infants. Diagnosis of food-induced colic can be established by implementation of several brief trials of hypoallergenic formula. Symptoms should resolve when the child is placed on the hypoallergenic formula and recur when the regular formula or breastfeeding resumes. A food-allergic cause is confirmed when two placebo-controlled, crossover, blinded trials of the suspected allergen results in symptoms during the allergen challenges and resolution during the placebo challenges. In infants with food allergen–induced colic, symptoms typically are short-lived, and repeat challenges should be carried out every 3 to 4 months.

Non–IgE-Mediated Gastrointestinal Food Allergy

Several gastrointestinal disorders are thought to result from cell-mediated hypersensitivities (see Table 81-6). Food protein-induced enterocolitis syndrome (FPIES) is a disorder most commonly seen in infants between 1 week and 3 months of age who present with protracted vomiting and diarrhea, which may result in dehydration.[125] A study from Israel reported a prevalence for milk-induced FPIES of 0.34% in a large (>14,000 infants), population-based birth cohort.[126] Vomiting usually occurs 1 to 4 hours after feeding, and continued exposure may result in bloody diarrhea, anemia, abdominal distention, and failure to thrive. Symptoms are most commonly provoked by cow's milk or soy protein–based formulas, and one case was attributed to food proteins passed in maternal breast milk.[127]

A similar enterocolitis syndrome has been reported in older infants and children due to egg, wheat, rice, oat, peanut, nuts, chicken, turkey, and fish sensitivity.[127] Hypotension occurs in about 15% of cases after allergen ingestion, and 10% to 15% of patients present with methemoglobinemia. In adults, shellfish sensitivity may provoke a similar syndrome with symptoms of severe nausea, abdominal cramps, and protracted vomiting. After an acute reaction, there is a prominent increase in the number of peripheral blood neutrophils, peaking at 4 to 6 hours from the onset of symptoms. Stools often contain occult blood, neutrophils, eosinophils, and Charcot-Leyden crystals. Skin-prick test results for the suspected foods are negative. Jejunal biopsies classically reveal flattened villi, edema, and increased numbers of lymphocytes, eosinophils, and mast cells. Although the immunopathogenic mechanism of this syndrome has not been elucidated, some studies suggest that food antigen–induced secretion of tumor necrosis factor-α (TNF-α) from local mononuclear cells may be responsible for the secretory diarrhea and hypotension.

Diagnosis can be established when elimination of the responsible allergen leads to resolution of symptoms within 72 hours and oral challenge provokes symptoms. However, secondary disaccharidase deficiency may uncommonly persist longer and may result in ongoing diarrhea for up to 2 weeks. OFCs consist of administering 0.3 to 0.6 g/kg of body weight of the suspected protein allergen. Vomiting usually develops within 1 to 4 hours of administering the challenge food. Diarrhea or loose stools often develop after 4 to 8 hours. In conjunction with a positive food challenge result, the peripheral blood absolute neutrophil count increases to at least 3500 cells/mm^3 within 4 to 6 hours of developing symptoms, and neutrophils and eosinophils may be found in the stools. Because about 15% of food antigen challenges lead to profuse vomiting, dehydration, and hypotension, they must be performed under medical supervision. One study suggested that the atopy patch test may be useful for the diagnosis of FPIES, but confirmatory studies are necessary.[128]

Food protein-induced proctocolitis, like the food-induced enterocolitis syndrome, usually manifests in the first few months of life. Although such reactions often are caused by cow's milk or soy protein hypersensitivity, most occur in breastfeeding infants. They typically do not appear ill, often have normally formed stools, and usually are discovered because of the presence of blood (gross or occult) in their stools. Blood loss is usually minor but occasionally can produce anemia. The diagnosis can be established when elimination of the responsible allergen leads to resolution of hematochezia, usually with dramatic improvement within 72 hours of appropriate food allergen elimination, but complete clearance and resolution of mucosal lesions may take up to 1 month. Reintroduction of the allergen leads to recurrence of symptoms within several hours to days. Lesions are confined to the distal large bowel. Sigmoidoscopy findings vary, ranging from areas of patchy mucosal injection to severe friability with small, aphthoid ulcerations and bleeding. Colonic biopsy reveals a prominent eosinophilic infiltrate in the surface and crypt epithelia and the lamina propria. In severe lesions with crypt destruction, neutrophils are prominent.

Cow's milk and soy protein-induced proctocolitis usually resolve within 6 months to 2 years of allergen avoidance, but occasional refractory cases are seen.

Dietary protein–induced enteropathy (excluding celiac disease) usually manifests in the first several months of life with diarrhea (mild to moderate steatorrhea in about 80%) and poor weight gain.[129] Symptoms include protracted diarrhea, vomiting in up to two thirds of patients, failure to thrive, and malabsorption, which is demonstrated by the presence of reducing substances in the stools, increased fecal fat, and abnormal D-xylose absorption. Cow's milk hypersensitivity is the most frequent cause of this syndrome, but it also has been associated with sensitivity to soy, egg, wheat, rice, chicken, and fish.

Diagnosis requires the identification and exclusion of the responsible allergen from the diet, which brings about a resolution of symptoms within several days to weeks. On endoscopy, a patchy villous atrophy is evident, and biopsy reveals a prominent mononuclear round cell infiltrate and a small number of eosinophils, which is not unlike celiac disease but usually is much less extensive. Colitis-like features are usually absent, but anemia occurs in about 40% of affected infants, and protein loss occurs in most. Complete resolution of the intestinal lesions may require 6 to 18 months of allergen avoidance. Unlike celiac disease, loss of clinical reactivity frequently occurs, but the natural history of this disorder has not been well studied.

Celiac disease is an extensive enteropathy that leads to malabsorption.[130] The disease occurs in adults and children at rates approaching 1% of the population. Total villous atrophy and extensive cellular infiltrates are associated with sensitivity to gliadin, the alcohol-soluble portion of gluten found in wheat, oat, rye, and barley. Celiac disease represents an interplay between the environment and genetics, with a strong association with human leukocyte antigen (HLA)-DQ2 (α1*0501, β1*0201), which is present in more than 90% of patients. The incidence of celiac disease is 1 case per 250 people in the United States according to the Celiac Disease Foundation. The striking increase in celiac disease that occurred in Sweden compared with genetically similar Denmark and the variation in prevalence associated with changes in patterns of gluten feeding in Sweden strongly implicated environmental factors (i.e., feeding practices) in the cause of this disorder. Introduction of gluten into infant diets before 4 months of age has been identified as a risk factor for celiac disease, whereas introduction after 6 months has been identified as a risk factor for wheat allergy. The intestinal inflammation in celiac disease is precipitated by exposure to gliadin. Gluten-specific T cells are found in the biopsies of these patients, and without exception, they respond to gluten-derived peptides bound to the disease-associated HLA-DQ2 or HLA-DQ8 molecules. Several gluten-derived peptides have been characterized and are the result of selective conversion of specific glutamine residues in gluten peptides into glutamic acid by tissue transglutaminase (tTGase). This deamidation creates epitopes that bind efficiently to DQ2 and are recognized by T cells. Most patients develop IgA antibodies against gliadin and tTGase. Virtually all celiac disease patients possess autoantibodies to distinct epitopes on the tTGase molecule, but the antibodies do not appear to be responsible for the pathology.

Initial symptoms often include diarrhea or frank steatorrhea, abdominal distention and flatulence, weight loss, and occasionally nausea and vomiting. Oral ulcers and other extraintestinal symptoms caused by malabsorption are not uncommon. Villous atrophy of the small bowel is a characteristic feature of celiac patients who ingest gluten. IgA antibodies to gluten are present in more than 80% of adults and children with untreated celiac disease. Patients usually have increased levels of IgG antibodies to a variety of foods, which is presumably the result of increased food antigen absorption.

Diagnosis depends on demonstrating biopsy evidence of villous atrophy and inflammatory infiltrate, resolution of biopsy findings after 6 to 12 weeks of gluten elimination, and recurrence of biopsy changes after a gluten challenge.[131] Revised diagnostic criteria have eliminated the requirement for a gluten challenge and instead place a greater focus on serologic studies. Quantification of IgA antigliadin and IgA antiendomysial antibodies may be used for screening with IgA anti-tTGase antibodies in patients older than 2 years of age. After the diagnosis of celiac disease is established, lifelong elimination of gluten-containing foods is necessary to control symptoms and to avoid the increased risk of malignancy.

CUTANEOUS FOOD ALLERGY

The skin is a frequent target organ in IgE- and non–IgE-mediated food hypersensitivity reactions (Table 81-7; see Table 81-5). Ingestion of food allergens may lead to the rapid onset of cutaneous symptoms or aggravate chronic conditions.

Cutaneous IgE-Mediated Food Allergy

Urticaria and angioedema are the most common acute symptoms of food-allergic reactions, although the prevalence of these reactions is unknown. Because the onset of symptoms follows within minutes of ingesting the responsible allergen, the cause-and-effect nature of the reaction is often obvious to the patient. Most individuals with these reactions do not seek medical assistance or necessarily report them to their physicians. The foods most commonly incriminated in adults are fish, shellfish, tree nuts, and peanut, and in children, they

TABLE 81-7 Cutaneous Food-Allergic Disorders

Disorder	Age Group	Characteristics	Diagnosis	Prognosis and Course
IgE-MEDIATED DISORDERS				
Acute urticaria and angioedema	Any	Pruritic, evanescent skin rash (hives) and swelling within minutes to 2 h after food ingestion; food identified as a culprit in 20%	History, positive SPT, and/or serum food-IgE level; confirmed by OFC if necessary	Varies, food-dependent; milk, soy, egg, and wheat typically outgrown; peanut, tree nuts, seeds, and shellfish typically persistent
Chronic urticaria and angioedema (rare)	Any	Hives and swelling for >6 wk; approximately 2% caused by food	History, positive SPT, and/or serum food-IgE level; confirmed by OFC if necessary	Varies
IgE AND NON–IgE-MEDIATED DISORDERS				
Atopic dermatitis	Infant and child; 90% start <5 yr	Relapsing pruritic vesiculopapular rash; generalized in infants, localized to flexor areas in older children; food allergy in about 35% of children with moderate to severe atopic dermatitis	History, SPT, and/or serum food-IgE level; elimination diet and OFC	60%-80% improve significantly or allergy resolves by adolescence
NON–IgE-MEDIATED DISORDERS				
Contact dermatitis	Any; more common in adults	Relapsing pruritic eczematous rash, often on hands or face; often occurs in occupational contact with food stuff	History, patch testing	Varies
Dermatitis herpetiformis	Any	Intensely pruritic vesicular rash on extensor surfaces and buttocks	Biopsy diagnostic, shows IgA granule deposits at the dermal-epidermal junction; resolves with dietary gluten avoidance	Lifelong

Modified from Nowak-Węgrzyn A, Sampson HA. Adverse reactions to foods. Med Clin North Am 2006;90:97-127.
Ig, Immunoglobulin; *OFC*, oral food challenge; *SPT*, skin-prick test;

include egg, milk, peanut, and nuts. Acute urticaria from contact with foods is thought to be common, but the true prevalence is unknown. Foods most often incriminated in acute cases include raw meats, fish, shellfish, milk, raw egg, vegetables, and fruits.[1] Most studies of patients with chronic urticaria and angioedema (i.e., symptoms lasting more than 6 weeks) indicate that allergy to foods or food additives are rarely (2% to 4%) implicated.

Diagnosis is based on the demonstration of food-specific IgE antibodies (i.e., skin test or in vitro IgE), resolution of skin symptoms with complete elimination of the putative food from the diet, and development of symptoms after challenge.

Mixed IgE- and Non–IgE-Mediated Cutaneous Food Allergy

Atopic dermatitis usually begins in early infancy (90% younger than 1 year of age). It is characterized by a typical distribution, extreme pruritus, chronically relapsing course, and association with asthma and allergic rhinitis.[132]

The role of allergen-specific IgE antibodies in the pathogenesis of atopic dermatitis involves several cell types. The numbers of Langerhans cells, which are the professional antigen-presenting cells (APCs) in the skin, are increased in the lesions of atopic dermatitis and display allergen-specific IgE antibodies on their surface. The FcεR1s on Langerhans cells, through bound antigen-specific IgE antibodies, play a unique role as nontraditional receptors. These IgE-bearing Langerhans cells are up to 1000 times more efficient than non–IgE-bearing APCs at presenting allergen to T cells (primarily Th2 cells) and activating T cell proliferation. Infiltrating T lymphocytes in acute eczematous lesions express predominantly Th2 cytokines, such as IL-4, IL-5, IL-13, and IL-17, whereas T cells in chronic lesions predominantly express IL-5, IL-13, and IL-22. This profile contrasts with classic delayed cell-mediated responses, such as the tuberculin response, in which cells express primarily mRNA for IFN-γ and IL-2 but not for IL-4 and IL-5.

OFCs in children with atopic dermatitis and food allergy induce sharp increases in plasma histamine concentrations but no increase in plasma tryptase levels, activation of eosinophils, and elaboration of eosinophil products. T lymphocytes bearing milk-specific antigens that can home to the skin have been identified in the circulation of children with IgE-mediated milk-induced skin symptoms, and these T cells are not present in patients with milk-induced gastrointestinal disease.[133] Food antigen–specific T cells have been cloned from active skin lesions and normal skin of patients with atopic dermatitis. Peripheral blood mononuclear cells from food-allergic children with atopic dermatitis elaborate an IgE-dependent HRF that primes basophils and possibly other IgE-bearing cells and that has been correlated with disease activity.[134] Spontaneous generation of HRF decreased to background levels over 6 to 9 months when the food allergens were identified and removed from the diet. Using density-gradient centrifugation, circulating eosinophils changed within 24 hours from a prechallenge normodense profile to a postchallenge hypodense profile in three patients studied, suggesting acute release of eosinophil-priming cytokines such as IL-5 or granulocyte-macrophage colony-stimulating factor (GM-CSF) (unpublished data). Biopsies obtained at the site of a challenge-induced morbilliform lesion 8 to 14 hours after a positive challenge revealed eosinophil infiltration and deposition of major basic protein. A murine model of food-induced atopic dermatitis–like skin lesions from oral feeding has been described.[135]

In one study, 35% to 40% of children with moderate to severe atopic dermatitis presenting to a university-based dermatologist were found to be food allergic after allergy evaluations and DBPCFCs.[16] An earlier study demonstrated a direct correlation between disease severity and the likelihood of food allergy. In a follow-up study of 34 children with atopic dermatitis, 17 children with food allergy placed on an appropriate allergen elimination diet experienced marked, significant improvement in their eczematous rash over the 4-year follow-up period compared with non–food-allergic children and food-allergic children not adhering to an allergen-elimination diet.[136] In a prospective, blinded, randomized, controlled trial of egg elimination in young children with atopic dermatitis and positive for egg-specific IgE, Lever and colleagues demonstrated a significant decrease in the area of affected skin and symptom scores in children avoiding egg compared with controls.[137] In a series of almost 500 children with atopic dermatitis and food allergy, approximately one third of symptomatic food hypersensitivities were outgrown in 2 to 3 years.[138] The probability of developing tolerance appeared to depend on the food antigen responsible; development of tolerance to soy was common, whereas development of tolerance to peanut was rare. Results of skin-prick tests often became negative or remained unchanged, but concentrations of allergen-specific IgE dropped significantly. The pathogenic role of food allergy in adults with atopic dermatitis remains requires study.

Diagnosis is based on demonstration of food-specific IgE antibodies or occasionally on food-specific patch tests, elimination diets, and OFCs.[1] At the time of first evaluation, skin symptoms provoked by a DBPCFC usually consist of a markedly pruritic, erythematous, morbilliform rash that develops in sites for which atopic dermatitis has a predilection. Urticarial lesions are rarely seen. However, urticaria is frequently seen in follow-up challenges conducted 1 to 2 years later in patients who had adhered to an appropriate allergen elimination diet and had experienced clearing of their eczema but who remained food sensitive. Attempts at reintroducing food should be under a physician's supervision.[115] Although the history may not suggest other food-induced complaints, food challenges can provoke intestinal symptoms (e.g., nausea, abdominal cramping, vomiting, diarrhea) in almost half of patients; upper respiratory symptoms (e.g., laryngeal edema, sensation of itching and tightness in the throat; persistent throat clearing with a dry, hacking cough; hoarseness) in about one third; and wheezing in about 10% of positive challenges. When absorption studies are performed (e.g., lactulose-rhamnose, lactulose-mannitol), most patients are found to have malabsorption even though gastrointestinal complaints are minimal.

Non–IgE-Mediated Cutaneous Food Allergy

Food-induced contact dermatitis is seen frequently among food handlers, especially among those who handle raw fish, shellfish (e.g., snow crabs), meats, and eggs. Patch tests can be used if necessary to confirm the diagnosis.

Dermatitis herpetiformis (DH) is a chronic, blistering skin disorder associated with a gluten-sensitive enteropathy. It is characterized by a chronic, intensely pruritic papulovesicular rash symmetrically distributed over the extensor surfaces and buttocks.[139] The histology of the intestinal lesion is virtually identical to that seen in celiac disease, but villous atrophy and inflammatory infiltrates are usually milder, and the T cell lines isolated from intestinal biopsy specimens of DH patients produce significantly more IL-4 than T cell lines isolated from celiac disease patients. Like patients with celiac disease, virtually all DH patients have circulating IgA antibodies against tTGase, the quantity of which appears to correlate with the extent of the jejunal mucosal lesions.

Diagnosis of DH depends on the presence of the characteristic skin lesions and demonstration of IgA deposition at the dermal–epidermal junction of the skin. Although many patients have minimal or no gastrointestinal complaints, biopsy of the small bowel usually reveals intestinal involvement. Elimination of gluten from the diet usually leads to resolution of skin symptoms and normalization of intestinal findings over several months. Administration of sulfones, the mainstay of therapy, leads to rapid resolution of skin symptoms but has virtually no effect on intestinal symptoms.

RESPIRATORY FOOD ALLERGY

Acute respiratory symptoms caused by food allergy represent pure IgE-mediated reactions, whereas chronic respiratory symptoms represent a mix of IgE-mediated and non–IgE-mediated symptoms (Table 81-8; see Table 81-5). Upper and lower respiratory reactions have been provoked in some children by DBPCFCs, with spirometry demonstrating significant reductions in forced vital capacity (FVC), forced expiratory volume in 1 second (FEV_1), and maximum end-expiratory flow (MMEF) values during positive food challenges.

Rhinoconjunctivitis alone is infrequently a manifestation of food allergy, and when present, it is typically accompanied by other allergic symptoms. Within minutes to 2 hours of ingestion, food allergens may induce typical signs and symptoms of rhinoconjunctivitis, including periocular erythema, pruritus, and tearing; nasal congestion, pruritus, and sneezing; and rhinorrhea. During a DBPCFC, the histamine level found in nasal lavage fluid may be increased up to 10-fold with the onset of nasal symptoms in some children. Children with atopic disorders and food allergy often experience nasal symptoms during OFCs. Of 480 children referred to Bock and colleagues for evaluation of adverse food reactions, about 16% experienced respiratory symptoms (e.g., sneezing, rhinorrhea, nasal obstruction, wheezing, cough) during a DBPCFC, but only 2% had symptoms confined to the respiratory tract alone.[140] Approximately 25% of 112 patients with histories of adverse food reactions occurring after 10 years of age developed respiratory symptoms after an OFC, and most were nasal symptoms caused by fruit or vegetable sensitivities.[141] Despite the notion that milk ingestion frequently leads to nasal congestion in young infants, the objective evidence from oral milk challenges shows that only 0.08% to 0.2% of infants develop nasal symptoms after a milk challenge.[142]

In our evaluations of children with atopic dermatitis, nasal symptoms typically develop within 15 to 90 minutes of initiating the DBPCFC and last about 0.5 to 2 hours. Nasal and periocular pruritus are commonly followed by prolonged bursts of sneezing and copious rhinorrhea. Levels of nasal fluid histamine and eosinophil cationic protein were found to increase significantly in children experiencing nasal symptoms.

Asthma or isolated wheezing alone is an infrequent manifestation of food allergy. Although ingestion of food allergens is rarely the main aggravating factor in chronic asthma, some evidence suggests that food antigens can provoke bronchial hyperreactivity.[143] In surveys of children with asthma attending pulmonary clinics, food-induced respiratory reactions were demonstrated in about 6% to 8.5% of children.[17] Bock and

TABLE 81-8 Respiratory Food-Allergic Disorders

Disorder	Age Group	Characteristics	Diagnosis	Prognosis and Course
IgE-MEDIATED DISORDERS				
Allergic rhinoconjunctivitis	Any	Ocular pruritus, conjunctival injection and watery discharge, nasal pruritus, congestion, rhinorrhea, sneezing within minutes to 2 h after food ingestion or inhalation; cutaneous and gastrointestinal manifestations typical	History, SPT, and/or serum food-IgE level; OFC	Varies
Acute bronchospasm	Any	Cough, wheezing, dyspnea on food ingestion or inhalation; possible risk factor for severe anaphylaxis; cutaneous and gastrointestinal manifestations typical	History, SPT, and/or serum food-IgE level; OFC	Varies
IgE AND NON–IgE-MEDIATED DISORDERS				
Asthma	Any	Chronic cough, wheezing, dyspnea; food allergy is risk factor for intubation in children who have asthma	History, SPT, and/or serum food-IgE level; OFC	Varies
NON–IgE-MEDIATED DISORDERS*				
Pulmonary hemosiderosis (Heiner syndrome)	Infants, children (rare)	Chronic cough, hemoptysis, lung infiltrates, wheezing, anemia; described in cow's milk– and buckwheat-allergic infants	History, SPT, and serum food-IgE negative, but milk and buckwheat IgG precipitins positive; lung biopsy with deposits of IgG and IgA	Unknown

Modified from Nowak-Węgrzyn A, Sampson HA. Adverse reactions to foods. Med Clin North Am 2006;90:97-127.
Ig, Immunoglobulin; *OFC*, oral food challenge; *SPT*, skin-prick test.
*Presumed.

colleagues found that about 25% of 279 children referred for evaluation with histories of food-induced wheezing or asthma experienced wheezing as one of the symptoms during a DBPCFC.[140] Similarly, a study of 88 children with atopic dermatitis and asthma identified acute bronchospasm in 15% of patients (i.e., dyspnea, cough, and wheezing) during a DBPCFC, and 8% had a greater than a 20% decline in FEV_1.[144] In a study of 26 asthmatic patients with food allergies, 12 developed mild, acute bronchospasm (i.e., cough or wheezing) during a DBPCFC, and 7 (58%) of the 12 had a significant increase in airway reactivity, as demonstrated by a greater than a twofold decrease in their FEV_1 values after challenge with methacholine at a provocative dose that induces a 20% decrease in FEV_1 (PD_{20}).[143] Asthmatic reactions to airborne food allergens have been reported when susceptible individuals are exposed to vapors or steam emitted from cooking food (e.g., fish, mollusks, crustaceans, eggs, garbanzo beans).[145] One study suggested that children with asthma who are sensitized to food allergens are at greater risk for severe asthma, as judged by hospitalizations, emergency visits, days missed from school, and rescue medication use.[146]

Diagnosis of food-induced respiratory disease is based on a patient's history, evidence of food-specific IgE (e.g., positive skin test results, in vitro IgE tests to food antigens), and OFCs. DBPCFCs after strict elimination of suspected food allergens are usually the only way to confirm the diagnosis of food-induced wheezing. Because many factors can exacerbate wheezing, elimination diets alone typically are not useful. Whether prechallenge and postchallenge studies of airway hyperreactivity should be performed remains to be established.

Non–IgE-Mediated Respiratory Food Allergy

Food-induced pulmonary hemosiderosis (i.e., Heiner syndrome) is a rare syndrome of recurrent episodes of pneumonia associated with pulmonary infiltrates and hemorrhage, hemosiderosis, gastrointestinal blood loss, iron-deficiency anemia, and failure to thrive. It was first reported in infants by Heiner and coworkers.[147] Hemosiderin-laden macrophages may be found in morning aspirates of the stomach or seen in biopsy specimens of the lung. Heiner syndrome is most often associated with a non–IgE-mediated hypersensitivity to cow's milk, but reactivity to egg, pork, and buckwheat have also been reported. Although peripheral blood eosinophilia and multiple serum precipitins to cow's milk are a relatively constant feature, the immunologic mechanisms responsible for this disorder are unknown.

Diagnosis is based on the elimination of the precipitating allergen and subsequent resolution of symptoms. Characteristic laboratory data, including precipitating IgG antibodies to cow's milk (or the responsible antigen), are also necessary for diagnosis.

FOOD-INDUCED GENERALIZED ANAPHYLAXIS

Food allergies are the single leading cause of generalized anaphylaxis seen in hospital emergency departments in the United States and account for at least one third of cases.[5] In addition to the cutaneous, respiratory, and gastrointestinal symptoms described earlier, patients may develop cardiovascular symptoms, including hypotension, vascular collapse, and cardiac dysrhythmias, presumably due to massive mediator release by mast cells. However, most food-induced anaphylactic reactions are not associated with major increases in serum levels of β-tryptase. In a series of 12 fatal or near-fatal anaphylactic reactions, all patients experienced severe respiratory compromise, 10 of 12 had nausea and vomiting, and only 7 of 12 patients (or 1 of 6 fatal reactions) had cutaneous symptoms.[148] About one third of patients developed a biphasic reaction and one fourth experienced prolonged symptoms, typically lasting 2 to 3 days. It is not known why foods provoke different constellations of symptoms in different individuals.

Factors that appear to be associated with severe reactions include the presence of asthma, a history of severe reactions, denial of symptoms, and failure to initiate therapy expeditiously. Surveys of food-induced anaphylactic deaths found that anaphylactic reactions to foods affected both sexes equally, most victims were adolescents or young adults, and almost all individuals with a food allergy had a history of some type of reaction to the food culprit that caused the fatal reaction.[149,150] Among the subjects for whom data were available, virtually all were known to have asthma, very few had epinephrine available for use at the time of their reaction, and about 10% of those who received epinephrine in a timely fashion did not survive. Peanuts or tree nuts were responsible for more than 85% of the fatalities in the United States.

Food-Dependent, Exercise-Induced Anaphylaxis

Among patients with exercise-induced anaphylaxis, approximately 30% to 50% report associated food triggers. Food-dependent, exercise-induced anaphylaxis (FDEIA) occurs only when the patient exercises within 2 to 4 hours of ingesting a food, but in the absence of exercise, the patient can ingest the food without any apparent reaction.[1] Patients usually have asthma and other atopic disorders, positive skin-prick test results for the food that provokes their symptoms, and occasionally a history of reacting to the food when they were younger. This disorder appears to be more common in females than males and most prevalent in the late teens to mid-30s.[151] The exact mechanism of this disorder is unknown, but several foods have been implicated, including wheat (i.e., omega-5 gliadin portion), shellfish, fruit, milk, celery, and fish.[152]

Diagnosis is based on an unequivocal history of food ingestion followed by exercise, the rapid onset (within 1 to 2 hours) of classic IgE-mediated symptoms, and the demonstration of food-specific IgE antibodies by skin-prick testing or in vitro tests for IgE. Lacking this evidence, a physician-supervised food challenge is usually warranted to ensure that the suspected food is truly responsible for the anaphylactic reaction.[153] Challenges should be done in a hospital setting by a physician experienced in the treatment of anaphylactic reactions.

Other Food-Induced Hypersensitivity Reactions

Ingestion of pasteurized, whole cow's milk by infants, especially those younger than 6 months of age, frequently leads to occult gastrointestinal blood loss and occasionally to *iron-deficiency anemia*.[154] Substitution of infant formula (including cow's milk–derived formulas that have been subjected to extensive heating) for whole cow's milk usually normalizes fecal blood loss within 3 days. These findings have reignited interest in the possible role of food allergy in inflammatory bowel disease (i.e., Crohn disease and ulcerative colitis). Although considerable circumstantial evidence makes such hypotheses attractive, proof is needed.

Given the presence of food antigen–immune complexes in many individuals after meals and mast cells in joint synovium, several investigators have suggested that arthritis may be caused by food hypersensitivity. Three small clinical trials using elemental diets in adults with active rheumatoid arthritis reported modest and transient improvements in pain and health assessment questionnaire scores at 3 to 4 weeks.[155] These findings suggest that individual patients may benefit from dietary interventions, but there is insufficient evidence to support the routine use of elemental diets in the management of rheumatoid arthritis.

In several disorders, symptoms have been associated with reactivity to ingested foods, but the associated immune response is unclear. Some investigators have claimed that certain neurologic disorders result from adverse food reactions and suggested that oligoantigenic diets may be useful in the treatment of migraines and epilepsy. A single study reported that 15% of 80 adults with frequent migraine headaches had clearing of their symptoms when placed on a specific food elimination diet (which did not correlate with skin test results) and had exacerbations of their symptoms during a double-blind challenge with a single food.[156] This study has not been replicated.

Diagnosis and Management of Food Allergy

FOOD ALLERGY GUIDELINES

Diagnosis and management of food allergy can vary between clinical practice settings. To promote the best clinical practices, the National Institute of Allergy and Infectious Diseases (NIAID) sponsored clinical guidelines for the diagnosis and management of food allergy in the United States.[5] An expert panel and coordinating committee representing 34 professional organizations, federal agencies, and patient advocacy groups developed the guidelines during a 2-year period. The 43 guidelines were based on an independent literature review and expert clinical opinion. The guidelines provide concise recommendations on how to diagnose, manage, and treat food allergy. They also identify gaps in the current scientific knowledge and provide guidance on points of controversy in patient management (Table 81-9).

The World Allergy Organization (WAO) Special Committee on Food Allergy published the Diagnosis and Rationale for Action against Cow's Milk Allergy (DRACMA) in 2008.[157]

TABLE 81-9 National Institute of Allergy and Infectious Diseases–Sponsored Expert Panel Report on the Diagnosis and Management of Food Allergy in the United States

Key Points	Guidelines and Comments
Definitions	Food allergy is an adverse health effect arising from a specific immune response. Food allergies result in immunoglobulin E (IgE)–mediated, immediate reactions (i.e., anaphylaxis) and a variety of chronic diseases (e.g., eosinophilic esophagitis, food protein-induced enterocolitis syndrome) in which IgE may not play an important role.
Epidemiology and natural history	
Children	Food allergy is more common in children than adults. Among the most common food allergies in children, milk, egg, wheat, and soy allergies often resolve in childhood; peanut, tree nut, fish, and shellfish allergies can resolve but are more likely to persist. Peanut allergy prevalence has increased over several decades and now affects 1% to 2% of young children.
Adults	Adult food allergies can reflect persistence of childhood allergies or de novo sensitization to food allergens encountered after childhood. A food allergy that starts in adult life tends to persist. Among adults, shellfish (2.5%), fish (0.5%), peanut (0.6%), and tree nut (0.5%) allergies are the most common. Adults and some children experience cross-reactivity between certain aeroallergens and foods (e.g., oral allergy/pollen food allergy syndrome) detailed in the guidelines. Milk, egg, wheat, and soy allergies often resolve in childhood; peanut, tree nut, fish, and shellfish allergies can resolve but more likely persist.
Comorbidities	Food allergies may coexist with asthma, atopic dermatitis, eosinophilic esophagitis, and exercise-induced anaphylaxis. Food allergy is associated with severe asthma, increased risk of severe exacerbations, and increased hospitalization rates. Food allergies disrupt the quality of life. Food allergy is not a common trigger of eczema in adults. Eosinophilic esophagitis, which involves localized eosinophilic inflammation of the esophagus, is a chronic, remitting-relapsing condition associated with sensitization to foods. In some patients, avoidance of specific foods results in normalization of histopathology. In children, it manifests with feeding disorders, vomiting, reflux symptoms, and abdominal pain. In adolescents and adults, it most often manifests with dysphagia and esophageal food impactions. One third of patients with exercise-induced anaphylaxis report reactions triggered by foods; exercise-induced anaphylaxis has natural history marked by frequent recurrence of episodes.
Risk factors for severe anaphylaxis	Fatal food-allergic reactions are usually caused by peanut, tree nuts, and seafood but also have resulted from milk, egg, seeds, and other foods. Fatalities have been associated with age (teenagers and young adults), delayed treatment with epinephrine, and comorbid asthma. Severity of future allergic reactions is not accurately predicted by the history. There are no laboratory tests to predict severity of future reactions. Food taken on empty stomach, exercise, alcohol, nonsteroidal antiinflammatory drugs, and antacid agents may increase severity of an allergic reaction. Therapy with β-blockers may decrease effectiveness of epinephrine in anaphylaxis.

TABLE 81-9 National Institute of Allergy and Infectious Diseases–Sponsored Expert Panel Report on the Diagnosis and Management of Food Allergy in the United States—cont'd

Key Points	Guidelines and Comments
Diagnosis	Food allergy is suspected when typical symptoms (e.g., urticaria, edema, wheezing, mouth itch, cough, nausea, vomiting, anaphylaxis) occur within minutes to hours of food ingestion. A detailed history of the reaction to each incriminated food is essential for proper diagnosis. Children younger than 5 years of age with moderate to severe atopic dermatitis should be considered for evaluation for milk, egg, peanut, wheat, and soy allergies if one or both of the following conditions are present: • Persistent atopic dermatitis despite optimized management and topical therapy • Reliable history of an immediate reaction after ingestion of a specific food A medically supervised food challenge is considered the most specific test for food allergy. Tests for food-specific IgE levels assist in the diagnosis but should not be relied as the sole means to diagnose food allergy. The medical history and examination are recommended to aid in the diagnosis. Food-specific IgE testing has limitations: • Positive test results are not intrinsically diagnostic, and reactions sometimes occur despite negative test results. • Testing food panels without considering the history is often misleading. Several tests are not recommended, including food-specific IgG/IgG_4, total IgE, applied kinesiology, and electrodermal testing.
Prevention	The recommendations follow the 2008 American Academy of Pediatrics clinical report.[175] Breastfeeding is encouraged for all infants, hydrolyzed infant formulas are suggested for infants at risk,* and complementary foods, including potential allergens, are not restricted after 4 to 6 months of age (not applicable for infants experiencing allergic reactions). Maternal diet during pregnancy should be healthy and balanced; evidence to support avoidance of potential food allergens is lacking.
Management†	
Avoidance	Education about food avoidance is essential to prevent reactions.
Immunizations	Patients with egg allergy can be immunized with influenza vaccines containing a low dose of egg protein. Yellow fever and rabies vaccines are contraindicated in persons with a history of urticaria, angioedema, asthma, or anaphylaxis to egg proteins. Allergy evaluation and testing can provide insight into the potential risk for an individual.
Anaphylaxis	Management of anaphylaxis relies on prompt administration of epinephrine, observation for 4 to 6 hours or longer after treatment, education on avoidance, early recognition and treatment, medical identification jewelry, and follow-up with a primary health care provider and consideration of consultation with an allergist-immunologist. Prescription for epinephrine autoinjectors and advice for patient education include having two doses available, switching from 0.15- to 0.3-mg fixed-dose autoinjectors at approximately 25 kg (55 lb) in the context of patient-specific circumstances, having a written emergency plan, and providing supporting educational material.[176,177]

Modified from Boyce J, Assa'ad AH, Burks AW, et al. Guidelines for the diagnosis and management of food allergy in the United States: summary of the NIAID-sponsored expert panel report. J Allergy Clin Immunol 2010;126(Suppl):S1-58.

*At-risk infants are defined as having one or more immediate family members (e.g., parent, sibling) with atopic disorder.

†Several Web-based resources on food allergies are available for medical professionals and patients: National Institute of Allergy and Infectious Diseases (www.niaid.nih.gov/topics/foodAllergy); National Institute for Health and Clinical Excellence (http://guidance.nice.org.uk/CG116); World Allergy Association (WAO) Diagnosis and Rationale for Action against Cow's Milk Allergy (DRACMA) Guidelines (http://www.worldallergy.org/publications/WAO_DRACMA_guidelines.pdf); Consortium of Food Allergy Research (https://web.emmes.com/study/cofar/EducationProgram.htm); Food Allergy Research and Education (http://www.foodallergy.org); Kids with Food Allergies Foundation Community (www.kidswithfoodallergies.org) (all accessed March 11, 2013).

Clinical practice guidelines on food allergies in children and young people were developed by the National Institute for Health and Clinical Excellence (NICE). These guidelines are intended for use predominantly in primary care within the National Health Service and community settings in England, Wales, and Northern Ireland. The European Academy of Allergy and Clinical Immunology (EAACI) created a task force that is currently developing guidelines for the diagnosis and management of food allergies that will be complementary with the NIAID U.S. Food Allergy Guidelines, which are available online (http://www.niaid.nih.gov/topics/foodallergy) in a full format, an executive summary, and a lay-language summary for patients, families, and caregivers.

The diagnostic approach to food allergy begins with the medical history and physical examination. These assessments guide the selection of the laboratory tests (Fig. 81-1). The value of the medical history largely depends on the patient's recollection of symptoms and the examiner's ability to differentiate between disorders provoked by food hypersensitivity and other causes (see Table 81.1). In some cases, it may be useful in diagnosing food allergy (e.g., acute events such as systemic anaphylaxis after isolated ingestion of shrimp), but history alone should never be used to make a diagnosis.

In several series, less than 50% of reported food-allergic reactions could be verified by DBPCFCs.[5] Information required to establish that a food-allergic reaction occurred and to construct an appropriate blinded challenge at a later date include the following: the food presumed to have provoked the reaction, the quantity of the suspected food ingested, the length of time between ingestion and development of symptoms, whether similar symptoms developed on other occasions when the food was eaten, whether other factors (e.g., exercise, alcohol, drugs) are necessary, and how long since the last reaction to the food occurred. In chronic disorders (e.g., atopic dermatitis, asthma,

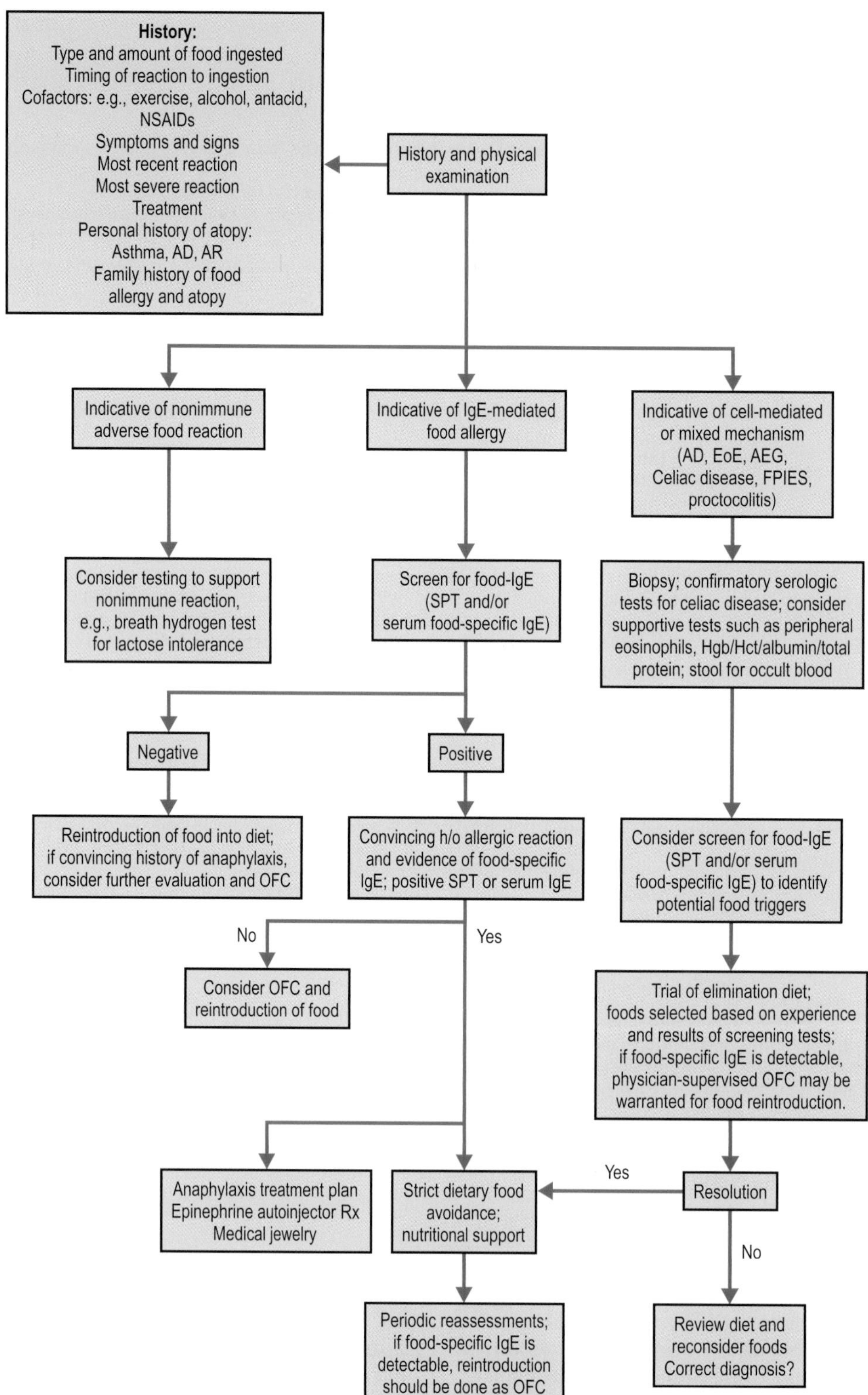

Figure 81-1 Current approach to the diagnosis and management of food allergy. *AD*, Atopic dermatitis; *AEG*, allergic eosinophilic gastroenteritis; *AR*, allergic rhinitis; *EoE*, eosinophilic esophagitis; *FPIES*, food protein–induced enterocolitis syndrome; *Hct*, hematocrit; *Hgb*, hemoglobin; *IgE*, immunoglobulin E; *NSAIDs*, nonsteroidal antiinflammatory drugs; *OFC*, oral food challenge; *Rx*, treatment; *SPT*, skin-prick test. *(Modified from Nowak-Węgrzyn A, Sampson HA. Adverse reactions to foods. Med Clin North Am 2006;90:97-127.)*

chronic urticaria), the history is often an unreliable indicator of the offending allergen.

Diet diaries are frequently discussed as an adjunct to history. Patients are instructed to keep a chronologic record of all foods ingested over a specified period, including items placed in the mouth but not swallowed, such as chewing gum. Any symptoms experienced by the patient are also recorded. The diary is then reviewed to determine whether there are any relationships between foods ingested and symptoms experienced. Occasionally, this method detects an unrecognized association between a food and a patient's symptoms. Unlike the medical history, it collects information on a prospective basis and does not depend on a patient's memory. This approach should be used selectively because it often causes patients and families to focus obsessively on foods instead of other potential triggers of their reactions.

Elimination diets are frequently used in the diagnosis and management of adverse food reactions. Foods suspected of provoking allergic disorders are completely omitted from the diet. The success of these diets depends on the identification of the correct allergens, the ability of the patient to maintain a diet completely free of all forms of the offending allergens, and the assumption that other factors do not provoke similar symptoms during the period of study. Unfortunately, these conditions are rarely met. In a young infant reacting to cow's milk formula, resolution of symptoms after substitution with a soy formula or casein hydrolysate (e.g., Alimentum, Nutramigen) or with an elemental amino acid–based formula (e.g., Neocate, EleCare) is highly suggestive of cow's milk or other food allergy, respectively, but it also could be caused by lactose intolerance. Although avoidance of suspected food allergens is recommended before blinded challenges, elimination diets alone are rarely diagnostic of food allergy, especially in chronic disorders such as atopic dermatitis or asthma.

Skin-prick tests are reproducible and frequently used to screen patients with suspected IgE-mediated food allergies. Glycerinated food extracts (1 : 10 or 1 : 20) and appropriate positive (e.g., histamine) and negative (e.g., saline) controls are applied by the prick or puncture technique. The criteria for interpreting skin-prick tests were established by Bock and colleagues[158] about 35 years ago. Any food allergens eliciting a wheal with a diameter at least 3 mm greater than the negative control are considered to be positive; all other results are considered to be negative. Investigators have been evaluating the utility of using the mean wheal diameter as a predictor of clinical reactivity. Hill and coworkers[159] reported that skin-prick tests inducing mean wheal diameters greater than 8 mm were diagnostic of milk, egg, and peanut allergies and are more than 95% predictive of clinical reactivity. To make such testing universally applicable, standardization of skin test reagents and testing procedures will be necessary. Until then, a positive skin-prick test should be interpreted as indicating the *possibility* that the patient has symptomatic reactivity to the specific food, whereas negative skin test results confirm the absence of IgE-mediated reactions (negative predictive accuracy is greater than 95%) if good-quality food extracts are used.[5]

The skin-prick test may be considered an excellent means of excluding IgE-mediated food allergies, but it can only suggests the presence of clinical food allergies. There are some exceptions to this general statement, First, IgE-mediated sensitivity to several fruits and vegetables (e.g., apples, oranges, bananas, pears, melons, potatoes, carrots, celery) is frequently not detected with commercially prepared reagents, presumably due to the lability of the responsible allergen. Second, commercial extracts sometimes lack the appropriate allergen to which an individual is reactive, as demonstrated by the use of fresh foods for skin test reagents. Third, children younger than 1 year of age may have IgE-mediated food allergy in the absence of positive skin test results, and infants younger than 2 years of age may have smaller wheals, presumably due to a lack of skin reactivity. Fourth, a positive skin test result for a food that when ingested in the absence of other foods, provokes a serious systemic anaphylactic reaction may be considered diagnostic.

Intradermal skin testing is more sensitive than the skin-prick test but is much less specific than a DBPCFC.[158] In Bock's study, no patient with a positive intradermal skin test result for a food and a concomitant negative skin-prick test result had a positive result for the DBPCFC.[158] Intradermal skin testing increases the risk of inducing a systemic reaction compared with skin-prick testing and is therefore not recommended.

There has been increasing interest in the use of the atopy patch test for the diagnosis of non–IgE-mediated food allergy in several disorders. Unfortunately, the lack of standardized reagents and method limits the utility of this approach. In one large study of children with atopic dermatitis, the investigators concluded that the patch test added little diagnostic benefit compared with standard diagnostic tests.[160]

In vitro allergen-specific IgE tests (e.g., enzyme-linked immunosorbent assay [ELISA], CAP System fluorescence enzyme-labeled assay [FEIA] and UniCAP, Fisher Thermo Scientific, Uppsala, Sweden; Magic Lite immunochemiluminometric assay, ALK-Abelló, Harsholm, Denmark) are used for measuring serum for IgE-mediated food allergies. In the past 10 years, the quantitative measurement of food-specific IgE antibodies (i.e., CAP System FEIA or UniCAP) has been shown to be more predictive of symptomatic IgE-mediated food allergy than other methods.[161] Food-specific IgE levels exceeding the diagnostic values (Table 81-10) indicate that patients are more than 95% likely to experience an allergic reaction if they ingest the specific food. The IgE levels can be monitored, and if they fall to less than 2 kU_A/L for egg, milk, or peanut, the patient without recent severe reactions should be challenged again to determine whether he or she has outgrown the food allergy.[4] Periodic evaluations should be offered to children with peanut allergy, and an OFC for peanut should be considered in patients who have not had reactions in the past 1 to 2 years and who have a serum peanut IgE level of less than 2.0 kU_A/L.

Component-resolved diagnosis (CRD) is based on individual natural or recombinant allergens that are purified. Using advanced microtechnology, qualified amounts of allergens can be spotted on activated biochip (e.g., ISAC microarray) surfaces, and minute quantities of serum are needed to detect IgE antibody to almost any number of specific allergens in a single-step process. CRD potentially offers superior specificity due to the purity of the components compared with whole-food extracts. OFCs were used in several studies to evaluate the clinical applications of CRD in cases of food allergy.

Nicolaou and colleagues correlated peanut sensitization with the outcome of the OFC for 8-year-old children within a population-based cohort.[68] The prevalence of peanut sensitization was 12%, and among those sensitized, 22% were diagnosed with clinical peanut allergy. Children with peanut allergy had higher fold-change values (i.e., calculated expression level estimates of the sample against the negative controls) to major peanut components Ara h 1 to 3, whereas the peanut-tolerant

TABLE 81-10 Food-Specific IgE Serum Concentrations Highly Predictive of Clinical Reactivity

Allergen	Diagnostic Decision Level kU_A/L*	Sensitivity (%)	Specificity (%)	Positive Predictive Value (%)	Negative Predictive Value (%)
Egg white	7	61	95	98	38
Infants ≤2 yr[178]	0.35	91	77	95	68
Ovomucoid for baked egg[55]	10.8	55	96	88	80
Milk	15	57	94	95	53
Infants ≤1 yr[179]	5	30	99	95	64
Peanut	14	57	99	99	36
Fish	20	25	100	99	89
Soybean	30	44	94	73	82
Wheat	26	61	92	74	87
Tree nuts[180]	15	Other values were not calculated and are not available		95	

Additional data from references 178, 179, 180.
*kU_A/L = allergen specific kilo units per liter.

children had higher values to cross-reactive carbohydrate determinants and grass components (Phl p 1, 4, 5b). The groups did not have different responses for Ara h 8 or Bet v 1. One study found that children with detectable serum specific IgE against peanut Ara h 2 had low chances of tolerating peanut despite a low peanut-specific IgE concentration.[162]

Children with suspected egg allergy (n = 108) underwent blinded challenges to raw and heated egg (at 90° C or 194° F for 60 minutes).[55] An egg white–specific IgE concentration greater than 7 kU_A/L was most useful in the diagnosis of allergy to uncooked egg white, and an ovomucoid-specific IgE level greater than 11 kU_A/L was superior in predicting reactions to heated egg white. The negative decision point based on 95% clinical sensitivity was 0.6 for uncooked egg white, and the negative decision point was 1.2 kU_A/L for heated egg white. In 68 children evaluated with a blinded food challenge for suspected egg allergy, IgE levels in response to egg allergens were tested with the immunosolid-phase allergen chip (ISAC) 103 microarray.[163] Forty-four (94%) of 47 ovomucoid-negative patients tolerated boiled egg, whereas 20 (95%) of 21 ovomucoid-positive patients reacted to raw egg. In the analysis of 145 oral challenges serving as reference parameters for CRD using microarray technology for suspected allergy to cow's milk (n = 85) and hen's egg (n = 60), CRD was not capable of replacing OFC, nor did testing with singular allergen components prove to be superior to in vitro testing for whole antigen.[164] However, CRD may complement OFC by identifying optimal candidates (i.e., with a more favorable probability of passing the challenge) for the more labor-intensive diagnostic tests. However, the utility of CRD requires validation with OFC in large, prospective studies.

Basophil histamine release (BHR) assays have usually been reserved for use in research settings, but the semi-automated methods using small amounts of whole blood are being promoted for screening multiple food allergens.[165] One such method was employed in a study comparing BHR assays with skin-prick tests, food-specific IgE, food antigen–induced intestinal mast cell histamine release, and food challenges in suspected food-allergic children. As demonstrated in earlier studies, the food allergen–induced BHR correlated most closely with serum food-specific IgE results. In the few children challenged in this study, the BHR assay did not appear to be any more predictive of clinical sensitivity than the skin-prick test or food-specific IgE, but further studies are warranted.

IPEC was first used for the diagnosis of food allergy more than 60 years ago. IPEC in 30 patients with food allergy, which was previously documented by double-blind challenge, provoked reactions on the gastric mucosa in all patients.[105] Tissue histamine and stainable mast cells in biopsies of the site were decreased compared with prechallenge samples. Skin-prick and food-specific IgE test results were positive in only about half of these patients. Although the sensitivity of IPEC appears to be superior to skin tests, food-specific IgE assays, and BHR assays, especially in patients with gastrointestinal allergy, the specificity of IPEC in skin test–positive, nonreactive patients has not been evaluated. Patients often experience systemic symptoms, suggesting this procedure may be no safer than oral challenges.

The DBPCFC has been labeled the gold standard for the diagnosis of food allergies.[5] Many investigators have used DBPCFCs successfully in children and adults to examine a variety of food-related complaints. In clinical practice, open (unblinded) and single-blinded OFCs are frequently used. The selection of foods to be tested in an OFC is usually based on history and skin test or in vitro IgE test results. The diagnostic OFC is discussed further in Chapter 83.

LIMITATIONS OF DIAGNOSTIC TESTS AND TREATMENT FOR FOOD ALLERGY

There are no controlled trials supporting the diagnostic value of food-specific IgG or IgG_4 antibody levels, food antigen–antibody complexes, evidence of lymphocyte activation (e.g., ^3H uptake, IL-2 production, leukocyte inhibitory factor production), or sublingual or intracutaneous provocation.[5]

There is no cure for food allergy. Management relies on food avoidance, nutritional advice, and timely treatment of acute reactions. These issues and approaches to prevention and future treatments for food allergy are discussed in Chapter 84.

Natural History of Food Allergy

The prevalence of food hypersensitivity is greatest in the first few years of life.[3] Most young children outgrow their food hypersensitivity (i.e., become tolerant) within a few years, except in most cases of peanut, tree nut, and seafood allergy.

Most children outgrow milk allergy, and those with a milder phenotype of milk allergy become tolerant by school age. In a prospective, population-based study, most milk-allergic children lost their milk allergy by 3 years of age: 50% by 1 year, 70% by 2 years, and 85% by 3 years.[166] All children with negative skin-prick test results to milk at 1 year of age lost their sensitivity by their third birthday, whereas 25% of those with positive skin test results remained milk allergic at 3 years of age. In contrast, among children with a more severe phenotype (i.e., multiple food allergies, asthma, and allergic rhinitis), 21% remained allergic to milk by 16 years of age.[14] The highest serum concentration of cow's milk–specific IgE for each patient (defined as the peak cm-IgE level), was highly predictive of outcome ($P < .001$), with few children whose peak milk-specific IgE concentration exceeded 50 kU_A/L outgrowing the milk allergy by their teenage years. Clinically, reactivity to baked milk appears to be a useful marker of a more severe milk allergy. Children who were initially reactive to baked milk were 28 times less likely to become tolerant to unheated milk compared with children tolerant to baked milk over a median of 37 months (range, 8 to 75 months; $P < .001$).[47,48]

Similar to milk allergy, 66% of egg-allergic children become food tolerant by 5 years of age.[167] However, among those with a more severe phenotype, 32% continued to avoid egg at the age of 16 years.[13] A patient's highest recorded egg IgE level, presence of other atopic disease, and presence of other food allergy were significantly related to egg allergy persistence. In contrast to milk allergy, children reactive to baked egg have excellent chances of outgrowing their egg allergy.[168]

Approximately 20% of children with peanut allergy and 9% of children with tree nut allergy become tolerant to these foods with age.[169,170] Unlike milk and egg allergy, peanut allergy occasionally recurs in children who appear to have outgrown their reactivity.[1] Risk of recurrence appears to be approximately 10% among children who refuse to eat peanuts on a regular basis, compared with no recurrences in children eating peanuts regularly. The possibility of peanut allergy recurrence should be discussed before undertaking the OFC to peanut and before indicating that patients should ingest peanut frequently after a negative OFC result. Epinephrine should be carried for several months after a negative result until the patient has proven tolerance to multiple ingestions of regular servings of peanuts and peanut-containing foods. It appears that the natural history of allergy to seeds, fish, and shellfish are similar to nuts.

Among 133 children evaluated in a food allergy referral center and followed for a median time of 5 years (range, 1 to 19 years), rates of resolution were 25% by 4 years, 45% by 6 years, and 69% by 10 years of age. By 6 years of age, 59% of children with a peak soy IgE level of less than 5 kU_A/L, 53% of children with a peak specific IgE level of 5 to 9.9 kU_A/L, 45% of children with a peak specific IgE level of 10 to 49.9 kU_A/L, and 18% of children with a peak specific IgE level of greater than 50 kU_A/L had outgrown the soy allergy ($P < .01$ for trend).[171]

In a population of 103 children with IgE-mediated wheat allergy in a food allergy referral center, rates of resolution were 29% by 4 years, 56% by 8 years, and 65% by 12 years of age. Higher wheat IgE levels were associated with poorer outcomes. The peak wheat IgE level recorded was a useful predictor of persistent allergy ($P < .001$), although many children, even those with the highest levels of wheat IgE, outgrew wheat allergy.[172].

FOOD ALLERGY IN ADULTS

Although younger children are more likely to outgrow their food allergies, older children and adults also may lose their reactivity if the responsible food allergen is identified and eliminated from the diet. Approximately one third of children and adults lose their clinical reactivity after 1 to 2 years of allergen avoidance. Skin-puncture test results typically remain positive and do not predict which patients will lose their clinical reactivity. Monitoring food allergen-specific IgE levels may be useful in predicting when patients outgrow their allergy. A significant drop in the specific IgE level to cow's milk and egg by 50% over 1 to 2 years has been identified as a favorable prognostic factor in children.[173] The severity of the initial reaction does not appear to correlate with the ultimate likelihood of losing clinical reactivity, but the degree of compliance with the allergen avoidance diet and the food responsible for the reaction do affect the outcome.

Most non–IgE-mediated gastrointestinal food allergies occur in infants and are outgrown in the first 2 to 3 years of life. However, allergic eosinophilic esophagitis is frequently seen in adults, and the number of young children and adolescents affected appears to be increasing. Long-term studies have not been completed, and the prognosis of this disorder is unknown. Although most cases of dietary protein–induced enteropathy are outgrown, celiac disease is a lifelong sensitivity, and gluten-containing grains must be avoided for life. No formal studies on the natural history of non–IgE-mediated cutaneous or respiratory disorders have been undertaken, but these sensitivities are thought to be long-lasting.

FOOD ALLERGY AS A MARKER OF ATOPIC PREDISPOSITION

In many children, food allergy coexists with other atopic conditions, such as atopic dermatitis, asthma, and allergic rhinitis. Sensitization to egg white in children with atopic dermatitis and a family history of atopy is associated with a 70% risk for respiratory allergic disease (i.e., asthma or allergic rhinitis) at 5 years of age.[174] Individuals with past and current food allergy should be considered at high risk for asthma and environmental allergy.

Summary

Ingested foods represent the greatest foreign antigenic load confronting the human immune system. Most individuals develop tolerance to food antigens, which gain easy access to the body. However, when tolerance fails to develop, the immune system responds with an allergic reaction.

Although allergic reactions to milk were first described by Hippocrates more than 2000 years ago, it is only the past 2 decades that food allergy has emerged as an important public health problem for people of all ages in societies with a Western lifestyle. Inadvertent ingestion of food allergens may provoke various gastrointestinal, cutaneous, and respiratory symptoms or systemic anaphylaxis with shock in up to 8% of children younger than 5 years of age and approximately 3.5% of the general population.

Food Allergy Guidelines have been established to facilitate uniform approaches to diagnosis and management. Although investigations have characterized food allergy disorders to some extent, our understanding of the basic immunopathologic mechanisms remains incomplete. The rigorous scientific methods now being applied in this field provide hope that the pathogenesis of these disorders will be elucidated and that new forms of therapy will become available in the next few years.

REFERENCES

Definitions and Historical Perspective

1. Sicherer SH, Sampson HA. Food allergy: recent advances in pathophysiology and treatment. Annu Rev Med 2009;60:261-77.
2. Branum AM, Lukacs SL. Food allergy among children in the United States. Pediatrics 2009; 124:1549-55.
3. Sicherer SH. Epidemiology of food allergy. J Allergy Clin Immunol 2011;127:594-602.
4. Nowak-Węgrzyn A, Assa'ad AH, Bahna SL, et al. Work group report: oral food challenge testing. J Allergy Clin Immunol 2009;123(Suppl):S365-83.
5. Boyce J, Assa'ad AH, Burks AW, et al. Guidelines for the diagnosis and management of food allergy in the United States: summary of the NIAID sponsored expert panel report. J Allergy Clin Immunol 2010;126(Suppl):S1-58.
6. Prausnitz C, Kustner H. Studies on supersensitivity. Centrabl Bakteriol 1921;86:160-9.

6a. Geha RS, Beiser A, Ren C, et al. Multicenter, double-blind, placebo-controlled, multiple-challenge evaluation of reported reactions to monosodium glutamate. J Allergy Clin Immunol 2000;106:973-80.

7. Loveless MH. Milk allergy: a survey of its incidence; experiments with a masked ingestion test. J Allergy 1950;21:489-99.
8. Loveless MH. Allergy for corn and its derivatives: experiments with a masked ingestion test for its diagnosis. J Allergy 1950;21:500-9.
9. Goldman AS, Sellars WA, Halpern SR, et al. Milk allergy: II. Skin testing of allergic and normal children with purified milk proteins. Pediatrics 1963;32:572-9.
10. May CD. Objective clinical and laboratory studies of immediate hypersensitivity reactions to foods in asthmatic children. J Allergy Clin Immunol 1976;58:500-15.
11. Fiocchi A, Brozek J, Schunemann H, et al. World Allergy Organization (WAO) Diagnosis and Rationale for Action against Cow's Milk Allergy (DRACMA) guidelines. Pediatr Allergy Immunol 2010;21(Suppl 21):1-125.

Epidemiology

12. Osborne NJ, Koplin JJ, Martin PE, et al. Prevalence of challenge-proven IgE-mediated food allergy using population-based sampling and predetermined challenge criteria in infants. J Allergy Clin Immunol 2011;127:668-76.
13. Savage JH, Matsui EC, Skripak JM, Wood RA. The natural history of egg allergy. J Allergy Clin Immunol 2007;120:1413-7.
14. Skripak JM, Matsui EC, Mudd K, Wood RA. The natural history of IgE-mediated cow's milk allergy. J Allergy Clin Immunol 2007;120: 1172-7.
15. Sheikh A, Alves B. Hospital admissions for acute anaphylaxis: time trend study. BMJ 2000; 320:1441.
16. Eigenmann PA, Sicherer SH, Borkowski TA, Cohen BA, Sampson HA. Prevalence of IgE-mediated food allergy among children with atopic dermatitis. Pediatrics 1998;101:E8.
17. Novembre E, de MM, Vierucci A. Foods and respiratory allergy. J Allergy Clin Immunol 1988;81(Pt 2):1059-65.

Prevalence of Food Allergy

18. Hu U, Chen J, Li H. Comparison of food allergy prevalence among Chinese infants in Chongqing, 2009 versus 1999. Pediatr Int 2010; 52:820-4.
19. Lin RY, Anderson AS, Shah SN, Nurruzzaman F. Increasing anaphylaxis hospitalizations in the first 2 decades of life: New York State, 1990-2006. Ann Allergy Asthma Immunol 2008;101: 387-93.
20. Yocum MW, Butterfield JH, Klein JS, et al. Epidemiology of anaphylaxis in Olmsted County: a population-based study. J Allergy Clin Immunol 1999;104:452-6.
21. Decker WW, Campbell RL, Manivannan V, et al. The etiology and incidence of anaphylaxis in Rochester, Minnesota: a report from the Rochester Epidemiology Project. J Allergy Clin Immunol 2008;122:1161-5.
22. Sicherer SH, Furlong TJ, Maes HH, et al. Genetics of peanut allergy: a twin study. J Allergy Clin Immunol 2000;106(Pt 1):53-6.
23. Lack G, Penagos M. Early feeding practices and development of food allergies. Nestle Nutr Workshop Ser Pediatr Program 2011;68: 169-83.
24. Prescott S, Nowak-Węgrzyn A. Strategies to prevent or reduce allergic disease. Ann Nutr Metab 2011;59(Suppl 1):28-42.
25. Du TG, Katz Y, Sasieni P, et al. Early consumption of peanuts in infancy is associated with a low prevalence of peanut allergy. J Allergy Clin Immunol 2008;122:984-91.

Pathogenesis and Etiology

26. Vickery BP, Scurlock AM, Jones SM, Burks AW. Mechanisms of immune tolerance relevant to food allergy. J Allergy Clin Immunol 2011;127: 576-84.
27. Michael JG. The role of digestive enzymes in orally induced immune tolerance. Immunol Invest 1989;18:1049-54.
28. Walzer M. Studies in absorption of undigested proteins in human beings: I. A simple direct method of studying the absorption of undigested protein. J Immunol 1927;14:143-74.
29. Brunner M, Walzer M. Absorption of undigested proteins in human beings: the absorption of unaltered fish proteins in adults. Arch Intern Med 1928;42:173-9.
30. Gray I, Walzer M. Studies in mucous membrane hypersensitiveness: III. The allergic reaction of the passively sensitized rectal mucous membrane. Am J Digest Dis 1938;4:707-11.
31. Hoffman KM, Ho DG, Sampson HA. Evaluation of the usefulness of lymphocyte proliferation assays in the diagnosis of cow's milk allergy. J Allergy Clin Immunol 1997;99:360-6.
32. Strid J, Hourihane J, Kimber I, Callard R, Strobel S. Epicutaneous exposure to peanut protein prevents oral tolerance and enhances allergic sensitization. Clin Exp Allergy 2005;35: 757-66.
33. Brown SJ, Asai Y, Cordell HJ, et al. Loss-of-function variants in the filaggrin gene are a significant risk factor for peanut allergy. J Allergy Clin Immunol 2011;127:661-7.

Food Allergens

34. Radauer C, Bublin M, Wagner S, Mari A, Breiteneder H. Allergens are distributed into few protein families and possess a restricted number of biochemical functions. J Allergy Clin Immunol 2008;121:847-52.
35. Masilamani M, Commins S, Shreffler W. Determinants of food allergy. Immunol Allergy Clin North Am 2012;32:11-33.
36. Jenkins JA, Breiteneder H, Mills EN. Evolutionary distance from human homologs reflects allergenicity of animal food proteins. J Allergy Clin Immunol 2007;120:1399-405.
37. Breiteneder H, Radauer C. A classification of plant food allergens. J Allergy Clin Immunol 2004;113:821-30.
38. Wal JM. Bovine milk allergenicity. Ann Allergy Asthma Immunol 2004;93(Suppl 3):S2-11.
39. Roth-Walter F, Berin MC, Arnaboldi P, et al. Pasteurization of milk proteins promotes allergic sensitization by enhancing uptake through Peyer's patches. Allergy 2008;63: 882-90.
40. Goldman AS, Anderson DW Jr, Sellers WA, et al. Milk allergy: I. Oral challenge with milk and isolated milk proteins in allergic children. Pediatrics 1963;32:425-43.
41. Bellioni-Businco B, Paganelli R, Lucenti P, et al. Allergenicity of goat's milk in children with cow's milk allergy. J Allergy Clin Immunol 1999;103:1191-4.
42. Werfel SJ, Cooke SK, Sampson HA. Clinical reactivity to beef in children allergic to cow's milk. J Allergy Clin Immunol 1997;99: 293-300.
43. Bleumink E, Young E. Identification of the atopic allergen in cow's milk. Int Arch Allergy Appl Immunol 1968;34:521-43.
44. Jarvinen KM, Beyer K, Vila L, et al. B-cell epitopes as a screening instrument for persistent cow's milk allergy. J Allergy Clin Immunol 2002;110:293-7.
45. Vila L, Beyer K, Jarvinen KM, et al. Role of conformational and linear epitopes in the achievement of tolerance in cow's milk allergy. Clin Exp Allergy 2001;31:1599-606.
46. Chatchatee P, Jarvinen KM, Bardina L, et al. Identification of IgE and IgG binding epitopes on beta- and kappa-casein in cow's milk allergic patients. Clin Exp Allergy 2001;31: 1256-62.
47. Nowak-Węgrzyn A, Bloom KA, Sicherer SH, et al. Tolerance to extensively heated milk in children with cow's milk allergy. J Allergy Clin Immunol 2008;122:342-7.
48. Kim JS, Nowak-Węgrzyn A, Sicherer SH, et al. Dietary baked milk accelerates the resolution of cow's milk allergy in children. J Allergy Clin Immunol 2011;128:125-31.
49. Benhamou AH, Caubet JC, Eigenmann PA, et al. State of the art and new horizons in the diagnosis and management of egg allergy. Allergy 2010;65:283-9.
50. Caubet JC, Kondo Y, Urisu A, Nowak-Węgrzyn A. Molecular diagnosis of egg allergy. Curr Opin Allergy Clin Immunol 2011;11:210-5.
51. Urisu A, Ando H, Morita Y, et al. Allergenic activity of heated and ovomucoid-depleted egg white. J Allergy Clin Immunol 1997;100: 171-6.
52. Lemon-Mule H, Sampson HA, Sicherer SH, et al. Immunologic changes in children with egg allergy ingesting extensively heated egg. J Allergy Clin Immunol 2008;122:977-83.
53. Cooke SK, Sampson HA. Allergenic properties of ovomucoid in man. J Immunol 1997;159: 2026-32.
54. Jarvinen KM, Beyer K, Vila L, et al. Specificity of IgE antibodies to sequential epitopes of hen's egg ovomucoid as a marker for persistence of egg allergy. Allergy 2007;62:758-65.
55. Ando H, Moverare R, Kondo Y, et al. Utility of ovomucoid-specific IgE concentrations in predicting symptomatic egg allergy. J Allergy Clin Immunol 2008;122:583-8.

56. Martos G, Lopez-Exposito I, Bencharitiwong R, Berin MC, Nowak-Węgrzyn A. Mechanisms underlying differential food allergy response to heated egg. J Allergy Clin Immunol 2011; 127:990-7.
57. Burks AW, Williams LW, Helm RM, et al. Identification of a major peanut allergen, Ara h I, in patients with atopic dermatitis and positive peanut challenges. J Allergy Clin Immunol 1991;88:172-9.
58. Burks AW, Williams LW, Connaughton C, et al. Identification and characterization of a second major peanut allergen, Ara h II, with use of the sera of patients with atopic dermatitis and positive peanut challenge. J Allergy Clin Immunol 1992;90(Pt 1):962-9.
59. Rabjohn P, Helm EM, Stanley JS, et al. Molecular cloning and epitope analysis of the peanut allergen Ara h 3. J Clin Invest 1999;103: 535-42.
60. Hourihane JO, Bedwani SJ, Dean TP, Warner JO. Randomised, double blind, crossover challenge study of allergenicity of peanut oils in subjects allergic to peanuts. BMJ 1997;314: 1084-8.
61. Chruszcz M, Maleki SJ, Majorek KA, et al. Structural and immunologic characterization of Ara h 1, a major peanut allergen. J Biol Chem 2011;286:39318-27.
62. Burks AW, Shin D, Cockrell G, et al. Mapping and mutational analysis of the IgE-binding epitopes on Ara h 1, a legume vicilin protein and a major allergen in peanut hypersensitivity. Eur J Biochem 1997;245:334-9.
63. Shin DS, Compadre CM, Maleki SJ, et al. Biochemical and structural analysis of the IgE binding sites on Ara h1, an abundant and highly allergenic peanut protein. J Biol Chem 1998;273:13753-9.
64. Nowak-Węgrzyn A, Sampson HA. Future therapies for food allergies. J Allergy Clin Immunol 2011;127:558-73, quiz 574-5.
65. Shreffler WG, Charlop-Powers Z, Castro RR, et al. The major allergen from peanut, Ara h 1, is a ligand of DC-SIGN [abstract]. J Allergy Clin Immunol 2006;117:S87.
66. de Leon MP, Drew AC, Glaspole IN, et al. IgE cross-reactivity between the major peanut allergen Ara h 2 and tree nut allergens. Mol Immunol 2007;44:463-71.
67. Koppelman SJ, Wensing M, Ertmann M, Knulst AC, Knol EF. Relevance of Ara h1, Ara h2 and Ara h3 in peanut-allergic patients, as determined by immunoglobulin E Western blotting, basophil-histamine release and intracutaneous testing: Ara h2 is the most important peanut allergen. Clin Exp Allergy 2004; 34:583-90.
68. Nicolaou N, Poorafshar M, Murray C, et al. Allergy or tolerance in children sensitized to peanut: prevalence and differentiation using component-resolved diagnostics. J Allergy Clin Immunol 2010;125:191-7.
69. Koppelman SJ, de Jong GA, Laaper-Ertmann M, et al. Purification and immunoglobulin E-binding properties of peanut allergen Ara h 6: evidence for cross-reactivity with Ara h 2. Clin Exp Allergy 2005;35:490-7.
70. Koppelman SJ, Hefle SL, Taylor SL, de Jong GA. Digestion of peanut allergens Ara h 1, Ara h 2, Ara h 3, and Ara h 6: a comparative in vitro study and partial characterization of digestion-resistant peptides. Mol Nutr Food Res 2010; 54:1711-21.
71. Mittag D, Akkerdaas J, Ballmer-Weber BK, et al. Ara h 8, a Bet v 1-homologous allergen from peanut, is a major allergen in patients with combined birch pollen and peanut allergy. J Allergy Clin Immunol 2004;114:1410-7.
72. Kleine-Tebbe J, Vogel L, Crowell DN, Haustein UF, Vieths S. Severe oral allergy syndrome and anaphylactic reactions caused by a Bet v 1-related PR-10 protein in soybean, SAM22. J Allergy Clin Immunol 2002;110:797-804.
73. Mittag D, Vieths S, Vogel L, et al. Soybean allergy in patients allergic to birch pollen: clinical investigation and molecular characterization of allergens. J Allergy Clin Immunol 2004;113:148-54.
74. Ito K, Sjolander S, Sato S, et al. IgE to Gly m 5 and Gly m 6 is associated with severe allergic reactions to soybean in Japanese children. J Allergy Clin Immunol 2011;128:673-5.
75. Bush RK, Taylor SL, Nordlee JA, Busse WW. Soybean oil is not allergenic to soybean-sensitive individuals. J Allergy Clin Immunol 1985;76(Pt 1):242-5.
76. Sicherer SH, Munoz-Furlong A, Godbold JH, Sampson HA. US prevalence of self-reported peanut, tree nut, and sesame allergy: 11-year follow-up. J Allergy Clin Immunol 2010;125: 1322-6.
77. Ahn K, Bardina L, Grishina G, Beyer K, Sampson HA. Identification of two pistachio allergens, Pis v 1 and Pis v 2, belonging to the 2S albumin and 11S globulin family. Clin Exp Allergy 2009;39:926-34.
78. Hourihane JO, Kilburn SA, Dean P, Warner JO. Clinical characteristics of peanut allergy. Clin Exp Allergy 1997;27:634-9.
79. Maloney JM, Rudengren M, Ahlstedt S, Bock SA, Sampson HA. The use of serum-specific IgE measurements for the diagnosis of peanut, tree nut, and seed allergy. J Allergy Clin Immunol 2008;122:145-51.
80. Lehrer SB, Ayuso R, Reese G. Seafood allergy and allergens: a review. Mar Biotechnol 2003;5:339-48.
81. Van DT, Elsayed S, Florvaag E, Hordvik I, Endresen C. Allergy to fish parvalbumins: studies on the cross-reactivity of allergens from 9 commonly consumed fish. J Allergy Clin Immunol 2005;116:1314-20.
82. Griesmeier U, Vazquez-Cortes S, Bublin M, et al. Expression levels of parvalbumins determine allergenicity of fish species. Allergy 2010; 65:191-8.
83. Bernhisel-Broadbent J, Scanlon SM, Sampson HA. Fish hypersensitivity: I. In vitro and oral challenge results in fish-allergic patients. J Allergy Clin Immunol 1992;89:730-7.
84. Roberts G, Golder N, Lack G. Bronchial challenges with aerosolized food in asthmatic, food-allergic children. Allergy 2002;57:713-7.
85. Jeebhay MF, Cartier A. Seafood workers and respiratory disease: an update. Curr Opin Allergy Clin Immunol 2010;10:104-13.
86. Munoz-Furlong A, Sampson HA, Sicherer SH. Prevalence of self-reported seafood allergy in the US. J Allergy Clin Immunol 2004;113: S100.
87. Shek LP, Cabrera-Morales EA, Soh SE, et al. A population-based questionnaire survey on the prevalence of peanut, tree nut, and shellfish allergy in 2 Asian populations. J Allergy Clin Immunol 2010;126:324-31.
88. Lehrer SB, McCants ML, Salvaggio JE. Identification of crustacea allergens by crossed radioimmunoelectrophoresis. Int Arch Allergy Appl Immunol 1985;77:192-4.
89. Reese G, Ayuso R, Carle T, Lehrer SB. IgE-binding epitopes of shrimp tropomyosin, the major allergen Pen a 1. Int Arch Allergy Immunol 1999;118:300-1.
90. Ayuso R, Lehrer SB, Reese G. Identification of continuous, allergenic regions of the major shrimp allergen Pen a 1 (tropomyosin). Int Arch Allergy Immunol 2002;127:27-37.
91. Ayuso R, Grishina G, Ibanez MD, et al. Sarcoplasmic calcium-binding protein is an EF-hand-type protein identified as a new shrimp allergen. J Allergy Clin Immunol 2009;124: 114-20.
92. Reese G, Ayuso R, Lehrer SB. Tropomyosin: an invertebrate pan-allergen. Int Arch Allergy Immunol 1999;119:247-58.
93. Salcedo G, Quirce S, az-Perales A. Wheat allergens associated with Baker's asthma. J Investig Allergol Clin Immunol 2011;21: 81-92.
94. Tatham AS, Shewry PR. Allergens to wheat and related cereals. Clin Exp Allergy 2008;38: 1712-26.
95. Palosuo K, Varjonen E, Nurkkala J, et al. Transglutaminase-mediated cross-linking of a peptic fraction of omega-5 gliadin enhances IgE reactivity in wheat-dependent, exercise-induced anaphylaxis. J Allergy Clin Immunol 2003;111:1386-92.
96. Matsuo H, Morita E, Tatham AS, et al. Identification of the IgE-binding epitope in omega-5 gliadin, a major allergen in wheat-dependent exercise-induced anaphylaxis. J Biol Chem 2004;279:12135-40.
97. Jones SM, Magnolfi CF, Cooke SK, Sampson HA. Immunologic cross-reactivity among cereal grains and grasses in children with food hypersensitivity. J Allergy Clin Immunol 1995;96:341-51.
98. Hoffmann-Sommergruber K, Mills EN. Food allergen protein families and their structural characteristics and application in component-resolved diagnosis: new data from the Euro-Prevall project. Anal Bioanal Chem 2009;395: 25-35.
99. Commins SP, Platts-Mills TA. Anaphylaxis syndromes related to a new mammalian cross-reactive carbohydrate determinant. J Allergy Clin Immunol 2009;124:652-7.
100. Commins SP, James HR, Kelly LA, et al. The relevance of tick bites to the production of IgE antibodies to the mammalian oligosaccharide galactose-alpha-1,3-galactose. J Allergy Clin Immunol 2011;127:1286-93.
101. Sicherer SH. Clinical implications of cross-reactive food allergens. J Allergy Clin Immunol 2001;108:881-90.

Pathophysiologic Mechanisms of Food Allergy

102. Vadas P, Gold M, Perelman B, et al. Platelet-activating factor, PAF acetylhydrolase, and severe anaphylaxis. N Engl J Med 2008;358: 28-35.
103. Shreffler WG, Lencer DA, Bardina L, Sampson HA. IgE and IgG4 epitope mapping by microarray immunoassay reveals the diversity of immune response to the peanut allergen, Ara h 2. J Allergy Clin Immunol 2005;116: 893-9.
104. Wang J, Lin J, Bardina L, et al. Correlation of IgE/IgG4 milk epitopes and affinity of milk-specific IgE antibodies with different phenotypes of clinical milk allergy. J Allergy Clin Immunol 2010;125:695-702.
105. Reimann HJ, Ring J, Ultsch B, Wendt P. Intragastral provocation under endoscopic control (IPEC) in food allergy: mast cell and histamine

changes in gastric mucosa. Clin Allergy 1985; 15:195-202.
106. Buisseret PD, Youlten LF, Heinzelmann DI, Lessof MH. Prostaglandin-synthesis inhibitors in prophylaxis of food intolerance. Lancet 1978;1:906-8.
107. Untersmayr E, Jensen-Jarolim E. The effect of gastric digestion on food allergy. Curr Opin Allergy Clin Immunol 2006;6:214-9.
108. Untersmayr E, Vestergaard H, Malling HJ, et al. Incomplete digestion of codfish represents a risk factor for anaphylaxis in patients with allergy. J Allergy Clin Immunol 2007;119: 711-7.
109. Varshney P, Steele PH, Vickery BP, et al. Adverse reactions during peanut oral immunotherapy home dosing. J Allergy Clin Immunol 2009; 124:1351-2.
110. Caffrey EA, Sladen GE, Isaacs PE, Clark KG. Thrombocytopenia caused by cow's milk. Lancet 1981;2:316.
111. Paganelli R, Levinsky RJ, Brostoff J, Wraith DG. Immune complexes containing food proteins in normal and atopic subjects after oral challenge and effect of sodium cromoglycate on antigen absorption. Lancet 1979;1:1270-2.
112. Lunardi C, Bambara LM, Biasi D, et al. Elimination diet in the treatment of selected patients with hypersensitivity vasculitis. Clin Exp Rheumatol 1992;10:131-5.

Clinical Manifestations of Food Allergy

113. Berin MC, Mayer L. Immunophysiology of experimental food allergy. Mucosal Immunol 2009;2:24-32.
114. Turner MW, Barnett GE, Strobel S. Mucosal mast cell activation patterns in the rat following repeated feeding of antigen. Clin Exp Allergy 1990;20:421-7.
115. Flinterman AE, Knulst AC, Meijer Y, Bruijnzeel-Koomen CA, Pasmans SG. Acute allergic reactions in children with AEDS after prolonged cow's milk elimination diets. Allergy 2006; 61:370-4.
116. Eyermann C. X-ray demonstration of colonic reactions in food allergy. J Missouri Med Assoc 1927;24:129-32.
117. Rowe A Jr, Rowe AH. Atopic dermatitis in infants and children. J Pediatr 1951;39:80-6.
118. Fries JH, Zizmor J. Roentgen studies in children with alimentary disturbances due to food allergy. Am J Dis Child 1937;54:1239-51.
119. Pollard H, Stuart G. Experimental reproduction of gastric allergy in human beings with controlled obseravtions on the mucosa. J Allergy 1942;13:467-73.
120. Moller C. Effect of pollen immunotherapy on food hypersensitivity in children with birch pollinosis. Ann Allergy 1989;62:343-5.
121. Liacouras CA, Furuta GT, Hirano I, et al. Eosinophilic esophagitis: updated consensus recommendations for children and adults. J Allergy Clin Immunol 2011;128:3-20, quiz 21-2.
122. Rothenberg ME, Spergel JM, Sherrill JD, et al. Common variants at 5q22 associate with pediatric eosinophilic esophagitis. Nat Genet 2010; 42:289-91.
123. Kagalwalla AF, Sentongo TA, Ritz S, et al. Effect of six-food elimination diet on clinical and histologic outcomes in eosinophilic esophagitis. Clin Gastroenterol Hepatol 2006; 4:1097-102.
124. Teitelbaum JE, Fox VL, Twarog FJ, et al. Eosinophilic esophagitis in children: immunopathological analysis and response to fluticasone propionate. Gastroenterology 2002;122:1216-25.
125. Powell GK. Milk- and soy-induced enterocolitis of infancy. J Pediatr 1978;93:553-60.
126. Katz Y, Goldberg MR, Rajuan N, Cohen A, Leshno M. The prevalence and natural course of food protein-induced enterocolitis syndrome to cow's milk: a large-scale, prospective population-based study. J Allergy Clin Immunol 2011;127:647-53.
127. Leonard SA, Nowak-Węgrzyn A. Food protein-induced enterocolitis syndrome: an update on natural history and review of management. Ann Allergy Asthma Immunol 2011;107: 95-101.
128. Fogg MI, Brown-Whitehorn TA, Pawlowski NA, Spergel JM. Atopy patch test for the diagnosis of food protein-induced enterocolitis syndrome. Pediatr Allergy Immunol 2006;17: 351-5.
129. Savilahti E. Food-induced malabsorption syndromes. J Pediatr Gastroenterol Nutr 2000; 30:S61-6.
130. Green PH, Cellier C. Celiac disease. N Engl J Med 2007;357:1731-43.
131. Ludvigsson JF, Green PH. Clinical management of coeliac disease. J Intern Med 2011; 269:560-71.
132. Novak N, Leung DY. Advances in atopic dermatitis. Curr Opin Immunol 2011;23:778-83.
133. Beyer K, Castro R, Feidel C, Sampson HA. Milk-induced urticaria is associated with the expansion of T cells expressing cutaneous lymphocyte antigen. J Allergy Clin Immunol 2002;109:688-93.
134. Sampson HA, Broadbent KR, Bernhisel-Broadbent J. Spontaneous release of histamine from basophils and histamine-releasing factor in patients with atopic dermatitis and food hypersensitivity. N Engl J Med 1989;321: 228-32.
135. Li XM, Kleiner G, Huang CK, et al. Murine model of atopic dermatitis associated with food hypersensitivity. J Allergy Clin Immunol 2001;107:693-702.
136. Sampson HA. Food allergy. Part 2: diagnosis and management. J Allergy Clin Immunol 1999;103:981-9.
137. Lever R, MacDonald C, Waugh P, Aitchison T. Randomised controlled trial of advice on an egg exclusion diet in young children with atopic eczema and sensitivity to eggs. Pediatr Allergy Immunol 1998;9:13-9.
138. Sicherer SH, Sampson HA. Food hypersensitivity and atopic dermatitis: pathophysiology, epidemiology, diagnosis, and management. J Allergy Clin Immunol 1999;104(Pt 2): S114-22.
139. Cardones AR, Hall RP III. Pathophysiology of dermatitis herpetiformis: a model for cutaneous manifestations of gastrointestinal inflammation. Dermatol Clin 2011;29:469-77, x.
140. Bock SA, Atkins FM. Patterns of food hypersensitivity during sixteen years of double-blind, placebo-controlled food challenges. J Pediatr 1990;117:561-7.
141. Kivity S, Dunner K, Marian Y. The pattern of food hypersensitivity in patients with onset after 10 years of age. Clin Exp Allergy 1994;24: 19-22.
142. Bock SA. Prospective appraisal of complaints of adverse reactions to foods in children during the first 3 years of life. Pediatrics 1987;79: 683-8.
143. James JM, Bernhisel-Broadbent J, Sampson HA. Respiratory reactions provoked by double-blind food challenges in children. Am J Respir Crit Care Med 1994;149:59-64.
144. James JM, Eigenman PA, Eggleston PA, Sampson HA. Airway reactivity changes in asthmatic patients undergoing blinded food challenges. Am J Respir Crit Care Med 1996; 153:597-603.
145. James JM, Crespo JF. Allergic reactions to foods by inhalation. Curr Allergy Asthma Rep 2007;7:167-74.
146. Wang J, Visness CM, Sampson HA. Food allergen sensitization in inner-city children with asthma. J Allergy Clin Immunol 2005;115: 1076-80.
147. Heiner DC, Sears JW. Chronic respiratory disease associated with multiple circulating precipitins to cow's milk. Am J Dis Child 1960;100:500-2.
148. Sampson HA, Mendelson L, Rosen JP. Fatal and near-fatal anaphylactic reactions to food in children and adolescents. N Engl J Med 1992;327:380-4.
149. Bock SA, Munoz-Furlong A, Sampson HA. Fatalities due to anaphylactic reactions to foods. J Allergy Clin Immunol 2001;107:191-3.
150. Bock SA, Munoz-Furlong A, Sampson HA. Further fatalities caused by anaphylactic reactions to food, 2001-2006. J Allergy Clin Immunol 2007;119:1016-8.
151. Robson-Ansley P, Toit GD. Pathophysiology, diagnosis and management of exercise-induced anaphylaxis. Curr Opin Allergy Clin Immunol 2010;10:312-7.
152. Palosuo K, Alenius H, Varjonen E, et al. A novel wheat gliadin as a cause of exercise-induced anaphylaxis. J Allergy Clin Immunol 1999; 103(Pt 1):912-7.
153. Nakamura K, Inomata N, Ikezawa Z. Dramatic augmentation of wheat allergy by aspirin in a dose-dependent manner. Ann Allergy Asthma Immunol 2006;97:712-3.
154. Sampson HA, Anderson JA. Summary and recommendations: classification of gastrointestinal manifestations due to immunologic reactions to foods in infants and young children. J Pediatr Gastroenterol Nutr 2000;30: S87-94.
155. Mangge H, Hermann J, Schauenstein K. Diet and rheumatoid arthritis: a review. Scand J Rheumatol 1999;28:201-9.
156. Vaughan TR. The role of food in the pathogenesis of migraine headache. Clin Rev Allergy 1994;12:167-80.

Diagnosis and Management of Food Allergy

157. Fiocchi A, Schunemann HJ, Brozek J, et al. Diagnosis and Rationale for Action Against Cow's Milk Allergy (DRACMA): a summary report. J Allergy Clin Immunol 2010;126: 1119-28.
158. Bock SA, Lee WY, Remigio L, Holst A, May CD. Appraisal of skin tests with food extracts for diagnosis of food hypersensitivity. Clin Allergy 1978;8:559-64.
159. Sporik R, Hill DJ, Hosking CS. Specificity of allergen skin testing in predicting positive open food challenges to milk, egg, and peanut in children. Clin Exp Allergy 2000;30:1540-6.
160. Mehl A, Rolinck-Werninghaus C, Staden U, et al. The atopy patch test in the diagnostic workup of suspected food-related symptoms in children. J Allergy Clin Immunol 2006; 118:923-9.
161. Sampson HA. Utility of food-specific IgE concentrations in predicting symptomatic food

allergy. J Allergy Clin Immunol 2001;107: 891-6.
162. Nicolaou N, Murray C, Belgrave D, et al. Quantification of specific IgE to whole peanut extract and peanut components in prediction of peanut allergy. J Allergy Clin Immunol 2011;127:684-5.
163. Alessandri C, Zennaro D, Scala E, et al. Ovomucoid (Gal d 1) specific IgE detected by microarray system predict tolerability to boiled hen's egg and an increased risk to progress to multiple environmental allergen sensitisation. Clin Exp Allergy 2012;42: 441-50.
164. Ott H, Baron JM, Heise R, et al. Clinical usefulness of microarray-based IgE detection in children with suspected food allergy. Allergy 2008;63:1521-8.
165. Shreffler WG. Evaluation of basophil activation in food allergy: present and future applications. Curr Opin Allergy Clin Immunol 2006;6:226-33.

Natural History of Food Allergy

166. Host A, Halken S. A prospective study of cow milk allergy in Danish infants during the first 3 years of life. Allergy 1990;45:587-96.
167. Wood RA. The natural history of food allergy. Pediatrics 2003;111(Pt 3):1631-7.
168. Leonard SA, Sampson HA, Sicherer SH, et al. Dietary baked egg accelerates resolution of egg allergy in children. J Allergy Clin Immunol 2012;13:473-80.
169. Skolnick HS, Conover-Walker MK, Koerner CB, et al. The natural history of peanut allergy. J Allergy Clin Immunol 2001;107:367-74.
170. Fleischer DM, Conover-Walker MK, Matsui EC, Wood RA. The natural history of tree nut allergy. J Allergy Clin Immunol 2005;116: 1087-93.
171. Savage JH, Kaeding AJ, Matsui EC, Wood RA. The natural history of soy allergy. J Allergy Clin Immunol 2010;125:683-6.
172. Keet CA, Matsui EC, Dhillon G, et al. The natural history of wheat allergy. Ann Allergy Asthma Immunol 2009;102:410-5.
173. Shek LP, Soderstrom L, Ahlstedt S, Beyer K, Sampson HA. Determination of food specific IgE levels over time can predict the development of tolerance in cow's milk and hen's egg allergy. J Allergy Clin Immunol 2004;114: 387-91.
174. Lau S, Nickel R, Niggemann B, et al. The development of childhood asthma: lessons from the German Multicentre Allergy Study (MAS). Paediatr Respir Rev 2002;3:265-72.
175. Greer FR, Sicherer SH, Burks AW; American Academy of Pediatrics Committee on Nutrition, American Academy of Pediatrics Section on Allergy and Immunology. Effects of early nutritional interventions on the development of atopic disease in infants and children: the role of maternal dietary restriction, breastfeeding, timing of introduction of complementary foods, and hydrolyzed formulas. Pediatrics 2008;121:183-91.
176. Sampson HA, Munoz-Furlong A, Bock SA, et al. Symposium on the definition and management of anaphylaxis: summary report. J Allergy Clin Immunol 2005;115:584-91.
177. Simons FE, Ardusso LR, Bilo MB, et al. World Allergy Organization anaphylaxis guidelines: summary. J Allergy Clin Immunol 2011;127: 587-93.
178. Boyano MT, García-Ara C, Esteban MM, et al. Validity of specific IgE antibodies in children with egg allergy. Clin Exp Allergy 2001;31: 1464-9.
179. Garcia-Ara C, Boyano-Martinez T, Diaz-Pena JM, et al. Specific-IgE levels in the diagnosis of immediate hypersensitivity to cow's milk protein in the infant. J Allergy Clin Immunol 2001;107:185-90.
180. Clark AT, Ewan PW. Interpretation of tests for nut allergy in one thousand patients, in relation to allergy or tolerance. Clin Exp Allergy 2003;33:1041-5.

82 Reactions to Food and Drug Additives

ROBERT K. BUSH | STEVE L. TAYLOR

OUTLINE

SUMMARY OF IMPORTANT CONCEPTS

» Adverse reactions to food or drug additives only occur in a limited segment of the population.
» With few exceptions, reactions to food or drug additives are not IgE mediated.
» IgE-mediated reactions can occur to food and drug additives derived from foods that are commonly allergenic.
» The likelihood of IgE-mediated reactions to such food and drug additives is dependent on the residual level of allergenic protein in the additive.
» Few additives have been identified as causing significant reactions; appropriate methods to substantiate reported reactions have not been conducted.
» Sulfite additives are a well-documented cause of asthma affecting approximately 5% of asthma patients.
» Proper diagnosis of a food or drug reaction often requires a double-blind placebo-controlled challenge.

Introduction

Many substances are added to foods and pharmaceutical products for a wide variety of technical functions. The U.S. Food and Drug Administration (FDA) recognizes more than 3000 substances allowed for addition to foods in the United States. Similarly, pharmaceutical products contain an enormous number of additives or "inactive ingredients," many of which can be found in the *United States Pharmacopeia*. Approximately 773 chemical agents are approved for use in drug products by the FDA.

Food additives serve many functions and can be nutrients or agents for coloring, flavoring, or antimicrobial purposes (Box 82-1). Many food ingredients serve more than one technical function; for example, sugar can serve as a sweetener, a bulking agent, and a preservative. With a few exceptions, such as sugar, the intake of specific food additives is rather small. Although many additives may be used in any given food product, the additives are typically minor ingredients of the composite food.

Additives in pharmaceuticals also serve numerous functions. Drug additives serve as agents of coloring, flavoring, emulsification, thickening, binding, and preservation (Box 82-2). Unlike in foods, the inert ingredients in pharmaceutical products often make up the majority of the product, because active pharmaceutical ingredients are frequently present as a small fraction of the product's total mass.

Labeling of Additives

In the United States, food labels provide an ingredient statement that identifies virtually all the intended ingredients in the food product. Some standardized foods (e.g., mayonnaise, ice cream) with well-known defined compositions are not required to have an ingredient statement, although in practice many do. The ingredient statement lists the ingredients in the composite food product in descending order of predominance. By U.S. regulation, virtually all intentionally added ingredients must be declared on the ingredient statement. However, a few groups of ingredients are allowed to be declared collectively without a listing of all the individual components (e.g., spices, natural/artificial flavors). Because numerous individual flavors are often added to a food product in extremely small quantities, the individual listing of these ingredients would add substantially to the length of the ingredient statement.

In the United States the Food Allergen Labeling and Consumer Protection Act mandates that any ingredient derived from a commonly allergenic food (defined as peanut, tree nuts such as almond and walnut, soybeans, wheat, milk, egg, fish, and crustacean shellfish such as shrimp, crab, and lobster) must be labeled clearly by source.[1] Examples of proper labeling would be "lactose (milk)" and "soybean lecithin." Source labeling of such ingredients is required regardless of the function of the ingredient. Thus, although flavors may still be labeled collectively, the presence of any flavors derived from commonly allergenic sources must be declared. An example would be "natural flavoring (milk and fish)." The only exemptions from the allergen source labeling provisions are provided for highly refined oils and ingredients that are exempted by notification or petition to FDA. Thus far, no exemptions by notification or petition have been approved by the FDA. Also, highly refined oils would still be labeled in most cases unless they are included in flavorings or some other collectively labeled category.

Labeling regulations differ in other parts of the world, although regulations to require source labeling of ingredients derived from commonly allergenic foods are also in force in some other countries. A list of food additives allowed for use in the United States is available at the FDA web site www.fda.gov/food/foodingredientspackaging/foodadditives. Similarly, a list

BOX 82-1 CATEGORIES OF FOOD ADDITIVES WITH EXAMPLES

Starches/complex carbohydrates	Cornstarch, modified starch
Preservatives (antimicrobials)	Potassium sorbate, sodium benzoate
Preservatives (antioxidants)	Butylated hydroxyanisole/ hydroxytoluene (BHA/BHT)
Preservatives (antibrowning)	Potassium metabisulfite, sulfur dioxide
Nutrients	Vitamin A, ferrous sulfate
Flavors	Ethyl vanillin, cinnamic aldehyde
Anticaking agents	Sodium aluminosilicate
Emulsifying agents	Lecithin
Sequestrants	Citric acid
Stabilizers and gums	Tragacanth gum, xanthan gum
Acidulents	Phosphoric acid, hydrochloric acid
Flavor enhancers	Monosodium glutamate
Colors	Tartrazine, annatto
Enzymes	Papain
Leavening agents	Sodium bicarbonate

BOX 82-2 CATEGORIES OF DRUG ADDITIVES WITH EXAMPLES

Encapsulation agents	Carboxymethyl cellulose, gelatin
Emulsifiers/solvents	Dextran, gums, egg albumin, polyoxyethylated castor oil
Synthetic sweeteners	Saccharin, aspartame
Vehicles	Oils, alcohols, propylene glycol
Stabilizers/antioxidants	Ethylenediamine, sulfites
Dyes	Tartrazine, sunset yellow, ponceau red, xanthene dyes
Preservatives	Benzoates, parabens, thimerosal, chlorobutamel
Adjuvants	Aluminum hydroxide, zinc oxide

of color additives for use in foods, drugs, and cosmetics can be found at www.fda.gov/forindustry/coloradditives.

The added ingredients in over-the-counter (OTC) pharmaceutical products are declared in an ingredient statement on the package or in an insert. For prescription drugs, information on the added ingredients is provided in the package insert.

Prevalence of Reactions to Additives

Many food and drug additives have been reported to cause adverse reactions, ranging from lethargy to severe asthma and anaphylaxis. Many of the food and drug additives listed in Boxes 82-1 and 82-2 have been reported to cause adverse reactions. However, many of these reactions have not been verified by appropriate diagnostic challenge procedures. Several food and drug additives have been extensively studied, including synthetic colorants, sulfites, monosodium glutamate (MSG), aspartame, and benzoates.

The prevalence of food allergies and food additive–induced sensitivities has been assessed in several large studies. In a Dutch study that started with a survey of 1483 adults and proceeded through clinical challenge trials, only three individuals were identified with food additive sensitivities,[2] amounting to 0.2% of the population. In a large Danish study of food additive–induced sensitivities that started with a survey of 4274 schoolchildren, an intolerance to food additives confirmed by double-blind challenge occurred in 2% of the children selected from the survey on the basis of atopic history, but in only 0.13% of the entire surveyed population.[3]

Young and colleagues[4] evaluated the prevalence of sensitivities to food additives among a British population using a combination of a survey questionnaire given to 18,582 individuals and a series of mixed-additive challenges conducted at home with self-reporting of symptoms. The researchers estimated the prevalence of adverse reactions to food additives as 0.01% to 0.23%. In a Berlin study of the prevalence of food reactions, a questionnaire was answered by 4093 persons, and those with self-reported food reactions were followed up by telephone and clinical investigation including double-blind placebo-controlled (DBPC) food challenges. The prevalence of adverse reactions to food additives (a mixture of various colors, preservatives, antioxidants, and flavor enhancers) was estimated at 0.18%.[5] Although this estimate is somewhat higher than in the earlier Dutch and Danish studies, the German study included more food additives and higher doses.

In a study of 54 Koreans age 1 to 44 with a variety of allergic diseases (asthma, rhinitis, atopic dermatitis, chronic urticaria) challenged with a mixture of seven common additives versus placebo, five (9.3%) responded to the food additives, two (3.7%) to both placebo and the additives, and three (5.5%) reacted to the placebo.[6] The authors concluded that there were no statistically significant differences among the groups.

Overall, adverse reactions to food additives may affect 0.01% to 0.23% of the general population, but the prevalence may be much higher (2% to 7%) in patients with atopic disease.[7]

Additionally, food ingredients derived from commonly allergenic sources have the potential to elicit allergic reactions if they contain sufficient quantities of allergenic proteins. The prevalence of allergic reactions to foods is estimated at 3.5% to 4.0% of the U.S. population,[8] and presumably many of these individuals would be susceptible to reactions to ingredients containing residual allergenic proteins.

The frequency of adverse reactions to drug additives is also unknown but is less common than food additive reactions. Adverse reactions to vaccine additives have been recently reviewed.[9] Many agents causing adverse reactions in drugs exist as single case reports. When used in a corticosteroid solution, cellulose derivatives (carboxymethylcellulose) have caused three cases of anaphylactic shock.[9] Emulsifying agents such as gums (arabic and tragacanth) have caused urticaria when administered in antihistamines and corticosteroid tablets.[10] Individuals have developed anaphylaxis to gelatin in vaccines. In some, skin-prick tests to the vaccine have been positive, and specific IgE antibodies to gelatin were in the patient's serum.[10,11] Sulfites used as antioxidants in drugs are well recognized as causing asthma and other reactions. Ethylenediamine is associated primarily with contact dermatitis, and sensitization occurs through cutaneous exposure. Ethylenediamine is also a component of aminophylline and has produced urticaria, exfoliative dermatitis, and anaphylaxis in sensitized individuals. Likewise, thimerosal, a preservative, often acts as a contact sensitizer but has caused anaphylaxis when administered in intravenous heparin solutions.[10] Benzalkonium chloride in bronchodilator solutions may cause bronchoconstriction when inhaled.[12] Overall, the role of excipients in drugs as a cause of adverse reactions remains unknown.

Some additives have been linked to occupational asthma.[13] Food and pharmaceutical additives are most frequently linked to chronic disorders such as asthma, chronic urticaria, and atopic dermatitis. Allergic contact dermatitis may also occur.[14,15] Because these illnesses are chronic in many patients and tend to flare episodically, establishing a causative role for food or pharmaceutical additives can be difficult.

Additive Challenge Studies: Urticaria and Asthma

PATIENTS WITH URTICARIA

Challenge studies are used to confirm a reported adverse reaction to a food or drug additive.[16] The initial history should ascertain the nature and severity of the symptoms and the interval between exposure and occurrence of urticaria. Further information should include whether symptoms are reproduced on subsequent exposure to the food or drug additive in question. Also, an approximation of the amount consumed should be obtained as well as any association with extenuating circumstances (e.g., exercise, alcohol consumption).

Patient Selection

The need for a diagnostic food or drug additive challenge depends on the circumstances. When an acute episode has occurred, the process becomes easier because a cause-and-effect relationship can be established. For the clinician, a diagnostic challenge for acute urticaria may be helpful in recommending appropriate avoidance procedures. For the researcher, a diagnostic challenge may be useful in establishing the role of a new agent in provoking urticaria and angioedema.

With chronic urticaria and angioedema, diagnostic challenge procedures become more difficult because the episodes of urticaria and angioedema occur sporadically over time, which makes false-positive results more likely. Epidemiologists might challenge all available patients with chronic urticaria to determine the prevalence of food additive reactions. The clinician might evaluate only patients with histories suggestive of food additive–induced urticaria or only those whose urticaria improves with an additive-free diet.

If the urticaria is active at the time of the study, patients are more likely to react in a positive manner to the challenge. If the urticarial reaction is quiescent, the patient is more likely to have a negative challenge.

Protocol Design

Before initiating a challenge procedure, consideration must be given to the severity of the likely reaction. If a patient has experienced anaphylaxis, all necessary equipment to resuscitate the patient must be available. Likewise, trained personnel should be available, and the procedure conducted in the morning when assistance is more likely available.

Antihistamines and Baseline. The use of medications, particularly antihistamines, can influence the result; it must be decided whether to continue or withhold antihistamines. Withholding antihistamines immediately before or within 24 hours of the challenge can increase the likelihood of false-positive reactions, whereas continuation of antihistamines may block the reaction and make false-negative reactions more likely. The longer the interval between the last dose of antihistamine and the challenge, the more likely is the subject to experience breakthrough urticaria, particularly if the placebo is given first and closer to the protective effects of the last antihistamine dose.[11] If it is decided to discontinue antihistamines, H_1 antihistamines of short duration of activity should be withheld for a minimum of 48 hours, hydroxyzine withheld for at least 72 hours, and second-generation antihistamines withheld for up to 1 week. Oral corticosteroids can be continued and usually are not thought to affect the reaction.

Alternatively, it may be appropriate to continue antihistamines at the lowest effective dose to stabilize the underlying chronic urticaria at a tolerable level. The dose of antihistamine chosen should improve patient comfort without abolishing urticaria. This dose of antihistamine should not be sufficient to affect the results of the additive challenge (i.e., produce a false-negative result).

Thus it is important to establish a stable baseline before a food or drug additive challenge. Furthermore, it must be established that the patient responds consistently to the challenge. This may require several blinded challenges with the active agent and placebo controls.

Figure 82-1 shows a sample format for conducting a challenge procedure. The procedure should be conducted in the morning after an overnight fast, and the food or drug additive agent in question should be withheld at least 48 hours before the challenge.

Blinded Placebo Challenge. The initial challenge procedure may consist of a single-blind challenge using a placebo control. If there is no objective finding, such as appearance of urticaria on two occasions, then the presumptive diagnosis is not correct. If a positive response is observed on single-blind challenge, either on one or both occasions, double-blind challenges may be necessary for confirmation. If only subjective symptoms such as pruritus occur, it may be necessary to repeat the challenge with three active and three placebo challenges.

A presumptive diagnosis of an adverse reaction to the additive can be made if a patient has objective findings such as urticaria and angioedema during a DBPC challenge in which a positive response occurs (urticaria) with the active food or drug additive and a negative response occurs with the placebo. However, because of the evanescent nature of urticaria, it may be appropriate to repeat the challenge with either additional active agents or placebo controls, to ensure that the reaction is consistent and reproducible. If an equivocal reaction occurs with the placebo, a third challenge may be necessary with either active or placebo control.

Dosages. The maximal amounts of food additives used for placebo-controlled trials are listed in Box 82-3. If a provoking dose has been reported in the literature, it is usually recommended that the starting dose be approximately one log lower than the lowest dose known to cause a reaction. If the provoking dose is not known, it may be calculated based on estimates of the quantity ingested obtained from the patient's history. The doses are usually administered in opaque capsules; however, it may be appropriate to consider liquid or solution challenges if this more closely mimics the natural exposure. Once the starting dose is obtained, incremental twofold increasing doses are typically administered at times varying from 30 to 60 minutes.

Controls. Studies of food additive–associated urticarial reactions include a surprising number done without appropriate placebo controls. Studies with properly controlled conditions indicate that food additives are an uncommon cause of chronic urticaria and angioedema.[13] The time interval between the last dose of antihistamine and the administration of a placebo in a

Previous reaction suspected of being due to food/drug additive ______

Date: ______

Sx ______

______

______

Time from ingestion of suspected agent to first sx ______

Time from appearance of first sx to peak of sx ______

Treatment received ______

______

______

______

Skin tests: Additive: ______ Results: Positive Negative

Other relevant illnesses: ______

______

______

Medications taken on day of challenge: ______

______

______

CHALLENGE SUBSTANCE: ______

BASELINE BP ______ BASELINE FEV_1 ______ (L): ______ (% PREDICTED)

CHALLENGE

Time given	Dose	Time evaluated	BP	FEV_1 (L)	Reaction

I understand that this challenge procedure may cause an allergic reaction in me, including, but not limited to swelling, itching, hives, asthma, wheezing or anaphylaxis (severe allergic reaction). I agree that this test is indicated and necessary.

Patient: ______

Parent or Guardian: ______

Witness: ______

Figure 82-1 Food/drug additive challenge information form. *(From Bock SA, Sampson HA, Atkins FM, et al: Double-blind, placebo-controlled food challenge (DBPCFC) as an office procedure: a manual. J Allergy Clin Immunol 1988;82:986.)*

challenge sequence should be carefully considered. If the placebo is administered closer to the last dose of an antihistamine, it may lead to false-positive responses if the protective effect of the antihistamine is lost during the course challenge. Using multiple placebos randomly interspersed during the challenge enhances the design of the study and eliminates the bias of the loss of the protective effect of the antihistamine.

It is also important to blind both subjects and observers and to avoid unspoken signals of concern and apprehension that may inadvertently lead to positive responses.

When conducting DBPC trials over 2 separate days, the placebo day must take place over the same interval as the day on which the active challenge is given, because urticaria may vary throughout the challenge.

Criteria for Positive Reactions. For evaluating urticaria, a scoring system based on the "rule of nines" may be used.[17] The body is divided into areas of 9% that are scored as 0 (no urticaria), 1 (25% of areas involved), 2 (50% involved), 3 (75% involved), or 4 (confluence of urticaria in areas involved). A

BOX 82-3 SUGGESTED MAXIMUM DOSES FOR CHALLENGE ADDITIVES

Tartrazine/FD&C dyes	50 mg
Sulfites	200 mg
Monosodium glutamate	2.5-5 g
Aspartame	150 mg
Parabens/benzoates	100 mg
BHA/BHT	100 mg
Nitrates/nitrites	100 mg

From Simon RA. Additive-induced urticaria: experience with monosodium glutamate (MSG). J Nutr 2000;130:1063S.

score of 9, or a 30% increase from the baseline urticaria, is considered a positive challenge.

If the blinded challenge procedures are negative, a final open feeding without reaction after negative challenge is considered appropriate to confirm the diagnosis.

ASTHMATIC PATIENTS

As with urticaria, an initial history describing the symptoms and the interval between exposure and onset of symptoms is important in establishing the role of food or drug additives in asthma. Furthermore, symptoms should be reproducible when the patient is exposed to the offending agent, as well as the amount consumed. Before performing challenges, a general physical examination, pulmonary function tests, and where applicable, skin tests and radioallergosorbent tests (RASTs) may be helpful in determining whether an IgE mechanism is involved in the adverse reaction to the food or drug additive. Challenges may be used to confirm a diagnosis when the history is equivocal or only suggestive. Single-blind challenges can be used as a screening approach, and if negative on two occasions, can exclude the possibility that the food or drug additive is the culprit. DBPC challenges may be necessary when the results of a single-blind challenge are equivocal or when conducting research protocols.

Patient Selection

As with urticaria, unstable asthma can lead to false-positive challenge results. Similarly, using medications that can block the reaction can lead to false-negative results. Asthma must be stable at the time of the challenge. For adults, a forced expiratory volume in 1 second (FEV_1) of greater than 1.5 L or greater than 70% of the predicted or prior best FEV_1 is required.[17] Occasionally, patients may need a course of oral or inhaled corticosteroids before the challenge to obtain stability. For safety, proper precautions must be in place. Venous access may be necessary if there is a risk of anaphylaxis. Equipment and trained personnel for resuscitation and initiation of endotracheal intubation and mechanical ventilation should be available. Procedures should be conducted in the morning when assistance is most readily available.

On the day of challenge, patients need to withhold inhaled or oral β_2-agonists. Inhaled salmeterol needs to be withheld for a minimum of 24 hours. Similarly, inhaled anticholinergics should be avoided on the day of the procedure. First-generation antihistamines should be withheld for 24 to 72 hours and chromones (cromolyn, nedocromil) for 48 hours. Second-generation antihistamines may need to be discontinued for 1 week.

Patients can continue to receive theophylline, which usually does not interfere with challenges. The effect of leukotriene modifiers has not been studied. Likewise, continuing or increasing doses of inhaled or oral corticosteroids may be necessary to maintain stable lung function, because unstable pulmonary function can lead to false-positive results.

Protocol Design

For initial screening or to establish the dosages for a double-blind procedure, an open single-blind protocol can be used. Because so few patients with asthma are likely to react to an additive challenge (except for sulfites), a single-blind challenge simplifies the process. More importantly, a single-blind challenge can individualize doses, whereas a double-blind protocol cannot. During each step of an active challenge, the dose is incrementally increased twofold. If a patient has a 10% to 15% decrease in FEV_1 with a dose of the agent, the usual incremental increase can be halved to lessen the risk of a severe reaction. This would not be possible with a double-blind protocol.

Dosages. Food or drug additive challenges are usually conducted using opaque capsules, but a liquid or solution challenge can be used if it more closely mimics the natural exposure. The maximum dosages recommended for several food and drug additives are listed in Box 82-3. Protocols for sulfite challenges are listed in Boxes 82-4 and 82-5. As with challenges for urticaria, it is recommended that the starting dose be one log lower than the lowest dose known to cause a reaction. If the provoking dose is unknown, an estimate may be obtained on the basis of the person's prior exposure.

Controls. If a single-blind challenge is positive, the challenge should be repeated in a DBPC manner. The initial dose in the double-blind protocol can be based on the patient's previously established provoking dose, or up to a twofold lower dose, accompanied by at least two placebo challenges. The challenges with placebo should take place over the same interval as the active challenge, to rule out decreases in pulmonary function being caused by the withholding of bronchodilator therapy.

Criteria for Positive Reactions. Stable baseline pulmonary function is necessary to initiate the challenge. Three consistent FEV_1 maneuvers with values within 5% of each other are necessary. Patients with unstable asthma may develop bronchoconstriction when performing forceful expiratory maneuvers. Therefore, several efforts may be necessary to establish a stable baseline.

Pulmonary function is measured before the challenge and before the next scheduled dose, or sooner if symptoms develop. A 20% or greater decrease in the FEV_1 from the baseline is considered a positive response. For most clinical applications, the FEV_1 is chosen as the gold standard for measuring pulmonary function. This is because the FEV_1, when properly performed, is highly reproducible. Some investigators have used measurements of airway resistance or specific airway conductance for challenges in asthmatic patients. These measurements are technically more difficult and subject to more variability than FEV_1 and thus more difficult to interpret, requiring larger changes in the magnitude of response to be considered positive.

BOX 82-4 CAPSULE AND NEUTRAL-SOLUTION METABISULFITE CHALLENGE*

Preparing patient and collecting preliminary data

Withhold short-acting aerosol sympathomimetics and cromolyn/nedocromil sodium for 8 hours and short-acting antihistamines for 24 to 48 hours before pulmonary function testing.

Measure pulmonary function: Forced expiratory volume in 1 second (FEV_1) must be 70% or greater of predicted normal value and 1.5 L or greater in adults. (Test contraindicated in patients with an FEV_1 below those levels. Standards for children have not been defined.)

Performing single-blind challenge

Administer placebo (powdered sucrose) in capsule form. Measure FEV_1.

Administer capsules containing 1, 5, 25, 50, 100, and 200 mg of potassium metabisulfite at 30-minute intervals. Measure FEV_1 30 minutes after administering each dose and if the patient becomes symptomatic.

If no response, administer 1, 10, and 25 mg of potassium metabisulfite in water-sucrose solution at 30-minute intervals. Measure FEV_1 30 minutes after each dose and if symptoms occur. Positive response is indicated by a decrease in FEV_1 of 20% or more.

Performing double-blind challenge

Perform challenge and placebo procedures on separate days, in random order.

Placebo day: Administer only sucrose in capsules and solution. Measure FEV_1 30 minutes after each dose and if patient becomes symptomatic.

Challenge day: Same protocol as single-blind challenge day.

From Bush RK. Sulfite and aspirin sensitivity: who is most susceptible? J Respir Dis 1987;8:23.

*Protocol used in the University of Wisconsin prevalence study. Perform this test only where the capability for managing severe asthmatic reactions exists.

BOX 82-5 ACID-SOLUTION METABISULFITE CHALLENGE*

Preparing patient and collecting preliminary data

Withhold aerosol sympathomimetics and cromolyn sodium for 8 hours and antihistamines for 24 to 48 hours before pulmonary function testing.

Measure pulmonary function: Forced expiratory volume in 1 second (FEV_1) must be greater than or equal to 70% of predicted normal value and greater than or equal to 1.5 L in adults. (Test contraindicated in patients with an FEV_1 below those levels. Standards for children have not been defined.)

Performing bisulfite challenge

Dissolve 0.1 mg of potassium metabisulfite in 20 mL of a sulfite-free lemonade crystal solution. Have the patient swish the solution around for 10 to 15 seconds, then swallow.

Measure FEV_1 10 minutes after the first dose. Then, administer 0.5, 1, 5, 10, 15, 25, 50, 75, and 100† per 20 mL of the solution at 10-minute intervals. Measure FEV_1 10 minutes after each incremental increase in dose. Positive response is signified by a decrease in FEV_1 of 20% or more.

From Bush RK: Sulfite and aspirin sensitivity: who is most susceptible? J Respir Dis 1987;8:23.

*Protocol investigated by the Bronchoprovocation Committee-American Academy of Allergy, Asthma and Immunology. Perform this test only where the capability for managing severe asthmatic reactions exists.

†Doses in excess of 100 mg are likely to produce nonspecific bronchial reactions in asthmatic patients because of the high levels of free sulfur dioxide (SO_2) generated.

In patients who have failed to respond in a DBPC challenge, open feeding without reaction is necessary to verify the negative response.

Of the thousands of food and drug additives, relatively few have been identified as causing significant adverse reactions. Often, appropriate methods to substantiate the relationship between the additive and the reported adverse reaction have not been conducted.

Food Colorants

Numerous synthetic colorants are allowed for use in foods.[18] These synthetic colorants fall into two general structural categories: the azo dyes and the nonazo dyes. Adverse reactions have been reported to only a few of these colorants, primarily tartrazine.[19]

SYNTHETIC COLORANTS (DYES)

Tartrazine

Numerous studies have examined the role of tartrazine, also known as FD&C Yellow #5, in various food sensitivity reactions, but especially in asthma and chronic urticaria. (FD&C refers to the 1938 U.S. Food, Drug, and Cosmetic Act.) Although some showed a possible causative role for tartrazine in urticaria and angioedema,[20] a cause-and-effect role for tartrazine in other illnesses has not been established. A literature review concluded that tartrazine-induced asthma does not occur even among aspirin-sensitive asthmatic patients thought to be at higher risk for tartrazine sensitivity.[19] Further, routine tartrazine exclusion from the diet of asthmatic patients is of little value.[21] Several methodologic flaws in earlier studies were responsible for the positive associations in these studies between tartrazine and asthma or urticaria.

Tartrazine has been frequently linked to chronic urticaria. Lockey[22] was the first to associate tartrazine with urticaria by identifying three patients who had experienced urticaria after ingestion of yellow color–coated drugs. His later, supposedly confirmatory studies consisted of nonblinded, uncontrolled trials with dilute solutions of tartrazine. Since then, many more studies have examined tartrazine in urticaria, although methodologic flaws make interpretation of the results difficult. Many positive reactions often observed in some studies are likely false-positive reactions resulting from the order effect of always administering the placebo first and the high likelihood of breakthrough urticaria from withdrawal of antihistamines. Many clinical trials were conducted with single-blind or open challenges, which increases the difficulty in interpreting the results, especially if medications are withheld. Several were conducted with a double-blind challenge design, but even these studies could have been compromised if patients always received placebo before tartrazine. However, the percentage of positive responders was lower in the double-blind challenge trials. In virtually all the studies on tartrazine in chronic urticaria, either antihistamines were withheld or no information was provided on medication status during challenge, which raises the question of breakthrough urticaria. Other complicating factors included using a mixture of colors, so positive reactions could not be attributed to any one substance.

The La Jolla/Scripps group conducted the first DBPC challenge trial of tartrazine in patients with chronic urticaria and a history suggestive of possible tartrazine sensitivity in whom antihistamines were not withheld.[19] Only 1 of 24 patients developed urticaria on single-blind challenge, and this reaction was confirmed on double-blind challenge. A comparatively large challenge dose of 50 mg of tartrazine was used to provoke this response, whereas earlier studies used smaller amounts (0.1 to 25 mg). This same group later indicated that 0 of 65 patients with chronic urticaria reacted to double-blind challenges with 50 mg of tartrazine.[23] In summary, despite numerous reports that tartrazine can provoke chronic urticaria, convincing evidence is lacking.

Interpreting whether tartrazine has a role in causing asthma is difficult because of methodologic flaws. In several studies of tartrazine-induced asthma, medications were withheld, and thus the withdrawal of medications could have been a significant contributing factor in the development of asthma. In most studies, when critical medications were continued during challenge, the frequency of positive asthmatic responses to tartrazine was almost zero. Only a few studies have identified more than one case of tartrazine-induced asthma while medications were continued and double-blind challenges were used.[24,25] Continued use of bronchodilators during challenge of aspirin-sensitive asthmatic patients was critical to avoiding false-positive responses.[26]

The definitive study involved 43 aspirin-tolerant and 194 aspirin-sensitive asthmatic patients.[19] β-Agonists, cromolyn, and antihistamines were withheld, but theophylline, bronchodilators, and inhaled and systemic corticosteroids were continued during challenge. The studies were single-blind, but all positive reactions were confirmed by double-blind challenges. None of the patients reacted to tartrazine at doses up to 50 mg. This evidence suggests that tartrazine does not provoke asthma.

Tartrazine has also been implicated as a possible factor in persistent rhinitis, although few studies have addressed this hypothesis. A group of 226 patients with persistent rhinitis were evaluated by DBPC challenge after 1 month of an additive-free diet.[27] Challenges with up to 40 mg of tartrazine elicited both objective (sneezing, rhinorrhea) and subjective (nasal blockage, nasal itching) symptoms of rhinitis, together with a 20% or greater reduction in nasal peak inspiratory flow rate in 2 of 20 patients who reported improvement on the additive-free diet.[26] As further evidence, of 26 Brazilians with various atopic diseases, none reacted to 35 mg of tartrazine in a DBPC challenge.[28]

Tartrazine has been linked to atopic dermatitis in only a few studies. However, mixtures of food colors were used in several of these studies, so positive results cannot necessarily be attributed to tartrazine.[5] Also, the medication status of patients involved in these studies was not revealed. Of 12 children with atopic dermatitis and a history suggestive of tartrazine provocation, multiple tartrazine (50 mg) challenges corresponded consistently to the highest symptom score in only one patient.[29] This single patient was probably sensitive to tartrazine, although the challenge dose was high compared with typical dietary exposures. A few cases of tartrazine-induced purpura have been noted.[23]

The overall prevalence of tartrazine sensitivity in the population cannot be estimated from current information. Prevalence of sensitivity to tartrazine, amaranth, sunset yellow, and carmoisine was estimated at 0 to 0.12% of more than 18,000 surveyed, but the study included self-reporting of symptoms and mixed additives for challenges.[4] However, prevalence of tartrazine sensitivity seems quite low.

Sunset Yellow

Sunset yellow, also known as FD&C Yellow #6, has been linked to food sensitivities much less often than tartrazine. Sunset yellow has been implicated in several isolated cases of gastrointestinal illness confirmed by blinded challenges. As with tartrazine, sunset yellow has also been implicated in urticaria and angioedema, although these studies had many of the same methodologic flaws previously discussed regarding tartrazine. Simon et al.[23] failed to identify a single reactor to sunset yellow among a total of 65 patients with chronic urticaria who were subjected to DBPC food challenge under conditions in which antihistamines were likely not withheld. Six of 15 patients experienced worsening of their atopic dermatitis on double-blind challenge with an additive mixture, but sunset yellow was only 1 of 22 common food additives included in the challenge trial.[30] Sunset yellow has also been implicated in childhood asthma.[31] However, the asthmatic reactions were not confirmed clinically with actual measurements of lung function, and the medication status of these children was not revealed. Sunset yellow has been implicated in one case each of purpura and orofacial granulomatosis. Again, prevalence of sunset yellow sensitivity in the population appears low.[4]

Other Synthetic Colors

Several other synthetic food colors are occasionally implicated in urticaria, angioedema, asthma, and atopic dermatitis. These synthetic colors include amaranth (FD&C Red #2), erythrosine (FD&C Red #3), brilliant blue (FD&C Blue #1), ponceau 4R, carmoisine, quinoline yellow, patent blue, azorubin, new coccine, indigo carmine (FD&C Blue #2), brilliant black BN, and fast green (FD&C Green #3). Studies of these food colors have had the same methodologic flaws previously discussed for tartrazine. Thus, there is no compelling evidence for the involvement of these colors in urticaria, angioedema, asthma, or atopic dermatitis. New coccine has been implicated in three cases of purpura, but this finding appears to be an isolated report. A single case of leukocytoclastic vasculitis has been ascribed to ponceau red 4R and confirmed by a placebo-controlled oral challenge with 50 mg of the dye. Erythrosine was implicated as a possible factor in persistent rhinitis in 7 of 226 patients.[27] A case of orofacial granulomatosis has also been linked to ingestion of carmoisine. Prevalence of sensitivities to green S, quinoline yellow, and indigo carmine was 0 to 0.11%.[4]

NATURAL FOOD COLORANTS

Natural colorants allowed for use in foods include annatto, carmine, carotene, turmeric, paprika, beet extract, and grape skin extract. These colorants have no role in pharmaceutical applications. Several studies have reported positive reactions following challenges with mixtures of natural colors[3,31] or natural and synthetic colors.[32] The natural colorants involved in these challenges were annatto, betanin, curcumin, turmeric, β-carotene, canthaxanthin, and beet extract. The reactions were asthma, urticaria, atopic dermatitis, colic, and vomiting. No one color can be identified as the causative factor when challenges are conducted with mixtures.

Annatto

Annatto is obtained as an extract from the seeds of the fruit of the Central and South American tree *Bixa orellana.* Bixin, the principal pigment in annatto, is a carotenoid. Although the extracts are red, annatto is often used to impart an orange or deep-yellow color to the finished food.

Case reports of probable IgE-mediated sensitivity to annatto have noted patient reactions to crackers,[33] cheese,[34] and breakfast cereal.[35] Clinical reactions to annatto have been confirmed by positive skin-prick tests, basophil activiation, and IgE binding.[34,35] An IgE-binding protein was identified through sulfite-polyacrylamide gel electrophoresis (SDS-PAGE) and immunoblotting.[35] This is not surprising since annatto is derived from a seed extract. Prevalence of annatto sensitivity was estimated at 0.01% to 0.07%.[4]

Carmine

Carmine and cochineal extract are red and derived from dried female cochineal insects, *Dactylopius coccus* Costa, which are parasites of the prickly pear cactus. An aqueous-alcoholic extract of the dried insects is made and concentrated by removing the alcohol, to obtain the color additive, cochineal extract. The principal coloring agent is carminic acid. Carmine is the aluminum or calcium-aluminum lake of the coloring principals, primarily carminic acid, obtained by aqueous cochineal extraction.

Carmine is widely used in cosmetics but has only a few cases of dermatologic reactions attributed to it. A case of severe anaphylactic shock possibly resulted from the cutaneous use of carmine.[36] Unfortunately, no follow-up was done to confirm the role of carmine in this patient.

A few cases of contact dermatitis to carmine have been reported.[37] Cases of urticaria and angioedema with positive skin-prick tests and serum specific IgE to carmine have been described in the literature.[38,39] Five cases of anaphylaxis were associated with ingestion of campari through positive skin tests and specific IgE.[40] Anaphylaxis to carmine in generic azithromycin was also reported.[38] Cases of occupational asthma have been reported as well.[41,42]

Because the extract is from insects, carmine contains proteins capable of eliciting IgE-mediated reactions. Several IgE-binding proteins have been identified,[28] and a major 38-kD cochineal allergen has been molecularly cloned and has sequence homology to phospholipases.[43]

Sulfites

Sulfites or sulfiting agents used as food or drug additives include sulfur dioxide (SO_2), sodium and potassium metabisulfite ($Na_2S_2O_5$, $K_2S_2O_5$), sodium and potassium bisulfite ($NaHSO_3$, $KHSO_3$), and sodium sulfite (Na_2SO_3). These can also occur naturally in many foods, particularly fermented beverages such as wines.[44]

USES IN FOODS

Sulfites are added to many different types of foods for several technical purposes (Table 82-1). Because sulfites have a wide variety of applications as food additives, the levels of use and residual sulfite concentrations found in foods can be wide ranging (Box 82-6). Some of the more highly sulfited food substances (e.g., dried fruit, wine) pose the greatest hazard to sulfite-sensitive individuals. Sulfites are extremely reactive in food systems. A dynamic equilibrium exists between free sulfites and many bound forms of sulfites. The fate of sulfites added to foods depends on the nature of each individual food.[44] At an acidic pH (less than 4.0), SO_2 can be released as a gas from food or solutions containing sulfites.

TABLE 82-1 Technical Attributes of Sulfites in Foods

Sulfite Attribute	Food Applications
Inhibition of enzymatic browning	Fresh fruits and vegetables* Salads* Guacamole* Shrimp (black spot formation) Prepeeled raw potatoes
Inhibition of nonenzymatic browning	Dehydrated potatoes Dried fruits Other dehydrated vegetables
Antimicrobial actions	Wines Corn wet milling to make cornstarch, corn syrup
Dough conditioning	Frozen pie crust Frozen pizza crust
Antioxidant action	No major U.S. applications
Bleaching effect	Maraschino cherries Hominy

From Taylor SL, Bush RK, Nordlee JA. Sulfites. In: Metcalfe DD et al, editors: Food allergy: adverse reactions to foods and food additives. Boston: Blackwell Scientific; 1996, p. 348.
*No longer allowed by the U.S. Food and Drug Administration.

Sulfites react with a variety of food constituents.[44] Some reactions are readily reversible; others are virtually irreversible. Before this use was banned by the FDA in 1986, high concentrations of sulfite (500 to 1000 ppm) were recommended to prevent enzymatic browning in lettuce. Because lettuce is composed mostly of cellulose and water, most sulfite added to lettuce exists as free inorganic sulfite.[45] Most other foods contain substances that readily react with sulfites, and therefore bound forms of sulfite predominate. The presence of free sulfite in lettuce may explain why sulfite-sensitive individuals reacted so vigorously to sulfited lettuce in salad bars before its ban.

USES IN DRUGS

Sulfites are added to a number of pharmaceutical products. Table 82-2 lists common drugs used by asthmatic patients that contain sulfites. Because of concerns over sulfite-induced asthma, sulfites have been removed from many drugs, especially those intended for asthmatic patients. Sulfites are routinely added to epinephrine. The level of sulfites in pharmaceutical products generally varies from 0.1% to 1.0%, although a few products may contain higher levels. In a few patients, paradoxic bronchoconstriction was caused by sulfiting agents used to stabilize bronchodilator medications.[46] Sulfites in epinephrine have had no reported adverse effects; therefore epinephrine should never be denied or avoided by sulfite-sensitive asthmatic patients because it may prove lifesaving.[47] Sulfite-sensitive individuals should be alerted to possible sulfites in medications, except epinephrine, and seek alternative formulations.

REACTIONS TO SULFITES

Clinical Manifestations

A host of adverse reactions and symptoms have been attributed to sulfiting agents.[48,49] Many of the responses have not been

BOX 82-6 ESTIMATED TOTAL SO_2 LEVEL AS CONSUMED FOR SOME SULFITED FOODS

≥100 ppm

- Dried fruit (excluding dark raisins and prunes)
- Lemon juice (nonfrozen)
- Lime juice (nonfrozen)
- Wine
- Molasses
- Sauerkraut juice
- Grape juice (white, white/pink/red sparkling)
- Pickled cocktail onions

50-99.9 ppm

- Dried potatoes
- Wine vinegar
- Gravies, sauces
- Fruit topping
- Maraschino cherries

10.1-49.9 ppm

- Pectin
- Shrimp (fresh)
- Corn syrup
- Sauerkraut
- Pickled peppers
- Pickles/relishes
- Cornstarch
- Hominy
- Frozen potatoes
- Maple syrup
- Imported jams and jellies
- Fresh mushrooms

≤10 ppm

- Malt vinegar
- Canned potatoes
- Beer
- Dry soup mix
- Soft drinks
- Instant tea
- Pizza dough (frozen)
- Pie dough
- Sugar (especially beet sugar)
- Gelatin
- Coconut
- Fresh fruit salad
- Domestic jams and jellies
- Crackers
- Cookies
- Grapes
- High-fructose corn syrup

From Taylor SL, Bush RK, Nordlee JA. Sulfites. In: Metcalfe DD et al, editors. Food allergy: averse reactions to foods and food additives. Boston: Blackwell Scientific; 1996, p. 348.
SO_2, Sulfur dioxide; *ppm*, parts per million.

documented by appropriate diagnostic challenges, although more robust evidence links sulfites to asthma and anaphylaxis.[50]

Reactions suggestive of a hypersensitivity response have been observed, including allergic contact dermatitis confirmed by patch testing.[51,52] Several cases of angioedema and urticaria have been reported.[53-55] In contrast, Simon,[56] using a rigorously blinded, placebo-controlled trial with objective criteria for positive reactions, was unable to demonstrate positive reactions to encapsulated metabisulfite (200 mg maximum dose) in 75 patients with chronic urticaria, anaphylaxis, or both and a history suggestive of sulfite sensitivity. Whereas some individuals may develop urticaria or anaphylactoid reactions as reactions to sulfites, the frequency with which these occur is extremely rare at best and requires confirmation by rigorously double-blinded challenges.

TABLE 82-2 Antiallergy/Antiasthma Medications Containing Additives

Medication	Manufacturer	Additive
INJECTABLE EPINEPHRINE		
Epi-Pen	Dey Laboratories	Sulfites
TwinJect	Verus Pharmaceuticals	Sulfites
Adrenalin	Monarch	Sulfites
Epinephrine	Multiple manufacturers	Sulfites
ISOPROTENEROL SOLUTIONS		
Isoproteranol	Elkins-Sinn	Sulfites
Isuprel	Sanofi-Winthrop	Sulfites
INJECTABLE CORTICOSTEROID		
Decadron	Merck	Sulfites
Dexamethasone	Multiple manufacturers	Sulfites
IPRATROPIUM/ALBUTEROL MDI		
Combivent	Boehringer-Ingelheim	Soy lecithin
Combivent Respimat		BAC
NASAL CORTICOSTEROID		
Numerous		BAC

BAC, Benzalkonium chloride; *MDI*, metered-dose inhaler.

Anaphylactic-like (anaphylactoid) events have been described in several individuals,[57-60] although appropriate confirmatory testing was not performed in many cases. An individual with sulfite-induced anaphylaxis had a positive skin test to sulfite, and histamine was released from basophils on incubation with sulfites; multiple single-blind placebo-controlled oral challenges reproduced the patient's symptoms.[58] Three patients had systemic anaphylaxis symptoms confirmed by sulfite challenges with positive skin tests to sulfites, two of whom had positive Prausnitz-Kustner transfer tests.[59]

Systemic reactions have been attributed to intravenous and inhalation administration of pharmaceuticals containing sulfiting agents.[48,61]

Sodium metabisulfite has also been associated with persistent rhinitis. A group of 226 patients with persistent rhinitis were evaluated by DBPC challenge after 1 month of an additive-free diet.[27] Challenges with up to 20 mg $Na_2S_2O_5$ elicited both objective (sneezing, rhinorrhea) and subjective (nasal blockage, nasal itching) symptoms of rhinitis, together with a 20% or greater reduction in nasal peak inspiratory flow rate in 6 of 20 patients who reported improvement with the additive-free diet.[27]

Sulfiting agents do not appear to play a role in patients with idiopathic anaphylaxis.[62] Similarly, sulfites do not appear to enhance the likelihood of anaphylaxis in patients with systemic mastocytosis.[62] Overall, the risk of adverse reactions to sulfiting agents for nonatopic, nonasthmatic individuals appears to be low. Properly performed DBPC challenges need to be undertaken in suspected reactions to confirm whether sulfite sensitivity is responsible.

More definitive evidence indicates that sulfites can provoke acute bronchospasm and severe asthma. Kochen[63] first suggested that ingestion of sulfited food can cause asthma; a child experienced cough and wheeze when exposed to dehydrated sulfited fruits in sealed plastic bags. Subsequently, Freedman[64] demonstrated that ingestion of sulfite solutions could induce changes in pulmonary function in individuals with a history of wheezing after ingestion of sulfited drinks. Later studies showed that exposure to potassium metabisulfite in controlled challenges was capable of causing significant bronchoconstriction, and that intravenous administration could lead to respiratory arrest.[65,66] Subsequent evidence confirmed that exposure to sulfiting agents through ingestion of sulfited beverages or foods and medications can lead to severe bronchoconstriction. Furthermore, fatal reactions to sulfite exposure are possible.[67] The bulk of available evidence indicates that severe bronchoconstriction, hypotension with loss of consciousness, and death can occur in response to sulfiting agents in some patients, particularly those with more severe, persistent asthma.

Prevalence

The prevalence of adverse reactions to sulfiting agents is not precisely known. Of 203 adult patients with asthma and no history of sulfite sensitivity receiving capsule and neutral-solution sulfite challenges, 120 were not receiving oral or inhaled corticosteroids, and 83 were using inhaled or oral steroids daily.[68] In this prevalence study, only one patient with milder asthma had a 20% or greater decline in FEV_1 after single-blind and confirmatory double-blind challenge. The response rate in the more severe asthma group was higher, estimated at 8.4%. The prevalence of sulfite sensitivity among all the patients with asthma was less than 3.9%. Patients with more persistent asthma appeared to be most at risk for having sulfite sensitivity.

Pediatric studies are limited, although sulfite-sensitive asthma was reported in a 2-year-old.[69] In 29 children age 5½ to 14 years with moderate to severe asthma challenged with sodium metabisulfite capsules or solutions, 66% had a greater than 20% decrease in peak expiratory flow rate.[70] However, avoidance diets did not result in significant improvement in patients' asthma.[70] In contrast, another study found that only 4 of 56 children with asthma (7%) responded to challenges with sulfite in capsules, and only 2 of 56 (3.5%) reacted to oral metabisulfite solution.[71] The prevalence of sulfite sensitivity may increase with age in severely asthmatic children.[72] Whether sulfite sensitivity is really more frequent in children and is age dependent remains to be established. Differences in challenge procedures, such as capsule versus acidic solutions, may account for some differences between studies.

Nonetheless, the overall presence of sulfite sensitivity, particularly in adult asthmatic patients, is small but significant. Having severe, persistent asthma appears to pose an additional risk for sensitivity, particularly in adults.

Mechanisms of Sensitivity

The mechanisms of sulfiting agent sensitivity are not known. On inhalation of less than 1.0 part per million (ppm) of sulfur dioxide, patients with asthma respond with significant bronchoconstriction.[73] Furthermore, inhalation of SO_2 itself and bisulfite (HSO_3^-) but not sulfite (SO_3) causes bronchoconstriction in patients with asthma.[74] Of 15 individuals challenged with doubling concentrations of SO_2 gas or a metabisulfite solution, all reacted to the metabisulfite solution, and 14 reacted to SO_2 inhalation.[75] This study concluded that the mechanism of sulfite sensitivity involves more than generated SO_2 alone. Some patients with asthma respond to either oral or inhalation challenge with sulfite, but inhalation is more likely to produce a bronchoconstrictive response.[76] Ten patients with asthma and sulfite sensitivity reacted to an acidic metabisulfite solution when administered as a mouthwash or a swallowed liquid, but not through a nasogastric tube.[77] No reaction occurred when they held their breath while swallowing the solution; some individuals likely respond to inhaled SO_2 while swallowing. SO_2 inhalation may activate airway irritant receptors and lead to cholinergic-mediated bronchoconstriction.

Other mechanisms of sulfite sensitivity may be involved. Direct evidence for IgE-mediated reactions is lacking, although some individuals have positive intradermal skin tests to metabisulfite, which can activate basophils in vitro.[78] Deficiencies in tissue sulfite oxidase levels may be involved in sulfite sensitivity.[77] However, congenital sulfite oxidase deficiency causes a severe neurologic disorder (encephalopathy) but not asthma.[79]

Diagnosis

Patient history alone is insufficient to establish the diagnosis of sulfite sensitivity. In addition, a positive sulfite challenge does not always correlate with the patient's history.[68] Therefore the diagnosis of sulfite sensitivity should be made only in individuals who demonstrate an objective response on appropriate challenge. Skin-prick and intradermal testing has identified some patients with positive challenge responses.[60,80] However, others with equally severe bronchospasm or other reactions have had negative skin tests. No standardized procedure has yet been established for sulfiting agent challenges. Patients may be challenged with capsules, neutral solutions, or acidic solutions of metabisulfite[81] (see Boxes 82-4 and 82-5). Currently, a capsule is the preferred vehicle because most sulfite exposure is likely to occur to bound forms in foods rather than in free form. Solutions may be considered for patients who have reacted to beverages such as sulfited wine.

Positive single-blind challenges should always be confirmed by a double-blind procedure. To overcome potential order effect (positive response to sulfites the day after negative placebo challenge day), the order of administration of active and placebo challenges should be randomized, and a third challenge day with either active or placebo capsules should be considered.

Treatment

Sulfite-sensitive individuals should avoid sulfite-treated foods and drugs that have triggered the response. Because an individual can have varying sensitivity to different sulfited foods, multiple challenges might be necessary to determine which sulfite-containing foods are tolerated. Clearly, all sulfite-sensitive asthmatic patients should be instructed to avoid highly sulfited foods with more than 100 ppm of SO_2 equivalents (see Box 82-6). Individuals with lower thresholds may be better advised to avoid all sulfited foods from their diet, although adherence to such diets can be extremely difficult. Packaged foods containing more than 10 ppm residual SO_2 equivalents must have the presence of sulfites written on the label. Sulfite-sensitive consumers need to be aware that the terms sulfur dioxide, sodium/potassium bisulfite, sodium/potassium metabisulfite, and sodium sulfite are all sulfites or sulfiting agents. Whereas avoidance of prepared and packaged foods is relatively straightforward, avoidance of sulfites in restaurant foods is more difficult. Some unlabeled sulfited foods remain in restaurants despite the FDA ban on their use on fresh fruits and vegetables. The major contributing problem is sulfited potatoes. Therefore, sulfite-sensitive individuals should be instructed to avoid all potato products in restaurants, except baked potatoes with skins intact.

Challenge studies with sulfited foods have been conducted in sulfite-sensitive patients with asthma. Clinical challenges with acidic solutions of sulfite in lemon juice or other vehicles demonstrate these to be more hazardous than other forms of sulfited foods.[77] Furthermore, it has been conclusively demonstrated that sulfited lettuce (banned under current FDA regulations) can trigger asthmatic reactions in sulfite-sensitive individuals.[82] Foods where sulfites exist primarily in the bound form, such as shrimp, are less likely to induce responses. To establish an appropriate avoidance diet as discussed earlier, patients may need to be challenged with individual foods to determine which ones they can tolerate.

When possible, sulfite-sensitive individuals should avoid pharmaceutical agents that contain sulfites. Some bronchodilator solutions, subcutaneous lidocaine, and intravenous corticosteroids may pose a risk for sensitive subjects (see Table 82-2). Package inserts should always be consulted for the most current information.

When patients experience bronchoconstriction as a consequence of sulfite exposure, inhaled bronchodilator medications that do not contain sulfites are the treatment of choice. If a patient exhibits hypotension or other evidence of a severe systemic reaction, injectable epinephrine is appropriate, even though the solution may contain sulfite as a preservative.

Agents that may block the response to sulfite, including cromolyn sodium, atropine, doxepin, and vitamin B_{12}, have been studied in only limited numbers of individuals.[83] Therefore these drugs remain investigational and cannot be recommended as standard therapy. Strict avoidance remains the fundamental approach to sulfite sensitivity.

REGULATORY RESTRICTIONS

The FDA banned the use of sulfites in fresh fruits and vegetables other than potatoes in 1986. Labeling is required of packaged products and alcoholic beverages containing sulfite residues in excess of 10 ppm. No regulations restrict the use of sulfites in medications, but pharmaceutical corporations have attempted to reduce sulfite-containing medications used for asthma treatment. Nevertheless, sulfite-sensitive patients and their physicians need to be alert to avoid inadvertent exposure.

Other Additives Known or Suspected to Cause Reactions

MONOSODIUM GLUTAMATE

A popular flavor enhancer, MSG occurs naturally but is also added to many foods. It is the sodium salt of one of the most common amino acids in the human body. In general, no clear consistent relationship seems to exist between MSG ingestion and the development of asthma, MSG symptom complex (Chinese restaurant syndrome), migraine headache, urticaria, angioedema, or rhinitis.[84-86] Further, mouse models of asthma fail to demonstrate any effects of MSG on the development of asthma or provocation of acute attacks.[87] Cases of orofacial granulomatosis have been ascribed to MSG,[88] but these were basically anecdotal reports with no confirmation by challenge.

Monosodium glutamate has been associated with persistent rhinitis. A group of 226 patients with persistent rhinitis were evaluated by DBPC challenge after 1 month of an additive-free diet.[27] Challenges with up to 400 mg of MSG elicited both objective (sneezing, rhinorrhea) and subjective (nasal blockage/itching) symptoms of rhinitis, together with a 20% or greater reduction in nasal peak inspiratory flow rate in 8 of 20 who reported improvement with the additive-free diet. Avoidance of MSG by adult patients with chronic asthma does not appear to have clinical value.[89]

ASPARTAME

Aspartame is a nonnutritive sweetener extensively used in food and beverage applications. Numerous anecdotal reports of adverse reactions to aspartame have included headaches and various neuropsychiatric symptoms, including seizures.[90] However, no clear symptom complex ever emerged from these complaints. Furthermore, careful evaluation of individuals with self-reported aspartame sensitivity through single-blind and double-blind challenges failed to identify a single aspartame reactor in 61 evaluated.[91] In a randomized DBPC crossover study, aspartame was no more likely than placebo to elicit urticaria or angioedema.[92] In a DBPC challenge study of 65 patients with chronic urticaria, none responded to doses of aspartame up to 150 mg.[93]

PROTEIN HYDROLYSATES

Protein hydrolysates are typically processed from the protein fractions of soybeans, wheat, corn, milk, peanuts, yeast, and gelatin. Soybean, wheat, and peanuts in particular are common allergenic foods. If the proteins are completely hydrolyzed to a mixture of amino acids, the allergens are destroyed, and the protein hydrolysates may be safe for individuals with allergies to the source food. Commercially, protein hydrolysates vary in the degree of hydrolysis from minimally hydrolyzed (5% to 10% of peptide bonds broken) to virtually completely hydrolyzed. The protein hydrolysates with a high degree of hydrolysis are often used in foods as flavor enhancers. The protein hydrolysates with lesser degrees of hydrolysis are used for texture improvement, water binding, emulsification, and flavor enhancement. On U.S. labels, the source of the protein hydrolysate must be identified unless the hydrolysate is part of the flavoring formulation. Additionally, the source of the protein hydrolysate must be identified if derived from a commonly allergenic source. The hydrolysates made from yeast are typically called "yeast autolysate" or autolyzed yeast.

Casein and whey hydrolysates are often used in hypoallergenic infant formulas. However, IgE-mediated allergic reactions occasionally occur with extensively hydrolyzed casein formulas in highly sensitized infants.[94] An infant formula based on partially hydrolyzed whey protein caused much more frequent reactions.[95] Protein fragments made by partial digestion of β-lactoglobulin with pepsin or pepsin and trypsin are able to bind to IgE from patients with cow's milk allergy.[96] Commercial hydrolysates also contain IgE-binding peptide fragments.[97]

Hydrolysates from other sources may also elicit allergic reactions. A commercial hydrolyzed soybean protein and an acid-hydrolyzed soy sauce made from soy protein were able to bind serum IgE from soybean-allergic individuals.[98] In contrast, an extensively hydrolyzed peanut protein hydrolysate sold as a flavor enhancer was unable to bind to IgE from peanut-allergic patients.[99] A case of contact urticaria from protein hydrolysates in a hair conditioner has been reported.[100]

BENZOATES/PARABENS

Sodium benzoate and benzoic acid are widely used antimicrobial preservatives in foods. The methyl, ethyl, n-propyl, n-butyl, and n-heptyl esters of para-hydroxybenzoic acid (the butyl ester is not used in foods), also known collectively as the parabens, are used on a much more limited basis as preservatives in foods. But, the parabens are extensively used as preservatives in pharmaceuticals and cosmetics. *p*-Hydroxybenzoic acid is also known as salicylic acid, which is structurally related to aspirin, a well-known cause of sensitivity disorders.

Sodium benzoate (100 mg) exacerbated atopic dermatitis after DBPC food challenge in three of six patients.[101] Sodium benzoate and *p*-hydroxybenzoic acid have also been identified as possible causes of purpura in a small number of patients.[102] Sodium benzoate does not appear to be causal in asthma,[103] whereas the parabens have not been thoroughly evaluated for their role in asthma. Most studies evaluating the role of benzoates and parabens in asthma lacked proper placebo controls or blinding techniques.[104] Thus any role for benzoate or parabens in asthma remains unproved. Benzoates also do not appear to be causal in urticaria or anaphylaxis.[103] For the parabens, data are insufficient for adequately judging whether any allergic reactions can be attributed to their oral use.[103] Contact dermatitis is a well-recognized reaction to parabens in sunscreens, eye drops, and shampoos from cutaneous application.[105,106]

Benzoate and *p*-hydroxybenzoate have also been associated with persistent rhinitis. A single case of perennial rhinitis induced by benzoates was confirmed on repeated double-blind challenge.[107] Challenges with up to 200 mg of benzoate or *p*-hydroxybenzoate elicited both objective and subjective symptoms, with 20% or greater reduction in nasal peak inspiratory flow rate in 19 of 20 who reported improvement with the additive-free diet.[27]

Although estimated prevalence of reactions to sodium benzoate was 0.01% to 0.11%, Young and coworkers[4] conducted challenges with mixtures of aspirin and benzoate. Because aspirin is a well-established sensitizing substance, the majority of these reactions could have been caused by aspirin, not benzoate.

SORBATE/SORBIC ACID

Sorbic acid and its potassium salt are widely used antimicrobial preservatives in foods, especially for preventing mold growth. Sorbates have been infrequently implicated in reactions. Many studies on sorbate have the same methodologic flaws as described for tartrazine. Among 226 patients with chronic urticaria challenged with 50 to 200 mg of sorbic acid, none had responses.[108] Sorbic acid can also cause contact urticaria in the perioral region, especially in children who smear sorbate-containing foods around their face. Rarely, sorbic acid has caused contact dermatitis.[109]

BHA/BHT

Butylated hydroxyanisole (BHA) and butylated hydroxytoluene (BHT) are popular antioxidants used in a variety of food products. As with benzoates, there is little evidence that BHA or BHT evoke any allergic reactions.[103]

NITRATES/NITRITES

Sodium nitrate and sodium nitrite are used as curing agents in meat products. Few reactions have been attributed to nitrate or nitrite, and most reports are compromised by methodologic flaws. Among 226 patients with chronic urticaria challenged with 100 mg of nitrate/nitrite, none had reactions.[108] Sodium nitrite provoked chronic urticaria in five patients in DBPC food challenge.[110] Simon[93] was unable to identify any reactors to nitrates or nitrites in 65 patients with chronic urticaria. A 22-year-old man had anaphylaxis after ingesting nitrates and nitrites, as confirmed by DBPC challenge.[111] A patient with chronic generalized pruritus responded to 10 mg of sodium nitrate in double-blind challenge, but no repeat challenge was performed.[109] Further studies are needed to confirm the role of nitrates and nitrites in these generalized reactions.

FLAVORING AGENTS

Numerous flavoring substances are used in foods and pharmaceuticals. Many flavoring formulations contain hundreds of different chemical compounds. On food ingredient labels, natural and artificial flavors typically appear as the final ingredient on the list because flavors are the least prevalent components of the formulated product.

Few reports of allergic reactions to flavors exist. IgE-mediated allergic reactions from flavoring ingredients in typical food products are even fewer.[112,113] Flavorings that contain allergenic proteins are rare. Four milk-allergic patients had reactions to foods labeled as nondairy or "pareve" (no meat or milk products), involving consumption of hot dogs and bologna (two cases each).[114] In all these situations, traces of milk protein were identified in the food product. The milk protein emanated from hydrolyzed sodium caseinate, part of the product's natural flavoring. Two patients had allergic reactions after ingesting an unsuspected source of cow's milk protein in dill pickle–flavored potato chips; the ingredient label listed "dill pickle seasoning" but did not identify the presence of milk or milk products.[115] One patient had a life-threatening systemic allergic reaction from ingestion of a soup mix found to contain peanut flour as part of the natural flavoring.[116] Although the only examples in the literature involve milk and peanuts, similar reactions might occur to soybeans, eggs, seafood, and other allergenic materials used occasionally in the formulation of certain flavorings.[112] However, the level of allergen resulting from flavors would be extremely low, even in the few flavorings in which allergenic materials are used.[112]

On rare occasions, flavoring substances can cause contact sensitization in the oral cavity. Most of these episodes involve products that are in prolonged contact with the oral cavity, such as chewing gum, toothpaste, hard candy, cigarettes, or denture products.[113] Balsam of Peru is one of the few flavoring agents that can elicit contact sensitization reactions,[117] but it is not a common flavoring ingredient. Other known offending substances include anethole, anise oil, cinnamon and cinnamic compounds, eugenol, menthol, peppermint oil, and spearmint oil.[113] Anaphylaxis from mint (menthe) in toothpaste occurred in a patient who had a positive skin-prick test to peppermint oil.[118] In an isolated case of angioedema and gastrointestinal distress, the patient had a positive patch test to a fragrance mix containing cinnamic derivatives and reacted to fragrance-containing foods in DBPC challenge.[119] These substances rarely cause reactions unless they are used in products that have prolonged contact with the oral cavity and are present in relatively high concentrations.

LECITHIN

Lecithin generally refers to a complex, naturally occurring mixture of phosphatides. Lecithin is used as an emulsifier in both food and pharmaceutical applications. The primary source of lecithin is soybeans, although lecithin may also be made from eggs, rice, sunflower seeds, and rapeseed. Although primarily phospholipids, soy lecithin can contain soy protein and soy allergen residues.[120,121] Despite the widespread use of lecithin as a food ingredient, allergic reactions to soy lecithin have been described only on occasion.[122,123] Lecithin contains rather low levels of residual protein. Soy lecithin contains between 230 and 1300 mg/kg of soy protein, and lower levels of protein are found in sunflower seed and egg lecithins.[121] Because lecithin is typically used in small amounts in many food applications, exposure to allergenic proteins is likely below the threshold for eliciting a reaction in most allergic individuals.

PAPAIN

Papain is a proteolytic enzyme occasionally used in food processing. An IgE-mediated allergic reaction to papain in a meat tenderizer was systemic and required epinephrine.[124] In 500 allergy patients with no prior history suggestive of papain allergy, 5 of 475 with seasonal pollen allergies had positive skin tests in DBPC food challenges to papain, and none of the 25 patients without pollen allergies had similar responses.[125]

GUMS

Many different types of gums are used in foods and pharmaceuticals. The major gums are guar, tragacanth, xanthan, carrageenan, acacia (gum Arabic), locust bean, and alginate. Several of these gums are legumes, including guar, tragacanth, locust bean, and acacia; other members of the legume family, such as peanut, are intensely allergenic. The gums are primarily composed of complex polysaccharides but occasionally contain residues of proteins.

Gums are a known cause of occupational asthma, particularly guar gum. Allergic reactions from the ingestion of gums are much less frequent. Anaphylaxis resulted from ingestion of guar gum in several foods and beverages.[126] Positive basophil activation was reported, although the presence of specific IgE to guar gum could not be demonstrated.

Several cases of allergic reactions to gum tragacanth have been reported.[127,128] Carrageenan has been implicated in a case of anaphylaxis resulting from its use in a barium enema.[129] A single case of allergic sensitization to gum Arabic (acacia gum) has been described.[130] Several patients experienced flares of chronic urticaria after taking thyroid tablets containing acacia gum.[131] These patients and 9 of 14 additional subjects with chronic urticaria but not taking the tablets had IgE antibodies against acacia extract, although challenges were not conducted. Allergic sensitization to carob bean gum was confirmed by challenge in an infant.[132]

LACTOSE

Lactose is the disaccharide that occurs naturally in cow's milk. Commercial lactose can contain residues of proteins, although the level of proteins in lactose is unknown. Lactose is a common ingredient in many pharmaceutical applications and is a common food ingredient. After several milk-allergic individuals with asthma complained of having reactions to their inhalers, milk protein was identified in the lactose used as an excipient in dry powder inhalers.[133] An allergic reaction to milk protein occurred from lactose contained in inhaled corticosteroid.[134] A case of urticaria attributed to lactose may have actually been triggered by contaminating milk proteins.[135]

GELATIN

Gelatin is typically derived from beef or pork. Kosher gelatin is made from the skin of several fish, including cod. Gelatin is usually considered a protein with rather low allergenic potential. The major sources of gelatin, beef and pork, are rarely allergenic. However, kosher gelatin is obtained from a frequently allergenic source, fish. The allergens in fish are localized in the edible muscle tissue. The gelatin is obtained from the fish skins, although remnants of muscle tissue are likely to adhere to the skin. Parvalbumin, the major fish allergen, is essentially not present in gelatin from well-washed fish skins.[136] The fate of any fish muscle allergens in the gelatin-making process is unknown, although the process involves significant modifications of protein structure.

Beef and pork gelatin is often used as a vaccine expander, and allergic reactions to injected pharmaceutical preparations containing gelatin have been reported.[4,137] Presumably these reactions were primarily associated with beef and pork gelatin. Both IgE-mediated and cell-mediated allergic reactions have occurred.[136] Gelatin (presumably beef and pork) contained in a hemostatic sponge used in a surgical procedure was also implicated in an allergic reaction.[138] Allergic reactions to gelatin used as a food ingredient are rarely reported. In 26 children with allergic reactions to vaccines, seven had allergic reactions to gelatin-containing foods (two before and five after vaccination).[139]

Cross-reactions occur between beef and pork gelatin and gelatins derived from other mammalian species because of IgE to α-galactose.[140] However, IgE to fish gelatin is rarely observed in individuals with known gelatin allergies. In a study of 10 fish-allergic patients, three had specific IgE to fish gelatin, suggesting that fish gelatin might be an allergen in patients with fish allergy.[141] However, after DBPC oral challenge of 30 codfish-allergic individuals, none reacted to food-grade fish gelatin, up to a cumulative dose of 3.61 g.[142] One did experience a reproducible but mild subjective reaction on challenge with a cumulative dose of 7.61 g of fish gelatin; the other 29 patients did not. The basis for this reaction is uncertain.

INULIN

Inulin is a fructan polysaccharide found in many different types of plants, such as chicory, artichoke, salsify, and Jerusalem artichoke. Inulin is often used intradermally for tests of renal function. No allergic reactions have been reported to inulin as a pharmaceutical agent. Increasingly, inulin is also used as a food ingredient because of its ability to stimulate the growth of beneficial intestinal bacteria, particularly the bifidobacteria. Anaphylaxis to inulin occurred after ingestion of salsify, artichokes, and several inulin-containing foods.[143] Positive skin-prick tests to inulin-containing foods, a positive DBPC food challenge, and evidence of specific IgE to an inulin-protein compound have been documented.[143]

WHEAT STARCH

Starch is a common food ingredient usually derived from corn, which is rarely an allergenic food source. However, starch is occasionally derived from wheat. Wheat starch contains trace residues of wheat proteins, although allergic reactions to wheat starch remain undocumented. Starch granules contain unique proteins that may not be allergenic, but commercial wheat starch might also contain residues of proteins from other wheat fractions that are allergenic. Anaphylaxis to chemically modified starch has been described, but the source of the starch was not defined.[144]

EDIBLE OILS

Edible oils are frequently derived from commonly allergenic foods such as peanut, soybean, and sunflower seed, although oils may also come from less commonly allergic foods, such as corn, olive, or safflower seed. However, peanut oil,[145] soybean oil,[146] and sunflower seed oil[147] can be safely ingested by individuals allergic to the source product from which the oil is derived, because highly refined oils contain extremely low levels of detectable allergen. Less well-refined and cold-pressed oils can contain protein residuals and may be hazardous for consumption by allergic individuals.[148] Gourmet oils made from allergenic sources such as sesame seeds or tree nuts may also contain protein residues and are likely to be hazardous to consumers with allergies to the source food.[149,150] The allergenicity of edible oils has been extensively reviewed.[151]

LYSOZYME

Lysozyme is an enzyme that is able to lyse (dissolve) bacterial cell membranes and thus serve as an antimicrobial agent in foods. Lysozyme occurs naturally in egg white, but the purified enzyme is used on occasion as an additive in other foods, especially soft cheeses. Lysozyme is a well-documented egg white allergen.[152] Allergic reactions have been reported from ingestion of cheeses containing lysozyme as an additive.[152] Allergic reactions have also been described from pharmaceutical uses of lysozyme.[153-155]

OTHER DRUG ADDITIVES

Benzalkonium chloride (BAC)[156] is a preservative used in albuterol and metaproterenol nebulizer solutions in the United States and in beclomethasone and ipratropium nebulizer solutions in other countries.[11] BAC has been reported to cause paradoxic bronchoconstriction in 60% of asthmatic patients. The reaction is frequently accompanied by cough and a burning sensation and occasionally by facial flushing and pruritus. It can be blocked by prior use of β_2-agonists, cromolyn, and partially by histamine H_1 receptor antagonists. The mechanism may involve non–IgE-mediated mast cell mediator release. Reduction in the concentration of commercial nebulizer solutions has reduced the likelihood of reactions.[11] Other potential BAC-containing sources include nasal saline, nasal corticosteroids, and nasal decongestant solutions. Whereas BAC can induce paradoxic bronchoconstriction, EDTA in bronchodilator solutions does not cause decreases in lung function.[157]

Benzyl alcohol is a common preservative in many injectable drugs and solutions and is a rare cause of contact dermatitis or angioedema.[156] Toxicity to high doses has occurred in newborns and resulted in mortality from intraventricular hemorrhage.[156]

Propylene glycol is used as a drug solubilizer in a number of topical, oral, and injectable medications. In infants, high doses can lead to lactic acidosis, hyperosmolality, and seizures. Of 487 patients with contact dermatitis, 4.5% reacted to propylene glycol.[156]

REFERENCES

Labeling of Additives

1. Taylor SL, Hefle SL. Food allergen labeling in the USA and Europe. Curr Opin Allergy Clin Immunol 2006;6:186-90.

Prevalence of Reactions to Additives

2. Niestijl-Jansen JJ, Kardinaal AF, Huijbers G. Prevalence of food allergy and intolerance in the adult Dutch population. J Allergy Clin Immunol 1993;4:446.
3. Fuglsang G, Madsen C, Halken S. Adverse reactions to food additives in children with atopic symptoms. Allergy 1994;49:39.
4. Young E, Patel S, Stoneham M, Rona R, Wilkinson JD. The prevalence of reaction to food additives in a survey population. J R Coll Physicians Lond 1987;21:241-7.
5. Zuberbier T, Edenharter G, Worm M, et al. Prevalence of adverse reactions to food in Germany: a population study. Allergy 2004;59:338-45.
6. Park HW, Park CH, Park SH, et al. Dermatologic adverse reactions to 7 common food additives in patients with allergic diseases: a double-blind, placebo-controlled study. J Allergy Clin Immunol 2008;121:1059-61.
7. Randhawa S, Bahna SL. Hypersensitivity reactions to food additives. Curr Opin Allergy Clin Immunol 2009;9:278-83.
8. Taylor SL, Hefle SL. Food allergies and intolerances. In: Shils ME, Shike M, Ross AC, Caballero B, Cousins RJ, editors. Modern nutrition in health and disease, 10th ed. Philadelphia: Lippincott Williams & Wilkins; 2005. p. 1512-30.
9. Leventhal JS, Berger EM, Brauer JA, Cohen DE. Hypersensitivity reactions to vaccine constituents: a case series and review of the literature. Dermatitis 2012;23:102-9.
10. Barbaud A. Place of excipients in drug-related allergy. Clin Rev Allergy Immunol 1995;13:253-63.
11. Kelso JM. The gelatin story. J Allergy Clin Immunol 1999;103:200-2.
12. Simon RA. Adverse reactions to food and drug additives. Immunol Allergy Clin North Am 1996;1996:137.
13. Simon RA. Adverse reactions to food additives. Curr Allergy Asthma Rep 2003;3:62-6.
14. Kaaman AC, Boman A, Wrangsjo K, Matura M. Contact allergy to sodium metabisulfite: an occupational problem. Contact Dermatitis 2010;63:110-2.
15. Nguyen SH, Dang TP, MacPherson C, Maibach H, Maibach HI. Prevalence of patch test results from 1970 to 2002 in a multi-centre population in North America (NACDG). Contact Dermatitis 2008;58:101-6.

Additive Challenge Studies: Urticaria and Asthma

16. Chapman JA, Bernstein IL, Lee RE, et al. Food allergy: a practice parameter. Ann Allergy Asthma Immunol 2006;96:S1-68.
17. Metcalfe DD, Sampson HA. Workshop on experimental methodology for clinical studies

of adverse reactions to foods and food additives. J Allergy Clin Immunol 1990;86:421-42.

Food Colorants

18. Newsome RL. Natural and synthetic coloring agents. In: Branen AL, Davidson PM, Salminen S, editors. Food additives. New York: Marcel Dekker; 1990.
19. Stevenson DD, Simon RA, Lumry WR, et al. Pulmonary reactions to tartrazine. Pediatr Allergy Immunol 1992;3:222.
20. Nettis E, Colanardi MC, Ferrannini A, Tursi A. Suspected tartrazine-induced acute urticaria/angioedema is only rarely reproducible by oral rechallenge. Clin Exp Allergy 2003;33:1725-9.
21. Ardern KD, Ram FS. Tartrazine exclusion for allergic asthma. Cochrane Database Syst Rev 2001:CD000460.
22. Lockey SD. Allergic reactions due to F D and C Yellow No. 5, tartrazine, an aniline dye used as a coloring and identifying agent in various steroids. Ann Allergy 1959;17:719-21.
23. Simon RA, Bosso JV, Daffern PD, et al. Prevalence of sensitivity to food/drug additives in patients with chronic idiopathic urticaria (CIUA). J Allergy Clin Immunol 1998;101: 154.
24. Spector SL, Wangaard CH, Farr RS. Aspirin and concomitant idiosyncrasies in adult asthmatic patients. J Allergy Clin Immunol 1979; 64:500-6.
25. Virchow C, Szczeklik A, Bianco S, et al. Intolerance to tartrazine in aspirin-induced asthma: results of a multicenter study. Respiration 1988;53:20-3.
26. Weber RW, Hoffman M, Raine Jr DA, Nelson HS. Incidence of bronchoconstriction due to aspirin, azo dyes, non-azo dyes, and preservatives in a population of perennial asthmatics. J Allergy Clin Immunol 1979;64:32-7.
27. Pacor ML, Di Lorenzo G, Martinelli N, et al. Monosodium benzoate hypersensitivity in subjects with persistent rhinitis. Allergy 2004; 59:192-7.
28. Pestana S, Moreira M, Olej B. Safety of ingestion of yellow tartrazine by double-blind placebo controlled challenge in 26 atopic adults. Allergol Immunopathol 2010;38:142-6.
29. Devlin J, David TJ. Tartrazine in atopic eczema. Arch Dis Child 1992;67:709-11.
30. Worm M, Vieth W, Ehlers I, Sterry W, Zuberbier T. Increased leukotriene production by food additives in patients with atopic dermatitis and proven food intolerance. Clin Exp Allergy 2001;31:265-73.
31. Ward NI. Assessment of chemical factors in relation to child hyperactivity. J Nutr Environ Med 1997;7:333.
32. Juhlin L. Recurrent urticaria: clinical investigation of 330 patients. Br J Dermatol 1981;104: 369-81.
33. Myles I, Beakes D. An allergy to goldfish? Highlighting the labeling laws for food additives. World Allergy Organiz J 2009;2:314-6.
34. Ebo DG, Ingelbrecht S, Bridts CH, Stevens WJ. Allergy for cheese: evidence for an IgE-mediated reaction from the natural dye annatto. Allergy 2009;64:1558-60.
35. Nish WA, Whisman BA, Goetz DW, Ramirez DA. Anaphylaxis to annatto dye: a case report. Ann Allergy 1991;66:129-31.
36. Park GR. Anaphylactic shock resulting from casualty simulation: a case report. J R Army Med Corps 1981;127:85-6.
37. Shaw DW. Allergic contact dermatitis from carmine. Dermatitis 2009;20:292-5.
38. Greenhawt M, McMorris M, Baldwin J. Carmine hypersensitivity masquerading as azithromycin hypersensitivity. Allergy Asthma Proc 2009;30:95-101.
39. Yamakawa Y, Oosuna H, Yamakawa T, Aihara M, Ikezawa Z. Cochineal extract–induced immediate allergy. J Dermatol 2009;36:72-4.
40. Wüthrich B, Kägi MK, Stücker W. Anaphylactic reactions to ingested carmine (E120). Allergy 1997;52:1133-7.
41. Anibarro B, Seone J, Vila C, Mugica V, Lombardero M. Occupational asthma induced by inhaled carmine among butchers. Occup Med Environ Health 2003;16:133-7.
42. Tabar-Purroy AI, Alvarez-Puebla MJ, Acero-Sainz S, et al. Carmine (E-120)–induced occupational asthma revisited. J Allergy Clin Immunol 2003;111:415-9.
43. Ohgiya Y, Arakawa F, Akiyama H, et al. Molecular cloning, expression, and characterization of a major 38-kd cochineal allergen. J Allergy Clin Immunol 2009;123:1157-62.

Sulfites

44. Taylor SL, Higley NA, Bush RK. Sulfites in foods: uses, analytical methods, residues, fate, exposure assessment, metabolism, toxicity, and hypersensitivity. Adv Food Res 1986;30:1-76.
45 Martin LB, Nordlee JA, Taylor SL. Sulfite residues in restaurant salads. J Food Prot 1986; 49:126.
46. Koepke JW, Christopher KL, Chai H, Selner JC. Dose-dependent bronchospasm from sulfites in isoetharine. JAMA 1984;251:2982-3.
47. Smolinske SC. Review of parenteral sulfite reactions. J Toxicol Clin Toxicol 1992;30:597-606.
48. Bush RK, Taylor SL, Busse W. A critical evaluation of clinical trials in reactions to sulfites. J Allergy Clin Immunol 1986;78:191-202.
49. Vally H, Misso NL, Madan V. Clinical effects of sulfite additives. Clin Exp Allergy 2009;39: 1643-51.
50. Reus K, Houben G, Stam M, Dubois A. Food additives as a cause of medical symptoms: relationship shown between sulfites and asthma and anaphylaxis; results of a literature review. Ned Tijdschr Geneeskd 2000;144:1836-9.
51. Madan V, Walker SL, Beck MH. Sodium metabisulfite allergy is common but is it relevant? Contact Dermatitis 2007;57:173-6.
52. Harrison DA, Smith AG. Concomitant sensitivity to sodium metabisulfite and clobetasone butyrate in Trimovate cream. Contact Dermatitis 2002;46:310.
53. Belchi-Hernandez J, Florido-Lopez JF, Estrada-Rodriguez JL, et al. Sulfite-induced urticaria. Ann Allergy 1993;71:230-2.
54. Wüthrich B. Sulfite additives causing allergic or pseudo-allergic reactions. In: Miyamoto T, Okuda M, editors. Progress in allergy and clinical immunology. Seattle: Hogrefe & Huber; 1992.
55. Wüthrich B, Kägi MK, Hafner J. Disulfite-induced acute intermittent urticaria with vasculitis. Dermatology 1993;187:290-2.
56. Simon RA. Update on sulfite sensitivity. Allergy 1998;53:78-9.
57. Prenner BM, Stevens JJ. Anaphylaxis after ingestion of sodium bisulfite. Ann Allergy 1976;37:180-2.
58. Sokol WN, Hydick IB. Nasal congestion, urticaria, and angioedema caused by an IgE-mediated reaction to sodium metabisulfite. Ann Allergy 1990;65:233-8.
59. Yang WH, Purchase EC, Rivington RN. Positive skin tests and Prausnitz-Kustner reactions in metabisulfite-sensitive subjects. J Allergy Clin Immunol 1986;78:443-9.
60. Twarog FJ, Leung DY. Anaphylaxis to a component of isoetharine (sodium bisulfite). JAMA 1982;248:2030-1.
61. Schwartz HJ. Sensitivity to ingested metabisulfite: variations in clinical presentation. J Allergy Clin Immunol 1983;71:487-9.
62. Meggs WJ, Atkins FM, Wright R, et al. Failure of sulfites to produce clinical responses in patients with systemic mastocytosis or recurrent anaphylaxis: results of a single-blind study. J Allergy Clin Immunol 1985;76:840-6.
63. Kochen J. Sulfur dioxide, a respiratory tract irritant, even if ingested. Pediatrics 1973;52: 145-6.
64. Freedman BJ. Asthma induced by sulphur dioxide, benzoate and tartrazine contained in orange drinks. Clin Allergy 1977;7:407-15.
65. Stevenson DD, Simon RA. Sensitivity to ingested metabisulfites in asthmatic subjects. J Allergy Clin Immunol 1981;68:26-32.
66. Baker GJ, Collett P, Allen DH. Bronchospasm induced by metabisulphite-containing foods and drugs. Med J Aust 1981;2:614-7.
67. Tsevat J, Gross GN, Dowling GP. Fatal asthma after ingestion of sulfite-containing wine. Ann Intern Med 1987;107:263.
68. Bush RK, Taylor SL, Holden K, Nordlee JA, Busse WW. Prevalence of sensitivity to sulfiting agents in asthmatic patients. Am J Med 1986; 81:816-20.
69. Frick WE, Lemanske Jr RF. Oral sulfite sensitivity and provocative challenge in a 2 year old. J Asthma 1991;28:221-4.
70. Towns SJ, Mellis CM. Role of acetyl salicylic acid and sodium metabisulfite in chronic childhood asthma. Pediatrics 1984;73:631-7.
71. Peroni DG, Boner AL. Sulfite sensitivity. Clin Exp Allergy 1995;25:680-1.
72. Vanderbossche LE, Hop WC, deJonste JC. Bronchial responsiveness to inhaled metasulfite in asthmatic children increases with age. Pediatr Immunol 1993;16:236.
73. Boushey HA. Bronchial hyperreactivity to sulfur dioxide: physiologic and political implications. J Allergy Clin Immunol 1982;69: 335-8.
74. Fine JM, Gordon T, Sheppard D. The roles of pH and ionic species in sulfur dioxide– and sulfite-induced bronchoconstriction. Am Rev Respir Dis 1987;136:1122-6.
75. Field PI, McClean M, Simmul R, Berend N. Comparison of sulphur dioxide and metabisulphite airway reactivity in subjects with asthma. Thorax 1994;49:250-6.
76. Schwartz HJ, Chester EH. Bronchospastic responses to aerosolized metabisulfite in asthmatic subjects: potential mechanisms and clinical implications. J Allergy Clin Immunol 1984;74:511-3.
77. Delohery J, Simmul R, Castle WD, Allen DH. The relationship of inhaled sulfur dioxide reactivity to ingested metabisulfite sensitivity in patients with asthma. Am Rev Respir Dis 1984;130:1027-32.
78. Garcia-Ortega P, Scorza E, Teniente A. Basophil activation test in the diagnosis of sulphite-induced immediate urticaria. Clin Exp Allergy 2010;40:688-90.
79. Bindu PS, Christopher R, Mahadevan A, Bharath RD. Clinical and imaging observations in isolated sulfite oxidase deficiency. J Child Neurol 2011;26:1036-40.
80. Boxer MB, Bush RK, Harris KE, et al. The laboratory evaluation of IgE antibody to

metabisulfites in patients skin test positive to metabisulfites. J Allergy Clin Immunol 1988;82:622-6.
81. Bush RK. Sulfite and aspirin sensitivity: who is most susceptible? J Respir Dis 1987;8:23.
82. Taylor SL, Bush RK, Selner JC, et al. Sensitivity to sulfited foods among sulfite-sensitive subjects with asthma. J Allergy Clin Immunol 1988;81:1159-67.
83. Simon R, Goldfarb G, Jacobsen D. Blocking studies in sulfite intolerance in children: a blocking study with cyanocobalamin. J Allergy Clin Immunol 1984;73:136.

Other Additives Known or Suspected to Cause Reactions

84. Jinap S, Hajeb P. Glutamate. Its applications in food and contribution to health. Appetite 2010;55:1-10.
85. Williams AN, Woessner KM. Monosodium glutamate "allergy": menace or myth? Clin Exp Allergy 2009;39:640-6.
86. Freeman M. Reconsidering the effects of monosodium glutamate: a literature review. J Am Acad Nurse Pract 2006;18:482-6.
87. Yoneda J, Chin K, Torii K, Sakai R. Effects of oral monosodium glutamate in mouse models of asthma. Food Chem Toxicol 2011;49: 299-304.
88. Oliver AJ, Rich AM, Reade PC, Varigos GA, Radden BG. Monosodium glutamate–related orofacial granulomatosis: review and case report. Oral Surg Oral Med Oral Pathol 1991; 71:560-4.
89. Zhou Y, Yang M, Dong BR. Monosodium glutamate avoidance for chronic asthma in adults and children. Cochrane Database Syst Rev 2012;6:CD004357.
90. Garriga MM, Metcalfe DD. Aspartame intolerance. Ann Allergy 1988;61:63-9.
91. Garriga MM, Berkebile C, Metcalfe DD. A combined single-blind, double-blind, placebo-controlled study to determine the reproducibility of hypersensitivity reactions to aspartame. J Allergy Clin Immunol 1991;87: 821-7.
92. Geha R, Buckley CE, Greenberger P, et al. Aspartame is no more likely than placebo to cause urticaria/angioedema: results of a multicenter, randomized, double-blind, placebo-controlled, crossover study. J Allergy Clin Immunol 1993;92:513-20.
93. Simon RA. Additive-induced urticaria: experience with monosodium glutamate (MSG). J Nutr 2000;130:1063S-6S.
94. Hill DJ, Cameron DJ, Francis DE, Gonzalez-Andaya AM, Hosking CS. Challenge confirmation of late-onset reactions to extensively hydrolyzed formulas in infants with multiple food protein intolerance. J Allergy Clin Immunol 1995;96:386-94.
95. Ellis MH, Short JA, Heiner DC. Anaphylaxis after ingestion of a recently introduced hydrolyzed whey protein formula. J Pediatr 1991; 118:74-7.
96. Schwartz HR, Nerurkar LS, Spies JR, Scanlon RT, Bellanti JA. Milk hypersensitivity: RAST studies using new antigens generated by pepsin hydrolysis of beta-lactoglobulin. Ann Allergy 1980;45:242-5.
97. Van Beresteijn EC, Meijer RJ, Schmidt DG. Residual antigenicity of hypoallergenic infant formulas and the occurrence of milk-specific IgE antibodies in patients with clinical allergy. J Allergy Clin Immunol 1995;96: 365-74.
98. Herian AM, Taylor SL, Bush RK. Allergenicity of various soybean products as determined by RAST inhibition. J Food Sci 1993;58:385.
99. Nordlee JA, Taylor SL, Jones RT, Yunginger JW. Allergenicity of various peanut products as determined by RAST inhibition. J Allergy Clin Immunol 1981;68:376-82.
100. Niinimaki A, Niinimaki M, Makinen-Kiljunen S, Hannuksela M. Contact urticaria from protein hydrolysates in hair conditioners. Allergy 1998;53:1078-82.
101. Van Bever HP, Docx M, Stevens WJ. Food and food additives in severe atopic dermatitis. Allergy 1989;44:588-94.
102. Kubba R. Anaphylactoid purpura caused by tartrazine and benzoates. Br J Dermatol 1975; (Suppl II):61.
103. Reus KEH, Houben GF, Stam M, Dubois AEJ. [Food additives as the cause of medical complaints: connection with asthma and anaphylaxis demonstrated only for sulfite: results of a literature study]. Ned Tijdschr Geneeskd 2000;144:1836-9.
104. Jacobsen DW. Adverse reactions to benzoates and parabens. In: Metcalfe DD, Sampson HA, Simon RA, editors. Food allergy–adverse reactions to foods and food additives. Boston: Blackwell Scientific; 1991.
105. Vilaplana J, Romaguera C. Contact dermatitis from parabens used as preservatives in eyedrops. Contact Dermatitis 2000;43:248.
106. Cooper SM, Shaw S. Allergic contact dermatitis from parabens in a tar shampoo. Contact Dermatitis 1998;39:140.
107. Asero R. Chronic generalized pruritus caused by nitrate intolerance. J Allergy Clin Immunol 1999;104:1110-1.
108. Volonakis M, Katsarou-Katsari A, Stratigos J. Etiologic factors in childhood chronic urticaria. Ann Allergy 1992;69:61-5.
109. Raison-Peyron N, Meynadier JM, Meynadier J. Sorbic acid: an unusual cause of systemic contact dermatitis in an infant. Contact Dermatitis 2000;43:247-8.
110. Moneret-Vautrin DA, Einhorn C, Tisserand J. [Role of sodium nitrite in histamine urticaria of dietary origin]. Ann Nutr Aliment 1980;34: 1125-32.
111. Hawkins CA, Katelaris CH. Nitrate anaphylaxis. Ann Allergy Asthma Immunol 2000;85: 74-6.
112. Taylor SL, Dormedy ES. Flavorings and colorings. Allergy 1998;53:80-2.
113. Taylor SL, Dormedy ES. The role of flavoring substances in food allergy and intolerance. Adv Food Nutr Res 1998;42:1-44.
114. Gern JE, Yang E, Evrard HM, Sampson HA. Allergic reactions to milk-contaminated "nondairy" products. N Engl J Med 1991;324: 976-9.
115. St Vincent JC, Watson WT. Unsuspected source of cow's milk protein in food. JAMA 1994;93: 209.
116. McKenna C, Klontz KC. Systemic allergic reaction following ingestion of undeclared peanut flour in a peanut-sensitive woman. Ann Allergy Asthma Immunol 1997;79:234-6.
117. Veien NK, Hattel T, Justesen O, Norholm N. Oral challenge with balsam of Peru. Contact Dermatitis 1985;12:104-7.
118. Paiva M, Piedade S, Gaspar A. Toothpaste-induced anaphylaxis due to mint (Mentha) allergy. Allergy 2009;65:1196-204.
119. Ricciardi L, Saitta S, Isolla S, Aglio M, Gangemi S. Fragrances as a cause of food allergy. Allergol Immunopathol 2007;35:276-7.
120. Gu X, Beardslee T, Zeece M, Sarath G, Markwell J. Identification of IgE-binding proteins in soy lecithin. Int Arch Allergy Immunol 2001; 126:218-25.
121. Paschke A, Zunker K, Wigotzki M, Steinhart H. Determination of the IgE-binding activity of soy lecithin and refined and non-refined soybean oils. J Chromatogr B Biomed Sci Appl 2001;756:249-54.
122. Palm M, Moneret-Vautrin DA, Kanny G, Denery-Papini S, Fremont S. Food allergy to egg and soy lecithins. Allergy 1999;54: 1116-7.
123. Renaud C, Cardiet C, Dupont C. Allergy to soy lecithin in a child. J Pediatr Gastroenterol Nutr 1996;22:328-9.
124. Mansfield LE, Bowers CH. Systemic reaction to papain in a nonoccupational setting. J Allergy Clin Immunol 1983;71:371-4.
125. Mansfield LE, Ting S, Haverly RW, Yoo TJ. The incidence and clinical implications of hypersensitivity to papain in an allergic population, confirmed by blinded oral challenge. Ann Allergy 1985;55:541-3.
126. Bridts CH, Ebo DG, DeClerck LS, Stevens WJ. Anaphylaxis due to the ingestion of guar gum. J Allergy Clin Immunol 2002;109:S221.
127. Danoff D, Lincoln L, Thomson DMP, Gold P. "Big Mac attack." N Engl J Med 1978;298: 1095-6.
128. Gelfand HH. The allergenic properties of the vegetable gums: a case of asthma due to tragacanth. J Allergy 1943;14:203-19.
129. Tarlo SM, Dolovich J, Listgarten C. Anaphylaxis to carrageenan: a pseudo-latex allergy. J Allergy Clin Immunol 1995;95:933-6.
130. Fotisch K, Fah J, Wuthrich B, et al. IgE antibodies specific for carbohydrates in a patient allergic to gum arabic *(Acacia senegal)*. Allergy 1998;53:1043-51.
131. Muthiah R, Kagen S, Zondlo A, et al. Hidden allergens in medications: allergy to acacia in Synthroid tablets. J Allergy Clin Immunol 1997;99:S492.
132. Savino F, Muratore MC, Silvestro L, Oggero R, Mostert M. Allergy to carob gum in an infant. J Pediatr Gastroenterol Nutr 1999;29:475-6.
133. Nowak-Wegrzyn A, Shapiro GG, Beyer K, Bardina L, Sampson HA. Contamination of dry powder inhalers for asthma with milk proteins containing lactose. J Allergy Clin Immunol 2004;113:558-60.
134. Sa AB, Oliveira LCL, Miyagi KVM, et al. Reaction due to milk proteins contaminating lactose added to inhaled corticosteroid. J Allergy Clin Immunol 2011;127:241.
135. Grimbacher B, Peters T, Peter HH. Lactose intolerance may induce severe chronic eczema. Int Arch Allergy Immunol 1997;113:516-8.
136. Kumagai T, Yamanaka T, Wataya Y, et al. Gelatin-specific humoral and cellular immune responses in children with immediate- and nonimmediate-type reactions to live measles, mumps, rubella, and varicella vaccines. J Allergy Clin Immunol 1997;100:130-4.
137. Koppelman SJ, Nordlee JA, Lee PW, et al. Parvalbumin in fish skin–derived gelatin. Food Addit Contam 2012;29:1347-55.
138. Sakaguchi M, Nakayama T, Inouye S. Food allergy to gelatin in children with systemic immediate-type reactions, including anaphylaxis, to vaccines. J Allergy Clin Immunol 1996;98:1058-61.
139. Khoriaty E, McClain CD, Permaul P, Smith ER, Rachid R. Intraoperative anaphylaxis induced by the gelatin component of thrombin-soaked

Gelfoam in a pediatric patient. Ann Allergy Asthma Immunol 2012;108:209-10.
140. Mullins RJ, James H, Platts-Mills TA, Cummins S. Relationship between red meat allergy and sensitization to gelatin and galactose-α-1,3-galactose. J Allergy Clin Immunol 2012;129:1334-42.
141. Sakaguchi M, Toda M, Ebihara T, et al. IgE antibody to fish gelatin (type I collagen) in patients with fish allergy. J Allergy Clin Immunol 2000;106:579-84.
142. Hansen TK, Poulsen LK, Stahl SP, et al. A randomized, double-blinded, placebo-controlled oral challenge study to evaluate the allergenicity of commercial, food-grade fish gelatin. Food Chem Toxicol 2004;42:2037-44.
143. Franck P, Moneret-Vautrin DA, Morisset M, et al. Anaphylactic reaction to inulin: first identification of specific IgEs to an inulin protein compound. Int Arch Allergy Immunol 2005;136:155-8.
144. Ebo DG, Schuerwegh A, Stevens WJ. Anaphylaxis to starch. Allergy 2000;55:1098-9.
145. Hourihane JO, Bedwani SJ, Dean TP, Warner JO. Randomised, double blind, crossover challenge study of allergenicity of peanut oils in subjects allergic to peanuts. BMJ 1997;314:1084-8.
146. Bush RK, Taylor SL, Nordlee JA, Busse WW. Soybean oil is not allergenic to soybean-sensitive individuals. J Allergy Clin Immunol 1985;76:242-5.
147. Halsey AB, Martin ME, Ruff ME, Jacobs FO, Jacobs RL. Sunflower oil is not allergenic to sunflower seed–sensitive patients. J Allergy Clin Immunol 1986;78:408-10.
148. Olszewski A, Pons L, Moutete F, et al. Isolation and characterization of proteic allergens in refined peanut oil. Clin Exp Allergy 1998;28:850-9.
149. Teuber SS, Brown RL, Haapanen LA. Allergenicity of gourmet nut oils processed by different methods. J Allergy Clin Immunol 1997;99:502-7.
150. Kanny G, De Hauteclocque C, Moneret-Vautrin DA. Sesame seed and sesame seed oil contain masked allergens of growing importance. Allergy 1996;51:952-7.
151. Hefle SL, Taylor SL. Allergenicity of edible oils. Food Technol 1999;53:62.
152. Frémont S, Kanny G, Nicolas JP, Moneret-Vautrin DA. Prevalence of lysozyme sensitization in an egg-allergic population. Allergy 1997;52:224-8.
153. Campi P, Pichler WJ, de Weck AL. Allergic reactions to egg lysozyme. N Engl Reg Allergy Proc 1988;9:254.
154. Pichler WJ, Campi P. Allergy to lysozyme/egg white–containing vaginal suppositories. Ann Allergy 1992;69:521-5.
155. Artesani MC, Donnanno S, Cavagni G, Calzone L, D'Urbano L. Egg sensitization caused by immediate hypersensitivity reaction to drug-containing lysozyme. Ann Allergy Asthma Immunol 2008;101:105.
156. Anerican Academy of Pediatrics. "Inactive" ingredients in pharmaceutical products: update. Pediatrics 1997;99:268.
157. Asmus MJ, Barros MD, Liang J, Chesrown SE, Hendeles L. Pulmonary function response to EDTA, an additive in nebulized bronchodilators. J Allergy Clin Immunol 2001;107:68-72.

83

Oral Food Challenge Testing

ROBERT A. WOOD

CONTENTS

SUMMARY OF IMPORTANT CONCEPTS

» Oral food challenges are an important element in the management of food allergies in patients, and they remain the most accurate tests for the diagnosis of food allergy.

» The basic methodology underlying all oral food challenges is administration of the suspect food in gradually increasing doses under close observation in a medical setting.

» Variations in challenge methodology include the inclusion of placebo controls, blinding, and different dosing strategies.

» Challenges should be terminated and treatment administered at the first sign that a reaction is occurring.

» Oral food challenges carry the potential for significant risk, but these risks can be minimized by appropriate dosing and by performing challenges in a controlled setting with experienced personnel.

Introduction

Although diagnostic testing methods for food hypersensitivity have improved over time, in vivo and in vitro methods are sufficiently limited that oral food challenge (OFC) testing remains an essential element in the diagnosis and management of food allergy. The double-blind, placebo-controlled food challenge (DBPCFC) remains the gold standard for the diagnosis of food allergy.[1,2] OFC indications, methodologies, and risks are reviewed in this chapter.

Indications for Oral Challenge Testing

Oral challenge testing should be considered for clinical and research purposes. As shown in the algorithm in Figure 83-1, in the clinical setting, challenges are typically done for three major reasons. First, OFCs are used to establish an accurate diagnosis when the diagnosis remains unclear after other standard diagnostic methods have been tried, including obtaining the patient's history, skin testing, measurement of specific immunoglobulin E (IgE) levels, and elimination diets. However, if a patient recently experienced an acute, severe reaction to the first peanut exposure and has a strongly positive skin test result or a markedly elevated peanut-specific IgE level, an OFC to peanut would not be necessary or appropriate.[2-10]

In a second scenario, if a patient has a chronic allergic condition, such as atopic dermatitis or allergic gastrointestinal disease; skin tests or specific IgE levels that are not in the diagnostic range; and an unclear response to an elimination diet, one or more challenge tests may be appropriate. Allergen component–based testing, especially for peanut, has been shown to better predict challenge outcome,[9,10] as have algorithms that combine both clinical and laboratory data.[11]

In a third situation, OFCs are frequently used to determine whether a patient with a known food allergy has developed tolerance to that food. For example, in a patient with a known allergy to egg or peanut who has remained reaction free over some period (usually a minimum of 1 year) and for whom test results suggest that the allergy might have been outgrown,[12-15] a challenge should be considered to determine the degree of tolerance. Although complete tolerance is the goal, if a reaction occurs during the challenge, the information can be used to guide the patient and family regarding the approach to the diet, such as the need for strict avoidance of the problem food or to establish some liberalization of the diet.

The data obtained from failed OFCs may help the physician to counsel patients regarding the risks they may encounter with accidental exposures, particularly for those who experienced a significant reaction with a very small dose. However, challenges typically do not provide information that can completely predict the risk of future reactions, because challenges are conducted by giving gradually increasing doses of the food and are normally stopped at the first sign of a reaction, after which medications are immediately administered. This protocol may not mimic the real-world situation, in which a single large dose may be ingested, early signs of a reaction may not be recognized, and medications may not be readily available.

In the clinical setting, in addition to the potential for risk and the chances of success, decision making about challenges is largely based on the preferences of the patient and family and the importance of the food to the diet. Clinicians typically are much quicker to do an OFC to a major food item, such as milk, egg, or wheat, even if the chances of success are less, because it would be advantageous to be able to reintroduce that food into the diet. It is also important to recognize that a food that is unimportant to one family might be extremely important to another. For example, one family may not care if lentils are ever introduced into the diet, but for another family practicing a vegetarian diet, lentils might be an extremely important food. Different patients also have very different tolerances for risk. Some are comfortable with the risks that a challenge entails, and others are so anxious that they may decide to defer a challenge until the chance of success is almost guaranteed.

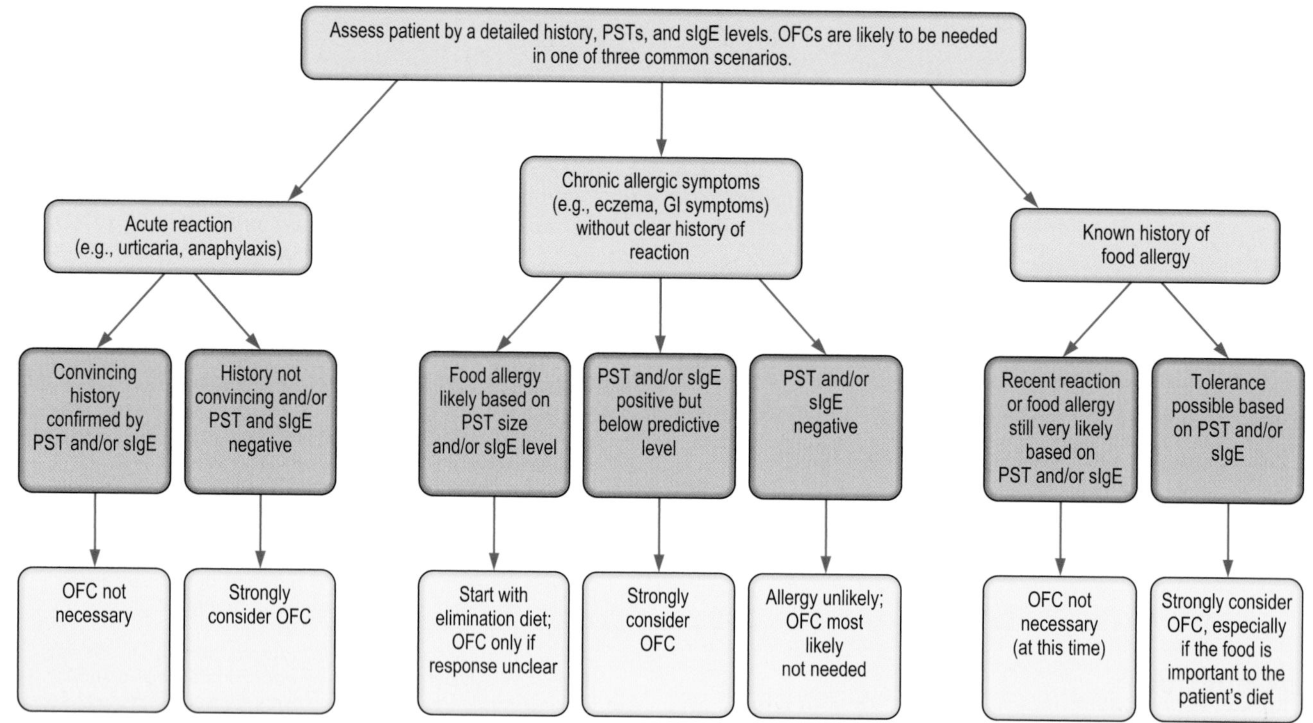

Figure 83-1 Oral food challenge decision-making algorithm. *GI*, Gastrointestinal; *OFC*, oral food challenge; *PST*, prick skin test; *sIgE*, specific IgE.

In the research setting, food challenges have been used with great success for many indications. First, they have been used to assess the accuracy of other diagnostic methods, including skin tests, patch tests, and allergen-specific IgE levels.[2-16] Second, they have been used to assess threshold doses for different food allergens,[17-22] providing essential data to establish guidelines for the food industry and the potential risks of low-level allergen exposure. Third, they have been used to determine the effects of food processing on the allergenicity of different foods.[23-31] Fourth, they have been used to assess the efficacy of potential treatments for food allergy.[32-37] As food allergy research moves rapidly in the direction of treatment, this indication for OFCs will continue to increase in importance.

Methodology

The general concepts underlying all oral challenge procedures are the same. The food in question is introduced in gradually increasing doses under observation in a controlled setting. Major differences among the various methods that are employed include the use of blinding and variations in dosing strategy.

OPEN CHALLENGES

An open challenge refers to an OFC in which the suspect food is administered without blinding or use of a placebo. The limitations of open challenges include the chance of bias on the part of the patient and the observer. This bias most often results in false-positive challenge results, with some authorities suggesting a false-positive rate of up to 30%[2] This is a common problem when the patient has significant anxiety about the challenge or when the patient's prior symptoms have been more subjective in nature. When a patient has only subjective complaints during a challenge, such as abdominal pain or pruritus, with no objective signs of reaction, the interpretation of the challenge outcome can be difficult. However, this difficulty can be markedly reduced when experienced observers conduct challenges.

Despite these limitations, open challenges still have significant utility in the clinical setting for several reasons. First, an open challenge can be the first approach when the probability of a negative outcome is estimated to be high, such as when studying an adverse reaction believed to be IgE mediated and the food skin test is negative. Second, when an open challenge result is negative, it is likely to be accurate and may obviate the need for a DBPCFC. Third, in infants and young children, for whom the impact of anxiety and other psychological factors is likely to be minimal, the risk of bias is significantly reduced, and open challenges may be appropriate as a first-line challenge procedure. Fourth, for practical reasons, open challenges are significantly easier to perform because food preparation is far simpler than for a blinded challenge, and the entire challenge can be performed with a single visit. Busy practitioners can perform many more open challenges than DBPCFCs.

SINGLE-BLIND CHALLENGES

In a single-blind challenge, the patient is blinded to the challenge material, but the observer is not. Single-blind challenges have the potential limitation of observer bias, and the only advantage they provide is a minor reduction in the personnel needed for food preparation because the same individual can prepare the challenge foods and act as an observer in the challenge. Single-blind challenges therefore have little role in clinical and research settings.

DOUBLE-BLIND, PLACEBO-CONTROLLED CHALLENGES

The DBPCFC remains the gold standard for the diagnosis of food allergy because the patient and observer biases are minimized. It is the preferred method for all scientific protocols and for the clinical evaluation of patients who present with a history of delayed reactions, chronic symptoms, or primarily subjective symptoms, such as abdominal pain, pruritus, chronic fatigue, multiple chemical sensitivities, or headache. The practical limitations of DBPCFCs include considerable time requirements for staff in the preparation of adequately blinded challenge materials and the requirement for two visits to accomplish both segments of the blinded challenge.[2,38] Suggestions for foods, placebos, and vehicles for DBPCFCs to several common food allergens are presented in Table 83-1. An open challenge should be performed after the successful completion of the DBPCFC, which requires an additional time commitment for the patient and staff. In some circumstances, depending on the comfort levels of the family and the physician and the willingness of the patient to eat another serving of food, this open challenge can be conducted at home, but in other instances, it is best done under observation.

Capsules are an effective method for blinding in DBPCFCs. However, capsule challenges may carry increased risk and are therefore not routinely recommended.[1] Two factors may increase the risk. First, in many patients the first signs of a reaction occur in the mouth and throat. They are sometimes just a complaint about localized pruritus, in which case the challenge is usually continued. In other instances, swelling or erythema may be readily visible, in which case the challenge should be terminated. Second, the capsules may not be consistently absorbed, such that a larger dose than necessary may be administered before a reaction is evident, possibly leading to a far more severe reaction.

Although it is the best available test to diagnose food allergy, even the DBPCFC is not perfect, and estimated false-positive and false-negative rates are between 1% and 3%.[39,40] The use of an open challenge after the blinded challenge helps to reduce or eliminate false-negative results, but all challenges need to be interpreted with care. Increasing the number of challenges with multiple active and placebo challenges can improve accuracy, but this approach usually is not practical and may increase risk by providing more doses of the active substance.[41] A final challenge may be conducted on a subsequent day, and one study demonstrated that more than 10% of negative challenge results prove positive when the entire provocative dose is given as a single challenge on a separate day.[42] The likely explanation for this phenomenon is that there may be an element of desensitization during a graded challenge, leading false-negative results.

TABLE 83-1 Foods and Vehicles for Double-Blind, Placebo-Controlled Food Challenges

Food	Challenge Material	Placebo	Vehicle
Egg	Dried egg white	Cornstarch, oat flour, rice flour	Applesauce, oatmeal, pudding, mashed potato
Milk	Dried milk, milk	Soy milk or formula, cornstarch, wheat or rice flour	Formula (soy, hydrolyzed, or elemental), soy or rice milk (chocolate), applesauce, pudding
Peanut	Peanut flour, peanut butter, crushed peanuts	Oat or wheat flour, soy butter	Hamburger, other meat patties, chili, oatmeal, pudding, cookies, candy
Soy	Soy flour, soy milk or formula	Flour (wheat, oat, rice, corn), safe formula	Formula (hydrolyzed or elemental), rice milk (chocolate), applesauce, oatmeal, pudding
Wheat	Wheat flour	Oat, rice, or corn flour	Applesauce, oatmeal, pudding
Tree nuts	Crushed nut or nut butter	Oat or wheat flour, soy or peanut butter	Applesauce, oatmeal, pudding

CHALLENGE SETTINGS AND PROCEDURES

Food challenges may be conducted at home without medical supervision only if the physician determines that there is no risk of a severe reaction. This approach may be appropriate for patients who present with complaints that are usually not associated with food allergy and when skin or in vitro testing results have been negative. It may also be appropriate to do a home reintroduction of a food that has been temporarily discontinued as part of an elimination diet but had been present in the diet previously. However, if there has been prolonged avoidance lasting weeks to a few months, the pattern of reactivity might have changed, and a home introduction may no longer be safe.[43] If a child with atopic dermatitis and a positive skin test result for egg undergoes a 3-week trial off egg, reintroducing egg at home would be safe in most cases, although no challenge may be needed if there was a dramatic improvement in the atopic dermatitis on the avoidance diet. However, if the family is likely to have difficulty interpreting the results of the home introduction or the avoidance has been prolonged, reintroduction should be done as a formal challenge under observation. If there is even a remote chance of a severe or anaphylactic reaction, challenges should be conducted only with a physician's supervision.

Oral food challenges should be performed in an environment that maximizes comfort and safety. The risks and benefits of the challenge should be discussed in detail; in most settings, informed consent should be obtained. The personnel involved in challenge procedures must be specially trained in the management of acute allergic reactions, and these trained personnel should continuously monitor patients undergoing challenge. Medications and equipment for resuscitation must be readily available. At a minimum, supplies should include injectable epinephrine, intravenous fluids, oral and parenteral antihistamines, oral and parenteral corticosteroids, inhaled or nebulized β-agonists, oxygen, and resuscitation equipment. If a severe reaction is suspected, the challenge should be performed in an inpatient setting or intensive care unit. The need for latex-free surroundings should be considered. Ideally, challenges should be conducted in a setting in which patients and their families can be comfortable and relaxed. Particularly for anxious children, activities to help provide distraction are a great benefit.

Before proceeding with a challenge, patients should have an examination with stable baseline values and should not have significant symptoms of atopic dermatitis, rhinoconjunctivitis, urticaria, or other symptoms evaluated during food challenges. They should have no wheezing or repetitive cough before the challenge, and they should not have been treated for a significant asthma exacerbation within a minimum of 1 week before undergoing the challenge. They must have no current illness (e.g., fever, vomiting, diarrhea) at the time of the challenge. Before challenges, patients should discontinue antihistamines and bronchodilators for appropriate periods, based on their elimination half-lives and duration of action. The challenge food should be provided gradually at 10- to 20-minute intervals or longer, should begin with a dose unlikely to trigger a reaction, and should progress stepwise with escalating doses, with an option to repeat doses or delay doses longer if symptoms may be developing (e.g., subjective signs of a reaction). Vital signs (e.g., heart rate, blood pressure, respiratory rate) should be monitored at the start and end of the challenge, with a brief examination focusing on the oral mucosa, skin, and respiratory system before each dose. Pulse oximetry, spirometry, or assessment of peak expiratory flow may be used when deemed appropriate. Challenges should be stopped and medications administered in the event of any significant objective symptoms; for example, a challenge may be continued if there are only one or two hives, especially where the food might have touched the skin. Challenges may also be stopped for subjective symptoms, such as significant abdominal pain, at the discretion of the supervising personnel. All challenge procedures, including the baseline examination, doses administered, vital signs, subjective complaints, objective signs, medications given, the discharge examination, and discharge instructions, should be fully documented in the patient's medical record. An example of a food challenge data collection form is provided in Figure 83-2.

Placebo and active challenges should ideally be separated by at least 24 hours, but when late reactions are not expected, both challenges can be performed on the same day. If a reaction needing treatment occurs, the next challenge should not be performed until the symptoms have resolved and enough time has elapsed for the effects of any medications that were administered to no longer be an issue.

Intravenous access before challenge initiation should be considered for all challenges but may not be necessary for most. It should be obtained routinely in patients deemed to be at high risk for a severe systemic reaction and for all patients with a history of food protein–induced enterocolitis syndrome.[44]

Oral Food Challenge Data Collection Form

Name ______________________ Record number ______________ Date __________

Food to be challenged ______________________

Current medications and last dose taken:

______________________ ______________________

______________________ ______________________

		Food		Signs and symptoms							
Dose #	Time	Dose %	Vol (mL or g)	Oral	Skin	Nose	Cough	Wheeze	Abd/GI	Medications given	Notes
1		1	1								
2		4	4								
3		10	10								
4		15	15								
5		20	20								
6		25	25								
7		25	25								

Suggested challenge dosing regimen (for a liquid challenge totalling 100 mL). The dosing is shown here as percent of total that can be calculated as weight or volume depending upon the substance being used. For example, if the total weight of a final challenge is 20 grams, then 1% = 200 mg.

Figure 83-2 Sample Oral Food Challenge Data Collection Form.

In all instances, the personnel and equipment to establish intravenous access should be available at all times during the challenge.

Most patients can be challenged in an outpatient setting, although in some instances, an inpatient setting is preferable. Each physician needs to consider the specifics of the outpatient setting in making this decision, including access to emergency care if needed and the availability of trained staff for observing challenges and treating reactions. In most challenges, patients can be discharged after an observation period of at least 2 hours after the last dose given, provided no reaction has occurred. The observation period must be adjusted based on the reaction history and the current signs and symptoms of the patient. The patient must be discharged with specific information and satisfactory arrangements for care if a late reaction occurs. If a patient experiences a severe reaction, observation for a minimum of 4 hours is recommended, and some patients need to be hospitalized for continued treatment or more prolonged observation in the event of more severe or persistent symptoms.

If the patient reports a history of reactions only in special situations, such as with exercise, with intake of concomitant drugs (e.g., aspirin), or only when the food has been processed in a certain way, specific challenge protocols should be considered. However, many of these reactions, such as food-dependent, exercise-induced anaphylaxis, can be severe, and these specialized protocols should be undertaken only by physicians with expertise in conducting challenge procedures.

Patients with a diagnosis of food protein–induced enterocolitis syndrome deserve special consideration.[44] Reactions with this syndrome are often severe, frequently including hypotension. All such challenges should be done with intravenous access established because the primary treatment for these reactions is fluid resuscitation. Some patients may also benefit from intravenous corticosteroids. Reactions are typically delayed by at least 1 hour after ingestion and more commonly by 2 to 3 hours, and observation times must be adjusted accordingly. In some medical centers, a complete blood count is obtained before and after these challenges because an increase in the leukocyte count is common.[44]

On discharge from all challenges, patients should be given detailed instructions about how the food should or should not be introduced in the diet and information on the signs and symptoms that may indicate a problem with that food in the future. Foods usually can be introduced in unlimited quantities after a successful challenge, although most patients should eat no more than one serving per day for the first several days. After failed challenges, specific challenge dietary instructions should be provided, which may range from continued strict avoidance for those with significant reactions after small doses to the introduction into the diet of small amounts of the food, such as milk or egg in baked products, for patients with lesser reactions after larger doses. In some cases, such as for those with resolved peanut allergy, it may be important to maintain the food in the diet on a regular basis to lower the risk of a recurrence of the allergy[45,46] and to continue to keep self-injectable epinephrine on hand until tolerance has been documented over a minimum of 6 months.

DOSING STRATEGIES

Although the general approach to dosing is similar from one protocol to another, there is no consensus about a single best strategy.[1,2,38,47-50] In all challenges, the food is given in gradually increasing amounts. For most IgE-mediated reactions, typical total doses administered are 8 to 10 g of the dry food or 100 mL of wet food, doubling the amounts for meat or fish.[2,38,47-50] Doses are typically given every 10 to 20 minutes over 1 to 2 hours, although the dosing interval can be lengthened if clinically indicated. For example, if a child has had prior severe reactions to a food, a 30- or 40-minute interval between doses may be selected. If capsules are chosen for blinding in a DBPCFC, the interval should be extended to a minimum of 30 minutes because absorption may be delayed, which can lead to more severe reactions if a larger dose than necessary was administered before the first signs of a reaction. It is reasonable to delay individual doses or to repeat prior doses if a reaction is suspected but not yet confirmed.

One common dosing scheme is to divide the total challenge into seven incremental doses: 1%, 4%, 10%, 15%, 20%, 25%, and 25% (Table 83-2; see Fig. 83-2). For patients deemed to be at higher risk for a severe reaction, it may be prudent to begin with one or more smaller doses, such as 0.1% or 0.5%. This may be appropriate for challenges conducted in the research setting, such as for a treatment study enrolling more-sensitive patients, compared with the clinical setting, in which less-sensitive patients are undergoing challenges. Some centers also begin with a labial challenge by placing a small amount of the challenge material on the lower lip for 1 to 2 minutes and observing for localized (or systemic) signs of a reaction.[51,52] The development of a contiguous rash on the cheek or chin, edema of the lip with rhinitis or conjunctivitis, or any systemic reaction is considered a positive test result, whereas negative labial challenges are typically followed by an OFC.

Several attempts have been made to define optimal starting doses for challenges based on studies of threshold doses. This approach could maximize safety and help to identify each patient's threshold for reactivity for the food. Unfortunately, studies of threshold doses have provided inconsistent results, and data are not available for most foods. From a practical standpoint, Sicherer and colleagues[51] evaluated 513 positive challenges to six common foods in children with atopic dermatitis, with starting doses ranging from 100 mg to 500 mg (usually 500 mg). The proportion of children who experienced a reaction at the first dose was 49% for egg, 55% for milk, 26% for peanut, 25% for wheat, 28% for soy, and 17% for fish. Eleven percent of these first-dose reactions were categorized as severe, and none of the reactions was predictable based on skin

TABLE 83-2 Suggested Challenge Dosing Regimen for a Liquid Challenge Totaling 100 mL

Dose	Time (min)	Percentage (%)*	Volume (mL)
1	0	1	1
2	15	4	4
3	30	10	10
4	45	15	15
5	60	20	20
6	75	25	25
7	90	25	25

*Dosing is shown as a percentage of the total that can be calculated as weight or volume, depending on the substance being used. For example, if the total weight of a final challenge is 20 g, 1% = 200 mg.

test results or specific IgE levels. Based on these results, the investigators recommended starting doses of 100 mg or less for these foods.

A position paper issued by the European Academy of Allergology and Clinical Immunology recommended that all challenges be initiated at a dose below the likely threshold for that food. The group proposed the following starting doses, based on published data and personal experience: peanut, 0.1 mg; milk, 0.1 mL; egg, 1 mg; wheat, 100 mg; soy, 1 mg; cod, 5 mg; shrimp, 5 mg; and hazelnut, 0.1 mg.[1,19-21] Although these doses maximize safety and can provide more information regarding an individual's threshold of reactivity, their inclusion adds several doses to the protocol and therefore lengthens the challenge to some degree. The potential benefits of this approach should be considered for each patient or research protocol.

Risk and Treatment of Oral Food Challenges

Several studies have focused on the types of reactions that occur and the types of treatment needed in positive (failed) OFCs.[52-56] The expected food-induced reactions involve some combination of cutaneous, gastrointestinal, respiratory, and cardiovascular reactions. Skin and gastrointestinal reactions are most common, and severe or life-threatening reactions are rare. Many patients describe localized pruritus in the mouth, throat, or ears as their first symptom, and these symptoms do not automatically mean that the challenge must stop, because they are often transient and may occur in challenges that are otherwise successful. Distinct behavioral changes are common, especially in young children. Children typically change suddenly from happy and playful to quiet and frightened with the onset of a reaction. These signs should always be taken seriously, because they likely herald the onset of a reaction.

Reibel and coworkers[52] reported a series of 178 positive food challenges to cow's milk, egg, wheat, and soy. One hundred twenty patients (67%) needed medical intervention, including 65% given oral medication and 35% given parenteral therapy. The researchers found a strong correlation between the level of specific IgE and the need for medical intervention, defining high-risk cutoffs of 17.5 kU/L for milk, wheat, and soy and 3.5 kU/L for egg. They recommended establishing intravenous access in children with specific IgE levels of 17.5 kU/L to milk or wheat or of 3.5 kU/L to egg.

Perry and associates[53] analyzed the outcome of 584 challenges to milk, egg, peanut, soy, and wheat. Of the 584 challenges, 253 (43%) resulted in an allergic reaction (Tables 83-3 and 83-4). Among those who reacted, there were 197 (78%) cutaneous, 108 (43%) gastrointestinal, 66 (26%) oral, 67 (26%) lower respiratory, and 62 (25%) upper respiratory reactions. No patients had cardiovascular symptoms. There was no difference between the five foods in the severity of failed challenges or the type of treatment required, and no relationships were detected between specific IgE levels or the dose ingested and reaction severity. Twenty-one percent of reactions resolved without treatment, and all others were reversed with short-acting antihistamines with or without epinephrine, β-agonists, or corticosteroids (Table 83-5). James and colleagues[54] studied respiratory reactions in 320 children with atopic dermatitis undergoing DBPCFCs, 55% of whom had asthma. Positive challenges occurred in 205 (64%) of the 320 patients evaluated, and 121 (59%) of these 205 patients experienced respiratory reactions, with nasal, laryngeal, or pulmonary symptoms in 34 (17%). Eighty-eight of the patients were monitored with spirometry, and of these, 13 (15%) developed lower respiratory symptoms, including wheezing during DBPCFC, and 6 had a more than 20% decrease in forced expiratory volume in 1 second (FEV_1). In the largest series reported, Järvinen and coworkers[55] analyzed 1273 challenges with specific attention to anaphylaxis and the need for epinephrine. A total of 436 (34%) of the OFCs resulted in a reaction. Epinephrine was administered in 50 challenges (11% of positive challenges, 3.9% overall), including 16% of failed challenges to egg, 12% to milk, 26% to peanut, and 4.3% to tree nuts. Reactions requiring epinephrine occurred in older children and were more often caused by peanuts. There was no difference in the prevalence of asthma, history of anaphylaxis,

TABLE 83-3 System Involvement in Positive Food Challenges

System	Milk (*n* = 90)	Egg (*n* = 56)	Peanut (*n* = 71)	Soy (*n* = 21)	Wheat (*n* = 15)	Total (*n* = 253)
Skin	68 (75%)	43 (77%)	55 (77%)	16 (76%)	15 (100%)*	197 (78%)
Oral	23 (26%)	12 (21%)	27 (38%)†	3 (14%)	1 (7%)	66 (26%)
Upper respiratory	16 (18%)	15 (27%)	25 (35%)†	4 (19%)	2 (13%)	62 (25%)
Lower respiratory	24 (27%)	19 (34%)	15 (21%)	4 (19%)	5 (33%)	67 (26%)
Gastrointestinal	37 (41%)	31 (55%)	28 (39%)	9 (43%)	3 (20%)	108 (43%)
Cardiovascular	0 (0%)	0 (0%)	0 (0%)	0 (0%)	0 (0%)	0 (0%)

From Perry TT, Matsui EC, Conover-Walker MK, Wood RA. The risk of oral food challenges. J Allergy Clin Immunol 2004;114:1164-8.
*P = .03 for probability of system involvement compared with all other foods.
†$P \leq .01$ for probability of system involvement compared with all other foods.

TABLE 83-4 Severity of Positive Food Challenges

Severity	Milk (*n* = 90)	Egg (*n* = 56)	Peanut (*n* = 71)	Soy (*n* = 21)	Wheat (*n* = 15)	Total (*n* = 253)
Mild	33 (37%)	18 (32%)	28 (39%)	9 (43%)	10 (67%)	98 (39%)
Moderate	33 (37%)	17 (30%)	25 (35%)	8 (38%)	0 (0%)	83 (33%)
Severe	24 (27%)	21 (38%)	18 (25%)	4 (19%)	5 (33%)	72 (28%)

From Perry TT, Matsui EC, Conover-Walker MK, Wood RA. The risk of oral food challenges. J Allergy Clin Immunol 2004;114:1164-8.

TABLE 83-5 Treatment Required for Positive Food Challenges

Treatment	Milk (*n* = 90)	Egg (*n* = 56)	Peanut (*n* = 71)	Soy (*n* = 21)	Wheat (*n* = 15)	Total (*n* = 253)
None	22 (24%)	11 (20%)	9 (13%)	7 (33%)	3 (20%)	52 (21%)
Antihistamine	68 (76%)	44 (79%)	62 (87%)	13 (62%)	12 (80%)	199 (77%)
Epinephrine	5 (6%)	10 (18%)	7 (10%)	3 (14%)	3 (20%)	28 (11%)
Steroids	2 (2%)	6 (11%)	4 (6%)	1 (5%)	1 (7%)	14 (6%)
Albuterol	2 (2%)	2 (3.4%)	5 (7%)	0 (0%)	2 (13%)	11 (4%)

From Perry TT, Matsui EC, Conover-Walker MK, Wood RA. The risk of oral food challenges. J Allergy Clin Immunol 2004;114:1164-8.

specific IgE level, or amount of food administered. Two doses of epinephrine were required in 3 of 50 patients, and there was only one biphasic reaction. No reaction resulted in life-threatening respiratory or cardiovascular compromise.

A series of 869 challenges to milk, egg, wheat, and soy in predominantly young children (median age, 1.2 years) focused on the relationship between the eliciting dose and reaction severity.[56] All challenges started at 3 to 5 mg of protein, and reaction severity was graded from I to V. No grade V reactions occurred, but grade IV reactions were seen at all eliciting doses, including the initial 3- to 5-mg dose for 10% of children allergic to milk or egg.

Although there are no published data for comparison, the risks of challenges are likely to be similar in adults and children. However, cardiovascular reactions may become more common with increasing age. No patients in any of the pediatric studies developed hypotension or other cardiovascular symptoms, but this may not be the case for adults. However, the overall approach to challenge is the same for children and adults.

The risk of challenges can be minimized by following several guidelines (Box 83-1). First, the starting dose and challenge protocol should be adjusted for individual patients who may be at higher risk for a severe reaction. Second, experienced observers who are present throughout the challenge, continually interacting with and reexamining the patient at regular intervals, can dramatically reduce risk. Third, the challenge should be stopped as soon as any observer is convinced that a reaction is occurring. Although there is a risk that stopping too early may result in a false-positive result, the risk of waiting too long or of giving an extra dose is much more significant. Fourth, all medications that might be needed should be prepared in appropriate doses before starting the challenge so that they can be administered without delay. Fifth, the challenge should be performed in a setting in which all measures that might be needed to treat a severe reaction are readily available.

Challenges should be terminated when the observer is reasonably convinced that a reaction is occurring, and treatment should be administered as indicated. Some challenges may have only minor, localized signs and symptoms, in which case treatment may not be necessary. In most instances, however, treatment with at least an antihistamine is warranted. Other therapies, including intramuscular epinephrine, oral or parenteral corticosteroids, inhaled or nebulized β-agonists, a histamine H_2 antagonist, oxygen, and intravenous fluids, should be administered at the discretion of the treating physician. Although there may be a greater role for cautious observation than there would be after accidental ingestions, it is still critical that reactions be treated as aggressively as necessary to prevent progression to something more severe or dangerous. Patients can be made much more comfortable in many instances with more aggressive treatment. Some physicians have recommended the use of activated charcoal in failed food challenges, although this has not become a standard clinical practice in most centers.

Although all OFCs carry risk, they remain an essential tool in the management of patients with suspected food allergy. Given the enormous nutritional and social benefits that can result from a negative challenge, these risks are reasonable when the risk-to-benefit ratio is carefully considered for each patient and challenges are performed under the guidance of an experienced practitioner in a properly equipped setting.

BOX 83-1 STEPS TO MINIMIZE CHALLENGE RISKS

- Adjust the starting dose and challenge protocol for individual patients who may be at higher risk for severe reactions.
- Use experienced observers who have been trained to do food challenges and are present throughout the challenge, continually interacting with and reexamining the patient at regular intervals.
- Stop the challenge as soon as the observer is convinced that a reaction is occurring.
- Prepare all medications that may be needed before the challenge so that they can be administered without delay.
- Perform challenges only in settings where all measures that might be needed to treat a severe reaction are readily available.

REFERENCES

Introduction

1. Bindslev-Jensen C, Ballmer-Weber BK, Bengtsson U, et al. European Academy of Allergology and Clinical Immunology. Standardization of food challenges in patients with immediate reactions to foods—position paper from the European Academy of Allergology and Clinical Immunology. Allergy 2004;59:690-7.
2. Nowak-Wegrzyn A, Assa'ad AH, Bahna SL, et al. Adverse Reactions to Food Committee of American Academy of Allergy, Asthma & Immunology. Work Group report: oral food challenge testing. J Allergy Clin Immunol 2009; 123:S365-83.

Indications for Oral Challenge Testing

3. Niggemann B, Reibel S, Wahn U. The atopy patch test (APT)—a useful tool for the diagnosis of food allergy in children with atopic dermatitis. Allergy 2000;55:281-5.
4. Sampson HA, Ho DG. Relationship between food-specific IgE concentrations and the risk of positive food challenges in children and adolescents. J Allergy Clin Immunol 1997;100: 444-51.
5. Sampson HA. Utility of food-specific IgE concentrations in predicting symptomatic food allergy. J Allergy Clin Immunol 2001;107:891-6.
6. Boyano MT, Garcia-Ara C, Diaz-Pena JM, et al. Validity of specific IgE antibodies in children

with egg allergy. Clin Exp Allergy 2001;31: 1464-9.
7. Nicolaou N, Poorafshar M, Murray C, et al. Allergy or tolerance in children sensitized to peanut: prevalence and differentiation using component-resolved diagnostics. J Allergy Clin Immunol 2010;125:191-7.
8. Vissers YM, Jansen AP, Ruinemans-Koerts J, Wichers HJ, Savelkoul HF. IgE component-resolved allergen profile and clinical symptoms in soy and peanut allergic patients. Allergy 2011;66:1125-7.
9. DunnGalvin A, Daly D, Cullinane C, et al. Highly accurate prediction of food challenge outcome using routinely available clinical data. J Allergy Clin Immunol 2011;127:633-9.
10. Perry TT, Matsui EC, Conover-Walker MK, et al. The relationship of allergen-specific IgE levels and oral food challenge outcome. J Allergy Clin Immunol 2004;114:144-9.
11. Skolnick HS, Conover-Walker MK, Barnes-Koerner C, et al. The natural history of peanut allergy. J Allergy Clin Immunol 2001;107: 367-74.
12. Fleischer DM, Conover-Walker MK, Christie L, et al. The natural progression of peanut allergy: resolution and possible recurrence. J Allergy Clin Immunol 2003;112:183-9.
13. Wood RA. The likelihood of remission of food allergy in children: when is the optimal time for challenge? Curr Allergy Asthma Rep 2012;12: 42-7.
14. Rancé F, Juchet A, Brémont F, Dutau G. Correlations between skin prick tests using commercial extracts and fresh foods, specific IgE, and food challenges. Allergy 1997;52:1031-5.
15. Taylor SL, Hefle SL, Bindslev-Jensen C, et al. Factors affecting the determination of threshold doses for allergenic foods: how much is too much? J Allergy Clin Immunol 2002;109: 24-30.
16. Taylor SL, Hefle SL, Bindslev-Jensen C, et al. A consensus protocol for the determination of the threshold doses for allergenic foods: how much is too much? Clin Exp Allergy 2004;34: 689-95.
17. Taylor SL, Moneret-Vautrin DA, Crevel RW, et al. Threshold dose for peanut: risk characterization based upon diagnostic oral challenge of a series of 286 peanut-allergic individuals. Food Chem Toxicol 2010;48:814-9.
18. Hourihane JO, Kilburn SA, Nordlee JA, et al. An evaluation of the sensitivity of subjects with peanut allergy to very low doses of peanut protein: a randomized, double-blind, placebo-controlled food challenge study. J Allergy Clin Immunol 1997;100:596-600.
19. Wensing M, Penninks A, Hefle SL, et al. The range of minimum provoking doses in hazelnut-allergic patients as determined by double-blind placebo controlled food challenges (DBPCFCs). Clin Exp Allergy 2002;32: 1757-62.
20. Bindslev-Jensen C, Briggs D, Osterballe M. Can we determine a threshold level for allergenic foods by statistical analysis of published data in the literature? Allergy 2002;57:741-6.
21. Ballmer-Weber BK, Vieths S, Lüttkopf D, Heuschmann P, Wüthrich B. Celery allergy confirmed by double-blind, placebo-controlled food challenge: a clinical study in 32 subjects with a history of adverse reactions to celery root. J Allergy Clin Immunol 2000;106: 373-8.
22. Ortolani C, Ballmer-Weber BK, Hansen KS, et al. Hazelnut allergy: a double-blind, placebo-controlled food challenge multicenter study. J Allergy Clin Immunol 2000;105:577-81.
23. Bernhisel-Broadbent J, Strause D, Sampson HA. Fish hypersensitivity. II: Clinical relevance of altered fish allergenicity caused by various preparation methods. J Allergy Clin Immunol 1992; 90:622-9.
24. Fiocchi A, Restani P, Riva E, et al. Heat treatment modifies the allergenicity of beef and bovine serum albumin. Allergy 1998;53:798-802.
25. Ballmer-Weber BK, Hoffmann A, Wüthrich B, et al. Influence of food processing on the allergenicity of celery: DBPCFC with celery spice and cooked celery in patients with celery allergy. Allergy 2002;57:228-35.
26. Ballmer-Weber BK, Wüthrich B, Wangorsch A, et al. Carrot allergy: double-blinded, placebo-controlled food challenge and identification of allergens. J Allergy Clin Immunol 2001;108: 301-7.
27. Morisset M, Moneret-Vautrin DA, Maadi F, et al. Prospective study of mustard allergy: first study with double-blind placebo-controlled food challenge trials (24 cases). Allergy 2003;58: 295-9.
28. Hansen TK, Poulsen LK, Stahl Skov P, et al. A randomized, double-blinded, placebo-controlled oral challenge study to evaluate the allergenicity of commercial, food-grade fish gelatin. Food Chem Toxicol 2004;42:2037-44.
29. Nowak-Wegrzyn A, Bloom KA, Sicherer SH, et al. Tolerance to extensively heated milk in children with cow's milk allergy. J Allergy Clin Immunol 2008;122:342-7.
30. Jones SM, Pons L, Roberts JL, et al. Clinical efficacy and immune regulation with peanut oral mmunotherapy. J Allergy Clin Immunol 2009; 124:292-300.
31. Skripak JM, Nash SD, Rowley H, et al. A randomized, double-blind, placebo-controlled study of milk oral immunotherapy for cow's milk allergy. J Allergy Clin Immunol 2008;122: 1154-60.
32. Blumchen K, Ulbricht H, Staden U. Oral peanut immunotherapy in children with peanut anaphylaxis. J Allergy Clin Immunol 2010;126: 83-91.
33. Nowak-Wegrzy A, Sampson HA. Future therapies for food allergies. J Allergy Clin Immunol 2011;127:558-73.
34. Varshney P, Jones SM, Scurlock AM, et al. A randomized controlled study of peanut oral immunotherapy (OIT): clinical desensitization and modulation of the allergic response. J Allergy Clin Immunol 2011;127:654-60.
35. Keet CA, Frischmeyer-Guerrerio PA, Thyagarajan A, et al. The safety and efficacy of sublingual and oral immunotherapy for milk allergy. J Allergy Clin Immunol 2012;129: 448-55.
36. Cochrane SA, Salt LJ, Wantling E, et al. Development of a standardized low-dose double-blind placebo-controlled challenge vehicle for the EuroPrevall project. Allergy 2012;67:107-13.
37. Sampson HA. Food allergy. Part 2: diagnosis and management. J Allergy Clin Immunol 1999; 103:981-9.

Methodology

38. Caffarelli C, Petroccione T. False negative food challenges in children with suspected food allergy. Lancet 2001;358:1871-2.
39. Briggs D, Aspinall L, Dickens A, Bindsley-Jensen C. Statistical model for assessing the proportion of subjects with subjective sensitisations in adverse reactions to foods. Allergy 2001;56 (Suppl. 67):83-5.
40. Niggemann B, Lange L, Finger A, et al. Accurate oral food challenge requires a cumulative dose on a subsequent day. J Allergy Clin Immunol 2012;130:261-3.
41. Barbi E, Gerarduzzi T, Longo G, Ventura A. Fatal allergy as a possible consequence of long-term elimination diet. Allergy 2004;59:668-9.
42. Sicherer S. Food protein-induced enterocolitis syndrome: case presentations and management lessons. J Allergy Clin Immunol 2005;115: 149-56.
43. Busse PJ, Nowak-Wegrzyn AH, Noone SA, Sampson HA, Sicherer SH. Recurrent peanut allergy. N Engl J Med 2002;347:1535-6.
44. Fleischer DM, Conover-Walker MK, Matsui EC, Wood RA. Peanut allergy: recurrence and its management. J Allergy Clin Immunol 2005;116: 1087-93.
45. Bindslev-Jensen C. Standardization of double-blind, placebo-controlled food challenges. Allergy 2001;56(Suppl. 67):75-7.
46. Koletzko S, Niggemann B, Arato A, et al. Diagnostic approach and management of cow's milk protein allergy in infants and children: ESPGHAN GI Committee practical guidelines. J Pediatr Gastroenterol Nutr 2012;55:221-9.
47. Järvinen KM, Sicherer SH. Diagnostic oral food challenges: Procedures and biomarkers. J Immunol Methods 2012;383:30-8.
48. Rancé F, Deschildre A, Villard-Truc F, et al. SFAIC and SP2A Workgroup on OFC in Children. Oral food challenge in children: an expert review. Eur Ann Allergy Clin Immunol 2009; 41:35-49.
49. Rancé F, Dutau G. Labial food challenge in children with food allergy. Pediatr Allergy Immunol 1997;8:41-4.
50. Rancé F, Kanny G, Dutau G, Moneret-Vautrin DA. Food hypersensitivity in children: clinical aspects and distribution of allergens. Pediatr Allergy Immunol 1999;10:33-8.
51. Sicherer SH, Morrow EH, Sampson HA. Dose-response in double-blind, placebo-controlled oral food challenges in children with atopic dermatitis. J Allergy Clin Immunol 2000;105: 582-6.
52. Reibel S, Röhr C, Ziegert M, et al. What safety measures need to be taken in oral food challenges in children? Allergy 2000;55:940-4.
53. Perry TT, Matsui EC, Conover-Walker MK, Wood RA. The risk of oral food challenges. J Allergy Clin Immunol 2004;114:1164-8.

Risk and Treatment of Oral Food Challenges

54. James JM, Bernhisel-Broadbent J, Sampson HA. Respiratory reactions provoked by double-blind food challenges in children. Am J Respir Crit Care Med 1994;149:59-64.
55. Järvinen KM, Amalanayagam S, Shreffler WG, et al. Epinephrine treatment is infrequent and biphasic reactions are rare in food-induced reactions during oral food challenges in children. J Allergy Clin Immunol 2009;124:1267-72.
56. Rolinck-Werninghaus C, Niggemann B, Grabenhenrich L, Wahn U, Beyer K. Outcome of oral food challenges in children in relation to symptom-eliciting allergen dose and allergen-specific IgE. Allergy 2012;67:951-7.

84 Food Allergy Management

SCOTT H. SICHERER | GIDEON LACK | STACIE M. JONES

CONTENTS

SUMMARY OF IMPORTANT CONCEPTS

» Avoidance of food allergens requires educating patients and caregivers about concerns, including reading ingredient labels, avoiding cross-contact with allergen, and obtaining safe meals in various circumstances.
» Appropriate management of food-induced anaphylaxis requires education about recognizing symptoms and treating promptly with epinephrine.
» IgE-mediated food allergy is increasing in the developed world. Strategies to prevent food allergy such as delayed weaning and delayed exposure to food allergens have recently been called into question.
» Evidence suggests early cutaneous exposure to food protein through a disrupted skin barrier leads to allergic sensitization, and early oral exposure to food allergen may induce tolerance.
» New therapies for food allergy employ both allergen-specific and allergen-nonspecific approaches, with great promise for effective treatment associated with successful immunomodulation.
» Because of safety concerns and long-term efficacy parameters that are still being evaluated, therapies for food allergy are still considered investigational.

Introduction

Food allergy is common and potentially fatal.[1-3] Successful management requires avoidance of the offending food and preparation to treat allergic reactions and anaphylaxis. Current treatment relies on education about allergen avoidance and prompt treatment with epinephrine, but both these approaches are prone to pitfalls resulting in frequent allergic reactions that are undertreated.[4] The apparent increase in food allergy and a lack of definitive therapies underscore a need for improved prevention and treatment. Risk factors are being identified that may inform better prevention strategies because studies indicate that past prevention strategies based on allergen avoidance may have failed.[5] Numerous treatment strategies are under investigation, including allergen-specific and allergen-nonspecific therapies that are already changing the approach to treating food allergies from passive avoidance to active desensitization and immunomodulation.[6]

Practical Management

Management of diagnosed food allergies requires avoidance of the offending allergens and prompt treatment of an allergic reaction.[7] Food allergen avoidance is challenging because food is necessary for sustenance and allergens are ubiquitous. Patients and caregivers must understand food-labeling laws, prevention of cross-contact of safe foods with allergens, and means of acquiring safe meals in settings such as restaurants and schools. Adding to the complexity of avoidance is the possibility of exposure to food allergens in occupational settings, in nonfood items such as cosmetics and medications, and through non-ingestion exposures by skin contact or inhalation. Nutritional concerns arise when multiple foods are removed from the diet. Successful emergency management requires prompt recognition and treatment of an allergic reaction or anaphylaxis.

The daily burden of managing food allergies seriously impacts quality of life.[8] Successful management requires detailed education of patients and caregivers about avoidance and treatment.

FOOD ALLERGEN AVOIDANCE STRATEGIES

General Approach to Avoidance

Allergen avoidance should be prescribed based on a confirmed diagnosis.[7] Avoidance education must include all persons responsible for obtaining or preparing foods. Educational materials are available through a variety of resources, including Food Allergy Research & Education (www.foodallergy.org) and the Consortium of Food Allergy Research (www.cofargroup.org); the latter organization has validated materials addressing avoidance of specific foods (e.g., milk, egg, wheat, soy) and general approaches to avoidance in different settings.[9]

Strict avoidance is typically prescribed to avoid any risk of allergic reaction, although it may not always be necessary. Examples where ingestion of the allergenic protein may be acceptable include raw fruits and vegetables in persons with mild symptoms of pollen-food–related syndrome; extensively heated forms of milk or egg (e.g., bakery goods) in persons who tolerate them despite reacting to whole forms[10]; and maternal ingestion of allergens when breastfeeding allergic infants who show no evidence of reactions. Patients who tolerate these forms of exposure are identified through their medical history or by medically supervised oral food challenge. Caution is needed because anaphylaxis can occur in some persons. The risk or benefit of allowing exposure to tolerated forms of the allergen should be individualized. There is no evidence that strict food avoidance (compared with less strict avoidance) has an effect on the rate of natural remission.[7] Avoidance of foods

TABLE 84-1 Options for Allergen Avoidance in Select Circumstances

Circumstance	Options	Risk or Benefit*
Raw fruits and vegetables causing oral symptoms (pollen related)	Allow ingestion on case-by-case basis based on preference and severity.	Small risk of systemic reaction or anaphylaxis.
Products with extensively heated (baked-in) egg or milk in persons with allergy to whole forms	Allow ingestion if tolerated by history or challenge (caution for possible anaphylaxis).	Unclear whether this approach speeds, hinders, or has no influence on recovery. Risk of reaction despite initial apparent tolerance. Possible risk of chronic inflammation from exposure.
Maternal ingestion of an allergen while breastfeeding, when same allergen caused a reaction when ingested by infant.	Allow mother to continue previously ingested amounts if infant showed no sign of acute or chronic reaction.	May risk reaction. No data on influence on natural course. Variations in dose ingested may alter the risk.
Allergy to peanut, not tree nuts	Allow ingestion of tolerated tree nuts.	Cross-contact or misidentification may lead to reactions. New onset of allergy to allowed food is possible, although degree of risk uncertain.
Allergy to some but not all tree nuts	Allow peanut in forms that are free from tree nuts. Allow ingestion of tolerated tree nuts.	As above, with less risk for commercial peanut butter and various commercial products with isolated nut ingredients (e.g., almond in almond milk).
Allergy to some but not all fish	Allow tolerated fish. Allow canned fish that are tolerated.	Risk of cross contact, misidentification, or new onset of allergy. Less risk for processed (canned) fish.
Allergy to some but not all shellfish	Allow tolerated shellfish.	Risk of cross-contact, misidentification, or new onset of allergy.
Allergy to some but not all botanically related foods (e.g., fruits, legumes, vegetables, grains)	Allow tolerated types.	See Chapter 81 for risk. Many options to ingest "related" foods if proved tolerated with lower risk of cross-contact, misidentification, or new onset of allergy.

*Individual quality of life or nutritional benefits are assumed. Decisions are individualized based on patient preferences, physician judgment, risk assessment, and past history.

that are related and may have cross-reactive proteins can be individualized according to risk of clinical cross-reactivity (see Chapter 81). Table 84-1 summarizes options for the approach to avoidance of dietary allergens.

Labeling of Manufactured Products

Patients must understand labeling laws to avoid allergen ingestion.[7] In the United States the Food Allergen Labeling and Consumer Protection Act (FALCPA) of 2004 requires that milk, egg, peanut, tree nuts, fish, crustacean shellfish, wheat, and soy be declared on ingredient labels using plain English words. These foods and food categories are often referred to as "major allergens." The law does not apply to any other foods or to noncrustacean seafood. The common names used to identify the foods may be listed within the ingredient list or in a separate statement (e.g., "contains peanut"). Although not required, if a "contains statement" is used, all the major allergens must be included. The law also requires that the specific type of allergen within a category be named, such as "walnut" or "shrimp." FALCPA applies to foods manufactured in or imported into the United States; it does not apply to agricultural products (e.g., fresh meat, eggs, poultry, fruits, vegetables) or alcoholic beverages, which may use food proteins as ingredients or processing agents. The law is subject to revisions, as described at http://www.fda.gov/Food/FoodSafety/FoodAllergens.

Labeling laws vary among countries, and some have none. Many countries have laws that include more than just the eight food allergen groups currently covered by the U.S. laws. For example, the European Union (EU) enacted legislation in 2005 requiring that six allergens not covered in U.S. laws be listed: rye, barley, oats, celery, mustard, and sesame seeds.

The FALCPA of 2004 does not regulate the use of advisory labeling, including statements describing the potential presence of unintentional ingredients in food products; such declarations are done voluntarily in the United States, and approaches are evolving internationally. Although many terms are used (e.g., "may contain," "manufactured on equipment with") to describe possible cross-contact, these do not convey risk.[11] Therefore, general advice is to avoid products with these advisories.[7] Nonetheless, there may be lower thresholds that would pose virtually no risk, and improved labeling based on studies of thresholds and adequate testing of final products may be possible.[12] Consumers should be aware that food proteins may be a component of nonfood items (Table 84-2).

Cross-Contact

Cross-contact (cross-contamination) of an otherwise safe food with an allergen is a concern for food preparation in commercial facilities, in restaurants and food establishments, and at home. Examples of cross-contact include a knife used to spread peanut butter then contaminating jelly; shared grills, pans, food processors, and other equipment used without thorough cleaning between preparation of different foods; dipping ice cream scoops from one flavor to the next; using a fryer for both shrimp and potatoes; and preparing foods in a workspace not cleaned between preparations. Patients and caregivers must be educated about these concerns and address them when obtaining or preparing meals.

TABLE 84-2 Examples of Food Allergens in Unexpected and Nonfood Items

Product type	Examples	Relevance
Cosmetics	Almond or milk in shampoos or ointments	Contact urticaria or dermatitis is possible. Some derivatives (e.g., shea nut butter) may have negligible protein.
Pet food	Milk, egg, fish, soy, etc.	Animal lick may cause contact urticaria. Fish food on fingers may transfer to eyes or mouth causing symptoms.
Medications	Lactose in dry powder inhaler (DPI) or tablets may have trace milk.	Case reports of reactions to casein identified in DPI, relevance in pills/pharmaceutical grade lactose unclear.
	Soy lecithin, egg lecithin	Relevance of potential trace protein in lecithin (fatty derivative) unclear, likely low risk.
Vaccines	Egg (influenza, yellow fever), possibly milk (DPT)	See Chapter 85
Nutrition supplements	glucosamine-chondroitin supplements (shark cartilage or shrimp shell), chitosan or chitin products (derived from Crustacean shell)	Relevance uncertain, likely low risk.
Saliva (kissing)	Residual protein from meals.	Relevant for intimate contact
Transfusion	Packed red blood cells, plasma (containing allergens from donor ingestion).	Risk presumably low, theoretically higher for products that include serum proteins rather than washed blood products.

Manner of Exposure (Skin Contact, Inhalation, Ingestion)

The primary concern regarding avoidance of an allergen relates to *ingestion*. Although exposures through skin contact or inhalation are unlikely to cause anaphylaxis, skin rashes and respiratory symptoms may occur.[13] For young children, there is a concern that skin contact could lead to ingestion (e.g., sucking fingers). Food odors may be caused by volatile organic compounds that lack appreciable proteins and present minimal allergic risk (e.g., odor of peanut butter would not trigger anaphylaxis)[14] or may include proteins when the food is aerosolized (e.g., during cooking, with powdery forms). In the latter situation (e.g., in proximity to boiling milk, frying fish, or powdered milk), respiratory or skin symptoms could occur.[13] Noningestion reactions occur in occupational settings as well (e.g., food handlers). Bakers' asthma describes airborne sensitivity to wheat flour. Individuals with bakers' asthma can typically tolerate wheat ingestion.

Persons with occupational allergy caused by foods may need to wear gloves and masks or find alternative employment. Aside from occupational exposures, individuals with food allergies may need to avoid situations where the food allergen is aerosolized nearby. Young children may need to be supervised around food allergens to avoid hand-to-mouth contact. Standard cleaning procedures (soap and water and wiping with friction) should suffice to remove allergens from surfaces.[15] Antibacterial foams and gels do not remove allergens from hands. Allergic reactions from kissing are common because allergen can be transferred in saliva.[16] Skin contact with the saliva is unlikely to cause a severe reaction, but intimate kissing is similar in risk to ingestion, and a partner may need to avoid the allergen.

Restaurants, Food Establishments, Travel

Restaurants and other food establishments, such as bakeries or ice cream stores, present challenges for food-allergic individuals. Consumers should identify themselves as allergic so that instructions about avoidance are not misperceived as being taste preferences. Clear communication is crucial because those preparing the foods may have limited understanding of the needs of an allergic consumer. For example, in a study of 100 employees of various food establishments in New York City, only 22% correctly responded to basic questions on whether fryer heat destroyed allergens, whether an allergic consumer could eat small amounts of an allergen, or whether removing an allergen from a finished meal was safe (e.g., removing nuts from a salad).[17] It may be prudent for consumers to review concerns such as cross-contact and hidden ingredients with the relevant personnel. All persons handling the food should be involved in discussions about meal preparation. This could prevent errors, such as a "prep" worker adding butter to a food that appears dry. Consumers may present written materials that describe the allergies ("chef cards"), and food establishments may follow guidelines; both are available from several sources, including Food Allergy Research & Education (www.foodallergy.org). Buffets or specialty or ethnic restaurants (e.g., seafood, Asian) may pose high risks and should be avoided depending on the consumer's specific allergies.

Traveling with food allergies requires considerations beyond obtaining meals safely in restaurants. Allergic reactions to peanut and tree nuts have been reported on commercial airliners, but the studies rely heavily on self-report.[18] Overall, exposure to the cabin air seems unlikely to trigger severe reactions for most persons with food allergies. Travelers with food allergies should avoid eating potentially unsafe airline foods and carry safe alternatives. Adults traveling with young children with food allergies might inspect crevices around their seats and wipe surfaces to avoid ingestion of residual allergens by toddlers. Some airlines may provide additional accommodations when requested in advance (e.g., flight with no peanuts served). Vacation choices, including all-inclusive resorts, cruises, and international travel, are circumstances in which advance planning is required because meals are prepared by others. Potentially less risky alternatives include accommodations with a kitchenette so that some meals can be self-prepared.

Avoidance for Schools and Camp

School-based strategies must be practical and must focus on policies to avoid ingestion of the allergen and promptly recognize and treat anaphylaxis.[19] There are currently no controlled studies evaluating the effectiveness of potential avoidance strategies. Allergen avoidance may vary depending on the age of the children, with more supervision, cleaning, and containment of allergen needed for younger children. Risk-taking behaviors among adolescents with food allergy, such as eating unsafe foods and delaying treatment of a reaction, are likely contributing factors to the observation that this age-group is at increased risk for fatal allergic reactions.[3,20] Therefore, peer and patient education is suggested to improve safety for adolescents.

Allergists can encourage parents to request to meet with key school staff members who have responsibility for the care of their child and to work cooperatively with schools to ensure their child's safety. Key staff members may include the school nurse, principal, directors of transportation and food service, and classroom teachers. Avoidance strategies and emergency management must also be communicated to personnel who may not have primary responsibilities for the student, such as coaches, specialty teachers (art, music), substitute teachers, and field trip personnel. These individuals should also be familiar with emergency plans, should be trained to use epinephrine autoinjectors, and should recognize indicators for activating the emergency medical response system.

It may be helpful to counsel parents about the degree and manner of exposure that might be dangerous for a specific child, such as ingestion versus inhalation or touching food residues, so that parents are appropriately vigilant without becoming needlessly hypervigilant or anxious about avoidance strategies. Care must be taken not to ostracize or physically separate the child with food allergies. For example, an "allergen-aware" table should include the child's friends who are eating safe meals. Experts have not espoused blanket "bans" on foods, particularly because peanut butter, milk, egg, and other common allergens may be a protein staple of another child's diet. In specific cases, individual schools or classrooms might pursue these options. For example, removal of highly allergenic foods from the vicinity of very young children or children with significant developmental disabilities might be warranted when transfer of the allergen among the children is likely. Schools may choose to ban children from bringing food from home to share with classmates for celebratory functions and may offer acceptable alternative options. Table 84-3 provides suggestions to reduce accidental ingestion of allergens.

Management of food allergy is similar for schools and camps. However, the persons providing supervision in camps may be young and inexperienced, necessitating additional safeguards, such as additional supervision at mealtimes or having more experienced supervisors available when away from first-aid and nursing services.

Nutritional Issues

Allergen avoidance diets can result in failure to thrive and deficiencies in specific macronutrients and micronutrients.[21] These concerns, in addition to the daily lifestyle impact of following avoidance diets, underscore the importance of having an accurate diagnosis to allow the broadest diet possible. Additionally, food aversion and anxiety may result in insufficient nutrient intake. Food allergy–related disorders such as eosinophilic esophagitis may be associated with poor appetite and early satiety, and children with untreated food allergy–related atopic dermatitis may experience malabsorption and increased energy needs from skin damage. Therefore, addressing nutritional concerns may require a multifaceted approach, including consultation with a registered dietitian. Nutritional counseling and regular growth monitoring are recommended for children with food allergies.[7]

TABLE 84-3 Preventive Measures to Reduce Risk of Allergen Ingestion in School Settings

Setting	Measures
School-wide	Institute policy on no food sharing or trading Educate teachers, including substitutes, coaches, special program teachers, and cafeteria staff. Consider allergen-safe cafeteria tables or schools, depending on student ages and needs (supervision, selective allergen exclusion) Enforce strict no-bullying policies.
Selected classroom	Allow no food in craft projects. Reduce food rewards, and provide a substitute. Maintain safe, nonperishable snacks as substitute, if needed. Consider "bans," depending on food (peanut) and age. Encourage handwashing.
School bus	Permit no eating or food parties. Have communication device for emergency calls. Allow younger child to sit at front.

Nutritional deficits caused by allergen-restricted diets include poor caloric intake (proteins, carbohydrates, fats) and insufficient vitamins, minerals, and trace elements. Many sources of protein, including milk, egg, soy, fish, shellfish, peanut, and tree nuts, are also common allergens. The *acceptable macronutrient distribution range* (AMDR) for protein is 5% to 20% for children 1 to 3 years of age, 10% to 30% for children 4 to 18 years of age, and 10% to 35% for adults. Quality proteins that include essential amino acids are typically obtained from meats. Complementary foods (e.g., rice, beans) may be needed for those who are vegetarian or meat allergic. The AMDR for fat is 25% to 35% of total energy intake for older children and adults (30% to 40% for children 1 to 3 years of age). Essential fatty acids (linoleic and linolenic) are found in fish. However, essential fatty acids are also available in vegetable oils such as canola, corn, soy, and olive. The diet should consist of a blend of saturated fats, which are usually obtained from animal origin, but also monosaturated and polyunsaturated fats, which are components of vegetable oils. The AMDR for carbohydrate is 45% to 65% of total caloric intake. Carbohydrates, particularly grains, contribute to dietary fiber, iron, thiamine, niacin, riboflavin, and folic acid. Micronutrients include vitamins, minerals and trace elements. The U.S. Department of Agriculture maintains documents regarding dietary recommendations via www.usda.gov or www.choosemyplate.gov. Table 84-4 describes nutritional concerns and possible solutions for diets devoid of some of the key common allergens.

EMERGENCY MANAGEMENT

The emergency management of food-induced anaphylaxis is similar to the treatment of anaphylaxis from any cause (see Chapter 77). Any food can potentially trigger anaphylaxis, but peanut, tree nuts, fish, shellfish, and milk appear to account for

TABLE 84-4 Nutritional Concerns and Substitutions for Diets Devoid of Select Allergens*

Allergen	Key Nutrients	Substitutions
Milk	Protein, fat, calcium, vitamin A, vitamin D, vitamin B_{12}.	Meats, fish, or poultry (protein, fat, vitamin B_{12}); fortified soy drinks (calcium, protein, vitamins D and B_{12}), legumes (protein), avocado (fat), enriched milks from rice, almond, oat or fortified juices (calcium; vitamins D, A, and B_{12}), dark-green leafy vegetables (vitamin A)†
Soy	Protein, thiamine, folate, magnesium, phosphorus, zinc, riboflavin, iron	Meat (protein, thiamine, phosphorous, iron); other legumes (protein, thiamine, folate, iron); fish (protein, phosphorous, iron); dark-green leafy vegetables (riboflavin, folate); whole grains (thiamine, riboflavin, folate, magnesium, iron); alternative fortified "milks" (see above)
Wheat	Carbohydrates, fiber, niacin, riboflavin, iron, folate	Enriched flours, including rice, oat, corn, and potato (carbohydrates, niacin, thiamine, riboflavin, iron, folate); fruits and vegetables (fiber, carbohydrates); meat (niacin, iron, thiamine); leafy green vegetables (riboflavin, folate)
Egg	Protein, vitamin B_{12}, selenium, biotin	Meat/fish (protein, vitamin B_{12}, selenium), soy (protein, biotin)

*This table cannot be used in isolation to construct adequate nutritional plans.

†Adults can obtain calcium and vitamin D from nondairy sources (fortified juices, alternative "milks" and supplements). However, infants and children require a replacement source of fat and protein and fortified juices or rice milk are otherwise insufficient; complete fortified nutritional formulas (soy, casein hydrolysates, amino acid based, etc.) may suffice, but children avoiding milk/soy may benefit from more complete dietary assessments. A diet devoid of egg, peanut, fish, or shellfish is typically easily substituted with other protein sources.

most of the episodes leading to fatalities.[2,3,20] Prompt recognition of anaphylaxis and treatment with epinephrine are crucial for a good outcome. In a study of 45 episodes of anaphylaxis in children, those who received epinephrine early were less likely to require hospital admission (14% vs. 47%, respectively; $P<.05$).[22] Box 84-1 lists risk factors for fatal food-induced anaphylaxis and comorbid conditions that increase risk.[2,3,7] The treatment of severe reactions caused by food protein–induced enterocolitis is different and involves intravenous hydration and corticosteroids, although proof for the efficacy of the latter is lacking.

Recognition of Reactions

Patients diagnosed with potentially severe food allergies, and their caretakers, must be educated regarding recognition of reactions. Signs, symptoms, and time course should be reviewed, as well as when and how to inject epinephrine and alert emergency services. Anaphylaxis caused by food allergy may occur without urticaria or skin symptoms in up to 20% of patients, which may account for delays in treatment leading to poor outcomes.[20] Additionally, biphasic reactions, with recurrence of symptoms several hours after resolution of initial reactions, are described in 1% to 20% of patients.[7] Given the possibility of biphasic reactions, victims of food-induced anaphylaxis should remain under medical observation for 4 to 6 hours or longer after anaphylaxis to ensure that symptoms have subsided.

BOX 84-1 RISKS FOR FATAL FOOD ANAPHYLAXIS AND COMORBID CONDITIONS

Risks Associated with Fatal Food Anaphylaxis

- Delayed treatment with epinephrine
- Allergy to peanut, tree nuts, fish, or shellfish
- Adolescent or young adult
- Asthma
- Cardiovascular disease in middle-aged or older patient
- Lack of skin symptoms

Comorbid Conditions Associated with Increased Food Anaphylaxis Risk or that Affect Severity or Treatment

- Asthma
- Mastocytosis
- Chronic lung disease
- Medications
  - β-Adrenergic antagonists
  - Angiotensin-converting enzyme (ACE) inhibitors
  - α-Adrenergic blockers

Treatment with Epinephrine and Antihistamines

Although antihistamines are indicated to treat symptoms such as urticaria or oral pruritus, dependence on antihistamines is a common reason for delaying anaphylaxis treatment with epinephrine,[23] which may result in an increased risk of a progressively severe reaction.[3,20] Patients and caregivers should be counseled on the appropriate use of self-injectable epinephrine and not to depend on antihistamines or bronchodilators for treatment of anaphylaxis. Repeated doses of epinephrine may be needed in 10% to 20% of episodes of food-induced anaphylaxis.[4] Prompt transfer to a facility capable of managing anaphylaxis should be sought. Patients and families should understand that although subsequent reactions are not necessarily more severe than initial reactions, they may be. For example, initial mild reactions to peanut may be followed by more severe reactions on subsequent exposures. Likewise, specific IgE levels do not predict the severity of a reaction. Epinephrine autoinjectors may be prescribed for anyone diagnosed with a food allergy but should be prescribed for patients with a prior history of anaphylaxis, those with food allergy and asthma, and those with a known food allergy to potent allergens such as peanut, tree nuts, fish, and shellfish.[7] In a survey of whether an epinephrine autoinjector is required for persons with pollen-food–related syndrome, of 122 allergists, 67% prescribed on a case-by-case basis depending on symptoms.[24]

Emergency Plans and Special Considerations for School

Patients with potentially severe food allergies should be given a written emergency plan that describes when to inject epinephrine and instructions on how to self-inject. The prescriptions of epinephrine, plans for monitoring expiration dates of autoinjectors, avoidance measures, and follow-up instructions are detailed in Chapter 77. Autoinjector dosing is limited because only two doses are available, but generally the 0.15-mg dose is recommended for children weighing 10 to 25 kg (22 to 55 lb) and the 0.3-mg dose for those over 25 kg.[7]

There are special considerations for treating children in schools or camps. The family must notify the school about the child's potentially life-threatening food allergy and provide written treatment plans, including the child's name, identifying information (child's picture, if provided), specifics about the food allergies, symptoms and treatments, instructions to activate emergency services, and medical and family contact information. In some circumstances, a child may be allowed to carry autoinjectors and to self-inject, but a supervising adult should have the primary responsibility to recognize and treat anaphylaxis. In the school setting, this is ideally a health professional, but a delegate might be needed. Epinephrine autoinjectors should be available promptly in the event of anaphylaxis. Children should be encouraged to wear medical identification jewelry.

Because 25% of anaphylaxis episodes in schools occur without a previous diagnosis,[25] a prescription for unassigned epinephrine for general use, consistent with district regulations and state laws, should be considered. When to inject epinephrine can be confusing for lay personnel. The safety of the drug should be emphasized such that injections should be given if there is suspicion of anaphylaxis. It may be advisable to inject epinephrine at the time of first symptoms if an allergen was ingested that previously caused anaphylaxis, or before symptoms if an allergen was ingested that previously caused anaphylaxis with cardiovascular collapse.[26]

Food Allergy Risk Factors and Prevention

Recent epidemiologic studies in the United Kingdom (UK) and North America suggest that prevalence rates of food allergy in children have increased (see Chapter 81). Food allergy prevention through allergen avoidance during pregnancy, breastfeeding, and infancy had been considered an effective public health policy to prevent allergies, although epidemiologic data to support this approach were minimal. However, allergen avoidance appears to have failed to reduce IgE-mediated food allergy. Studies that have identified risk factors for food allergy may inform better prevention strategies (Table 84-5). Other data suggest that early oral exposure leads to the induction of tolerance. Novel strategies to prevent food allergy in infants need to be tested in randomized controlled trials (RCTs).

TABLE 84-5 Changes in Notions about Allergy Prevention through Diet[7,59,60,84,89,90]

Prior Notion/ Recommendation (for those at risk for atopy)	Recent Notions/Recommendations
Avoid peanut during pregnancy.	No proof of effectiveness.
Avoid food allergens during lactation.	Possible reduction in atopic dermatitis, no evidence regarding food allergy.
Breastfeeding exclusively for 3-4 months.	May protect for atopy, but evidence is modest; lack of evidence for food allergy prevention.
Alternative hypoallergenic formulas.	May protect for atopy, but evidence is modest; lack of evidence for food allergy prevention.
Delay complementary foods until 4-6 months.	Lack of evidence to prevent atopic disease.
Avoid allergens: milk to age 1 year; egg to 2 years; and peanut, nuts, and fish to 3 years.	Early introduction of allergenic foods at 4-6 months may protect against development of food allergy, but firm evidence is lacking.

PREVALENCE OF FOOD ALLERGY

An understanding of risk factors for food allergy requires controlled studies on prevalence. Data suggest an increase in prevalence over the past 10 to 15 years.[1] The methodologic challenges to determining the correct prevalence of food allergy are discussed in Chapter 83. There are also geographic associations with food allergy. A validated questionnaire-based survey showed that the prevalence of peanut allergy was increased tenfold in Jewish children in the UK compared with Jewish children in Israel.[27] Furthermore, different patterns of immunologic reactivity to different component allergens within peanut have been observed in different countries.[28] These geographic differences could be caused by environmental differences such as patterns of allergen exposure or the preparation of food, but they could also result from genetic differences in geographically diverse groups. Du Toit and associates[27] suggest that differences in peanut allergy between the UK and Israel result from environmental rather than genetic factors.

HEREDITARY, GENETIC, AND MOLECULAR RISK FACTORS

Family History

A child has a sevenfold increase in the risk of peanut allergy if there is a parent or sibling with peanut allergy.[29] In monozygotic twins, a child has a 64% likelihood of peanut allergy if the twin sibling has peanut allergy.[30] Although it is unlikely that genetic risk factors could account for the recent increase in food allergy, it is likely that genetic factors may predispose to its development. The contribution of HLA background has not been carefully studied.

Gender

Several studies report that gender could be related to food allergy, particularly peanut and tree nut allergies. Sicherer and coworkers[31] found that the male/female ratio of peanut allergic children is almost 3:1; in adults the male/female ratio is less than 1. A cross-sectional study by questionnaire in more than 16,000 individuals found that prevalence of peanut allergy was significantly higher in young males under 4 years of age than in females; by adolescence the male/female ratio was equal; and during adulthood almost twice as many females had peanut allergy as males.[32] Thus a number of studies suggest a reversal in the male/female ratio for food allergy during and after adolescence, possibly mediated through endocrine changes.

Ethnicity

Utilizing specific IgE data from a large survey, Liu and associates[33] showed the risk of possible and likely food allergy was increased in non-Hispanic blacks (odds ratio [OR] 3.06; 95%

confidence interval [CI] 2.14 to 4.36) compared with white individuals. For example, the prevalence of likely food allergy to shrimp in non-Hispanic blacks was 2.3% versus 0.3% in non-Hispanic whites. Kumar and others[34] showed that black children were more likely to be sensitized to multiple foods than white children. As assessed by genetic ancestry informative markers, African ancestry is a notable risk factor for increased risk of peanut sensitization at levels associated with clinical reactivity.

These findings could result from a lack of recognition and diagnosis of symptoms or from differential access to health care in ethnic minorities. Studying the link between food allergy and ethnicity, Branum and associates[35] found that food allergy increased between 1997 and 2007 most significantly among Hispanic children, despite black non-Hispanic children having the highest rates of detectable IgE antibodies to food. Food allergen IgE levels were highest in non-Hispanic whites despite this population having the lowest prevalence of detectable IgE antibodies to foods. Whereas discrepancy between rates of reported clinical food allergy and rates of sensitization to foods can be explained by differential health care access in different communities, another explanation is that increased IgE levels to food is not indicative of food allergy but only indicates sensitization. Thus, increased levels of IgE found in certain ethnic groups may not reflect true food allergy and may only indicate sensitization. Few data exist on this issue, and community-based studies in different ethnic populations with oral food challenges are required to clarify the relationship among clinical reactivity, ethnicity, and immunoglobulin E.

Genetic Polymorphisms

Gene polymorphisms in interleukin-10 (IL-10)[36] and IL-13[37] have been identified in association with food allergy, but these studies will need to be replicated in different populations. Two single-nucleotide polymorphisms (SNPs) in the CD14 gene region have been studied in a population of 53 peanut-allergic individuals and 64 peanut-tolerant siblings.[38] Variations in the two important SNPs of CD14 (rs2569190 and rs2569193) were associated with the presence of peanut allergy.

More recent studies point to important gene-environment interactions in the development of food sensitization. In a prospective birth cohort study of 970 children, Hong and coworkers[39] showed that children who were ever breastfed (including exclusively breastfed children) were at 1.5 times higher risk of food sensitization than never-breastfed children. However, the association was altered by rs425648 in the IL-12 receptor β_1 gene (IL-12 rβ_1). Breastfeeding increased the risk of food sensitization in children carrying the GG genotype but significantly decreased the risk of food sensitization in breastfed infants carrying the GT/TT genotype. Similar interactions were observed for SNPs in the TSLP gene and the Toll-like receptor gene (TLR9).

Atopic Dermatitis and Filaggrin Loss-of-Function Mutations

Hill and Hosking[40] showed a greater frequency of sensitization and allergy to foods with increasing severity of atopic dermatitis (AD) and established a relative risk (RR) of 5.9 for IgE-mediated food allergy in an infant with severe eczema. Several recent studies have confirmed that loss-of-function mutations within the filaggrin (*FLG*) gene are associated with development of AD.[41,42] *FLG* was also studied as a candidate gene in the etiology of peanut allergy.[43] The six most prevalent *FLG* mutations were studied in these European groups. Loss-of-function mutations showed a significant association with peanut allergy (OR 5.3; CI 2.8 to 10.2). This association was closely replicated in a Canadian cohort in the same study. The association of *FLG* mutation with peanut allergy was highly significant ($P = .0008$) even after controlling for coexistent AD. This study indicates a role for epithelial barrier dysfunction in the pathogenesis of peanut allergy (see later).

CHANGES IN DIET

Changes in diet over the past decades and differences in macronutrient and micronutrient dietary content could explain the increase in allergies. There are four hypotheses related to this notion: obesity, dietary fat, antioxidants, and vitamin D.

Obesity

The coinciding trend in increasing atopy with increasing childhood obesity has been well studied, especially in the context of asthma. Obesity induces an inflammatory state associated with an increased risk of atopy and could theoretically lead to an increased risk for food allergy. Visness and associates[44] demonstrated that atopy (defined by any positive specific IgE measurement) was increased in obese compared with normal-weight children. This association was driven primarily by allergic sensitization to foods (OR for food sensitization = 1.59; 95% CI 1.28 to 1.98). Elevated C-reactive protein levels as a measure of inflammation were associated with total IgE levels, atopy, and food sensitization.

Dietary Fat

Data suggest that reduction in consumption of animal fats and corresponding increase in the use of margarine and vegetable oils has led to an increase in allergies. Advocates of this hypothesis argue that the consumption of omega-6 (ω-6) polyunsaturated fatty acids (e.g., linoleic acid) has increased, and through reduced consumption of oily fish, there has been a reduction in ω-3 polyunsaturated fatty acids (e.g., eicosapentaenoic acid).[45,46] ω-6 Fatty acids lead to the production of prostaglandin E_2 (PGE_2), whereas ω-3 fatty acids inhibit synthesis of PGE_2. PGE_2 reduces interferon-γ (IFN-γ) production by T lymphocytes, thus resulting in increased IgE production by B lymphocytes. A systematic review identified 10 reports satisfying inclusion criteria for a meta-analysis on the influence of ω-3 and ω-6 oils on allergic sensitization and concluded that "supplementation with Omega 3 and Omega 6 oils is unlikely to play an important role in the strategy for the primary prevention of sensitization or allergic disease."[47]

Antioxidants

The antioxidant hypothesis suggests that a decrease in consumption of fresh fruit and vegetables containing antioxidants might account for allergies. However, dietary trends are conflicting; the intake of some antioxidants has increased, and others have decreased. Epidemiologic, animal, molecular, and immunologic evidence suggests associations between antioxidants and asthma.[48] However, no such data are currently available for food allergy.

Vitamin D

Epidemiologic data suggest that excessive vitamin D or vitamin D deficiency results in increased allergies. The first observations derived from farming communities in Germany, where less vitamin D supplementation was used in foods and a lower prevalence of allergies in children was found. Allergies increased coinciding with vitamin D supplementation intervention programs to prevent rickets in childhood.[49] Likewise, two independent cohort studies showed that infants who had vitamin D supplementation were at increased risk of food allergy.[50,51]

Conversely, the vitamin D deficiency hypothesis argues that inadequate vitamin D (associated with more time indoors and lack of sunlight) is responsible for the increase in allergies. Camargo and coworkers[52] found a strong north-south gradient for EpiPen (Dey, Napa, Calif.) prescriptions in the United States. Vassallo and associates[53] showed that season of birth is a risk factor for food allergy and that infants born during the winter had a higher risk of developing food allergy. Nwaru and others[54] found that maternal intake of vitamin D during pregnancy was associated with a decreased risk of food sensitization.

HYGIENE HYPOTHESIS

The hygiene hypothesis proposes that the lack of early childhood exposure to infectious agents, gut flora, and parasites increases susceptibility to allergic diseases by modulating immune system development. Limited data for the hygiene hypothesis exist with respect to food allergy.

A Norwegian birth cohort study found that cesarean birth was associated with a sevenfold increased risk of perceived reactions to eggs, fish, or nuts.[55] A meta-analysis found six studies that showed cesarean delivery mildly increased the risk of food allergy or food atopy (OR 1.32; 95% CI 1.12 to 0.55).[56] However, in a study evaluating 503 infants, the mode of delivery at birth bore no relationship to sensitisation or food allergy.[57]

Early colonization of the infant by colonic microflora could protect against the development of allergic disease. Such observations have led to strategies to alter commensal gut flora through administration of either probiotics or prebiotics. Although some studies of probiotics reported some protective effect against development of eczema, no reduction in food sensitization was shown.[58]

EXPOSURE TO FOOD ALLERGENS

Important questions remain about exposure to food allergens in the maternal and infant diet. Until 2008, the American Academy of Pediatrics (AAP) recommended that infants whose family history placed them at increased risk of atopy should avoid peanuts through their first three birthdays and common food allergens until the first (milk), second (egg), or third (tree nuts and fish) birthdays.[59] According to these recommendations, mothers should avoid peanuts during pregnancy and breastfeeding and additional allergens during lactation. In the UK, similar recommendations were in place with respect to peanut avoidance; however, these recommendations were withdrawn in the United States[60] and in the UK.[61]

Evidence on which to base advice for weaning infants is lacking. The World Health Organization (WHO) strategy to prevent allergy is to promote exclusive breastfeeding during the first 6 months of the infant's life to delay weaning onto solids.[62] However, there is no convincing evidence that exclusive breastfeeding beyond 4 months of age has any effect on reducing atopic disease. Observational cohort studies show that breastfeeding[63] and prolonged breastfeeding[64] are associated with an increased risk of asthma and eczema. Although such studies do not eliminate the possibility of *reverse causality* (high-risk infants with eczema are deliberately breastfed longer), they raise the question as to whether exposure to solids in infancy could prevent food allergy.

Although some evidence suggests that breastfeeding for 3 to 4 months compared with formula feeding may prevent the occurrence of AD and wheezing in childhood, evidence is conflicting as to whether this prevents the development of cow's milk or other food allergies. Since a large proportion of infants are not exclusively breastfed in the first 3 to 4 months of life (with large geographic and societal variations), there has been interest in whether extensively hydrolyzed milk formula or non–cow's milk–based formulas (e.g., soy or rice formula) may prevent the development of allergic disease. Most of these studies have concentrated on AD and asthma, and food allergy has not been carefully delineated as an end point. A Cochrane review concluded that "there is limited evidence that prolonged feeding with a hydrolysed formula compared to a cow's milk formula reduces infant and childhood cow's milk allergy."[65] However, a large prospective randomized interventional study found that different hydrolyzed formula (especially extensively hydrolyzed casein formula) reduced the incidence of AD at 36 months of age in a high-risk group of infants.[66] This study did not include food allergy as a specific end point. There is a lack of evidence that early consumption of soy formula prevents the development of food allergy in high-risk or normal populations.[60]

Food Allergen Exposure Revisited

Studies eliminating food allergens during pregnancy, lactation, and infancy have consistently failed to reduce long-term IgE-mediated food allergy in children.[67] Three possible explanations for this failure exist. First, allergen reduction measures have not been sufficient in previous studies, and dietary elimination was not sufficiently stringent. Although plausible, it seems unlikely that "complete" allergen avoidance could successfully prevent food allergy as a public health measure; despite rigorous dietary supervision, meticulous elimination studies have failed to achieve a reduction in food allergy.[67,68] Second, food sensitization does not occur because of consumption but through other routes of exposure. This is supported by a number of murine studies showing that allergic sensitization to antigen occurs after cutaneous exposure and has been suggested in recent clinical studies. Third, the paradigm of allergen avoidance is flawed; animal data and some observational clinical data support early oral exposure as a means of preventing the development of allergy.

Dual-Allergen Exposure Hypothesis

The view that allergic sensitization to food occurs through oral exposure and that prevention of food allergy is best accomplished through elimination diets has been questioned. It is proposed that allergic sensitization to food can occur through low-dose cutaneous sensitization and that early consumption of food protein induces oral tolerance. The timing and balance of cutaneous and oral exposure determine whether a child develops allergy or tolerance (Fig. 84-1).

Data Suggesting Cutaneous Sensitization. The molecular basis for the increased skin permeability in eczema is the loss of function or null mutations in the gene encoding for filaggrin.

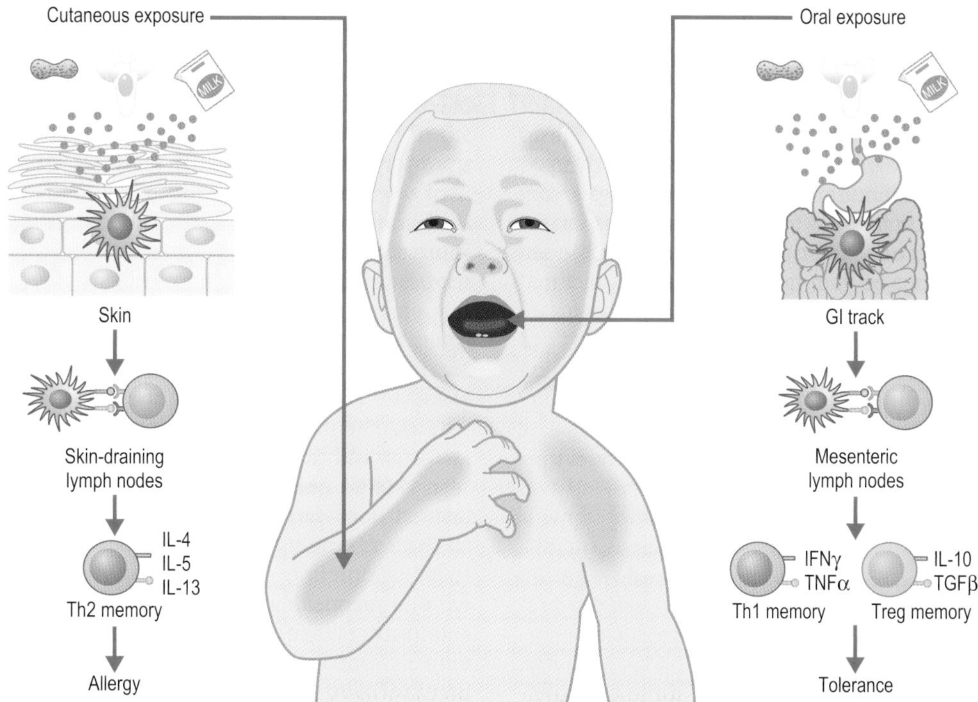

Figure 84-1 Dual-allergen-exposure hypothesis for pathogenesis of food allergy. Tolerance occurs as a result of oral exposure to food, and allergic sensitization results from cutaneous exposure. *GI*, Gastrointestinal; *IFN-γ*, interferon-γ; *TGF-β*, transforming growth factor beta; *Th2*, T helper type 2 lymphocyte; *TNF-α*, tumor necrosis factor alpha; *Treg*, T regulatory lymphocyte. *(Modified from Lack G. Epidemiologic risks of food allergy. J Allergy Clin Immunol 2008;121:1331-6.)*

This protein is important for epidermal differentiation, desquamation, and barrier function and has been recognized as the strongest genetic contributor to eczema.[69-72] Filaggrin protein deficiency is also associated with increased transepidermal water loss, and this measurable functional impairment of the skin barrier precedes development of eczema.[73]

In different studies, 14% to 56% of cases of eczema carry one or more *FLG* null mutations, and the presence of a *FLG* null allele represents a 1.2- to 13-fold increased risk of developing AD.[74] Low-dose exposure to environmental food proteins on tabletops, hands, and dust may occur.[15] Such proteins can penetrate the disrupted skin barrier and are taken up by Langerhans cells, which leads to helper T cell type 2 (Th2) responses and IgE.[69] This may explain the association between the presence of early eczema in infancy and subsequent development of food allergy and also different rates of food allergy in different countries and changes in food allergy over time. Thus, one would expect to see allergic sensitization in communities where infants avoid peanut consumption despite high overall consumption of peanut and its presence in the environment (UK, United States, Canada, Australia). In countries where consumption and consequently environmental exposure are high, but where infants eat peanut regularly, one would not expect to see peanut allergy (southern and western Africa, Asia).

In animal models, exposure of mice to ovalbumin or peanut on abraded skin leads to significant specific IgE responses.[75,76] Food allergy to hen egg ovalbumin (OVA) was demonstrated in a murine model for loss-of-function mutations in the *FLG* gene.[41] Topical application of the allergen OVA in these flaky-tailed mice resulted in cutaneous inflammatory infiltrates and sensitization, as measured by specific IgE to OVA. Wild-type mice did not have elevated levels of total serum IgE and did not generate a specific IgE or IgG response to OVA. This model is distinct from other models of murine cutaneous exposure with normal *FLG* expression. In flaky-tailed mice, application of allergen to the skin results in an allergen specific IgE response without any pre-existing cutaneous inflammation or abrasion. This provides strong evidence that filaggrin protein deficiency and consequent skin barrier dysfunction is sufficient to allow cutaneous penetration of allergen and the development of sensitization.

In human subjects in a prospective birth cohort study, low-dose exposure to peanut in the form of arachis oil applied to inflamed skin on infants was associated with increased risk of peanut allergy at age 5 years.[77] A cross-sectional study evaluating the relevant route of peanut exposure in the development of allergy used a questionnaire to determine maternal peanut consumption during pregnancy, breastfeeding, and the first year of life, as well as peanut consumption among all household members.[78] The median weekly household peanut consumption in the peanut allergic cases was significantly elevated (18.8 g; $n = 133$) compared with controls without allergy (6.9 g; $n = 150$) and high-risk controls (1.9 g; $n = 160$) ($P < .0001$). A dose-response relationship was observed between environmental (nonoral) peanut exposure and the development of peanut allergy. These findings suggest that high levels of environmental exposure to peanut during infancy may promote sensitization, whereas low levels appear protective in atopic children. Early oral exposure to peanut in infants with high environmental peanut exposure may have had a protective effect against the development of peanut allergy. This supports the hypothesis that peanut sensitization occurs as a result of environmental exposure.

Data Suggesting Oral Tolerance. Numerous studies have demonstrated that early high-dose oral exposure confers clinical and immunologic tolerance to food allergens. In murine models a single oral dose of allergen (β-lactoglobulin, OVA, or peanut) is sufficient to achieve tolerance and prevent subsequent allergic sensitization.[79-81] In human subjects, oral exposure to nickel through orthodontic braces before ear piercing protects against nickel allergy.[82,83] Conversely, delaying initial exposure to cereal grain until after 6 months of life has been associated with an increased risk of IgE-mediated food allergy.[84]

In Western societies that avoid peanuts during pregnancy and infancy, the rate of peanut allergy is relatively high.[85] In regions where peanut is consumed in high amounts during infancy (Middle East, Southeast Asia, and Africa), peanut allergy is reportedly rare.[86-88] In a recent cross-sectional study among Israeli ($n = 5615$) and UK ($n = 5171$) Jewish children, the prevalence of PA was tenfold higher in the UK (1.85%) than in Israel (0.17%) ($P < .001$).[27] This study also found that peanut is introduced earlier and is eaten more frequently and in larger quantities in Israel than in the UK. These findings raise the question of whether early introduction of peanut during infancy prevents the development of peanut allergy. Two recent observational cohort studies demonstrated an association between oral exposure to cow's milk in the first two weeks of life and tolerance to milk,[89] and in an Australian cohort study[90] introduction of egg before six months of age appeared to protect against egg allergy, even after controlling for confounding variables.

The immune response to peanut in peanut allergic children is seen primarily in the cutaneous lymphocyte antigen (CLA) skin-homing memory T lymphocyte population and not in the $\alpha_4\beta_7$ gut-homing lymphocytes; conversely, peanut-tolerant patients have a mixed CLA/$\alpha_4\beta_7$ response to peanut antigen.[91] The observation that the CLA-positive memory T lymphocyte population was activated by peanut in the peanut-allergic patients was not influenced by the presence of AD and was allergen specific. Although these data are consistent with the dual-allergen exposure hypothesis, there are no direct clinical data to support it.

TRIALS USING ORAL TOLERANCE INDUCTION TO PREVENT FOOD ALLERGIES

Some theories suggest that early introduction of foods such as peanut or egg leads to tolerance and protects against developing food allergy. These theories are being tested in two RCTs. The LEAP Study (Learning Early About Peanut Allergy, www.leapstudy.co.uk) includes 640 high-risk children who were enrolled at age 4 to 11 months. Each child was randomized to an avoidance group (complete avoidance of peanut-containing foods) or a consumption group (consume a peanut snack three times a week; 6 g of peanut protein/wk). The proportion of each group that develops peanut allergy by 5 years of age will be compared to determine which approach best prevents peanut allergy. The study will reach completion in 2013.

The EAT Study (Enquiring About Tolerance, www.eatstudy.co.uk) is researching the effect of early introduction of complementary foods with breastfeeding. Infants ($n = 1302$) are randomized to one of two groups. In one group ($n = 651$), six allergenic foods are introduced from 3 months of age while the infant continues to breastfeed (early introduction group). The other group ($n = 651$) follows current UK government weaning advice: aim for exclusive breastfeeding for 6 months (standard weaning group). The children will be monitored until 3 years of age to see whether early diet has an effect in reducing the prevalence of food allergy, as determined by double-blind, placebo-controlled food challenges.

ADDITIONAL CHALLENGES FOR IDENTIFYING PREVENTION STRATEGIES

Interventional studies have an advantage over observational studies in determining the role of early food and micronutrient exposure in the development of allergies. RCTs represent the "gold standard" of clinical medicine, especially when findings are replicated and shown to be consistent in meta-analyses. However, positive RCTs are easier to interpret than negative studies. The pathogenesis of food allergy is likely to be multifactorial, and the induction of oral tolerance likely depends on several conditions. Exposure to food proteins in the gastrointestinal (GI) tract may require an optimal microenvironment to meet the necessary conditions for induction of tolerance, such as immune factors (e.g., cytokines, antibodies, Tregs) whose function may depend on vitamin D, as well as bacterial colonization. Thus, in animal models, oral tolerance induction with a single dose of food protein protects against the development of allergies. However, oral tolerance cannot be induced in germ-free mice; tolerance requires the presence of both intestinal microflora and food antigen.[92] Each factor is necessary, but neither is sufficient for the development of tolerance. For example, if foods or micronutrients are introduced into the diet of young Western infants with reduced microbial exposure, no effect may be seen, but caution is needed before concluding causal irrelevance. A Western-urban lifestyle is associated with numerous changes in the way foods are presented to young infants. It may be important that food allergens be presented to the GI tract in the context of breast milk, which contains numerous immunomodulatory factors.[93]

Future Therapeutic Strategies

The apparent rising prevalence of food allergies, lack of effective prevention strategies, and inadequate treatment that relies on allergen avoidance and injection of epinephrine for anaphylaxis have considerably increased the urgency to develop effective treatments. Both allergen-specific therapies and more generalized immunomodulatory approaches are under investigation in animal and human models of food allergy.

Because it is important to delineate the responses to therapeutic interventions, the terms *desensitization* and *tolerance* are often used to better define the clinical and immunologic state during therapy. Desensitization refers to a change in threshold dose of ingested allergen required to induce allergic symptoms after food exposure occurring while on therapy. This is a reversible state typically induced by allergen exposure, in which effector cells are rendered less reactive or nonreactive by administration of allergen. In contrast, tolerance refers to the long-lasting effects of treatment, presumably due to effects on T cell responsiveness that persist after the treatment is stopped. The immunomodulatory effects of desensitization can be seen early in the course of immunotherapy; however, evidence suggests that the length of time to reach tolerance varies with the type and amount of specific allergen, the duration of therapy, and the individual patient. The overall goal of effective immunotherapy is long-term tolerance induction through active

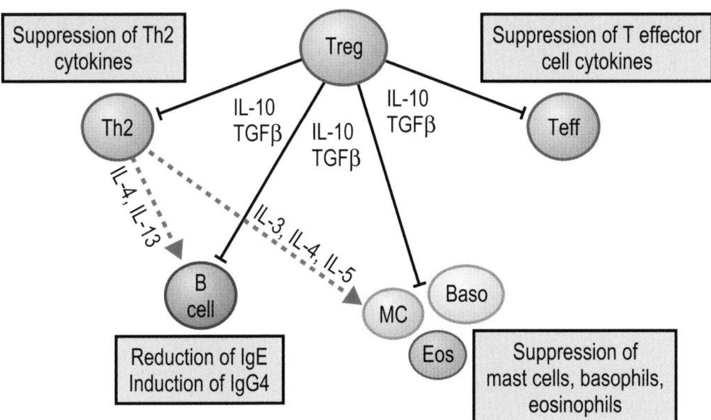

Figure 84-2 Food allergy treatments modulate the food allergic response through activation of regulatory T cells and suppression of a variety of effector cell types. *Baso,* Basophil; *Eos,* eosinophil; *IL,* interleukin; *MC,* mast cell; *Teff,* T effector lymphocyte; *TGF-β,* transforming growth factor beta; *Th2,* T helper type 2 lymphocyte; *Treg,* T regulatory lymphocyte.

immunomodulation to promote regulatory T cell development and immunologic skewing away from the classic Th2 response seen with many of the emerging therapies (Fig. 84-2).

TRADITIONAL IMMUNOTHERAPY AND NEED FOR ALTERNATIVES

Traditional subcutaneous immunotherapy (SCIT) has proved highly effective in patients with IgE-mediated respiratory disease and insect sting allergy, and it represents the only routinely administered antigen-specific immunotherapy prescribed for allergic disease.[94] SCIT for food allergy was first used at the beginning of the 20th century. Subsequent studies have brought the utility and safety of SCIT for food allergy into question. Although some evidence for decreased clinical responsiveness has been demonstrated in studies using SCIT for peanut allergy, an unacceptably high rate of systemic reactions prevented further development of this therapy.[95,96]

Because SCIT has proven unsafe for the treatment of food allergy, novel immunotherapeutic strategies designed to alter the immune response to food allergens are currently under investigation. Strategies include allergen-nonspecific and allergen-specific immunotherapy (Table 84-6). The remainder of this chapter examines the current evidence base for these emerging therapies, which primarily target IgE-mediated food allergy. These therapies are currently investigational but hold great promise for the future.

TABLE 84-6 Emerging Therapies for Food Allergy*

Therapy	Use	Stage of Study	Allergen Studied
ALLERGEN-NONSPECIFIC THERAPY			
Anti-IgE therapy	Treatment	Human phase I-II	Peanut, milk
Traditional Chinese medicine	Treatment	Human phase I-II	Peanut, tree nut, fish, shellfish, sesame
Probiotics	Prevention	Longitudinal study	Nonspecific
Prebiotics	Prevention	Longitudinal study	Nonspecific
Trichuris suis egg therapy	Treatment	Preclinical	Peanut
Lactococcus lactis expressing IL-10 or IL-12	Treatment	Preclinical	Milk
Toll-like receptor 9	Treatment	Preclinical	Peanut
ALLERGEN-SPECIFIC THERAPY			
Subcutaneous IT	Treatment	Human phase I (aborted due to safety)	Peanut
Oral IT	Treatment	Human phase I-III	Peanut, milk, egg, fish, fruits
Heated antigen	Treatment	Human phase I-II	Egg, milk
Sublingual IT	Treatment	Human phase I-II	Peanut, milk, hazelnut, kiwi, peach
Epicutaneous IT	Treatment	Human phase I-II	Peanut, milk
Recombinant protein IT with adjuvants	Treatment	Human phase I	Peanut
Recombinant protein IT	Treatment	Preclinical	Peanut
Plasmid DNA IT	Treatment	Preclinical	Peanut
Peptide IT	Treatment	Preclinical	Peanut, egg
ISS-ODN IT	Treatment	Preclinical	Peanut
Human Fc-FC fusion proteins	Treatment	Preclinical	Peanut
Engineered allergen	Treatment	Preclinical	Egg, peanut, milk, fish, fruits
Mannoside-conjugated BSA	Treatment	Preclinical	BSA
Antigen-fixed leukocytes	Treatment	Preclinical	Peanut

IL, Interleukin; *IT,* immunotherapy.
*For detailed information on clinical trials, see clinicaltrials.gov.

ALLERGEN-NONSPECIFIC THERAPIES

Allergen-nonspecific therapies are designed to have a global impact on the immune response. The therapies discussed may have clinical utility as monotherapies or as adjuncts to allergen-specific immunotherapy to enhance the immune response or improve safety.

Humanized Monoclonal Anti-IgE

The development of monoclonal anti-IgE antibodies was at the forefront of biologic therapies for allergic disease. Omalizumab, a recombinant, humanized, monoclonal anti-IgE antibody is approved by the U.S. Food and Drug Administration (FDA) for the treatment of allergic asthma and has demonstrated efficacy when used with "rush" immunotherapy for allergic rhinitis[97] and as adjunctive therapy to minimize systemic immunotherapy reactions in patients with allergic asthma.[98] Anti-IgE therapy has been used in two clinical trials for peanut allergy. In the first, the antibody Hu-901 led to a mean increase in reaction threshold to peanut during oral food challenge (OFC) of 2627 mg in the highest-dose group.[99] However, about 25% of participants were nonresponders. The second, multicenter RCT using omalizumab to treat peanut allergy was initiated in 26 subjects but was stopped prematurely because of safety issues during OFC.[100] Only 14 subjects randomized to receive omalizumab (0.016 mg/kg/IgE [IU/mL]) or placebo every 2 to 4 weeks for 20 to 22 weeks completed the study and had follow-up OFC. Tolerability to 1000 mg or more of peanut flour occurred more often in omalizumab-treated subjects (44%) than placebo-treated subjects (20%), but 55.6% and 80% in each group, respectively, did not achieve the prespecified tolerability (≥1000 mg) during OFC. Clinical trials are in progress to evaluate anti-IgE as a monotherapy or as an adjunct to oral immunotherapy.[101]

Traditional Chinese Medicine

The health benefits of traditional Chinese medicine (TCM), a component of which includes herbal therapies, have been anecdotally reported for generations. To evaluate scientifically the impact of herbal medications on food allergy responses, experiments were conducted in a mouse model of peanut allergy.[102,103] The herbal formula FAHF-2 was developed as a formulation of nine Chinese herbs. In preclinical studies, FAHF-2 blocked peanut-induced anaphylaxis during and after the development peanut hypersensitivity, with effectiveness sustained for up to 6 months after therapy. Suppression of allergic symptoms correlated with immunologic changes of reduced specific IgE, basophil, mast cell, and Th2 cytokine responses and increased specific IgG2 responses, which are thought to be mediated via $CD8^+$ T cells activation and IFN-γ.[104] During a subsequent phase I study,[105] subjects received FAHF-2 tablets or placebo three times daily for 1 week. FAHF-2 treatment was well tolerated (minor GI symptoms in 2/19 subjects) and led to reductions in IL-5 levels, which suggests immunomodulation occurred. A phase II clinical trial is in progress.

Probiotics and Prebiotics

Probiotics are ingested, live, health-promoting microbes that modify intestinal microbial populations to benefit the host. Probiotic dietary supplements, typically with *Lactobacillus* and *Bifidobacterium* species, have been used in clinical trials to evaluate the preventive impact on atopic disease and the impact on active disease. The immunomodulatory effects of probiotics may include increased synthesis of IgA and IL-10, with reciprocal suppression of tumor necrosis factor alpha (TNF-α) and other inflammatory cytokines, inhibition of allergen-induced T cell activation, activation of regulatory T cells (Tregs), and enhanced Toll-like receptor 4 (TLR4) signaling.[106]

In murine models, probiotics have shown immunomodulatory effects associated with protection from respiratory and oral allergy.[107] However, the use of probiotics in clinical trials has not been associated with strong, long-term preventive or treatment effects on atopy. In a study of 112 pregnant women, probiotics were ingested from 4 to 8 weeks prenatally through 6 months postnatally. Infants from the treatment group had reduced eczema compared with controls (36.4% vs. 62.9%; $P = 0.029$) at 12 months, but there were no differences in total IgE levels or sensitization to food allergens.[108] Similar findings were reported in two additional longitudinal prevention studies.[109,110] In a study of probiotics for treatment, 131 children age 6 to 24 months with at least two episodes of wheezing and a family history of atopy were treated with 6 months of probiotic therapy or placebo. No differences were seen in atopic disease events, but active treatment was associated with sensitization to fewer aeroallergens.[111]

Prebiotics are oligosaccharides that promote probiotic colonization of the GI tract. In a trial of 830 infants at low risk for atopy, reduced prevalence of AD at year 1 was reported among prebiotic-treated subjects versus controls (5.7% vs. 9.7%; $P = 0.04$).[112] In another study of 134 infants with parental atopy, infants randomized to 6 months of placebo-supplemented formula showed higher incidence for AD, wheezing, and urticaria (27.9%, 20.6%, and 10.3%, respectively) than those randomized to prebiotic-supplemented formula (13.6%, 7.6%, and 1.5%) ($P < .05$).[113]

Other allergen-nonspecific therapies, such as *Lactococcus lactis* supplementation and TLR9 agonists, have shown some benefit in allergic animal models, but no clinical trials have been conducted for food allergy to date.[6] *Trichuris suis* egg therapy has shown benefit in clinical trials for autoimmune disorders such as Crohn disease, ulcerative colitis, and multiple sclerosis and in a murine model of food allergy. Side effects have limited the overall benefit for allergic disease to date.[6]

ALLERGEN-SPECIFIC IMMUNOTHERAPY

Because allergen-specific immunotherapy is directed at a specific allergen-driven response, these therapies offer a focused target and should be associated with significant immunomodulation (Table 84-7).

Oral Immunotherapy

Oral immunotherapy (OIT) has been studied for several years in clinical trials and has the largest evidence base for effectiveness among emerging therapies for food allergy. Although still investigational, OIT is associated with a robust response to therapy, but with limitations related to side effect profiles. Early open-label trials have shown a beneficial response to OIT with a variety of allergens, including milk, egg, and fish, with evidence of clinical desensitization in up to 80% of patients treated.[114,115]

The concepts of clinical desensitization and tolerance have been more fully explored in recent studies. Current OIT protocols are typically conducted using an allergen flour ingested in a food vehicle and consist of the following three phases:

1. Modified rush desensitization, with 6 to 8 doses of allergen given under observation in rapid succession during day 1 to obtain a relative "desensitized state."

TABLE 84-7 Immunologic Changes in IgE-mediated Food Allergy Compared with Effective Immunotherapy

Immune Parameters	Food Allergy	Effective Immunotherapy
Serum IgE	↑	↓
Serum IgG4	↔	↑
Mast cell reactivity	↑	↓
Basophil activation	↑	↓
Helper T cell (Th2) cytokines	↑	↓
Regulatory T cell activation	↓	↑

2. Dosing buildup, with a daily dose of the food protein at home with scheduled dose escalations under observation every 1 to 2 weeks until a target dose is reached.
3. Home maintenance therapy, with daily ingestion of a target dose (typically for years).

These phases are usually followed by OFC to assess clinical desensitization (while receiving therapy) and functional tolerance (while off therapy on diet restriction). Clinical desensitization has been well documented in open-label studies for peanut,[116-118] milk,[119,120] and egg,[121,122] with success rates ranging from 75% to 100% after 1 to 2 years of therapy. Desensitization has been associated with immunomodulation with reduced markers of mast cell (skin tests) and basophil activation, changes in IgE and IgG profiles, reduced Th2 cytokine profile, and activation of Tregs.

Results from recent multicenter RCTs have confirmed OIT may be a successful approach.[123-125] In a peanut allergy study, 28 children (ages 1 to 16 years) were randomized to receive peanut OIT (target dose of 4000 mg) versus placebo OIT during 1 year of therapy.[123] Active OIT ($n = 16$ children) was associated with increased peanut protein consumption compared with placebo OIT ($n = 9$) at the 12-month OFC (5000 vs. 280 mg; $P < .001$). The peanut OIT group showed decreased skin prick test (SPT) size ($P < .001$), IL-5 ($P = .01$) and IL-13 ($P = .02$) and increased peanut-specific IgG4 ($P < .001$) and Tregs ($P = .04$). Specific-IgE increased initially ($P < .01$) but showed only a trend toward reduction after 12 months. Similar findings were noted during a trial of milk OIT in 20 milk-allergic children (ages 6 to 21 years) randomized to milk OIT (target dose of 500 mg in 12 children) versus placebo OIT (7 children) for about 6 months of therapy.[124] After OIT, the change in milk reaction threshold was 5100 mg in the OIT group ($P = .002$) compared with no change in the placebo group ($P = .16$). During open-label extension, 13 subjects further increased their dosing to 7000 mg of daily milk over 13 to 75 weeks.[126] Median milk-specific IgE decreased (29.9 kUa/L to 11.9 kUa/L; $P = .0355$), and milk-specific IgG4 increased (3.9 μg/mL to 101.3 μg/mL; $P = .001$).

In a Consortium of Food Allergy Research (CoFAR) study, 55 egg-allergic children (ages 5 to 18 years) were randomized to egg OIT versus placebo for 2 years (with placebo crossover after month 10), with desensitization OFC performed at 10 and 22 months.[125] None of the placebo-treated subjects versus 55% of egg OIT-treated subjects passed the 5-g OFC at 10 months ($P < .001$); median consumed dose was 5000 mg with egg OIT versus 250 mg with placebo. Further desensitization was noted after 22 months, with 75% of subjects passing a 10,000-mg OFC. Desensitization was associated with changes from baseline in the egg OIT group, such as decreased egg-specific IgE by 10 months ($P = .02$), increased egg-specific IgG4 ($P = .005$), reduced basophil activation ($P = .04$), and reduced SPT size at month 22 ($P = .009$).

These studies highlight the efficacy of allergen-specific OIT in inducing clinical desensitization and treatment-specific immunomodulation.

The prevailing question is whether OIT induces *tolerance*, not just desensitization. Long-lasting tolerance has not been evaluated in any study to date; however, several studies have evaluated short-term tolerance through a more functional definition of tolerance as tested by OFC 4 to 8 weeks after cessation of therapy.[120,122,125] These assessments have provided evidence for functional tolerance induction in a subpopulation of subjects. In an open-label study of six egg-allergic children (ages 3 to 13 years), OIT dosing and duration were determined by individual egg-IgE level.[122] After 33 months of OIT and a median dose of 2400 mg, all six children passed a tolerance OFC and introduced egg into their diet. Similarly, after 33 to 70 months of peanut OIT (maintenance dose = 2000 to 4000 mg), 11 of 19 participants (58%) passed a tolerance OFC (personal communication, AW Burks and SM Jones, June 2012). All had decreased specific-IgE ($P = .0001$) and SPT ($P = .02$) with increased specific IgG4 ($P = .0001$) relative to baseline.

In a trial comparing milk sublingual immunotherapy (SLIT) versus SLIT plus OIT over 60 weeks, investigators found a more robust response in OIT-treated subjects.[120] Tolerance OFCs were performed after 1 and 6 weeks off therapy in subjects demonstrating desensitization at week 60. Of SLIT/OIT subjects, 10% failed the tolerance OFC at 1 week, and 20% failed the tolerance OFC at 6 weeks. Eight of SLIT/OIT treatment subjects (40%) demonstrated tolerance associated with immunomodulation. In the COFAR egg OIT trial, 11 of 40 (27.5%) children passed a tolerance OFC after 4 to 6 weeks off therapy at 24 months[125] and continued egg ad libitum through 30 to 36 months. Of the immune markers measured, small SPT size and increases in egg-specific IgG4 levels were associated with sustained unresponsiveness.

In combination, the results from several studies suggest functional tolerance induction is possible in at least a portion of participants; however, further study is needed to determine the duration of tolerance and the persistence of immunomodulation.

Clinical trials using OIT have focused primarily on single-allergen delivery to impact single-food allergy. In a multisensitized mouse model of tree nut allergy, OIT with a single tree nut had efficacy in causing desensitization to multiple tree nuts.[127] Clinical studies are ongoing to evaluate this approach and OIT with multiple allergens.

Although OIT has demonstrated significant clinical successes, safety remains a concern for wide-scale implementation. OIT trials have been conducted through study protocols under close monitoring by experienced research staff in clinical research centers with necessary rescue equipment/procedures in place. Generally, side effects are mild to moderate, predominantly oropharyngeal, and easily treated.[117,123-125,128] However, more severe reactions have been reported, including generalized urticaria/angioedema, wheezing/respiratory distress, laryngeal edema, and repetitive emesis.

In the first wide-scale safety report of OIT for peanut allergy, investigators reported symptoms in 93% of participants during initial escalation (maximum 50 mg), in 46% during buildup, and in 3.5% during home dosing (300 mg).[128] Treatment was given in 0.7% of home doses, and epinephrine was administered to two subjects during home dosing. In a follow-up study by the same group, two subjects withdrew during initial escalation (maximum 6 mg) and 47% experienced side effects requiring antihistamines; two events required epinephrine.[123] Symptoms were noted after 1.2% of 407 buildup doses. Sixteen of 19 active OIT subjects reached a daily 4000-mg maintenance dose with minimal side effects. Similarly, in the milk OIT study, 45.4% of OIT doses versus 11.2% of placebo doses were associated with clinical reactions, most of which were mild and oropharyngeal.[124] Epinephrine was administered after 4 doses. In a recent egg OIT study, 75% of 11,860 OIT doses during year 1 were symptom free versus 96% of 4018 placebo doses.[125]

Of participants treated with OIT, about 20% experienced dose-limiting GI side effects, preventing continuation of therapy.[129] Viral infections, menses, and exercise have been associated with lowering the reaction threshold for subjects receiving stable OIT dosing.[130] These further complicate the risk of current dosing regimens and often require dose adjustments to compensate for illness.[117] The implementation of rush OIT protocols, designed to shorten the interval to maintenance therapy, has been associated with increased adverse symptoms in milk OIT[119,131] and peanut OIT.[117] Pretreatment with omalizumab before and during OIT reduced side effects (mean frequency for all reactions = 1.6%) and reduced the time to the 2000-mg daily dose (7 to 11 weeks) in a pilot study of 11 milk-allergic subjects.[101] One subject withdrew from treatment. Nine of 10 subjects reached 1000 mg on day 1 and 9 of 10 reached 2000 mg after 7 to 11 weeks. One participant received epinephrine during rush OIT.

Additional studies are needed to improve the safety profile before OIT can be sanctioned for widespread use.

Extensively Heated Milk and Egg Protein. A possible alternative or treatment adjunct to OIT is the use of crude, heated allergen. Because high-temperature cooking of egg and milk proteins results in conformational changes of native protein structure and reduced IgE binding, some children with milk or egg allergy may tolerate baked products.

Two clinical trials have been conducted in milk-allergic[132] and egg-allergic[133] children. The results suggest that up to 80% of milk-allergic or egg-allergic children can safely ingest extensively heated milk products in a muffin or egg products in a waffle. OFC was done to confirm the allergy and ability to tolerate the baked product. Children able to consume 1 to 3 servings of heated product daily were noted to experience accelerated tolerance development[10] compared with an age-matched allergic cohort. Side effects were negligible, and no subjects who tolerated the baked product required epinephrine during OFC, although 35% of baked milk-reactive subjects and 19% of baked egg-reactive subjects did. Clinical successes were associated with reduced specific IgE and SPT, increased specific IgG4, and activated Tregs.[10,133,134] Similar findings were noted in ovalbumin-sensitized mice treated with heated OVA or ovomucoid.[135] Heat treatment reduced allergenicity of the egg antigens through enhanced GI digestibility and reduced absorption in a form capable of triggering basophils.

These findings suggest that ingestion of extensively heated egg or milk products may serve as a safe and efficacious treatment modality. Questions remain about the dose required for efficacy, degree of heating needed, role of the food matrix in the observed response, ability of heated proteins to induce lasting tolerance, and role of heated allergens as treatment adjuncts to other forms of immunotherapy.

Sublingual Immunotherapy

Sublingual immunotherapy has shown efficacy for treatment of inhalant allergies and asthma. SLIT has clinical advantages similar to SCIT but lower risks for severe, fatal reactions. Minor side effects, consisting of oral pruritus and swelling, are often reported but are rarely of significance. SLIT employs a liquid concentrate administered sublingually in small, increasing doses in a controlled setting coupled with home dosing to reach a target maintenance dose. Although the mechanism of action is not fully elucidated, data suggest that it is similar to that in other forms of immunotherapy.

Use of SLIT for food allergy was first reported in an adult with severe anaphylaxis to kiwi fruit.[136] Other groups have reported successful therapy with SLIT for hazelnut,[137] peach,[138] milk[120,139] and peanut[140,141] allergies. In the study of hazelnut allergy, 23 adults were randomized to hazelnut or placebo SLIT consisting of a 4-day buildup phase followed by 3 months of maintenance therapy.[137] The tolerated dose of hazelnut increased from a mean of 2.29 g at baseline to 11.56 g at OFC with active SLIT (P = .02) versus 3.49 to 4.14 g with placebo SLIT (P not specified). Systemic symptoms were noted in only 0.2% of total doses. Oropharyngeal symptoms were observed in 7.4% of subjects, many of whom had oral allergy syndrome at baseline.

The RCT providing perhaps the strongest evidence to date employed SLIT in 18 peanut-allergic children (ages 1 to 11 years).[140] Participants were randomized to receive SLIT using crude peanut or placebo extracts. Those receiving peanut SLIT were escalated from 0.25 μg to 2000 mg biweekly for 6 months, then continued maintenance therapy for an additional 6 months before OFC. Peanut SLIT subjects safely ingested 20 times more peanut during OFC than controls (1710 vs. 85 mg, respectively; P = .011). Side effects were predominantly oropharyngeal, with 11.5% of peanut SLIT subjects having oropharyngeal reactions compared with 8.6% of placebo subjects. Epinephrine was not administered during the trial. Immunologic changes from baseline to OFC at about 12 months included decreased SPT size (P = .02), basophil activation (P = .009), and IL-5 levels (P = .015) and increased peanut-specific IgG4 (P = .014). Specific IgE was elevated during the first 4 months (P = .002), then declined steadily through 12 months (P = .003). This study demonstrates that peanut SLIT can safely induce some level of desensitization and SLIT-induced immunomodulation in children.

In a peanut SLIT trial from the CoFAR group, 70% of adolescent and adult subjects receiving peanut SLIT had a response to therapy compared to 15% of placebo SLIT subjects.[141] The amount of peanut consumed in the peanut SLIT group increased from 3.5 mg at baseline to 496 mg at week 44 of the OFC, with 95.2% of doses being symptom-free, excluding local oral/pharyngeal symptoms. Median peanut-IgE levels declined among peanut SLIT subjects while basophil activation did not change.

In an open-label treatment trial comparing SLIT to SLIT plus OIT for milk allergy, 30 subjects were randomized to three treatment arms: SLIT alone (7-mg target dose), SLIT pretreatment with low-dose OIT (1000-mg target dose), and SLIT pretreatment with higher-dose OIT (2000-mg target dose).[120] After 60 weeks of therapy, subjects in the SLIT group demonstrated a 40-fold increase in reaction threshold compared with a 54-fold and a 159-fold increase in SLIT/OIT (high) and SLIT/OIT (low), respectively (P = .053; SLIT vs. OIT). No differences in symptoms were noted; however, OIT dosing was associated with more multisystem symptoms, more treatment with β-agonists and antihistamines, and more epinephrine use.

Although both OIT and SLIT can confer benefits to patients, the therapies differ in dosing limitations, effectiveness, side effects, and immunomodulation (Table 84-8). Further study is needed to improve antigen delivery using SLIT while maintaining its preferable safety profile, with better understanding of nuances in antigen delivery to the gut-associated lymphoid tissue (via OIT) compared with the submucosal lymphoid tissue (via SLIT). Even when effective, these forms of therapy will not likely be applicable across all ages and risk categories of food allergies, and thus specific paradigms and alternate treatments are needed.

TABLE 84-8 Comparison of Oral Immunotherapy (OIT) and Sublingual Immunotherapy (SLIT)

	OIT	SLIT
Typical daily dose	300-4000 mg	2-7 mg
Predominant side effects	Oral, gastrointestinal (systemic increases with infection, exercise, menses)	Oropharyngeal
Desensitization	Large effect	Lesser effect
Functional tolerance	Effective in subset of patients	Unknown to date
Immunomodulation	Significant	Modest

Epicutaneous Immunotherapy

Epicutaneous immunotherapy (EPIT) has been used safely and effectively for grass pollen–induced allergic rhinitis.[142] The current evidence base for the use of EPIT in food allergy is limited to one trial in milk-allergic infants and children and preclinical studies using allergic mouse models. EPIT acts by delivering a small dose of allergenic protein directly to the epidermal layer of the skin.[143] In mouse studies with OVA linked to Alexa488 and applied through EPIT technology, allergens were taken up by Langerhans and dendritic cells in skin and trafficked to regional lymph nodes to trigger an altered allergen-specific T cell response.[143] Mice treated with EPIT or SCIT versus placebo (or nothing) showed reduced airway hyperresponsiveness and allergen-specific IgE levels and increased allergen-specific IgG2a.[144] No differences were detected between EPIT and SCIT.

A 3-month double-blind, placebo-controlled pilot study of EPIT was conducted in milk-allergic infants and children (3 months to 15 years).[145] Nineteen participants were randomized to milk or placebo EPIT; 16 were evaluable by a second OFC on day 90. The cumulative dose of cow's milk consumed during OFC trended higher in the milk EPIT group (1.77 ± 2.98 mL to 23.61 ± 28.61 mL) versus the placebo group (4.36 ± 5.87 mL to 5.44 ± 5.88 mL) ($P = .13$). Adverse events, without anaphylaxis, were reported more often in the milk EPIT group compared with controls (24 vs. 8 events, respectively) and were mostly mild skin reactions. Additional studies of EPIT are in progress for peanut allergy.

Modified or Recombinant Allergen Immunotherapy

Food allergens can be modified by site-directed mutagenesis to reduce IgE-binding sites while retaining T cell epitopes that provide an immunomodulatory signal to activate regulatory or other effector T cells. Animal studies have been conducted using recombinant/mutated allergens alone or with bacterial adjuvants. In a mouse model of peanut allergy, two studies of recombinant/modified allergens have been conducted using heat-killed *Listeria monocytogenes* (HKLM) and heat-killed *Escherichia coli* (HKE) as adjuvants.[146,147] In the first study, allergic mice were treated with subcutaneous doses of modified peanut proteins (Ara h1, 2, 3) with HKLM during 3 weekly injections.[147] Compared with sham-treated mice, those with combination treatment demonstrated reduced anaphylaxis and decreased IgE, IL-5, and IL-13 and increased IFN-γ. The same investigators also used HKE to produce engineered/mutated Ara h1, 2, 3 (HKE-EMP123) that was rectally administered to peanut-allergic mice over 3 weeks.[146] Treated animals had reduced symptoms scores at OFC and desensitization for 10 weeks after therapy. Histamine release, peanut-specific IgE, and Th2 cytokines were also reduced, and peanut-specific IgG2 levels were increased. A phase I clinical trial using HKE-EMP123 is in progress in peanut-allergic adults.

Peptide Vaccine

Peptide immunotherapy uses small peptide fragments rather than whole allergen, a concept that should prevent immune activation with regard to anaphylaxis but may provide epitopes for suppressive T cell activity. Peptide immunotherapy has shown utility in early clinical trials for cat allergy and bee sting allergy. Peptide immunotherapy with the immunodominant epitopes of OVA has also been used in animal models of food allergy.[148] Mice treated with subcutaneous peptide injections were protected from anaphylaxis on OVA challenge and exhibited decreased histamine levels, OVA-specific IgE, and Th2 cytokines and increased IFN-γ. They also had higher levels of mRNA transcripts for forkhead box P3 protein (FOXP3) and transforming growth factor beta (TGF-β) in the intestine, which suggests modification of the local mucosal immune response. Another study employed immunodominant T cell epitope peptide delivery by OIT in egg-allergic mice.[149] Reduced clinical symptoms and changes in immunologic parameters were noted when both single-peptide and multipeptide OIT was given. There are no current clinical trials using peptide therapy for food allergy.

Plasmid DNA Immunotherapy

In animal model systems, plasmid DNA can be used to deliver allergenic genes of interest to provide immunomodulation. In peanut-allergic mice, Ara h2 complexed with chitosan was delivered orally by plasmid DNA nanoparticles.[150] Treatment with the plasmid DNA complex lowered anaphylaxis scores during challenge, reduced histamine, and elevated specific IgG2. Another group delivered nanoparticle pDNA containing TGF-β/chitosan complexes in OVA-sensitized mice[151] and showed increased OVA-specific IgA and reduced specific IgE. Plasmid DNA studies are limited to preclinical trials to date but provide intriguing data for potential future application in humans.

Other allergen-specific approaches in early, preclinical studies include cytokine-modulated immunotherapy, immunostimulatory sequence-conjugated protein-modulated immunotherapy, human immunoglobulin fusion proteins, sugar-conjugated BSA, and antigen-fixed leukocytes.[6,152] These show promise for future clinical applications.

Summary

Current therapy for food allergy requires education about avoidance in a variety of settings and instructions on when and how to treat inevitable allergic reactions. These approaches require constant vigilance and affect quality of life. Increasing attention has therefore focused on primary prevention and improved therapies, with a shift in our approach to the prevention of food allergy. Previous guidelines on food allergen avoidance during pregnancy, breastfeeding, and infancy have been questioned. The relationship between allergen exposure and development of food allergy is complex. Allergen exposure through a disrupted skin barrier may be involved in establishing allergy, whereas allergen exposure through the gastrointestinal mucosa may be involved in establishing tolerance. Immune responses to such allergen exposures are likely to be modulated by nonspecific factors, such as GI microflora, infectious exposure, other dietary factors, and possibly sunlight exposure.

Interventional trials in progress and in the next few years should help to determine the relative contribution of these different factors and allow us to reduce the burden caused by food allergy. Advances in our understanding of the immunologic mechanisms underlying food allergy and the complexities of the mucosal immune response have resulted in substantial progress toward definitive therapeutic options for food-allergic individuals. Current therapeutic strategies are focused on harnessing oral tolerance to modulate the allergic response using antigen-specific and antigen-nonspecific approaches. Although significant gains and positive clinical and immunomodulatory insights have been appreciated, these approaches are often associated with significant risk and unanswered long-term safety and efficacy questions. Ongoing studies will fill our current therapeutic knowledge gaps and carefully move toward broader clinical application in the future.

REFERENCES

Introduction

1. Sicherer SH. Epidemiology of food allergy. J Allergy Clin Immunol 2011;127:594-602.
2. Bock SA, Muñoz-Furlong A, Sampson HA. Fatalities due to anaphylactic reactions to foods. J Allergy Clin Immunol 2001;107:191-3.
3. Bock SA, Muñoz-Furlong A, Sampson HA. Further fatalities caused by anaphylactic reactions to food, 2001-2006. J Allergy Clin Immunol 2007;119:1016-8.
4. Jarvinen KM, Sicherer SH, Sampson HA, Nowak-Wegrzyn A. Use of multiple doses of epinephrine in food-induced anaphylaxis in children. J Allergy Clin Immunol 2008;122: 133-8.
5. Lack G. Epidemiologic risks for food allergy. J Allergy Clin Immunol 2008;121:1331-6.
6. Nowak-Wegrzyn A, Sampson HA. Future therapies for food allergies. J Allergy Clin Immunol 2011;127:558-73.

Practical Management

7. Boyce JA, Assa'ad A, Burks AW, et al. Guidelines for the diagnosis and management of food allergy in the United States: report of the NIAID-sponsored expert panel. J Allergy Clin Immunol 2010;126(Suppl. 6):S1-58.
8. Lieberman JA, Sicherer SH. Quality of life in food allergy. Curr Opin Allergy Clin Immunol 2011;11:236-42.
9. Sicherer SH, Vargas PA, Groetch ME, et al. Development and validation of educational materials for food allergy. J Pediatr 2012;160: 651-6.
10. Kim JS, Nowak-Wegrzyn A, Sicherer SH, et al. Dietary baked milk accelerates the resolution of cow's milk allergy in children. J Allergy Clin Immunol 2011;128:125-31.
11. Hefle SL, Furlong TJ, Niemann L, et al. Consumer attitudes and risks associated with packaged foods having advisory labeling regarding the presence of peanuts. J Allergy Clin Immunol 2007;120:171-6.
12. Madsen CB, Hattersley S, Allen KJ, et al. Can we define a tolerable level of risk in food allergy? Report from a EuroPrevall/UK Food Standards Agency workshop. Clin Exp Allergy 2012;42:30-7.
13. Roberts G, Golder N, Lack G. Bronchial challenges with aerosolized food in asthmatic, food-allergic children. Allergy 2002;57:713-7.
14. Simonte SJ, Ma S, Mofidi S, Sicherer SH. Relevance of casual contact with peanut butter in children with peanut allergy. J Allergy Clin Immunol 2003;112:180-2.
15. Perry TT, Conover-Walker MK, Pomes A, Chapman MD, Wood RA. Distribution of peanut allergen in the environment. J Allergy Clin Immunol 2004;113:973-6.
16. Maloney JM, Chapman MD, Sicherer SH. Peanut allergen exposure through saliva: assessment and interventions to reduce exposure. J Allergy Clin Immunol 2006;118:719-24.
17. Ahuja R, Sicherer SH. Food-allergy management from the perspective of restaurant and food establishment personnel. Ann Allergy Asthma Immunol 2007;98:344-8.
18. Greenhawt MJ, McMorris MS, Furlong TJ. Self-reported allergic reactions to peanut and tree nuts occurring on commercial airlines. J Allergy Clin Immunol 2009;124(3):598-9.
19. Young MC, Muñoz-Furlong A, Sicherer SH. Management of food allergies in schools: a perspective for allergists. J Allergy Clin Immunol 2009;124:175-82.
20. Sampson HA, Mendelson LM, Rosen JP. Fatal and near-fatal anaphylactic reactions to food in children and adolescents. N Engl J Med 1992;327:380-4.
21. Groetch ME. Diets and nutrition. In: Metcalfe DD, Sampson HA, Simon RA, editors. Food allergy: adverse reactions to foods and food additives. Boston: Blackwell; 2008. p. 482-97.
22. Gold MS, Sainsbury R. First aid anaphylaxis management in children who were prescribed an epinephrine autoinjector device (EpiPen). J Allergy Clin Immunol 2000;106:171-6.
23. Simons FE, Clark S, Camargo CA Jr. Anaphylaxis in the community: learning from the survivors. J Allergy Clin Immunol 2009;124: 301-6.
24. Ma S, Sicherer SH, Nowak-Wegrzyn A. A survey on the management of pollen-food allergy syndrome in allergy practices. J Allergy Clin Immunol 2003;112:784-8.
25. McIntyre CL, Sheetz AH, Carroll CR, Young MC. Administration of epinephrine for life-threatening allergic reactions in school settings. Pediatrics 2005;116:1134-40.
26. American Academy of Allergy, Asthma and Immunology. Anaphylaxis in schools and other childcare settings. AAAAI Board of Directors. J Allergy Clin Immunol 1998;102: 173-6.

Food Allergy Risk Factors and Prevention

27. Du Toit G, Katz Y, Sasieni P, et al. Early consumption of peanuts in infancy is associated with a low prevalence of peanut allergy. J Allergy Clin Immunol 2008;122:984-91.
28. Vereda A, van Hage M, Ahlstedt S, et al. Peanut allergy: Clinical and immunologic differences among patients from 3 different geographic regions. J Allergy Clin Immunol 2011;127: 603-7.
29. Hourihane JO, Dean TP, Warner JO. Peanut allergy in relation to heredity, maternal diet, and other atopic diseases: results of a questionnaire survey, skin prick testing, and food challenges. BMJ 1996;313(7056):518-21.
30. Sicherer SH, Furlong TJ, Maes HH, Desnick RJ, Sampson HA, Gelb BD. Genetics of peanut allergy: a twin study. J Allergy Clin Immunol 2000;106:53-6.
31. Sicherer SH, Muñoz-Furlong A, Sampson HA. Prevalence of peanut and tree nut allergy in the United States determined by means of a random digit dial telephone survey: a 5-year follow-up study. J Allergy Clin Immunol 2003;112:1203-7.
32. Emmett SE, Angus FJ, Fry JS, Lee PN. Perceived prevalence of peanut allergy in Great Britain and its association with other atopic conditions and with peanut allergy in other household members. Allergy 1999;54:380-5; 891 [erratum].
33. Liu AH, Jaramillo R, Sicherer SH, et al. National prevalence and risk factors for food allergy and relationship to asthma: results from the National Health and Nutrition Examination Survey 2005-2006. J Allergy Clin Immunol 2010;126:798-806.
34. Kumar R, Tsai HJ, Hong X, et al. Race, ancestry, and development of food-allergen sensitization in early childhood. Pediatrics 2011;128:e821-9.
35. Branum AM, Lukacs SL. Food allergy among children in the United States. Pediatrics 2009;124:1549-55.
36. Campos Alberto EJ, Shimojo N, Suzuki Y, et al. IL-10 gene polymorphism, but not TGF-β1 gene polymorphisms, is associated with food allergy in a Japanese population. Pediatr Allergy Immunol 2008;19:716-21.
37. Liu X, Beaty TH, Deindl P, et al. Associations between specific serum IgE response and 6 variants within the genes IL4, IL13, and IL4RA in German children: the German Multicenter Atopy Study. J Allergy Clin Immunol 2004;113:489-95.
38. Dreskin SC, Ayars A, Jin Y, Atkins D, Leo HL, Song B. Association of genetic variants of CD14 with peanut allergy and elevated IgE levels in peanut allergic individuals. Ann Allergy Asthma Immunol 2011;106:170-2.
39. Hong X, Wang G, Liu X, et al. Gene polymorphisms, breast-feeding, and development of food sensitization in early childhood. J Allergy Clin Immunol 2011;128:374-81.
40. Hill DJ, Hosking CS. Food allergy and atopic dermatitis in infancy: an epidemiologic study. Pediatr Allergy Immunol 2004;15:421-7.
41. Fallon PG, Sasaki T, Sandilands A, et al. A homozygous frameshift mutation in the

mouse *Flg* gene facilitates enhanced percutaneous allergen priming. Nat Genet 2009;41:602-8.
42. Sandilands A, Terron-Kwiatkowski A, Hull PR, et al. Comprehensive analysis of the gene encoding filaggrin uncovers prevalent and rare mutations in ichthyosis vulgaris and atopic eczema. Nat Genet 2007;39:650-4.
43. Brown SJ, Asai Y, Cordell HJ, et al. Loss-of-function variants in the filaggrin gene are a significant risk factor for peanut allergy. J Allergy Clin Immunol 2011;127:661-7.
44. Visness CM, London SJ, Daniels JL, et al. Association of obesity with IgE levels and allergy symptoms in children and adolescents: results from the National Health and Nutrition Examination Survey 2005-2006. J Allergy Clin Immunol 2009;123:1163-9.
45. Devereux G, Seaton A. Diet as a risk factor for atopy and asthma. J Allergy Clin Immunol 2005;115:1109-17.
46. Black PN, Sharpe S. Dietary fat and asthma: is there a connection? Eur Respir J 1997;10:6-12.
47. Anandan C, Nurmatov U, Sheikh A. Omega 3 and 6 oils for primary prevention of allergic disease: systematic review and meta-analysis. Allergy 2009;64:840-8.
48. Allan K, Kelly FJ, Devereux G. Antioxidants and allergic disease: a case of too little or too much? Clin Exp Allergy 2010;40:370-80.
49. Wjst M. Another explanation for the low allergy rate in the rural Alpine foothills. Clin Mol Allergy 2005;3:7.
50. Milner JD, Stein DM, McCarter R, Moon RY. Early infant multivitamin supplementation is associated with increased risk for food allergy and asthma. Pediatrics 2004;114:27-32.
51. Hypponen E, Sovio U, Wjst M, et al. Infant vitamin d supplementation and allergic conditions in adulthood: northern Finland birth cohort 1966. Ann NY Acad Sci 2004;1037:84-95.
52. Camargo CA Jr, Clark S, Kaplan MS, Lieberman P, Wood RA. Regional differences in EpiPen prescriptions in the United States: the potential role of vitamin D. J Allergy Clin Immunol 2007;120:131-6.
53. Vassallo MF, Banerji A, Rudders SA, et al. Season of birth and food allergy in children. Ann Allergy Asthma Immunol 2010;104:307-13.
54. Nwaru BI, Ahonen S, Kaila M, et al. Maternal diet during pregnancy and allergic sensitization in the offspring by 5 yrs of age: a prospective cohort study. Pediatr Allergy Immunol 2010;21:29-37.
55. Eggesbo M, Botten G, Stigum H, Nafstad P, Magnus P. Is delivery by cesarean section a risk factor for food allergy? J Allergy Clin Immunol 2003;112:420-6.
56. Bager P, Wohlfahrt J, Westergaard T. Caesarean delivery and risk of atopy and allergic disease: meta-analyses. Clin Exp Allergy 2008;38:634-42.
57. Sicherer SH, Wood RA, Stablein D, et al. Maternal consumption of peanut during pregnancy is associated with peanut sensitization in atopic infants. J Allergy Clin Immunol 2010;126:1191-7.
58. Dotterud CK, Storro O, Johnsen R, Oien T. Probiotics in pregnant women to prevent allergic disease: a randomized, double-blind trial. Br J Dermatol 2010;163:616-23.
59. American Academy of Pediatrics. Committee on Nutrition. Hypoallergenic infant formulas. Pediatrics 2000;106:346-9.
60. Greer FR, Sicherer SH, Burks AW. Effects of early nutritional interventions on the development of atopic disease in infants and children: the role of maternal dietary restriction, breastfeeding, timing of introduction of complementary foods, and hydrolyzed formulas. Pediatrics 2008;121:183-91.
61. http://cot.food.gov.uk/pdfs/cotstatement200807peanut.pdf
62. World Health Organization. Global strategy for infant and young child feeding: the optimal duration of exclusive breast feeding. Fifty-fourth World Health Assembly. Provisional agenda item 13.1.1. Geneva: WHO; 2001.
63. Sears MR, Greene JM, Willan AR, et al. Long-term relation between breastfeeding and development of atopy and asthma in children and young adults: a longitudinal study. Lancet 2002;360(9337):901-7.
64. Bergmann RL, Diepgen TL, Kuss O, et al. Breastfeeding duration is a risk factor for atopic eczema. Clin Exp Allergy 2002;32:205-9.
65. Osborn DA, Sinn J. Formulas containing hydrolysed protein for prevention of allergy and food intolerance in infants. Cochrane Database Syst Rev 2006;(4):CD003664.
66. Von Berg A, Koletzko S, Filipiak-Pittroff B, et al. Certain hydrolyzed formulas reduce the incidence of atopic dermatitis but not that of asthma: three-year results of the German Infant Nutritional Intervention Study. J Allergy Clin Immunol 2007;119:718-25.
67. Zeiger RS, Heller S. The development and prediction of atopy in high-risk children: follow-up at age seven years in a prospective randomized study of combined maternal and infant food allergen avoidance. J Allergy Clin Immunol 1995;95:1179-90.
68. Arshad SH, Bateman B, Sadeghnejad A, Gant C, Matthews SM. Prevention of allergic disease during childhood by allergen avoidance: the Isle of Wight Prevention Study. J Allergy Clin Immunol 2007;119:307-13.
69. Dubrac S, Schmuth M, Ebner S. Atopic dermatitis: the role of Langerhans cells in disease pathogenesis. Immunol Cell Biol 2010;88:400-9.
70. Smith FJ, Irvine AD, Terron-Kwiatkowski A, et al. Loss-of-function mutations in the gene encoding filaggrin cause ichthyosis vulgaris. Nat Genet 2006;38:337-42.
71. Brown SJ, McLean WH. Eczema genetics: current state of knowledge and future goals. J Invest Dermatol 2009;129:543-52.
72. Palmer CN, Irvine AD, Terron-Kwiatkowski A, et al. Common loss-of-function variants of the epidermal barrier protein filaggrin are a major predisposing factor for atopic dermatitis. Nat Genet 2006;38:441-6.
73. Flohr C, England K, Radulovic S, et al. Filaggrin loss-of-function mutations are associated with early-onset eczema, eczema severity and transepidermal water loss at 3 months of age. Br J Dermatol 2010;163:1333-6.
74. Brown SJ, Irvine AD. Atopic eczema and the filaggrin story. Semin Cutan Med Surg 2008;27:128-37.
75. Saloga J, Renz H, Larsen GL, Gelfand EW. Increased airways responsiveness in mice depends on local challenge with antigen. Am J Respir Crit Care Med 1994;149:65-70.
76. Strid J, Hourihane J, Kimber I, Callard R, Strobel S. Disruption of the stratum corneum allows potent epicutaneous immunization with protein antigens resulting in a dominant systemic Th2 response. Eur J Immunol 2004;34:2100-9.
77. Lack G, Fox D, Northstone K, Golding J. Factors associated with the development of peanut allergy in childhood. N Engl J Med 2003;348:977-85.
78. Fox AT, Sasieni P, Du TG, Syed H, Lack G. Household peanut consumption as a risk factor for the development of peanut allergy. J Allergy Clin Immunol 2009;123:417-23.
79. Frossard CP, Hauser C, Eigenmann PA. Antigen-specific secretory IgA antibodies in the gut are decreased in a mouse model of food allergy. J Allergy Clin Immunol 2004;114:377-82.
80. Marth T, Strober W, Kelsall BL. High-dose oral tolerance in ovalbumin TCR-transgenic mice: systemic neutralization of IL-12 augments TGF-β secretion and T cell apoptosis. J Immunol 1996;157:2348-57.
81. Strid J, Thomson M, Hourihane J, Kimber I, Strobel S. A novel model of sensitization and oral tolerance to peanut protein. Immunol 2004;113:293-303.
82. Kerosuo H, Kullaa A, Kerosuo E, et al. Nickel allergy in adolescents in relation to orthodontic treatment and piercing of ears. Am J Orthod Dentofac Orthop 1996;109:148-54.
83. Mortz CG, Lauritsen JM, Bindslev-Jensen C, Andersen KE. Nickel sensitization in adolescents and association with ear piercing, use of dental braces and hand eczema. The Odense Adolescence Cohort Study on Atopic Diseases and Dermatitis (TOACS). Acta Derm Venereol 2002;82:359-64.
84. Poole JA, Barriga K, Leung DY, et al. Timing of initial exposure to cereal grains and the risk of wheat allergy. Pediatrics 2006;117:2175-82.
85. Lack G. The concept of oral tolerance induction to foods. Nestle Nutr Workshop Ser Pediatr Program 2007;59:63-8.
86. Green R, Luyt D. Clinical characteristics of childhood asthmatics in Johannesburg. S Afr Med J 1997;87:878-82.
87. Hill DJ, Hosking CS, Heine RG. Clinical spectrum of food allergy in children in Australia and South-East Asia: identification and targets for treatment. Ann Med 1999;31:272-81.
88. Lee BW, Shek LP, Gerez I, Soh SE, Van Bever HP. Food allergy: lessons from Asia. World Allergy Org J 2008;1:129-33.
89. Katz Y, Rajuan N, Goldberg MR, et al. Early exposure to cow's milk protein is protective against IgE-mediated cow's milk protein allergy. J Allergy Clin Immunol 2010;126:77-82.
90. Koplin JJ, Osborne NJ, Wake M, et al. Can early introduction of egg prevent egg allergy in infants? A population-based study. J Allergy Clin Immunol 2010;126:807-13.
91. Chan SMH, Stephens AC, Fox AT, Grieve AP, Lack G. Cutaneous lymphocyte antigen and alpha-4 beta-7 T lymphocyte responses are associated with peanut allergy and tolerance in children. Allergy 2012;67:336-42.
92. Sudo N, Sawamura S, Tanaka K, et al. The requirement of intestinal bacterial flora for the development of an IgE production system fully susceptible to oral tolerance induction. J Immunol 1997;159:1739-45.

93. Field CJ. The immunological components of human milk and their effect on immune development in infants. J Nutr 2005;135:1-4.

Traditional Immunotherapy and Need for Alternatives

94. Akdis CA, Akdis M. Mechanisms of allergen-specific immunotherapy. J Allergy Clin Immunol 2011;127:18-27.
95. Oppenheimer JJ, Nelson HS, Bock SA, Christensen F, Leung DYM. Treatment of peanut allergy with rush immunotherapy. J Allergy Clin Immunol 1992;90:256-62.
96. Nelson HS, Lahr J, Rule R, Bock A, Leung D. Treatment of anaphylactic sensitivity to peanuts by immunotherapy with injections of aqueous peanut extract. J Allergy Clin Immunol 1997;99:744-51.

Allergen-Nonspecific Therapies

97. Casale TB, Busse WW, Kline JN, et al. Omalizumab pretreatment decreases acute reactions after rush immunotherapy for ragweed-induced seasonal allergic rhinitis. J Allergy Clin Immunol 2006;117:134-40.
98. Massanari M, Nelson H, Casale T, et al. Effect of pretreatment with omalizumab on the tolerability of specific immunotherapy in allergic asthma. J Allergy Clin Immunol 2010;125: 383-9.
99. Leung DY, Sampson HA, Yunginger JW, et al. Effect of anti-IgE therapy in patients with peanut allergy. N Engl J Med 2003;348:986-93.
100. Sampson HA, Leung DY, Burks AW, et al. A phase II, randomized, double-blind, parallel-group, placebo-controlled oral food challenge trial of Xolair (omalizumab) in peanut allergy. J Allergy Clin Immunol 2011;127:1309-10.
101. Nadeau KC, Schneider LC, Hoyte L, Borras I, Umetsu DT. Rapid oral desensitization in combination with omalizumab therapy in patients with cow's milk allergy. J Allergy Clin Immunol 2011;127:1622-4.
102. Qu C, Srivastava K, Ko J, et al. Induction of tolerance after establishment of peanut allergy by the Food Allergy Herbal Formula-2 is associated with up-regulation of interferon-γ. Clin Exp Allergy 2007;37:846-55.
103. Srivastava KD, Qu C, Zhang T, et al. Food Allergy Herbal Formula-2 silences peanut-induced anaphylaxis for a prolonged posttreatment period via IFN-γ-producing CD8+ T cells. J Allergy Clin Immunol 2009;123: 443-51.
104. Li XM, Brown L. Efficacy and mechanisms of action of traditional Chinese medicines for treating asthma and allergy. J Allergy Clin Immunol 2009;123:297-306.
105. Wang J, Patil SP, Yang N, et al. Safety, tolerability, and immunologic effects of a food allergy herbal formula in food allergic individuals: a randomized, double-blinded, placebo-controlled, dose escalation, phase 1 study. Ann Allergy Asthma Immunol 2010;105(1):75-84.
106. Prescott SL, Bjorksten B. Probiotics for the prevention or treatment of allergic diseases. J Allergy Clin Immunol 2007;120(2):255-62.
107. Lyons A, O'Mahony D, O'Brien F, MacSharry J, Sheil B, Ceddia M et al. Bacterial strain-specific induction of Foxp3+ T regulatory cells is protective in murine allergy models. Clin Exp Allergy 2010;40(5):811-9.
108. Kim JY, Kwon JH, Ahn SH, Lee SI, Han YS, Choi YO et al. Effect of probiotic mix *(Bifidobacterium bifidum, Bifidobacterium lactis, Lactobacillus acidophilus)* in the primary prevention of eczema: a double-blind, randomized, placebo-controlled trial. Pediatr Allergy Immunol 2010;21:e386-93.
109. Kalliomaki M, Salminen S, Poussa T, Arvilommi H, Isolauri E. Probiotics and prevention of atopic disease: 4-year follow-up of a randomised placebo-controlled trial. Lancet 2003;361(9372):1869-71.
110. Kopp MV, Hennemuth I, Heinzmann A, Urbanek R. Randomized, double-blind, placebo-controlled trial of probiotics for primary prevention: no clinical effects of *Lactobacillus* GG supplementation. Pediatrics 2008;121:e850-6.
111. Rose MA, Stieglitz F, Koksal A, et al. Efficacy of probiotic *Lactobacillus* GG on allergic sensitization and asthma in infants at risk. Clin Exp Allergy 2010;40:1398-405.
112. Gruber C, van Stuijvenberg M, Mosca F, et al. Reduced occurrence of early atopic dermatitis because of immunoactive prebiotics among low-atopy-risk infants. J Allergy Clin Immunol 2010;126:791-7.
113. Arslanoglu S, Moro GE, Schmitt J, et al. Early dietary intervention with a mixture of prebiotic oligosaccharides reduces the incidence of allergic manifestations and infections during the first two years of life. J Nutr 2008;138: 1091-5.

Allergen-Specific Immunotherapy

114. Patriarca G, Nucera E, Roncallo C, et al. Oral desensitizing treatment in food allergy: clinical and immunological results. Aliment Pharmacol Ther 2003;17:459-65.
115. Meglio P, Bartone E, Plantamura M, Arabito E, Giampietro PG. A protocol for oral desensitization in children with IgE-mediated cow's milk allergy. Allergy 2004;59(9):980-7.
116. Jones SM, Pons L, Roberts JL, et al. Clinical efficacy and immune regulation with peanut oral immunotherapy. J Allergy Clin Immunol 2009;124:292-300.
117. Blumchen K, Ulbricht H, Staden U, et al. Oral peanut immunotherapy in children with peanut anaphylaxis. J Allergy Clin Immunol 2010;126:83-91.
118. Anagnostou K, Clark A, King Y, et al. Efficacy and safety of high-dose peanut oral immunotherapy with factors predicting outcome. Clin Exp Allergy 2011;41:1172-4.
119. Longo G, Barbi E, Berti I, et al. Specific oral tolerance induction in children with very severe cow's milk-induced reactions. J Allergy Clin Immunol 2008;121:343-7.
120. Keet CA, Frischmeyer-Guerrerio PA, Thyagarajan A, et al. The safety and efficacy of sublingual and oral immunotherapy for milk allergy. J Allergy Clin Immunol 2012;129: 448-55.
121. Buchanan AD, Green TD, Jones SM, et al. Egg oral immunotherapy in nonanaphylactic children with egg allergy. J Allergy Clin Immunol 2007;119:199-205.
122. Vickery BP, Pons L, Kulis M, et al. Individualized IgE-based dosing of egg oral immunotherapy and the development of tolerance. Ann Allergy Asthma Immunol 2010;105:444-50.
123. Varshney P, Jones SM, Scurlock AM, et al. A randomized controlled study of peanut oral immunotherapy: clinical desensitization and modulation of the allergic response. J Allergy Clin Immunol 2011;127:654-60.
124. Skripak JM, Nash SD, Rowley H, et al. A randomized, double-blind, placebo-controlled study of milk oral immunotherapy for cow's milk allergy. J Allergy Clin Immunol 2008; 122:1154-60.
125. Burks AW, Jones SM, Wood RA, et al. Oral immunotherapy for treatment of egg allergy in children. N Engl J Med 2012;367: 233-43.
126. Narisety SD, Skripak JM, Steele P, et al. Open-label maintenance after milk oral immunotherapy for IgE-mediated cow's milk allergy. J Allergy Clin Immunol 2009;124: 610-2.
127. Kulis M, Li Y, Lane H, Pons L, Burks W. Single-tree nut immunotherapy attenuates allergic reactions in mice with hypersensitivity to multiple tree nuts. J Allergy Clin Immunol 2011;127:81-8.
128. Hofmann AM, Scurlock AM, Jones SM, et al. Safety of a peanut oral immunotherapy protocol in children with peanut allergy. J Allergy Clin Immunol 2009;124:286-91.
129. Vickery BP, Scurlock AM, Steele P, et al. Early and persistent gastrointestinal side effects predict withdrawal from peanut oral immunotherapy. J Allergy Clin Immunol 2011;126, AB87.
130. Varshney P, Steele PH, Vickery BP, et al. Adverse reactions during peanut oral immunotherapy home dosing. J Allergy Clin Immunol 2009; 124:1351-2.
131. Pajno GB. Oral desensitization for milk allergy in children: state of the art. Curr Opin Allergy Clin Immunol 2011;11:560-4.
132. Nowak-Wegrzyn A, Bloom KA, Sicherer SH, et al. Tolerance to extensively heated milk in children with cow's milk allergy. J Allergy Clin Immunol 2008;122:342-7.
133. Lemon-Mule H, Sampson HA, Sicherer SH, et al. Immunologic changes in children with egg allergy ingesting extensively heated egg. J Allergy Clin Immunol 2008;122:977-83.
134. Shreffler WG, Wanich N, Moloney M, Nowak-Wegrzyn A, Sampson HA. Association of allergen-specific regulatory T cells with the onset of clinical tolerance to milk protein. J Allergy Clin Immunol 2009;123:43-52.
135. Martos G, Lopez-Exposito I, Bencharitiwong R, Berin MC, Nowak-Wegrzyn A. Mechanisms underlying differential food allergy response to heated egg. J Allergy Clin Immunol 2011;127: 990-7.
136. Mempel M, Rakoski J, Ring J, Ollert M. Severe anaphylaxis to kiwi fruit: immunologic changes related to successful sublingual allergen immunotherapy. J Allergy Clin Immunol 2003;111:1406-9.
137. Enrique E, Pineda F, Malek T, et al. Sublingual immunotherapy for hazelnut food allergy: a randomized, double-blind, placebo-controlled study with a standardized hazelnut extract. J Allergy Clin Immunol 2005;116:1073-9.
138. Fernandez-Rivas M, Garrido FS, Nadal JA, et al. Randomized double-blind, placebo-controlled trial of sublingual immunotherapy with a Pru p 3 quantified peach extract. Allergy 2009;64:876-83.
139. De Boissieu D, Dupont C. Sublingual immunotherapy for cow's milk protein allergy: a preliminary report. Allergy 2006;61:1238-9.
140. Kim EH, Bird JA, Kulis M, et al. Sublingual immunotherapy for peanut allergy: clinical and immunologic evidence of desensitization. J Allergy Clin Immunol 2011;127:640-6.
141. Fleischer DM, Burks AW, Vickery BP, et al. Sublingual immunotherapy for peanut allergy: a randomized, double-blind, placebo-controlled multicenter trial. J Allergy Clin Immunol 2013; (in press).

142. Senti G, Graf N, Haug S, et al. Epicutaneous allergen administration as a novel method of allergen-specific immunotherapy. J Allergy Clin Immunol 2009;124:997-1002.
143. Dioszeghy V, Mondoulet L, Dhelft V, et al. Epicutaneous immunotherapy results in rapid allergen uptake by dendritic cells through intact skin and downregulates the allergen-specific response in sensitized mice. J Immunol 2011;186:5629-37.
144. Mondoulet L, Dioszeghy V, Ligouis M, et al. Epicutaneous immunotherapy on intact skin using a new delivery system in a murine model of allergy. Clin Exp Allergy 2010;40:659-67.
145. Dupont C, Kalach N, Soulaines P, et al. Cow's milk epicutaneous immunotherapy in children: a pilot trial of safety, acceptability, and impact on allergic reactivity. J Allergy Clin Immunol 2010;125:1165-7.
146. Li XM, Srivastava K, Grishin A, et al. Persistent protective effect of heat-killed *Escherichia coli* producing "engineered," recombinant peanut proteins in a murine model of peanut allergy. J Allergy Clin Immunol 2003;112:159-67.
147. Li XM, Srivastava K, Huleatt JW, et al. Engineered recombinant peanut protein and heat-killed *Listeria monocytogenes* coadministration protects against peanut-induced anaphylaxis in a murine model. J Immunol 2003;170: 3289-95.
148. Yang M, Yang C, Mine Y. Multiple T cell epitope peptides suppress allergic responses in an egg allergy mouse model by the elicitation of forkhead box transcription factor 3- and transforming growth factor-beta-associated mechanisms. Clin Exp Allergy 2010;40:668-78.
149. Rupa P, Mine Y. Oral immunotherapy with immunodominant T-cell epitope peptides alleviates allergic reactions in a Balb/c mouse model of egg allergy. Allergy 2012;67:74-82.
150. Roy K, Mao HQ, Huang SK, Leong KW. Oral gene delivery with chitosan-DNA nanoparticles generates immunologic protection in a murine model of peanut allergy. Nat Med 1999;5:387-91.
151. Li F, Wang L, Jin XM, et al. The immunologic effect of TGF-β1 chitosan nanoparticle plasmids on ovalbumin-induced allergic BALB/c mice. Immunobiology 2009;214:87-99.
152. Smarr CB, Hsu CL, Byrne AJ, Miller SD, Bryce PJ. Antigen-fixed leukocytes tolerize Th2 responses in mouse models of allergy. J Immunol 2011;187:5090-8.

85 Adverse Reactions to Vaccines for Infectious Diseases

JOHN M. KELSO | MATTHEW J. GREENHAWT

CONTENTS

SUMMARY OF IMPORTANT CONCEPTS

» Whereas mild, self-limited adverse reactions to vaccines are common, serious complications are rare. In most cases, the risk of an adverse outcome from the disease itself is greater than the risk from repeat vaccination.

» Immunoglobulin E (IgE)-mediated adverse reactions to vaccines may be due to the immunizing agent itself or, more often, to some other protein constituent such as gelatin. Skin testing may be helpful in determining the cause of such reactions.

» A number of rare, non–IgE-mediated events are associated with specific vaccines and may preclude further doses.

» Suggested long-term adverse sequelae of vaccination, such as atopy or autism, have not been substantiated after careful epidemiologic studies.

» When a serious adverse event possibly related to vaccination occurs, it should be reported to the Vaccine Adverse Event Reporting System (VAERS). Such reactions should be investigated to determine the cause and to make recommendations to the individual patient regarding subsequent immunizations.

Putting Adverse Reactions to Vaccines in Perspective

SUCCESS OF VACCINES

The Centers for Disease Control and Prevention (CDC) recently compiled a list of the greatest public health achievements of the twentieth century.[1] At the top of the list is vaccination. Table 85-1 summarizes the impact of vaccines on dramatically reducing or even eliminating the morbidity associated with infectious diseases. These improvements constitute remarkable accomplishments, and it is against this background of enormous benefit that adverse reactions to vaccines must be evaluated.

RARITY OF SERIOUS REACTIONS

In the overall picture, the rarity of serious adverse reactions to vaccines also should be considered. During calendar years 1999 to 2008, 2.05 billion doses of all vaccines were distributed in the United States (CDC, written communication, September 13, 2011). The Vaccine Adverse Event Reporting System (VAERS) received 177,883 reports during this time frame (CDC, written communication, September 8, 2011). Some reports involve reactions after the administration of more than one vaccine at a single visit. These data yield a reporting rate of 8.7 per 100,000 doses distributed.

EVOLUTION OF AN IMMUNIZATION PROGRAM

When an infectious disease is responsible for widespread morbidity and mortality, the adverse events caused by a vaccine developed to combat the disease may be more readily accepted. Once the vaccine leads to a dramatic decline in the disease, however, vaccine side effects become relatively more apparent and less acceptable. A theoretical evolution of an immunization program has been described,[2] as depicted in Fig. 85-1: Before vaccine availability, incidence of the disease is high (stage 1). As a program of vaccination against the disease is begun, incidence of disease decreases while vaccine use increases (stage 2). Some incidence of adverse events attributable to the vaccine will, of course, reflect its usage. The number of vaccine adverse events initially is small in relation to the number of disease cases, but as the natural disease is largely eliminated because of widespread vaccine usage, this same number of vaccine adverse events becomes large by comparison with disease cases (stage 3). Attention to these vaccine adverse events may lead to a loss of confidence in the vaccine and lower vaccination rates, with resultant resurgence in disease. If confidence is restored, vaccination rates increase (stage 4). Eventually, high vaccination rates may lead to the eradication of the disease, and vaccination may be stopped, eliminating vaccine-related adverse events (stage 5).

CONSEQUENCES OF NOT VACCINATING

The risk of adverse events after vaccination must be put in the context of the consequences of not vaccinating vulnerable

TABLE 85-1 Decrease in Reports of Vaccine-Preventable Diseases in the United States

Disease	Baseline Twentieth Century Annual Morbidity*	No. of Cases Reported for 2009†	Percent Decrease
Diphtheria	175,885	0	100.0%
Haemophilus influenzae type b	20,000	38	99.8%
Measles	503,282	71	100.0%
Mumps	152,209	1991	98.7%
Pertussis	147,271	16,858	88.6%
Poliomyelitis	16,316	1	100.0%
Rubella	47,745	3	100.0%
Congenital rubella syndrome	823	2	99.8%
Smallpox	48,164	0	100.0%
Tetanus	1314	18	98.6%

*Centers for Disease Control and Prevention (CDC). Impact of vaccines universally recommended for children—United States, 1990-1998. MMWR Morb Mortal Wkly Rep 1999;48:243-8.
†Centers for Disease Control and Prevention (CDC). Summary of notifiable diseases: United States, 2009. MMWR Morb Mortal Wkly Rep 2011;58:1-100.

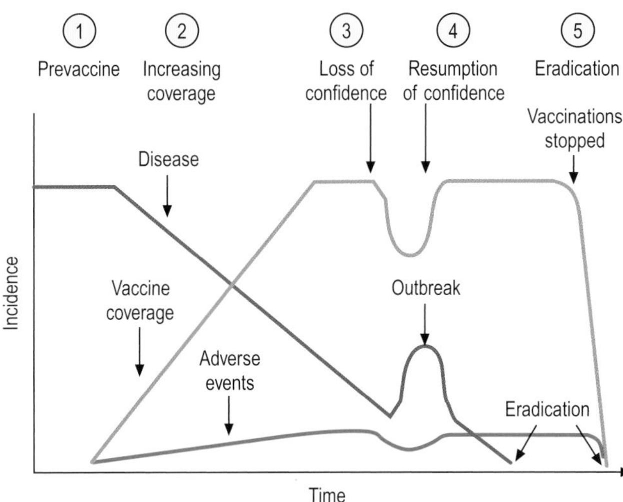

Figure 85-1 Evolution of an immunization program. *(Modified from Chen RT, Rastogi SC, Mullen JR, et al. The Vaccine Adverse Event Reporting System [VAERS]. Vaccine 1994;12:542-50.)*

populations as well. In this country, many states allow exemptions from childhood immunizations based on philosophical objection. As indicated by reports to the CDC surveillance system, children who were not vaccinated against measles were 35 times more likely to contract the disease than those vaccinated.[3] Concerns about the old whole-cell pertussis vaccine led to antivaccine campaigns in several countries.[4] As a result, vaccine coverage declined, and pertussis disease rates surged 10- to 100-fold. A rubella outbreak occurred in Nebraska in 1999.[5] In all 83 cases, the patients either were unvaccinated or had an unknown vaccination status. At least one infant with congenital rubella syndrome was born to one of the affected women. A polio outbreak occurred in the Dominican Republic and Haiti in 2000 and 2001.[6] In all 21 cases, which included two fatalities, the patients were either unvaccinated or inadequately vaccinated. Military recruits in the United States previously received routine vaccination against adenovirus. When the sole manufacturer of the vaccine ceased production, the incidence of adenoviral respiratory illness escalated, leading to two deaths.[7] In the United Kingdom, concern over alleged side effects of measles-mumps-rubella (MMR) vaccine in the late 1990s led to a marked decline in vaccination rates, with a resultant marked increase in measles outbreaks in the early 2000s.[8]

MONITORING FOR VACCINE-RELATED ADVERSE EVENTS

VAERS has been in place in the United States since 1990.[2] Established by the CDC and the U.S. Food and Drug Administration (FDA), VAERS is a passive surveillance system; that is, it relies on reporting by health care providers and parents or patients. A report to VAERS is actually a report of a suspected association between vaccine administration and an adverse event. Thus, although VAERS provides important data for evaluation of potential causality between a vaccine and a subsequent event, more thorough epidemiologic evaluation requires that the number of subjects vaccinated without the subsequent event be known, and that the number not vaccinated with and without the subsequent event also be known. To meet this need, the CDC has established the Vaccine Safety Datalink (VSD), which monitors the immunization and medical records of more than half a million children enrolled in several large staff model health maintenance organizations (HMOs).[9] Another active surveillance system, the Immunization Monitoring Program, Active (IMPACT), has been established in Canada.[10] These postlicensure surveillance systems are particularly important, because prelicensure studies may not include enough subjects to detect rare adverse events.[11]

Immunoglobulin E–Mediated Reactions to Vaccines

Anaphylaxis after vaccination is rare. The VSD, described previously, reviewed the diagnosis codes for medical encounters after the administration of more than 7.5 million doses of vaccines to a cohort of 2.2 million children and adolescents.[12] Depending on which anaphylaxis or allergy codes were included in the evaluation, the risk of anaphylaxis was estimated to be 0.65 to 1.53 per 1 million doses. The National Vaccine Injury Compensation Program (VICP) provides compensation to patients who claim injury or death as a result of vaccination.[13] A review of the VICP database found 9 cases of anaphylaxis, including 5 deaths, associated with 8 different vaccines over the 10-year period 2000 to 2009.[14]

There is a distinction between how to evaluate patients who have already had an apparent allergic reaction to a vaccine and those with a history of apparent allergic reactions to vaccine constituents. For those who have already reacted to a vaccine, it is important to determine whether or not the reaction was immunoglobulin E (IgE)-mediated and if so, to determine the culprit allergen. This evaluation involves skin tests with the suspect vaccine and skin tests or serum-specific IgE antibody tests to vaccine constituents. For those who have reacted to a vaccine constituent such as gelatin, egg, latex, or yeast, but not

BOX 85-1 GELATIN-CONTAINING VACCINES

Vaccine	Gelatin Content (per stated dose)
Influenza (Fluzone, Sanofi Pasteur)	250 µg per 0.5 mL
Influenza (FluMist, MedImmune)	2000 µg per 0.2 mL
Measles, mumps, rubella (MMRII, Merck)	14,500 µg per 0.5 mL
Measles, Mumps, Rubella, Varicella (ProQuad, Merck)	11,000 µg per 0.5 ml
Rabies (RabAvert, Novartis)	12,000 µg per 1.0 mL
Typhoid Vaccine Live Oral Ty21a (VIVOTIF, Berna)	capsule
Varicella (VARIVAX, Merck)	12,500 µg per 0.5 mL
Yellow fever (YF-VAX, Sanofi Pasteur)	7500 µg per 0.5 mL
Zoster (ZOSTAVAX, Merck)	15,580 µg per 0.65 mL

to vaccination itself, whether or not skin testing is required before vaccine administration depends on the particular vaccine constituent allergy and the particular vaccine.

IMMUNOGLOBULIN E–MEDIATED REACTIONS TO VACCINE CONSTITUENTS OTHER THAN THE IMMUNIZING AGENT

Gelatin

Gelatin is added to many vaccines as a stabilizer (Box 85-1). The first case report of an allergic reaction to the gelatin component of a vaccine described a classic anaphylactic reaction in a young woman on receiving an MMR immunization. Her medical history included the development of a swollen tongue and itchy throat within minutes of eating gelatin in any form.[15] Laboratory evaluation revealed that the only component of the vaccine to which she made IgE antibody was gelatin. Subsequent reports from Japan evaluated 26 children who experienced allergic reactions to measles, mumps, or rubella vaccines containing gelatin: 24 of the 26 made IgE antibody to gelatin, whereas none of 26 control children who had been vaccinated uneventfully made such antibodies.[16] Similar reports involving MMR vaccine followed from other countries,[17] and reports regarding other gelatin-containing vaccines, including varicella,[18,19] Japanese encephalitis,[20] and influenza[21] also were rendered. Vaccine manufacturers in Japan and Germany removed gelatin or changed to a less allergenic gelatin in vaccines, with a resultant decline in reported cases of allergic reactions after immunizations.[22-24] A new Japanese encephalitis vaccine does not contain gelatin.[25] A history of allergy to the ingestion of gelatin should be sought before the administration of any gelatin-containing vaccine. A negative history, however, may not exclude an allergic reaction to gelatin injected with the vaccine.[16] Most persons who produce IgE antibody to gelatin and immediate-type allergic reactions to gelatin-containing vaccines attributable to those antibodies have not reported allergic reactions to the ingestion of gelatin prior to vaccination, although some may do so afterward. Presumably, the different route of exposure, injection versus ingestion, accounts for this fact.[26] The incidence of gelatin allergy among vaccine recipients suffering anaphylactic reactions has been higher in Japan[16] than in other countries.[17,27] A strong association has been recognized between gelatin allergy and human leukocyte antigen (HLA)-DR9, an HLA type unique to Asians, suggesting a genetic susceptibility to gelatin allergy.[28] A subsequent report found additional both positive and negative associations between certain HLA types and gelatin allergy.[29] This type of HLA analysis might shed light on the risk for allergic reactions to other vaccines.

Persons who react to gelatin on ingestion should be evaluated by an allergist before vaccine administration. If the history is consistent with an immediate-type allergic reaction to gelatin and this is confirmed by skin tests or serum-specific IgE antibody tests to gelatin, it is prudent to skin test such patients with gelatin-containing vaccines before administration. If the vaccine skin test results are negative, the vaccine can be given in the usual manner but the patient should be observed for at least 30 minutes afterward. If the vaccine skin test results are positive, the vaccine can be administered in graded doses.

Egg

Concern has been raised over the administration of vaccines "grown in eggs" to egg-allergic recipients. A report in 1983 described two egg-allergic children who suffered allergic reactions to measles vaccine,[30] seeming to support the need for caution. However, a subsequent review of the reported cases of anaphylaxis induced by measles or MMR vaccine found no other cases in egg-allergic recipients.[15] Furthermore, hundreds of egg-allergic children had been administered the vaccines without adverse reaction. Measles and mumps vaccines are grown in chick embryo fibroblast cultures (as opposed to "eggs") and contain negligible or no egg protein.[31] Follow-up studies in which measles or MMR vaccine was administered in the normal manner to egg-allergic children without adverse reaction have confirmed the safety of this approach.[32,33] Current recommendations indicate that MMR vaccine can be given routinely to children with egg allergy without previous skin testing.[34]

Egg protein is present in higher amounts in influenza vaccines than in MMR vaccine[31] and could in theory cause reactions in egg-allergic recipients. Numerous studies, however, have demonstrated that influenza vaccine can be safely administered to even severely egg-allergic recipients,[35-41] probably owing to the very low amount of egg protein (ovalbumin) contained in recent years' vaccines.[42-44] In an attempt to vaccinate egg-allergic patients, protocols had called for skin testing with the vaccine and, if the skin test results were positive, either withholding the vaccine or administering it in divided doses. However, results of studies using such protocols indicate that vaccine skin testing is not predictive of reactions,[35,36,38,40,41] and that trivalent inactivated influenza vaccine (TIV) can be administered safely as a single dose.[37,38,40,41] Based on review of these data, statements from the CDC's Advisory Committee on Immunization Practices (ACIP) and the American Academy of Pediatrics (AAP) Committee on Infectious Diseases ("Red Book") specifically recommend that patients with egg allergy receive influenza vaccine with some precautions.[45,46] Patients with a history of only hives after egg ingestion can receive TIV at their primary care provider's office, whereas persons with a history of more severe reactions after egg ingestion should be referred to an allergist to receive TIV. Clinicians who administer TIV to any egg-allergic individual must have available the proper medications and resuscitative equipment to treat potential anaphylaxis and must observe the patient for 30 minutes after the vaccination to monitor for signs or symptoms of such a reaction. LAIV, although containing the lowest amount of ovalbumin per dose, has not been formally studied for safety in egg-allergic individuals; accordingly, only TIV should be

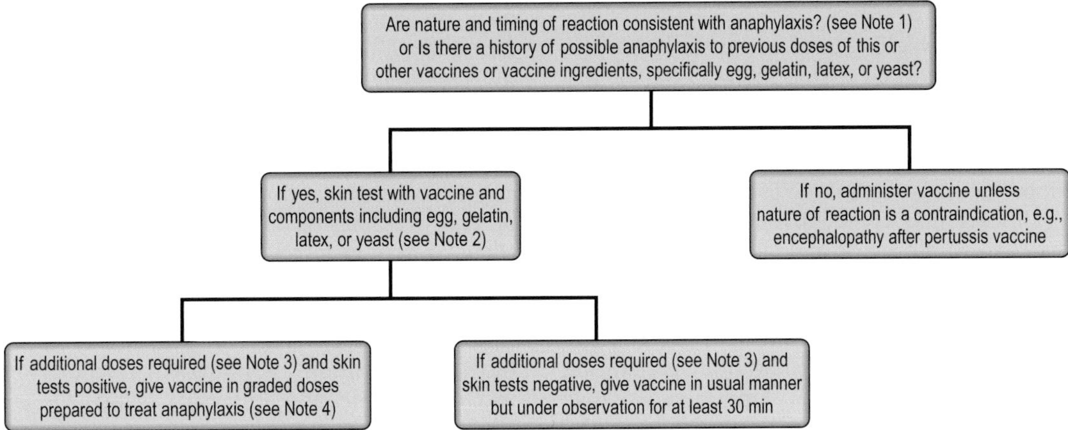

Figure 85-2 Suggested approach to suspected immediate-type allergic reactions to vaccines.
Note 1. Are nature and timing of reaction consistent with a systemic IgE-mediated reaction?
Probable systemic IgE-mediated reaction: reaction occurring within 4 hours of vaccine administration to include signs and/or symptoms from more than one of the following systems:
- Dermatologic: urticaria, flushing, angioedema, pruritus
- Respiratory: rhinoconjunctivitis (red, watery, itchy eyes, stuffy, runny, itchy nose, sneezing), upper airway edema (change in voice, difficulty swallowing, difficulty breathing, stridor), bronchospasm/asthma (cough, wheeze, shortness of breath, chest tightness)
- Cardiovascular: hypotension, tachycardia, palpitations, light-headedness, loss of consciousness (NOTE: hypotension or loss of consciousness with pallor and bradycardia is much more likely to be due to a vasovagal reaction)
- Gastrointestinal: cramping, nausea, vomiting, diarrhea

Possible systemic IgE-mediated reaction:
- Signs and/or symptoms from only one system (as above)
- Signs and/or symptoms from more than one system (as above) but occurring more than 4 hours after vaccination

Note 2. Skin tests with vaccine and components including egg, gelatin, latex, or yeast
Vaccine skin tests:
- Prick test with full-strength vaccine; consider 1:10 dilution if patient has a history of life-threatening reaction.
- If results of prick test with full-strength vaccine are negative, perform intradermal testing with 0.02 mL of vaccine at a 1:100 dilution.
- NOTE: Vaccine skin tests may cause false (or clinically irrelevant) positive reactions. Thus, if skin testing gives a positive reaction, also perform on normal control subjects.

Vaccine component skin tests:
- Prick tests with commercial extracts of egg (influenza and yellow fever vaccines) or *Saccharomyces cerevisiae* yeast (hepatitis B and quadrivalent human papillomavirus vaccines)
- Prick test with sugared gelatin (e.g., Jell-O): dissolve 1 teaspoon of gelatin powder in 5 mL of normal saline. Vaccines that contain gelatin: influenza (some brands), measles, mumps, rabies (some brands), rubella, typhoid (capsule), varicella, yellow fever, zoster (see Box 85-1)
- Prick test with latex: soak 2 fingers of latex glove or a toy balloon in 5 mL of normal saline. Vaccines that contain latex in packaging: available at http://www.cdc.gov/vaccines/pubs/pinkbook/downloads/appendices/B/latex-table.pdf
- In vitro assays for specific IgE antibody to egg, gelatin, latex, and yeast also are commercially available as an alternative or complement to skin testing.

Note 3. If fewer than the recommended number of doses are received, consider measuring level of IgG antibodies to immunizing agent (see Table 85-2). If the measured level is associated with protection from disease, consider withholding additional doses, although magnitude and duration of immunity may be less than if all doses received.
Note 4. Vaccine administration in graded doses:
- With a vaccine for which the usual dose is 0.5 mL, administer graded doses of vaccine at 15-minute intervals: 0.05 mL of 1:10 dilution, 0.05 mL of full strength, 0.10 mL of full strength, 0.15 mL of full strength, 0.20 mL of full strength.

administered to egg-allergic patients. LAIV also is contraindicated in any individual with asthma. If the patient has a history of reaction to the influenza vaccine itself, as opposed to a history of a reaction to the ingestion of eggs, evaluation as outlined in Figure 85-2 is appropriate.

Yellow fever vaccine is cultured in chicken embryos and contains egg protein.[31] Anaphylactic reactions in egg-allergic persons have been reported.[47-49] Additional cases have been reported in persons whose egg-allergic status is not known.[50] Patients presenting for yellow fever vaccination are routinely asked if they are allergic to eggs. Of note, however, allergy to a heat-labile egg protein has been described.[51] The affected patient ate cooked eggs without difficulty and denied egg allergy when asked before receiving her yellow fever vaccine. She nonetheless developed an urticarial reaction to the vaccination. Subsequent skin tests were positive for raw egg and vaccine. The vaccine, which is not heated during manufacturing, would still contain egg proteins that would otherwise be destroyed by heat. Clearly, then, the clinical history may not identify all persons allergic to egg proteins present in yellow fever or other vaccines. Chicken proteins other than those found in chicken egg may be present in yellow fever vaccine and may be responsible for reactions in chicken-allergic recipients.[52] A history of allergy after the ingestion of egg, raw or cooked, should be sought before the administration of yellow fever vaccine, and persons with a positive history should be evaluated by an allergist before vaccine administration. Such patients should first be skin tested with yellow fever vaccine. If the vaccine skin test results are negative, the vaccine can be given in the usual manner, but the patient should be observed for at least 30 minutes afterward. If the vaccine skin test results are positive, the vaccine can be administered in graded doses.

Latex

Package inserts for many vaccines used in the United States indicate that the vial stoppers and syringe plungers contain dry natural rubber and include cautionary statements regarding possible risks for latex-allergic vaccine recipients. Storage of liquid in a vial in which the liquid is in contact with a natural rubber latex stopper can cause the release of latex allergens into the solution.[53] This solution could, in theory, subsequently cause a reaction when administered to a latex-allergic patient. There is a single case report of a latex-allergic patient who suffered an anaphylactic reaction after administration of hepatitis B vaccine drawn through a rubber stopper.[54] She had no reaction to a subsequent dose administered without puncturing the stopper. However, other vaccine vial stoppers and syringe plungers are made of synthetic rubber and pose no risk to latex-allergic persons. A search of 167,223 reports in the VAERS database through 2003 revealed 28 reports of immediate-type allergic reactions to various vaccines in patients also reported to be latex-allergic.[55] Some of these reactions may possibly have been due to latex allergy; however, in view of the large number of immunizations administered every year in the United States, the reported risk of allergic reactions possibly due to latex contamination of vaccines appears to be very small. The latex content of vaccine packaging is updated regularly by the CDC (current data are available at www.cdc.gov/vaccines/pubs/pinkbook/pink-appendx.htm).[56]

Patients with a history of latex-precipitated anaphylaxis can safely receive vaccines from vials with nonlatex stoppers. If the only available preparation has a latex stopper, the stopper should be removed and the vaccine drawn up directly from the vial without passing the needle through the stopper. If the only available vaccine contains latex in the packaging that cannot be avoided, such as in a prefilled syringe, the vaccine can still be administered, but the patient should be observed for at least 30 minutes afterward.

Yeast

Recombinant hepatitis B virus (HBV) vaccines are prepared by harvesting hepatitis B surface antigen from cultures of *Saccharomyces cerevisiae* (common baker's or brewer's yeast), and the final vaccine products contain up to 5% yeast protein.[57,58] Before licensure, clinical trials were performed to address whether residual yeast proteins in the vaccines could induce anaphylaxis, including testing for IgE anti-yeast antibody levels.[59,60] Approximately 1% to 2% of subjects had anti-yeast IgE antibodies before immunization but demonstrated no significant rise in IgE after receiving HBV vaccine. A search of 180,895 reports to VAERS through 2004 revealed 15 cases that mentioned a history of "allergy" to yeast and also described potential anaphylactic reactions.[61] Eleven of these cases involved HBV vaccine, but four involved other vaccines that do not contain yeast protein. Some of these reactions could have been due to yeast allergy; however, allergy to yeast is quite rare.[62] The small number of reports to VAERS suggests that yeast-associated anaphylaxis after administration of HBV vaccine in sensitized patients appears to be a rare event. Quadrivalent human papillomavirus vaccine (HPV4) also contains residual yeast protein.[63]

If the patient has a history of immediate-type allergy to baker's or brewer's yeast and a positive skin test response to *S. cerevisiae*, an appropriate precaution is skin testing with yeast-containing vaccines before administration. If the results of vaccine skin tests are negative, the vaccine can be given in the usual manner, but the patient should be observed for at least 30 minutes afterward. If the vaccine skin test results are positive, the vaccine can be administered in graded doses.

Milk

A recent publication described eight children who developed anaphylaxis within 1 hour of receiving diphtheria, tetanus, and pertussis vaccines (DTaP or Tdap).[64] Six had a history of past allergic reactions to cow's milk, and all had very high levels of milk-specific serum IgE. These vaccines may contain trace (nanogram) quantities of residual casein from the medium in which they are produced. The results of this report require further investigation.[65] Anaphylactic reactions to DTaP or Tdap vaccines are rare, and a majority of patients with cow's milk allergy tolerate them without reaction. It is recommended that all patients, including those with milk allergy, continue to receive these vaccines on schedule,[64,65] but perhaps with some additional observation after vaccination in those with very high levels of milk sensitivity.

REACTIONS TO SPECIFIC VACCINES

Diphtheria

Many recipients of diphtheria vaccine generate IgE antibody to the vaccine[66-68]; however, most go on to receive subsequent doses uneventfully.[67] Local reactions to subsequent doses may be more frequent in persons who have made anti-diphtheria IgE,[68] but generalized reactions have been reported only rarely.[69-71]

One interesting case involved a generalized urticarial reaction after administration of a conjugate *Haemophilus influenzae* type b (Hib) vaccine in which the conjugate protein CRM 197 is a mutant diphtheria protein.[72] Subsequent skin testing revealed positive reactions to the vaccine in question but not to other Hib vaccines using different conjugate proteins. This case demonstrates the importance of determining which vaccine component is responsible for a reaction. The child in this report may safely receive other Hib vaccines with different conjugate proteins, yet he may react to pneumococcal and meningococcal conjugate vaccines because they contains the same CRM 197 conjugate protein to which he is allergic.

Haemophilus influenzae *Type b*

Reports of reactions consistent with anaphylaxis have been rare after Hib vaccination.[73,74] Only one report has demonstrated IgE antibody to an Hib vaccine component, which was not the Hib polysaccharide but rather the protein in a conjugate vaccine (see preceding section on diphtheria).[72]

Hepatitis B

Based on the report described earlier regarding HBV vaccine–associated anaphylaxis in reportedly yeast-allergic patients,[61] an Institute of Medicine report has concluded that "evidence convincingly supports a causal relationship between hepatitis B vaccine and anaphylaxis in yeast-sensitive individuals"[69]; however, no IgE antibody testing is described. The CDC estimates the rate of anaphylaxis among vaccine recipients to be 1 per 600,000 vaccine doses.[75]

Human Papillomavirus Vaccine

Anaphylaxis induced by the human papillomavirus (HPV) vaccine has been reported to occur at rates ranging from 1 per 1 million[76] to 2.6 per 100,000[77] doses, but the allergic nature of these events has not been confirmed with skin tests.[78] Syncope due to vasovagal reactions also is common in the adolescent age group, in which the vaccine is administered,[79,80] and could have been confused with anaphylaxis.

Influenza

In 1976, the CDC coordinated a nationwide surveillance system to monitor adverse events associated with the administration of that year's influenza vaccine to 48,161,019 recipients.[81] A total of 11 cases of anaphylaxis (0.024 case per 100,000 vaccinees), none of which were fatal, and none of which occurred in persons known to be allergic to eggs, were reported. One anecdotal report from the 1970s noted an "anaphylactic death after influenza immunization," but no details were provided.[82] A review of all VAERS reports from 1990 to 2005, during which 747 million doses of influenza vaccine were administered, revealed 4 reports of death occurring shortly after influenza vaccination that identified anaphylaxis as the cause,[83] but information was not provided on egg allergy or on any evaluation conducted to determine whether these were allergic reactions. An IOM report revealed only 22 published cases overall of influenza vaccine "presenting temporality and clinical symptoms consistent with anaphylaxis."[69] Isolated cases of anaphylaxis without defined etiology also have been reported after intranasal administration of live attenuated influenza vaccine (LAIV).[84] Thus the rate of anaphylaxis after influenza vaccination is very low, with little evidence to support egg allergy as the cause of such events. The use of this vaccine in egg-allergic patients is described earlier under "Egg."

Japanese Encephalitis

Japanese encephalitis vaccine can cause typical immediate-type allergic reactions, consisting of urticaria with or without wheezing, occurring 5 to 60 minutes after vaccination.[20,85,86] Most affected patients have anti-gelatin IgE, which is not found in those immunized uneventfully. These allergic reactions presumably are due to gelatin allergy, as has been described with other gelatin-containing vaccines.[15-19]

Japanese encephalitis vaccine also has been particularly likely to cause an unusual, late-onset urticaria and angioedema reaction.[25] Reports from several countries have placed the incidence of such reactions as high as 1% among the recipients of this vaccine. The median interval between vaccination and onset of the reaction is 2 to 3 days.[87-89] Although the reactions usually are confined to the skin, some cases have involved hypotension or respiratory distress.[89,90] One death occurred 60 hours after Japanese encephalitis vaccination (and 12 hours after plague vaccination); however, the cause of death and relationship, if any, to vaccination could not be determined.[87] Two studies have suggested that a prior history of urticaria, asthma, rhinitis, or eczema increases the risk for these late-onset reactions.[87,91]

A new inactivated Vero cell culture–derived Japanese encephalitis vaccine has replaced the previous inactivated mouse brain–derived vaccine.[25] The new vaccine does not contain gelatin. Whether the new vaccine will carry a lower rate of adverse reactions is yet to be determined.

Measles-Mumps-Rubella

There are many reports of anaphylactic reactions to MMR vaccine.[15-17,27,30,92-99] Tens of millions of doses are distributed each year, however, making the incidence of such reactions on the order of 2 to 10 per 1 million.[17,27] As noted previously, allergy to gelatin added to the vaccine as a stabilizer has been determined to be the likely cause in 27% to 92% of cases.[16,17,27] As detailed earlier, no relationship has been found between anaphylactic reactions to MMR vaccine and egg allergy.

Meningococcus

Anaphylactic reactions to meningococcal polysaccharide or polysaccharide-protein conjugate vaccines have been very rare, on the order of 1 per 1 million doses.[100,101]

Pertussis

Natural infection with pertussis causes the production of anti-pertussis IgE in many recipients.[102,103] Immunization with either whole-cell or acellular pertussis vaccine results in the production of anti-pertussis IgE in about one third of the recipients after the primary series and in as many as two thirds after a booster.[104,105] The production of these antibodies appears unrelated to atopic status[105,106] or alum content.[104] Although the presence of the IgE antibodies may predispose recipients to local reactions to subsequent doses of the vaccine,[105] they have not generally predisposed to systemic reactions.[105,106] A single case report describes an anaphylactic reaction after the third dose of diphtheria-pertussis-tetanus (DPT) vaccine in an infant.[107] A skin test with the DPT vaccine gave a positive reaction, whereas a skin test with diphtheria-tetanus (DT) vaccine yielded a negative result, implicating the pertussis component.

Immunization to pertussis vaccine also has been examined for the possibility that it would enhance IgE production to allergens.[108,109] In neither children nor adults did pertussis vaccine increase the level of IgE antibody to common aeroallergens.

Pneumococcus

Two separate reports have described anaphylaxis in children who received 23-valent pneumococcal vaccine when IgE antibodies to the vaccine were demonstrated.[110,111] A postlicensure surveillance study was conducted after the introduction of 7-valent pneumococcal conjugate vaccine.[112] A total of 14 of the 4154 VAERS reports received described anaphylactic episodes. In 9 of these episodes, the subject received other vaccines at the same time, so the reaction could have been due to the other vaccines. In this same group, 12 patients were receiving the pneumococcal vaccine for the first time, making an allergic reaction to the immunizing agent unlikely, although not ruling out a reaction to some other vaccine constituent to which the vaccinees had been previously exposed.

Rabies

A few cases consistent with immediate-type allergic reactions to human diploid cell rabies vaccine (HDVC) have been reported, but without any confirmatory laboratory data regarding IgE antibody.[113] Of interest, a number of cases consistent with serum sickness have been reported,[113-117] and many of these have been associated with IgE antibody to a vaccine constituent,[115,116] even though such reactions generally are thought to be immunoglobulin G (IgG) immune complex–related.[117] The timing of the reactions varies, with onset of symptoms from 2 to 21 days after vaccine administration. The symptoms have included those typical of serum sickness such as arthralgia, fever, and malaise, and urticaria has been a prominent feature. The rabies virus used in the vaccine is inactivated with beta-propiolactone (BPA).[115] The cell culture medium in which the virus is grown, however, contains human albumin, among other ingredients, and the BPA added to inactivate the virus also alters the albumin. This BPA-altered albumin has been shown to stimulate the production of specific IgE antibody in vaccine recipients who go on to report the serum sickness–like reaction to subsequent doses.[115,116] How IgE antibody could result in this clinical picture is not adequately explained.

The more recently approved purified chick embryo cell (PCEC) rabies vaccine also has been associated with cases of anaphylaxis.[118] Two of the reported patients had anaphylaxis to both PCEC and HDCV, suggesting cross-reactivity. PCEC (but not HDCV) contains gelatin, and another patient who had anaphylaxis after PCEC was found to have anti-gelatin IgE. The serum sickness–like reactions reported with HDCV appear to be less common with PCEC.[118]

Tetanus

As with diphtheria toxoid, many recipients of tetanus vaccine generate specific IgE antibodies to the toxoid.[66-68,119-121] The production of these IgE antibodies may be related to the aluminum adjuvant.[120] Most persons go on to receive subsequent doses without systemic reaction.[67,120,121] A number of anaphylactic reactions, however, have been reported after tetanus toxoid administration.[69,122-126]

Varicella

A report describing the first 3 years of postlicensure safety surveillance for varicella vaccine found 30 cases consistent with anaphylaxis, a rate of 1 to 3 per 1 million doses distributed.[127,128] Reports from Japan[18] and the United States[19] have implicated gelatin allergy as the cause of some of these reactions.

Yellow Fever

Before 1999, the only reports of anaphylaxis induced by yellow fever vaccine dated from the 1940s and described only three patients.[47-49] A 1999 report reviewed VAERS data over a 7-year period and identified 40 cases of probable or possible anaphylaxis to yellow fever vaccine and estimated the rate of such reactions at 7 per 1 million doses.[50] A subsequent report found an additional 28 cases.[129] Other anaphylactic reactions to yellow fever vaccine almost certainly have occurred in the 50 years between reports of such reactions. This association underscores the importance of vaccine safety surveillance systems such as VAERS to establish the occurrence and frequency of rare reactions. It also emphasizes the importance of consistent reporting to VAERS by clinicians administering vaccines. The possible association between reactions to yellow fever vaccine and egg allergy is discussed previously. The vaccine also contains gelatin, which has been proved to be responsible for many allergic reactions to other vaccines.

SUGGESTED APPROACH TO A SUSPECTED IMMUNOGLOBULIN E–MEDIATED REACTION TO A VACCINE

A suggested approach to a suspected IgE-mediated reaction to a vaccine is outlined in Figure 85-2. The first step in the evaluation is to determine if the nature and timing of the reaction are consistent with a systemic IgE-mediated reaction. Although many schemes have been used to classify such reactions,[130,131] that proposed in Note 1 to Figure 85-2 seems reasonable and is similar to schemes used in the evaluation of vaccine reactions.[27,55,61] Pertinent, too, is a history of similar reactions to the same or other vaccines, or to vaccine constituents. The various elements that make up a vaccine are clearly labeled in manufacturer package inserts. If the reaction occurred with the first dose of a vaccine, the chance that the immunizing agent itself is the allergen is greatly diminished. The clinician also should inquire about allergic reactions to food, because influenza and yellow fever vaccines contain egg protein,[31,35,42-44,132] HBV and HPV4 vaccines contain yeast,[57,58,63] and many vaccines contain gelatin (see Box 85-1). Patients also should be asked about immediate-type allergic reactions to latex, because many vaccines contain latex in the packaging.[56]

Once a history has been obtained of a vaccine reaction occurring shortly after administration that is consistent with mast cell degranulation, it is appropriate to determine whether future doses of the suspect vaccine, or of other vaccines with common components, are required for the particular patient. If a patient's reaction occurred with a vaccine in which only one dose is normally given, or to the final dose in a series, a reasonable approach might be to simply label the patient allergic" to the vaccine in question without further testing. In view of the potential for cross-reaction with common components in other vaccines and with certain foods, however, a more thorough evaluation, even if no further doses are required, is appropriate.

Many vaccines are given as a series, because recipients occasionally require several doses to achieve a "protective" response. Some recipients, however, may generate an adequate response with fewer than the usual number of doses. In this circumstance, it may be reasonable to determine the level of immune response in terms of antibody level achieved in a particular patient by the doses already received. Protective levels of specific antibody to the immunizing agent have been determined for many vaccines, and some are routinely available in commercial reference laboratories (Table 85-2). If a patient can be determined to have already mounted a sufficient antibody response to be considered protected, then consideration can be given to omitting further doses of the vaccine. Of note, however, the level of protective antibody may not persist as long in persons vaccinated with fewer than the usual number of doses. Antibody levels may need to be checked again at some interval, particularly if the patient, because of travel or other reasons, may have an increased chance of exposure to the particular infectious agent.

To determine whether or not the vaccine was responsible for the patient's apparent allergic reaction, skin testing with the vaccine should be performed.[133] The vaccine should first be tested by the skin prick method. Full-strength vaccine can be used, unless the history of reaction was truly life-threatening, in which case beginning even the prick test with dilute vaccine is appropriate. If results of the full-strength prick test are negative, with appropriate positive and negative controls, an intradermal test with the vaccine diluted 1 : 100 should be performed, again with appropriate controls.[134] If the intradermal skin test result is negative, the chance that the patient has IgE antibody to any vaccine constituent is negligible, and the vaccine can be administered in the usual manner.[135] It is prudent, nonetheless, in a patient with a history suggestive of an anaphylactic reaction, to administer the vaccine under observation with epinephrine and other treatments available.

A number of caveats are applicable to the interpretation of positive results on skin testing for reactivity to vaccines. As

TABLE 85-2 Levels of Antibody Associated with Protection from Vaccine-Preventable Diseases

Vaccine	Protective Level of IgG Antibody
Diphtheria	≥0.1 IU/mL[13]
Haemophilus influenzae type b	≥0.15 µg/mL*
Hepatitis A	≥10 mIU/mL†
Hepatitis B surface antibody	≥10 mIU/mL‡
Measles (rubeola)	≥120 PRN titer[152]
Polio (inactivated)	≥1:8 neutralizing antibody titer§
Rabies	≥0.5 IU VNA/mL‖
Rubella	≥10 IU/mL[161]
Tetanus	≥0.1 IU/mL[13]
Yellow fever	≥0.7 IU/mL*

IgG, immunoglobulin G; *IU*, international unit; *mIU*, milli-international units; *PRN*, plaque reduction neutralization; *VNA*, virus-neutralizing antibodies.
*Data from Plotkin SA. Immunologic correlates of protection induced by vaccination. Pediatr Infect Dis J 2001;20:63-75.
†Data from Fiore AE, Feinstone SM, Bell BP. Hepatitis A vaccines. In: Plotkin SA, Orenstein WA, Offit PA, editors. Vaccines. 5th ed. Philadelphia: Elsevier; 2008.
‡Data from Centers for Disease Control and Prevention. Epidemiology and prevention of vaccine-preventable diseases. 11th ed. Washington, D.C.: Public Health Foundation; 2009.
§Data from Vidor E, Plotkin SA. Poliovirus vaccine—inactivated. In: Plotkin SA, Orenstein WA, Offit PA, editors. Vaccines. 6th ed. Philadelphia: Elsevier; 2013.
‖Data from Rupprecht CE, Plotkin SA. Rabies vaccines. In: Plotkin SA, Orenstein WA, Offit PA, editors. Vaccines. 6th ed. Philadelphia: Elsevier; 2013.

with any skin test reagent, and particularly with materials not standardized for skin testing such as vaccines, false-positive (irritant) results and clinically irrelevant positive results may occur.[134] No negative or positive predictive values for interpreting skin testing to vaccines or vaccine components have been established. DPT vaccines induce the production of IgE antibodies in a substantial percentage of recipients, who go on to receive subsequent doses without systemic reaction.[67,105,121] Among children with egg allergy but no history of reaction to vaccines, some with positive results on skin prick testing to influenza vaccine have been given the vaccines uneventfully.[35,36,38,40,41] Also, some healthy children and adults with positive intradermal skin test results to influenza vaccine, 1:100, have been given the vaccine uneventfully.[38,136] Thus, if a patient with a suspected IgE-mediated reaction to a vaccine has a positive skin test result, the same vaccine skin test should be conducted in several control subjects who have received the vaccine without adverse reaction. If the control subjects also exhibit positive results, the patient's positive skin test response may or may not be clinically relevant. Although the aforementioned considerations complicate the interpretation of vaccine skin tests, if the test result is positive, particularly in a patient with a history of an allergic reaction to the vaccine, the patient must be assumed to indeed be allergic. Intradermal skin tests with certain vaccines, such as tetanus toxoid, also can induce delayed-type hypersensitivity responses.

If the suspect vaccine contains egg (influenza and yellow fever), gelatin (see Box 85-1), latex (see list at http://www.cdc.gov/vaccines/pubs/pinkbook/downloads/appendices/B/latex-table.pdf), or yeast (HBV and HPV4 vaccines) proteins, the patient also should be skin prick–tested for these allergens. Egg and yeast (*S. cerevisiae*) extracts for skin testing are commercially available. Gelatin can be prepared by dissolving 1 level teaspoon of any sugared gelatin powder (for example, Jell-O) in 5 mL of normal saline to create a skin prick test solution.[15] In vitro assays for specific IgE antibody to egg, gelatin, latex, and yeast also are commercially available as an alternative or complement to skin testing.

If results of vaccine or vaccine component skin testing are positive, the vaccine may still be administered, if necessary, using a graded-dose protocol.[34,137] This protocol was developed for the administration of egg-containing vaccines to egg-allergic recipients but has been used for other vaccines as well.[52,125]

Non–Immunoglobulin E–Mediated Reactions to Vaccines

Virtually all vaccines can cause minor, self-limited side effects. These include local (injection site) reactions such as pain, warmth, tenderness, swelling, and erythema, as well as mild systemic reactions such as fever. Such reactions are not contraindications to further doses of any vaccine.[13]

NON–IMMUNOGLOBULIN E–MEDIATED REACTIONS TO VACCINE CONSTITUENTS OTHER THAN THE IMMUNIZING AGENT

Neomycin

Approximately 1% of the general population demonstrates delayed-type hypersensitivity by patch testing to neomycin.[138] There are very rare reports of apparent immediate-type allergic reactions to topical neomycin, but none in relation to vaccination. If the patient gives a history of an immediate-type reaction, it is appropriate to investigate before immunization with vaccine containing this antibiotic. For those patients reporting a delayed-type contact dermatitis to neomycin, immunization may proceed in the usual fashion. The only anticipated reaction is formation of a small, temporary papule at the injection sites—for which associated risk is clearly outweighed by the benefit of the vaccination.[139]

Thimerosal

As with neomycin, delayed-type hypersensitivity to thimerosal is reported[140]; rarely, immediate-type reactivity may be seen. Although patients with delayed-type thimerosal sensitivity on patch testing may exhibit large local reactions to vaccination with thimerosal-containing vaccines,[141,142] the vast majority tolerate such immunizations uneventfully.[140,143-145] A single case report has described a generalized maculopapular rash attributed to thimerosal in an influenza vaccine.[146] A single instance of an immediate-type reaction that may have been caused by thimerosal in a vaccine also has been reported.[147] Risks associated with thimerosal in terms of its mercury content are discussed further on.

Aluminum

Aluminum-containing vaccines may cause formation of persistent nodules palpable at the injection site, probably as a consequence of a delayed-type hypersensitivity to aluminum.[148-150]

REACTIONS TO SPECIFIC VACCINES

Measles-Mumps-Rubella

Transient rashes occur in 5% of measles vaccine recipients, which may represent vaccine-induced modified measles.[151] Measles or MMR vaccine causes a late-onset fever 5 to 12 days after administration in as many as 15% of recipients.[34,75,151] Coincident with this fever is an increased risk of febrile seizures (in excess of 25 to 34 febrile seizures per 100,000 children vaccinated), although without long-term sequelae.[69,152,153] For reasons that are not clear, when the MMR vaccine is given in a combination preparation with varicella vaccine (i.e., MMRV), the risk of febrile seizures is double that associated with administration of the MMR and varicella vaccines by separate injections at the same visit (one additional febrile seizure per 2500 children vaccinated).[154] This increased risk has been documented only for the first dose of the vaccines, typically given between 12 and 15 months of age, and not for the second dose, typically given between 4 and 6 years of age. For this reason, the preferred strategy is to administer the MMR and varicella vaccines by separate injections at the same visit for the first dose, and combined as MMRV vaccine for the second dose.[154]

Measles, rubella, and MMR vaccines can cause thrombocytopenia within 2 months of vaccination.[75,155-157] Prospective studies put the risk of this complication as high as 1 in 30,000, whereas passive surveillance (VAERS) puts the risk at 1 in 1 million.[75,156,157] The low platelet counts usually are without serious consequence, but hemorrhage may rarely occur.[155,157,158] Although thrombocytopenia may be more likely in patients who have had idiopathic thrombocytopenic purpura or thrombocytopenia as a result of a previous vaccine, this risk may not preclude a subsequent dose, because the rate of thrombocytopenia with natural infection with rubella or measles is 10 times higher than that with the vaccine.[75,156,157] Determining immunity by antibody titers generated to previous doses of the vaccine may help the clinician make an informed decision.[34,75,157]

Rubella vaccine causes transient arthralgia in up to 15% of adult female vaccine recipients, with much lower rates among children and men.[69,159] The mechanism of the arthritis is direct infection of the joints by the virus, as in natural infection.[160]

Pertussis

Pertussis vaccine, given in combination with diphtheria and tetanus toxoids, has generated concern in terms of serious adverse reactions including seizures, encephalopathy, hypotonic-hyporesponsive episodes, and inconsolable crying. The incidence of these reactions decreased dramatically with conversion from whole-cell (DTP) to acellular (DTaP) pertussis vaccines.[34,161-163] DTP vaccine caused febrile seizures in up to 0.06% of recipients.[163] The VSD project (described previously under "Monitoring for Vaccine-Related Adverse Events") attributed an additional six to nine febrile seizures per 100,000 children to DTP vaccination.[152] The reactions were more common among children with a personal or family history of seizures[34,161] but were not associated with epilepsy (recurring, nonfebrile seizures)[152,164] or neurodevelopmental sequelae.[152] The rate of fever and seizures is substantially lower with DTaP vaccine.[162,165]

DTP vaccine caused episodes of inconsolable crying lasting more than 3 hours in 1% of recipients.[34] No sequelae were reported,[34,75] and such episodes are substantially less frequent after DTaP.[161] Hypotonic/hyporesponsive episodes (HHEs) are defined as the sudden onset of hypotonia, hyporesponsiveness, and pallor or cyanosis occurring within 48 hours of an immunization.[159,166] The vast majority of cases occurred after vaccination with pertussis-containing vaccines (0.06% after DTP),[165] and in children younger than 2 years of age.[166] A follow-up study of data for 215 HHE cases reported to VAERS found the event to be benign, self-limited, and nonrecurrent.[166] HHE is much less frequent after DTaP.[165-167]

A number of neurologic central nervous system (CNS) adverse events more severe than febrile seizures or HHE were reported after DTP vaccination.[159] These reactions were termed encephalopathy and were described as "a severe, acute [CNS] disorder unexplained by another cause, which may be manifested by major alterations of consciousness or by generalized or focal seizures that persist for more than a few hours without recovery within 24 hours."[34] The incidence of such reactions was estimated at 0 to 10.5 per 1 million doses of DTP.[159] Evidence indicates that such reactions may have had permanent sequelae, such as chronic nervous system dysfunction.[168] Still unresolved is whether these children would have gone on to chronic nervous system dysfunction even without the acute vaccine reaction.[168] The active IMPACT surveillance network in Canada found no cases of encephalopathy attributable to DTaP vaccine among 6.5 million doses administered.[34] Because febrile seizures, prolonged crying, and HHE are not known to have permanent sequelae, they are not absolute contraindications to subsequent pertussis vaccination, particularly if the risk of pertussis infection is high, as during an outbreak or in foreign travel.[34,75] Encephalopathy reactions are an absolute contraindication to further pertussis vaccination.[34,75]

Polio

When polio struck more than 21,000 people each year in the United States, a few cases caused by the oral polio vaccine (OPV) itself may have seemed less consequential. With the eradication of natural disease in the Western Hemisphere, however, the eight or nine vaccine-associated paralytic poliomyelitis (VAPP) cases per year became all of the cases. Thus, beginning in the year 2000, the routine use of OPV was discontinued in the United States in favor of an all-IPV schedule,[169] which led to the elimination of VAPP.[170] OPV continues to be used elsewhere in the world, and VAPP continues to be a problem in those areas.[171]

Rotavirus

In 1998, an oral vaccine against rotavirus was introduced and recommended for routine vaccination of infants. In the first several months of its widespread use, however, numerous reports of intussusception were reported through the VAERS.[172] After careful review of the cases of intussusception, all of which occurred within 1 to 2 weeks after vaccination, the recommendation for the use of the vaccine and the vaccine itself were withdrawn.[173] In 2006 and 2008, two new live, oral, rotavirus vaccines were licensed and recommended for routine use in infants in the United States after large-scale safety studies designed specifically to evaluate the risk for intussusception found no increased risk with the new vaccines.[174] Postmarketing studies have suggested that there may be some increased risk of intussusception with the new vaccines, but at a rate far lower than with the older vaccine.[175] However, this risk is far outweighed by the benefits of vaccination.[176]

Tetanus

Owing to increasing rates of pertussis in adolescents and adults, new vaccines were recommended in 2006 for persons 11 to 64 years of age to provide not only booster doses for tetanus and diphtheria (Td) but for pertussis as well (Tdap).[177,178] The recommended interval between doses of Td had been 10 years, with shorter intervals thought to be associated with increased rates of Arthus reactions.[179] In a recent study, however, the rates of injection site reactions to Tdap were no different in those vaccinated less than 2 years than in those vaccinated more than 2 years after previous Td.[180] Another study found no higher rates of injection site reactions whether a Tdap-containing vaccine was administered 1 month after a Td-containing vaccine or placebo.[181] Thus, with the pertussis disease burden continuing to be substantial, it is now recommended that Tdap be given to all adolescents and adults (including those 65 years of age and older) regardless of interval since the last Td.[182]

Varicella

A few varicella-like lesions appear at the injection site in about 4% of varicella vaccine recipients, and generalized varicella-like rashes appear in as many as another 4%.[183] Although premarketing trials described these generalized rashes as also consisting of only a handful of lesions, postmarketing surveillance describes these rashes, perhaps at a lower rate, as containing many more lesions.[184] Analysis of varicelliform rashes after vaccinations has revealed that they can result either from wild-type virus, representing natural infection, or from the vaccine strain of virus, representing attenuated disease caused by the live attenuated vaccine virus. Rashes caused by wild-type virus (60%) appear from 1 to 24 days (median, 8 days) after vaccination and consist of 10 to 1000 lesions (median, 100 lesions). Those caused by vaccine-strain virus appear from 5 to 42 days (median 21 days) after vaccination and consist of 1 to 500 lesions (median, 51).[128,184,185] Similarly, a typical dermatomal herpes zoster rash may rarely appear after varicella vaccination and may contain either wild-type or vaccine-strain virus.[127,128,184,185]

Although varicella disease (chickenpox) itself can be more severe in children with atopic dermatitis, the varicella vaccine can be safely administered to children with atopic dermatitis without an increased risk of complications.[186] Humoral and cellular immune responses to the vaccine are similar in children with and without atopic dermatitis.[187]

Yellow Fever

Vaccine-associated encephalitis can rarely occur in recipients of yellow fever vaccine.[188] This risk appears to be greatest in infants younger than 9 months of age, in whom the rate may be as high as 4 per 1000.[188] This has resulted in recommendations that the vaccine not be given to any infant younger than 6 months of age and to those 6 to 9 months of age only if the risk of exposure is high.[34]

The yellow fever vaccine has recently been associated with a very severe multisystem illness in adults with features strikingly similar to yellow fever disease itself.[189] This adverse reaction, now termed yellow fever vaccine–associated viscerotropic disease (YEL-AVD), has occurred exclusively in first-time vaccine recipients and carries a 65% mortality rate.[189] Most cases of YEL-AVD have occurred in patients who are not known to be immunocompromised; however, a history of a thymus disorder and age 60 years or greater have been identified as risk factors, making these clinical a contraindication and a precaution, respectively.[189] The cause of these reactions is still unknown, but this vaccine should not be given to patients unless they are at risk for acquiring yellow fever, typically by traveling to an area where the disease is endemic. An inactivated and thus presumably safer vaccine is being developed.[190]

Adverse Reactions to Vaccines for Biologic Agents Used as Weapons

A number of biologic agents that would only very rarely be encountered otherwise have been developed as weapons of war or terrorism.[191] Vaccines have been developed for many of these agents but normally are recommended only for very limited groups at increased risk of exposure, such as laboratory workers or military members. Although the potential for exposure of wider segments of the population has long been recognized as a potential threat, the worldwide increase in terrorist events has increased this likelihood. Consequently, these vaccines may be administered to larger numbers of people, and a larger absolute number of adverse reactions can be expected.

Anthrax

Anthrax vaccine adsorbed (AVA) is prepared from a cell-free filtrate of an avirulent form of *Bacillus anthracis*.[192] It contains "protective antigen" and other cell products adsorbed to aluminum hydroxide as an adjuvant. The vaccination schedule consists of intramuscular injections at 0 and 4 weeks and 6, 12, and 18 months, with annual boosters. Intramuscular administration results in fewer local reactions than with the previously recommended subcutaneous route, which often resulted in the development of persistent subcutaneous nodules.[193] The vaccine is contraindicated in persons with a history of a severe generalized or systemic reaction to a previous dose.[192] The Institute of Medicine reviewed reports of adverse reactions after anthrax vaccination and "found no evidence that vaccine recipients face an increased risk of experiencing life-threatening or permanently disabling adverse events immediately after receiving AVA, when compared with the general population. Nor did it find any convincing evidence that vaccine recipients face elevated risk of developing adverse health effects over the longer term."[194]

Smallpox

The global eradication of smallpox by vaccination is a magnificent success story. The last case of the disease, which had plagued humankind for millennia, occurred in 1977, and the world was declared free of smallpox in 1980.[195] The only known repositories of smallpox virus are the CDC in the United States and the Institute of Virus Preparations in Russia.[196] The potential use of smallpox as a weapon of war or terror has heightened the possibility that smallpox vaccination would once again be required.

The causative agent of smallpox is variola virus. Smallpox vaccine is live vaccinia virus, a related orthopoxvirus, which does not normally produce disease in humans, yet does stimulate an immune response cross-protective for variola.[197] The vaccine, typically given only once, is administered by a multiple-puncture technique with a bifurcated needle. The expected response to the vaccine is formation of a papule at the site of vaccination within 3 to 5 days, which subsequently becomes vesicular and then pustular. A scab forms subsequently and then separates within 2 to 3 weeks, leaving a scar. Fever is common, and lymphadenopathy can occur.[198] Complication rates for vaccinia (smallpox) vaccination are much higher among primary (first-time) vaccinees than among persons being revaccinated.[199] The most frequent complication is autoinoculation (with an incidence of 1 case among 2000 vaccinees) to other sites, such as the face or genitals. Most such lesions heal spontaneously. Generalized vaccinia (1 in 5000 vaccinees) describes a blood-borne spread of the vaccine virus, with development of lesions distant to the site of inoculation about a week after vaccination. This condition also usually is self-limited. Eczema vaccinatum (1 in 25,000 vaccinees) may occur in vaccine recipients who have eczema or other chronic skin conditions or even a history of such conditions in the past. Lesions develop at the site of current or former skin conditions. Although this complication also usually is mild, it can be severe or even fatal. Progressive vaccinia (1 in 500,000 vaccinees) occurs in persons with underlying immune deficiency. Rather than the usual healing at the site of vaccination, progressive enlargement of the lesion and ultimate necrosis occur. Secondary lesions with necrosis may develop as well. This condition also can be fatal. Postvaccination encephalitis (1 case in 125,000 vaccinees) may occur approximately 1 or 2 weeks after vaccination. The fatality rate for this complication is 25%, and another 25% of affected patients are left with permanent neurologic sequelae.[199] A more recently recognized complication of smallpox vaccination is myopericarditis (1 in 8000 vaccinees).[200,201] As with other complications, the rate is higher among primary vaccinees.[200] Follow-up evaluation of patients with myopericarditis has demonstrated a good prognosis with normalization of the electrocardiogram (ECG), echocardiogram, and treadmill testing.[202] Nonetheless, this serious complication has led to the inclusion of cardiac disease as a relative contraindication to smallpox vaccination.[203]

Relative contraindications to vaccinia (smallpox) vaccination include the presence or history of eczema or other chronic skin condition, immunosuppression, pregnancy or breastfeeding, age younger than 18 years, cardiac disease, and known allergy to a component of the vaccine.[204] Household contacts with current eczema or a history of this or other chronic skin condition, or immunosuppression, or who are pregnant, also are at increased risk of complications as a result of accidental inoculation from the vaccinated individual.[204] In the case of actual smallpox exposure, the risk of the disease and its sequelae may outweigh the risk of vaccine complications, even in those with relative contraindications.

Vaccinia Immunoglobulin

Similar to other specific immunoglobulin preparations, vaccinia immunoglobulin (VIG) is harvested from the plasma of persons who have been vaccinated with vaccinia virus. VIG may be of help in ameliorating some complications of vaccinia immunization, including eczema vaccinatum, progressive vaccinia, and severe generalized vaccinia.[198] It also may be used for autoinoculation to the eye or eyelid, but it is specifically contraindicated in vaccinia keratitis, where it may promote scarring. VIG is not effective in postvaccination encephalitis or in the treatment of smallpox itself. When indicated for complications of vaccinia vaccination, VIG is available through the CDC.[198] Both intramuscular and intravenous preparations are available.

Other Biologic Agents Used as Weapons

A number of other biologic agents have been developed for use as weapons, including the agents of plague, tularemia, botulism, Q fever, viral encephalitides, and hemorrhagic fevers.[191] Manufacture of a licensed plague vaccine was discontinued in 1999. The vaccine was effective against bubonic but not pneumonic plague, the latter being the primary form of plague as a biologic weapon.[205] Investigational vaccines are in development for protection against the agents of other potential biologic weapons.[192]

Controversies Regarding Long-Term Consequences of Vaccination

ATOPY

In regard to immunity, evidence suggests that all humans are born relatively skewed toward Th2 responsiveness and that, by a process of "immune deviation," most switch to greater Th1 responsiveness in infancy and early childhood.[206] This switch may require early Th1-stimulating microbial exposures and may involve immune suppression by regulatory T cells. A "hygiene hypothesis" has been advanced whereby a lack of such early childhood microbial exposure would contribute to the prevalence of atopic (i.e., Th2) diseases.[206]

Because immunization prevents natural infection, it has been suggested that vaccines may contribute to the hygienic environment that permits atopic immune responsiveness. Because both natural disease and vaccination lead to immune responses, this theory requires that the differences in immune response would allow disease to protect from, and vaccination to promote, subsequent atopy. Furthermore, different infections and vaccines promote different types of immune responsiveness (relative dominance of Th1 or Th2).

Investigators in Japan examined the prevalence of atopic diseases and total IgE and cytokine profiles among school children in relation to their tuberculin delayed-type hypersensitivity (DTH) skin reaction after immunization with bacille Calmette-Guérin (BCG).[207] They found that a strong DTH response was "protective," reducing atopy by more than half, and suggested that a modification of immune profiles by BCG vaccination led to the decrease in atopy. Alternatively, this finding may simply represent the lesser Th1 responsiveness of children already skewed to Th2. Studies from Sweden and Turkey found no relationship between BCG vaccination and development of atopic sensitization or disease.[208,209] Also, in a prospective study of children in Germany either vaccinated with BCG or not, no long-term decrease in total or specific IgE or clinical atopy was observed in the vaccinated group.[210] A systematic review and meta-analysis have concluded that "BCG vaccination is unlikely to be associated with protection against the risk of allergic sensitization and disease."[211]

A study of children in Africa showed decreased allergen skin test reactivity in those who had had natural measles infection.[212] A larger study, however, actually found a slightly increased incidence of atopic diseases among children who had had measles infection.[213]

A retrospective study of health records found an increase in atopic disease among children vaccinated with whole-cell pertussis vaccine.[214] By contrast, a prospective trial of vaccines containing diphtheria and tetanus, with or without pertussis, found no increase in the diagnosis of atopic disease or the rate of positive allergen skin tests in the group that received pertussis vaccine.[215]

The number of potential confounding variables in studies of vaccination and atopy in various populations in various countries is enormous. This variability has been addressed in a very large multinational study, the International Study of Asthma and Allergies in Childhood.[216] This study evaluated symptoms of atopy by questionnaire in 6- to 7-year-old and 13- to 14-year-old children in 56 countries. Immunization rates were evaluated for the birth year of the groups. In contrast with the theory that immunization causes atopy, they actually found some weak inverse correlations between DTP and measles immunization in the 13-year-old children and symptoms of atopy. Furthermore, a thorough systematic review of the evidence relating childhood immunization to allergic disease concluded that "infant vaccines do not increase the risk of allergic disease."[217] Overall, the bulk of the evidence would thus seem to refute the idea that immunization causes atopy.[218]

AUTISM

Measles-Mumps-Rubella Vaccine

On the basis of data for a case series of 12 children, a suggestion had been made that autism might be related to MMR immunization.[219] This contention led to a careful analysis by several groups. In a study in the United Kingdom, researchers identified children with autism from disability and special school registries and linked their data with computerized immunization records. They found no change in the rate of autism cases after the introduction of MMR vaccine and no temporal association between vaccination and diagnosis.[220] Another group of investigators in California examined MMR immunization rates and autism caseloads and similarly found no correlation.[221]

The Institute of Medicine conducted exhaustive reviews on the matter in 2001 and again in 2011 and concluded that "the evidence favors a rejection of a causal relationship between MMR vaccine and autism."[69,222] Finally, a study of all 537,303 children born in Denmark over an 8-year period compared immunization status and medical diagnoses in national databases and found no association between MMR vaccination and autism or autistic-spectrum disorder.[223] The original study suggesting a link between MMR and autism has been formally retracted.[224]

Thimerosal

Because mercury is neurotoxic, in 1997 the FDA undertook a review of mercury-containing vaccines.[225] Thimerosal (50% mercury by weight) has been used for decades as an additive to several vaccines as a bactericidal agent. It was determined that infants receiving recommended vaccines in the first few months of life might be receiving an amount of mercury, in the form of thimerosal, exceeding federal guidelines on permissible exposure. Although no harmful effects of the exposure to mercury in vaccines had been reported, recommendations were made to reduce or eliminate the thimerosal content of vaccines. As a result, thimerosal has been removed from or reduced to trace amounts in all vaccines routinely recommended for children.[226] Subsequent studies carefully evaluated the risk of the previous exposure to thimerosal in vaccines and the subsequent development of neurologic disorders, particularly autism. Systematic reviews of these studies have concluded that there is no relationship between the receipt of thimerosal-containing vaccines and autism.[227,228]

AUTOIMMUNE DISEASES

For a number of diseases that are accepted as or suspected of being autoimmune in nature, such as Guillain-Barré syndrome, multiple sclerosis, type 1 diabetes, optic neuritis, and transverse myelitis, a temporal association with vaccination has been reported, suggesting that the vaccine may have caused the disease.[69] Because these conditions so rarely occur in association with vaccination, a review by the Institute of Medicine has concluded that for the vast majority, the "evidence is inadequate to accept or reject a causal relationship."[69]

Vaccination Relative to Immunocompromise and Immunoglobulin Preparations

IMMUNOCOMPROMISE

Several issues of importance are recognized regarding vaccinations in immunocompromised persons, that is, those with primary or secondary immune deficiency diseases or those with immunosuppression caused by disease or treatment. The first of these issues is safety, which largely relates to the administration of live vaccines (Box 85-2). Live attenuated vaccines have the potential to cause vaccine strain–induced disease.[34] The disease also may be attenuated but may be fulminant, particularly in immunocompromised recipients. The course of the vaccine-related disease often mirrors natural infection. The live vaccines routinely recommended for administration to immunocompetent persons include intranasal influenza, MMR, oral rotavirus, varicella, and zoster vaccines. Other available live vaccines are BCG, oral typhoid, vaccinia (smallpox), and yellow fever. Replication of the infective agents in live vaccines poses little or no risk to immunocompetent patients but can lead to disseminated disease; accordingly, these vaccines are contraindicated in the immunocompromised.[34,229] Exceptions to this

BOX 85-2 LIVE VERSUS NON-LIVE VACCINES

Live Vaccines	Non-Live (Killed, Subunit, Toxoid) Vaccines
Bacille Calmette-Guérin (BCG)	Diphtheria, tetanus, acellular pertussis (DTaP, Tdap)
Influenza (intranasal)	Diphtheria-tetanus (DT, Td)
Measles-mumps-rubella (MMR)	Hepatitis A
Oral poliovirus (OPV)	Hepatitis B
Rotavirus	*Haemophilus influenzae* type b (Hib) conjugates
Typhoid (oral)	Human papillomavirus (HPV)
Vaccinia (smallpox)	Inactivated poliovirus (IPV)
Varicella	Influenza (injectable)
Yellow fever	Japanese encephalitis
Zoster	Meningococcal
	Meningococcal conjugate
	Pneumococcal
	Pneumococcal conjugate
	Rabies
	Typhoid (injectable)

rule are that MMR, varicella, and rotavirus vaccines should be considered for human immunodeficiency virus (HIV)-infected persons who are not severely immunosuppressed.[34] Another issue relative to immunization of the immunocompromised is efficacy. Non-live vaccines may be safe to give to persons with impaired immunity, yet they may not be effective because they rely on an immune response for effect (see Box 85-2).[34,229] Recommendations regarding the vaccination of persons with primary and secondary immunodeficiencies are summarized in Table 85-3.

Immunization is sometimes used diagnostically in the evaluation of suspected immunodeficiency. Persons with antibody deficiencies are susceptible to infection not because of a low level of an antibody class or subclass, but rather because of the inability to make functional protective antibodies to particular pathogens. It is therefore useful in the evaluation of patients suspected of antibody deficiency to measure levels of specific antibodies to immunizing antigens. Because most people have already been immunized against diphtheria and tetanus, the level of antibodies to these agents provides information on the ability to make antibodies to protein antigens. Measuring levels of antipneumococcal antibodies before and after immunization with the 23-valent pneumococcal vaccine provides information on the ability to make antibody to polysaccharide antigens.[230] Many patients have now been immunized with 7- or 13-valent pneumococcal protein-conjugate vaccines. If this is the case, their antibody responses to the serotypes in the conjugate vaccines represent a response to protein antigens. To assess their responses to polysaccharide antigens, they must be given the 23-valent polysaccharide vaccine; titers to serotypes present only in the polysaccharide vaccine are then measured before and after immunization.[230]

In certain clinical circumstances, such as in patients already on intravenous immunoglobulin (IVIG) antibody replacement therapy, the measurement of antibodies to vaccines is not helpful, because these antibodies are abundant in the IVIG donor pool and cannot be distinguished from recipient antibodies. A novel approach has been developed for use in this situation: vaccination with a "neoantigen"—that is, an antigen (bacteriophage phi X 174) to which neither the donors to the IVIG pool nor the recipient would have been exposed.[231,232]

IMMUNOGLOBULIN PREPARATIONS

Immunoglobulin preparations interfere with the desired immune response to parenteral live viral vaccines,[13,34] presumably because these preparations contain antibodies to the immunizing virus, or because of other immunomodulation.

TABLE 85-3 Vaccination of Persons with Primary and Secondary Immunodeficiencies

Primary	Specific Immunodeficiency	Contraindicated Vaccine(s)*	Risk-Specific Recommended Vaccine(s)*	Effectiveness and Comments
B lymphocyte (humoral)	Severe antibody deficiencies (e.g., X-linked agammaglobulinemia, common variable immunodeficiency)	OPV† Smallpox LAIV BCG Ty21a (live typhoid) Yellow fever	Pneumococcal Consider measles and varicella vaccination	Effectiveness of any vaccine is uncertain if it depends only on the humoral response (e.g., PPSV, MPSV4) IVIG interferes with immune response to measles vaccine and possibly varicella vaccine
	Less severe antibody deficiencies (e.g., selective IgA deficiency, IgG subclass deficiency)	OPV† BCG Yellow fever Other live vaccines appear to be safe	Pneumococcal	All vaccines likely effective; immune response might be attenuated
T lymphocyte (cell-mediated and humoral)	Complete defects (e.g., severe combined immunodeficiency [SCID] disease, complete DiGeorge syndrome)	All live vaccines‡,§,‖	Pneumococcal	Vaccines might be ineffective
	Partial defects (e.g., most patients with DiGeorge syndrome, Wiskott-Aldrich syndrome, ataxia-telangiectasia)	All live vaccines‡,§,‖	Pneumococcal Meningococcal Hib (if not administered in infancy)	Effectiveness of any vaccine depends on degree of immune suppression
Complement	Persistent complement, properdin, or factor B deficiency	None	Pneumococcal Meningococcal	All routine vaccines likely effective
Phagocytic function	Chronic granulomatous disease, leukocyte adhesion defect, and myeloperoxidase deficiency	Live bacterial vaccines‡	Pneumococcal¶	All inactivated vaccines safe and likely effective Live viral vaccines likely safe and effective

TABLE 85-3 Vaccination of Persons with Primary and Secondary Immunodeficiencies—cont'd

Primary	Specific Immunodeficiency	Contraindicated Vaccine(s)*	Risk-Specific Recommended Vaccine(s)*	Effectiveness and Comments
Secondary	HIV infection/AIDS	OPV[†] Smallpox BCG LAIV Withhold MMR and varicella in severely immunocompromised persons Yellow fever vaccine might have a contraindication or a precaution depending on clinical parameters of immune function**	Pneumococcal Consider Hib (if not administered in infancy) and meningococcal vaccination	MMR, varicella, rotavirus, and all inactivated vaccines, including inactivated influenza, might be effective[††]
	Malignant neoplasm, transplantation, immunosuppressive or radiation therapy	Live viral and bacterial, depending on immune status[‡,§]	Pneumococcal	Effectiveness of any vaccine depends on degree of immune suppression
	Asplenia	None	Pneumococcal Meningococcal Hib (if not administered in infancy)	All routine vaccines likely effective
	Chronic renal disease	LAIV	Pneumococcal Hepatitis B[‡‡]	All routine vaccines likely effective

From National Center for Immunization and Respiratory Diseases. General recommendations on immunization—recommendations of the Advisory Committee on Immunization Practices (ACIP). MMWR Recomm Rep 2011;60:1-64.

AIDS, acquired immunodeficiency syndrome; *BCG,* bacille Calmette-Guérin; *CDC,* Centers for Disease Control and Prevention; *Hib, Haemophilus influenzae* type b; *HIV,* human immunodeficiency virus; *IVIG,* intravenous immunoglobulin; *LAIV,* live attenuated influenza vaccine; *MMR,* measles-mumps-rubella; *MPSV4,* quadrivalent meningococcal polysaccharide vaccine; *OPV,* oral poliovirus vaccine (live); *PCV,* pneumococcal conjugate vaccine; *PPSV,* pneumococcal polysaccharide vaccine; *TIV,* trivalent inactivated influenza vaccine.

*Other vaccines that are universally or routinely recommended should be given if not contraindicated.

†OPV is no longer available in the United States.

‡Live bacterial vaccines: BCG and oral Ty21a *Salmonella typhi* vaccine.

§Live viral vaccines: MMR, MMRV, OPV, LAIV, yellow fever, zoster, rotavirus, varicella, and vaccinia (smallpox). Smallpox vaccine is not recommended for children or the general public.

‖Regarding T lymphocyte immunodeficiency as a contraindication for rotavirus vaccine, data are available only for severe combined immunodeficiency.

¶Pneumococcal vaccine is not indicated for children with chronic granulomatous disease beyond age-based universal recommendations for PCV. Children with chronic granulomatous disease are not at increased risk for pneumococcal disease.

**Symptomatic HIV infection or $CD4^+$ T lymphocyte count below 200/mm^3, or less than 15% of total lymphocytes for children younger than 6 years of age, is a contraindication to yellow fever vaccine administration. Asymptomatic HIV infection with $CD4^+$ T lymphocyte count of 200 to 499/mm^3 for persons 6 years of age and older or 15% to 24% of total lymphocytes for children younger than 6 years of age is a precaution for yellow fever vaccine administration. Details of yellow fever vaccine recommendations are available from the CDC, as follows: Staples JE, Gershman M, Fischer M; Centers for Disease Control and Prevention (CDC). Yellow fever vaccine: recommendations of the Advisory Committee on Immunization Practices (ACIP). MMWR Recomm Rep 2010;59:1-27.

††HIV-infected children should receive immunoglobulin after exposure to measles and may receive varicella and measles vaccine if $CD4^+$ T lymphocyte count is 15% or greater.

‡‡Indicated based on the risk from dialysis-based blood-borne transmission.

Immunoglobulin preparations given within 2 weeks after live virus vaccination could prevent adequate immunization. Suggested intervals after first giving an immunoglobulin preparation until vaccination are listed in Table 85-4.[13]

Vaccination during Pregnancy and Breastfeeding

A theoretical risk of causing disease in the fetus is recognized for administration of a live vaccine to a pregnant woman, although smallpox is the only vaccine known to have done so.[13] Nonetheless, pregnant women should not receive any live vaccines[13] (see Box 85-2). HPV vaccine also should not be administered during pregnancy, because it has not been studied to determine the risk of adverse effects.[233] Inactivated (injectable) influenza vaccine is specifically indicated in pregnancy, and other vaccines such as tetanus (Td or Tdap) and hepatitis B should be administered in pregnancy if otherwise indicated.[13,233]

Non-live vaccines (see Box 85-2) pose no risk to breastfeeding women or their babies.[13] Most live vaccines (see Box 85-2) also are safe, with the exception of vaccinia (smallpox) and yellow fever (YF) vaccines.[13] It is not known whether or not the vaccinia virus is excreted in human breast milk; however, because of the risk of contact transmission from the vaccine site, breastfeeding mothers should not receive the smallpox vaccine.[204] There have been two reports of probable transmission of vaccine-strain yellow fever virus from breastfeeding mothers to their infants.[234,235] The CDC has concluded that "until more information is available, YF vaccine should be avoided in breastfeeding women. However, when travel of nursing mothers to a YF-endemic area cannot be avoided or postponed, these women should be vaccinated."[190]

TABLE 85-4 Recommended Intervals between Administration of Antibody-Containing Products and Measles- or Varicella-Containing Vaccine, by Product and Indication for Vaccination

Product/Indication	Dose (with IgG content) and Administration Route*	Recommended Interval before Measles- or Varicella-Containing Vaccine† Administration (months)
Tetanus immunoglobulin	250 units (10 mg IgG/kg) IM	3
Hepatitis A immunoglobulin		
Contact prophylaxis	0.02 mL/kg (3.3 mg IgG/kg) IM	3
International travel	0.06 mL/kg (10 mg IgG/kg) IM	3
Hepatitis B immunoglobulin	0.06 mL/kg (10 mg IgG/kg) IM	3
Rabies immunoglobulin	20 IU/kg (22 mg IgG/kg) IM	4
Varicella immunoglobulin	125 units/10 kg (60-200 mg IgG/kg) IM, maximum 625 units	5
Measles prophylaxis immunoglobulin		
Standard (i.e., nonimmunocompromised) contact	0.25 mL/kg (40 mg IgG/kg) IM	5
Immunocompromised contact	0.50 mL/kg (80 mg IgG/kg) IM	6
Blood transfusion		
RBCs, washed	10 mL/kg, negligible IgG/kg IV	None
RBCs, adenine-saline added	10 mL/kg (10 mg IgG/kg) IV	3
Packed RBCs (hematocrit 65%)‡	10 mL/kg (60 mg IgG/kg) IV	6
Whole blood (hematocrit 35-50%)‡	10 mL/kg (80-100 mg IgG/kg) IV	6
Plasma/platelet products	10 mL/kg (160 mg IgG/kg) IV	7
Cytomegalovirus IGIV	150 mg/kg maximum	6
IVIG		
Replacement therapy for immune deficiencies§	300-400 mg/kg IV§	8
Immune thrombocytopenic purpura treatment	400 mg/kg IV	8
Postexposure varicella prophylaxis‖	400 mg/kg IV	8
Immune thrombocytopenic purpura treatment	1000 mg/kg IV	10
Kawasaki disease	2 g/kg IV	11
Monoclonal antibody to respiratory syncytial virus F protein (Synagis [MedImmune])¶	15 mg/kg IM	None

From National Center for Immunization and Respiratory Diseases. General recommendations on immunization—recommendations of the Advisory Committee on Immunization Practices (ACIP). MMWR Recomm Rep 2011;60:1-64.

HIV, Human immunodeficiency virus; *IgG*, immune globulin G; *IM*, intramuscular; *IV*, intravenous; *IVIG*, intravenous immunoglobulin; *MMRV*, measles-mumps-rubella-varicella; *RBCs*, red blood cells.

*This table is not intended for determining the correct indications and dosages for using antibody-containing products. Unvaccinated persons might not be protected fully against measles during the entire recommended interval, and additional doses of immunoglobulin or measles vaccine might be indicated after measles exposure. Concentrations of measles antibody in an immunoglobulin preparation can vary by manufacturer's lot. Rates of antibody clearance after receipt of an immunoglobulin preparation also might vary. Recommended intervals are extrapolated from an estimated half-life of 30 days for passively acquired antibody and an observed interference with the immune response to measles vaccine for 5 months after a dose of 80 mg IgG/kg.

†Does not include zoster vaccine. Zoster vaccine may be given with antibody-containing blood products.

‡Assumes a serum IgG concentration of 16 mg/mL.

§Measles and varicella vaccinations are recommended for children with asymptomatic or mildly symptomatic HIV infection but are contraindicated for persons with severe immunosuppression from HIV or any other immunosuppressive disorder.

‖The investigational VariZIG, similar to licensed varicella-zoster immunoglobulin (VZIG), is a purified human immunoglobulin preparation made from plasma containing high levels of antivaricella antibodies (IgG). The interval between VariZIG and varicella vaccine (Var or MMRV vaccine) is 5 months.

¶Contains antibody only to respiratory syncytial virus.

Summary of Recommendations

The dramatic reduction or elimination of many diseases by vaccination is perhaps the greatest public health achievement in history. Whereas mild, self-limited adverse reactions to vaccines are common, serious complications or long-term sequelae are rare. In virtually all cases, the risk of an adverse outcome from the disease itself is far greater than the risk from vaccination.

When a serious adverse event possibly related to vaccination occurs, it should be investigated to determine the cause and to make recommendations to the individual patient regarding subsequent immunizations. Adverse reactions may or may not be IgE-mediated and may be due to the immunizing agent itself or to some other vaccine constituent. Serious reactions also should be reported even if the clinician is not certain of the relationship of the reaction to vaccination. Public health agencies and vaccine manufacturers need these reports to quantify rare adverse vaccine reactions and to further improve vaccine safety. New vaccines continue to be developed and recommended for use, including the newly approved vaccines for HPV, rotavirus, and zoster infections. Postmarketing surveillance and reporting may reveal as-yet unknown adverse events associated with these immunizations.

REFERENCES

Putting Adverse Reactions to Vaccines in Perspective

1. Ten great public health achievements—United States, 2001-2010. MMWR Morb Mortal Wkly Rep 2011;60:619-23.
2. Chen RT, Rastogi SC, Mullen JR, et al. The Vaccine Adverse Event Reporting System (VAERS). Vaccine 1994;12:542-50.
3. Salmon DA, Haber M, Gangarosa EJ, et al. Health consequences of religious and philosophical exemptions from immunization laws: individual and societal risk of measles. JAMA 1999;282:47-53.
4. Gangarosa EJ, Galazka AM, Wolfe CR, et al. Impact of anti-vaccine movements on pertussis control: the untold story. Lancet 1998;351: 356-61.
5. Danovaro-Holliday MC, LeBaron CW, Allensworth C, et al. A large rubella outbreak with spread from the workplace to the community. JAMA 2000;284:2733-9.
6. Update: Outbreak of poliomyelitis—Dominican Republic and Haiti, 2000-2001. MMWR Morb Mortal Wkly Rep 2001;50: 855-6.
7. Two fatal cases of adenovirus-related illness in previously healthy young adults—Illinois, 2000. MMWR Morb Mortal Wkly Rep 2001; 50:553-5.
8. Jansen VA, Stollenwerk N, Jensen HJ, et al. Measles outbreaks in a population with declining vaccine uptake. Science 2003;301: 804.
9. DeStefano F; Vaccine Safety Datalink Research Group. The Vaccine Safety Datalink project. Pharmacoepidemiol Drug Saf 2001;10:403-6.
10. Scheifele DW, Halperin SA; CPS/Health Canada, Immunization Monitoring Program, Active (IMPACT). Immunization Monitoring Program, Active: a model of active surveillance of vaccine safety. Semin Pediatr Infect Dis 2003;14:213-9.
11. Jacobson RM, Adegbenro A, Pankratz VS, Poland GA. Adverse events and vaccination—the lack of power and predictability of infrequent events in pre-licensure study. Vaccine 2001;19:2428-33.

Immunoglobulin E–Mediated Reactions to Vaccines

12. Bohlke K, Davis RL, DeStefano F, et al. Epidemiology of anaphylaxis among children and adolescents enrolled in a health maintenance organization. J Allergy Clin Immunol 2004; 113:536-42.
13. General recommendations on immunization—recommendations of the Advisory Committee on Immunization Practices (ACIP). MMWR Morb Mortal Wkly Rep 2011;60:1-64.
14. Johann-Liang R, Josephs S, Dreskin SC. Analysis of anaphylaxis cases after vaccination: 10-year review from the National Vaccine Injury Compensation Program. Ann Allergy Asthma Immunol 2011;106:440-3.
15. Kelso JM, Jones RT, Yunginger JW. Anaphylaxis to measles, mumps, and rubella vaccine mediated by IgE to gelatin. J Allergy Clin Immunol 1993;91:867-72.
16. Sakaguchi M, Nakayama T, Inouye S. Food allergy to gelatin in children with systemic immediate-type reactions, including anaphylaxis, to vaccines. J Allergy Clin Immunol 1996;98:1058-61.
17. Patja A, Makinen-Kiljunen S, Davidkin I, Paunio M, Peltola H. Allergic reactions to measles-mumps-rubella vaccination. Pediatrics 2001;107:E27.
18. Sakaguchi M, Yamanaka T, Ikeda K, et al. IgE-mediated systemic reactions to gelatin included in the varicella vaccine. J Allergy Clin Immunol 1997;99:263-4.
19. Singer S, Johnson CE, Mohr R, Holowecky C. Urticaria following varicella vaccine associated with gelatin allergy. Vaccine 1999;17:327-9.
20. Sakaguchi M, Yoshida M, Kuroda W, et al. Systemic immediate-type reactions to gelatin included in Japanese encephalitis vaccines. Vaccine 1997;15:121-2.
21. Lasley MV. Anaphylaxis after booster influenza vaccine due to gelatin allergy. Pediatr Asthma Allergy Immunol 2007;20:201-5.
22. Nakayama T, Aizawa C. Change in gelatin content of vaccines associated with reduction in reports of allergic reactions. J Allergy Clin Immunol 2000;106:591-2.
23. Kuno-Sakai H, Kimura M. Removal of gelatin from live vaccines and DTaP—an ultimate solution for vaccine-related gelatin allergy. Biologicals 2003;31:245-9.
24. Zent O, Hennig R. Post-marketing surveillance of immediate allergic reactions: polygeline-based versus polygeline-free pediatric TBE vaccine. Vaccine 2004;23:579-84.
25. Fischer M, Lindsey N, Staples JE, Hills S. Japanese encephalitis vaccines: recommendations of the Advisory Committee on Immunization Practices (ACIP). MMWR Morb Mortal Wkly Rep 2010;59:1-27.
26. Kelso JM. The gelatin story. J AllergyClin Immunol 1999;103:200-2.
27. Pool V, Braun MM, Kelso JM, et al. Prevalence of anti-gelatin IgE antibodies in people with anaphylaxis after measles-mumps rubella vaccine in the United States. Pediatrics 2002; 110:e71.
28. Kumagai T, Yamanaka T, Wataya Y, et al. A strong association between HLA-DR9 and gelatin allergy in the Japanese population. Vaccine 2001;19:3273-6.
29. Sakaguchi M, Nakayama T, Kaku H, et al. Analysis of HLA in children with gelatin allergy. Tissue Antigens 2002;59:412-6.
30. Herman JJ, Radin R, Schneiderman R. Allergic reactions to measles (rubeola) vaccine in patients hypersensitive to egg protein. J Pediatr 1983;102:196-9.
31. O'Brien TC, Maloney CJ, Tauraso NM. Quantitation of residual host protein in chicken embryo-derived vaccines by radial immunodiffusion. Appl Microbiol 1971;21:780-2.
32. James JM, Burks AW, Roberson PK, Sampson HA. Safe administration of the measles vaccine to children allergic to eggs. N Engl J Med 1995;332:1262-6.
33. Baxter DN. Measles immunization in children with a history of egg allergy. Vaccine 1996;14: 131-4.
34. Red book—Report of the committee on infectious diseases. 28th ed. Elk Grove Village, Ill.: American Academy of Pediatrics; 2009.
35. James JM, Zeiger RS, Lester MR, et al. Safe administration of influenza vaccine to patients with egg allergy. J Pediatr 1998;133: 624-8.
36. Chung EY, Huang L, Schneider L. Safety of influenza vaccine administration in egg-allergic patients. Pediatrics 2010;125:e1024-30.
37. Gagnon R, Primeau MN, Des Roches A, et al. Safe vaccination of patients with egg allergy with an adjuvanted pandemic H1N1 vaccine. J Allergy Clin Immunol 2010;126:317-23.
38. Greenhawt MJ, Chernin AS, Howe L, Li JT, Sanders G. The safety of the H1N1 influenza A vaccine in egg allergic individuals. Ann Allergy Asthma Immunol 2010;105:387-93.
39. Owens G, Macginnitie A. Higher-ovalbumin-content influenza vaccines are well tolerated in children with egg allergy. J Allergy Clin Immunol 2011;127:264-5.
40. Howe LE, Conlon AS, Greenhawt MJ, Sanders GM. Safe administration of seasonal influenza vaccine to children with egg allergy of all severities. Ann Allergy Asthma Immunol 2011;106: 446-7.
41. Webb L, Petersen M, Boden S, et al. Single-dose influenza vaccination of patients with egg allergy in a multicenter study. J Allergy Clin Immunol 2011;128:218-9.
42. Waibel KH, Gomez R. Ovalbumin content in 2009 to 2010 seasonal and H1N1 monovalent influenza vaccines. J Allergy Clin Immunol 2010;125:749-51, 51.e1.
43. Li JT, Rank MA, Squillace DL, Kita H. Ovalbumin content of influenza vaccines. J Allergy Clin Immunol 2010;125:1412-3.
44. McKinney KK, Webb L, Petersen M, Nelson M, Laubach S. Ovalbumin content of 2010-2011 influenza vaccines. Journal of Allergy and Clinical Immunology 2011;127:1629-32.
45. Prevention and control of influenza with vaccines: Recommendations of the Advisory Committee on Immunization Practices (ACIP), 2011. MMWR Morb Mortal Wkly Rep 2011;60:1128-32.
46. American Academy of Pediatrics Committee on Infectious Diseases. Recommendations for prevention and control of influenza in children, 2011-2012. Pediatrics 2011;128:813-25.
47. Swartz HF. Systemic allergic reaction induced by yellow fever vaccine. J Lab Clin Med 1943;28:1663-7.
48. Sprague H, Barnard J. Egg allergy: significance in typhus and yellow fever immunization. US Navy Med Bull 1945;45:71-4.
49. Rubin S. An allergic reaction following typhus-fever vaccine and yellow-fever vaccine due to egg yolk sensitivity. J Allergy 1946;17:21-3.
50. Kelso JM, Mootrey GT, Tsai TF. Anaphylaxis from yellow fever vaccine. J Allergy Clin Immunol 1999;103:698-701.
51. Kelso JM. Raw egg allergy—a potential issue in vaccine allergy. J Allergy Clin Immunol 2000; 106:990.
52. Kelso JM, Cockrell GE, Helm RM, Burks AW. Common allergens in avian meats. J Allergy Clin Immunol 1999;104:202-4.
53. Primeau M-N, Adkinson NF, Hamilton RG. Natural rubber pharmaceutical vial closures release latex allergens that produce skin reactions. J Allergy Clin Immunol 2001;107: 958-62.
54. Lear JT, English JS. Anaphylaxis after hepatitis B vaccination. Lancet 1995;345:1249.
55. Russell M, Pool V, Kelso JM, Tomazic-Jezic VJ. Vaccination of persons allergic to latex: a review of safety data in the Vaccine Adverse Event Reporting System (VAERS). Vaccine 2004;23:664-7.
56. Latex in vaccine packaging. In: Atkinson W, Wolfe S, Hamborsky J, editors. Centers for Disease Control and Prevention. Epidemiology

and prevention of vaccine-preventable diseases. 12th ed. Washington, D.C.: Public Health Foundation; 2011.
57. ENGERIX-B package insert. Research Triangle Park, N.C.: GlaxoSmithKline; 2010.
58. RECOMBIVAX HB package insert. Whitehouse Station, N.J.: Merck & Co.; 1998.
59. Wiedermann G, Scheiner O, Ambrosch F, et al. Lack of induction of IgE and IgG antibodies to yeast in humans immunized with recombinant hepatitis B vaccines. Int Arch Allergy Appl Immunol 1988;85:130-2.
60. West DJ. Clinical experience with hepatitis B vaccines. Am J Infect Control 1989;17:172-80.
61. DiMiceli L, Pool V, Kelso JM, Shadomy SV, Iskander J; Team VAERS. Vaccination of yeast sensitive individuals: review of safety data in the US vaccine adverse event reporting system (VAERS). Vaccine 2006;24:703-7.
62. Baur X, Degens PO, Sander I. Baker's asthma: still among the most frequent occupational respiratory disorders. J Allergy Clin Immunol 1998;102:984-97.
63. GARDASIL package insert. Merck, 2011.
64. Kattan JD, Konstantinou GN, Cox AL, et al. Anaphylaxis to diphtheria, tetanus, and pertussis vaccines among children with cow's milk allergy. J Allergy Clin Immunol 2011;128:215-8.
65. Slater JE, Rabin RL, Martin D. Comments on cow's milk allergy and diphtheria, tetanus, and pertussis vaccines. J Allergy Clin Immunol 2011;128:434.
66. Nagel J, Svec D, Waters T, Fireman P. IgE synthesis in man. I. Development of specific IgE antibodies after immunization with tetanus-diphtheria (Td) toxoids. J Immunol 1977;118:334-41.
67. Nagel JE, White C, Lin MS, Fireman P. IgE synthesis in man. II. Comparison of tetanus and diphtheria IgE antibody in allergic and nonallergic children. J Allergy Clin Immunol 1979;63:308-14.
68. Mark A, Bjorksten B, Granstrom M. Immunoglobulin E responses to diphtheria and tetanus toxoids after booster with aluminium-adsorbed and fluid DT-vaccines. Vaccine 1995;13:669-73.
69. IOM (Institute of Medicine). Adverse effects of vaccines: evidence and causality. Washington, D.C.: The National Academies Press; 2011.
70. Martin-Munoz MF, Pereira MJ, Posadas S, et al. Anaphylactic reaction to diphtheria-tetanus vaccine in a child: specific IgE/IgG determinations and cross-reactivity studies. Vaccine 2002;20:3409-12.
71. Skov PS, Pelck I, Ebbesen F, Poulsen LK. Hypersensitivity to the diphtheria component in the Di-Te-Pol vaccine. A type I allergic reaction demonstrated by basophil histamine release. Pediatr Allergy Immunol 1997;8:156-8.
72. Nelson M, Oakes H, Smith L. Anaphylaxis complicating routine childhood immunization: *Haemophilus influenzae* b conjugated vaccine. Pediatr Asthma Allergy Immunol 2000;14:315.
73. Stratton KR, Howe CJ, Johnston RB. Adverse events associated with childhood vaccines: evidence bearing on causality. Washington, D.C.: National Academy Press; 1994.
74. Milstien JB, Gross TP, Kuritsky JN. Adverse reactions reported following receipt of *Haemophilus influenzae* type b vaccine: an analysis after 1 year of marketing. Pediatrics 1987;80:270-4.
75. Centers for Disease Control and Prevention. Update: vaccine side effects, adverse reactions, contraindications, and precautions. Recommendations of the Advisory Committee on Immunization Practices (ACIP). MMWR Morb Mortal Wkly Rep 1996;45:1-35.
76. Halsey NA. The human papillomavirus vaccine and risk of anaphylaxis. CMAJ 2008;179:509-10.
77. Brotherton JM, Gold MS, Kemp AS, et al. Anaphylaxis following quadrivalent human papillomavirus vaccination. CMAJ 2008;179:525-33.
78. Kang LW, Crawford N, Tang ML, et al. Hypersensitivity reactions to human papillomavirus vaccine in Australian schoolgirls: retrospective cohort study. BMJ 2008;337:a2642.
79. Slade BA, Leidel L, Vellozzi C, et al. Postlicensure safety surveillance for quadrivalent human papillomavirus recombinant vaccine. JAMA 2009;302:750-7.
80. Syncope after vaccination—United States, January 2005-July 2007. MMWR Morb Mortal Wkly Rep 2008;57:457-60.
81. Retailliau HF, Curtis AC, Storr G, et al. Illness after influenza vaccination reported through a nationwide surveillance system, 1976-1977. Am J Epidemiol 1980;111:270-8.
82. Bierman CW, Shapiro GG, Pierson WE, et al. Safety of influenza vaccination in allergic children. J Infect Dis 1977;136:S652-5.
83. Vellozzi C, Burwen DR, Dobardzic A, et al. Safety of trivalent inactivated influenza vaccines in adults: background for pandemic influenza vaccine safety monitoring. Vaccine 2009;27:2114-20.
84. Vasu N, Ghaffari G, Craig ET, Craig TJ. Adverse events associated with intranasal influenza vaccine in the United States. Ther Adv Respir Dis 2008;2:193-8.
85. Sakaguchi M, Inouye S. Two patterns of systemic immediate-type reactions to Japanese encephalitis vaccines. Vaccine 1998;16:68-9.
86. Sakaguchi M, Nakashima K, Takahashi H, et al. Anaphylaxis to Japanese encephalitis vaccine. Allergy 2001;56:804-5.
87. Berg SW, Mitchell BS, Hanson RK, et al. Systemic reactions in U.S. Marine Corps personnel who received Japanese encephalitis vaccine. Clin Infect Dis 1997;24:265-6.
88. Takahashi H, Pool V, Tsai TF, Chen RT. Adverse events after Japanese encephalitis vaccination: review of post-marketing surveillance data from Japan and the United States. The VAERS Working Group. Vaccine 2000;18:2963-9.
89. Plesner AM, Ronne T. Allergic mucocutaneous reactions to Japanese encephalitis vaccine. Vaccine 1997;15:1239-43.
90. Ruff TA, Eisen D, Fuller A, Kass R. Adverse reactions to Japanese encephalitis vaccine. Lancet 1991;338:881-2.
91. Plesner A, Ronne T, Wachmann H. Case-control study of allergic reactions to Japanese encephalitis vaccine. Vaccine 2000;18:1830-6.
92. Aukrust L, Almeland TL, Refsum D, Aas K. Severe hypersensitivity or intolerance reactions to measles vaccine in six children. Clinical and immunological studies. Allergy 1980;35:581-7.
93. Van Asperen PP, McEniery J, Kemp AS. Immediate reactions following live attenuated measles vaccine. Med J Aust 1981;2:330-1.
94. McEwen J. Early-onset reaction after measles vaccination. Further Australian reports. Med J Aust 1983;2:503-5.
95. Pollock TM, Morris J. A 7-year survey of disorders attributed to vaccination in North West Thames region. Lancet 1983;1:753-7.
96. Puvvada L, Silverman B, Bassett C, Chiaramonte LT. Systemic reactions to measles-mumps-rubella vaccine skin testing. Pediatrics 1993;91:835-6.
97. Thurston A. Anaphylactic shock reaction to measles vaccine. J R Coll Gen Pract 1987;37:41.
98. Kalet A, Berger DK, Bateman WB, Dubitsky J, Covitz K. Allergic reactions to MMR vaccine. Pediatrics 1992;89:168-9.
99. Fasano MB, Wood RA, Cooke SK, Sampson HA. Egg hypersensitivity and adverse reactions to measles, mumps, and rubella vaccine. J Pediatr 1992;120:878-81.
100. Ball R, Braun MM, Mootrey GT; Vaccine Adverse Event Reporting System Working Group. Safety data on meningococcal polysaccharide vaccine from the Vaccine Adverse Event Reporting System. Clin Infect Dis 2001;32:1273-80.
101. Granoff DM, Feavers IM, Borrow R. Meningococcal vaccines. In: Plotkin SA, Orenstein WA, editors. Vaccines. 4th ed. Philadelphia: Saunders; 2004.
102. Hedenskog S, Bjorksten B, Blennow M, Granstrom G, Granstrom M. Immunoglobulin E response to pertussis toxin in whooping cough and after immunization with a whole-cell and an acellular pertussis vaccine. Int Arch Allergy Appl Immunol 1989;89:156-61.
103. Torre D, Issi M, Chelazzi G, Fiori GP, Sampietro C. Total serum IgE levels in children with pertussis. Am J Dis Child 1990;144:290-1.
104. Duchen K, Granstrom M, Hedenskog S, Blennow M, Bjorksten B. Immunoglobulin E and G responses to pertussis toxin in children immunised with adsorbed and non-adsorbed whole cell pertussis vaccines. Vaccine 1997;15:1558-61.
105. Edelman K, Malmstrom K, He Q, et al. Local reactions and IgE antibodies to pertussis toxin after acellular diphtheria-tetanus-pertussis immunization. Eur J Pediatr 1999;158:989-94.
106. Odelram H, Granstrom M, Hedenskog S, Duchen K, Bjorksten B. Immunoglobulin E and G responses to pertussis toxin after booster immunization in relation to atopy, local reactions and aluminium content of the vaccines. Pediatr Allergy Immunol 1994;5:118-23.
107. Turktas I, Ergenekon E. Anaphylaxis following diphtheria-tetanus-pertussis vaccination—a reminder. Eur J Pediatr 1999;158:434.
108. Gifford CG, Gonsior EC, Villacorte GV, Bewtra A, Townley RG. Pertussis booster vaccination and immediate hypersensitivity. Ann Allergy 1985;54:483-5.
109. Assa'ad A, Lierl M. Effect of acellular pertussis vaccine on the development of allergic sensitization to environmental allergens in adults. J Allergy Clin Immunol 2000;105:170-5.
110. Ponvert C, Ardelean-Jaby D, Colin-Gorski AM, et al. Anaphylaxis to the 23-valent pneumococcal vaccine in child: a case-control study based on immediate responses in skin tests and specific IgE determination. Vaccine 2001;19:4588-91.
111. Ponvert C, Scheinmann P, de Blic J. Anaphylaxis to the 23-valent pneumococcal vaccine: a

second explored case by means of immediate-reading skin tests with pneumococcal vaccines. Vaccine 2010;28:8256-7.
112. Wise RP, Iskander J, Pratt RD, et al. Postlicensure safety surveillance for 7-valent pneumococcal conjugate vaccine. JAMA 2004;292:1702-10.
113. Centers for Disease Control and Prevention. Systemic allergic reactions following immunization with human diploid cell rabies vaccine. MMWR Morb Mortal Wkly Rep 1984;33:185-7.
114. Dreesen DW, Bernard KW, Parker RA, Deutsch AJ, Brown J. Immune complex-like disease in 23 persons following a booster dose of rabies human diploid cell vaccine. Vaccine 1986;4:45-9.
115. Swanson MC, Rosanoff E, Gurwith M, et al. IgE and IgG antibodies to beta-propiolactone and human serum albumin associated with urticarial reactions to rabies vaccine. J Infect Dis 1987;155:909-13.
116. Anderson MC, Baer H, Frazier DJ, Quinnan GV. The role of specific IgE and beta-propiolactone in reactions resulting from booster doses of human diploid cell rabies vaccine. J Allergy Clin Immunol 1987;80:861-8.
117. Fishbein DB, Yenne KM, Dreesen DW, et al. Risk factors for systemic hypersensitivity reactions after booster vaccinations with human diploid cell rabies vaccine: a nationwide prospective study. Vaccine 1993;11:1390-4.
118. Dobardzic A, Izurieta H, Woo EJ, et al. Safety review of the purified chick embryo cell rabies vaccine: Data from the Vaccine Adverse Event Reporting System (VAERS), 1997-2005. Vaccine 2007;25:4244-51.
119. Matuhasi T, Ikegami H. Elevation of levels of IgE antibody to tetanus toxin in individuals vaccinated with diphtheria-pertussis-tetanus vaccine. J Infect Dis 1982;146:290.
120. Cogne M, Ballet JJ, Schmitt C, Bizzini B. Total and IgE antibody levels following booster immunization with aluminum absorbed and nonabsorbed tetanus toxoid in humans. Ann Allergy 1985;54:148-51.
121. Aalberse RC, van Ree R, Danneman A, Wahn U. IgE antibodies to tetanus toxoid in relation to atopy. Int Arch Allergy Immunol 1995;107:169-71.
122. Brindle MJ, Twyman DG. Allergic reactions to tetanus toxoid. A report of four cases. BMJ 1962;5285:1116-7.
123. Zaloga GP, Chernow B. Life-threatening anaphylactic reaction to tetanus toxoid. Ann Allergy 1982;49:107-8.
124. Lleonart-Bellfill R, Cisteró-Bahima A, Cerdà-Trias MT, Olivé-Pérez A. Tetanus toxoid anaphylaxis. DICP 1991;25:870.
125. Carey AB, Meltzer EO. Diagnosis and "desensitization" in tetanus vaccine hypersensitivity. Ann Allergy 1992;69:336-8.
126. Mayorga C, Torres MJ, Corzo JL, et al. Immediate allergy to tetanus toxoid vaccine: determination of immunoglobulin E and immunoglobulin G antibodies to allergenic proteins. Ann Allergy Asthma Immunol 2003;90:238-43.
127. Wise RP, Salive ME, Braun MM, et al. Postlicensure safety surveillance for varicella vaccine. JAMA 2000;284:1271-9.
128. Chaves SS, Haber P, Walton K, et al. Safety of varicella vaccine after licensure in the United States: experience from reports to the vaccine adverse event reporting system, 1995-2005. J Infect Dis 2008;197(Suppl 2):S170-7.
129. Lindsey NP, Schroeder BA, Miller ER, et al. Adverse event reports following yellow fever vaccination. Vaccine 2008;26:6077-82.
130. Sampson HA, Munoz-Furlong A, Campbell RL, et al. Second symposium on the definition and management of anaphylaxis: summary report—Second National Institute of Allergy and Infectious Disease/Food Allergy and Anaphylaxis Network Symposium. J Allergy Clin Immunol 2006;117:391-7.
131. Ruggeberg JU, Gold MS, Bayas JM, et al. Anaphylaxis: Case definition and guidelines for data collection, analysis, and presentation of immunization safety data. Vaccine 2007;25:5675-84.
132. Zeiger RS. Current issues with influenza vaccination in egg allergy. J Allergy Clin Immunol 2002;110:834-40.
133. Wood RA, Berger M, Dreskin SC, et al. An algorithm for treatment of patients with hypersensitivity reactions after vaccines. Pediatrics 2008;122:e771-7.
134. Wood RA, Setse R, Halsey N. Irritant skin test reactions to common vaccines. J Allergy Clin Immunol 2007;120:478-81.
135. Seitz CS, Brocker EB, Trautmann A. Vaccination-associated anaphylaxis in adults: diagnostic testing ruling out IgE-mediated vaccine allergy. Vaccine 2009;27:3885-9.
136. Anolik R, Spiegel W, Posner M, Jakabovics E. Influenza vaccine testing in egg sensitive patients. Ann Allergy 1992;68:69.
137. Murphy KR, Strunk RC. Safe administration of influenza vaccine in asthmatic children hypersensitive to egg proteins. J Pediatr 1985;106:931-3.

Non–Immunoglobulin E–Mediated Reactions to Vaccines

138. Prystowsky SD, Allen AM, Smith RW, et al. Allergic contact hypersensitivity to nickel, neomycin, ethylenediamine, and benzocaine. Relationships between age, sex, history of exposure, and reactivity to standard patch tests and use tests in a general population. Arch Dermatol 1979;115:959-62.
139. Rietschel RL, Bernier R. Neomycin sensitivity and the MMR vaccine. JAMA 1981;245:571.
140. Cox NH, Forsyth A. Thiomersal allergy and vaccination reactions. Contact Dermatitis 1988;18:229-33.
141. Rietschel RL, Adams RM. Reactions to thimerosal in hepatitis B vaccines. Dermatol Clin 1990;8:161-4.
142. Noel I, Galloway A, Ive FA. Hypersensitivity to thiomersal in hepatitis B vaccine. Lancet 1991;338:705.
143. Aberer W. Vaccination despite thimerosal sensitivity. Contact Dermatitis 1991;24:6-10.
144. Audicana MT, Munoz D, del Pozo MD, et al. Allergic contact dermatitis from mercury antiseptics and derivatives: study protocol of tolerance to intramuscular injections of thimerosal. Am J Contact Dermat 2002;13:3-9.
145. Kirkland LR. Ocular sensitivity to thimerosal: a problem with hepatitis B vaccine? South Med J 1990;83:497-9.
146. Lee-Wong M, Resnick D, Chong K. A generalized reaction to thimerosal from an influenza vaccine. Ann Allergy Asthma Immunol 2005;94:90-4.
147. Zheng W, Dreskin SC. Thimerosal in influenza vaccine: an immediate hypersensitivity reaction. Ann Allergy Asthma Immunol 2007;99:574-5.
148. Kaaber K, Nielsen AO, Veien NK. Vaccination granulomas and aluminium allergy: course and prognostic factors. Contact Dermatitis 1992;26:304-6.
149. Bergfors E, Trollfors B, Inerot A. Unexpectedly high incidence of persistent itching nodules and delayed hypersensitivity to aluminium in children after the use of adsorbed vaccines from a single manufacturer. Vaccine 2003;22:64-9.
150. Bergfors E, Bjorkelund C, Trollfors B. Nineteen cases of persistent pruritic nodules and contact allergy to aluminium after injection of commonly used aluminium-adsorbed vaccines. Eur J Pediatr 2005;164:691-7.
151. Strebel PM, Papania MJ, Dayan GH, Halsey NA. Measles vaccine. In: Plotkin SA, Orenstein WA, Offit PA, editors. Vaccines. Philadelphia: Elsevier; 2008.
152. Barlow WE, Davis RL, Glasser JW, et al. The risk of seizures after receipt of whole-cell pertussis or measles, mumps, and rubella vaccine. N Engl J Med 2001;345:656-61.
153. Vestergaard M, Hviid A, Madsen KM, et al. MMR vaccination and febrile seizures: evaluation of susceptible subgroups and long-term prognosis. JAMA 2004;292:351-7.
154. Marin M, Broder KR, Temte JL, Snider DE, Seward JF. Use of combination measles, mumps, rubella, and varicella vaccine: recommendations of the Advisory Committee on Immunization Practices (ACIP). MMWR Recomm Rep 2010;59:1-12.
155. Beeler J, Varricchio F, Wise R. Thrombocytopenia after immunization with measles vaccines: review of the vaccine adverse events reporting system (1990 to 1994). Pediatr Infect Dis J 1996;15:88-90.
156. Watson JC, Hadler SC, Dykewicz CA, Reef S, Phillips L. Measles, mumps, and rubella—vaccine use and strategies for elimination of measles, rubella, and congenital rubella syndrome and control of mumps: recommendations of the Advisory Committee on Immunization Practices (ACIP). MMWR Recomm Rep 1998;47:1-57.
157. Mantadakis E, Farmaki E, Buchanan GR. Thrombocytopenic purpura after measles-mumps-rubella vaccination: a systematic review of the literature and guidance for management. J Pediatr 2010;156:623-8.
158. Jadavji T, Scheifele D, Halperin S. Thrombocytopenia after immunization of Canadian children, 1992 to 2001. Pediatr Infect Dis J 2003;22:119-22.
159. Howson CP, Fineberg HV. Adverse events following pertussis and rubella vaccines. Summary of a report of the Institute of Medicine. JAMA 1992;267:392-6.
160. Plotkin SA, Reef SE. Rubella vaccine. In: Plotkin SA, Orenstein WA, Offit PA, editors. Vaccines. 5th ed. Philadelphia: Elsevier; 2008.
161. Edwards KM, Decker MD. Pertussis vaccines. In: Plotkin SA, Orenstein WA, Offit PA, editors. Vaccines. 5th ed. Philadelphia: Elsevier; 2008.
162. Rosenthal S, Chen R, Hadler S. The safety of acellular pertussis vaccine vs whole-cell pertussis vaccine. A postmarketing assessment. Arch Pediatr Adolesc Med 1996;150:457-60.
163. Cody CL, Baraff LJ, Cherry JD, Marcy SM, Manclark CR. Nature and rates of adverse reactions associated with DTP and DT immunizations in infants and children. Pediatrics 1981;68:650-60.
164. Shields WD, Nielsen C, Buch D, et al. Relationship of pertussis immunization to the onset of

neurologic disorders: a retrospective epidemiologic study. J Pediatr 1988;113:801-5.
165. Le Saux N, Barrowman NJ, Moore DL, et al. Decrease in hospital admissions for febrile seizures and reports of hypotonic-hyporesponsive episodes presenting to hospital emergency departments since switching to acellular pertussis vaccine in Canada: a report from IMPACT. Pediatrics 2003;112:e348.
166. DuVernoy TS, Braun MM. Hypotonic-hyporesponsive episodes reported to the Vaccine Adverse Event Reporting System (VAERS), 1996-1998. Pediatrics 2000;106: E52.
167. Heijbel H, Ciofi degli Atti MC, Harzer E, et al. Hypotonic hyporesponsive episodes in eight pertussis vaccine studies. Dev Biol Stand 1997;89:101-3.
168. Stratton KH, Howe CJ, Johnston RB. DPT vaccine and chronic nervous system dysfunction: a new analysis. Washington, D.C.: National Academy Press; 1994.
169. Prevention of poliomyelitis: recommendations for use of only inactivated poliovirus vaccine for routine immunization. Committee on Infectious Diseases. American Academy of Pediatrics. Pediatrics 1999;104:1404-6.
170. Alexander LN, Seward JF, Santibanez TA, et al. Vaccine Policy Changes and Epidemiology of Poliomyelitis in the United States. JAMA 2004;292:1696-701.
171. Minor P. Vaccine-derived poliovirus (VDPV): impact on poliomyelitis eradication. Vaccine 2009;27:2649-52.
172. Intussusception among recipients of rotavirus vaccine—United States, 1998-1999. MMWR Morb Mortal Wkly Rep 1999;48:577-81.
173. Withdrawal of rotavirus vaccine recommendation. MMWR Morbi Mortal Wkly Rep 1999; 48:1007.
174. Prevention of rotavirus disease: updated guidelines for use of rotavirus vaccine. Pediatrics 2009;123:1412-20.
175. Patel MM, López-Collada VR, Bulhões MM, et al. Intussusception risk and health benefits of rotavirus vaccination in Mexico and Brazil. N Engl J Med 2011;64:2283-92.
176. Greenberg HB. Rotavirus vaccination and intussusception—act two. N Engl J Med 2011;364:2354-5.
177. Broder KR, Cortese MM, Iskander JK, et al. Preventing tetanus, diphtheria, and pertussis among adolescents: use of tetanus toxoid, reduced diphtheria toxoid and acellular pertussis vaccines recommendations of the Advisory Committee on Immunization Practices (ACIP). MMWR Morb Mort Wkly Rep 2006; 55:1-34.
178. Kretsinger K, Broder KR, Cortese MM, et al. Preventing tetanus, diphtheria, and pertussis among adults: use of tetanus toxoid, reduced diphtheria toxoid and acellular pertussis vaccine recommendations of the Advisory Committee on Immunization Practices (ACIP) and recommendation of ACIP, supported by the Healthcare Infection Control Practices Advisory Committee (HICPAC), for use of Tdap among health-care personnel. MMWR Morb Mortal Wkly Rep 2006;55:1-37.
179. Wassilak SGF, Roper MH, Kretsinger K, Orenstein WA. Tetanus toxoid. In: Plotkin SA, Orenstein WA, Offit PA, editors. Vaccines. 5th ed. Philadelphia: Elsevier; 2008.
180. Talbot EA, Brown KH, Kirkland KB, et al. The safety of immunizing with tetanus-diphtheria-acellular pertussis vaccine (Tdap) less than 2 years following previous tetanus vaccination: Experience during a mass vaccination campaign of healthcare personnel during a respiratory illness outbreak. Vaccine 2010;28: 8001-7.
181. Beytout J, Launay O, Guiso N, et al. Safety of Tdap-IPV given one month after Td-IPV booster in healthy young adults: a placebo-controlled trial. Hum Vaccin 2009;5:315-21.
182. Updated recommendations for use of tetanus toxoid, reduced diphtheria toxoid and acellular pertussis (Tdap) vaccine from the Advisory Committee on Immunization Practices, 2010. MMWR Morb Mortal Wkly Rep 2011;60: 13-5.
183. Gershon AA, Takahashi M, Seward JF. Varicella vaccine. In: Plotkin SA, Orenstein WA, Offit PA, editors. Vaccines. 5th ed. Philadelphia: Elsevier; 2008.
184. Sharrar RG, LaRussa P, Galea SA, et al. The postmarketing safety profile of varicella vaccine. Vaccine 2000;19:916-23.
185. Galea SA, Sweet A, Beninger P, et al. The safety profile of varicella vaccine: a 10-year review. J Infect Dis 2008;197(Suppl 2):S165-9.
186. Kreth HW, Hoeger PH; Members of the VZV-AD study group. Safety, reactogenicity, and immunogenicity of live attenuated varicella vaccine in children between 1 and 9 years of age with atopic dermatitis. Eur J Pediatr 2006;165:677-83.
187. Schneider L, Weinberg A, Boguniewicz M, et al. Immune response to varicella vaccine in children with atopic dermatitis compared with nonatopic controls. J Allergy Clin Immunol 2010;126:1306-7.e2.
188. Monath TP, Cetron MS, Teuwen DE. Yellow fever vaccine. In: Plotkin SA, Orenstein WA, Offit PA, editors. Vaccines. 5th ed. Philadelphia: Elsevier; 2008.
189. Staples JE, Gershman M, Fischer M. Yellow fever vaccine: recommendations of the Advisory Committee on Immunization Practices (ACIP). MMWR Recomm Rep 2010;59: 1-27.
190. Monath TP, Fowler E, Johnson CT, et al. An inactivated cell-culture vaccine against yellow fever. N Engl J Med 2011;364:1326-33.

Adverse Reactions to Vaccines for Biologic Agents Used as Weapons

191. Franz DR, Jahrling PB, Friedlander AM, et al. Clinical recognition and management of patients exposed to biological warfare agents. JAMA 1997;278:399-411.
192. Wright JG, Quinn CP, Shadomy S, Messonnier N. Use of anthrax vaccine in the United States: recommendations of the Advisory Committee on Immunization Practices (ACIP), 2009. MMWR Recomm Rep 2010;59:1-30.
193. Pittman PR, Kim-Ahn G, Pifat DY, et al. Anthrax vaccine: immunogenicity and safety of a dose-reduction, route-change comparison study in humans. Vaccine 2002;20:1412-20.
194. Joellenbeck LM, Zwanziger LL, Durch JS, Strom BL. The anthrax vaccine: is it safe? Does it work? Washington, D.C.: National Academy Press; 2002.
195. Fenner F, Henderson D, Arita I. Smallpox and its eradication. Geneva: World Health Organization; 1988.
196. Henderson DA, Inglesby TV, Bartlett JG, et al. Smallpox as a biological weapon: medical and public health management. Working Group on Civilian Biodefense. JAMA 1999;281: 2127-37.
197. Centers for Disease Control and Prevention. Vaccinia (smallpox) vaccine: recommendations of the Immunization Practices Advisory Committee (ACIP). MMWR Recomm Rep 2001;50:1.
198. Centers for Disease Control and Prevention. Smallpox vaccination and adverse reactions. Guidance for clinicians. MMWR Recomm Rep 2003;52:1-28.
199. Centers for Disease Control and Prevention. Smallpox response plan and guidelines. 2002. Available at: http://www.bt.cdc.gov/agent/smallpox/response%2Dplan/#toc.
200. Arness MK, Eckart RE, Love SS, et al. Myopericarditis following smallpox vaccination. Am J Epidemiol 2004;160:642-51.
201. Casey CG, Iskander JK, Roper MH, et al. Adverse events associated with smallpox vaccination in the United States, January-October 2003. JAMA 2005;294:2734-43.
202. Eckart RE, Love SS, Atwood JE, et al. Incidence and follow-up of inflammatory cardiac complications after smallpox vaccination. J Am Coll Cardiol 2004;44:201-5.
203. Centers for Disease Control and Prevention. Supplemental recommendations on adverse events following smallpox vaccine in the pre-event vaccination program: recommendations of the Advisory Committee on Immunization Practices. MMWR Morb Mortal Wkly Rep 2003;52:282-4.
204. Centers for Disease Control and Prevention. Smallpox (vaccinia) vaccine contraindications. 2003. Available at: http://emergency.cdc.gov/agent/smallpox/vaccination/pdf/contraindications-clinic.pdf.
205. Inglesby TV, Dennis DT, Henderson DA, et al. Plague as a biological weapon: medical and public health management. Working Group on Civilian Biodefense. JAMA 2000;83:2281-90.

Controversies Regarding Long-Term Consequences of Vaccination

206. Romagnani S. Immunologic influences on allergy and the Th1/Th2 balance. J Allergy Clin Immunol 2004;113:400.
207. Shirakawa T, Enomoto T, Shimazu S, Hopkin JM. The inverse association between tuberculin responses and atopic disorder. Science 1997;275:77-9.
208. Alm JS, Lilja G, Pershagen G, Scheynius A. Early BCG vaccination and development of atopy. Lancet 1997;350:400-3.
209. Eifan AO, Akkoc T, Ozdemir C, Bahceciler NN, Barlan IB. No association between tuberculin skin test and atopy in a bacillus Calmette-Guérin vaccinated birth cohort. Pediatr Allergy Immunol 2009;20:545-50.
210. Gruber C, Kulig M, Bergmann R, et al; Group MASS. Delayed hypersensitivity to tuberculin, total immunoglobulin E, specific sensitization, and atopic manifestation in longitudinally followed early bacille Calmette-Guérin-vaccinated and nonvaccinated children. Pediatrics 2001;107:E36.
211. Arnoldussen DL, Linehan M, Sheikh A. BCG vaccination and allergy: a systematic review and meta-analysis. J Allergy Clin Immunol 2011;127:246-53, 53.e1-21.
212. Shaheen SO, Aaby P, Hall AJ, et al. Measles and atopy in Guinea-Bissau. Lancet 1996;347: 1792-6.
213. Paunio M, Heinonen OP, Virtanen M, et al. Measles history and atopic diseases: a population-based cross-sectional study. JAMA 2000;283:343-6.

214. Farooqi IS, Hopkin JM. Early childhood infection and atopic disorder. Thorax 1998;53:927-32.
215. Nilsson L, Gruber C, Granstrom M, Bjorksten B, Kjellman NI. Pertussis IgE and atopic disease. Allergy 1998;53:1195-201.
216. Anderson HR, Poloniecki JD, Strachan DP, et al. Immunization and symptoms of atopic disease in children: results from the International Study of Asthma and Allergies in Childhood. Am J Public Health 2001;91:1126-9.
217. Koppen S, de Groot R, Neijens HJ, et al. No epidemiological evidence for infant vaccinations to cause allergic disease. Vaccine 2004;22:3375-85.
218. Sanchez-Solis M, Garcia-Marcos L. Do vaccines modify the prevalence of asthma and allergies? Exp Rev Vaccines 2006;5:631-40.
219. Wakefield AJ, Murch SH, Anthony A, et al. Ileal-lymphoid-nodular hyperplasia, non-specific colitis, and pervasive developmental disorder in children. Lancet 1998;351:637-41.
220. Taylor B, Miller E, Farrington CP, et al. Autism and measles, mumps, and rubella vaccine: no epidemiological evidence for a causal association. Lancet 1999;353:2026-9.
221. Dales L, Hammer SJ, Smith NJ. Time trends in autism and in MMR immunization coverage in California. JAMA 2001;285:1183-5.
222. Stratton K, Gable A, Shetty P. Immunization safety review: measles-mumps-rubella vaccine and autism. Washington, D.C.: National Academy Press; 2001.
223. Madsen KM, Hviid A, Vestergaard M, et al. A population-based study of measles, mumps, and rubella vaccination and autism. N Engl J Med 2002;347:1477-82.
224. Retraction—Ileal-lymphoid-nodular hyperplasia, non-specific colitis, and pervasive developmental disorder in children. Lancet 2010;375:445.
225. Thimerosal in vaccines—an interim report to clinicians. American Academy of Pediatrics. Committee on Infectious Diseases and Committee on Environmental Health. Pediatrics 1999;104:570-4.
226. Thimerosal content in some US licensed vaccines. 2011. Available at: http://www.vaccinesafety.edu/thi-table.htm.
227. Immunization safety review: vaccines and autism. Washington, D.C.: National Academy Press; 2004.
228. Parker SK, Schwartz B, Todd J, Pickering LK. Thimerosal-containing vaccines and autistic spectrum disorder: a critical review of published original data. Pediatrics 2004;114:793-804.

Vaccination Relative to Immunocompromise and Immunoglobulin Preparations

229. Moss W, Lederman H. Immunization of the immunocompromised host. Clin Focus Primary Immune Defic 1998;1:1-8.
230. Bonilla FA, Bernstein IL, Khan DA, et al. Practice parameter for the diagnosis and management of primary immunodeficiency. Ann Allergy Asthma Immunol 2005;94:S1-63.
231. Ochs HD, Davis SD, Wedgwood RJ. Immunologic responses to bacteriophage phi-X 174 in immunodeficiency diseases. J Clin Invest 1971;50:2559-68.
232. Pyun KH, Ochs HD, Wedgwood RJ, et al. Human antibody responses to bacteriophage phi X 174: sequential induction of IgM and IgG subclass antibody. Clin Immunol Immunopathol 1989;51:252-63.

Vaccination during Pregnancy and Breastfeeding

233. Centers for Disease Control and Prevention. Guidelines for vaccinating pregnant women: Recommendations of the Advisory Committee on Immunization Practices (ACIP). 2013.
234. Transmission of yellow fever vaccine virus through breast-feeding—Brazil, 2009. MMWR Morb Mortal Wkly Rep 2010;59:130-2.
235. Kuhn S, Twele-Montecinos L, MacDonald J, Webster P, Law B. Case report: probable transmission of vaccine strain of yellow fever virus to an infant via breast milk. CMAJ 2011;183:E243-5.

WITHDRAWN

SECTION H

Therapeutics

86 Allergen Control for Prevention and Management of Allergic Diseases

ADNAN CUSTOVIC | EUAN TOVEY

CONTENTS

SUMMARY OF IMPORTANT CONCEPTS

- High exposure to allergens can worsen inflammation and trigger asthma symptoms in sensitized individuals.
- Current understanding of "personal exposure" to inhalant allergens is not yet based on precise measurements or knowledge of exposure, seriously limiting development of effective tools for reducing exposure.
- Most of the currently used allergen avoidance methods have been tested under artificial experimental conditions, with limited data on clinical effectiveness.
- There is a diversity of opinions about the role of currently available inhalant allergen control methods in the management of asthma, and guidelines differ in their recommendations.
- A pragmatic approach to allergen avoidance views single avoidance measures as ineffective and uses a comprehensive allergen control regimen with regular removal of accumulating allergen; tailors the intervention to patient's sensitization and exposure status; starts intervention as early in natural history of disease as possible; and advises pet removal for patients with allergy symptoms on exposure.
- The development of allergen sensitization is influenced by allergen exposure, but also by other environmental exposures (e.g., endotoxin) and the genetic predisposition of the individual.
- No evidence-based advice is currently available on the effectiveness of inhalant allergen avoidance in primary prevention of allergic disease.

Introduction

Allergen avoidance is essential in the management of patients with allergy. In food allergy, avoidance of offending foods is the most important aspect of the overall treatment strategy. However, opinions differ on the role of inhalant allergen control for prevention and management of asthma and other allergic diseases, and guidelines offer differing recommendations.[1] For example, the 2007 U.S. National Heart, Lung, and Blood Institute (NHLBI) guidelines for the diagnosis and management of asthma recommend evaluation and identification of the role relevant allergens—suggesting that inhaled allergens are the most important factor for both children and adults—and advise asthmatic patients to reduce exposure to allergens to which they are sensitive. The 2010 Global Initiative for Asthma (GINA) strategy for asthma management and prevention is more cautious and recommends that measures should be taken to avoid allergens where possible, suggesting that avoiding allergens completely is usually impractical and very limiting to the patient. Both GINA and British guidelines on the management of asthma (2011 revision) question the effectiveness of the currently used measures to create a low-allergen environment in homes and suggest that single interventions have limited or no benefit.

This chapter discusses these discrepant opinions on the role of inhalant allergen avoidance in treatment and prevention of asthma, rhinitis, and eczema, providing guidance on a pragmatic approach to allergen control measures to ensure a low-allergen environment is achieved and maintained. Identification of patients who may benefit from such interventions is a major focus.

Rationale for Allergen Control

The following premises are often used as a rationale for the use of allergen control for prevention and management of allergic disease:

1. Sensitization to inhalant allergens is a strong risk factor for asthma, and the magnitude of risk increases with increasing titers of IgE antibodies.[2,3]
2. Domestic allergen exposure in early life increases the risk of the subsequent development of sensitization[4] and asthma.[5]
3. High allergen exposure among sensitized individuals with established allergic disease exacerbates symptoms and worsens the underlying inflammatory process.[6,7]
4. Complete cessation of allergen exposure may lead to the improvement in disease control.

For example, patients with hay fever have no symptoms in the absence of exposure to pollen. Also, relocation of atopic asthmatic patients into the low-allergen environment of high-altitude facilities improves markers of asthma severity.[8] Further, for patients with occupational asthma, removal from exposure improves asthma symptoms and lung function compared with reducing exposure or continued exposure in the workplace.[9]

ALLERGEN EXPOSURE

Development of Sensitization and Asthma

Our understanding of the role of allergen exposure in the development of sensitization and allergic disease, as well as its effect on severity and exacerbation in patients with established disease, has changed and evolved over the last 25 years.[1] Whereas initially allergen exposure was considered a major factor in the development of both sensitization and asthma in a simple dose-response manner,[5] subsequent evidence has proved that the relationship among allergen exposure, sensitization, and asthma is much more complex. Some longitudinal studies have demonstrated a linear dose-response relationship between mite and cat allergen exposure in early life and subsequent development of specific sensitizations,[4] but others have not confirmed this relationship.[10,11] In contrast, a protective effect of high cat allergen exposure on cat sensitization has also been reported,[12] suggesting that the dose-response relationship between allergen exposure and sensitization may differ among allergens, dose ranges and exposure patterns[13] (e.g., linear for mite and cockroach, bell-shaped for mouse and cat). Only one longitudinal study reported a significant relationship between early life mite allergen exposure and increased risk of asthma,[5] whilst most others did not find such association.[4,10,11,14]

A complex relationship between genetic predisposition, dust mite allergen exposure and endotoxin exposure has been reported, which suggested that although increasing allergen exposure was associated with increased risk of sensitization, the size of the effect was markedly reduced at higher endotoxin exposure among children with specific genotype (CC homozygotes at *CD14/-159*)[15] (Fig. 86-1). Therefore, because development of allergen-specific sensitization is influenced not only by allergen exposure but also by other environmental exposures (including endotoxin) as well as the individual's genetic predisposition, the effects of allergen control could vary greatly between individuals with different genetic predispositions.[16] This complex interaction between environmental exposures and genotype is further illustrated by the opposite effect of day care attendance on asthma development in children with different genetic variants in the *TLR2* gene.[17] Also, cat ownership substantially increases the risk of early life eczema only in children with filaggrin loss-of-function genetic variants.[18] This

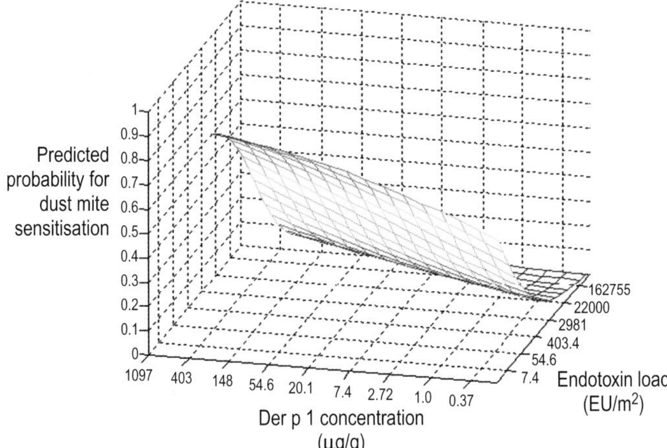

Figure 86-1 Fitted predicted probability for sensitization to mite at age 5 years in relation to environmental endotoxin load and Der p 1 exposure in children with CC genotype in the promoter region of the CD14 gene (*CD14/-159* C to T) derived from the logistic regression analysis. *(From Simpson A et al. Endotoxin exposure, CD14, and allergic disease: an interaction between genes and the environment. Am J Respir Crit Care Med 2006;174:386-92.)*

mounting body of evidence suggests that only individuals with particular susceptibility may benefit from a specific intervention, and that the same intervention for individuals with different susceptibility may cause harm.

Asthma Severity and Exacerbations

In allergic asthmatic patients, markers of asthma severity such as increased airway hyperresponsiveness (AHR), peak expiratory flow rate (PEFR) variability, and diminished lung function are associated with high exposure to sensitizing allergen,[6,7] emphasizing the contribution of allergen exposure to the ongoing chronic disease process. On the other hand, the main cause of asthma exacerbations are respiratory viral infections,[19] suggesting that respiratory viruses rather than allergens are major acute determinants of asthma attacks. However, most patients are exposed to respiratory viruses and allergens contemporaneously, and rather than being mutually exclusive, viruses, allergic sensitization, and allergen exposure interact in increasing the risk of exacerbation in childhood and adult asthma.[20,21] As further indirect evidence of this interaction, anti-IgE (omalizumab) treatment greatly reduced the seasonal exacerbations of asthma during the fall and spring (presumably caused by viral infection).[22]

Evidence that high exposure to allergens can worsen inflammation and trigger asthma symptoms in sensitized individuals is used as a foundation for the proposal that allergen avoidance should lead to the improvement in asthma control. Such an intervention is a cornerstone of the management of occupational asthma; however, even in this model where identification and complete avoidance of the offending allergen are feasible, only complete cessation of exposure *early* in the natural history of the disease results in resolution of symptoms. If exposure continues longer, asthma may become a self-perpetuating process, and even complete cessation of exposure to the causal allergen may fail to impact the progression and severity of the disease. The duration of this "window of opportunity" during which removal from exposure is effective differs among individuals, adding another level of complexity. Thus the supposition that high domestic allergen exposure appears to contribute to the chronicity and severity of asthma does not translate directly into the effectiveness of allergen control, either in treatment or in prevention of disease.

All the previous findings indirectly suggest that important principles of allergen control should aim to achieve a complete cessation of allergen exposure and commence the intervention early in the natural history of the disease. The application of effective control measures, which can ensure that a low-allergen environment is achieved and maintained over a prolonged period, and the identification of patients who may benefit from such intervention as early in the natural history of the disease as possible are the cornerstones of a clinically successful intervention strategy.

Allergen Control Measures

Knowledge about the aerodynamic characteristics and distribution of different allergens is important for understanding personal exposure and designing effective methods to reduce exposure. The majority of mite and cockroach allergens are contained within relatively large particles (>10 µm in diameter), whereas a significant portion of airborne cat and dog allergen is carried on small particles (<5 µm). This may partly account for the difference in clinical presentation of allergic asthma. Asthmatic patients sensitized to mite and cockroach are usually unaware of the relationship between exposure to allergen and symptoms, whereas those allergic to cat or dog often develop wheezing or cough within minutes of entering a home with a pet, presumably by inhalation of relatively large amounts of allergen on small particles that penetrate deep into the respiratory tract.

Application of this information to allergen control measures is important. For example, air filtration units may be useful in removing airborne pet allergens from the ambient air but will have little effect on mite or cockroach allergens. Removal of aeroallergens from the air in a bedroom or living room does not translate directly to a major reduction in overall personal allergen exposure of the individuals living in that space. It is also unclear whether the almost-continuous indoor exposure to small particles carrying a minority of the total mite or cockroach allergens provides a subclinical challenge to help maintain airway inflammation.

Our understanding of what represents "personal exposure" to allergens is based predominantly on assumptions and beliefs rather than precise measurements and scientific knowledge about the nature and sources of exposure. For example, common assumptions are that most exposure to mite allergens occurs overnight in bed, that levels of inhalant allergens are dust reservoirs (e.g., mattress, carpet), and that aeroallergens measured in the ambient air are good markers of personal exposure. Recent data based on continuous measurement of personal aeroallergen throughout the day and night suggest that for some people, or for some occasions, the majority of daily domestic aeroallergen exposure does not occur in bed but rather from the disturbance of allergen on other domestic surfaces and clothing.[1] This is consistent with another recent study of personal aeroallergen exposures, including from nondomestic sources.[23] Further extrapolations are then made about the measurement of "effectiveness" of various measures to reduce exposure; it is also assumed, for example, that control of mite allergen exposure in bed measured by the amount of allergen recovered by vacuuming the mattress equates to reduction in personal exposure. Most of these assumptions are not based on solid evidence and at best represent oversimplification of the dynamic nature and multiple factors contributing to acute and chronic individual inhaled aeroallergen exposure. As a result, most current recommendations on allergen avoidance have been tested under highly artificial experimental conditions, with experimental designs aiming predominantly to differentiate between different consumer products (e.g., vacuum cleaners, bed covers, air cleaners) using proxy measures of exposure, usually reservoir allergen concentrations or allergen recovered from air by static air samplers. The effect of most of these measures on personal inhaled allergen exposure is largely unknown.[1]

A further problem is that different products are often advertised directly to consumers, without the requirement to provide a solid evidence base about their clinical effectiveness. A review of 50 web sites of various asthma foundations and consumer groups found that almost one third were associated with promotion of proprietary products for allergen avoidance, some with their own "certification programs" and only two expressing uncertainty about the clinical effectiveness of these products.[1] At present, we lack substantial experimentally based models of how and when most domestic allergen exposure occurs, which limits the development of effective tools for reducing exposure.

MEASURES TO REDUCE DUST MITE ALLERGENS[24]

Encasings. The most recommended method to reduce allergen exposure in bed is to cover the mattress, comforter (duvet), and pillows with encasings that are impermeable to mite allergens (e.g., finely woven fabrics). Measuring the amount of allergen recovered by vacuuming the bed assesses their effectiveness, but the effect on the overall personal inhaled aeroallergen exposure, particularly over time, is unknown.

Bedding. Current advice is to wash bedding regularly, if possible in a hot cycle above 131°F (55°C) to kill the mites. However, there is no consistent information on the effectiveness of different laundry procedures or the duration of these effects.

Carpets. The effect of carpet removal and replacement with hard flooring (wooden or linoleum) on airborne and inhaled aeroallergens is contentious and likely complex due to a number of factors relevant to particle aerosolization, including electrostatic charge, cleaning frequency, and type of floor. Also, replacement with hard flooring will likely minimize the reservoirs but requires routine cleaning. If carpets remain in place, methods to reduce mite allergen levels include exposing carpets to sunlight, steam cleaning, use of acaricides or tannic acid, or freezing with liquid nitrogen. However, all these methods are only partially effective in reducing reservoir allergen levels, and the effect on personal exposure is unknown.

Vacuum Cleaners. In the experimental allergen exposure chamber, vacuum cleaners with built-in high-efficiency particulate air (HEPA) filters and double-thickness bags do not leak allergens. However, real-life studies using intranasal air samplers to monitor personal exposure during vacuum cleaning of floors showed an increase in the amount of allergens inhaled while using high-efficiency vacuum cleaners,[25] suggesting that experimental chamber data alone are insufficient to justify the recommendations or certification of high-efficiency vacuum cleaners to allergy sufferers.

Controlling Humidity. Reducing humidity is recommended for control of mite population in the whole living dwelling. However, reducing the relative humidity of the indoor air alone may not be sufficient to reduce humidity in the mite microhabitats within the home (e.g., middle of mattress, deep in carpet). This approach depends on the local climate and housing design. For example, central mechanical ventilation heat-recovery units are effective in reducing indoor humidity in the geographic areas where outdoor humidity is low and home insulation is good, but have not proved effective in areas of high humidity and poor insulation. The effect of air humidity on the dynamics of airborne particles has rarely been studied.

Clearly, a major reduction in mite allergen levels in homes can be achieved only by a comprehensive strategy that combines the most appropriate measures applicable to individual households and a particular geographic area; simple, single measures are unlikely to attain desired effect. A comprehensive allergen control regimen combining a number of the previous measures, with an emphasis on regular removal of allergen, can achieve and maintain a low-allergen environment for a prolonged period,[26] but its effect on the long-term personal aeroallergen exposure amongst individuals living in this environment remains to be accurately modelled.

PET ALLERGEN AVOIDANCE MEASURES

Pet removal is the only appropriate advice to patients with pet allergy who experience symptoms on exposure.[24] Even after permanent removal of an animal, it can take many months for allergen levels in the reservoirs within the home to fall. Despite the advice by health professionals, however, a sizable proportion of these pet-sensitized individuals decide to keep their animal. Suggested measures to control allergen levels with pet in situ include the use of high-efficiency vacuum cleaners (see earlier).

Air Filtration. Air-cleaning units with HEPA filters can reduce the airborne concentration of cat and dog allergens in homes with pets. However, although experimental measurements suggest substantial reduction in airborne allergen levels, field studies using measurements of personal inhaled allergen exposure are much less convincing.[27]

Pet Washing. Washing pets reduces the levels of allergens in fur and dander samples, but the levels return to the starting values within days. It is unlikely that a modest reduction in allergen recovered from pet fur will relate into any clinical benefit.

COCKROACH ALLERGEN REDUCTION

Physical and chemical procedures can be used to control cockroach populations in infested houses. Identification of species, food and water sources, and hiding places are all helpful. Sealing cracks and holes in plasterwork and floors can restrict cockroach access. Several pesticides are available, in gel or bait form. Before applying an insecticide, general cleaning should remove all possible food sources, and further cleaning should be delayed for a week to avoid removal of insecticides.

CLINICAL EFFECTIVENESS

Attempts to replicate clinical benefits observed in the studies at high-altitude facilities, often attributed to allergen avoidance, by using allergen control measures in patient homes have led to conflicting results.[28] The controversy is not whether allergen avoidance works; as demonstrated earlier, a complete absence of exposure usually results in a remission of some allergic symptoms (e.g., seasonal allergic rhinitis) or improvement in others (e.g., occupational asthma).[28] The practical questions not yet resolved are how to achieve a sufficient real-life reduction in personal inhaled allergen exposure and how to identify patients who will benefit from an effective intervention.

With respect to domestic pets and based on clinical experience, it is generally accepted that cat- or dog-allergic patients should see significant clinical improvement associated with the absence of contact with the sensitizing pet. It is also clear that a randomized double-blind study of pet removal from home is not feasible. One small, prospective, nonrandomized nonblinded observational study of 20 symptomatic patients with newly diagnosed pet-allergic asthma who were keeping a pet in their home found that removal of pets from homes reduced airway responsiveness more than optimal pharmacotherapy alone.[29] Thus the advice to pet-sensitized pet owners to remove the pet from home will always be based on common sense rather than the evidence obtained within the context of a rigorous trial.

CLINICAL EFFECTS OF CONTROL MEASURES

Systematic Reviews

Mite Avoidance in Asthma. A recent update of the Cochrane meta-analysis reported no effect of the current chemical and physical methods aimed at reducing exposure to dust mite allergens and concluded that these interventions cannot be recommended to patients with mite-sensitive asthma[30] (Table 86-1). A total of 3002 patients were recruited in 54 trials, of which 36 assessed physical methods (26 mattress covers), 10 chemical methods, and eight a combination of chemical and physical methods.[30] The most plausible explanation for the lack of clinical effect is that the allergen control methods used did not adequately reduce personal aeroallergen exposure. Also, mite-sensitive asthmatic patients are usually sensitized to other allergens, questioning whether a focus on one allergen is the most appropriate approach to allergen control.

Mite Avoidance in Patients with Rhinitis or Eczema. A Cochrane systematic review of nine randomized controlled trials of mite avoidance measures in the management of perennial allergic rhinitis involving 501 participants concluded that most studies completed by 2011 were small and of poor methodologic quality, making it difficult to generate definitive recommendations.[31] However, this review was more cautious than that on asthma, suggesting interventions that achieve substantial reductions in dust mite load may offer some benefit in reducing rhinitis symptoms.

There are, as yet, no systematic reviews assessing the effect of mite avoidance measures in patients with eczema.

Pet Avoidance in Patients with Asthma. Cochrane Airways Group systematic review on the effect of cat and dog allergen avoidance with the pet in home emphasized the paucity of evidence on the clinical effectiveness of pet allergen avoidance.[32] With limited data available, no meta-analysis was possible. Only two small studies (22 and 35 participants) met the inclusion criteria. Both investigated the effectiveness of air filtration units and reported no significant differences between the active intervention and control on any of the primary and secondary outcomes. The authors concluded that the available trials were too small to provide unequivocal evidence for or against the use of air filtration units in the management of pet-allergic asthma.[32]

Studies of Single Interventions

The largest randomized double-blind placebo-controlled trial assessing the effectiveness of mite-impermeable bed covers as a single intervention involved over 1000 adults with physician-diagnosed asthma using inhaled corticosteroids (ICS) and found no benefits of the intervention in any of the primary or secondary outcome measures (morning PEFR during first 6 months, proportion of patients able to discontinue ICS during second 6 months, symptom scores, quality of life).[33] The patients for this study were selected regardless of allergen sensitization and mite allergen exposure. However, two thirds had positive

TABLE 86-1 Comparison of House-dust Mite Reduction versus Control, Outcome Morning Peak Expiratory Flow Rate

Review: House-dust mite control measures for asthma
Comparison: 01 House-dust mite reduction versus control
Outcome: 05 Peek expiratory flow rate (PEFR) incoming

Study	Treatment (n)	Mean (SD)	Control (n)	Mean (SD)	Standardized Mean Difference (Fixed) 95% CI	Weight (%)	Standardized Mean Difference (Fixed) 95% CI
01 CHEMICAL METHODS							
Bahir 1997	13	262.00 (82.00)	17	262.00 (82.00)		1.9	0.0 [−0.72, 0.72]
Chang 1996	12	411.00 (75.00)	14	383.00 (100.00)		1.6	0.30 [−0.47, 1.08]
Dietemann 1993	11	67.88 (11.28)	12	75.37 (10.46)		1.4	−0.66 [−1.51, 0.18]
Reiser 1990	23	92.00 (20.00)	23	100.00 (18.00)		2.9	−0.41 [−1.00, 0.17]
Subtotal (95% CI)	59		66			7.8	−0.21 [−0.53, 0.15]
Test for heterogeneity: chi-square = 3.58; df = 3; *P* = .31; I² = 16.2%							
Test for overall effect: *z* = 1.14; *P* = .3							
02 PHYSICAL METHODS: PARALLEL-GROUP STUDIES							
Cinti 1996	10	98.20 (22.70)	10	91.80 (15.80)		1.3	0.31 [−0.57, 1.20]
Fang 2001	19	349.00 (96.00)	16	304.00 (117.00)		2.2	0.41 [−0.26, 1.09]
Halken 2003	26	358.00 (96.00)	21	342.00 (86.00)		3.0	0.17 [−0.40, 0.75]
Lee 2003	22	88.60 (13.66)	20	89.43 (17.33)		2.7	−0.05 [−0.66, 0.55]
Luczynska 2003	16	367.00 (156.00)	15	388.00 (75.00)		2.0	−0.17 [−0.87, 0.54]
Rijssenbeek 2002	16	435.00 (115.00)	14	440.00 (115.00)		1.9	−0.04 [−0.76, 0.68]
Sheikh 2002	23	16.38 (25.62)	20	13.68 (43.14)		2.7	0.08 [−0.52, 0.68]
Walshaw 1996	22	407.00 (112.00)	20	369.00 (114.00)		2.7	0.33 [−0.28, 0.94]
Woodcock 2003	313	429.30 (91.70)	315	436.20 (88.80)		40.3	−0.08 [−0.23, 0.08]
De Vries 2007	47	457.00 (145.00)	45	464.00 (111.00)		5.9	−0.05 [−0.46, 0.36]
Van den Bemt 2004	26	431.00 (115.00)	26	385.00 (109.00)		3.3	0.32 [−0.23, 0.86]
Subtotal (95% CI)	540		522			68.0	0.00 [−0.12, 0.12]
Test for heterogeneity: chi-square = 5.99; df = 10; *P* = .82; I² = 0.0%							
Test for overall effect: *z* = 0.00; *P* = 1							
03 PHYSICAL METHODS: CROSSOVER STUDIES							
Antonicelli 1991	9	443.00 (106.00)	9	445.00 (117.00)		1.2	−0.02 [−0.94, 0.91]
Burr 1976	32	335.00 (111.00)	32	329.00 (118.00)		4.1	0.05 [−0.44, 0.54]
Mitchell 1980	10	67.00 (15.00)	10	64.30 (12.70)		1.3	0.19 [−0.69, 1.06]
Warburton 1994	12	350.00 (101.00)	12	344.00 (97.00)		1.5	0.06 [−0.74, 0.86]
Warner 1993	14	232.60 (88.00)	14	231.30 (97.00)		1.8	0.01 [−0.73, 0.75]
Subtotal (95% CI)	77		77			9.9	0.06 [−0.26, 0.37]
Test for heterogeneity: chi-square = 0.12; df = 4; *P* = 1; I² = 0.0%							
Test for overall effect: *z* = 0.34; *P* = 1							
04 COMBINATION METHODS							
Carswell 1996	23	99.60 (17.80)	26	98.90 (14.50)		3.1	0.04 [−0.52, 0.60]
Cloosterman 1999	76	544.00 (132.00)	81	529.00 (126.00)		10.1	0.12 [−0.20, 0.43]
Dorward 1988	9	388.00 (106.00)	9	392.00 (71.00)		1.2	−0.04 [−0.97, 0.88]
Subtotal (95% CI)	108		116			14.4	0.09 [−0.18, 0.35]
Test for heterogeneity: chi-square = 0.13; df = 2; *P* = .94; I² = 0.0%							
Test for overall effect: *z* = 0.65; *P* = .5							
Total (95% CI)	784		781			100.0	0.00 [−0.10, 0.10]
Test for heterogeneity: chi-square = 11.66; df = 22; I² = 0.0%							
Test for overall effect: *z* = 0.03; *P* = 1							

-4.0 -2.0 0 2.0 4.0
Favors control Favors treatment

From Gotzsche PC, Johansen HK. House dust mite control measures for asthma. Cochrane Database Syst Rev 2008;(2): CD001187, with permission. Copyright Cochrane Collaboration.

mite-specific IgE, and approximately one in four beds had very high mite allergen levels (greater than 10 μg/g of major mite allergen Der p 1). Post hoc analysis of the subgroup of 130 patients with high mite-specific IgE (≥10 kU_A/L) and high baseline mite allergen exposure (>10 μg/g Der p 1 in mattress dust) showed no differences in outcomes between the active and the placebo group. Although the reservoir allergen concentration in the intervention group was significantly reduced at 6 months, the difference was not sustained at 12 months. This trial demonstrated convincingly that a single simple intervention with allergen-impermeable encasings for the mattress, comforter, and pillows is ineffective in the long-term management of asthma in adults, even in patients highly allergic to dust mite *and* exposed to high levels of mite allergens—the subpopulation of adult asthmatic patients in whom this type of intervention would be expected to have a beneficial effect.

Similarly, the results of the largest randomized double-blind placebo-controlled study of bed encasings in patients with perennial allergic rhinitis and positive nasal challenge to mite extract demonstrated no beneficial effect of the intervention.[34]

In contrast, a relatively small study of 60 mite-sensitized children with physician-diagnosed asthma and positive specific dust mite bronchial challenge exposed to a high level of mite allergen in their beds reported that ICS was safely reduced by approximately 50% in the active group (polyurethane mattress and pillow encasings with advice to families to wash blankets or duvets every 3 months), with no effect in the control group.[35] The beneficial effect was not apparent until the encasings had been in place for 6 months and was maintained 12 months.[35] These data suggest that there may be a differential response to allergen control between adults and children.

Multifaceted Interventions

Studies of multifaceted interventions tailored toward patients' individual needs reported different outcomes from single interventions, with evidence of improvement in asthma control.[36,37] Of note, these studies were not included in the previously mentioned systematic reviews of interventions aimed at reducing exposure to a single allergen (e.g., dust mite).

The largest multifaceted intervention in children, the U.S. Inner-City Asthma Study, adopted a number of wide-ranging, comprehensive environmental interventions tailored to the child's allergen sensitization and exposure status.[37] A total of 937 children age 5 to 11 years with physician diagnosed, poorly controlled asthma and at least one positive skin test were recruited from seven inner cities with high levels of poverty; more than half the households had an annual income less than $15,000. Despite having moderate/severe asthma, with either a hospital admission or two unscheduled visits to an emergency department (ED) or a physician in the preceding 6 months, less than half the participants were taking antiinflammatory agents. A tailor-made intervention was devised using data on the child's sensitization and level of allergen exposure. The comprehensive environmental control regimen also included the education of the parent/caregiver, and advice was provided on the reduction of passive smoke exposure when appropriate. Mattress and pillow encasings and a high-filtration vacuum cleaner were supplied to all homes. Further products required for the tailored intervention (e.g., a HEPA air filter for the reduction in passive smoke exposure) were supplied free of charge. Because of the complexity of the intervention, no attempt was made to introduce placebo devices into control homes. Children in the intervention group had significantly fewer days with asthma symptoms than the controls; this effect was apparent within 2 months of starting the study and was sustained throughout the 2-year study period (Fig. 86-2, *A*). The number of ED visits was also reduced, with other secondary outcome measures showing either a statistically significant improvement or a trend toward improvement in the active group. Statistical modeling indicated that for mite and cockroach allergen, the increase in symptom-free days was seen predominantly in children with greater than 50% reductions in home allergen levels.[37]

This important study demonstrated that allergen levels can be reduced in poor, inner-city homes and also estimated the size of the potential beneficial effect: a multifaceted environmental intervention costing approximately $2000 per child was associated with an additional 34 symptom-free days over 2 years. Although estimated to be cost-effective in the context of the U.S. health care system, the cost-effectiveness of such intervention cannot be directly translated to other countries with different health care services and usually lower pharmacologic costs.

A recent study of environmental control using nocturnal temperature-controlled laminar airflow treatment found that this device, which displaces aeroallergens from the breathing zone, improves quality of life and reduces airway inflammation in adults and children with atopic asthma, without significant adverse effects[38] (Fig. 86-2, *B*).

IDENTIFICATION OF PATIENTS LIKELY TO BENEFIT FROM INTERVENTION

In a clinical practice and in most studies of allergen control, allergic sensitization is usually considered only as a dichotomous variable; individuals are assigned as sensitized or not based on arbitrary cutoff points on either skin tests or measurement of specific serum IgE. At a population level, however, a sizable proportion of such defined "atopic" individuals have no evidence of symptoms of allergic diseases. Recent studies suggest that atopy may include several endotypes that differ in their association with asthma.[39] If this hypothesis is confirmed, detectable serum IgE or positive skin tests should be viewed as intermediate phenotypes of different atopic vulnerabilities. For this to be clinically useful, biomarkers are needed to differentiate accurately between different "atopy endotypes" and discriminate asymptomatic from clinically relevant sensitization. Application of these findings to allergen control is unclear, but novel diagnostic tests and biomarkers are urgently needed to help identify asthmatic patients whose atopy is contributing to disease severity and those likely to benefit from a comprehensive and targeted allergen avoidance.[28] Until such tests are developed, allergen-specific IgE antibody quantification or the size of the skin test response may be a better tool to help identify asthmatic patients likely to benefit from allergen control, versus the mere presence or absence of sensitization.

Allergen Control in Disease Prevention

The consistent finding of an association between allergic sensitization and childhood asthma raises the question as to whether successful allergen control that results in a major reduction in exposure to aeroallergens early in life can reduce the risk of subsequent development of sensitization and symptoms of allergic disease. This question is being addressed by several "primary prevention" studies, although by design these long-term studies will take many years to report definitive findings.[40-42]

At least seven ongoing studies with published results to date are described here. All these primary prevention studies have by necessity focused on children at high risk of developing allergic disease. However, the definition of "high risk" differed among studies (e.g., both parents atopic, single parent atopic, mother with asthma). Furthermore, it is important to emphasize that all the studies used different allergen control approaches and were of a different design (e.g., four included dietary intervention in addition to environmental control). In addition, the studies used different definitions of "primary outcomes" and assessed those at different ages. As a consequence, results between studies are not directly comparable.

Isle of Wight was the first study to implement an intervention designed to reduce exposure to inhalant allergens as part

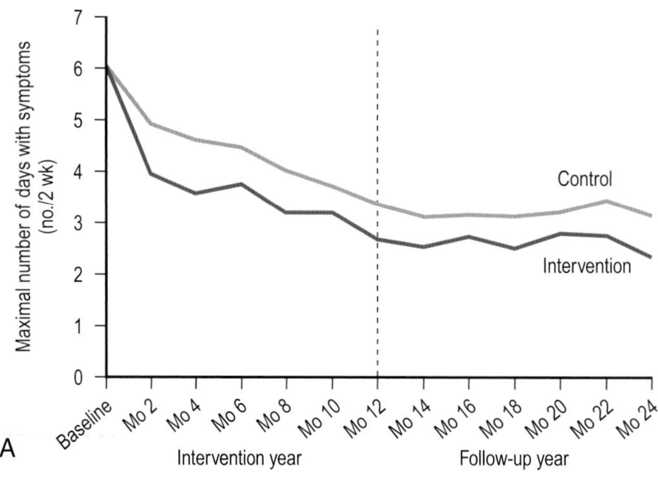

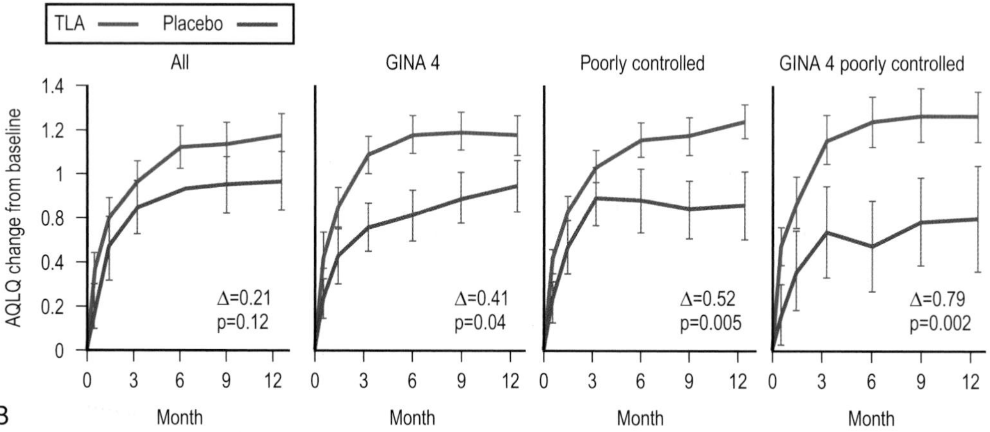

Figure 86-2 A, Mean maximal number of days with symptoms for every 2-week period before follow-up assessment during 2 years of study. Difference between groups was significant in both the intervention year (*P* <.001) and the follow-up year (*P* <.001). **B,** Change in Asthma Quality of Life Questionnaire (*AQLQ*) score during 1 year of temperature-controlled laminar airflow *(TLA)* or placebo treatment in the whole population (*All*): those with highest asthma treatment intensity at baseline (*GINA 4,* Global Initiative for Asthma), those with poor asthma control at baseline (Asthma Control Test, ACT <18), or both (GINA 4, ACT <18). (**A** *from Morgan WJ et al. Results of a home-based environmental intervention among urban children with asthma. N Engl J Med 2004;351:1068-80;* **B** *from Boyle RJ et al. Nocturnal temperature controlled laminar airflow for treating atopic asthma: a randomised controlled trial. Thorax 2012;67:215-21.)*

of a primary prevention program in 120 children (58 intervention, 62 control).[43] The intervention included avoidance of both food and dust mite allergens. Breastfeeding mothers were to avoid allergenic foods, and these foods were not introduced into the infant's diet until after 9 months of age. Infants who were not breastfed were given a hydrolyzed formula. Environmental control measures consisted of the application of acaricide to carpets and upholstered furniture. Infants in both groups slept on polyvinyl-covered mattresses with a vented head area. A reduction in sensitization and in wheeze was reported at age 1 year, but by 2 and 4 years differences in respiratory symptoms failed to reach statistical significance. At age 8 years, sensitization to mite was reduced by more than 50% in the active group, despite only modest reductions in mite allergen levels. Children in the active group were significantly less likely to have current wheeze, nocturnal cough, wheeze with AHR, and atopy. Thus, despite only a modest reduction in mite allergen levels, the combined intervention resulted in a marked reduction in important clinical signs and symptoms suggestive of childhood asthma. Because of the study design, however, it is impossible to determine which part of the intervention program is responsible for the effect.

In the Canadian Primary Prevention Study (CaPPS) the multifaceted intervention included measures to reduce exposure to both inhalant and food allergens. Compliance with mattress encasings and acaricides (applied by the study nurses) was excellent, but despite advice, carpet use and pet ownership did not decline. At age 2 years, probable asthma was significantly reduced in the active group. At age 7 the prevalence of physician-diagnosed asthma was significantly lower in the intervention group than in the control group (14.9% vs. 23.0%).[44] The prevalence of allergic rhinitis, eczema, atopy, and AHR did not differ between the two groups. Thus in CaPPS the multifaceted intervention program appeared effective in reducing the prevalence of asthma in high-risk children at 7 years of age.

In the Study on the Prevention of Allergy in Children in Europe (SPACE) the multifaceted intervention was directed toward both inhalant and food allergens. Mite avoidance focused on the infant's bed, with application of mattress covers. Mothers were advised to breastfeed children, and a hypoallergenic formula was recommended as an alternative. Parents were advised to delay the introduction of potentially allergenic foods. Compliance with the measures was reported to be good. At age 1 year, there was a reduction in sensitization to mites, but no difference in the proportion of children who had ever wheezed (21% in both groups). At age 2 years, no differences were found between the control and intervention group in the prevalence of mite sensitization (8.4% control vs. 6.1% intervention) or the development of respiratory symptoms (wheezing 10.3% vs. 10.7%; nocturnal cough 12.5% vs. 12.5%) or allergic diseases (asthma 3.5% vs. 5.1%; eczema 20.0% vs. 19.6%; rhinitis 28.9% vs. 25.8%).[45] Thus in SPACE, mite avoidance did not have a protective effect on the development of mite sensitization or symptomatic allergy in children at age 2 years.

The Childhood Asthma Prevention Study (CAPS), a multicenter, parallel-group RCT in Sydney, Australia. Families at risk (no cat in home) were randomized into one of four study groups (mite avoidance with placebo dietary intervention, $n = 155$; mite avoidance with active dietary intervention, $n = 153$; active dietary intervention alone, no mite avoidance, $n = 159$; placebo dietary intervention, no mite avoidance, $n = 149$). Of 616 children randomized in this study, 516 were evaluated at 5 years of age. The mite avoidance intervention resulted in a 61% reduction in allergen concentrations in the child's bed, but no difference between the randomized groups were observed in prevalence of asthma, wheeze, or atopy. However, prevalence of eczema was higher in the active mite avoidance group (26% vs. 19%). The prevalence of asthma, wheezing, eczema, or atopy did not differ between the diet groups.[46] Thus in the CAPS study, dust mite avoidance measures and dietary fatty acid modification during infancy and early childhood did not prevent the onset of asthma, eczema, or atopy in high-risk children by age 5 years.

In the Primary Prevention of Asthma in Children Study (PREVACS) in the Netherlands, a total of 476 children were recruited during the prenatal period and randomized to either a control group (receiving usual care) or an intervention group with families receiving instruction from nurses on how to reduce exposure of newborns to mite, pet, and food allergens and passive smoking. At 2 years of age the intervention group had fewer asthma-like symptoms (e.g., wheezing, shortness of breath, nighttime cough) than the control group. However, no significant differences in total or specific IgE were found between the groups. Furthermore, the incidence of asthma-like symptoms during the first 2 years of life was similar in both groups, although subanalysis revealed a significant reduction in the intervention group among females (but not males). This intervention was not effective in reducing asthma-like symptoms in high-risk children during the first 2 years of life, although some modest effect was observed at age 2 years.[47]

The Prevention and Incidence of Asthma and Mite Allergy Study (PIAMA) is a multicenter population-based cohort trial of more than 4000 children in The Netherlands. Nested within this cohort is an intervention study among 810 high-risk infants who were randomly allocated to receive active mite-proof encasings for the mattress and pillows of the parental and infant beds or cotton placebo encasings in a double-blind manner. Early intervention with mite-impermeable mattress covers was successful in reducing exposure to mite allergens. However, it only temporarily reduced the risk of asthma symptoms in early life (at 2 years), but at age 8 there was no reduction in risk of wheeze, hay fever, eczema, or allergic sensitization.[48]

The Manchester Asthma and Allergy Study (MAAS) is a population-based birth-cohort study of more than 1000 children, with a nested intervention study in the high-risk group. Participants were recruited from the antenatal clinics, and children with two atopic parents who had no pets in their home were randomly allocated before birth to a stringent environmental control (n = 145) or normal regimen (n = 146). The comprehensive environmental control regimen included fitting mite-proof encasings to the parental mattress, comforter, and pillows by the 16th week of pregnancy; washing bedding weekly at over 55° C; and supplying high-filtration vacuum and acaricide (Acarosan) to apply to dust reservoirs with high mite allergen levels. Just before the birth of the child, custom-made cot and carry cot mattresses of allergen-impermeable fabric were supplied to the family, carpets removed from the nursery, and a vinyl cushion floor fitted; a washable toy was also supplied. A significant and sustained reduction in exposure to mite, cat, and dog allergens was observed in the homes of children in the active group. At age 1 year there was slightly more atopy in the intervention than the control group (17% vs. 14%), but this did not reach statistical significance. Asthma-like symptoms were consistently lower in the intervention versus control group, reaching statistical significance for attacks of severe wheeze with shortness of breath, for prescribing medication for wheezy attacks, and for wheeze after playing or exertion. No difference between the groups was seen for eczema. Counterintuitively, 3-year-old children in the intervention group were significantly *more* frequently sensitized to dust mite than controls (risk ratio 2.85).[49] However, lung function assessed by specific airway resistance was significantly better in the intervention group. Furthermore, improvement in lung function in the environmental intervention group between birth and age 3 years likely resulted from some aspect of the environmental control regimen, because there was no difference between the groups in infant lung function at age 4 weeks. Thus in MAAS, stringent environmental control was associated with increased risk of mite sensitisation, but better lung function at age 3 years.

Summary

Although the general consensus is that allergen control should lead to an improvement of symptoms in susceptible patients with allergic disease, there is little evidence to support the use of simple physical or chemical methods as single interventions to control dust mite or pet allergen levels (e.g., mattress encasings, acaricides, HEPA filters). Although a multifaceted intervention in carefully selected patients could have some effect, this has not been addressed adequately in adult asthma; thus the current evidence is inadequate to advise this as a strategy for adult patients. In contrast, trials of allergen-impermeable bed encasings as a single intervention in asthmatic children reported benefits, as did a more comprehensive environmental intervention in children living in poor-quality housing. The apparent differences in response between adults and children may be analogous to occupational asthma, where prompt removal from exposure to a sensitizing allergen is associated with a better long-term outcome than removal after prolonged exposure. For rhinitis and eczema, the most recent well-designed studies on single mite avoidance measures failed to demonstrate a clear clinical benefit.

Until the unequivocal evidence for all age groups and all allergens is available, a pragmatic approach to environmental control should be followed. First, single avoidance measures are ineffective; use a comprehensive allergen control regimen to achieve a complete cessation of exposure, or as great a reduction in personal exposure as possible. Second, domestic interventions require attention to hardware to reduce exposure as well as removal of accumulating allergen (cleaning, laundry). Third, tailor the intervention to the patient's sensitization and exposure status. If unable to assess the exposure, use the level of allergen-specific IgE antibodies or size of skin test wheal as an indicator. Fourth, start the intervention as early in the natural history of the disease as possible.

Environmental control in the prevention of allergic disease has inconsistent and often confusing outcomes. Ongoing prevention cohorts provide much information, but much longer follow-up is required before we can ensure interventions cause no harm and confidently give advice. No single primary prevention strategy will be applicable to the whole population, only to individuals within the population with a particular susceptibility.[15,16] We need to move away from the concept of blanket advice aimed at the whole population to individualized measures for patients with specific susceptibilities who will benefit from a particular intervention.

REFERENCES

Introduction

1. Tovey ER, Marks GB. It's time to rethink mite allergen avoidance. J Allergy Clin Immunol 2011;128:723-7.

Rationale for Allergen Control

2. Stevens W, Addo-Yobo E, Roper J, et al. Differences in both prevalence and titre of specific immunoglobulin E among children with asthma in affluent and poor communities within a large town in Ghana. Clin Exp Allergy 2011;41:1587-94.
3. Simpson A, Soderstrom L, Ahlstedt S, et al. IgE antibody quantification and the probability of wheeze in preschool children. J Allergy Clin Immunol 2005;116:744-9.
4. Lau S, Illi S, Sommerfeld C, et al. Early exposure to house-dust mite and cat allergens and development of childhood asthma: a cohort study. Multicentre Allergy Study Group. Lancet 2000;356(9239):1392-7.
5. Sporik R, Holgate ST, Platts-Mills TA, Cogswell JJ. Exposure to house-dust mite allergen (Der p 1) and the development of asthma in childhood: a prospective study. N Engl J Med 1990;323:502-7.
6. Rosenstreich DL, Eggleston P, Kattan M, et al. The role of cockroach allergy and exposure to cockroach allergen in causing morbidity among inner-city children with asthma. N Engl J Med 1997;336:1356-63.
7. Langley SJ, Goldthorpe S, Craven M, et al. Exposure and sensitization to indoor allergens: association with lung function, bronchial reactivity, and exhaled nitric oxide measures in asthma. J Allergy Clin Immunol 2003;112:362-8.
8. Peroni DG, Piacentini GL, Costella S, et al. Mite avoidance can reduce air trapping and airway inflammation in allergic asthmatic children. Clin Exp Allergy 2002;32:850-5.
9. De Groene GJ, Pal TM, Beach J, et al. Workplace interventions for treatment of occupational asthma. Cochrane Database Syst Rev 2011;(5):CD006308.
10. Cullinan P, MacNeill SJ, Harris JM, et al. Early allergen exposure, skin prick responses, and atopic wheeze at age 5 in English children: a cohort study. Thorax 2004;59:855-61.
11. Tovey ER, Almqvist C, Li Q, Crisafulli D, Marks GB. Nonlinear relationship of mite allergen exposure to mite sensitization and asthma in a birth cohort. J Allergy Clin Immunol 2008;122:114-8.
12. Platts-Mills T, Vaughan J, Squillace S, Woodfolk J, Sporik R. Sensitisation, asthma, and a modified Th2 response in children exposed to cat allergen: a population-based cross-sectional study. Lancet 2001;357(9258):752-6.
13. Peng RD, Paigen B, Eggleston PA, et al. Both the variability and level of mouse allergen exposure influence the phenotype of the immune response in workers at a mouse facility. J Allergy Clin Immunol 2011;128:390-414.
14. Bertelsen RJ, Carlsen KC, Carlsen KH, et al. Childhood asthma and early life exposure to indoor allergens, endotoxin and beta(1,3)-glucans. Clin Exp Allergy 2010;40:307-16.
15. Simpson A, John SL, Jury F, et al. Endotoxin exposure, CD14, and allergic disease: an interaction between genes and the environment. Am J Respir Crit Care Med 2006;174:386-92.
16. Kerkhof M, Daley D, Postma DS, et al. Opposite effects of allergy prevention depending on CD14 rs2569190 genotype in 3 intervention studies. J Allergy Clin Immunol 2012;129:256-9.
17. Custovic A, Rothers J, Stern D, et al. Effect of day care attendance on sensitization and atopic wheezing differs by Toll-like receptor 2 genotype in 2 population-based birth cohort studies. J Allergy Clin Immunol 2011;127:390-7.
18. Bisgaard H, Simpson A, Palmer CN, et al. Gene-environment interaction in the onset of eczema in infancy: filaggrin loss-of-function mutations enhanced by neonatal cat exposure. PLoS Med 2008;5:e131.
19. Papadopoulos NG, Christodoulou I, Rohde G, et al. Viruses and bacteria in acute asthma exacerbations: a GA(2) LEN-DARE systematic review. Allergy 2011;66:458-68.
20. Green RM, Custovic A, Sanderson G, et al. Synergism between allergens and viruses and risk of hospital admission with asthma: case-control study. BMJ 2002;324(7340):763.
21. Murray CS, Poletti G, Kebadze T, et al. Study of modifiable risk factors for asthma exacerbations: virus infection and allergen exposure increase the risk of asthma hospital admissions in children. Thorax 2006;61:376-82.
22. Busse WW, Morgan WJ, Gergen PJ, et al. Randomized trial of omalizumab (anti-IgE) for asthma in inner-city children. N Engl J Med 2011;364:1005-15.

Allergen Control Measures

23. Raja S, Xu Y, Ferro AR, Jaques PA, Hopke PK. Resuspension of indoor aeroallergens and relationship to lung inflammation in asthmatic children. Environ Int 2010;36:8-14.
24. Custovic A, Murray CS, Gore RB, Woodcock A. Controlling indoor allergens. Ann Allergy Asthma Immunol 2002;88:432-41; quiz 442-3, 529.
25. Gore RB, Durrell B, Bishop S, et al. High-efficiency particulate arrest-filter vacuum cleaners increase personal cat allergen exposure in homes with cats. J Allergy Clin Immunol 2003;111:784-7.
26. Custovic A, Simpson BM, Simpson A, et al. Manchester Asthma and Allergy Study: low-allergen environment can be achieved and maintained during pregnancy and in early life. J Allergy Clin Immunol 2000;105:252-8.
27. Gore RB, Bishop S, Durrell B, et al. Air filtration units in homes with cats: can they reduce personal exposure to cat allergen? Clin Exp Allergy 2003;33:765-9.
28. Custovic A, Wijk RG. The effectiveness of measures to change the indoor environment in the treatment of allergic rhinitis and asthma: ARIA update [in collaboration with GA(2)LEN]. Allergy 2005;60:1112-5.
29. Shirai T, Matsui T, Suzuki K, Chida K. Effect of pet removal on pet allergic asthma. Chest 2005;127:1565-71.
30. Gotzsche PC, Johansen HK. House dust mite control measures for asthma: systematic review. Allergy 2008;63:646-59.
31. Nurmatov U, van Schayck CP, Hurwitz B, Sheikh A. House dust mite avoidance measures for perennial allergic rhinitis: an updated Cochrane systematic review. Allergy 2012;67:158-65.
32. Kilburn S, Lasserson TJ, McKean M. Pet allergen control measures for allergic asthma in children and adults. Cochrane Database Syst Rev 2003;(1):CD002989.
33. Woodcock A, Forster L, Matthews E, et al. Control of exposure to mite allergen and allergen-impermeable bed covers for adults with asthma. N Engl J Med 2003;349:225-36.
34. Terreehorst I, Hak E, Oosting AJ, et al. Evaluation of impermeable covers for bedding in patients with allergic rhinitis. N Engl J Med 2003;349:237-46.
35. Halken S, Host A, Niklassen U, et al. Effect of mattress and pillow encasings on children with asthma and house dust mite allergy. J Allergy Clin Immunol 2003;111:169-76.
36. Krieger J, Jacobs DE, Ashley PJ, et al. Housing interventions and control of asthma-related

indoor biologic agents: a review of the evidence. J Public Health Manag Pract 2010;16(5 Suppl): 11-20.
37. Morgan WJ, Crain EF, Gruchalla RS, et al. Results of a home-based environmental intervention among urban children with asthma. N Engl J Med 2004;351:1068-80.
38. Boyle RJ, Pedroletti C, Wickman M, et al Nocturnal temperature controlled laminar airflow for treating atopic asthma: a randomised controlled trial. Thorax 2012;67:215-21.
39. Simpson A, Tan VY, Winn J, et al. Beyond atopy: multiple patterns of sensitization in relation to asthma in a birth cohort study. Am J Respir Crit Care Med 2010;181:1200-6.

Allergen Control in Disease Prevention

40. Simpson A, Custovic A. Allergen avoidance in the primary prevention of asthma. Curr Opin Allergy Clin Immunol 2004;4:45-51.
41. Simpson A, Custovic A. The role of allergen avoidance in primary and secondary prevention. Pediatr Pulmonol Suppl 2004;26:225-8.
42. Simpson A, Custovic A. Prevention of allergic sensitization by environmental control. Curr Allergy Asthma Rep 2009;9:363-9.
43. Arshad SH, Bateman B, Matthews SM. Primary prevention of asthma and atopy during childhood by allergen avoidance in infancy: a randomised controlled study. Thorax 2003;58: 489-93.
44. Chan-Yeung M, Ferguson A, Watson W, et al. The Canadian Childhood Asthma Primary Prevention Study: outcomes at 7 years of age. J Allergy Clin Immunol 2005;116:49-55.
45. Horak F Jr, Matthew F, Ihorst G, et al. Effect of mite-impermeable mattress encasings and an educational package on the development of allergies in a multinational randomized controlled birth-cohort study: 24 months' results of the Study of Prevention of Allergy in Children in Europe. Clin Exp Allergy 2004;34:1220-5.
46. Marks GB, Mihrshahi S, Kemp AS, et al. Prevention of asthma during the first 5 years of life: a randomized controlled trial. J Allergy Clin Immunol 2006;118:53-61.
47. Schonberger HJ, Dompeling E, Knottnerus JA, et al. The PREVASC study: the clinical effect of a multifaceted educational intervention to prevent childhood asthma. Eur Respir J 2005; 25:660-70.
48. Gehring U, de Jongste JC, Kerkhof M, et al. The 8-year follow-up of the PIAMA intervention study assessing the effect of mite-impermeable mattress covers. Allergy 2012;67:248-56.
49. Woodcock A, Lowe LA, Murray CS, et al. Early life environmental control: effect on symptoms, sensitization, and lung function at age 3 years. Am J Respir Crit Care Med 2004;170:433-9.

87

Injection Immunotherapy for Inhalant Allergens

HAROLD S. NELSON

CONTENTS

SUMMARY OF IMPORTANT CONCEPTS

» Allergen immunotherapy is an effective treatment for both allergic rhinitis and allergic asthma.
» Clinical effectiveness requires administration of adequate doses of extracts; effective doses have been determined for many allergens in controlled studies.
» Immunotherapy induces an early and transient increase in regulatory T cells that decrease both T helper cell subset Th1 and Th2 responses to allergens. Later in immunotherapy, there is immune deviation from a predominantly Th2 to a predominantly Th1 response to the administered allergen.
» Immunotherapy induces disease modification, reducing new sensitizations, progression from rhinitis to asthma, and resulting in clinical improvement that persists for years after it is discontinued.
» Active investigation of modifications in allergen extracts and in their route of administration is under way, seeking to reduce the inconvenience and improve the safety of immunotherapy.

Historical Development

In 2011 the allergy community celebrated the one hundredth anniversary of the initial description of immunotherapy by Leonard Noon and John Freeman.[1-3] The practice of injection therapy for hay fever spread rapidly. Its use was extended to the treatment of perennial rhinitis and asthma with injections of extracts of additional pollens and of perennial allergens such as house dust and animal danders. In the 1950s and 1960s, adequately controlled studies were conducted in England by Frankland and Augustin[4] and in the United States by Lowell and Franklin[5,6] that established beyond any doubt that immunotherapy is an effective form of treatment. Throughout the previous century, immunotherapy was still practiced by the same method used by Noon: injections usually at weekly intervals of progressively greater concentrations of extract, followed by a period of years of injection of maintenance doses. In recent years, however, there have been renewed efforts either to administer the extract by a route less prone to cause systemic reactions or to modify the extract so that only a limited number of injections are required.

Clinical Efficacy of Allergen Immunotherapy

ALLERGIC RHINITIS

Well-controlled studies have confirmed the effectiveness of allergen immunotherapy in both seasonal[7] and perennial allergic rhinitis.[8] In a meta-analysis of data from 51 studies with 2871 participants receiving allergen injection therapy for seasonal allergic rhinitis,[9] 16 studies evaluated efficacy with extracts of mixed grass, 12 with ragweed, 6 with *Parietaria*, 5 with timothy grass, 4 with birch, 3 cedar, 2 orchard grass, 1 Bermuda grass, 1 *Juniperus ashei*, and 1 *Cocos* (coconut). The standardized mean difference (SMD) (95% CI) between active treatment and placebo in symptom scores was −0.73 (−0.97 to −0.50) and for medication scores, −0.57 (−0.82 to −0.33). The SMD for quality of life was −0.52 (−0.69 to −0.34).

BRONCHIAL ASTHMA

A number of placebo-controlled studies have established the effectiveness of allergen immunotherapy in carefully selected patients with asthma caused by grass pollen,[10] cats,[11] and house dust mites[12] (Figure 87-1). Two studies, one in children[13] and one in adults,[14] demonstrated a 50% reduction in inhaled corticosteroids compared with placebo after 2 years of immunotherapy with house dust mite extract. In a meta-analysis of data from 88 published reports of such therapy in 3459 subjects with asthma,[15] a majority of the studies were on monotherapy: 42 with extracts of house dust mites, 27 with pollens, 10 with domestic pet allergens, 2 with latex, and 2 with *Cladosporium.* Multiple allergens were administered in 6 studies. The SMD (95% CI) for symptom scores was −0.59 (−0.83, −0.35) and for medications, −0.53 (−0.80, −0.27). A significant reduction in allergen-specific bronchial hyperresponsiveness was observed, but no consistent effect on lung function was noted. However, other carefully conducted studies of seasonal[16] or perennial[17] asthma have yielded only limited[16] or no[17] evidence for clinical improvement in patients with asthma. These studies underscore the necessity for careful selection of patients and allergens for

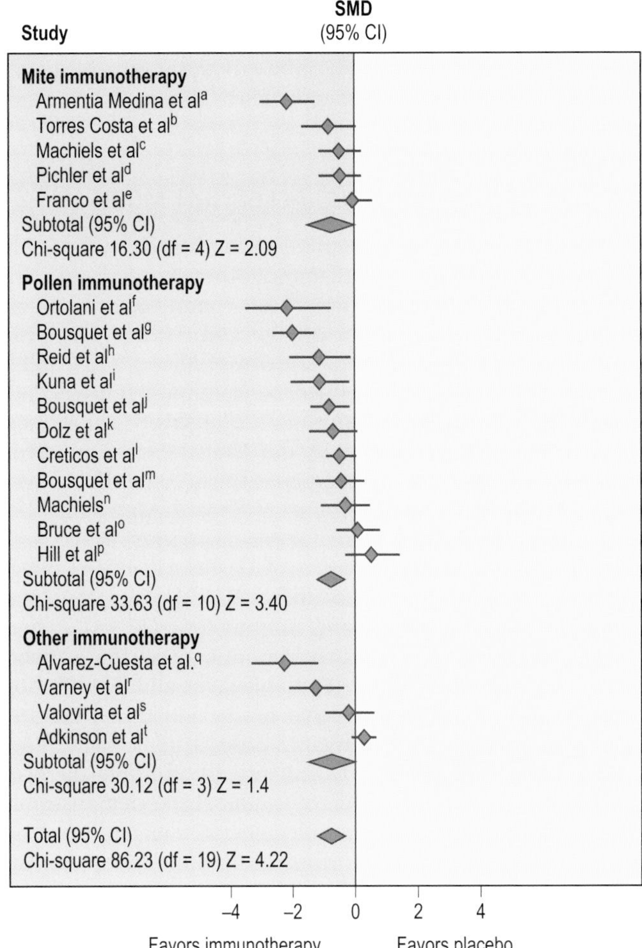

Figure 87-1 Odds ratios and 95% confidence intervals (CIs) for clinical improvement as evidenced by reduction in asthmatic symptoms after allergen immunotherapy in placebo-controlled studies. *df,* Degrees of freedom. *(Modified from Abramson M, Puy R, Weiner J. Immunotherapy in asthma: an updated systematic review. Allergy 1999;54:1022-41. Referenced studies: a, Armentia Medina et al. Allergo Immunopathol (Madr) 1995;23:211; b, Torres Costa et al. Allergy 1996;51:238; c, Machiels et al. J Clin Invest 1990;85:1024; d, Pichler et al. Allergy 1997;52:274; e, Franco et al. Allergo Immunopathol (Madr) 1995;23:58; f, Ortolani et al. J Allergy Clin Immunol 1984;73:283; g, Bousquet et al. J Allergy Clin Immunol 1990;85:490; h, Reid et al. J Allergy Clin Immunol 1986;78:590; i, Kuna et al. J Allergy Clin Immunol 1989;83:816; j, Bousquet et al. J Allergy Clin Immunol 1989;84:546; k, Dolz et al. Allergy 1996;51:489; l, Creticos et al. N Engl J Med 1996;334:501; m, Bousquet et al. Clin Allergy 1985;25:179; n, Machiels et al. Clin Exp Allergy 1990;20;653; o, Bruce et al. J Allergy Clin Immunol 1977;59:449; p, Hill et al. BMJ 1982;284:306; q, Alvarez-Cuesta et al. J Allergy Clin Immunol 1994;93:556; r, Varney et al. Clin Exp Allergy 1997;27:860; s, Valovirta et al. Ann Allergy 1986;57:173; t, Adkinson et al. N Engl J Med 1997;336:324.)*

treatment if immunotherapy is to be of benefit for this indication.

ATOPIC DERMATITIS

Atopic dermatitis has not traditionally been considered an indication for allergen immunotherapy, despite anecdotal accounts of clinical improvement with this treatment.[18-20] A randomized, 1-year, dose-response study of immunotherapy with house dust mite extract was undertaken in 89 adults with chronic atopic dermatitis who had at least a class 3 (≥3.5 KU/L specific IgE) in vitro assay for IgE to house dust mites.[21] The highest dose, administered weekly, was $\frac{1}{5}$ of the customary monthly maintenance dose used for treatment of respiratory allergies. The lower two doses were $\frac{1}{10}$ and $\frac{1}{1000}$ of the highest dose. After 1 year, symptom scores were significantly reduced with the two higher doses compared with the lowest dose, and the use of topical corticosteroids was significantly reduced in the highest-dose group. Although the results are encouraging, this study requires independent confirmation before the indication of immunotherapy is extended to include atopic dermatitis.

CLINICAL EFFICACY WITH SPECIFIC ALLERGENS

Pollens

Although asthma due to plant aeroallergens does occur and responds well to allergen immunotherapy,[10,16] pollen typically produces symptoms of rhinitis and conjunctivitis. The ability to make an accurate diagnosis of pollen rhinitis has made seasonal allergic rhinitis due to grass in England[4,7,10] and to ragweed in the United States[5,6] the most popular model for investigating the efficacy and mechanisms of allergen immunotherapy. Adequate doses of pollen extracts regularly reduce the clinical symptoms of allergic rhinitis[4-7] and, when present, asthma.[10]

House Dust Mites

The importance of house dust mite sensitivity in asthma is indicated by the increased risk for asthma in people with a positive result to mites on skin prick testing,[22-24] the correlation of symptoms to levels of house dust mite exposure in mite-sensitive patients with asthma,[25,26] and the decrease in asthma symptoms when house dust mite–sensitive patients are moved to an environment with minimal exposure to mite allergen.[27-29] It is not surprising then, that nearly half of the immunotherapy studies entered into the meta-analyses of data on immunotherapy for asthma were with house dust mite extracts.[15] Allergen immunotherapy for treatment of perennial rhinitis due to house dust mite allergy also has been effective.[8]

Domestic Pet Allergen

As with house dust mites, epidemiologic studies reveal that skin prick test reactivity to domestic pet allergen extracts conveys an increased risk for the occurrence of asthma.[22,24] Domestic pet allergen exposure is potentially avoidable. In the past, immunotherapy with domestic pet allergen extracts often was not considered appropriate except for people who are occupationally exposed.[30] The increasing number of studies of immunotherapy in patients allergic to these allergens, especially from cats, is an acknowledgment that even sensitive patients often will not eliminate exposure in their homes and to the widespread presence of cat allergens in public places[31] and even homes without cats.[32] Two studies have demonstrated that immunotherapy with cat allergen extract in patients without cats in the home can reduce asthma symptom medication scores[33] and nonspecific bronchial hyperresponsiveness to histamine,[34] supporting the importance of the ubiquitous presence of this allergen.

Fungi

Airborne fungal spores have been recognized as causing epidemic outbreaks[35] and life-threatening episodes[36] of asthma. From the standpoint of immunotherapy, fungi present several features that set them apart from the other inhalant allergens[37]: (1) there are hundreds of thousands of different species of fungi; (2) accurate information on exposure patterns to most fungal species is lacking; (3) fungal extracts are of very variable quality,[38,39] a characteristic that may relate in part to a high rate of somatic mutation and in part to their high content of proteolytic enzymes; and (4) for many genera of fungi, suitable extracts are lacking, because they do not grow in artificial media. A comparison of seven commercially available *Alternaria alternata* extracts revealed a fifty-fivefold difference in the quantity of the major allergen (Alt a 1) in extracts labeled as equivalent in potency.[39]

A few double-blind, controlled studies have focused on immunotherapy with standardized extracts of two of the most important outdoor seasonal fungi, *Cladosporium herbarum* and *Alternaria alternata.* Ten months of immunotherapy with *Cladosporium herbarum* in 30 asthmatic children significantly reduced medication use but not symptom scores,[40] whereas 5 to 7 months of immunotherapy in 22 asthmatic adults produced a significant reduction in symptom and medication scores from those for placebo.[41] One year of specific immunotherapy with a standardized *Alternaria* extract in 24 patients with rhinitis and/or asthma who were sensitive only to *Alternaria* significantly reduced symptom and medication scores and skin and nasal reactivity to *Alternaria.*[42] A 3-year placebo-controlled trial of *A. alternata* immunotherapy was completed in 45 children.[43] By the third season, symptoms in the actively treated children were reduced 63.5%, with significant improvement in quality of life.

With fungi, as with any allergen, the use of immunotherapy should be guided by the sensitivity and exposure of the patient, a pattern of symptoms consistent with the pattern of exposure, and the availability of an extract of sufficient quality to allow delivery of a therapeutically effective dose. These criteria will be satisfied for few fungi except *Alternaria* and *Cladosporium.* There is no justification for the use of mold mixes.

Cockroach

The combination of sensitivity and exposure to cockroach is now recognized as a major factor in the pathogenesis of inner city asthma[44] and probably is also widespread in warmer climates. Adequately controlled trials of immunotherapy with cockroach extracts are lacking, however. As with the fungal extracts, commercially available cockroach extracts tend to be of variable and low potency.[45,46]

Natural Rubber Latex

A placebo-controlled trial of immunotherapy was undertaken in subjects with cutaneous ($n = 8$) or respiratory ($n = 16$) symptoms caused by exposure to natural rubber latex.[47] After 6 months of therapy, there was improvement in both cutaneous and respiratory symptoms with active treatment. Systemic reactions, all responding promptly to treatment, were observed with 8% of doses with the latex extract. Although this study shows that immunotherapy for latex sensitivity can be successful, the rate of systemic reactions suggests caution in undertaking it. Furthermore, there is no approved latex extract in the United States, nor is there likely to be one. Therefore avoidance remains the mainstay of treatment on latex sensitivity.

Mixed Bacterial Vaccine

At one time it was common for patients to receive injections of a mixed respiratory bacterial vaccine. Its use was based on the observation that infections often triggered exacerbations of asthma, and on a belief that many patients had a true allergy to the bacterial antigens. The availability of antibiotics, plus convincingly negative results of controlled studies,[48] led to its abandonment.

EFFICACY WITH MULTIPLE ALLERGEN MIXES

Most of the double-blind, placebo-controlled studies that have demonstrated efficacy of immunotherapy in allergic rhinitis and bronchial asthma have been conducted with single allergen extracts. The Global Allergy and Asthma European Network (GA^{2}LEN)–European Academy of Allergy and Clinical Immunology (EAACI) guidelines for immunotherapy do not recommend the use of mixtures of allergens.[49] The typical immunotherapy prescription in the United States, however, contains multiple unrelated allergen extracts,[50] and the *Allergen Immunotherapy: A Practice Parameter Third Update* (AIPP)—prepared by a joint task force for the American Academy of Allergy, Asthma & Immunology (AAAAI), the American College of Allergy, Asthma & Immunology (ACAAI), and the Joint Council of Allergy, Asthma and Immunology (JCAAI)—supports the use of allergen mixtures, cautioning only that patients should be treated only with relevant allergens and that dilution limits the number of antigens that can be added to a maintenance concentrate if a therapeutic dose is to be delivered.[51] Some evidence suggests that treatment with multiple allergens may be successful. A number of studies have demonstrated efficacy with mixtures of two allergens.[52] Fewer studies have examined true multiallergen mixes in immunotherapy. In the studies of ragweed-allergic rhinitis conducted by Lowell and Franklin, however, patients were receiving extracts containing multiple allergens. Only the ragweed was removed[5] or reduced,[6] yet in both studies, the result of receiving less ragweed extract was an increase in ragweed pollen–induced symptoms. This observation indicates that the ragweed pollen extract had been effective even though combined with other allergen extracts. The results in asthmatic children reported by Johnstone and Crump[53] suggest that a mixture containing multiple unrelated allergens can be effective in treating asthma, whereas a study by Reid and colleagues[54] showed significant reduction in asthma symptoms in adults when grass extract was combined with multiple other allergens.

These four studies indicate that immunotherapy with multiple allergen mixes, when appropriate, can be effective so long as the number of allergens added does not lead to dilution of the individual constituents to ineffective concentrations.

SPECIFICITY OF ALLERGEN IMMUNOTHERAPY

The immunologic specificity of allergen immunotherapy has been clearly established. Lowell and Franklin removed ragweed from the allergen extract for one of each pair of patients, but all patients continued to receive tree, grass, or plantain pollens.[5] Despite continuing to receive other pollen extracts, the patients who did not receive ragweed pollen extract had significantly more symptoms during the ragweed season.

The specificity of allergen immunotherapy also has been addressed by Norman and Lichtenstein.[55] These investigators identified a group of patients with allergic rhinitis who were sensitive to both grass and ragweed. They treated half the patients with ragweed immunotherapy and then monitored all of their subjects through both ragweed and grass seasons.

Patients in the treatment group had markedly reduced symptoms compared with those in the placebo group during the ragweed season, but symptoms did not differ between the two groups during the grass pollen season. Thus, treatment with ragweed pollen extract had little or no effect on grass pollen–induced symptoms.

EVIDENCE OF DISEASE MODIFICATION

New Sensitizations

Three studies have reported that immunotherapy in monosensitized patients reduces the rate of development of new sensitivities as indicated by newly positive results on skin prick tests.[56-58] In the two largest studies, one in children 5 to 8 years of age sensitive only to house dust mites[57] and the other in more than 8 thousand adolescents and young adults monosensitized to a variety of allergens,[58] the reduction in new sensitization by 56% to 65% compared with the control group persisted without diminution for 3 years after 3 to 4 years of active treatment. One randomized controlled trial (RCT) of immunotherapy in polysensitized children failed to show any long-term effect on new sensitizations.[59]

Development of Asthma in Patients with Rhinitis Only

A multicenter study in Europe examined the effect of immunotherapy with birch and/or timothy grass for 3 years on the development of asthma in children 6 to 14 years of age who only had symptoms of rhinitis.[60] At the end of 3 years, children in the untreated control group were significantly (odds ratio [OR], 2.52) more likely to have developed clinical asthma than those who had received immunotherapy. Follow-up evaluation at 7 years after completion of immunotherapy indicated that the protective effect on the development of asthma was still significant.[61]

Persistence of Clinical Improvement After Cessation of Immunotherapy

Three studies have examined the persistence of clinical improvement after discontinuation of immunotherapy with grass pollen extract.[62-64] Specific immunotherapy to grass was discontinued after 3 to 4 years treatment in 108 patients who had responded well to treatment.[62] There was no control group. A progressive increase in the number of patients reporting a return of grass pollen symptoms was noted, which reached 31% by the third year but with no appreciable increase in the fourth and fifth years. A double-blind, placebo-controlled trial supported the findings in this open study.[63] Thirty-two patients who had received immunotherapy with grass pollen extract for 3 to 4 years were randomized to either continue to receive grass extract or to receive placebo injections for the following 3 years. They were compared with untreated patients with grass-induced allergic rhinitis. Both those continuing to receive active immunotherapy and subjects in the placebo group had significantly fewer symptoms and need for medication than the untreated control subjects, and scores in the active treatment and placebo groups were virtually identical. Furthermore, the subjects in both treatment groups exhibited similar persisting suppression of conjunctival sensitivity and of immediate and late cutaneous reactions to grass pollen extract.[63] In addition, 12-year follow-up data have been reported for an open study of grass immunotherapy in children. Compared with the control subjects, the treated children still displayed decreased symptom and medication scores during the grass season and fewer new sensitizations.[64]

Persistence of improvement also has been monitored after cessation of immunotherapy with house dust mite extract.[65] Injections were stopped in patients with asthma who had been receiving specific immunotherapy for periods of 12 to 96 months and who no longer required medication to control their symptoms. Over a 3-year period after discontinuation, approximately half experienced a relapse in symptoms. Although likelihood of relapse, as expected, correlated inversely with duration of immunotherapy, the inverse correlation with suppression of immediate skin test reactivity to house dust mite extract was even stronger.

EFFECT ON THE ORAL ALLERGY SYNDROME

The initial report that immunotherapy to cross-reacting inhalant allergens could reduce the symptoms of the oral allergy syndrome[66] has been repeatedly confirmed, particularly with symptoms on ingestion of apples in patients allergic to birch pollen.[67,68]

COMPARISON WITH TOPICAL NASAL CORTICOSTEROIDS

A preseasonal course of immunotherapy was compared with topical nasal corticosteroids in 41 birch-allergic patients, all with rhinitis and half with asthma.[69] Symptoms of rhinoconjunctivitis were significantly lower in the group receiving nasal corticosteroids, but medication use did not differ. Seasonal peak expiratory flows decreased and bronchial sensitivity to methacholine increased only in the nasal steroid group.

THE PHARMACOECONOMICS OF IMMUNOTHERAPY

Two studies have used the State of Florida Medicaid database to examine the possible cost benefits of allergen immunotherapy in children with newly diagnosed allergic rhinitis. The first study examined the health care utilization for 6 months before initiation of immunotherapy and during the 6 months following its discontinuation.[70] Although less than half of the 520 children received as much as 1 year of immunotherapy, highly significant reductions were achieved in pharmacy claims, outpatient visits, and hospital admissions in comparison with the data for similar children not receiving immunotherapy. The total costs were reduced from $1,212 to $917 even when the cost of the immunotherapy was included. A follow-up study compared 2771 children with newly diagnosed allergic rhinitis who received immunotherapy and 11,010 with newly diagnosed allergic rhinitis not receiving immunotherapy.[71] The outcome was health care utilization for the 18 months after initiation of immunotherapy. In the immunotherapy group, total expenses were $3,247 including the cost of immunotherapy, as compared with $4,872 in the control group. Further studies of this type are needed for patients with private health insurance and with bronchial asthma.

Immunologic Response to Inhalant Immunotherapy

Box 87-1 summarizes the changes that characterize the immunologic response to inhalant immunotherapy, as discussed next.

BOX 87-1 THE IMMUNOLOGIC RESPONSE TO IMMUNOTHERAPY

END-ORGAN RESPONSE

Decreased Early and Late Responses to Specific Allergen

Conjunctiva[1,11]
Skin: early[72-75]; late[76]
Nose[72,77]
Bronchi: early[34,79]; late[78]

Decreased Nonspecific Reaction to Bronchial Challenge

Histamine[34]
Methacholine[79]

Decreased Tissue Inflammation

Eosinophils[80-83]
Metachromatic cells[82,84]

HUMERAL RESPONSE

IgE

Early rise in specific IgE[85,86]
Suppression of seasonal rise in specific IgE[85]
Late decline in specific IgE[85,86]

IgG

Increase in specific IgG[87]
Early predominantly IgG1[89]
Late predominantly IgG4[89]

CELLULAR RESPONSE

Basophils

Nonspecific loss of responsiveness[92]

Lymphocytes and Peripheral Blood Mononuclear Cells

Decreased serum IL-2R[94]
Decreased lymphocyte proliferation[95]
Generation of specific suppressor cells[96,97]
Regulatory T lymphocytes
Increased expression of Foxp3[99]
Secreting IL-10[98,100,101]
Secreting TGF-β[98]

Evidence of Immune Deviation

Decreased stimulated release of Th2 cytokines
IL-4[105]
IL-13[105]
Preferential deletion of Th2 T cells[104]
Increased stimulated release of Th1 cytokines
IFN-γ[106,107,122]
Increased stimulated mRNA for Th1 cytokines
IFN-γ[108]
IL-12[109]

Other Immunologic Changes

Decrease in FcεRII/CD23 and B cell activation markers[116-119]
Decreased costimulatory molecules[120]
Decreased release of cytokines
IL-2[103]
TNF[110]
Histamine-releasing factors[111-114]
Platelet-activating factor[115]

IFN, Interferon; *IgE, IgG,* immunoglobulins E and G; *IL,* interleukin; *IL-2R,* interleukin type 2 receptor; *mRNA,* messenger RNA; *TGF-β,* growth factor-β; *TNF,* tumor necrosis factor.

END-ORGAN CHANGES

Sensitivity

Conjunctival. In his 1911 report, Noon noted marked changes in the conjunctival allergen threshold and used these changes to guide dosing.[1] Conjunctival allergen challenge continues to be a useful measure of efficacy of immunotherapy.[11]

Cutaneous. Similar to the change in conjunctival reactivity, a rapid reduction in the immediate skin reaction occurs.[72] It has been reported within a few weeks with cluster immunotherapy.[73-75] In addition to the reduction in the immediate cutaneous reaction, an even greater reduction in the late cutaneous reaction that develops 3 to 12 hours after injection of allergen.[76]

Mucosal. Reduction in the sensitivity to grass pollen on nasal challenge was demonstrated in patients treated with grass immunotherapy by a rush protocol followed by weekly maintenance injections.[72] Specific immunotherapy in ragweed-sensitive patients blocked the increase in nasal sensitivity to allergen challenge that occurred in the untreated patients during the ragweed pollen season—the so-called priming effect.[77] A year of conventional immunotherapy with house dust mite extract has been shown to significantly reduce the late bronchial response after inhalation challenge with house dust mite extract.[78] Immunotherapy with both cat dander[34] and house dust mite extract[79] for 3 years reduced both the specific and nonspecific (e.g., histamine and methacholine, respectively) sensitivity to bronchial challenge.

Inflammation

Eosinophils and metachromatic cells (basophils and mast cells) are the principal effector cells of the allergic response. The increased levels of eosinophils seen during natural allergen exposure have been shown to be reduced by allergen immunotherapy[80-84] as measured in nasal secretions,[80] bronchoalveolar lavage fluids,[81] and nasal mucosa.[82] Blocking of the seasonal increase in nasal basophils[82] and c-Kit$^+$ mast cells[84] also has been observed.

HUMERAL CHANGES

Immunoglobulin E

Immunotherapy produces initially an increase in specific IgE antibodies; however, the normal seasonal rise in specific IgE is blunted, whereas the postseasonal decline is unaffected.[85] These changes result in a progressive decline in specific IgE in the treatment group in comparison with the levels in the control population.[86]

Immunoglobulin G

In 1935 Cooke and associates reported that ragweed immunotherapy resulted in generation of an antibody that, when mixed with serum from a ragweed-allergic donor, would inhibit the immediate reaction to ragweed at a passive transfer site.[87] Levels of this antibody generally were not found to correlate with clinical improvement, however.[88]

With use of modern laboratory methods, it has been demonstrated that the allergen-specific IgG response is restricted with regard to subclass.[89] Immunotherapy results in a prompt rise in allergen-specific antibodies in the IgG1 and IgG4 but not the IgG2 and IgG3 subclasses. No correlation was found between preseasonal levels of either subclass of antibody and symptoms scores during the season.[89] A modest negative correlation has been found between clinical improvement with immunotherapy and two functional assays of IgG4 that measure competition between IgG4 and IgE antibodies for binding to the specific allergen.[90] Two years after immunotherapy was discontinued, the functional IgG antibody activity and clinical improvement persisted, whereas IgG1 and IgG4 antibody levels had fallen sharply.[91] These studies suggest that IgG antibodies may play some role in the clinical response to immunotherapy.

CELLULAR CHANGES

Basophils

Decreased sensitivity of basophils to release histamine in vitro on exposure to ragweed was reported in a group of children undergoing clinically effective ragweed immunotherapy in a double-blind, placebo-controlled study.[92] Subsequently, however, it was demonstrated that the decreased cell reactivity also occurred to a non–cross-reacting allergen.[93]

Lymphocytes and Peripheral Blood Mononuclear Cells

Suppressor Cells. Immunotherapy reduced serum interleukin-2 (IL-2) receptors[94] and diminished the proliferative response of peripheral blood lymphocytes to ragweed Amb a I.[95] The reduction in proliferation was allergen-specific. The observation of reduced proliferative response led to a search for allergen-specific suppressor cells induced by allergen immunotherapy.[96,97] It was demonstrated that immunotherapy generated allergen-specific cells that would suppress allergen-induced lymphocyte proliferative response[96] and the production of ragweed-specific IgE.

Regulatory T Cells. Evidence has been forthcoming that the normal immune system includes a population of professional regulatory T cells that inhibit the activation of conventional T cells in the periphery. These regulatory T cells can prevent the development of autoimmunity, as well as allergy.[98] Although the number of these $CD4^{+}CD25^{high}$ regulatory T cells was found to be increased in children with allergic asthma, their Foxp3 expression and suppressor activity were reduced.[99] By contrast, patients with allergic asthma on immunotherapy had normal Foxp3 expression and suppressor activity. In vitro, the reduced Foxp3 expression and suppressor activity could be induced by tumor necrosis factor-α (TNF-α) and restored to normal by an anti–TNF-α agent.[99]

The normal immune reaction to inhalant allergens was found to be characterized by suppressed lymphocyte proliferation, suppressed Th1 and Th2 responses to allergen stimulation and increased IL-10 and transforming growth factor-β (TGF-β) secretion by allergen-specific T cells.[98] In vitro suppression of IL-10 and TGF-β in lymphocyte cultures from healthy people resulted in increased lymphocyte proliferation to the allergen.[98] Patients who received immunotherapy to house dust mites developed increased production of IL-10 and TGF-β in allergen-stimulated cultures, along with suppression of the allergen-specific lymphocyte proliferation and decreased production of interferon-γ (IFN-γ), IL-5, and IL-13, which could be reversed in vitro by neutralization of IL-10 and TGF-β.[98] The production of IL-10 and TGF-β was found to be associated with a subset of $CD4^{+}CD25^{+}$ T lymphocytes. IL-10 is a general inhibitor of proliferative and cytokine responses in T cells. It inhibits IgE and enhances IgG4 production. TGF-β, on the other hand, induces an immunoglobulin isotype switch to IgA. The induction of $IL\text{-}10^{+}CD4^{+}CD25^{+}$ T cells by immunotherapy was confirmed in other studies[100,101]—a finding consistent with the induction of a regulatory T cell population by specific immunotherapy. Somewhat contradictory was the observation, after a year of sublingual immunotherapy with birch pollen extract, that the clearest increase in IL-10 mRNA expression in stimulated peripheral blood mononuclear cells (PBMCs) was in patients who did not benefit clinically from immunotherapy, whereas the least increase was found in those with the greatest reduction of symptoms.[102] When samples were examined that had been obtained from the patients at the time of first reaching maintenance levels of immunotherapy, however, the peak expression of allergen-induced IL-10 mRNA was associated with the most favorable outcome of immunotherapy. These results suggest that an early and transient increase in allergen-specific IL-10 expression in PBMCs is associated with the best therapeutic outcome.[102]

Immune Deviation. Two types of $CD4^{+}$ helper T lymphocytes have been described: Th2, preferentially secreting IL-4, and Th1, preferentially secreting IFN-γ in response to allergen stimulation.[103] Allergic and nonallergic individuals were found to have similar low levels of antigen-specific Th1 and type 1 T regulatory (Tr1) cells in their peripheral circulation, but the allergic subjects had increased numbers of allergen-specific Th2 cells.[104] With initiation of immunotherapy, a steady decrease in the Th2/Th1 and Th2/Tr1 ratios occurred with depletion of the allergen-specific Th2 cells, perhaps as a consequence of induced apoptosis of these cells, decreased release of IL-4 and IL-13 from allergen-stimulated peripheral blood lymphocytes,[105] or increased numbers of circulating $CD4^{+}$ T lymphocytes producing IFN-γ[106] or the IFN-γ/IL-4 ratio.[107]

After 1 year of immunotherapy with grass pollen extract or placebo, patients underwent nasal challenge with grass pollen extract, followed by nasal biopsy 24 hours later.[108] Subjects treated with specific immunotherapy had significantly fewer infiltrating $CD4^{+}$ T lymphocytes and total and activated eosinophils, and a significant increase was observed at 24 hours in cells expressing mRNA for IFN-γ in the treated patients.

Ten subjects from this same grass immunotherapy protocol were studied again after 4 years of treatment.[109] Skin biopsy specimens were obtained 24 hours after intradermal allergen injection. An increase in the number of cells with mRNA for IL-12 was noted. The number of $IL\text{-}12^{+}$ cells correlated positively with the number of cells with mRNA for IFN-γ and correlated negatively with those with mRNA for IL-4. Because IL-12 promotes Th1 and suppresses Th2 lymphocyte proliferation, the finding of increased IL-12–secreting cells would be consistent with a shift from an allergen-specific Th2 toward an allergen-specific Th1 response occurring as a result of immunotherapy.

Stimulated Release of Cytokines. Adherent monocytes from allergic asthmatic children released significantly increased amounts of IL-1 and TNF on stimulation with house dust mite allergen.[110] After 1 year of house dust mite immunotherapy, stimulated production of both cytokines was reduced, but the difference was significant only for TNF.

Spontaneous in vitro release of histamine was measured before and after 4 months of immunotherapy with a variety of allergen extracts.[111] Immunotherapy resulted in a significant reduction in spontaneous histamine release in the study cohort as a whole. Elevated levels of both spontaneous and allergen-induced histamine-releasing factor (HRF) have been demonstrated in subjects with ragweed-[112] and grass-allergic[113] rhinitis. Levels of both forms of HRF rose with pollen exposure in the placebo-treated patients but not in those receiving specific immunotherapy. Untreated asthmatic children allergic to house dust mites demonstrated increased levels of spontaneous and allergen-induced release of HRF; this was reduced in children who experienced clinical improvement with treatment with house dust mite extract.[114]

Plasma platelet-activating factor (PAF) levels were higher in asthmatic children who had not received or had responded poorly to specific immunotherapy but were reduced in good responders.[115]

Low-Affinity Immunoglobulin E Receptor (FcεRII) on B Lymphocytes. Expression of the low-affinity IgE receptor (FcεRII/CD23) is regulated by the Th2 cytokine IL-4. In two studies, house dust mite–sensitive asthmatic children were shown to have a significantly increased percentage of B lymphocytes expressing the low-affinity receptor for IgE over that in healthy children.[116,117] Immunotherapy with house dust mite extract resulted in a significant reduction in the percentage of B lymphocytes expressing FcεRII/CD23 in both studies. Furthermore, reduction in the severity of allergic symptoms and medication requirement during the following grass pollen season correlated closely with immunotherapy induced reduction in the proportion of FcεRII/CD23$^+$ B lymphocytes.[118] Grass immunotherapy also blocked the seasonal increase in B cell activation antigens (CD23, CD40, and human leukocyte antigen [HLA]-DR) observed during the pollen season in placebo-treated subjects.[119]

Costimulatory Molecules. Biopsy specimens of tissue involved in the late phase cutaneous reaction were obtained after 1 year of immunotherapy with birch pollen extract or placebo.[120] The magnitude of the late phase reactions was reduced in subjects receiving active immunotherapy relative to those in the placebo group. The active treatment group also had fewer T cells, macrophages, and cells expressing the costimulatory molecules CD80 and CD86 infiltrating the site. The investigators suggested that decreased costimulation might lead to diminished immune response after allergen exposure.

Antigen-Presenting Cells. Plasmacytoid dendritic cells (pDCs) express IgE receptors (e.g., FcεRI) for capturing allergen and inducing a Th2 response as well as expression of a Toll-like receptor (TLR) that responds to ligands derived from bacteria by producing IFN-α and IL-12, which promote a Th1 response.[121] Human blood pDCs from allergic individuals have been found to have impaired IFN-α production after TLR9 stimulation.[122] On reaching maintenance doses of subcutaneous immunotherapy, a fivefold increase in cytosine-phosphate-guanine DNA motif (CpG)-stimulated IFN-α from isolated pDCs occurred that was not accounted for by increased frequency of pDCs or expression of TLR9, suggesting that immunotherapy had restored dendritic cell TLR9-mediated innate immune function to normal levels.[122]

OVERVIEW OF THE IMMUNE RESPONSE TO IMMUNOTHERAPY

The immunologic responses to subcutaneous immunotherapy appear to be contradictory: In some studies, regulatory T cells are induced that suppress both Th1 and Th2 cytokine responses to specific allergen stimulation,[98,100-102] whereas other studies report an immune deviation from a Th2 to a Th1 response such that allergen stimulation of T cells results in increased synthesis of IL-12 and IFN-γ and decreased synthesis of IL-4.[106-109] It appears that the regulatory T cell response occurs very early in the course of subcutaneous immunotherapy.[100,102] Additional evidence points to waning of the regulatory T cell response with continued immunotherapy.[100,102] On the other hand, the clearest demonstration of immune deviation was in patients who had received high-dose subcutaneous immunotherapy for 3 to 4 years.[109] A prospective study of the immunologic response to sublingual immunotherapy (SLIT) supported the concept of the regulatory T cell response dominating early and the immune deviation from Th2 to Th1 dominating late in the course of immunotherapy.[123] After 4 weeks of SLIT, there were increased numbers of CD4$^+$CD25$^+$ T cells with increased Foxp3 and IL-10 and decreased IL-4 and IFN-γ mRNA expression. After 52 weeks of SLIT, by contrast, increased IFN-γ mRNA expression and reduced IL-4, IL-10, and Foxp3 mRNA expression were detected. A 3-year subcutaneous immunotherapy study demonstrated progressive decline in the number of allergen-specific Th2 cells with little change in the number of allergen-specific Th1 and Tr1 cells.[104]

CORRELATIONS WITH CLINICAL OUTCOME

Sensitivity to the allergen on titrated skin prick testing,[72,124] titrated conjunctival challenge,[124] and titrated nasal challenge[72] after immunotherapy has been shown to correlate with symptoms of rhinitis occurred during natural pollen exposure. Of note, an inverse correlation was reported between the number of cells positive for mRNA for IFN-γ in nasal biopsies 24 hours after nasal allergen challenge[108] and symptom and medication scores during the grass pollen season.

Practical Considerations in Allergen Immunotherapy

PATIENT SELECTION

Unlike with severe anaphylaxis to *Hymenoptera* envenomation, no absolute indications for specific immunotherapy with inhalant allergens are recognized. Even among allergy societies the recommended indications differ significantly. The AIPP directive[51] states that aeroallergen immunotherapy should be considered for patients who have symptoms of allergic rhinitis, rhinoconjunctivitis, or asthma after natural exposure to allergens and who demonstrate specific IgE antibodies to relevant allergens. Further considerations are the severity and duration of symptoms, medication requirements, and patient preference. The patient's asthma must be clinically stable before allergen immunotherapy is administered.[51] Guidelines jointly published by the GA²LEN and the EAACI gave similar indications for immunotherapy but in addition specified the availability of a standardized, high-quality allergen extract of the specific allergen intended to be used for immunotherapy.[49] Patients with mild allergic asthma are considered to be suitable candidates for immunotherapy provided that their asthma is under control and their forced expiratory volume at 1 minute (FEV_1) is greater than 70% of predicted.[49]

Appreciation of the disease-modifying action of immunotherapy in blocking the development of new sensitivities in monosensitized persons and in preventing asthma in children who have allergic rhinitis only has led to reexamination of the age at which immunotherapy can be initiated in children.[125] Favoring early institution of allergen immunotherapy is that it appears to be most effective against asthma in children and young adults.[126] Furthermore, the younger the patient, the greater the potential advantage of a treatment that may be stopped after 3 to 5 years with persisting benefit,[62,63,65] as opposed to pharmacotherapy, which must be continued indefinitely to maintain symptom relief. Whereas the GA²LEN/EAACI guide still states that "immunotherapy should in general not be offered to patients below the age of 5,"[49] the AIPP specifies that "immunotherapy can be initiated in young children less than 5 years of age if indicated" and notes that "indications are similar to those of other age groups."[51] The AIPP does caution, however, that "allergen immunotherapy for inhalant allergens is usually not considered in infants and toddlers because (1) there might be difficulty in communicating with the child regarding systemic reactions and (2) injections can be traumatic to very young children."[51]

WHO SHOULD WRITE A PRESCRIPTION FOR ALLERGEN IMMUNOTHERAPY?

In view of the complexity of the decision-making process as to whether allergen immunotherapy is indicated, along with the depth of knowledge required to formulate a proper allergen extract for treatment, it is clear that this should be undertaken only by a physician with special training in the field. The AIPP states that the physician should be trained and experienced in prescribing and administering immunotherapy.[51] The practice of some laboratories of performing in vitro testing and then recommending allergen immunotherapy on the basis of the results of the tests plus a questionnaire completed by the patient—the so-called remote practice of allergy—has been shown to result in unnecessary and inappropriate immunotherapy.[127]

FORMULATION OF AN ALLERGEN EXTRACT FOR SPECIFIC IMMUNOTHERAPY

Considerations in writing an allergy extract prescription are (1) which allergen extracts to include, on the basis of the patient's history and sensitivities, possible cross-allergenicities among the allergens, and compatibility of the extracts on mixing, and (2) how much of each allergen extract to include, based on doses that have been proved to be clinically effective and the potency of the allergen extracts available.

Patterns of Cross-allergenicity

If it is accepted that each allergen group should be present in the treatment extract in roughly similar amounts, then botanical cross-reactivity must be considered either in selecting the extracts to be included in the skin test panel or in formulating the treatment extract, or both. The general patterns of botanical cross-allergenicity are as follows: (1) there is rarely significant cross-allergenicity between families; (2) there is generally some degree of cross-allergenicity between tribes or genera of families; and (3) there is generally a high degree of cross-allergenicity between species of the same genus (see example in Box 87-2). Clinically significant cross-reactivity among the members of the same family is exemplified in the trees by the strong cross-allergenicity among members of the conifer family (cedar, cypress, juniper, arbor vitae).[128] Examples of species with strong cross-allergenicity within a genus, not suggested by the common names, are pecan and hickory in the genus *Carya* and poplar, cottonwood, and aspen in the genus *Populus.* Among the grasses, members of the Festucoideae, represented by the Northern pasture grasses, strongly cross-react but are allergenically unique and distinct from those of the Eragrostoideae represented primarily by Bermuda grass.[129] Pancoideae grasses, represented by Bahia and Johnson grasses, if locally important should be used for diagnosis and treatment.[130] Among the weeds, locally important varieties should be used for testing and treatment in the *Artemesia, Ambrosia,* and *Amaranthus* families, but the major Chenopodioideae species, Russian thistle and kochia, differ in antigenicity, and use of a mixture, rather than either alone, is most appropriate.[131,132]

Mixing Allergen Extracts

Fungal and some insect extracts have been shown to contain proteases that are capable of degrading the proteins in other extracts with which they may be mixed.[133] Many fungal extracts, as well as cockroach extracts, have been shown in mixture to cause loss of allergenic potency of a number of pollen, house dust mite, and dander extracts.[134-136] House dust mite extract

BOX 87-2 PATTERNS OF BOTANICAL CROSS-ALLERGENICITY

- There is rarely significant cross-allergenicity between families.
- There is generally some degree of cross-allergenicity between tribes or genera of a family, but this is variable.
- There is generally a high degree of cross-allergenicity between species of the same genus.

	Family	Genus	Species
Designation	Chenopodioideae	*Kochia scoparia* *Salsola pestifer*	
	Asteraceae		*Ambrosia artemisiifolia* *Ambrosia trifida*
Cross-reactivity	None	Partial	Marked

TABLE 87-1 Effective Maintenance Doses for Allergen Immunotherapy

Allergen	Reference(s)	Effective Dose	Less Effective or Ineffective
Short ragweed	Van Metre et al[143]	11 μg Amb a 1	
	Creticos et al[142]	12.4 μg Amb a 1	0.6 μg Amb a 1
	Creticos et al[141]	6.0 μg Amb a 1	
	Furin et al[80]	24.0 μg Amb a 1	2.0 μg Amb a 1
	Majchel[140]	24.0 μg Amb a 1	2.0 μg Amb a 1
Dermatophagoides	Haugaard et al[144]	7.0 μg Der p 1	0.7 μg Der p 1
	Olsen et al[12]	7.0 μg Der p 1 10.0 μg Der f 1	
Cat dander	Alvarez-Cuesta et al[33]	11.3 μg Fel d 1	
	Hedlin et al[34]	17.3 μg Fel d 1	
	Varney et al[11]	15.0 μg Fel d 1	
	Ewbank et al[73]	15.0 μg Fel d 1	3.0 μg Fel d 1
	Nanda[74]	15.0 μg Fel d 1	3.0 μg Fel d 1
Dog dander	Lent et al[75]	15.0 μg Can f 1	3.0 μg Can d 1
Grass	Varney et al[7]	18.6 μg Phl p 5	
	Walker et al[10]	20.0 μg Phl p 5	
	Dolz et al[168]	15.0 μg Dac q 5 and Lol p 5	
	Frew et al[145]	20.0 μg Phl p 5	2.0 μg Phl p 5

did not appear to cause degradation of these pollen extracts, consistent with the low protease content of U.S. mite extracts, which are made from mite bodies. Perhaps the best general rule for formulating extracts for immunotherapy is not to mix cockroach or any fungal extract with pollen, mite, or dander extracts.

Adequate Allergen Doses for Effective Immunotherapy

Many studies have addressed the issue of effective doses for allergen immunotherapy (Table 87-1). By general agreement, very-low-dose immunotherapy is not effective, and high doses are more effective than moderate doses. Quantifying these terms, however, is frustrated by the lack of widely accepted and meaningful measurements of potency.

Johnstone with coinvestigators Crump[53] and Dutton[137] placed 210 children with perennial asthma consecutively referred to a pediatric allergy clinic into one of four immunotherapy treatment groups. Children received either placebo injections or all of the inhalable allergens to which they exhibited positive results on skin testing but at a maximum concentration for each allergen of 1:10,000,000 w/v, 1:5,000 w/v, or 1:250 w/v. The outcome was assessed after 4 years of treatment ($n = 173$) and at the end of treatment on their reaching age 16 ($n = 130$), during which time they, their parents, and the evaluating physicians were unaware of the treatment group to which they had been randomized. Results did not differ between children receiving placebo and those receiving the lowest allergen dose (10^{-7}). After 4 years, 18% of children in the placebo and lowest dose groups, 58% of those in the 1:5000 w/v group, and 81% of those in the 1:250 w/v group were free of asthma.[53] When the children reached the age of 16 years, the results were placebo and lowest dose, 22%; 1:5000 w/v, 66%; and 1:250 w/v, 78% free of asthma.[137]

A study by Franklin and Lowell[6] confirmed the differences reported between high and intermediate doses of allergen reported by Johnstone. Twenty-five ragweed-sensitive subjects were paired by severity of symptoms. One in each group continued to receive the highest tolerated dose of ragweed extract (median dose, 0.3 mL of a 1:50 w/v concentration), whereas the other received a twentyfold lower concentration (median dose, 0.3 mL of 1:1000 w/v). During the ensuing ragweed pollen season, those in the group receiving the higher dose reported significantly fewer symptoms.

Standardized Extracts. Allergen extracts can be meaningfully standardized either for their total allergenic reactivity or for their content of one or more major allergens. In the United States, under the direction of the Center for Biologics Evaluation and Research of the Food and Drug Administration (FDA), both methods are used: total allergenic activity measured by titrated intradermal skin testing for grasses and house dust mites and major allergen content for short ragweed and cat dander. In Europe, each extract manufacturer sets its own internal standards, generally based on skin test reactivity and reported in the company's unique units.[138] Because these measures of potency are not interchangeable, the trend has been to express immunotherapy dosing in terms of the major allergen content of the maintenance dose.[139]

Ragweed. Studies at Johns Hopkins University examined the dose response in ragweed immunotherapy during natural ragweed exposure. Immunotherapy with maintenance doses of 2 μg of Amb a 1 was less effective than that using higher doses[80] and in one study provided no more symptom relief than placebo.[140] Consistent efficacy was observed with doses containing 6.0, 11, and 12.4 μg of Amb a 1,[141-143] suggesting that a maintenance dose containing 12 μg of Amb a 1 should be sufficient.

The total ineffectiveness of low-dose allergen immunotherapy was confirmed in a double-blind comparison of ragweed immunotherapy using the current standard method (with a median maintenance dose of 11 μg of Amb a 1), the so-called Rinkel method (with a median dose of 0.001 μg of Amb a 1), and placebo injections.[143] Rhinitis symptoms during the ragweed season were significantly decreased in the standard therapy group, but no difference was found between the groups receiving Rinkel therapy and placebo.

House Dust Mites. The dose response to a standardized extract of *Dermatophagoides pteronyssinus* was assessed by bronchial allergen challenge for efficacy and rate of systemic reactions for safety in 55 patients treated for 2 years.[144] The targeted maintenance doses contained 0.7 μg of Der p 1, 7 μg of Der p 1, and 21 μg of Der p 1. After 24 months, no significant change was observed in bronchial responsiveness to the mite extract in the placebo group, whereas the median provocative inhaled dose of mite extract for the three treatment groups increased by 0.9 doubling dilutions, 7.9 doubling dilutions, and 3.2 doubling dilutions, respectively. The systemic reaction rates in the three groups were 0.56%, 3.30%, and 7.10%, respectively. On the basis of risk versus benefit, it was suggested that a maintenance dose of 7.0 μg Der p 1 was appropriate for the typical house dust mite–sensitive patient with asthma. The effectiveness of this dose was confirmed in a 1-year, double-blind study in 23 adults with perennial asthma caused by house dust mite sensitivity. These patients received maintenance doses of 7.0 μg of Der p 1 or placebo, or 10.0 μg of Der f 1 or placebo.[12] Active treatment significantly reduced asthma symptoms and medication use and improved pulmonary function, whereas no significant changes were observed with placebo.

Domestic Pet Allergen. Specific content of Fel d 1 was known for two studies in which immunotherapy with a standardized cat allergen extract was effective in double-blind, placebo-controlled trials.[11,33] In a 1-year study, maintenance injections containing 13.2 μg of Fel d 1 resulted in patient-reported improvement in 81.3%, versus only 20.7% with placebo.[33] In the other study, 28 cat-sensitive adult patients received 3 months of maintenance injections with either a dose of cat extract containing 15 μg of Fel d 1 or placebo.[11] Efficacy was assessed by means of exposure for 7 hours in a home with three cats. Pretreatment and post treatment symptom scores were 61.6 and 17.1, for a significant reduction, in the active treatment group, versus 64.7 and 62.1 in the placebo group. Three years of treatment with a maintenance dose of cat extract containing 17.3 μg of Fel d 1 resulted in reduced bronchial sensitivity to both cat dander extract and histamine.[34]

Two studies of similar design have assessed the dose response to immunotherapy with cat hair and dander extract.[73,74] In each study, subjects were brought to maintenance in 4 weeks with use of a cluster schedule. Maintenance doses were expressed in the Fel d 1 content and consisted of placebo, 0.6 μg, 3.0 μg, and 15.0 μg. In the first study, outcome was assessed at 5 weeks, shortly after reaching maintenance.[73] In the second study, assessments were made at 5 weeks and again after 1 year of maintenance treatment.[74] Responses with doses containing 0.6 μg of Fel d 1 did not differ from those with placebo. Doses containing 3.0 μg produced suppression of skin prick test reactivity and rise in cat-specific IgG_4, but other responses, such as reduction in symptoms on nasal allergen challenge or decrease in $CD4^+$/$IL\text{-}4^+$ PBMCs, were observed only with the dose containing 15 μg of Fel d 1. A similar study was conducted with dog dander extract (AP Dog, Hollister-Stier Laboratories, Spokane, Washington).[75] Subjects received either placebo or dog dander extract that at maintenance contained 0.6 μg, 3.0 μg, or 15 μg of Can f 1. Again, maintenance dosing was achieved in 4 weeks with use of a cluster schedule, and assessment of the results of treatment was made after 5 weeks. Results were very similar to those with cat extract, with the lowest dose not differing from placebo, the middle dose inducing changes in skin prick tests and IgG_4 antibody, but the highest dose producing a broader pattern of immunologic changes.

Grass. Two studies with timothy grass extracts containing 18.6 μg of Phl p 5[7] or 20 μg of Phl p 5[10] resulted in dramatic reduction in symptoms and medication requirements for control of allergic rhinitis[7,10] and bronchial asthma.[10] A study comparing a dose of timothy grass extract containing 20 μg of Phl p 5 and one containing 2 μg with placebo was conducted in patients with grass-induced allergic rhinoconjunctivitis not adequately controlled by symptomatic treatment.[145] In comparison with placebo, the higher dose resulted in reduction in symptoms by 29% and medication by 32%; the reductions with the lower dose were 22% and 16%, respectively.

Birch. Effective treatment of allergic rhinitis and asthma caused by birch pollen has been reported with maintenance doses of birch pollen extract containing 3.28 μg,[146] 12 μg,[147] and 15 μg[148] of the major allergen Bet v 1 administered subcutaneously. Although comparison across studies is difficult, the results in these three studies do not establish a clear dose response over the range studied.

Nonstandardized Extracts. Nonstandardized extracts are seldom studied to establish effective doses, because they are variable in potency from manufacturer to manufacturer and from lot to lot for a single manufacturer. Nevertheless, representative extracts have been analyzed for their major allergen content, with the finding that the pollen extracts generally are similar in potency to the standardized grasses and short ragweed (2011 personal communication, G. Plunkett, PhD, ALK-Abello, Inc., Round Rock, Texas). On the other hand, the major allergen content of cockroach extracts[45,46] and fungal extracts[39,149] tends to be very variable and generally is quite low.

WRITING AN ALLERGEN EXTRACT PRESCRIPTION

The method of standardization that is used in the United States (bioequivalent allergen units and major allergen content in FDA units) does not allow direct use of information on dosing by major allergen content. However, representative lots of standardized extracts have been assessed for their major allergen content (Table 87-2). Although this information allows an approximation of proven doses, the range of major allergen content for extracts labeled with the same U.S. standardized potency is quite broad. Nevertheless, on the basis of the information available, the AIPP has recommended probable effective dose ranges for the standardized allergen extracts.[51] The AIPP also recommends dosing for unstandardized pollens with 0.5 mL of a 1:100 w/v or 1:200 w/v dose and cockroach and fungal extracts with the highest tolerated dose, on the basis of available data.[51]

Table 87-3 shows a representative allergen extract prescription written for doses of each allergen at maintenance that are in the range at which good clinical results have been reported (see Table 87-1). If more than one Northern pasture grass[129,150] or more than one ragweed[132] had been included, allowance would have been needed for cross-allergenicity by reducing the amount of each individual allergen extract. The relative weakness of the standardized cat extract is obvious by the large volume required to achieve the targeted dose.

TABLE 87-2 Representative Major Allergen Content of U.S. Standardized Extracts*

Allergen Extract	Expressed Potency	Major Allergen	Mean Content of Major Allergen	Minimum Content of Major Allergen	Maximum Content of Major Allergen
Kentucky blue grass	100,000 BAU/mL	Poa p 5	270 μg/mL	190 μg/mL	330 μg/mL
Timothy grass	100,000 BAU/mL	Phl p 5	600 μg/mL	260 μg/mL	865 μg/mL
Bermuda grass	10,000 BAU/mL	Cyn d 1	185 μg/mL	20 μg/mL	427 μg/mL
Short ragweed	1:10 w/v	Amb a 1	525 μg/mL	335 μg/mL	763 μg/mL
Dermatophagoides pteronyssinus	10,000 AU/mL	Der p1	62 μg/mL	38 μg/mL	98 μg/mL
D. pteronyssinus	10,000 AU/mL	Der p 2	63 μg/mL	28 μg/mL	104 μg/mL
D. farinae	10,000 AU/mL	Der f 1	73 μg/mL	21 μg/mL	140 μg/mL
D. farinae	10,000 AU/mL	Der f 2	85 μg/mL	51 μg/mL	140 μg/mL
Cat hair/epithelium	10,000 BAU/mL	Fel d 1	40 μg/mL	24 μg/mL	79 μg/mL
Birch	1:10 w/v	Bet v 1	415 μg/mL	234 μg/mL	688 μg/mL
Dog hair	1:10 w/v	Can f 1	5.4 μg/mL	0.5 μg/mL	7.2 μg/mL
AP Dog[†]	1:100 w/v	Can f 1	140 μg/mL	90 μg/mL	225 μg/mL

*Major allergen content of multiple lots of extracts manufactured between 2001 and 2011 by a single manufacturer. Data provided by G. Plunkett, PhD, ALK-Abello Inc., Round Rock, Texas.
[†]Acetone-precipitated dog dander. Available from Hollister-Stier Laboratories, Spokane, Wash.

TABLE 87-3 Allergen Immunotherapy Prescription Form

Allergen Extract	Target Dose of Major Allergen	Amount of Major Allergen Required in 10 mL*	Mean Concentration of Major Allergen in 1 mL of Stock Extract	Amount of Stock Extract to Be Added to 10-mL Vial
Short ragweed	12.0 μg Amb a 1	240 μg	525 μg/mL of 1:10 w/v	0.5 mL 1:10 w/v
Timothy grass	20 μg Phl p 5	400 μg	600 μg/mL of 100,000 BAU	0.7 mL 100,000 BAU/mL
Dermatophagoides pteronyssinus	7.0 μg Der p 1	140 μg	62 μg/mL of 10,000 AU	2.3 mL 10,000 AU/mL
Cat hair and dander	15 μg Fel d 1	300 μg	40 μg/mL of 10,000 AU	7.5 mL 10,000 AU/mL (reduced to 6.5 mL due to excess volume)
Diluent (0.03% HSA)				0 mL

An example of an allergen prescription for a 10-mL maintenance vial using amounts of extracts that will provide proven effective doses of the major allergens when 0.5 mL is given as a maintenance dose. Calculations are based on values given in Table 87-2 and Figure 87-2. In this example, the total extract added comes to 11 mL. Therefore, the amount of cat extract added should be reduced to 6.5 mL, because it is the weakest of the extracts.
HSA, Human serum albumin.
*Presuming maintenance injection of 0.05 mL.

Labeling the Treatment Vials

It is critical that the vials containing the allergen extract for treatment be clearly and completely labeled (Figure 87-2). The AIPP specifies what should appear in the label on the vial.[51] To ensure that injections are given from the correct treatment set, the label should contain the patient's name and some other identifying information such as registration number or birth date. To ensure that the correct vial from the treatment set is used, the vial number and dilution should be on the label, and consistent use of the following scheme for color-coding the caps is recommended: red, 1:1, most concentrated; yellow, 1:10 dilution of most concentrated; blue, 1:100 dilution; green, 1:1,000 dilution; and silver, 1:10,000 dilution. Additionally, the label should list the specific allergens contained in the mixture and the expiration date of the contents. The latter two requirements are particularly important when the vials are administered in another physician's office.

STORING AND HANDLING ALLERGEN EXTRACTS

Once an allergen extract has been prepared for administration, its components are subject to loss of potency, particularly when in more dilute concentrations.[151] This loss of potency can be retarded by the addition of preservatives such as 0.03% human serum albumin or glycerin in concentrations of 10% to 50%.[151] Fifty percent glycerin is by far the best preservative, but its use is limited by the pain that accompanies its injection.[152] Half of a group of volunteers reported definitely annoying discomfort with injection of 0.05 mL total dose of glycerin and 13% reported intolerable discomfort with injection of 0.20 mL total dose. The loss of potency is greatly accelerated by higher temperatures.[151] Accordingly, allergen extracts should be kept at refrigerator temperature at all times, except when actually in use. The accelerated loss of potency at high ambient temperatures does not, however, preclude shipping extracts without

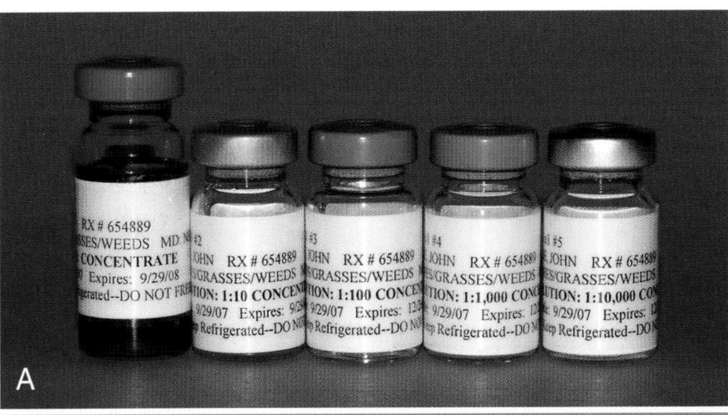

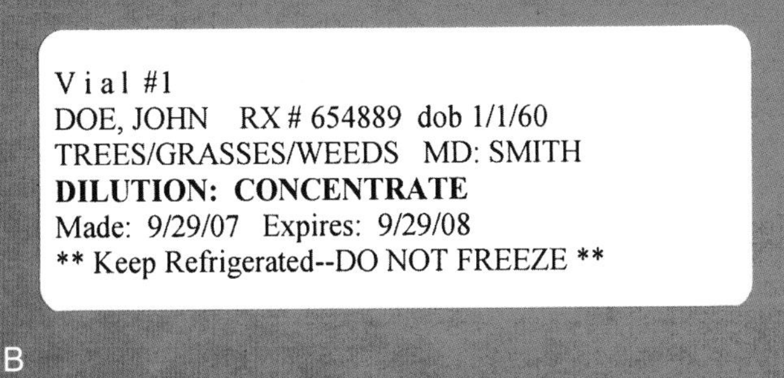

Figure 87-2 Labeling treatment vials. **A,** A treatment set with vials color-coded according to the recommendations of the *Allergen Immunotherapy: A Practice Parameter Third Update.*[144] The vials are capped from red (the most concentrated) through progressive tenfold dilutions marked yellow, blue, green, and silver, respectively. **B,** A representative treatment set label with all of the information recommended by the immunotherapy practice parameter third update.

refrigeration. Timothy grass extracts at concentrations of 10,000 BAU/mL and 100,000 BAU/mL were mailed round trip between San Antonio and Phoenix in August.[153] Temperatures were recorded at higher than 20° C (68° F) for 11 days and higher than 30° C (86° F) for 6 hours. Although some loss in potency of the 10,000 BAU/mL extract occurred under these conditions, the potency remained within the FDA release limits.

INJECTION SCHEDULES

The initial buildup to maintenance is conventionally achieved by twice-weekly to every other weekly injections of allergen extract.[154] Alternative schedules such as cluster[73-75,155] and rush[156,157] protocols also have been used. Box 87-3 presents a representative schedule for the conventional buildup phase of allergen immunotherapy; Box 87-4 provides a cluster dosing schedule. Clinical experience indicates that the 1 : 1,000 v/v dilution of the maintenance vial generally is a safe starting concentration.[158]

Once patients reach maintenance doses of their immunotherapy extract, it is customary to give the maintenance injections at less frequent intervals, typically decreasing over time to once-monthly injections.[51]

Rush Protocols

Clinical interest in rush protocols continues, because they greatly shorten the time required to reach maintenance.[156,157] These protocols have reduced the number of injections to 8 over a period of 3 days,[157] and even to 8 injections in a single day, in an approach termed "ultrarush."[159] Both protocols have resulted in systemic reactions in a large percentage of the asthmatic patients receiving such treatment. The incidence of systemic reactions was reduced from 73% to 27% by premedication with a combination of medications including antihistamines and oral corticosteroids[156] and from 36% to 7% by similar premedication plus exclusion from treatment any patients with reduced pulmonary function or termination of treatment after the occurrence of very large local reactions.[160] With rush protocols, patients have tolerated being placed directly on weekly maintenance injections without a high incidence of systemic reactions.

BOX 87-3 EXAMPLE OF A CONVENTIONAL ALLERGEN EXTRACT TREATMENT SCHEDULE

The following schedule should be used, with modification if necessary as outlined in the accompanying instructions.

INSTRUCTIONS FOR THE INJECTION OF ALLERGENIC EXTRACTS

Begin with vial #**4** and progress to vial #1, which is the most concentrated or "maintenance" solution. The injections should be given every **week.** Once maintenance is reached, the injection should be given every **3 to 4** weeks, with the following exceptions: **give weekly for first month and every 2 weeks for the second month.**

SCHEDULE

Vial #5	Vial #4	Vial #3	Vial #2	Vial #1
0.05 mL	0.05 mL	0.05 mL	0.05 mL	0.05 mL
0.10 mL	0.10 mL	0.10 mL	0.07 mL	0.07 mL
0.20 mL	0.20 mL	0.20 mL	0.10 mL	0.10 mL
0.40 mL	0.40 mL	0.40 mL	0.15 mL	0.15 mL
			0.25 mL	0.20 mL
			0.35 mL	0.30 mL
			0.50 mL	0.40 mL
				0.50 mL

The **bold underlined** entries are representative instructions that would be placed in the blank spaces in the schedule.

BOX 87-4 EXAMPLE OF A CLUSTER IMMUNOTHERAPY DOSING SCHEDULE

Visit 1*	0.10 mL	Vial # 4
	0.40 mL	Vial # 4
	0.10 mL	Vial # 3
Visit 2	0.20 mL	Vial # 3
	0.40 mL	Vial # 3
	0.07 mL	Vial # 2
Visit 3	0.10 mL	Vial # 2
	0.15 mL	Vial # 2
	0.25 mL	Vial # 2
Visit 4	0.35 mL	Vial # 2
	0.50 mL	Vial # 2
Visit 5	0.07 mL	Vial # 1
	0.10 mL	Vial # 1
Visit 6	0.15 mL	Vial # 1
	0.20 mL	Vial # 1
Visit 7	0.30 mL	Vial # 1
	0.40 mL	Vial # 1
Visit 8	0.50 mL	Vial # 1
Visit 9	0.50 mL	Vial # 1

*Visits may be once or twice weekly.

Cluster Protocols

Cluster immunotherapy also has been reported to be associated with a similar rate of reactions, with similar clinical efficacy to that of weekly injections.[155,161,162] The advantages of a cluster regimen are the capability to reach maintenance doses in 3 to 6 weeks (see Box 87-4),[73-75,161,162] with more rapid achievement of clinical improvement[161] and a reduction in the number of injections, number of office visits, and overall cost.[162]

Modification of Treatment Schedule

The proposed treatment schedule may require modification, most often because of missed visits, the first injection from a new vial of extract, or reactions to the previous injection. It does not appear to be necessary to reduce the dose for injections given during a pollen season[163,164] or with large local reactions to reduce the risk for a subsequent systemic reaction.[165,166] In two studies that monitored for systemic reactions in nearly 10,000 patients, no correlation was found between pollen season and the rate of systemic reactions, even when the patient was receiving the offending pollen.[163,164] In two large, prospective studies, no significant difference was noted in the rate of systemic reactions when adjustment in dose was and was not made for large local reactions.[165,166] Such adjustments are unnecessary, increase costs, and delay the patient's achieving clinical benefit from immunotherapy.

When dose adjustments are necessary, few studies have assessed the magnitude and effectiveness of the reduction. One retrospective study examined the modifications practiced in a large clinic.[167] The usual clinic protocol was to reduce by one dose for each week late beginning after 2 weeks and up to 8 weeks. With a gap of greater than 8 weeks, the dose reduction was the allergist's decision, the dose from a newly mixed vial was reduced 50%, and after a systemic reaction the dose was reduced tenfold. All three strategies were not associated with an increase in systemic reactions with the subsequent injection. Other strategies for dose modification are discussed in the AIPP.[51]

DURATION OF IMMUNOTHERAPY

Only a few studies have adequately addressed the question of the duration of inhalant allergen immunotherapy. Benefit can be demonstrated after a single series of preseasonal injections.[7] A general perception supported by prospective observations, however, is that the clinical benefits may increase with continuation of the same dose over several seasons.[168] In a group of patients with asthma treated with house dust mite immunotherapy until they became asymptomatic, the rate of relapse was significantly higher among those who received immunotherapy for less than 35 months.[65] Patients who had received immunotherapy with timothy grass extract for 3 or 4 years were randomized to continue receiving either monthly maintenance injections of timothy or placebo injections. Over the subsequent three grass pollen seasons, no difference in symptom or medication scores was found between those who continued to receive active treatment and those receiving placebo injections.[63]

A prospective study was conducted in patients with rhinitis and asthma who received immunotherapy with house dust mite extract. Half the subjects received immunotherapy for 3 years; the other half received it for 5 years.[169] Assessment at the end of 5 years revealed no difference between the two groups for asthma score or asthma- or rhinitis-related quality of life. A significant difference was found in favor of the 5-year treatment group for rhinitis symptoms. These studies suggest that 3 years of high-dose immunotherapy may be sufficient in many cases to provide long-lasting remission of symptoms.

REACTIONS TO ALLERGEN IMMUNOTHERAPY

A recognized complication of allergen immunotherapy is the occurrence of localized and systemic reactions. Three reviews of fatal reactions to injections of allergenic extracts conducted by an AAAI committee have emphasized the small but definite risk of death with this form of treatment.[170-172] The fatality rate in the United States during the period covered by the surveys was estimated to be about 1 per 2.5 million injections.[172] Recently, the first report of a prospective Web-based surveillance of reactions to immunotherapy has been forthcoming.[173] Data covering 1922 prescribers of injection immunotherapy showed no deaths and a systemic reaction rate of 10.2 per 10,000 injection visits. Of the systemic reactions, 74% were only cutaneous or upper respiratory, 23% were asthmatic, and 3% involved life-threatening respiratory compromise or hypotension.

Two studies monitored nearly 10,000 patients during both buildup and maintenance allergen immunotherapy.[163,164] The usual maintenance dose was 2400 protein nitrogen units (PNU) of allergen,[163] or 1 : 100 w/v of allergenic material.[164] The rate of systemic reactions over a 1-year observation period was 2.1%,[164] whereas observation over a 13-year period revealed systemic reactions in 2.9% of patients.[163] Reactions were more frequent during the initial buildup.[163,164] Although it has been suggested that patients are at increased risk for systemic reactions during their pollen seasons,[171] studies of large numbers of patients receiving immunotherapy have failed to demonstrate such a correlation.[163,164] One study, however, demonstrated a significantly increased occurrence of systemic reactions during the August–to-October peak for outdoor mold spores.[164]

In patients with asthma receiving rush immunotherapy with house dust mite extract, an asthma episode was the most common form of systemic reaction.[157] Patients whose initial FEV_1 was less than 80% of predicted were particularly subject to the development of bronchospasm.[157] This predilection has led to the recommendation that patients should not receive immunotherapy if their FEV_1 is below 70% of predicted even after medication.[160] Also likely to be of benefit is having patients with asthma perform peak expiratory flow maneuvers before their injection and again before leaving the clinic.

The interval between allergen extract injection and development of a systemic reaction is of considerable importance because it dictates how long the patient should remain in the physician's office after receiving treatment. The more severe reactions tend to occur earlier. Information was available on the timing of onset of 27 fatal reactions to allergen immunotherapy.[171,172] In 23 of the reactions, onset occurred before 20 minutes, but 4 were reported to have begun more than 30 minutes after injection. Based on a review of the literature, the AIPP recommends that the patient remain in the physician's office or medical clinic for 30 minutes after an injection.[51] Patients with asthma are at greater relative risk for a fatal reaction to allergen immunotherapy compared with patients who have only rhinitis.[170-172] This correlation is particularly strong if the asthma is labile or symptomatic at the time of the injection, requires oral corticosteroid treatment, or has resulted in hospitalization or emergency room visits, or if the patient has a complicating cardiovascular disease.[170-172] Additional factors that have been identified in patients experiencing fatal reactions are dosage errors,[171,172] first injection from a new vial of extract,[171,172] concomitant use of β-adrenergic blocking agents,[171] and administration of immunotherapy at home or in an unsupervised clinic.[171,172]

Two studies reported on the occurrence of biphasic systemic reactions associated with immunotherapy. In one study, they were reported after 10% of systemic reactions[174]; in the other, after 23%.[175] In both studies, the recurrent symptoms were mild, usually subsiding spontaneously and not requiring epinephrine or emergency department visits.

The occurrence of a local reaction to immunotherapy was not found to be predictive of the occurrence of a systemic reaction in two large studies.[165,166] It was concluded that local reactions do not require dose adjustments for the purpose of avoiding systemic reactions.

Pretreatment

Although pretreatment is not routinely used before immunotherapy, it has been shown to reduce systemic reactions in patients using rush, cluster, and conventional schedules.[156,160,176,177] Pretreatment for immunotherapy with oral corticosteroids, ketotifen, and theophylline,[160] or with oral corticosteroids, and the combination of histamine H_1 and H_2 antagonists,[156] reduced the systemic reaction rate during rush immunotherapy to less than half of that observed without pretreatment. A similar reduction in both number and severity of systemic reactions during cluster and conventional immunotherapy was reported with pretreatment with an antihistamine each day before initiation of injections.[176,177] Premedication with the leukotriene receptor antagonist montelukast reduced the occurrence of local reactions to immunotherapy.[178] The study was too small to assess the effect on systemic reactions.

NON–IMMUNOGLOBULIN E–MEDIATED ADVERSE REACTIONS TO ALLERGEN IMMUNOTHERAPY

The presence or subsequent development of antibodies of the IgG isotype to proteins used for injection suggests the possibility of formation of antigen-antibody complexes and induction of immune complex–mediated disease. However, no evidence for this was found in two studies in patients on long-term immunotherapy.[179,180]

ALLERGEN IMMUNOTHERAPY IN PREGNANCY

Concern for administering allergen immunotherapy during pregnancy centers on two possible adverse effects: the possibility of loss of a fetus through abortion during the course of a systemic reaction, due to contraction of uterine smooth muscle, and the potential for impairment of fetal development. The occurrence of a miscarriage resulting from a systemic reaction was documented in a case report.[181] On the other hand, two studies comprising nearly 200 women who received allergen immunotherapy, through one or more pregnancies, revealed no increase in rates of prematurity, toxemia, abortion, neonatal death, or congenital malformations.[182,183]

ADHERENCE TO ALLERGEN IMMUNOTHERAPY

The long duration of allergen immunotherapy using conventional schedules and conventional extracts is an important factor in discontinuation of treatment by the patient.[184,185] In two reports from private practices involving 532 subjects, 46% did not continue prescribed courses of allergen immunotherapy. The most common cause given by the patients was inconvenience.[184,185] Using the same definition of noncompliance, a large private practice reported a 34.8% rate of discontinuation among patients receiving injections at remote, nonallergist's offices, compared with only 10.8% among those receiving injections in the office of the prescribing allergist.[186]

Alternative Extracts and Methods of Administration

In addition to conventional allergen immunotherapy methods, a number of modified extracts and administration protocols are in clinical use or under investigation, as summarized in Box 87-5.

MODIFIED ALLERGEN EXTRACTS

A disadvantage of conventional allergen immunotherapy is the considerable investment in time and money required on the part of the patient to achieve and maintain effective doses of allergen extract. Therefore, as far back as 60 years ago, allergists began experimenting with methods to retard the absorption of allergen from the injection site and thereby decrease the number of injections required.[187]

A modification of allergen extracts widely used for several decades was termed "repository immunization." This approach consisted of mixing allergen extracts with mineral oil and an emulsifier.[187] Inconsistent clinical responses plus concerns over injection of mineral oil led to abandonment of this treatment.

Precipitation with alum was one of the first methods employed to retard absorption. A commercially available aqueous-extracted, aluminum-precipitated ragweed extract produces therapeutic and immunologic results equal to those obtained with aqueous ragweed extract.[188] The principal advantage of the aqueous-extracted, aluminum-precipitated extract is a marked reduction in systemic reactions while attaining the same clinical and immunologic results as with aqueous extracts.[189] A disadvantage is the limited number of allergens

BOX 87-5 MODIFICATIONS TO ALLERGEN EXTRACTS AND ROUTES OF ADMINISTRATION*

- Depot preparations
  - Aluminum adsorption
  - Tyrosine adsorption
  - Liposome-encapsulated
- Allergoids
- Recombinant technology
  - Unmodified major allergens
  - Mutated or deleted major allergens
  - T cell epitope peptides
- Toll-like receptor stimulation
  - 3-Deacylated monophosphoryl lipid A
  - CpG (type A and type B): combined with allergen or administered without allergen
- Intralymphatic
- Transcutaneous
- Transmucosal
  - Oral
  - Intranasal
  - Sublingual

*In clinical use or under investigation.

available and the absence of house dust mite and domestic pet allergen extracts.

Clinical studies have been conducted with 3-deacylated monophosphoryl lipid A, which induces a Th1 response.[190] The adjuvant has been combined with tyrosine-adsorbed glutaraldehyde-modified grass pollen extract in a treatment involving only four injections. In a study with over 1000 subjects, active treatment reduced symptom or medication scores by 13.4% over the four peak pollen weeks, with greater reductions (17.1%) in subjects with a history of severe rhinoconjunctivitis.[190]

As with preparation of vaccines of infectious agents, such as tetanus toxoid, allergenic proteins can be treated with formaldehyde[85] or with glutaraldehyde[191] to produce larger molecules with decreased ability to react with IgE antibodies.[85] These altered allergens are referred to as allergoids. Extensive trials were conducted with a ragweed allergoid at Johns Hopkins University[85] and a glutaraldehyde-modified ragweed at Northwestern.[191] Although studies with modified extracts have not continued in the United States, studies using allergoids continue in Europe,[192] where glutaraldehyde-polymerized extracts have been reported to allow safely administering 10 times the customary dose of extract[193] and to achieve maintenance doses with two injections separated by 30 minutes.[194] A regimen with only four doses to maintenance has been reported, with good clinical response, in birch-sensitive patients.[195,196]

Despite reported good clinical responses, a note of caution regarding allergoids is raised by a study that compared the allergenicity and immunogenicity of four commercially available allergoid products with three commercially available intact grass pollen allergen extracts.[197] The investigators found that the reduced allergenicity of the allergoids, measured by basophil activation, was matched by reduced immunogenicity demonstrated by T cell activation. On the basis of their results, they questioned the rationale behind chemical modification into allergoids.

Instead of binding the allergen to a carrier, encapsulation of unmodified house dust mite extracts in liposomes has been investigated.[198] Liposomes are lipid vesicles formed by one or more phospholipid bilayers that entrap the water-soluble extract in their internal aqueous compartment. They are biodegradable and stable and prolong the half-life of the encapsulated drug while acting as an adjuvant, inducing a Th1 response. The clinical effectiveness of this approach has not been established.

APPLICATION OF RECOMBINANT TECHNOLOGY

The development of recombinant technology offers the possibility of entirely new approaches to allergen immunotherapy. Most of the important allergens of the major inhalants have been identified, cloned, sequenced, and expressed in one of a variety of systems.[199] This technologic advance allows (1) production of virtually unlimited quantities of allergenic proteins, (2) expression of the allergenic protein in fragments, (3) expression of only limited portions of the protein as peptides, or (4) mutation or deletion of specific amino acids within the protein or its component peptides.

Unmodified Allergens

Unmodified purified major allergens have been employed for immunotherapy.[200-203] The immunologic response to injections of Antigen E (Amb a 1) were considered to be equivalent to those obtained with the whole unmodified extract of ragweed.[200] However, immunotherapy with the two major allergens of timothy grass was not as effective as those with a partially purified whole timothy grass pollen extract in a 3-year blinded study.[201] A mixture of five recombinant timothy grass pollen allergens was reported to reduce symptom medication scores but was not compared to the crude timothy grass pollen extract.[202] Native and recombinant Bet v 1 was compared with whole birch extract and placebo.[203] The clinical responses to all three active treatments were superior to those with placebo and not significantly different from each other.

Peptides

The concept that the clinical response to allergen immunotherapy reflects the induction of nonresponsiveness in Th2 lymphocytes led to the concept of immunotherapy with allergen-derived peptides representing T cell–activating epitopes, which do not react with IgE antibodies.[204] An early approach was to prepare fragments of the allergenic proteins by peptic digestion and fractionation by molecular exclusion chromatography.[205] The current approach to peptide therapy is to identify and sequence the major allergens, synthesize overlapping peptide segments of these major allergens, and identify those that contain dominant T cell epitopes while exhibiting very low or no IgE-binding activity.[206] This approach was adopted to develop peptide vaccines for ragweed pollen, containing epitopes from Amb a 1, and for cat dander, containing epitopes from Fel d 1. Clinical trials of these vaccines showed some reduction in symptoms in comparison with that associated with placebo regimens.[207] Administration of the higher doses of the peptides, however, caused respiratory symptoms several hours after injection.[207,208] Although these became less severe with repeated dosing, peptide-specific IgE developed in a number of patients, some of whom experienced reactions with succeeding injections.[207,208] As a result of problems with side effects, plus limited efficacy, development was halted.

Researchers at the National Heart and Lung Institute in London identified peptides derived from Fel d 1 that bound to 10 commonly expressed HLA-DR molecules.[209] They then identified immunodominant peptides by T cell proliferation and cytokine secretion and lack of IgE recognition by studying histamine-releasing activity. Studies were conducted using a mixture of 12 Fel d 1–derived peptides 16 to 17 amino acids in length encompassing most of the T cell epitopes of Fel d 1. Administration of these peptides suppressed PBMC proliferation and decreased production of IL-4, IL-13, and IFN-γ.[210] After peptide immunotherapy, $CD4^+$ T cells were generated that were able to actively suppress allergen-specific proliferative responses, and production of IL-10 was increased.[211] Cat-allergic asthmatic subjects received intradermal injections of the mixture. At follow-up evaluation 3 to 4 months after completion of the treatment, a significant reduction was observed in the late asthmatic response to inhaled cat allergen, with significant improvement in asthma-related quality of life.[212] This approach to immunotherapy is currently being pursued in clinical trials using peptides derived from cat, ragweed, house dust mite, and grass.[213]

Modified Allergens

A clinical trial has been conducted with genetically modified derivatives of the major birch pollen allergen, Bet v 1.[214,215] Two products were studied, one consisting of two fragments of Bet v 1 encompassing amino acids 1 to 73 and 74 to 159, respectively, and the other, a Bet v 1 trimer.[213] Both exhibited a greater than 100-fold reduction in allergenic activity. Treatment with the trimer led to an IgG response and a significant reduction in Bet v 1–specific Th2 responses in stimulated PBMCs. There were trends toward improvement in subjects' well-being, but they did not reach statistical significance for symptom or medication scores.[215] Other hypoallergenic variants of Bet v 1 are undergoing clinical trials.[216]

Among other modified allergens that have been reported are hybrid molecules derived from Der p 1 and Der p 2[217] and a mosaic protein derived from DNA coding for fragments of Phl p 1,[218] both having reduced IgE reactivity; a fusion protein of a bacterial surface layer protein and the major birch pollen allergen Bet v 1 that enhanced Th1 and regulatory T cell responses[219]; and a fusion protein comprising the major allergen of cat, Fel d 1 and the Fc portion of IgG1.[220] The allergen portion of this fusion protein binds to specific IgE on FcεR , whereas the Fcγ portion coaggregates inhibitory Fcγ RIIb driving inhibition of allergic reactivity.

TOLL-LIKE RECEPTOR STIMULATION

TLRs are cell surface or intracellular receptors that recognize pathogen-associated molecular patterns commonly found in bacteria and viruses. Agonists for two TLRs have been studied in conjunction with immunotherapy: (1) unmethylated CpG DNA motifs, which stimulate TLR9, and (2) lipopolysaccharides and a derivative, monophosphoryl lipid A (MPL), which stimulate TLR4.[221] They commonly consist of two 5′ purines, a CpG motif, and two 3′ pyrimidines. CpGs stimulate the innate immune system inducing the release of IFN-α and -β, IL-6, IL-12, and IL-18 primarily from monocytes and IFN-γ from NK cells.[222] This concerted response biases the adaptive arm of the immune system toward a Th1 response.[223] It was found that conjugating the allergen protein to the immunostimulatory sequence produced a greater immunologic response and significantly reduced the reactivity of the protein with IgE owing to steric interference.[224]

Clinical studies have been reported with the CpG/Amb a 1 preparation.[225,226] Twenty-five ragweed-allergic subjects received six escalating doses of ragweed Amb a 1–immunostimulating complex (AIC).[225] During the first peak ragweed pollen season, mean symptom score in the active treatment group was 13.2 versus 40.8 for the placebo-treated subjects, whereas without further treatment, the mean symptom score for this group was 13.9 versus 49.4 for the placebo group during the second ragweed season.

A study of AIC was conducted in 462 ragweed-allergic subjects during the 2004 and 2005 seasons.[226] Two thirds received one injection per week of AIC for 6 weeks (1.2 to 30 μg); the remainder, placebo. Half of the patients in the active treatment group received two booster injections of AIC before the 2005 season. There were no serious reactions to the injections. During the peak of the 2004 ragweed season the total nasal symptom scores (TNSSs) were reduced 21% in subjects in the active treatment group compared with those in the placebo treatment group ($P = .04$). During the peak of the 2005 ragweed season, compared to those receiving placebo, the TNSSs were reduced 13.5% in those who had received booster injections (P = not significant) and 28.5% in those who had not ($P = .02$). Compared to the placebo-treated subjects, fexofenadine use was 20% less in the booster group (P = not significant) and 38% less in the nonboosted group ($P = .04$).[226]

The CpG used in the foregoing studies was of the B type, selected because its phosphorothioate backbone provided greater stability than that afforded by the phosphodiester backbone of the A-type CpG. It was later found that incorporation of an A-type CpG (G10) into a viruslike particle (bacteriophage Qb coat protein) provided stability, leading to clinical studies with this compound.[227] Subcutaneous administration of an A-type CpG ODN (G10)-Qb in conjunction with house dust mite extract in an open trial demonstrated almost complete tolerance on conjunctival challenge and reduced immediate skin reactivity to house dust mite extract with active treatment. Subsequent studies have administered G10-Qb without accompanying allergen injection. A total of 299 subjects with perennial allergic rhinitis sensitive to house dust mites were randomized to receive either 6 weekly injections of viruslike particles containing a type-A CpG (CYT003-QbG10) at 0.5 mg or 1.0 mg, or placebo. The higher dose was more effective, reducing symptom and medication scores, improving rhinitis-related quality of life, and increasing conjunctival threshold all significantly more than with placebo.[228] Sixty-three subjects with asthma requiring maintenance inhaled corticosteroids were randomized to receive either CYT003-QbG10 or placebo and then underwent steroid tapering over a 12-week study.[229] There were significant differences in favor of active treatment for symptoms, pulmonary function, and quality of life.

ALTERNATIVE ROUTES OF ADMINISTRATION

Intralymphatic Route

The clinical and immunologic response to three monthly injections of grass pollen extract into an inguinal lymph node were compared with those with subcutaneous injection of the same extract for a period of 3 years in 112 subjects sensitive to grass.[230] The total dose by the intralymphatic route was more than 1000 times less than that given by subcutaneous injection. Systemic reactions were fewer and less severe with intralymphatic injection. A more rapid increase in tolerance to intranasal challenge with grass pollen extract as observed in the intralymphatic group, whereas after 3 years, no difference was found in clinical or immunologic outcomes between the two groups. Confirmatory studies are needed, but intralymphatic immunotherapy has several attractive features: It uses currently approved extracts, multiple allergen mixes can be administered, and no expensive development program is required to gain approval.

Transcutaneous Route

Two groups of investigators have reported results with transcutaneous (epicutaneous) application of grass pollen extract in adults[231,232] and children.[233] Patches with grass pollen extract were applied weekly for 6, 12, or 13 weeks and left in place for 8,[232] 48,[231] or 24[234] hours. In two studies, epidermal penetration was enhanced by stripping the site with tape[231,232]; in a third study, by inclusion of salicylic acid in the preparation. In all three studies, symptom scores were reduced in the active treatment group during the ensuing grass pollen season. In two of the studies, subjects were observed through a second pollen season without further treatment and with continued significant improvement.[231,232] In one study, 10 of 99 patients receiving active treatment experienced mild or moderate systemic reactions and were dropped from the series.[232] The transcutaneous route of immunotherapy has many attractive features, including home administration and benefit persisting for at least a second year without further treatment. Further studies are needed to define the best adjuvant for skin penetration and the optimal number and duration of patch applications. Until these methodologic questions are answered, this approach must be considered investigational.

COMBINATION TREATMENT WITH OMALIZUMAB

Because the concerns with safety and the limitations in the rapidity of dose escalation with immunotherapy both result from reactions of the injected allergens with specific IgE, reduction in the levels of IgE would be expected to be beneficial. This approach was used in a double-blind, placebo-controlled study using the monoclonal anti-IgE antibody omalizumab as an adjuvant to rush immunotherapy.[234] Subjects with ragweed-allergic rhinitis received 9 weeks of treatment with omalizumab or placebo, following which they underwent a 1-day rush immunotherapy protocol with ragweed extract or placebo. They then underwent further weekly dose increases and were monitored through the ragweed season. The addition of omalizumab resulted in a fivefold decrease in the risk of anaphylaxis caused by the rush immunotherapy, as well as a reduction in the rate of systemic reactions during the weekly buildup phase, from 9.7% to zero.

The protective effect of 3 months of pretreatment with omalizumab was examined in 248 patients whose perennial asthma was not completely controlled on inhaled corticosteroids, who were sensitive by skin prick testing to cats, dogs, or house dust mites, and who underwent specific immunotherapy to one or more of these allergens by cluster buildup followed by 7 weeks of maintenance injections.[235] Systemic reactions, all occurring during the cluster buildup, occurred in 26.2% of those who received placebo but in only 13.5% of those who had received omalizumab.

Conclusions

Allergen immunotherapy has been practiced with only minor changes for more than 100 years. The clinical effectiveness of adequate doses in appropriate patients for both allergic rhinitis and bronchial asthma has been repeatedly confirmed. Recent studies have revealed a broad antiinflammatory response with restoration of an immune response resembling that observed in nonallergic individuals. Studies also have confirmed a persisting beneficial effect after an adequate course of allergen immunotherapy is discontinued. These findings suggest that immunotherapy should be used more, rather than less, contrary to the current trend. Increased utilization is unlikely to occur, however, unless alternative extracts or methods of administration make immunotherapy safer and more convenient for the patient.

REFERENCES

Historical Development

1. Noon L. Prophylactic inoculation against hay fever. Lancet 1911;i:1572-3.
2. Freeman J. Further observations on the treatment of hay fever by hypodermic inoculations of pollen vaccine. Lancet 1911;ii:814-7.
3. Nelson HS. Some highlights of the first century of immunotherapy. Ann Allergy Asthma Immunol 2011;107:417-21.
4. Frankland AW, Augustin R. Prophylaxis of summer hay-fever and asthma: a controlled trial comparing crude grass-pollen extracts with the isolated main protein component. Lancet 1954;i:1055-7.
5. Lowell FC, Franklin W. A double-blind study of the effectiveness and specificity of injection therapy in ragweed hay fever. N Engl J Med 1965;273:675-9.
6. Franklin W, Lowell FC. Comparison of two dosages of ragweed extract in the treatment of pollenosis. JAMA 1967;201:915-7.

Clinical Efficacy of Allergen Immunotherapy

7. Varney VA, Gaga M, Frew AJ, et al. Usefulness of immunotherapy in patients with severe summer hay fever uncontrolled by antiallergic drugs. BMJ 1991;302:265-9.
8. Varney VA, Tabbah K, Mavroleon G, Frew AJ. Usefulness of specific immunotherapy in patients with severe perennial allergic rhinitis induced by house dust mite: a double-blind, randomized, placebo-controlled trial. Clin Exp Allergy 2003;33:1076-82.
9. Calderon MA, Alves B, Jacobson M, et al. Allergen injection immunotherapy for seasonal allergic rhinitis. Cochrane Database Syst Rev 2007;(1):CD001936.
10. Walker SM, Pajno GB, Lima MT, et al. Grass pollen immunotherapy for seasonal rhinitis and asthma: a randomized, controlled trial. J Allergy Clin Immunol 2001;107:87-93.
11. Varney VA, Edwards J, Tabbah K, et al. Clinical efficacy of specific immunotherapy to cat dander: a double-blind placebo-controlled trial. Clin Exp Allergy 1997;27:860-7.
12. Olsen OT, Larsen KR, Jacobsen L, Svendsen UG. A 1-year, placebo-controlled, double-blind house-dust-mite immunotherapy study in asthmatic adults. Allergy 1997;52:853-9.
13. Zielen S, Kardoa P, Madonini E. Steroid-sparing effects with allergen-specific immunotherapy in childen wih asthma: a randomized controlled trial. J Allergy Clin Immunol 2010;126:942-9.
14. Blumberga G, Groes L, Haugaard L, Dahl R. Steroid-sparing effect of subcutaneous SQ-standardized specific immunotherapy in moderate and severe house dust mite allergic asthmatics. Allergy 2006;61:843-8.
15. Abramson MJ, Puy RM, Weiner JM. Injection allergen immunotherapy for asthma. Cochrane Database Syst Rev 2010;(8):CD001186.
16. Creticos PS, Reed CE, Norman PS, et al. Ragweed immunotherapy in adult asthma. N Engl J Med 1996;334:501-6.
17. Adkinson NF Jr, Eggleston PA, Eney D, et al. A controlled trial of immunotherapy for asthma in allergic children. N Engl J Med 1997;336:324-31.
18. Ring J. Successful hyposensitization treatment in atopic eczema: results of a trial in monozygotic twins. Br J Dermatol 1982;107:597-602.
19. Zachariae H, Cramers M, Herlin T, et al. Non-specific immunotherapy and specific hyposensitization in severe atopic dermatitis. Acta Derm Venerol 1985;114:48-54.
20. Seidenari S, Mosca M, Taglietti M, et al. Specific hyposensitization in atopic dermatitis. Dermatologica 1986;172:229.
21. Werfel T, Breuer K, Rueff F, et al. Usefulness of specific immunotherapy in patients with atopic dermatitis and allergic sensitization to house dust mites: a multi-centre, randomized, dose-response study. Allergy 2006;61:202-5.
22. Sears MR, Burrows B, Flannery EM, et al. Atopy in childhood: I. Gender and allergen related risks for development of hay fever and asthma. Clin Exp Allergy 1993;23:941-8.
23. Peat JK, Tovey E, Mellis CM, et al. Importance of house dust mite and *Alternaria* allergens in childhood asthma. An epidemiological study in two climatic regions of Australia. Clin Exp Allergy 1993;23:812-20.
24. Gergen PJ, Turkeltaub PC. The association of individual allergen reactivity with respiratory disease in a national sample: data from the second National Health and Nutrition Examination Survey, 1976-80 (NHANES II). J Allergy Clin Immunol 1992;90:579-88.
25. Zock JP, Brunekreef B, Hazebroek-Kampschreur AA, Roosjen CW. House dust mite allergen in bedroom floor dust and respiratory healthy of children with asthmatic symptoms. Eur Respir J 1994;7:1254-9.
26. Vervloet D, Charpin D, Haddi E, et al. Medication requirements and house dust mite exposure in mite-sensitive asthmatics. Allergy 1991;46:554-8.
27. Valletta EA, Comis A, Del Col G, et al. Peak expiratory flow variation and bronchial hyperresponsiveness in asthmatic children during periods of antigen avoidance and reexposure. Allergy 1995;50:366-9.
28. Peroni DG, Boner AL, Vallone G, et al. Effective allergen avoidance at high altitude reduces

allergen-induced bronchial hyperresponsiveness. Am J Respir Crit Care Med 1994;149:1442-6.
29. Simon HU, Grotzer M, Nikokaizik WH, et al. High altitude climate therapy reduces peripheral blood T lymphocyte activation, eosinophilia, and bronchial obstruction in children with house dust mite allergic asthma. Pediatr Pulmonol 1994;17:304-11.
30. Patterson R. Clinical efficacy of allergen immunotherapy. J Allergy Clin Immunol 1979;64:155-8.
31. Custovic A, Taggart SCO, Woodcock A. House dust mite and cat allergen in different indoor environments. Clin Exp Allergy 1994;24:1164-8.
32. Ingram JM, Sporik R, Rose G, et al. Quantitative assessment of exposure to dog (Can f I), and cat (Fel d I) allergens: relation to sensitization and asthma in children living in Los Alamos, New Mexico. J Allergy Clin Immunol 1995;96:449-56.
33. Alvarez-Cuesta E, Cuesta-Herranz J, Puyana-Ruiz J, et al. Monoclonal antibody-standardized cat extract immunotherapy: risk-benefit effects from a double-blind placebo study. J Allergy Clin Immunol 1994;93:556-66.
34. Hedlin G, Graff-Lonnevig V, Heilbron H, et al. Immunotherapy with cat- and dog-dander extracts. V. Effects of 3 years of treatment. J Allergy Clin Immunol 1991;87:955-64.
35. Salvaggio J, Aukrust L. Mold-induced asthma. J Allergy Clin Immunol 1981;68:327-46.
36. O'Hollaren MT, Yunginger JW, Offord KP, et al. Exposure to an aeroallergen as a possible precipitating factor in respiratory arrest in young patients with asthma. N Engl J Med 1991;324:359-63.
37. Salvaggio JE, Burge HA, Chapman JA. Emerging concepts in mold allergy: what is the role of immunotherapy? J Allergy Clin Immunol 1993;92:217-22.
38. Yunginger JW, Jones RT, Gleich GJ. Studies on *Alternaria* allergens. II. Measurement of the relative potency of commercial *Alternaria* extracts by the direct RAST and by RAST inhibition. J Allergy Clin Immunol 1976;58:405-13.
39. Esch R. Manufacturing and standardizing fungal allergen products. J Allergy Clin Immunol 2004;113:210-5.
40. Dreborg S, Agrell B, Foucard T, et al. A double-blind, multicenter immunotherapy trial in children using a purified and standardized *Cladosporium herbarum* preparation. Allergy 1986;41:131-40.
41. Malling H-J, Dreborg S, Weeke B. Diagnosis and immunotherapy of mould allergy. V. Clinical efficacy and side effects of immunotherapy with *Cladosporium herbarum*. Allergy 1986;41:507-19.
42. Horst M, Hejjaoui A, Horst V, et al. Double-blind, placebo-controlled rush immunotherapy with a standardized *Alternaria* extract. J Allergy Clin Immunol 1990;85:460-72.
43. Kuna P, Kaczmarck J, Kupezyk M. Efficacy and safety of immunotherapy for allergies to *Alternaria alternata* in children. J Allergy Clin Immunol 2011;127:502-8.
44. Arruda LK, Vailes LD, Ferriani VPL, et al. Cockroach allergens and asthma. J Allergy Clin Immunol 2001;107:419-28.
45. Patterson MI, Slater JE. Characterization and comparison of commercially available German and American cockroach allergen extracts. Clin Exp Allergy 2002;32:721-7.
46. Slater JE, James R, Pongracie JA, et al. Biological potency of German cockroach allergen extracts determined in an inner city population. Clin Exp allergy 2007;37:1033-9.
47. Sastre J, Fernandez-Nieto M, Rico P, et al. Specific immunotherapy with a standardized latex extract in allergic workers: a double-blind, placebo-controlled study. J Allergy Clin Immunol 2003;111:985-94.
48. Fontana VJ, Salanitro AS, Wolfe HI, Moreno F. Bacterial vaccine and infectious asthma. JAMA 1965;193:895-90.
49. Zuberier T, Bachert C, Bousquet PJ, et al. GA^{2}LEN/EAACI pocket guide for allergen-specific immunotherapy for allergic rhinitis and asthma. Allergy 2010;65:1525-30.
50. Esch RF. Specific immunotherapy in the U.S.A. General concept and recent initiatives. Arbeiten aus dem Paul-Ehrlich-Institut. Band 94. 10th International Paul Ehrlich Seminar, Lubeck, 2002. p. 17-23.
51. Cox L, Nelson H, Lockey R. Allergen immunotherapy: a practice parameter third update. J Allergy Clin Immunol 2011;127:S1-55.
52. Nelson HS. Multi-allergen immunotherapy for allergic rhinitis and asthma. J Allergy Clin Immunol 2009;123:763-9.
53. Johnstone DE, Crump L. Value of hyposensitization therapy for perennial bronchial asthma in children. Pediatrics 1961;27:39-44.
54. Reid MJ, Moss RB, Hsu YP, et al. Seasonal asthma in northern California: allergic causes and efficacy of immunotherapy. J Allergy Clin Immunol 1986;78:590-600.
55. Norman PS, Lichtenstein LM. The clinical and immunologic specificity of immunotherapy. J Allergy Clin Immunol 1978;61:370-7.
56. Des Roches A, Paradis L, Menardo JL, et al. Immunotherapy with a standardized *Dermatophagoides pteronyssinus* extract. VI. Specific immunotherapy prevents the onset of new sensitizations in children. J Allergy Clin Immunol 1997;99;450-3.
57. Pajno GB, Barberio G, De Luca F, et al. Prevention of new sensitizations in asthmatic children monosensitized to house dust mite by specific immunotherapy. A six-year follow-up study. Clin Exp Allergy 2001;31:1392-7.
58. Purello-D'Ambrosio F, Gangemi S, Merendino RA, et al. Prevention of new sensitizations in monosensitized subjects submitted to specific immunotherapy or not. A retrospective study. Clin Exp Allergy 2001;31:1295-302.
59. Limb SL, Brown KC, Wood RA, et al. Long term immunologic effects of aeroallergen immunotherapy. Int Arch Allergy Immunol 2006;140:245-51.
60. Moller C, Dreborg S, Ferdousi HA, et al. Pollen immunotherapy reduces the development of asthma in children with seasonal rhinoconjunctivitis (the PAT study). J Allergy Clin Immunol 2002;109:251-6.
61. Jacobsen L, Niggemann B, Dreborg S, et al. Specific immunotherapy has long-term preventive effect on seasonal and perennial asthma: 10-year follow-up on the PAT study. Allergy 2007;62:943-8.
62. Ebner C, Kraft D, Ebner H. Booster immunotherapy (BIT). Allergy 1994;49:38-42.
63. Durham SR, Walker SM, Varga EM, et al. Long-term clinical efficacy of grass-pollen immunotherapy. N Engl J Med 1999;341:468-75.
64. Eng PA. Twelve-year follow-up after discontinuation of preseasonal grass pollen immunotherapy in childhood. Allergy 2006;61:198-201.
65. Des Roches A, Paradis L, Knani J, et al. Immunotherapy with a standardized *Dermatophagoides pteronyssinus* extract. V. Duration of the efficacy of immunotherapy after its cessation. Allergy 1996;51:30-3.
66. Kelso JM, Jones RT, Tellez R, Yunginger JW. Oral allergy syndrome successfully treated with pollen immunotherapy. Ann Allergy Asthma Immunol 1995;74:391-6.
67. Asero R. How long does the effect of birch pollen injection SIT on apple allergy last? Allergy 2003;58:435-8.
68. Bucher X, Pichler WJ, Dahinden CA, Helbling A. Effect of tree pollen specific subcutaneous immunotherapy on the oral allergy syndrome to apple and hazelnut. Allergy 2004;59:1272-6.
69. Rak S, Heinrich C, Jacobsen L, et al. A double-blinded, comparative study of the effects of short preseason specific immntherapy and topical steroids in patients with allergic rhinoconjunctivitis and asthma. J Allergy Clin Immunol 2001;108:921-8.
70. Hankin CS, Cox L, Lang D, et al. Allergy immunotherapy among Medicaid-enrolled children with allergic rhinitis: patterns of care, resource use, and costs. J Allergy Clin Immunol 2008;121:227-32.
71. Hankin CS, Cox L, Lang D, et al. Allergen immunotherapy and health care cost benefits for children with allergic rhinitis: a large-scale, retropective, matched cohort study. Ann Allergy Asthma Immunol 2010;104:79-85.

Immunologic Response to Inhalant Immunotherapy

72. Bousquet J, Maasch H, Martinot B, et al. Double-blind, placebo-controlled immunotherapy with mixed grass pollen allergoids. II. Comparison between parameters assessing the efficacy of immunotherapy. J Allergy Clin Immunol 1988;82:439-46.
73. Ewbank PA, Murray J, Sanders K, et al. A double-blind, placebo-controlled immunotherapy dose-response study with standardized cat extract. J Allergy Clin Immunol 2003;111:155-61.
74. Nanda A, O'Connor M, Anand M, et al. Dose dependence and time course of the immunologic response to administration of standardized cat allergen extract. J Allergy Clin Immunol 2004;114:1339-44.
75. Lent A, Harbeck R, Strand M, et al. Immunological response to administration of standardized dog allergen extract at differing doses. J Allergy Clin Immunol 2006;118:1249-56.
76. Nish WA, Charlesworth EN, Davis TL, et al. The effect of immunotherapy on the cutaneous late phase response to antigen. J Allergy Clin Immunol 1994;93:484-93.
77. Iliopoulos O, Proud D, Adkinson NF Jr, et al. Effects of immunotherapy on the early, late, and rechallenge nasal reaction to provocation with allergen: changes in inflammatory mediators and cells. J Allergy Clin Immunol 1991;87:855-66.
78. Van Bever HP, Bosmans J, De Clerck LS, Stevens WJ. Modification of the late asthmatic reaction by hyposensitization in asthmatic children allergic to house dust mite (*Dermatophagoides pteronyssinus*) or grass pollen. Allergy 1988;43:378-85.
79. Pichler CE, Helbling A, Pichler WJ. Three years of specific immunotherapy with house-dust-mite extracts in patients with rhinitis and asthma: significant improvement of allergen-

specific parameters and of nonspecific bronchial hyperreactivity. Allergy 2001;56:301-6.
80. Furin MJ, Norman PS, Creticos PS, et al. Immunotherapy decreases antigen-induced eosinophil cell migration into the nasal cavity. J Allergy Clin Immunol 1991;88:27-32.
81. Rak S, Bjornson A, Hakanson L, et al. The effect of immunotherapy on eosinophil accumulation and production of eosinophil chemotactic activity in the lung of subjects with asthma during natural pollen exposure. J Allergy Clin Immunol 1991;88:878-88.
82. Wilson DR, Iani AMA, Walker SM, et al. Grass pollen immunotherapy inhibits seasonal increases in basophils and eosinophils in the nasal epithelium. Clin Exp Allergy 2001;31:1705-13.
83. Wilson DR, Nuri-Aria KT, Walker SM, et al. Grass pollen immunotherapy: symptomatic improvement correlates with reductions in eosinophils and IL-5 mRNA expression in the nasal mucosa during the pollen season. J Allergy Clin Immunol 2001;107:971-6.
84. Nouri-Aria KT, Pilette C, Jacobson MR, et al. IL-9 and c-Kit+ mast cells in allergic rhinitis during seasonal allergen exposure: effects of immunotherapy. J Allergy Clin Immunol 2005;116:73-9.
85. Norman PS, Lichtenstein LM, Marsh DG. Studies on allergoids from naturally occurring allergens. IV. Efficacy and safety of long-term allergoid treatment of ragweed hay fever. J Allergy Clin Immunol 1981;68:460-70.
86. Sherman WB, Stull A, Cooke RA. Serologic changes in hay fever cases treated over a period of years. J Allergy 1940;11:225-44.
87. Cooke RA, Barnard JH, Hebald S, Stull A. Serological evidence of immunity with coexisting sensitization in a type of human allergy (hay fever). J Exp Med 1935;62:733-50.
88. Alexander HL, Johnson MC, Bukantz SC. Studies on correlation between symptoms of ragweed hay fever and titer of thermostable antibody. J Allergy 1948;19:1-8.
89. Djurup R, Osterballe O. IgG subclass antibody response in grass pollen-allergic patients undergoing specific immunotherapy. Prognostic value of serum IgG subclass antibody levels early in immunotherapy. Allergy 1984;39:433-41.
90. Shamji MH, Ljorring C, Francis JN, et al. Functional rather than immunoreactive levels of IgG4 correlate closely with clinical response to grass pollen immunotherapy. Allergy 2011;67:217-26.
91. James LK, Shamji MH, Walker SM, et al. Long-term tolerance after allergen immunotherapy is accompanied by selective persistence of blocking antibodies. J Allergy Clin Immunol 2011;127:509-16.
92. Sadan N, Rhyne MB, Mellits ED, et al. Immunotherapy of pollinosis in children. Investigation of the immunologic basis of clinical improvement. N Engl J Med 1969;280:623-7.
93. Lichtenstein LM, Levy DA. Is desensitization for ragweed hay fever immunologically specific? Int Arch Allergy 1972;42:615-26.
94. Hsieh KH. Decreased production of interleukin-2 receptors after immunotherapy to house dust. J Clin Immunol 1988;8:171-7.
95. Evans R, Pence H, Kaplan H, Rocklin RE. The effect of immunotherapy on humoral and cellular responses in ragweed hayfever. J Clin Invest 1976;57:1378-85.
96. Rocklin RE, Sheffer AL, Greineder DK, Melmon KL. Generation of antigen-specific suppressor cells during allergy desensitization. N Engl J Med 1980;302:1214-9.
97. Tamir R, Castracane JM, Rocklin RE. Generation of suppressor cells in atopic patients during immunotherapy that modulate IgE synthesis. J Allergy Clin Immunol 1987;79:591-8.
98. Jutel M, Akdis M, Budak F, et al. IL-10 and TGF-β cooperate in the regulatory T cell response to mucosal allergens in normal immunity and specific immunotherapy. Eur J Immunol 2003;33:1205-14.
99. Lin YL, Shieh CC, Wang JY. The functional insufficiency of human CD4+CD25high T-regulatory cells in allergic asthma is subjected to TNF-alpha modulation. Allergy 2008;63:67-74.
100. Francis NJ, Till SJ, Durham SR. Induction of IL-10+CD4+CD25+ T cells by grass pollen immunotherapy. J Allergy Clin Immunol 2003;111:11255-61.
101. Gardner LM, Thien FC, Douglass JA, et al. Induction of T regulatory cells by standardized house dust mite immunotherapy: an increase in CD4+CD25 interleukin-10+ T cells expressing peripheral tissue trafficking markers. Clin Exp Allergy 2004;34:1209-19.
102. Savolainen J, Jacobsen L, Valovirta E. Sublingual immunotherapy in children modulates allergen induced expression of cytokine mRNA in PBMC. Allergy 2006;61:1184-90.
103. Varney VA, Hamid QA, Gaga M, et al. Influence of grass pollen immunotherapy on cellular infiltration and cytokine mRNA expression during allergen-induced late-phase cutaneous responses. J Clin Invest 1993;92:644-51.
104. Wambre E, DeLong JH, James EA, et al. Differentiation stage determines pathologic and protective allergen-specific CD4+ T-cell outcomes during specific immunotherapy. J Allergy Clin Immunol 2012;129:544-51.
105. Gabrielsson S, Soderlund A Paulie, S, et al. Specific immunotherapy prevents increased levels of allergen-specific IL-4 and IL-13-producing cells during pollen season. Allergy 2001;56:293-300.
106. Lack G, Nelson HS, Amran D, et al. Rush immunotherapy results in allergen-specific alterations in lymphocyte function and interferon-gamma production in CD4+ T cells. J Allergy Clin Immunol 1997;99:530-8.
107. Majori. M, Caminati A, Corradi M, et al. T-cell cytokine pattern at three time points during specific immunotherapy for mite-sensitive asthma. Clin Exp Allergy 2000;30:341-7.
108. Durham SR, Ying S, Varney VA, et al. Grass pollen immunotherapy inhibits allergen-induced infiltration of CD4+ T lymphocytes and eosinophils in the nasal mucosa and increases the number of cells expressing messenger RNA for interferon-gamma. J Allergy Clin Immunol 1996;97:1356-65.
109. Hamid QA, Schotman E, Jacobson MR, et al. Increases in IL-12 messenger RNA+ cells accompany inhibition of allergen-induced late skin responses after successful grass pollen immunotherapy. J Allergy Clin Immunol 1997;99:254-60.
110. Wang JY, Lei HY, Hsieh KH. The effect of immunotherapy on interleukin-1 and tumor necrosis factor production of monocytes in asthmatic children. J Asthma 1992;29:193-201.
111. Wantke F, Gotz M, Janisch R. Spontaneous histamine release in whole blood in patients before and after 4 months of specific immunotherapy. Clin Exp Allergy 1993;23:992-5.
112. Kuna P, Alam R, Kuzminska B, Rozniecki J. The effect of preseasonal immunotherapy on the production of histamine-releasing factor (HRF) by mononuclear cells from patients with seasonal asthma: results of a double-blind, placebo-controlled, randomized study. J Allergy Clin Immunol 1989;83:816-24.
113. Brunet C, Bedard PM, Lavoie A, et al. Allergic rhinitis to ragweed pollen. II. Modulation of histamine-releasing factor production by specific immunotherapy. J Allergy Clin Immunol 1992;89:87-94.
114. Liao TN, Hsieh KH. Altered production of histamine-releasing factor (HRF) activity and responsiveness to HRF after immunotherapy in children with asthma. J Allergy Clin Immunol 1990;86:894-901.
115. Hsieh KH, Ng CK. Increased plasma platelet activating factor in children with acute asthmatic attacks and decreased in vivo and in vitro production of platelet activating factor after immunotherapy. J Allergy Clin Immunol 1993;91:60-7.
116. Gagro A, Rabatic S, Trescec A, et al. Expression of lymphocytes FcεRII/CD23 in allergic children undergoing hyposensitization. Int Arch Allergy Immunol 1993;101:203-8.
117. Kljaic-Turkalj M, Cvoriscec B, Tudoric N, et al. Decrease in CD23+ B lymphocytes and clinical outcome in asthmatic patients receiving specific rush immunotherapy. Int Arch Allergy Immunol 1996;111:188-94.
118. Jung CM, Prinz JC, Rieber EP, Ring J. A reduction in allergen-induced FcεR2/CD23 expression on peripheral B cells correlates with successful hyposensitization in grass pollinosis. J Allergy Clin Immunol 1995;95:77-87.
119. Hakansson L, Heinrich C, Rak S, Venge P. Activation of B-lymphocytes during pollen season. Effect of immunotherapy. Clin Exp Allergy 1998;28:791-8.
120. Plewako H, Arvidsson M, Oancca I, et al. The effect of specific immunotherapy on the expression of costimulatory molecules in late phase reaction of the skin in allergic patients. Clin Exp Allergy 2004;34:1862-7.
121. Bellinghausen I. Modification of the innate immune function of dendritic cells by allergen-specific immunotherapy. Clin Exp Allergy 2010;40:12-4.
122. Tversky JR, Bieneman AP, Chichester KL, et al. Subcutaneous allergen immunotherapy restores human dendritic cell innate immune function. Clin Exp Allergy 2010;40:94-102.
123. Bohle B, Kinaciyan T, Gerstmayr M, et al. Sublingual immunotherapy induces IL-10-producing T regulatory cells, allergen-specific T-cell tolerance, and immune deviation. J Allergy Clin Immunol 2007;120:707-13.
124. Lofkvist T, Agrell B, Dreborg S, Svensson G. Effects of immunotherapy with a purified standardized allergen preparation of *Dermatophagoides farinae* in adults with perennial allergic rhinoconjunctivitis. Allergy 1994;49:100-7.

Practical Considerations in Allergen Immunotherapy

125. Finegold I. Immunotherapy: when to initiate treatment in children. Allergy Asthma Proc 2007;28:698-705.
126. Bousquet J, Hejjaoui A, Clauzel AM, et al. Specific immunotherapy with a standardized *Dermatophagoides pteronyssinus* extract. II.

Prediction of efficacy of immunotherapy. J Allergy Clin Immunol 1988;82:971-7.
127. Nelson HS, Areson J, Reisman R. A prospective assessment of the remote practice of allergy. Comparison of the diagnosis of allergic disease and the recommendations for allergen immunotherapy by board-certified allergists and a laboratory performing in vitro assays. J Allergy Clin Immunol 1993;92:380-6.
128. Yoo T-J, Spitz E, McGerity JL. Conifer pollen allergy: studies of immunogenicity and cross antigenicity of conifer pollens in rabbit and man. Ann Allergy 1975;34:87-93.
129. Martin BG, Mansfield LE, Nelson HS. Cross-allergenicity among the grasses. Ann Allergy 1985;54:99-104.
130. Davies JM, Bright ML, Rolland JM, et al. Bahia grass pollen specific IgE is common in seasonal rhinitis patients but has limited cross-reactivity with ryegrass. Allergy 2005;60:251-5.
131. Asero R, Weber B, Mistrello G, et al. Giant ragweed specific immunotherapy is not effective in a proportion of patients sensitized to short ragweed: analysis of the allergenic differences between short and giant ragweed. J Allergy Clin Immunol 2005;116:1036-41.
132. Weber RW. Cross-reactivity of pollen allergens: impact on allegen immunotherapy. Ann Allergy Asthma Immunol 2007;99:203-11.
133. Esch RE. Role of proteases on the stability of allergic extracts. In: Klein R, editor. Regulatory control and standardization of allergenic extracts. Stuttgart: Gustav Fischer Verlag; 1990. p. 171-7.
134. Nelson HS, Iklé D, Buchmeier A. Studies of allergen extract stability: the effects of dilution and mixing. J Allergy Clin Immunol 1996;98: 382-8.
135. Grier TJ, LeFevre DM, Duncan EA, Esch RE. Stability of standardized grass, dust mite, cat and short ragweed allergens after mixing with mold or cockroach extracts. Ann Allergy Asthma Immunol 2007;99:151-60.
136. Grier TJ, LeFevre DM, Duncan EA, Esch RE. Stability and mixing compatibility of dog epithelia and dog dander allergens. Ann Allergy Asthma Immunol 2009;103:411-7.
137. Johnstone DE, Dutton A. The value of hyposensitization therapy for bronchial asthma in children—a 14-year study. Pediatrics 1968;42: 793-802.
138. Cox L, Jacobsen L. Comparison of allergen immunotherapy practice patterns in the United States and Europe. Ann Allergy Asthma Immunol 2009;103:451-60.
139. Nelson HS. The use of standardized extracts in allergen immunotherapy. J Allergy Clin Immunol 2000;106:41-5.
140. Majchel AM, Proud D, Friedhoff L, et al. The nasal response to histamine challenge: effect of the pollen season and immunotherapy. J Allergy Clin Immunol 1992;90:85-91.
141. Creticos PS, Adkinson NF Jr, Kagey-Sobotka A, et al. Nasal challenge with ragweed pollen in hay fever patients: effect of immunotherapy. J Clin Invest 1985;76:2247-53.
142. Creticos PS, Marsh DG, Proud D, et al. Responses to ragweed-pollen nasal challenge before and after immunotherapy. J Allergy Clin Immunol 1989;84:197-205.
143. Van Metre TE Jr, Adkinson NF, Amodio FJ, et al. A comparative study of the effectiveness of the Rinkel method and the current standard method of immunotherapy for ragweed pollen hay fever. J Allergy Clin Immunol 1979;66: 500-13.
144. Haugaard L, Dahl R, Jacobsen L. A controlled dose-response study of immunotherapy with standardized, partially purified extract of house dust mite: clinical efficacy and side effects. J Allergy Clin Immunol 1993;91:709-22.
145. Frew AJ, Powell RJ, Corrigan CJ, et al. Efficacy and safety of specific imunotheapy with SQ allergen extract in treatment-resistant seasonal allergic rhinoconjunctivitis. J Allergy Clin Immunol 2006;117:319-28.
146. Khinchi MS, Poulsen LK, Carat F, et al. Clinical efficacy of sublingual and subcutaneous birch pollen allergen-specific immunotherapy: a randomized, placebo-controlled, double-blind, double-dummy study. Allergy 2004;59: 45-53.
147. Pauli G, Larsen TH, Rak S, et al. Efficacy of recombinant birch pollen vaccine for the treatment of birch-allergic rhinoconjunctivitis. J Allergy Clin Immunol 2008;122:951-60.
148. Bodtger U, Poulsen LK, Jacobi HH, et al. The safety and efficacy of subcutaneous birch pollen immunotherapy—a one-year, randomized, double-blind, placebo-controlled study. Allergy 2002;57:297-303.
149. Vailes L, Sridhara S, Cromwell O, et al. Quantitation of the major fungal allergens, Alt a 1 and Asp f 1, in commercial allergenic products. J Allergy Clin Immunol 2001;107:641-6.
150. Leavengood DC, Renard RL, Martin BG, Nelson HS. Cross allergenicity among grasses determined by tissue threshold changes. J Allergy Clin Immunol 1985;76:789-94.
151. Nelson HS. Effect of preservatives and conditions of storage on the potency of allergy extracts. J Allergy Clin Immunol 1981;67:64-9.
152. Van Metre TE Jr, Rosenberg GL, Vaswani SK, et al. Pain and dermal reaction caused by injected glycerin in immunotherapy solutions. J Allergy Clin Immunol 1996;97:1033-9.
153. Moore M, Tucker M, Grier T, Quinn J. Effects of summer mailing on in vivo and in vitro relative potencies of standardized timothy grass extract. Ann Allergy Asthma Immunol 2010;104:147-51.
154. Malling HJ, Weeke B. Position paper: immunotherapy. Allergy 1993;48(Suppl. 14):9-35.
155. Van Metre TE Jr, Adkinson NF Jr, Amodio FJ, et al. A comparison of immunotherapy schedules for injection treatment of ragweed pollen hay fever. J Allergy Clin Immunol 1982;69: 181-93.
156. Portnoy J, Bagstad K, Kanarek H, et al. Premedication reduces the incidence of systemic reactions during inhalant rush immunotherapy with mixtures of allergenic extracts. Ann Allergy 1994;73:409-18.
157. Bousquet J, Hejjaoui A, Dhivert H, et al. Immunotherapy with a standardized *Dermatophagoides pteronyssinus* extract. III. Systemic reactions during the rush protocol in patients suffering from asthma. J Allergy Clin Immunol 1989;83:797-802.
158. Moyer DB, Nelson HS. Use of modified radioallergosorbent testing in determining initial immunotherapy doses. Otolaryngol Head Neck Surg 1985;93:335.
159. Sharkey P, Portnoy J. Rush immunotherapy: experience with a one-day schedule. Ann Allergy Asthma Immunol 1996;76:175-80.
160. Hejjaoui A, Dhivert H, Michel FB, Bousquet J. Immunotherapy with a standardized *Dermatophagoides pteronyssinus* extract. IV. Systemic reactions according to the immunotherapy schedule. J Allergy Clin Immunol 1990;85: 473-9.
161. Tabar AI, Echechipia S, Garcia BE, et al. Double-blind comparative study of cluster and conventional immunotherapy schedules and *Dermatophagoides pteronyssinus*. J Allergy Clin Immunol 2005;116:109-18.
162. Mauro M, Russello M , Alesina R, et al. Safety and pharmacoeconomics of a cluster administration of mite immunotherapy compared to the traditional one. Eur Ann Allergy Clin Immunol 2006;38;31-4.
163. Lin MS, Tanner E, Lynn J, Friday GA Jr. Nonfatal systemic allergic reactions induced by skin testing and immunotherapy. Ann Allergy 1993;71:557-62.
164. Tinkelman DG, Cole WQ III, Tunno J. Immunotherapy: a one-year prospective study to evaluate risk factors of systemic reactions. J Allergy Clin Immunol 1995;95:8-14.
165. Tankersley MS, Butler KK, Butler WK, Goetz DW. Local reactions during allergen immunotherapy do not require dose adjustment. J Allergy Clin Immunol 2000;106:840-3.
166. Kelso MJ. The rate of systemic reactions to immunotherapy injections is the same whether or not the dose is reduced after a local reaction. Ann Allergy Asthma Immunol 2004; 92:225-7.
167. Webber CM, Calabria CW. Assessing the safety of subcutaneous immunotherapy dose adjustments. Ann Allergy Asthma Immunol 2010; 105:369-75.
168. Dolz I, Martinez-Cocerac C, Bartolone JM, Cimmara M. A double-blind, placebo-controlled study of immunotherapy with grass pollen extract Alutard SQ during a 3-year period with initial rush immunotherapy. Allergy 1996;51:489-500.
169. Tabar AI, Arroabarren E, Echechipia S, et al. Three years of specific immunotherapy may be sufficient in house dust mite respiratory allergy. J Allergy Clin Immunol 2011;127: 57-63.
170. Lockey RF, Benedict IM, Turkeltaub PC, Bukantz SC. Fatalities from immunotherapy (IT) and skin testing (ST). J Allergy Clin Immunol 1987;79:660-77.
171. Reid MJ, Lockey RF, Turkeltaub PC, Platts-Mills TA. Survey of fatalities from skin testing and immunotherapy 1985-1989. J Allergy Clin Immunol 1993;92:6-15.
172. Bernstein DI, Wanner M, Borish L, Liss GM. Twelve-year survey of fatal reactions to allergen injections and skin testing: 1990-2001. J Allergy Clin Immunol 2004;113:1129-36.
173. Bernstein DL, Epstein T, Murphy-Barendts K, Liss GM. Surveillance of systemic reactions to subcutaneous immunotherapy injections: year 1 outcomes of the ACAAI and AAAAI collaborative study. Ann Allergy Asthma Immunol 2010;104:530-5.
174. Confino-Cohen R, Goldberg A. Allergen immunotherapy-induced biphasic systemic reactions: incidence, characteristics, and outcome: a prospective study. Ann Allergy Asthma Immunol 2010;104:73-8.
175. Scranton SE, Gonzalez EG, Waibei KH. Incidence and characteristics of biphasic reactions after allergen immunotherapy. J Allergy Clin Immunol 2009;123:493-8.
176. Nielsen L, Johnsen CR, Mosbech H, et al. Antihistamine premedication in specific cluster immunotherapy: a double-blind, placebo-controlled study. J Allergy Clin Immunol 1996;97:1207-13.
177. Ohashi Y, Nakai Y, Muraata K. Effect of pretreatment with fexofenadine on the safety of

immunotherapy in patients with allergic rhinitis. Ann Allergy Asthma Immunol 2006;96: 600-5.
178. Wohn S, Gamper S, Hemmer W, et al. Premedication with montelukast reduces local reactions of allergen immunotherapy. Int Arch Allergy Immunol 2007;144:137-42.
179. Stein MR, Brown GL, Lima JE, et al. A laboratory evaluation of immune complexes in patients on inhalant immunotherapy. J Allergy Clin Immunol 1978;62:211-6.
180. Levinson AI, Summers RJ, Lawley TJ, et al. Evaluation of the adverse effects of long-term hyposensitization. J Allergy Clin Immunol 1978;62:109-14.
181. Francis N. Abortion after grass pollen injection. J Allergy 1941;12:559-63.
182. Metzger WJ, Turner E, Patterson R. The safety of immunotherapy during pregnancy. J Allergy Clin Immunol 1978;61:268-72.
183. Shaikh WA. A retrospective study on the safety of immunotherapy in pregnancy. Clin Exp Allergy 1993;23:857-60.
184. Lower T, Henry J, Mandik L, et al. Compliance with allergen immunotherapy. Ann Allergy 1993;70:480-2.
185. Cohn JR, Pizzi A. Determinants of patient compliance with allergen immunotherapy. J Allergy Clin Immunol 1993;91:734-7.
186. Tinkelman D, Smith F, Cole WQ III, Silk HJ. Compliance with an allergen immunotherapy regimen. Ann Allergy Asthma Immunol 1995;74:241-6.

Alternative Extracts and Methods of Administration

187. Norman PS, Winkenwerder WL, D'Lugoff BC. Controlled evaluations of repository therapy in ragweed hay fever. J Allergy 1967;39: 82-92.
188. Norman PS, Winkenwerder WL, Lichtenstein LM. Trials of alum-precipitated pollen extracts in the treatment of hay fever. J Allergy Clin Immunol 1972;50:31-44.
189. Nelson HS. Long-term immunotherapy with aqueous and aluminum-precipitated grass extracts. Ann Allergy 1980;45:333-7.
190. DuBuske LH, Frew A, Horak F, et al. Ultrashort-specific immunotherapy successfully treats seasonal allergic rhinoconjunctivitis to grass pollen. Allergy Asthma Proc 2011;32:239-47.
191. Hendrix SG, Patterson R, Zeiss GR, et al. A multi-institutional trial of polymerized whole ragweed for immunotherapy of ragweed allergy. J Allergy Clin Immunol 1980;66: 486-94.
192. Corrigan CJ, Kettner J, Doemer C, Cromwell O. Efficacy and safety of preseasonally-specific immunotherapy with an aluminum-adsorbed six-grass pollen allergoid. Allergy 2005;60: 801-7.
193. Casanovas M, Sastre J, Fernandez-Nieto M, et al. Double-blind study of tolerability and antibody production of unmodified and chemically modified allergen vaccines of *Phleum pratense*. Clin Exp Allergy 2005;35: 1377-83.
194. Casanovas M, Martin R, Jimenez C, et al. Safety of an ultra-rush immunotherapy build-up schedule with therapeutic vaccines containing depigmented and polymerized allergen extracts. Int Arch Allergy Immunol 2006;139: 153-8.
195. Hoiby AS, Strand V, Robinson DS, et al. Efficacy, safety and immunological effects of a 2-year immunotherapy with Depigoid birch pollen extract: a randomized, double blind, placebo-contrrolled study. Clin Exp Allergy 2010;40:1062-70.
196. Pfaar O, Robinson DS, Sager A, Emuzyte R. Immunotherapy with depigmented-polymerized mixed tree pollen extract: a clinical trial and responder analysis. Allergy 2010;88:1614-21.
197. Henmar H, Lund G, Lund L, et al. Allergenicity, immunogenicity and dose-relationship of three intact allergen vaccines and four allergoid vaccines for subcutaneous grass pollen immunotherapy. Clin Exp Immunol 2008;153: 316-23.
198. Basomba A, Tabar AI, de Roas DHF, et al. Allergen vaccination with a liposome-encapsulated extract of *Dermatophagoides pteronyssinus*: a randomized, double-blind, placebo-controlled trial in asthmatic patients. J Allergy Clin Immunol 2002;109:943-8.
199. Chapman MD, Smith AM, Vailes LD, et al. Recombinant allergens for diagnosis and therapy of allergic disease. J Allergy Clin Immunol 2000;106:409-18.
200. Norman PS, Winkenwerder WL, Lichtenstein LM. Immunotherapy of hay fever with ragweed antigen E: comparison with whole pollen extract and placebo. J Allergy 1968;42:91-108.
201. Osterballe O. Immunotherapy with grass pollen major allergens. Clinical results from a prospective 3-year double blind study. Allergy 1982;37:379-88.
202. Jutel M, Jaeger L, Suck R, et al. Allergen-specific immunotherapy with recombinant grass pollen allergens. J Allergy Clin Immunol 2005;116:608-13.
203. Pauli G, Larsen TH, Rak S, et al. Efficacy of recombinant birch pollen vaccine for the treatment of birch-allergic rhinoconjunctivitis. J Allergy Clin Immunol 2008;122:951-60.
204. Yssel H, Fasler S, Lamb J, de Vries JE. Induction of non-responsiveness in human allergen-specific type 2 T helper cells. Curr Opinion Immunol 1994;6:847-52.
205. Michael JG, Litwin A, Hasert V, Pesce A. Modulation of the immune response to ragweed allergens by peptic fragments. Clin Exp Allergy 1990;20:669-74.
206. Wallner BP, Gefter ML. Peptide therapy for treatment of allergic diseases. Clin Immunol Immunopathol 1996;80:105-9.
207. Norman PS, Ohman JL Jr, Long AA, et al. Treatment of cat allergy with T-cell reactive peptides. Am J Respir Crit Care Med 1996;154: 1623-8.
208. Maguire P, Nicodemus C, Robinson D, Aaronson D, Umetsu DT. The safety and efficacy of ALLERVAX CAT in cat allergic patients. Clin Immunol 1999;93:222-31.
209. Moldaver D, Larché M. Immunotherapy with peptides. Allegy 2011;66;784-91.
210. Oldfield WL, Kay AB, Larche M. Allergen-derived T cell peptide-induced late asthmatic reactions precede the induction of antigen-specific hyporesponsiveness in atopic allergic asthamtic subjects. J Immunol 2001;167: 1734-9.
211. Verhoef A, Alexander C, Kay AB, Larche M. T cell epitope immunotherapy induces a CD 4+ T cell population with regulatory activity. PLOS Med 2005;2:253-61.
212. Alexander C, Tarzi M, Larche' M, Kay AB. The effect of Fel d 1-derived T-cell peptides on upper and lower airway outcome measurements in cat-allergic subjects. Allergy 2005; 60:1269-74.
213. Circassia trials. Available at: www.circassia.co.uk. (Accessed July 10, 2011.)
214. Gafvelin G, Thunberg S, Kronqvist M, et al. Cytokine and antibody responses in birch-pollen-allergic patients treated with genetically modified derivatives of the major birch pollen allergen Bet v 1. Int Arch Allergy Immunol 2005;38:59-66.
215. Purohit A, Niederberger V, Kronqvist M, et al. Clinical effects of immunotherapy with genetically modified recombinant birch pollen Bet v 1 derivatives. Allergy 2008;38:1514-25.
216. Valenta R, Niespodziana K, Focke-Tejkl M, et al. Recombinant allergens: what does the future hold? J Allergy Clin Immunol 2011;127: 860-4.
217. Asturias JA, Ibarrola I, Arilla MC, et al. Engineering of major house dust mite allergens Der p 1 and Der p 2 for allergen-specific immunotherapy. Clin Exp Allergy 2009;39:1088-98.
218. Ball T, Linhart B, Sonneckk K, et al. Reducing allergenicity by altering allergen fold: a mosaic protein of Phl p 1 for allergy vaccination. Allergy 2009;64:569-80.
219. Gerstmayr M, Ilk N, Schabussova I, et al. A novel approach to specific allergy treatment: the recombinant allergen-S-layer fusion protein rSbsC-Bet v 1 matures dendritic cells that prime Th0/Th1 and IL-10 producing regulatory T cells. J Immunol 2007;179: 7270-5.
220. Saxon A, Kepley C, Zhang K. "Accentuate the negative, eliminate the positive": engineering allergy therapeutics to block allergic reactivity through negative signaling. J Allergy Clin Immunol 2008;121:320-5.
221. Nguyen TH, Stokes JR, Casale TB. Future forms of immunotherapy and immunomodulators in allergic disease. Immunol Allergy Clin N Am 2011;31:343-65.
222. Broide D, Schwarze J, Tighe H, et al. Immunostimulatory DNA sequences inhibit IL-5, eosinophilic inflammation, and airway hyperresponsiveness in mice. J Immunol 1998;161: 7054-62.
223. Van Uden J, Raz E. Immunostimulatory DNA and applications to allergic disease. J Allergy Clin Immunol 1999;104:902-10.
224. Tighe H, Takabayashi K, Schwartz D, et al. Conjugation of immunostimulatory DNA to the short ragweed allergen Amb a 1 enhances its immunogenicity and reduces its allergenicity. J Allergy Clin Immunol 2000;106:124-34.
225. Creticos PS, Schroeder JT, Hamilton RG, et al. Immunotherapy with a ragweed-Toll-like receptor 9 agonist vaccine for allergic rhinitis. N Engl J Med 2006;355:1445-55.
226. Busse W, Gross G, Korenblat P, et al. Phase 2/3 study of the novel vaccine Amb a 1 immunostimulatory oligodeoxyribonucleotide conjugate AIC (Tolamba) in ragweed-allergic adults. Late-breaking abstracts. AAAAI Annual Meeting, Miami Beach, Fla., March 2006.
227. Senti G, Johansen P, Haug S, et al. Use of A-type CpG oligodeoxynucleotides as an adjuvant in allergen-specific immunoatherapy in humans: a phase I/IIa clinical trial. Clin Exp Allergy 2009;39:562-70.
228. Klimek L, Willers J, Hammann-Haenni A, et al. Assessment of clinical efficacy of CYT003-QbG10 in patients with allergic rhinoconjunctivitis: a phase IIb study. Clin Exp Allergy 2011;41:1305-12.
229. Renner WA. Cytos Biotechnology presents novel Toll-like receptor 9 agonist CYT003-QβG10 for the treatment of allergic asthma at

the 2010 Annual Conference of the European Respiratory Society. Available at: www.cytos.com.

230 Senti G, Vavricka BMP, Edrmann I, et al. Intralymphatic allergen administration renders specific immunotherapy faster and safer: a randomized controlled trial. Proc Natl Acad Sci U S A 2008;105:17908-12.

231. Senti G, Graf N, Haug S, et al. Epicutaneous allergen administration as a novel method of allergen-specific immunotherapy. J Allergy Clin Immunol 2009;124:997-1002.

232. Senti G, von Moos S, Tay F, et al. Epicutaneous allergen-specific immunotherapy ameliorates grass pollen-induced rhinoconjunctivitis: a double-blind, placebo-controlled dose escalation study. J Allergy Clin Immunol 2012;129:128-35.

233. Agostinis F, Forti S, Berardino D. Grass transcutaneous immunotherapy in children with seasonal rhinoconjunctivitis. Allergy 2010;65:410-1.

234. Casale TB, Busse WW, Kline JN, et al. Omalizumab pretreatment decreases acute reactions after rush immunotherapy for ragweed-induced seasonal allergic rhinitis. J Allergy Clin Immunol 2006;117:134-40.

235. Massanari M, Nelson H, Casale T, et al. Effect of pretreatment with omalizumab on the tolerability of specific immunotherapy in allergic asthma. J Allergy Clin Immunol 2010;125:383-9.

WITHDRAWN

88

Sublingual Immunotherapy for Inhalant Allergens

ROBYN E. O'HEHIR | ALESSANDRA SANDRINI | ANTHONY J. FREW

CONTENTS

SUMMARY OF IMPORTANT CONCEPTS

» Sublingual immunotherapy (SLIT) offers a safer, more convenient approach to desensitizing patients than standard injection immunotherapy.

» The immunologic mechanisms of successful SLIT are largely similar to those of injection allergen-specific immunotherapy.

» Dendritic cells play a key role in inducing tolerance, most likely through regulatory T cells.

» Three phases of tolerance can be identified: early tolerization of mast cells and basophils, followed by T cell tolerance and eventually B cell tolerance.

» SLIT effectively reduces symptoms and medication requirements that parallel immunologic changes (e.g., reduced T cell proliferation, immune deviation, Treg induction) and modifies the course of allergic disease, reducing the risk of asthma in pediatric rhinitis.

» Economic considerations are crucial in determining candidates for SLIT. Subcutaneous injection immunotherapy provides similar long-term benefits at a lower cost than SLIT, and standard therapy is a relatively inexpensive option for symptom control compared with SLIT.

Background

The history of modern immunotherapy started after the breakthrough discovery of anaphylaxis in 1902 by Richet and Portier, who first observed severe allergic reactions while studying the toxicity of jellyfish in dogs. They introduced the novel concept that the protective immune system could cause significant harm. Investigation of the phenomenon soon led to the insight that anaphylaxis itself could be prevented by vaccination-like regimens of repeated allergen exposure, leading to a state of "tolerance" or "specific desensitization."

With this insight, the field of clinical allergen-specific immunotherapy (SIT) was born. Protocols to desensitize humans were developed, especially using the subcutaneous route, with administration of cumulatively increasing quantities of a sensitizing allergen delivered in doses and at time points that avoid or minimize the risk of anaphylaxis. In time, this leads to clinical tolerance such that a severe reaction does not occur to the sensitizing allergen under conditions that previously provoked allergic reactions. Specific immunotherapy was initially developed for the treatment of allergic rhinitis, with subsequent protocol refinements allowing therapeutic application to asthma and anaphylactic allergy.

However, the risk of a severe allergic reaction during injection immunotherapy has somewhat restricted its use, especially in the asthmatic population. Safer forms of immunotherapy administration have been investigated over the years, and the sublingual route has been shown to be the safest and most effective alternative route.[1]

ALLERGEN EXTRACTS

Sublingual immunotherapy (SLIT) involves the administration of allergens to the oral mucosa. Over the past 2 decades, several studies investigated different preparations of aqueous allergen extracts for sublingual use, including sprays, drops, and more recently, fast-dissolving tablets. Historically, preparations were made by extracting allergens with ammonium bicarbonate solution, followed by ultrafiltration, sterilizing filtration, and lyophilization. Extracts are analyzed for potency by measuring global IgE binding by radioallergosorbent test (RAST) or enzyme-linked immunosorbent assay (ELISA) inhibition and major allergen content by ELISA.[2] Extracts are then reconstituted before use such that the "parent compound" immunologic activity is equal to 100 IR/ml (100 IR [index of reactivity] is defined as the concentration of reference extract that elicits skin-prick test wheal geometric mean diameter of 7 mm in 30 subjects sensitive to the corresponding allergen).

Allergen extract standardization by determination of total allergenic proteins and biologic activity is extremely important to improve clinical efficacy of allergen immunotherapy. Standardized extracts for SLIT subsequently became available as drops for house-dust mite (*Dermatophagoides farinae* and *D. pteronyssinus*), cat epithelia, weeds (ragweed, *Parietaria*, mugwort), grasses (Bermuda, ryegrass, timothy, meadow), and tree pollens (birch, hazel, olive, cypress). To improve reliability of dosing and compliance, standardized tablet formulations were developed, and grass pollen SLIT tablets became commercially available and approved for the treatment of allergic rhinitis in 2009. The tablet formulation increases the stability of the product and ensures standardization of doses.[3] In pharmacologic terms the two formulations are equivalent; ultimately both result in a sublingual solution of allergen extract. However, use of tablets simplifies SLIT administration because tablets are easier to take than drops and minimize potential risks of dose administration errors.

THERAPEUTIC REGIMENS

Several large clinical trials have shown SLIT to be clinically effective, improving allergic rhinitis and asthma symptoms and reducing requirements for rescue medication.[4-8] It is widely used in Europe, especially France, Germany, and Italy. The allergen is held under the tongue for 2 minutes to allow optimal contact with the oral mucosa before being swallowed.

Proposed regimens include a rapid progressive increase in dose (with drops) and even a start-up dose at maintenance levels with recent lyophilized grass pollen tablets. SLIT delivers high doses of allergens, at 50- to 100-fold the doses used for subcutaneous immunotherapy (SCIT),[9] with no adjuvant, and has been shown to be safe with a low incidence of significant side effects. In addition to the safer profile, SLIT is administered at home, an additional advantage over injection immunotherapy, which requires clinic visits.

Proposed duration of treatment vary across the studies, but overall therapy for more than 12 months seems to be more effective, with 3 years suggested when grass pollen tablets are used. Favorable cost-benefit analysis has been presented, although not all health care systems have been convinced. SLIT vaccines are relatively expensive, especially compared with standard drug treatment for allergic rhinitis, and thus needs to be targeted to patients with significant disease.

Mucosal Tolerance

In conceptual terms, it is advantageous for animals not to react immunologically to their food. Most proteins encountered at the mucosal surface are harmless, and even if organisms are pathogenic, the crucial issue is whether they are capable of invasion, so the fiercest immune reactions are reserved for foreign proteins that can penetrate the gut or airway. The amount of protein in pollen grains and other inhaled allergenic particles is very small compared to that of dietary components, helping to explain why all people are not tolerant of inhalant allergens.

It has long been known that IgE responses to allergens can be reduced or prevented by prior oral administration of the allergen. Most evidence has been obtained in animal models. Oral tolerance involves several separate processes, which contribute to varying degrees depending on the dose and frequency of administration. In mouse models, oral tolerance can be induced either by a single high dose of antigen or by repeated administration of lower doses. High-dose tolerance appears to involve clonal T cell anergy, in which T cells become unresponsive on reexposure to allergen, failing to proliferate or to produce interleukin-2 (IL-2), or may involve deletion of relevant T cells. In contrast, low-dose exposure is mediated by regulatory T cells (Tregs), which actively control tolerance, preventing responses to food antigens and bacterial microflora. Tolerance can also be induced by T helper type 3 (Th3) cells (originally described in experimental allergic encephalomyelitis), which use transforming growth factor-β1 (TGF-β1) to achieve tolerance.

Of particular relevance to allergy, the ability of mouse strains to develop IgE antibodies against injected allergens can be prevented by early dietary exposure to the relevant allergen. This form of primary tolerance is different from the situation that pertains in clinical allergy, where one wants to switch off an established allergic response, but may be a useful model for studying some aspects of SLIT. The precise mechanisms by which "oral tolerance" is induced remain unclear, but the route of allergen processing and presentation seems likely to be important factors in determining whether and how T cells respond.

Tolerance in humans may be induced by several mechanisms, including the induction of secretory immunoglobulin A (IgA) antibodies, which bind foreign proteins and prevent their entry into the body without causing local inflammation. Another, likely more relevant mechanism is the development of Tregs, which can mediate suppression by direct cell-cell contact or through soluble immunoregulatory cytokines, principally IL-10 and TGF-β1.[10-12] Tregs have also been shown to deplete T cell numbers and induce T cell anergy (unresponsiveness to standard specific triggers of proliferation). Unlike the intestinal mucosa, which has areas of organized mucosa-associated lymphoid tissue that serve as inductive sites for the immune response, the oral mucosa has no organized aggregates of lymphoid cells.

However, the process of tolerization does appear to occur at the local level. The development and regulation of T cell responses are initially controlled by dendritic cells (DCs), specialized antigen-presenting cells (APCs) that can integrate a range of local signals to direct and orchestrate the adaptive immune response. The interactions between DCs and T cells determine whether the eventual response is active or tolerant, while preventing uncontrolled or inappropriate inflammation. As such, the DC is a key player in the development of mucosal tolerance.[12] Various functional DC phenotypes have been identified that seem to drive Th1, Th2, or Th17 effector cells or Tregs. Induction of a tolerogenic phenotype of DCs would therefore seem to be a key immunologic event in SLIT (or any other form of mucosal tolerance). In mouse models of SLIT, both Th2- and Th17-type cells can be detected, whereas human oral mucosa shows good evidence for local induction of Th17 cells; it is less clear whether Th2 cells are induced in the oral mucosa.[11-13]

In humans the predominant DCs in uninflamed oral mucosa are conventional Langerhans cells (LCs), which belong to the myeloid DC lineage; plasmacytoid DCs are virtually absent. The density of mucosal DCs varies in different parts of the pharynx. The sublingual area is not particularly rich in DCs compared with other areas of the pharynx and the palate, although the immunologic implications of this difference have not been fully explored. Oral LCs differ from skin LCs in their expression of various surface molecules involved in innate and adaptive immune responses. Oral LCs constitutively express the high-affinity IgE receptor (FcεRI), the IgG receptors FcγRII and FcγRIII, as well as Toll-like receptor 4 (TLR4).[11] Oral LCs also express the costimulatory molecules CD80 and CD86. This pattern of surface marker expression suggests a relatively immature LC phenotype because these receptors for IgE and IgG are downregulated on activation. In vitro studies suggest that immature DCs tend to drive T cell responses toward tolerance; ligation of TLR4 on DCs has been shown to upregulate their expression of IL-10 and TGF-β1 and leads to the induction of Tregs. Human oral DCs cultured in vitro with grass pollen antigens showed similar patterns of cytokine response,

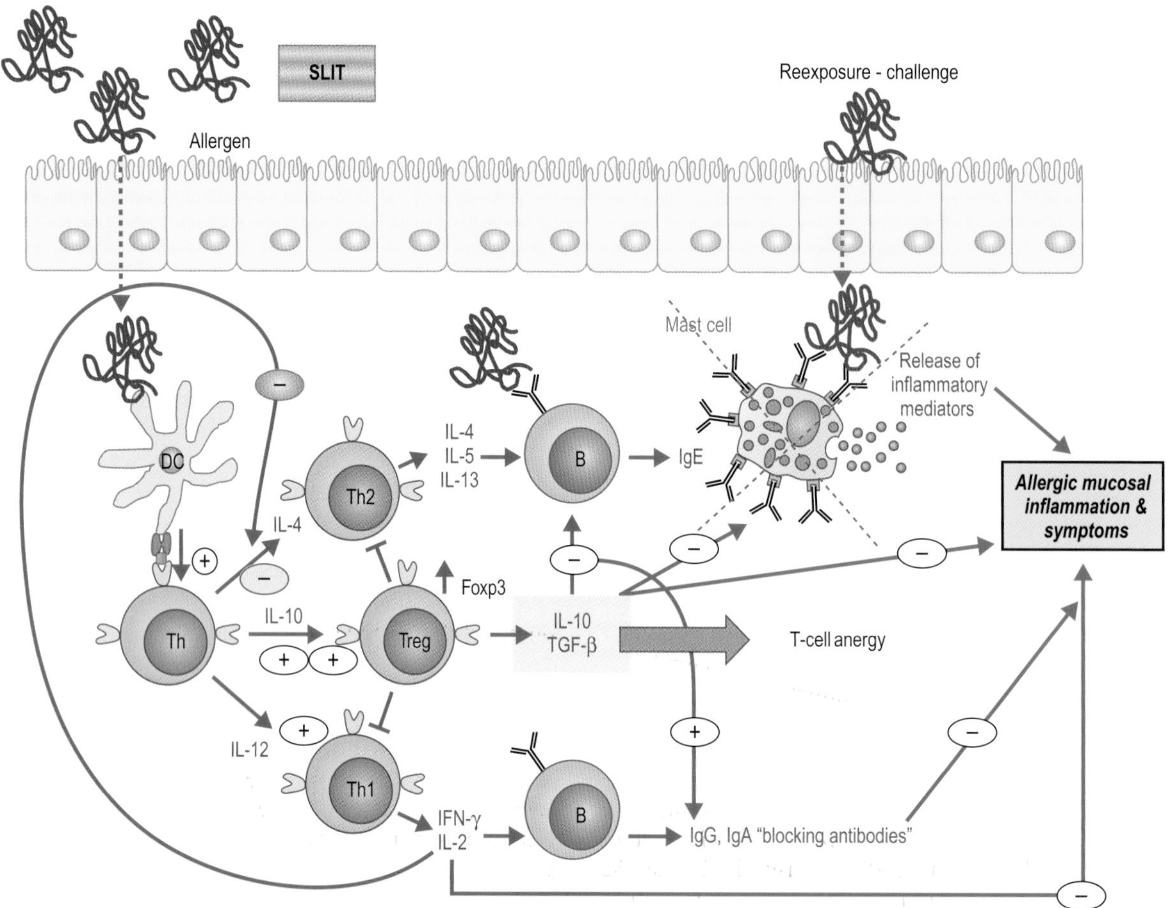

Figure 88-1 Immunologic mechanisms of specific sublingual immunotherapy (*SLIT*). Locally administered allergen using SLIT is taken up by mucosal dendritic cells (*DCs*) and then presented to T cells together with IL-12, biasing the response toward a Th1-like profile and away from the pro-IgE Th2 profile arbitrated by protolerogenic mechanisms mediated by the increased release of IL-10. There is enhanced secretion of interferon-γ (*IFN-γ*) and IL-2, which drive specific B cell production of nonpathogenic and protective IgG1 and IgG4 antibodies and decreased release of the Th2 pro-IgE cytokine IL-4. Oral mucosal DCs actively upregulate regulatory T cell (*Treg*) subtypes, including forkhead box P3 protein (*Foxp3*)–expressing T cells, contributing to T cell anergy mediated by IL-10 and transforming growth factor (*TGF-β*). These interconnected pathways lead to reduction in allergic inflammation and symptoms.

indicating their default tendency is toward tolerogenesis. Similarly, absorption of grass pollen antigen into human buccal mucosa attenuates the maturation of the mucosal LCs and enhances their ability to produce TGF-β1 and IL-10, which again supports the concept of DC-driven tolerance as the main mechanism of SLIT[11,12] (Fig. 88-1).

When allergens are placed in contact with the oral mucosa, a small amount of the allergenic material is absorbed into the mucosa (the rest is swallowed and digested, never reaching immunocompetent cells).[14] The fraction that is retained in the oral mucosa is taken up by DCs that migrate to the regional lymph nodes, as confirmed by radioactively labeled allergen studies.[15] Most of the radioactivity is absorbed after swallowing and appears in the plasma, peaking at 1 to 2 hours. Both standard allergens and chemically modified allergoids persist in the mouth for several hours, and small amounts can still be identified in the oral cavity up to 20 hours later. Absorption from sites other than the oral mucosa might also contribute to the immunologic stimulus from SLIT, although clinical data suggest little clinical benefit from allergens given orally and simply swallowed without a period of retention in the sublingual area.

Immunologic Mechanisms

The immunologic changes associated with successful SCIT have been studied in detail[16,17] (see Chapter 87). Molecular and cellular mechanisms include increased suppressor capacity of $CD4^+CD25^+$ forkhead box $P3^+$ protein ($Foxp3^+$) Tregs; enhanced suppressor activity of IL-10–secreting type 1 Tregs (Tr1); suppression of eosinophils, mast cells, and basophils; and antibody isotype switching from IgE to IgG4. Current data suggest that regulatory IL-10–producing Th1 cells are pivotal to the various changes induced by SIT. This may be driven by triggering TLRs on DCs, creating the necessary microenvironment for Tr1 induction. Chronic allergen exposure may then favor expansion of Th1-like Tr1 cells through IL-12 and IL-27 synthesis, as well as delta-4 expression on APCs. Recruitment of these cells into areas of inflammation will lead to amplification of local cytokine responses, including IL-12, IL-10, and TGF-β1. The IL-12 will skew any Th2 and Th17 cells toward the Th1 phenotype,[18] while IL-10 suppresses allergen-specific Th2 and Th17 responses, induces IgG4, and inhibits recruitment of mast cells, basophils, and eosinophils. Lastly, TGF-β1 blocks the Th2 response and decreases the activation of mast cells and eosinophils. Research in this area is now focused on identifying more efficient ways of inducing allergen-specific Tregs, including the use of appropriate immunologic adjuvants.

Most of these phenomena can also be found after SLIT[12,19,20] (Box 88-1 and see Fig. 88-1). In a murine model of SLIT, locally administered allergen was taken up by mucosal DCs and then presented to T cells together with IL-12, biasing the response toward a Th1-like profile and away from the pro-IgE Th2 profile. In human studies the immunologic response to SLIT is relatively modest, with smaller changes in specific IgE, specific IgG, and cytokines compared with those identified in patients treated with SCIT. However, induction of allergen-specific IgG4 is a consistent finding in most SLIT studies using large doses of allergen, as confirmed by a recent meta-analysis.[21] However, some studies reporting good clinical responses to SLIT have detected no change in allergen-specific IgE, IgG, or IgG4. This may partly reflect the timing of the immunologic analysis relative to the SLIT protocol, although doubts remain about the true relationship between changes in these immunologic measures and the delivery of clinical benefit.

T cell–proliferative responses to relevant allergens are reduced after SLIT.[22,23] An early study showed that after 4 weeks of birch pollen SLIT, higher frequencies of circulating $CD4^+CD25^+$ T cells were detected in conjunction with increased Foxp3 and IL-10 and decreased IL-4 and interferon-γ (IFN-γ) messenger RNA expression. T cell proliferation was greatly reduced after 4 and 52 weeks of treatment; at 4 weeks this effect could be reversed by depletion of $CD25^+$ cells or addition of anti–IL-10 antibodies, providing evidence of the important modulating role of Tregs and IL-10 in early SLIT. After 52 weeks, however, proliferation remained suppressed regardless of depletion of $CD25^+$ cells and addition of anti–IL-10 antibodies, suggesting that tolerance mechanisms other than active suppression by IL-10–producing Tregs are present during the later course of SLIT. In parallel, increased IFN-γ and reduction of IL-4, IL-10, and Foxp3 mRNA expression were detected. Neither TGF-β1 levels nor cell-cell contact–mediated suppression of $CD4^+CD25^+$ cells changed during the course of SLIT.[22] Inflammatory responses to allergen challenge are also attenuated.[24,25] For example, lower levels of intercellular adhesion molecule 1 (ICAM-1) protein in conjunctival fluid after provocation tests were found in patients receiving SLIT for house-dust mite (HDM) allergy than in control subjects.[25] Interestingly, SLIT appears to normalize the pattern of IL-10 production in response to allergen stimulation, restoring the response toward that seen in normal healthy subjects.

Subsequently, a randomized double-blind placebo-controlled trial of HDM SLIT provided further evidence that SLIT is associated with not only suppression of allergen-specific T cell proliferation and immune deviation, but also induction of functional regulatory T cells.[26] Clinically effective SLIT decreased allergen-induced $CD4^+$ T cell division and IL-5 production and increased IL-10 secretion (after 24 months of therapy) and serum Der p 2–specific IgG4. Recombinant human soluble TGF-β receptor II (sTGF-βRII)/Fc chimeric protein blocked immunotherapy-induced suppression of allergen-specific T cell proliferation after 6 months of therapy, whereas anti–IL-10R antibody did not restore HDM extract–induced proliferation, demonstrating the important role of the suppressive cytokine TGF-β as the mediator of early SLIT-induced suppression of the T cell responses to allergen. Significant increases in the proportions of Tregs were observed at 12 months of therapy, with a decline at 2 years, suggesting different phases of immunoregulatory mechanisms during treatment.[26]

Stimulation of IL-10–producing Tregs with SLIT has been further documented.[27] Allergen-induced Foxp3 mRNA expression was significantly increased after 2 years of grass pollen SLIT in children, and the changes in Foxp3 mRNA expression positively correlated with IL-10 and TGF-β mRNA during SLIT. An increase in allergen-induced IL-17 mRNA expression was also observed during SLIT treatment.[27]

In the recent large studies of SLIT with grass pollen tablets, the actively treated participants showed increased numbers of Foxp3-expressing peripheral blood mononuclear cells (PBMCs), together with elevated concentrations of allergen-specific IgG4 and IgA, and inhibition of IgE-facilitated allergen binding to B cells.[28] A recent pilot study evaluating the clinical efficacy and immunologic mechanisms of dual SLIT (HDM and timothy grass) demonstrated promotion of allergen-specific suppressive $CD4^+CD25(high)$-CD127(low)-$CD45RO^+$ $Foxp3^+$ memory Tregs with reduced DNA methylation of CpG sites within the Foxp3 locus.[29] An increase in allergen-specific IgG4 levels, reduced allergen-specific IgE levels, and subsequent basophil activation were also observed with dual SLIT. In another study, grass pollen SLIT–treated patients had increased expression of programmed cell death ligand (PDL1) on their B cells and monocytes during the pollen season, with concurrent reductions in IL-4,[30] suggesting a long-term effect on B cells.

Although considerable overlap seems to exist in the immune responses found in individual studies of SCIT and SLIT, some differences have been found between injection and sublingual SIT[31] in a comparative study of children sensitive to HDM (*D. pteronyssinus*) who received SLIT or SCIT over a 2-year period.[32] No differences were found between the sublingual and injection groups in terms of clinical outcomes or subjective evaluation, but increased specific IgE and IgG4 levels were detected only in the SCIT group, although the specific IgE/IgG4 ratio was reduced in both groups. Both groups showed an increase in CD4/CD8 ratio over the 2 years, but increases in $CD4^+CD25^+$ cells and decreases in $CD8^+CD25^+$ subsets in peripheral blood were only found in the SCIT group. Both groups showed reductions in intracellular cytokine production for tumor necrosis factor-α (TNF-α) and IL-2 production over time.[32] Therefore, although overlap exists, not all the phenomena reported after SCIT occur after SLIT. The existence of a different or additional mechanism for SLIT remains possible.

Recent studies have started to identify cellular markers of efficacy in SLIT.[33] If validated, these would be particularly helpful in guiding decisions on which patients to treat or continue to treat. For example, in a study of grass pollen SLIT, a series of markers associated with DCs were studied by

BOX 88-1 POSSIBLE MECHANISMS OF SUBLINGUAL IMMUNOTHERAPY

Induction of IgG (blocking) antibodies
Reduction in specific IgE (long term)
Reduced recruitment of effector cells
Altered helper T cell cytokine balance (shift to Th1 from Th2)
T cell anergy
B cell suppression
Increased regulatory T cell (Treg) function

quantitative polymerase chain reaction (PCR). Several markers were identified, linked to functional DC phenotypes that drive Th1 and Th17 differentiation. Expression of two of these markers, C1Q and STAB1, was increased in PBMCs from clinical responders to SLIT compared with PBMCs from nonresponders or placebo-treated patients. Increased expression of these two molecules may therefore represent an early indication that SLIT is likely to be effective. Further development of this concept may enable targeting of SLIT to patients who are most capable of responding.

Therapeutic Efficacy

Commercial SLIT allergen preparations may be lyophilized tablets or liquid extracts, which are usually given using a calibrated dropper. In contrast to injection SIT, SLIT regimens allow rapid buildup to the maintenance dose, and some preparations allow treatment to start with the same dose used for daily maintenance.

SIDE EFFECTS

Sublingual has a much safer profile than injection immunotherapy, but local side effects are common with SLIT, most frequently local irritation of the oral mucosa and sometimes local swelling. However, systemic reactions are extremely rare.[34] Caution is advised in patients who have experienced systemic side effects to other forms of SIT. Most local side effects seem to ease with repeated use, and these rarely lead patients to discontinue therapy. To avoid unnecessary discontinuation, patients should be supervised when they take their first doses. This allows any side effects to be discussed and set in context.

ALLERGIC RHINITIS

Several well-conducted clinical trials showed 30% to 40% reductions in symptom score and rescue medication use in patients with seasonal allergic rhinitis after SLIT.[5,7,8,21,35-37] Before these large studies, the data were less convincing; many trials were underpowered or of short duration. From these early studies, however, meta-analysis concluded that SLIT was effective, even if the magnitude of the benefit was difficult to determine. This meta-analysis has been superseded by a series of large clinical trials with modern commercial products, and a large body of evidence on the efficacy of SLIT now exists for pollen allergy.[7,36]

One of the first large studies of grass pollen SLIT was a double-blind placebo-controlled trial conducted with a timothy grass pollen tablet (Grazax ALK) to treat allergic rhinoconjunctivitis, given over 3 years to patients who only had clinically significant symptoms on exposure to grass pollen (those with clinically significant symptoms to other allergens were excluded).[6] The primary outcome measure was a combined symptom-medication score, assessed across the whole of the grass pollen season. There was a 33% difference in favor of active SLIT in the first season, which increased to 41% in the second and 36% in the third pollen season. The effect of SLIT on quality of life was also addressed, with a 21% improvement in quality-of-life scores (RQLQ) in those who received grass pollen tablets compared to those receiving placebo. Moreover, quality-of-life measures were 26% better with SLIT than antihistamines alone.

After 3 years, SLIT was discontinued, and follow-up maintained double-blind conditions, for a further two pollen seasons, to assess whether the treatment provided lasting benefit.[36] A clinically and statistically significant benefit persisted, with symptom-medication scores showing a 34% difference in the first and 27% in the second posttreatment year. The pollen counts were somewhat lower in the final year than in the previous 4 years, which may have artificially lowered the observed difference. Further follow-up is not planned; both morally and practically it was not possible to continue to study patients who had already gone untreated for 5 years. These extended clinical benefits were accompanied by persistent elevations in allergen-specific IgG4 and other treatment-associated antibody changes. A subsequent study of this same timothy grass preparation in 439 North American adults found differences of 18% to 26% in symptom-medication scores in favor of active therapy in the first year of treatment.

Overall the Grazax studies indicate that clinically significant benefits can be achieved in the first year of SLIT, but the magnitude of benefit does not seem to increase much in the second and third years. However, the years 2 and 3 of SLIT may well contribute to the durability of the response, which we can now say with confidence extends for at least 2 years after therapy, supporting open-label clinical practice reports of benefits up to 7 years after ceasing SLIT.

Another commercial grass pollen tablet, containing a mixture of pollens from five grasses (Oralair, Stallergenes), has also shown clinical benefit in a 3-year double-blind placebo-controlled study, performed in 633 subjects who started treatment either 2 or 4 months before the pollen season and continued until the end of each season.[38] By year 3 of treatment, differences of 34.6% to 36% were found in symptom scores, with no particular benefit for starting 4 months before the pollen season than just 2 months preseasonal SLIT. Local adverse effects became less troublesome with each successive year of treatment. These data are comparable to those in the timothy grass tablet study previously discussed,[6] although from a technical perspective, the mixed-grass pollen tablet study was better designed, planned from the outset as a 5-year study.[38] This study has also been extended into a posttreatment period. In the first year off therapy, among those who had started with more severe disease, the actively treated group showed a 34% difference in adjusted symptom scores. However, there was no detectable persisting benefit in the groups with milder disease.

These large trials have confirmed the clinical efficacy of tablet SLIT for grass pollen–induced allergic rhinitis and the persistence of benefit after cessation of therapy for at least 2 years after ceasing SLIT.[4,36,38-40] It seems unlikely that any longer-term studies will be conducted in the near future.

Pediatric Studies

Grass pollen SLIT has also been studied in children and adolescents. Both in Europe and North America, timothy grass pollen tablets were well tolerated and achieved levels of benefit comparable to those found in adults.[41,42] In the North American study, 89% of patients were sensitized to multiple allergens (more than in comparable European studies); in the first year of treatment, total symptom and medication scores were 26% less in the actively treated group, whereas quality-of-life scores for rhinitis were 18% better in the active group.[42] In the European study, 256 children age 5 to 16 years were recruited, 234 of whom completed the trial.[41] Combined symptom-medication scores showed a median difference of 34% over the whole season, with a 65% difference during the peak pollen season. A similar benefit in favor of active SLIT was observed for asthma symptoms (64% over whole season). Allergen-specific IgG4 levels increased in the actively treated group, as previously observed in studies of adults.

These positive outcomes for timothy grass pollen tablets contrast with earlier studies in children that found no benefit for grass pollen SLIT, using liquid preparations (administered as drops).[43] It remains unclear whether these discordant results reflect the way the SLIT was given (drops versus tablets) or perhaps a less severely affected group of children; SLIT appears to have more impact in those with more prominent symptoms. Furthermore, differences in delivered doses may have accounted for the discrepant results with earlier studies. A recent double-blind placebo-controlled trial in 207 children with single high-dose SLIT using an aqueous extract of grass pollen demonstrated clear benefit, improving symptoms, reducing medication requirements, and increasing number of well days.[44]

Other Allergens

Sublingual immunotherapy has been most extensively tested in grass pollen allergy, but tablet-based therapies are currently being developed for tree pollen allergy, HDM allergy, and animal dander. Earlier forms of SLIT, in small studies using liquid preparations (drops), have shown some clinical benefit with concurrent immunologic effects,[26] as described in the previous section. In this particular study, HDM SLIT reduced allergic rhinitis symptom scores after 1 year of treatment. In a recent systematic review, HDM SLIT had the highest standardized mean difference (SMD) favoring SLIT of −0.97 (95% CI −1.8, −0.3) and appeared more effective than treatment with other allergen types and even more effective than treatment with grass pollen, which was shown to have an SMD of −0.35 (−0.45, −0.24).[45]

However, the majority of trials with HDM SLIT are small, heterogeneity in this group is high, and level of significance is lower than in the recent review. Therefore caution is required when interpreting these findings; larger studies are awaited. HDM SLIT showed reduction of conjunctival sensitivity to *D. pteronyssinus* and also improved symptoms.[45] A recent U.S. study tested SLIT with *D. farinae* extract, given as drops, in adults.[46] The treatment was well tolerated, and changes were found in immunologic parameters (increased IgG4) consistent with other SLIT studies. The threshold response to inhaled *D. farinae* also increased, but the study was underpowered to demonstrate benefits on symptom-medication scores. A Korean study of HDM SLIT found that polysensitized patients responded as well as monosensitized patients, although there was no placebo group.[45] In a cautionary note, however, a Dutch study of HDM SLIT in primary care children detected no clinical benefit.[47] As with similar findings in grass pollen allergy, it remains unclear whether this lack of effect is caused by the type of preparation used for SLIT or the relatively mild degree of symptoms encountered in this particular study population.

Taking these data into consideration, further large-scale placebo-controlled studies are needed in well-defined patient groups before SLIT can be recommended for HDM allergy.

ASTHMA

The vast majority of studies with SLIT evaluated participants with allergic rhinitis with or without asthma. SLIT appears to reduce asthma symptoms and medication scores after 2 years of treatment,[26] observed across most studies of SLIT, especially for HDM allergy.[48] The magnitude of this effect seems comparable to the effect on allergic rhinitis symptoms, but somewhat smaller for medication scores, as suggested by a recent meta-analysis of studies of HDM SLIT.[48] There was significant inter-study heterogeneity, however, and more robust data are needed from large studies with objective, well-defined outcomes for asthma. An open, randomized controlled trial (RCT) evaluating the effect of birch pollen SLIT in the pollen seasons as an add-on therapy to the standard therapy compared with the addition of montelukast for persistent moderate asthma showed that bronchial and nasal symptom scores were lower at 3 and 5 years than baseline in the SLIT group. Airway hyperreactivity and bronchodilator use decreased significantly in both groups at 5 years, but only in the SLIT group at 3 years. Subjects who received SLIT demonstrated a significant decrease in nasal eosinophils from baseline and the montelukast group.[49]

Further larger studies are needed. SLIT is currently recommended for patients with allergic rhinitis, with or without asthma, but is not currently recommended specifically for treatment of asthma.

DURABILITY OF TREATMENT

A key question in deciding on how widely to use SLIT is how long the benefits of therapy extend beyond the period of treatment. Maintaining double-blind trials for years after completion of therapy is extremely difficult, both for the investigators and for the participants who go without treatment for years to answer the question properly. Evidence from long-term follow-up of open-label therapy showed that the longer the course of treatment, the longer the benefit persists.[50] Five years of SLIT gave benefits for at least 7 years,[51] whereas the benefit of 3 or 4 years of SLIT seemed to wear off more quickly.[36,52] The more recent, double-blind placebo-controlled studies allow assessment to continue for 2 years after completing therapy, although longer-term follow-up seems unlikely. Unfortunately, accurate cost-benefit analysis requires an estimate of the durability of therapy, so the lack of long-term data remains a problem.

Effects on Natural History of Allergic Disease

There is considerable interest in the possibility that SIT may modify the course of allergic disease. If proved, this effect would dramatically alter the economic argument in favor of SIT, since one could discount the costs of treatment against the costs of the future condition that has been avoided. Data have been presented in two areas: prevention of new sensitizations and prevention of asthma.

Atopic children typically have a limited range of sensitivities when they first present, but with time they go on to develop IgE against more allergens. Both injection and sublingual SIT have been shown to limit this tendency, but some caution is needed in interpreting the clinical benefit of this observation. Studies of HDM SIT and grass pollen SIT have shown 50% reductions in the probability of developing additional sensitivities. This benefit seems to be long-lasting and has been shown up to 12 years after completing SIT. In a comparable study of SLIT, only 3% of treated children acquired new sensitivities over

3 years, versus 34% of untreated children.[53] It seems unlikely that SIT with one allergen directly affects B cells that recognize unrelated allergens. However, SIT might reduce nasal inflammation and thereby alter the local environment to make it less likely that exposure to other allergens will lead to sensitization.

Allergen-specific immunotherapy has also been shown to modify the risk of developing asthma in children with allergic rhinitis.[54] Although only limited data support this proposition, an open but randomized study using SIT for birch or grass pollen allergy in 205 children age 6 to 14 years without previously diagnosed asthma has offered strongly supportive evidence. Three years after completing SIT, 45% of those who remained untreated had developed asthma, but only 26% of the treated group had clinical asthma. These results seem robust, and the differences were sustained over the next 7 years, without further SIT. In terms of the number needed to treat, using SIT in four children prevented one case of asthma developing. SLIT also seems capable of achieving this outcome. In a 3-year study of 89 children, 18 of 44 control subjects developed asthma, versus only 8 of 45 SLIT-treated children. A more formal trial of this concept is now under way (the GAP study) and will report in a few years.[55]

Specific immunotherapy may also modify the course of asthma that has become established. The most convincing data come from a 1950s randomized study that used uncharacterized mixed-allergen extracts.[55a] The methodology can be criticized, but the observed benefits were reasonably convincing, with about 70% of treated children having no asthma symptoms after 4 years of SIT, versus only 19% of untreated controls. Moreover, far fewer children in the treated group were classified as "severe" at age 16 than in the untreated group. Although conducting such a study would be difficult today, the data are useful in confirming the potential of SIT to reduce both the duration and the severity of asthma. No similar study has been done with modern injection SIT. However, a prospective, nonrandomized, open-label study of SLIT reported that asthmatic children who received SLIT were less likely to have asthma after 4 to 5 years than those receiving standard antiasthma medication, and the benefit was sustained for 5 years after completing SLIT. Further work is needed to confirm this in a larger study.

In summary, both subcutaneous and sublingual SIT appear to modify the course of allergic disease, by reducing the incidence of new sensitizations, and by either preventing the development of clinical asthma or speeding up its resolution. The mechanism remains unclear but likely involves a combination of immunologic effects and downstream changes to the structure and function of the small airways. Better data are needed, but if confirmed, these disease-modifying and preventive effects of SIT would have a major impact on any cost–benefit analysis.

Safety and Cost-Effectiveness

One of the main drivers for the development of SLIT was the awareness of risks associated with SCIT. Although SIT is usually quite safe in patients who do not have asthma, occasional serious adverse events do happen, but these are rarely fatal. In most reports the rate of serious systemic reactions in patients with rhinitis is about 1 in 500 injections. The major risk of fatal outcome is in patients with unstable asthma given SIT injections, whose risk of systemic reactions may be as high as 35%, although most reports cite a rate of about 1 in 20 injections.[56]

Most clinical trials of SLIT have reported local side effects, particularly itching of the mouth and palate.[56,57] However, few serious systemic side effects were reported in the major trials or in the earlier literature. Since these sublingual drugs became available, a small number of serious adverse events have been reported. The first report of anaphylaxis to SLIT was in a North American patient given a personalized mixture of *Alternaria*, cat, dog, grass, ragweed, and mixed-weed pollen.[58] This adverse event occurred with a nonstandardized regimen but raised legitimate concerns. More troublesome, another report described two patients who had systemic reactions to SLIT taken at home, after being prescribed SLIT because they had problems with conventional injection SIT.[59] Neither reaction was witnessed by medical personnel, so some doubt remains about their precise nature, but clearly caution is required if SLIT is considered for such patients. Normally the first dose of SLIT should be taken in the physician's office, particularly in patients who previously experienced problems with SIT. More often, grade 2 or 3 reactions are reported; in some series, up to 11.6% of patients had experienced wheezing or worsening of nasal symptoms after a SLIT dose, although the overall frequency of systemic adverse reactions was only 1 in 3000 doses.

Patients with autoimmune, malignant, or cardiac disease should not receive SIT. Those with autoimmune or malignant disease face the theoretic risk of exacerbating their condition while attempting to alter the immune system by SIT. Cardiac patients are excluded because they are less able to withstand the effects of systemic adverse reactions, and patients taking β-adrenergic blockers are excluded because they may not respond to epinephrine if this is needed to treat systemic adverse reactions. The same considerations are usually applied to SLIT, although the risks may be less than with injection SIT.

No discussion of new therapeutic options is complete without consideration of the economic aspects. Rhinoconjunctivitis is a common condition, and standard therapies such as antihistamines and even nasal corticosteroids are relatively inexpensive compared with forms of SIT. SLIT offers improvements that cannot be achieved by standard pharmacotherapy, but it is a relatively expensive option, whereas antihistamine therapy will be adjusted according to symptoms. Cost-effectiveness analysis requires assumptions on the likely durability of benefits and the period over which they impact relevant financial outcomes. Some evidence of cost-effectiveness has been presented from the principal study of grass pollen tablets (Grazax) in seven countries of northern Europe.[60] The outcome measure was quality-adjusted life years (QALY), indicating a cost of 13,000 to 18,000 euros ($17,000 to $25,000 USD) per QALY gained. The benefit comprised reductions in rescue medication and fewer hours lost from work (production loss). The analysis used a horizon of 9 years and assumed that the clinical benefit achieved in the first years of therapy would be sustained throughout. On this basis, tablet-based SLIT could be considered as cost-effective at current prices compared with standard thresholds applied by national regulatory bodies. Similar data have been presented for southern Europe centers from the same trial.

Future Directions

Future developments in SLIT may take several forms, including mucoadhesives, allergoids, adjuvants, and new allergens (latex, foods). The delivery of allergen may be improved by creating formulations that adhere to the mucosa and deliver the necessary amount of allergen more efficiently. These mucoadhesives could allow smaller amounts of allergen to be given, thereby reducing the risk of local side effects and adverse reactions. The efficiency of SLIT might also be improved by more persistent presence of the allergen. Experimental data from a mouse model of asthma suggest this may be effective, with various forms of mucoadhesives described, including chitosan particles and maltodextrin conjugates.[61] This approach has not yet been tested in humans.

As with injection SIT, it may be possible to use modified allergens. For example, allergoids retain the ability to stimulate T cells while having reduced binding to IgE. This should reduce side effects and has been tested in patients with grass pollen allergy, in whom it appears effective, both when given as SLIT year-round and when used preseasonally only for 10 weeks. Significant improvements were found in visual analog scores in the first season of SLIT, and reduction in medication use followed in the second year of SLIT.[62]

Adjuvants that selectively induce IL-10 could also enhance the efficacy of SLIT vaccines. A combination of dexamethasone and 1,25-dihydroxyvitamin D_3 inhibits lipopolysaccharide-induced DC maturation and induces IL-10 production by human and murine DCs, leading to differentiation of $CD4^+$ naïve T cells toward a Treg profile. Another adjuvant, *Lactobacillus plantarum,* induces DC maturation toward a mixed Th1/Treg pattern of differentiation. Both these adjuvants have enhanced the efficacy of SLIT in a mouse model of asthma.[63]

Summary

Allergen-specific immunotherapy has been used for more than 100 years to treat patients with allergic conditions. Treatment by the sublingual route is becoming increasingly popular in Europe and is now being adopted in the United States. SLIT appears to be as effective as SCIT for allergic rhinitis and is more convenient for patients. The precise mechanisms of SIT action remain uncertain. Both SCIT and SLIT are associated with induction of regulatory T cells, expression of IL-10 and TGF-β1, and secretion of allergen-specific IgG4. Additional mechanisms may also operate in SLIT. The major threat to future use of SLIT is the lack of comprehensive cost-effectiveness data, which is increasingly required by health care providers in deciding which treatments to fund. Future SLIT developments will include a wider range of allergens, adaptations with mucoadhesives and adjuvants to refine the mucosal response, and research into the durability of responses to determine cost-effectiveness.

REFERENCES

Background

1. Frew AJ. Sublingual immunotherapy. N Engl J Med 2008;358:2259-64.
2. Moingeon P. Sublingual immunotherapy: from biological extracts to recombinant allergens. Allergy 2006;61(Suppl 81):15-9.
3. Didier A. Future developments in sublingual immunotherapy. Allergy 2006;61(Suppl 81): 29-31.
4. Nelson HS, Nolte H, Creticos P, et al. Efficacy and safety of timothy grass allergy immunotherapy tablet treatment in North American adults. J Allergy Clin Immunol 2011;127:72-80.
5. Durham SR, Emminger W, Kapp A, et al. Long-term clinical efficacy in grass pollen–induced rhinoconjunctivitis after treatment with SQ-standardized grass allergy immunotherapy tablet. J Allergy Clin Immunol 2010; 125:131-8.
6. Dahl R, Kapp A, Colombo G, et al. Sublingual grass allergen tablet immunotherapy provides sustained clinical benefit with progressive immunologic changes over 2 years. J Allergy Clin Immunol 2008;121:512-8.
7. Dahl R, Kapp A, Colombo G, et al. Efficacy and safety of sublingual immunotherapy with grass allergen tablets for seasonal allergic rhinoconjunctivitis. J Allergy Clin Immunol 2006;118: 434-40.
8. Radulovic S, Wilson D, Calderon M, Durham S. Systematic reviews of sublingual immunotherapy (SLIT). Allergy 2011;66:740-52.
9. Moingeon P, Mascarell L. Induction of tolerance via the sublingual route: mechanisms and applications. Clin Dev Immunol 2012;2012:623474.

Mucosal Tolerance

10. Allam JP, Bieber T, Novak N. Dendritic cells as potential targets for mucosal immunotherapy. Curr Opin Allergy Clin Immunol 2009;9:554-7.
11. Novak N, Allam JP. Mucosal dendritic cells in allergy and immunotherapy. Allergy 2011;66 (Suppl 95):22-4.
12. Novak N, Bieber T, Allam JP. Immunological mechanisms of sublingual allergen-specific immunotherapy. Allergy 2011;66:733-9.
13. Allam JP, Novak N. Local immunological mechanisms of sublingual immunotherapy. Curr Opin Allergy Clin Immunol 2011;11:571-8.
14. Bagnasco M, Altrinetti V, Pesce G, et al. Pharmacokinetics of Der p 2 allergen and derived monomeric allergoid in allergic volunteers. Int Arch Allergy Immunol 2005;138:197-202.
15. Allam JP, Wurtzen PA, Reinartz M, et al. Phl p 5 resorption in human oral mucosa leads to dose-dependent and time-dependent allergen binding by oral mucosal Langerhans cells, attenuates their maturation, and enhances their migratory and TGF-β1 and IL-10-producing properties. J Allergy Clin Immunol 2010;126:638-45.

Immunologic Mechanisms

16. Jutel M, Akdis CA. Immunological mechanisms of allergen-specific immunotherapy. Allergy 2011;66:725-32.
17. Rolland JM, Gardner LM, O'Hehir RE. Functional regulatory T cells and allergen immunotherapy. Curr Opin Allergy Clin Immunol 2010;10:559-66.
18. Ebner C, Siemann U, Bohle B, et al. Immunological changes during specific immunotherapy of grass pollen allergy: reduced lymphoproliferative responses to allergen and shift from TH2 to TH1 in T-cell clones specific for Phl p 1, a major grass pollen allergen. Clin Exp Allergy 1997;27:1007-15.
19. O'Hehir RE, Sandrini A, Anderson GP, Rolland JM. Sublingual allergen immunotherapy: immunological mechanisms and prospects for refined vaccine preparation. Curr Med Chem 2007;14:2235-44.
20. Scadding G, Durham SR. Mechanisms of sublingual immunotherapy. Immunol Allergy Clin North Am 2011;31:191-209, viii.
21. Radulovic S, Calderon MA, Wilson D, Durham S. Sublingual immunotherapy for allergic rhinitis. Cochrane Database Syst Rev 2010;(12): CD002893.
22. Bohle B, Kinaciyan T, Gerstmayr M, et al. Sublingual immunotherapy induces IL-10-producing T regulatory cells, allergen-specific T-cell tolerance, and immune deviation. J Allergy Clin Immunol 2007;120:707-13.
23. Ciprandi G, Fenoglio D, Cirillo I, et al. Induction of interleukin 10 by sublingual immunotherapy for house dust mites: a preliminary report. Ann Allergy Asthma Immunol 2005;95: 38-44.
24. Fenoglio D, Puppo F, Cirillo I, et al. Sublingual specific immunotherapy reduces PBMC proliferations. Eur Ann Allergy Clin Immunol 2005;37:147-51.
25. Passalacqua G, Albano M, Fregonese L, et al. Randomised controlled trial of local allergoid immunotherapy on allergic inflammation in mite-induced rhinoconjunctivitis. Lancet 1998; 351(9103):629-32.
26. O'Hehir RE, Gardner LM, de Leon MP, et al. House dust mite sublingual immunotherapy: the role for transforming growth factor-beta and functional regulatory T cells. Am J Respir Crit Care Med 2009;180:936-47.
27. Nieminen K, Valovirta E, Savolainen J. Clinical outcome and IL-17, IL-23, IL-27 and Foxp3 expression in peripheral blood mononuclear cells of pollen-allergic children during sublingual immunotherapy. Pediatr Allergy Immunol 2010;21(1 Pt 2):e174-84.
28. Scadding GW, Shamji MH, Jacobson MR, et al. Sublingual grass pollen immunotherapy is associated with increases in sublingual Foxp3-expressing cells and elevated allergen-specific

immunoglobulin G4, immunoglobulin A and serum inhibitory activity for immunoglobulin E–facilitated allergen binding to B cells. Clin Exp Allergy 2010;40:598-606.
29. Swamy RS, Reshamwala N, Hunter T, et al. Epigenetic modifications and improved regulatory T-cell function in subjects undergoing dual sublingual immunotherapy. J Allergy Clin Immunol 2012;130:214-24.
30. Piconi S, Trabattoni D, Rainone V, et al. Immunological effects of sublingual immunotherapy: clinical efficacy is associated with modulation of programmed cell death ligand 1, IL-10, and IgG4. J Immunol 2010;185:7723-30.
31. Maggi E, Vultaggio A, Matucci A. T-cell responses during allergen-specific immunotherapy. Curr Opin Allergy Clin Immunol 2012;12:1-6.
32. Antunez C, Mayorga C, Corzo JL, Jurado A, Torres MJ. Two year follow-up of immunological response in mite-allergic children treated with sublingual immunotherapy: comparison with subcutaneous administration. Pediatr Allergy Immunol 2008;19:210-8.
33. Zimmer A, Bouley J, Le Mignon M, et al. A regulatory dendritic cell signature correlates with the clinical efficacy of allergen-specific sublingual immunotherapy. J Allergy Clin Immunol 2012; 129:1020-30.

Therapeutic Efficacy

34. Moingeon P, Mascarell L. Novel routes for allergen immunotherapy: safety, efficacy and mode of action. Immunotherapy 2012;4:201-12.
35. Calderon MA, Penagos M, Durham SR. Sublingual immunotherapy for allergic rhinoconjunctivitis, allergic asthma, and prevention of allergic diseases. Clin Allergy Immunol 2008; 21:359-75.
36. Durham SR, Emminger W, Kapp A, et al. SQ-standardized sublingual grass immunotherapy: confirmation of disease modification 2 years after 3 years of treatment in a randomized trial. J Allergy Clin Immunol 2012;129: 717-25.
37. Bousquet J, Schunemann HJ, Bousquet PJ, et al. How to design and evaluate randomized controlled trials in immunotherapy for allergic rhinitis: an ARIA-GA(2) LEN statement. Allergy 2011;66:765-74.
38. Didier A, Worm M, Horak F, et al. Sustained 3-year efficacy of pre- and co-seasonal 5-grass-pollen sublingual immunotherapy tablets in patients with grass pollen–induced rhinoconjunctivitis. J Allergy Clin Immunol 2011;128: 559-66.
39. Rak S, Yang WH, Pedersen MR, Durham SR. Once-daily sublingual allergen-specific immunotherapy improves quality of life in patients with grass pollen–induced allergic rhinoconjunctivitis: a double-blind, randomised study. Qual Life Res 2007;16:191-201.
40. Malling HJ, Montagut A, Melac M, et al. Efficacy and safety of 5-grass pollen sublingual immunotherapy tablets in patients with different clinical profiles of allergic rhinoconjunctivitis. Clin Exp Allergy 2009;39:387-93.
41. Bufe A, Eberle P, Franke-Beckmann E, et al. Safety and efficacy in children of an SQ-standardized grass allergen tablet for sublingual immunotherapy. J Allergy Clin Immunol 2009; 123:167-73.
42. Blaiss M, Maloney J, Nolte H, et al. Efficacy and safety of timothy grass allergy immunotherapy tablets in North American children and adolescents. J Allergy Clin Immunol 2011;127:64-71.
43. Roder E, Berger MY, Hop WC, et al. Sublingual immunotherapy with grass pollen is not effective in symptomatic youngsters in primary care. J Allergy Clin Immunol 2007;119:892-8.
44. Wahn U, Klimek L, Ploszczuk A, et al. High-dose sublingual immunotherapy with single-dose aqueous grass pollen extract in children is effective and safe: a double-blind, placebo-controlled study. J Allergy Clin Immunol 2012; 130:886-93.
45. Lee JE, Choi YS, Kim MS, et al. Efficacy of sublingual immunotherapy with house dust mite extract in polyallergen sensitized patients with allergic rhinitis. Ann Allergy Asthma Immunol 2011;107:79-84.
46. Bush RK, Swenson C, Fahlberg B, et al. House dust mite sublingual immunotherapy: results of a US trial. J Allergy Clin Immunol 2011;127: 974-81.
47. De Bot CM, Moed H, Berger MY, et al. Sublingual immunotherapy not effective in house dust mite-allergic children in primary care. Pediatr Allergy Immunol 2012;23:150-8.
48. Compalati E, Passalacqua G, Bonini M, Canonica GW. The efficacy of sublingual immunotherapy for house dust mites respiratory allergy: results of a GA2LEN meta-analysis. Allergy 2009;64:1570-9.
49. Marogna M, Colombo F, Spadolini I, et al. Randomized open comparison of montelukast and sublingual immunotherapy as add-on treatment in moderate persistent asthma due to birch pollen. J Investig Allergol Clin Immunol 2010;20:146-52.
50. Di Rienzo V, Marcucci F, Puccinelli P, et al. Long-lasting effect of sublingual immunotherapy in children with asthma due to house dust mite: a 10-year prospective study. Clin Exp Allergy 2003;33:206-10.
51. Marogna M, Spadolini I, Massolo A, Canonica GW, Passalacqua G. Long-lasting effects of sublingual immunotherapy according to its duration: a 15-year prospective study. J Allergy Clinl Immunol 2010;126:969-75.
52. Eifan AO, Shamji MH, Durham SR. Long-term clinical and immunological effects of allergen immunotherapy. Curr Opin Allergy Clin Immunol 2011;11:586-93.

Effects on Natural History of Allergic Disease

53. Marogna M, Tomassetti D, Bernasconi A, et al. Preventive effects of sublingual immunotherapy in childhood: an open randomized controlled study. Ann Allergy Asthma Immunol 2008;101: 206-11.
54. Novembre E, Galli E, Landi F, et al. Coseasonal sublingual immunotherapy reduces the development of asthma in children with allergic rhinoconjunctivitis. J Allergy Clin Immunol 2004;114:851-7.
55. Valovirta E. Effect of AIT in children including potential to prevent the development of asthma. Allergy 2011;66(Suppl 95):53-4.
55a. Johnstone DE, Dutton A. The value of hyposensitization therapy for bronchial asthma in children—a 14-year study. Pediatrics 1968;42: 793–802.

Safety and Cost-Effectiveness

56. Bernstein DI, Wanner M, Borish L, Liss GM. Twelve-year survey of fatal reactions to allergen injections and skin testing. J Allergy Clin Immunol 2004;113:1129–36.
57. Rodriguez-Perez N, Ambriz-Moreno Mde J, Canonica GW, Penagos M. Frequency of acute systemic reactions in patients with allergic rhinitis and asthma treated with sublingual immunotherapy. Ann Allergy Asthma Immunol 2008; 101:304-10.
58. Dunsky EH, Goldstein MF, Dvorin DJ, Belecanech GA. Anaphylaxis to sublingual immunotherapy. Allergy 2006;61:1235.
59. De Groot H, Bijl A. Anaphylactic reaction after the first dose of sublingual immunotherapy with grass pollen tablet. Allergy 2009;64: 963-4.
60. Bachert C, Vestenbaek U, Christensen J, Griffiths UK, Poulsen PB. Cost-effectiveness of grass allergen tablet (Grazax) for the prevention of seasonal grass pollen induced rhinoconjunctivitis: a Northern European perspective. Clin Exp Allergy 2007;37:772-9.

Future Directions

61. Saint-Lu N, Tourdot S, Razafindratsita A, et al. Targeting the allergen to oral dendritic cells with mucoadhesive chitosan particles enhances tolerance induction. Allergy 2009;64:1003-13.
62. Quercia O, Bruno ME, Compalati E, et al. Efficacy and safety of sublingual immunotherapy with grass monomeric allergoid: comparison between two different treatment regimens. Eur Ann Allergy Clin Immunol 2011;43: 176-83.
63. Van Overtvelt L, Lombardi V, Razafindratsita A, et al. IL-10-inducing adjuvants enhance sublingual immunotherapy efficacy in a murine asthma model. Int Arch Allergy Immunol 2008; 145:152-62.

Principles of Pharmacotherapeutics

H. WILLIAM KELLY | HENGAMEH H. RAISSY

CONTENTS

SUMMARY OF IMPORTANT CONCEPTS

» Individual patient response to drug therapy represents a confluence of pharmacology, pharmacokinetics, pathophysiology, age, gender, genetics, and patient adherence.

» Receptor theory is essential to understanding drug action and states that drugs act as agonists, antagonists, or inverse agonists of physiologic receptors and thus can only mimic, intensify, inhibit, or block normal physiologic responses.

» Dose response has two critical aspects: most drugs exhibit a log-linear dose to effect and a ceiling at about 80% of maximum, where further increases result in diminishing results, and pathophysiologic conditions can alter dose response.

» Drug efficacy and safety are not altered by making the drug more potent and merely determine the dose required to produce the pharmacologic effect; however, both can be improved by receptor targeting (delivery method, pharmacokinetic changes).

» Patient pathophysiology, comorbidities, and other therapies all can profoundly affect the dose-response curve of a drug for both efficacy and safety.

Introduction

This chapter provides an overview of the pharmacotherapeutic principles that affect the individual patient response to medication administration. Specific aspects of drugs used in the therapy of asthma and allergy are used to illustrate these principles. These examples are not meant to confer superiority of one product or one form of therapy over another, but rather to convey how knowledge of these principles is used to individualize patient therapy to achieve optimal outcomes. More in-depth discussions of the pharmacology, pharmacokinetics, and pharmacodynamics are found in the individual chapters for each drug class.

Factors affecting therapeutic response can be categorized broadly as either *drug* or *patient* factors. Drug factors include pharmacologic properties, structure-activity relationships, physicochemical properties (e.g., lipophilicity or hydrophilicity), formulation or delivery system, and mechanism of elimination from the body. Patient factors include both normal physiologic variables and pathophysiologic differences. Physiologic variables include age, gender, and genetic background, as well as normal diurnal patterns and dietary differences. Pathophysiologic differences include disease state and disease severity, concomitant diseases (comorbidities), and concurrent therapies. Figure 89-1 depicts the factors involved in determining the response to any given pharmacotherapeutic intervention.

Goals of Therapy

The general goal of therapy of any disease is to minimize the impact of the disease on the patient's life. This includes measures to relieve symptoms, prevent disease progression, prevent morbidity and mortality, and minimize the potential for adverse effects of the medication. Ideally, these goals would be achieved with the most convenient and affordable medication; however, the ultimate goal is to provide the most cost-effective therapy (i.e., therapy that provides greatest degree of health for cost). Realistically, the ideal goal of "normal health" (cure of the disease) may not be achievable in either asthma or other allergic disorders; therefore both the clinician and the patient often must make compromises to derive the best achievable outcome.

Although understanding of clinical pharmacologic principles is essential to the rational use of medications, achieving optimal therapeutic outcomes requires attention to a multitude of factors, including numerous psychosocial issues that can also affect success of therapy. Thus, to be successful, the goals of therapy need to be shared goals and the potential therapeutic options for achieving the therapeutic goal understood and agreed on by both the clinician and the patient. The specific goals for treating asthma and allergic rhinitis can be found elsewhere in this text. This discussion is intended to provide a basic blueprint for understanding the role and application of clinical pharmacologic principles in disease management.

Basic Principles of Clinical Pharmacology

Clinical pharmacology uses biopharmaceutical, pharmacokinetic, and pharmacodynamic principles to design optimal drug therapy regimens for individual patients. Although most physicians are familiar with the concept of serum drug concentration monitoring, the practice of clinical pharmacology or *pharmacotherapeutics* involves institution of therapy based on individual

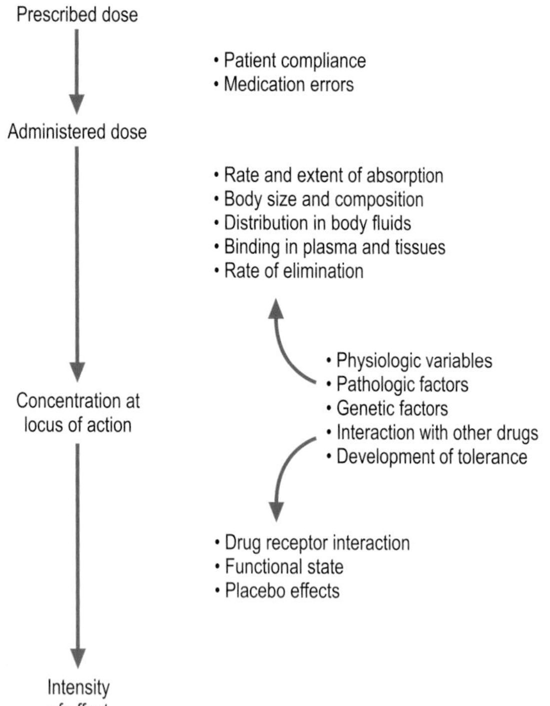

Figure 89-1 Factors that determine the relationship between prescribed dosage and outcome.

patient disease status and establishing and monitoring desired therapeutic outcomes. It is therefore important to understand patient physiologic variables and the influence of pathophysiologic differences on pharmacokinetics and pharmacodynamics.

For this discussion, *biopharmaceutics* refers to various physicochemical properties of drugs that affect how they are formulated and how the formulations affect dissolution, dosing, and drug delivery. *Pharmacokinetics* refers to the absorption, distribution, metabolism, and elimination characteristics of drugs. *Pharmacodynamics* is the study of the biologic effects of the drug or, more specifically, the efficacy and intensity of pharmacologic response relative to drug plasma concentration.

Pharmacodynamics

RECEPTOR THEORY

The relationship between drug concentration and pharmacologic response or effect is the essence of clinical pharmacology. The principal model to describe the relationship between drug concentration and response is that drugs or chemicals bind to or interact with macromolecules on cell surfaces (receptors) or in the cytoplasm to produce an effect. After receptor binding, the drug could activate and/or intensify a normal physiologic function and is termed an *agonist* (β_2-adrenergic agonists and glucocorticosteroids). Other drugs are devoid of any intrinsic activity but compete for the receptor for endogenous regulatory substances and are designated antagonists (anticholinergics and antihistamines). Through molecular biology techniques, most of the receptors of interest for asthma and allergy drugs (β_2-agonists, glucocorticosteroids, H_1 antihistamines, methylxanthines, leukotriene modifiers, and anticholinergics) have been identified and described, and much is still being learned about their molecular activity and interactions.[1,2]

It is now known that receptors have constitutive activity and can exist in an inactive conformation (R) or active conformation (R*) and that the R* conformation can provide intrinsic activity without drug or endogenous ligand binding.[3] Agonists work by stabilizing the R* conformation, thus increasing signaling.[4] In addition, it has been shown that many antagonists (e.g., H_1 antihistamines) actually act as *inverse agonists* by preferentially binding to the inactive R conformation and stabilizing it.[5,6] There are *partial* inverse agonists as well. Most drugs formerly known as "antagonists" actually exhibit some partial agonist or partial inverse-agonist activity. Although not all drugs or actions of drugs produce therapeutic effects through receptor agonism or antagonism, drugs cannot create new physiologic effects. Drugs produce therapeutic and toxicologic effects by mimicking, intensifying, or inhibiting normal cellular functions either selectively or nonselectively, or alternatively by producing cellular death.

Basic receptor theory assumes that the intensity of the pharmacologic or toxicologic response is proportional to the concentration of the drug at the receptor site and follows the laws of mass action, as described in the following equation[2]:

$$\text{C (drug concentration)} + \text{R (number of receptors)} \xrightarrow{k_1} \text{CR} \xrightarrow{k_2} \text{C} + \text{R}$$
$$\downarrow$$
$$\text{Effect} \qquad [89\text{-}1]$$

Equation 89-1 assumes reversible binding of the drug-receptor complex and that the maximum effect (E_{max}) occurs with occupation of all available receptors. The rate of association and disassociation of the drug-receptor complex are represented by k_1 and k_2. The applicable Equation 89-2 or 89-3 describes the hyperbolic relationship pictured in Figure 89-2, *A*, in which no drug produces no effect, 50% of E_{max} occurs when C equals the dissociation constant for the drug-receptor interaction ($K_d = k_2/k_1$, also referred to as the *affinity*), and the E_{max} is approached asymptotically as C increases above K_d (the E_{max} model).[2,3]

$$E = (E_{max})(C)/K_d + (C) \qquad [89\text{-}2]$$

Equation 89-2 is often reparameterized to give the Hill equation that was originally described to represent the association between oxygen and hemoglobin,[2] as follows:

$$E = (E_{max})(C)/EC_{50} + (C) \qquad [89\text{-}3]$$

where the EC_{50} is the effective concentration that produces half the maximal response. Figure 89-2, *B*, represents the effect plotted against the logarithm of the concentration. This provides a linear relationship with the log drug concentration and effect between 20% and 80% of E_{max}. Understanding specific aspects of the classic dose-response curves allows the clinician to derive a clear perspective of similarities and differences of drugs in similar pharmacologic classes (β_2-agonists) or physiologic classes (bronchodilators).

If the concentration-response curves depicted in Figure 89-2 represented three different drugs in the same pharmacologic class, drugs A and B would represent two drugs of equal efficacy but different potencies, and drug C would represent a drug of both a different potency and a different efficacy or intrinsic

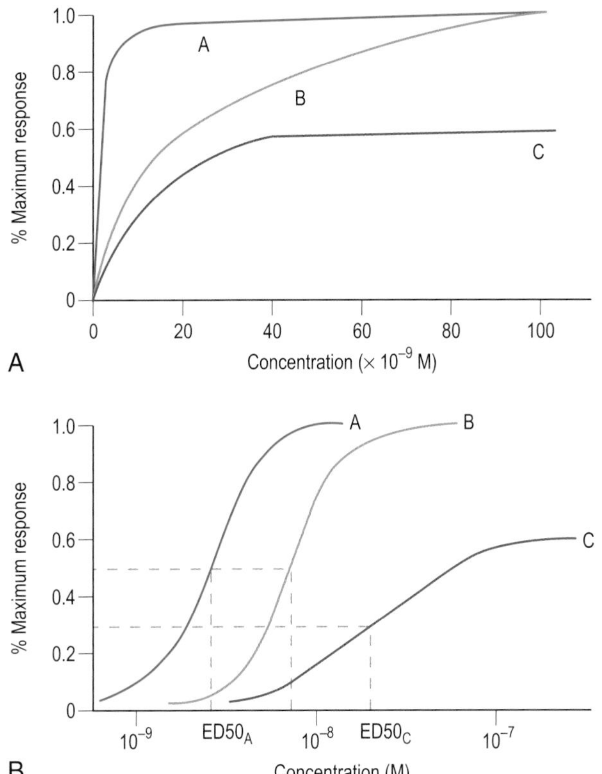

Figure 89-2 Representative dose-response curves. A and B represent the same curves on linear and log-linear scales, respectively. Individual curves *A* and *B* represent full agonists with different potencies and similar efficacy. Curve C represents a compound with both different potency and efficacy (partial agonist). All three curves could also represent the same agonist against different levels of functional antagonist. *ED50$_A$*, *ED50$_C$*, Effective dose that produces 50% of the maximal effect for either drug A or drug C (indicated by subscript letters).

activity (partial agonist).[7] Although drug C represents both decreased potency and only partial agonistic efficacy compared with drugs A and B, potency and efficacy are not necessarily linked.[1-3] For example, the β_2-agonist salmeterol is a partial agonist, with 60% of the efficacy of isoproterenol.[7] However, salmeterol is more potent in vitro than isoproterenol (EC_{50} of 53 nM and 200 nM, respectively).[7,8]

In contrast, the curves in Figure 89-2 could also represent the dose-response curves of differing activities for one drug at differing receptors (β_1- vs. β_2-receptors) or represent activity of the same drug-receptor at differing physiologic conditions, such as desensitization (B vs. C) or presence of increased concentrations of physiologic antagonist (A vs. B).

DIRECT- VERSUS INDIRECT-ACTING AGONISTS

Often agonist drugs act by stimulating the production of an intracellular intermediate or second messenger. The guanine nucleotide regulatory binding proteins (G proteins) comprise a superfamily of these intracellular receptors.[1] After binding to the membrane-bound portion of the receptor, a conformational change occurs, leading to intracellular binding to a G protein and the production of a second messenger. β_2-Adrenergic agonists and muscarinic agonists act in this manner.[3] Other drugs, such as glucocorticosteroids, first penetrate the plasma membrane and then bind to a specific receptor. The activated receptor complex is translocated to the nucleus, where it works by inducing gene transcription.[9]

Although both β_2-agonists and glucocorticosteroids obviously work indirectly at the subcellular level, indirect-acting drugs are operationally defined by whether the onset of activity occurs rapidly after receptor binding (direct) or whether there is a considerable disassociation (lag time) between receptor binding and pharmacologic response (indirect). For direct-acting agents, the onset of effect is primarily the function of the association constant (k_1; see Equation 89-1), assuming diffusion of the drug to the receptor site is not limited. Intensity and duration are a function of the affinity (K_d), which can also be expressed as the drug-receptor complex half-life.[2] For indirect-acting drugs, the onset of effect is more complex and may relate more directly to dose and binding affinity.[2]

STRUCTURE-ACTIVITY RELATIONSHIPS

Many drugs are chemical modifications of endogenous hormones or mediators. Chemical structural modifications can alter selectivity, efficacy, and potency of drugs. For example, changing a catecholamine to a resorcinol (isoproterenol to metaproterenol) decreases potency without altering efficacy or selectivity.[10] On the other hand, changing the N-terminal from dibutyl to a tertiary butyl group (metaproterenol to terbutaline) enhances β_2-receptor selectivity, decreases efficacy (partial agonist), and increases potency.[8,10] These changes can also significantly alter the pharmacokinetic properties of the drugs, which may have equally profound effects on the clinical efficacy and utility (i.e., long-acting inhaled β-agonists formoterol and salmeterol, with large, lipophilic side chains). Similarly, esterification of C17 and C21 increases lipophilicity of inhaled corticosteroids, increasing cell penetration, while C17 monoesterification enhances receptor binding (potency).[11]

Because of asymmetric substitution on the beta carbon of the side chain, all synthetic β_2-agonists exist as racemic mixtures of two optical isomers (i.e., the same chemical structure but mirror images). Levorotatory substitution (R configuration), as with naturally occurring catecholamines (L-epinephrine), confers significantly greater intrinsic activity because receptors are stereoselective.[12] For example, (*R*)-albuterol is approximately 100 times more potent than (*S*)-albuterol, whereas the ratio of activity for the (*R*) and (*S*) isomers of terbutaline, formoterol, and salmeterol are 1000:1, 1000:1, and 50:1, respectively.[12] There is no evidence that the less active isomer inhibits the effect of the more active isomers when the racemic mixture is administered, as would be expected from the marked difference in potency (i.e., binding affinity). However, some in vitro studies suggest that the therapeutically inactive isomers (distomers) are not inert and may have some pharmacologic effects that may be detrimental in asthma (see Chapter 95).[13] Examples of other asthma drugs that occur as racemic mixtures include zileuton, budesonide, and ipratropium bromide. Also, because most biologic systems are relatively stereoselective, each isomer may have distinctly different pharmacokinetic patterns.[12,13]

CLINICAL CORRELATES OF RECEPTOR THEORY

The concept of reversible binding and the law of mass action can be readily appreciated with the anticholinergics.[2] With increasing concentrations of acetylcholine, any given concentration of anticholinergic is less effective. Whether a similar mass-action tug-of-war occurs with inverse agonists such as antihistamines during times of a high pollen count is unclear.[6]

The log concentration-response nature of the dose-response curves helps explain why, with drugs such as theophylline with its narrow therapeutic index (Fig. 89-3), increasing the dose to achieve a concentration increase from 5 to 10 mg/L results in a significant clinical improvement but that increasing from 15 to 20 mg/L may result in a minimal additional improvement despite the same absolute increase in concentration (5 mg/L). When comparing drugs of different potency at the top of the dose-response curve, it becomes difficult to discern differences. Also, administering increased doses of drug near the maximum effect primarily increases the duration of effect without a discernible difference in intensity of effect.[2] However, this is a relatively inefficient method of prolonging duration compared to altering pharmacokinetic properties or dosing frequency.

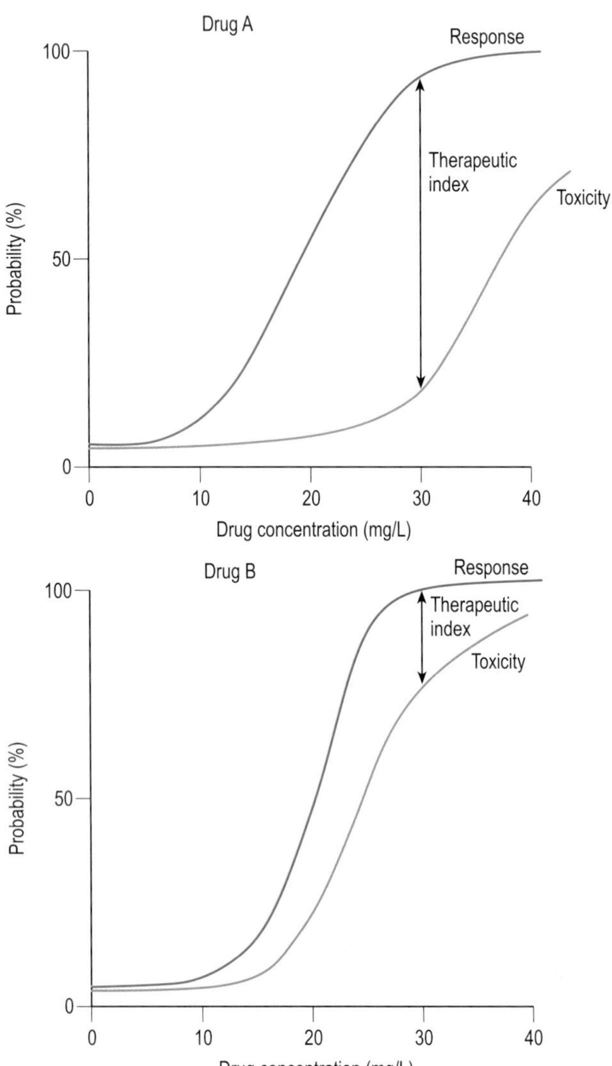

Figure 89-3 Relationship between drug concentration and therapeutic effect and toxic effect for drug A with a wide therapeutic index (*top*) and drug B with a narrow therapeutic index (*bottom*).

Pharmaceutics

Pharmaceutic formulations are designed to optimally deliver effective concentrations of the drug to the site of action. Development of the appropriate formulations depends on multiple factors, including the physicochemical, pharmacokinetic, and pharmacodynamic properties of the drugs. For example, oral formulations are of little use if the drug is not absorbed or has essentially no bioavailability as a result of first-pass metabolism by the liver (e.g., isoproterenol). On the other hand, it seems to make little sense to produce an inhaled formulation of a drug that is completely absorbed from both the gastrointestinal (GI) tract and the lung because it would be unlikely to produce a selective topical effect (e.g., methylprednisolone, dexamethasone). In addition, drugs in which high concentrations are required to achieve the therapeutic response (e.g., theophylline in mg/L) are not suitable for aerosol delivery. Large quantities of drug particles can produce irritation and bronchospasm, and existing metered-dose pressurized-canister technology cannot accommodate greater than 2-mg to 5-mg doses per actuation because of clogging of the stem valves and actuators.[14]

PARENTERAL FORMULATIONS

The principal advantage of parenteral formulations of systemically active drugs is the assurance of delivery regardless of the presence of vomiting or GI intolerance and the theoretic advantage of a more rapid response for direct-acting drugs with slow absorption. However, for indirect-acting drugs such as the glucocorticosteroids, no evidence exists for either a more rapid or more intense response from parenteral administration over oral administration.[9,15] In addition, some of the newer agents that are antibodies to immunoglobulin E (IgE) or interleukin-5 (IL-5) are digested by GI enzymes and thus require subcutaneous or intravenous administration.

Disadvantages of parenteral therapy include the need for intravenous access and possible adverse effects to excipients in the formulations. Acute bronchospasm has been reported after parenteral hydrocortisone administration, presumably caused by the succinate salt used to enhance solubility. Adverse effects secondary to β_2-agonists are significantly more common after parenteral than aerosol administration, and aerosol administration produces greater bronchodilation in patients with acute severe asthma.[16]

ORAL FORMULATIONS

Oral formulations have the greatest degree of patient acceptance but share the drawback of not being site selective, thus enhancing the risk of unwanted systemic effects. Oral formulations of drugs can be manipulated to overcome the disadvantages of gastric acid breaking down active drug (enteric coating), rapid drug elimination (extended release or repeated release), and palatability (flavoring or beaded coating). However, altered formulations have no effect on reducing first-pass metabolism. It is possible for excipients of oral formulations to produce unwanted effects (e.g., preservatives, dyes, or alcohol content of elixirs). Sustained-release formulations, such as theophylline or pseudoephedrine, provide the advantage of improved adherence to once-daily or twice-daily dosing regimens.[17] However, because the formulation producing the sustained release is proprietary, significant differences may exist among preparations.

AEROSOL FORMULATIONS

In asthma, which is localized to the lower airways, and in allergic rhinitis, which is localized to the nasal cavities and adjacent structures, it makes sense to target drug therapy to the affected organs. From a pharmacotherapeutic perspective, targeted therapy improves the *therapeutic index* of a drug, defined as the ratio of the dose that produces the therapeutic effect over that which produces toxicity. From a drug delivery perspective, aerosols present a unique set of challenges. No other drug delivery system is so highly dependent on patient technique for optimal delivery of the therapeutic dose[18] (see Chapter 66 for a more extensive review).

Formulation changes (suspension vs. solution, propellant), delivery device (nebulizer, metered-dose inhaler [MDI], or dry powder inhaler [DPI]) can all alter delivery.[14,18-20] The use of add-on spacer devices can alter dose-response characteristics by enhancing therapeutic effect, reducing topical adverse effects, or increasing or decreasing systemic activity.[14] When administered through an identical spacer device, respirable particles and delivery may be increased for one drug but reduced for another.[19] Extrapolation of data from one delivery device drug formulation combination is therefore not possible.

Pharmacokinetic Principles

Absorption, distribution, metabolism, and elimination all determine the delivery of active drug to the site of action or receptor. This relationship is shown in Figure 89-4; for systemically administered drugs, the concentration of "free" or non–protein-bound drug in the serum or plasma is in equilibrium with the drug concentration at the receptor site. This same relationship applies to the systemic activity from aerosolized drugs. The widespread availability of specific and sensitive drug assays has facilitated our understanding of the pharmacokinetics that determine efficacy and toxicity from numerous drugs.[21]

Routine therapeutic drug monitoring is primarily used for drugs with a low therapeutic index, such as theophylline. Drugs with a high safety profile (fewer acute, direct, pharmacologically based toxicities), such as the inhaled β_2-agonists, leukotriene receptor antagonists, H_1 antihistamines, and glucocorticosteroids, do not require routine serum concentration monitoring. The "therapeutic range" for any given drug is a statistical concept. It represents a combination of probability curves for therapeutic response and unacceptable toxicity (see Fig. 89-3).[21] The upper limit of the therapeutic range is most often defined by an unacceptable rate of toxicity, but may also be a result of a flat dose-response, as with the leukotriene receptor antagonists.

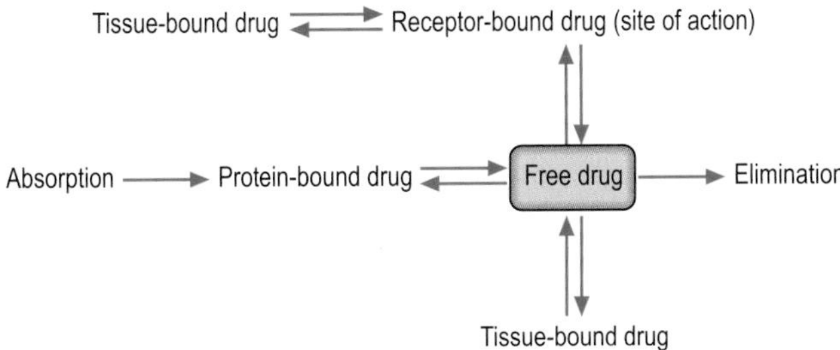

Figure 89-4 Schematic presentation of interrelationship among absorption, distribution, and elimination of a drug and its concentration at the site of action.

With the introduction of therapeutic drug monitoring, clinicians also became aware that much of the variability in response to standard dosages of drugs was caused by pharmacokinetic variability. As a result of this knowledge, pharmacokinetic and pharmacodynamic studies are now mandatory and are performed early in the drug development process. Unfortunately, the pharmacokinetics and pharmacodynamics of many widely used older drugs remain poorly defined. In addition, the U.S. Food and Drug Administration (FDA) has determined that for drugs to be used in children to treat diseases that are unlikely to be significantly different from those seen in adults, such as asthma and rhinitis,[22] only pharmacokinetic studies and limited safety and efficacy studies are needed. Thus, the physician can expect to receive essential pharmacokinetic information on newly available drugs in healthy volunteers, patients with the disease being treated, and patients with special circumstances (elderly, children, or individuals with impaired renal or hepatic function).

ABSORPTION

After administration of a dosage formulation, absorption describes the rate and extent entering the body.[23] The clinician is often concerned with the bioavailability of drugs, which refers to how much of a drug reaches the systemic circulation in relation to the reference standard of intravenous administration. The FDA primarily uses results of bioavailability studies rather than therapeutic efficacy studies to determine the equivalence of generic drugs, with the exception of drugs delivered by inhalers (pMDI and DPI). Bioavailability is substantially affected by processes such as metabolism because the drug passes through the GI wall, which contains cytochrome P-450 isozyme 3A4 (CYP3A4) and P-glycoprotein carrier protein, and the liver, which contains numerous other cytochrome P-450 isozymes.[23,24] These can result in first-pass metabolism after absorption of a drug from the GI lumen and are the primary method of limiting systemic activity of inhaled glucocorticosteroids.[25]

One of the main determinants of absorption, regardless of site, is *solubility*. In general, drugs in aqueous solution are absorbed more rapidly than suspensions or solid-dosage forms, in which the dissolution rate is usually the rate-limiting step. Thus, extended-release (ER) oral dosage forms are produced by slowing drug release from a matrix (ER albuterol) or coating with a substance that impedes dissolution (most ER theophyllines). Once in solution, the nonionized (more lipophilic) form of a drug is more rapidly absorbed. Regardless of ionization state, drugs will always be more rapidly absorbed from the intestine than the stomach because of the greater surface area of the intestinal lining. Thus, administering almost any drug with food, which delays gastric emptying, will slow absorption.[23] Coadministration with food may prevent dissolution, or the drug may be adsorbed to the food, decreasing bioavailability (e.g., zafirlukast). For ER oral drugs, the effect of coadministration with food is mixed, depending on the formulation. Fatty foods may increase the rate of dissolution of some drugs, producing "dose dumping," or may prevent the wetting and dissolution of others, with decreased bioavailability. Also, the absorption of theophylline undergoes diurnal variability, with slower absorption at night apparently caused primarily by the recumbent position.[17] This phenomenon can be exploited by dosing once-daily theophylline preparations at night.

Rate and extent of absorption can also affect the duration of action of aerosolized drugs. The large surface area of the airways and bypassing of the first-pass metabolism result in drugs being rapidly and completely absorbed from the lung. Some examples of this effect are the highly water-soluble cromolyn, nedocromil, and short-acting β_2-agonists. These drugs are rapidly absorbed through the parenchyma away from their site of action, limiting their duration of action to 2 to 6 hours. In contrast, the greater lipophilicity of the long-acting β_2-agonists formoterol and salmeterol prolongs their retention in lung tissue, increasing their duration of action to at least 12 hours.[26] Greater lipophilicity also prolongs the duration of local antiinflammatory effects of inhaled glucocorticosteroids.[11]

Absorption and first-pass metabolism can also affect the therapeutic index of aerosolized drugs. For example, 40% to 80% of a drug administered by MDI or DPI is deposited in the oropharynx and is swallowed, and 10% to 50% is delivered to the airways, depending on the preparation.[14] Drugs that are poorly absorbed, such as the strongly ionized quaternary amine ipratropium bromide, have a significantly greater therapeutic index than the tertiary amine atropine sulfate, which is completely bioavailable orally.[27] Drugs with high first-pass metabolism produce fewer systemic effects than drugs with a low first-pass metabolism because total systemic bioavailability is less. However, all the drug that reaches the airway is 100% available and capable of producing systemic effects. The use of an effective spacer device that significantly reduces oropharyngeal deposition would be expected to enhance the safety of drugs with significant oral bioavailability. This has been the case with high-dose inhaled beclomethasone. However, a spacer device is unlikely to enhance the topical/systemic activity ratio of fluticasone and may actually worsen it because fluticasone has an oral bioavailability of less than 1%.[25] Also, there appears to be minimal benefit other than reduced topical effects and improved coordination of delivery for drugs with poor oral absorption, such as nedocromil and cromolyn.

DISTRIBUTION

After absorption of a drug into the systemic circulation and extensively perfused organs (often called the central compartment), the drug distributes into less well-perfused tissue (peripheral compartment) and to its site of action (see Fig. 89-4). The rate of tissue diffusion depends on the physicochemical properties of the drug and blood flow to the specific tissue. If tissue distribution is rapid compared with absorption, then absorption is the rate-limiting step for onset and peak effect with direct-acting drugs. The extent of tissue distribution depends on serum protein and tissue binding, as well as the physicochemical properties of the drug.

The quaternary amine anticholinergics are not only poorly absorbed across membranes but also poorly distributed into the central nervous system (CNS).[27] The lack of CNS side effects with the newer nonsedating H_1 antihistamines mainly results from their lipophobic nature and affinity for CNS vascular endothelial P-glycoprotein producing lower concentrations in the brain, although improved selectivity for H_1 receptors also plays a role.[6] Increased lipophilicity of inhaled corticosteroids improves distribution of drug into tissue and cells, thus increasing their potency.[25] Again, diffusion may be the rate-limiting step to the onset of effect of direct-acting drugs. The slow onset of bronchodilation from salmeterol appears to be caused by slow diffusion through the cell membrane to the receptor site as a result of its lipophilic properties. On the other hand, formoterol has an onset of action similar to albuterol because of its greater hydrophilicity compared with salmeterol.[26]

The lack of tissue distribution resulting from high serum protein binding is thought to contribute to the low adverse effect profile for montelukast.[28] However, protein binding does not have a consistent effect on tissue distribution because it depends on the relative binding affinities between the serum proteins and tissues. For example, fluticasone and mometasone differ in protein binding (90% and 99%, respectively) but are similar in potency and pharmacokinetics and produce the same level of HPA-axis suppression at the same microgram doses.[11,25] For highly tissue-bound drugs such as the H_1 antihistamines, the redistribution rate out of the tissues may also be the primary determinant of duration of action, particularly for pharmacodynamic responses, such as suppression of cutaneous wheal and flare responses to histamine.[29]

The *volume of distribution* (Vd) is a clinical pharmacokinetic term that relates the amount of drug in the body at a given time to the plasma or serum concentration (Cp) observed after distribution is complete, as shown in the following equation:

$$\text{Vd} = \text{Amount of drug in body/Cp} \qquad [89\text{-}4]$$

After a single dose of a drug, the amount of drug is equivalent to the fraction of the dose that is bioavailable (F), and thus the Vd determines the increase in Cp after a single dose of the drug, as follows:

$$\Delta\text{Cp} = \text{F} \times \text{Dose/Vd} \qquad [89\text{-}5]$$

The Vd is also affected by the physiologic characteristics of the patient (hydration status and pH). The principal clinical utility of the Vd is that it helps determine an appropriate loading dose of a drug. If the Vd is known, the dose to achieve with any given increase in plasma concentration of a drug can be estimated.

ELIMINATION

After entry into the body, the process of elimination of drugs begins. Drugs that are relatively water soluble (e.g., atropine, cetirizine) may be excreted unchanged, either filtered by the renal glomeruli or actively secreted by organic acid or base transport systems in the renal tubules or bile ducts (e.g., cromolyn, nedocromil). However, because of their lipophilic nature, most drugs are first metabolized to more polar compounds and then excreted. These more polar metabolites may be active (e.g., cetirizine, the major metabolite of hydroxyzine)[6] or inactive.

The phase I metabolic biotransformation of drugs, which consists of introducing or exposing a functional group on the parent compound, is generally enzymatic and primarily occurs in the liver. Other organs, such as the lungs, kidneys, and GI tract, may also serve as significant sites of metabolism. The majority of drug biotransformations are catalyzed by the cytochrome P-450 (CYP) family of heme-containing membrane proteins localized in the smooth endoplasmic reticulum of tissues. Oxidative reactions catalyzed by these enzymes require the reduced form of nicotinamide adenine dinucleotide phosphate (NADP) and molecular oxygen. It is now known that the CYP mixed-function oxidase system consists of a superfamily of enzymes (12 P-450 gene families identified in humans) with varying specificity for xenobiotic substrates. Three isozyme families (CYP1, CYP2, and CYP3) encode the enzymes responsible for most drug biotransformations.[30]

The phase II conjugation reactions (glucuronidation, acetylation, and sulfation) resulting from a covalent linkage generally occur in the cytosolic fraction of the cell, although some glucuronyl transferases occur in the microsomal membrane as well. Conjugation reactions may or may not follow an initial phase I biotransformation.

As a result of low substrate specificity among P-450 isozymes, more than one may catalyze a given biotransformation; however, many drugs are primarily metabolized by one subfamily. For example, CYP3A4 is involved in the majority of all drug metabolic conversions, including a number of H_1 antihistamines, the leukotriene antagonists, and corticosteroids (Table 89-1). The level of specific enzyme activity is genetically determined.[30] Phenotypic differences in the ability to metabolize drugs through polymorphically controlled pathways not only determines rate of metabolism but also may put some patients at greater risk of toxicity from some drugs. For example, the metabolic clearance of the more active isomer of the anticoagulant *S*-warfarin is affected by CYP2C9 variants, with up to a tenfold difference in clearance rates between those homozygous for the wild-type CYP2C9*1 and CYP2C9*3 homozygotes, with the latter having a significantly increased risk of bleeding.[31] A common promoter polymorphism in the CYP1A2 at position -2964 is associated with significantly decreased clearance and elevated theophylline concentrations in Japanese men.[32] In the FDA-approved cancer drugs 6-mercaptopurine and irinotecan, enzymatic polymorphisms have clearly been demonstrated to put patients at risk for significant toxicity, and commercial assays are available to test for the polymorphisms.[33] This is a first step in providing truly individualized therapy.

Enzymatic biotransformation is also stereoselective, generally favoring more rapid inactivation of the eutomer.[12] Other factors that affect enzyme activity include disease state, age, the presence of enzyme inhibitors or inducers, and possibly gender. Although there is some P-450 enzymatic activity in the fetus, both phase I and II enzyme systems begin maturing over the first 2 weeks of life at differing rates. Then enzyme activity rapidly increases over the first year, and the most rapid metabolism is found in children 1 to 9 years old. Drug metabolism then declines during puberty to adult values, and finally cytochrome P-450 activity is generally reduced in elderly persons, although conjugation enzymes are maintained.[30]

CLEARANCE

Enzymatic activity, hepatic function, and renal function are the principal physiologic determinants of drug clearance. Clearance is the primary determinant for developing dosing regimens of systemic drugs for long-term administration. Clearance (Cl) is defined as the volume of blood or plasma that is completely cleared of drug over a unit of time. More clinically relevant is that the *steady-state concentration* (Cp_{ss}) of drug occurs when

TABLE 89-1 Major and Minor Cytochrome P-450 (CYP) Enzyme Substrates

Drug	1A2	2A6	2B6	2C8	2C9	2C19	2D6	2E1	3A4
Budesonide									X
Caffeine	X								
Dexamethasone									Minor
Fexofenadine									Minor
Fluticasone									X
Formoterol		Minor			Minor	Minor	Minor		
Loratadine							Minor		Minor
Methylprednisolone									Minor
Mometasone									Minor
Montelukast					X				X
Promethazine			X						X
Cetirizine									Minor
Salmeterol									X
Theophylline	X				Minor		Minor	X	X
Zafirlukast					X				
Zileuton	Minor								Minor
Chlorpheniramine									
Azelastine	Minor					Minor	Minor		Minor
Prednisone									Minor
Prednisolone									Minor
Codeine							X		Minor
Dextromethorphan		Minor			Minor	Minor	X	Minor	Minor
Acetaminophen	Minor	Minor			Minor		Minor	Minor	Minor
Albuterol									X
Aspirin					Minor				

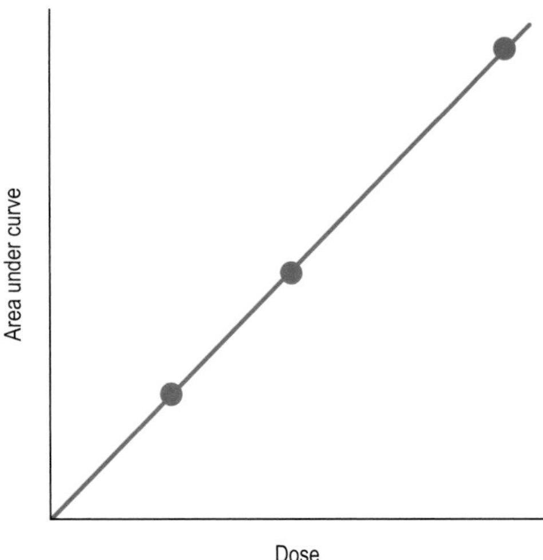

Figure 89-5 Representation of relationship between dose and area under the concentration time curves (or steady-state plasma concentrations) for a drug undergoing first-order elimination (linear kinetics).

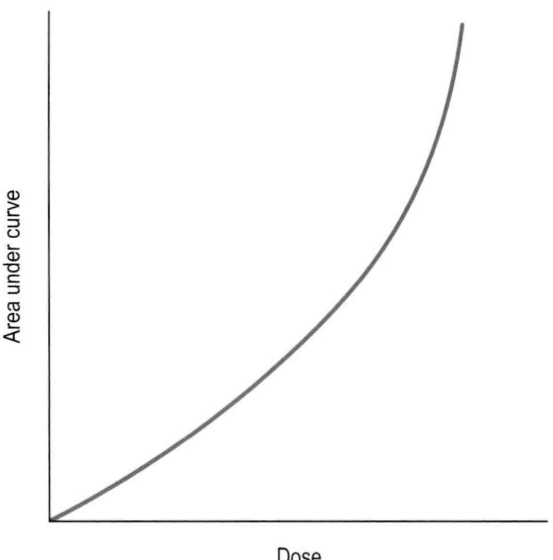

Figure 89-6 Representation of relationship between dose and area under the concentration time curves (or steady-state plasma concentrations) for a drug undergoing saturable elimination (nonlinear kinetics).

the dosing rate equals the rate of drug elimination, and the Cp_{ss} is determined by the clearance as follows:

$$Cp_{ss} = \text{Dosing rate}/\text{Cl} \quad [89\text{-}6]$$

For the vast majority of drugs, the clearance remains constant over the range of concentrations experienced clinically, even though the processes for clearing the drugs (enzymatic metabolism and active secretion) are potentially saturable processes. Thus, the amount of drug eliminated over a unit of time increases as the concentration increases, producing a constant percentage of drug lost per unit time (first-order elimination kinetics). In contrast, if saturation occurred, a constant amount of drug is eliminated per unit time (zero-order kinetics). In this case, clearance changes with serum concentrations.

For chronic dosing of drugs undergoing first-order elimination, it is easy to see that, with the clearance unchanging, any change in dosing rate will result in a proportional change in steady-state concentration. Figure 89-5 depicts what occurs with serum concentrations in first-order (linear kinetics) with increasing doses, and Figure 89-6 depicts what occurs with drugs undergoing saturable elimination (Michaelis-Menten or nonlinear kinetics). Theophylline, a drug with a narrow therapeutic index, occasionally exhibits nonlinear kinetics in the usual therapeutic range of serum concentrations, particularly in children.[17]

Clearance for a drug can be estimated by giving a continuous infusion and using Equation 89-6 after steady state has been reached, but it is more often estimated after a single intravenous dose of the drug, as follows:

$$\text{Cl} = \text{Dose}/\text{AUC} \quad [89\text{-}7]$$

where AUC is the total area under the serum concentration time curve (area under curve). Occasionally the clinician may see the term *oral clearance.* This refers to clearance calculated from oral dosing when absolute bioavailability is unknown, and it should not be confused with *actual* clearance. Drugs with a high first-pass effect will have higher oral clearance than actual clearance; however, the oral clearance would be the more appropriate value to use in determining oral dosage regimens for the drug.

HALF-LIFE

Drugs undergoing first-order elimination kinetics can be characterized by their half-life. The half-life is the time it takes to eliminate one half of the drug from the body or to reduce the serum concentration by one half. The elimination half-life of a drug depends on both the previously discussed physiologically defined pharmacokinetic variables, Vd and Cl, as follows:

$$\text{Cl (organ function)}/\text{Vd (physiologic status)} = 0.693/T_{1/2} = \text{KE} \quad [89\text{-}8]$$

where $T_{1/2}$ is half-life, 0.693 is the natural log constant, and KE, the elimination rate constant, is the slope of the log concentration time curve. Both physiologic variables affect the half-life. The Cl determines how much of the blood is cleared of drug, and the Vd determines how much drug is presented to the clearing organ in that unit of blood. As can be seen, only changes in clearance affect steady-state serum concentrations. Changes in Vd affect the time to reach steady-state concentrations but not the final concentration, which is determined by the dose and clearance. For example, a highly lipophilic inhaled corticosteroid will have the same steady-state serum concentration as a more hydrophilic one with a lower Vd if they have the same clearance.

The clinical utility of the half-life is threefold. First, it helps to determine a reasonable dosing interval for chronically administered drug. Second, the half-life, in conjunction with the absorption rate, determines the fluctuation of serum concentrations over the dosing interval. The elimination half-life will generally determine the pharmacologic duration of action of a drug unless the effect at the receptor lasts significantly longer. After one half-life, 50% of the drug is left; after two half-lives, 25% remains; after five half-lives, only 3.125% remains. Thus, clinically the drug is essentially eliminated from the body in five half-lives. Third, with continuous dosing, a drug will accumulate up to a steady-state concentration (Figure 89-7),

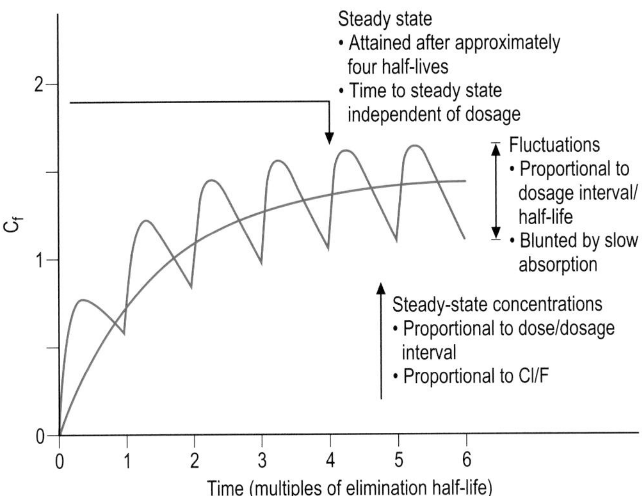

Figure 89-7 Fundamental pharmacokinetic profile for repeated administration of a first-order eliminated drug. *C_f*, Concentration of oral drug; *Cl*, clearance, *F*, bioavailable fraction of dose.

and this accumulation process is just the reverse of the elimination, in that 50% of steady state is achieved after one half-life, 75% after two half-lives, and 96.87% after five half-lives. This is the same time that it takes to reach any new steady state after a dosage change. Thus the clinician can use the half-life to determine when to evaluate the effects of a new dosage or whether using a loading dose or holding doses may be more prudent to effect faster change.

When using this information, the clinician can more logically decide how to begin dosing and how to monitor therapy. In drugs with extremely long half-lives, the use of loading doses may be appropriate.[23] It is important to remember that, although the concept of a loading dose is to reach steady state sooner, the drug only reaches steady state after five half-lives. Also, the steady-state concentration depends only on the maintenance dose and clearance, whereas the loading dose is estimated from the Vd. Thus, after a loading dose, the serum drug concentration will increase or decrease over the five half-lives to achieve the final steady-state concentration.

For drugs that undergo saturation kinetics, the total plasma clearance depends on the plasma concentration and is described by a form of the Michaelis-Menten equation:

$$\mathrm{Cl} = \mathrm{v_m}/(\mathrm{K_m} + \mathrm{Cp}) \quad [89\text{-}9]$$

where K_m represents the plasma concentration at which half the maximal rate of elimination (v_m) is reached. If plasma concentrations are much less than K_m, elimination will follow first-order kinetics and appear linear. Steady state can be estimated by the following equation:

$$\mathrm{Cp_{ss}} = \text{Dosing rate} \times \mathrm{K_m}/\mathrm{v_m} - \text{Dosing rate} \quad [89\text{-}10]$$

As the dosing rate approaches maximal elimination rate, the denominator approaches zero and Cp_{ss} increases disproportionately (see Fig. 89-6).

Pharmacodynamic Variability

With the advent of therapeutic drug monitoring and the individualizing of patient dosing in the 1970s and 1980s, it was widely assumed that the large variability in response was accounted for by pharmacokinetic differences. However, in recent years the study of pharmacokinetics in relation to pharmacodynamics has shown that pharmacodynamic variability plays an important role in interindividual and intraindividual response to drugs. Some of the factors that produce pharmacodynamic differences, such as tolerance and tachyphylaxis, have been well documented and mechanistically explained, whereas others, such as functional antagonism, the effect of inflammation on receptor activity, pharmacogenomics, and chronopharmacology, have been observed but less well investigated. Intact tissue or in vivo pharmacodynamics illustrates factors affecting response other than classic mass-action receptor theory. Receptors and tissues from the milieu of disease may respond quite differently.

PATHOPHYSIOLOGIC FACTORS

Pathophysiologic factors that alter response to drugs can include changes in both pharmacokinetics and pharmacodynamics. The pharmacokinetic changes are often obvious (e.g., decreased aerosol delivery during severe airways obstruction, decreased metabolic clearance of theophylline secondary to hypoxemia), whereas others are less obvious (e.g., increased CNS penetration of theophylline with acidosis and low serum albumin). However, alteration of the concentration-response or dose-response curves by pathophysiologic changes has drawn great interest in recent years.

Functional antagonism is a phenomenon used to explain changes in the dose-response characteristics of bronchodilators.[8] Functional antagonism is defined as the reciprocal relationship between two agonists with opposing action. Potential bronchodilators are often screened in vitro with isolated smooth muscle preparations that are contracted with low concentrations of histamine or an acetylcholine derivative. Increasing the contractile stimulus concentration increases the amount of the relaxing agonist required, thus shifting the dose-response curve to the right[34,35] (see Fig. 89-2, *B*). Partial agonists are more easily antagonized than full agonists; therefore the expression of shifting the dose-response curve depends on the contractile agonist used because partial-contractile agonists are less likely to induce the effect.[8] For example, β_2-agonist dose-response curves are readily shifted by methacholine but not leukotriene D_4 or serotonin despite equal degrees of bronchoconstriction.[36] In human bronchi, histamine and methacholine produce similar degrees of functional antagonism and shift the dose-response curves of β_2-agonists and theophylline to the right.[37,38] Clinical studies with both theophylline and β_2-agonists have shown diminished response in patients presenting with increased bronchospasm.[10,16,17]

Besides the increased release and production of functional antagonists, the airways inflammation in asthma has been implicated in altering the response to both β_2-agonists and corticosteroids through both direct and indirect mechanisms at the postreceptor level.[1,39] The proinflammatory cytokines released in asthma can produce heterologous desensitization to β_2-agonists and vasoactive intestinal peptide.[1] In addition, β_2-receptor numbers are decreased and β_2-agonist binding is decreased after antigen challenge. Studies have also shown that allergic inflammation, possibly through the production of local cytokines, reduces glucocorticoid receptor–binding affinity or glucocorticoid receptor–DNA binding.[39,40]

PATIENT FACTORS

Given the many variables already discussed that may account for altered response to drugs, the potential for true interindividual differences in response may be genetically determined or as yet undefined, and may also be gender or age based. Gene polymorphisms have been associated with altered responses to β_2-agonists, corticosteroids, and leukotriene modifiers (see Chapter 90).[41] Thus, even with similar clinical expression of disease and consistency of delivered dose or attainment of the same serum concentration, greatly differing responses occur. Single nucleotide polymorphisms (SNPs) at rs37972 and rs37973 that map to the glucocorticoid-induced transcript-1 gene (GLCCI1) were found to result in diminished response to inhaled glucocorticosteroids.[42] Subjects homozygous for the rs37973 mutant allele, about 16% of the population, obtained only about one third of the forced expiratory volume in 1 second (FEV_1) response to inhaled glucocorticosteroids as the subjects with the wild-type allele. In addition, SNPs of corticotropin-releasing factor receptor type 1, located on chromosome 17q21-22, a region linked to asthma, have been associated with response to inhaled glucocorticosteroids, particularly rs242941, which has been positively associated with an enhanced response in two asthmatic populations.[43]

Polymorphisms in two enzymes forming leukotrienes—5-lipoxygenase and leukotriene C_4 synthase—have been associated with diminished response to a 5-lipoxygenase inhibitor and a cysteinyl leukotriene receptor antagonist.[41]

CHRONOPHARMACOLOGY

Some have suggested that the timing of dosing may have a significant effect on therapeutic outcome.[44,45] Circadian rhythms in the body lead to changes in endogenous hormone secretion. Nonasthmatic healthy individuals have a circadian change in pulmonary function, and some asthmatic patients have an exaggerated decrease with a nadir at 4 to 5 AM and a peak in the early afternoon. Patients with nocturnal asthma have increased bronchial hyperresponsiveness and increased leukotriene excretion at night. The dosing of montelukast once nightly was designed to produce maximal drug concentration in the late-night and early-morning hours.[28] Both oral and inhaled corticosteroids lead to an improved response when administered as a single dose at 3 PM, without an increase in adrenal suppression compared with an 8 AM dose.[44,45] In addition, the dose-response curve to inhaled β_2-agonists is shifted to the right in patients awakening because of nocturnal asthma.[46] Although this may be explained by either functional antagonism or cytokine downregulation of β_2-receptors, the mechanism is still unknown.

TOLERANCE

Tolerance or *desensitization* of agonist receptors with continued stimulation is a well-described phenomenon in clinical pharmacology. Desensitization of β_2-adrenergic receptors has been the most extensively studied and is reviewed in more detail in Chapter 95. Desensitization of β_2-receptors may occur by at least three mechanisms: phosphorylation, sequestration, and downregulation.[1,10] *Phosphorylation* of the β_2-receptors follows short-term exposure (minutes) and results in a decreased binding affinity between drug and receptor. *Sequestration* also follows short-term exposure but requires drug occupancy and reverses immediately after dissociation of the drug from receptor. However, if the agonist remains coupled for a sufficient period of time (hours), *downregulation* occurs in which receptor numbers diminish. Interestingly, the susceptibility of β_2-receptors to downregulation appears to be genetically determined (see Chapter 95). In addition to the receptor-based mechanisms, a postreceptor mechanism of desensitization is now believed to be likely. Enhanced breakdown of cyclic adenosine monophosphate (cAMP) by an increase in phosphodiesterase (PDE) isozyme activity would account for the particularly rapid development of tolerance to β_2-agonists in inflammatory and immunocompetent cells.[8]

Clinically important aspects of β_2-receptor desensitization include (1) shortened duration of bronchodilator effect, (2) greater apparent desensitization in β_2-receptors in other tissues than bronchial smooth muscle (which may be a function of relative receptor numbers), (3) improvement of receptor affinity and reversal of downregulation by glucocorticoids, (4) apparent ability to easily overcome desensitization with increased dosage, and (5) apparent leveling off in the degree of desensitization over time.[1,10] Finally, it is important to realize that, because desensitization is a receptor phenomenon, cross-tolerance is the rule; thus changing or alternating β_2-agonists would not improve efficacy.

Although glucocorticoid resistance occurs, it is thought to be a result of inflammation and not agonist-induced tolerance.[39] Tolerance or desensitization has not been reported for drugs that work by inhibiting enzymatic breakdown, and theophylline, a phosphodiesterase inhibitor, has not been reported to induce tolerance.[17] Although other inverse agonists (β-blocking drugs) have resulted in increased receptor sensitization, this phenomenon has not been shown to occur with the H_1 antihistamines.[6]

Drug Interactions

Pharmacodynamic drug interactions may occur at the receptor or cellular level or at the functional level, whereas pharmacokinetic interactions are those occurring as a result of absorption, distribution, metabolism, or elimination changes. Some interactions may involve both pharmacodynamic and pharmacokinetic changes. Drug interactions may produce beneficial results, as well as potentially adverse effects. Numerous drugs with the potential for adverse consequences are frequently administered together without problems. Indeed, it is difficult to determine the risk of adverse consequences of drug interactions because the denominator (total number of patients receiving the combination) is largely unknown. Adverse drug reactions are increasingly recognized as a significant medical problem, leading to an estimated 700,000 emergency department visits and 117,318 hospitalizations per year in the United States in 2004-2005,[47] and the clinician needs to be cognizant of the possibility of enhancing adverse drug reactions through drug interactions.

Case reports and evaluation of spontaneous reporting systems, such as Medwatch used by the FDA, tend to exaggerate the significance of interactions because only the more severe reactions are reported. For example, a review of the FDA's spontaneous reporting system for 48 reports of adverse events in patients who received concomitant quinolone antibiotics (ciprofloxacin and norfloxacin) and theophylline found that 35% of patients experienced seizures.[48] On the other hand, a retrospective review of a Veterans Affairs (VA) Medical Center population revealed that 39 patients prescribed theophylline received 59 courses of ciprofloxacin and only one patient had an adverse outcome.[49] This dichotomy can contribute to the skepticism of the importance of drug interactions. However, the one patient with the adverse outcome required a 13-day hospitalization at a cost of $5492, which resulted in an overall increased cost of $93 for each prescription relevant to this potential drug interaction.

Drugs associated with severe toxicities and a narrow therapeutic index are more likely to be associated with significant drug interactions. In addition, drug interactions are more likely to be detected with drugs whose serum concentrations are routinely monitored in clinical practice. Adverse consequences from drug interactions can also occur as a result of severe exacerbation of disease resulting from the lost therapeutic effect from a drug. Many drug interactions go undetected in initial clinical trials unless there is reason to suspect a possible interaction. For example, how many patients received the combination of erythromycin and theophylline with or without adverse consequences before the publication of the interactions? However, once a mechanism and seriousness of a drug interaction is established, newer drugs in the class are tested for potential to produce drug interactions.

Erythromycin can produce life-threatening interactions with theophylline (seizures and death), yet a number of patients have received the combination without any problems. This may result from the variability of the interaction, initial dosage of theophylline, dosage of erythromycin, and interpatient variability in response to a given concentration of theophylline. Two studies have attempted to determine the magnitude of the problem with theophylline drug interactions. The first study looked at 913 patients receiving theophylline chronically who also had a prescription for either cimetidine (140 courses), erythromycin (93 courses), or ciprofloxacin (59 courses).[49] Only 2 of 292 (0.81%) patients with potential interactions were admitted for theophylline toxicity (one taking cimetidine and one ciprofloxacin). The other study evaluated the rate of exposure to theophylline drug interactions over 1 year in a state Medicaid population; 37% of patients (6619 total) taking theophylline were prescribed a potentially interacting drug.[50] The overall exposure rate to potential theophylline drug interactions was 17.8%. Thus, the apparent exposure to potentially clinically significant adverse drug interactions is high. Although the actual risk of a serious outcome appears low, the seriousness of the adverse effects warrants preventive measures to reduce the risk.

PHARMACODYNAMIC INTERACTIONS

Pharmacodynamic interactions are often used to benefit patients, such as the use of corticosteroids to upregulate β_2-receptor numbers and improve binding affinity, the additive bronchodilation from anticholinergics, and the enhanced efficacy of adding long-acting inhaled β_2-agonists to inhaled corticosteroids, which may partially be caused by the β_2-agonists priming the glucocorticoid receptor.[3] However, pharmacodynamic interactions may also be harmful, such as with the use of nonselective β-blockers in asthmatic patients or the potential additive hypokalemia produced by diuretics and β_2-agonists. Although ciprofloxacin inhibits the metabolism of theophylline, any seizures that occur may be caused by either elevated theophylline concentrations in the CNS or a pharmacodynamic interaction, specifically to quinolone-induced inhibition of γ-aminobutyric acid receptor binding, which may lower the seizure threshold.[48]

PHARMACOKINETIC INTERACTIONS

The vast majority of drug interactions fall into the pharmacokinetic category. Drugs that are most likely to undergo significant interactions are those drugs that are primarily eliminated by hepatic metabolism. Understanding which of the P-450 isozymes is involved in the metabolism of a drug enhances the capability to predict interactions. Table 89-1 lists which isozymes metabolize common allergy, asthma, and cough medications. Inhibitors or inducers can produce a clinically significant interactions by affecting the primary CYP isozyme (ritonavir inhibiting CYP3A4 leading to increasing fluticasone and budesonide concentrations) or by moderately inhibiting a number of isozymes involved (cimetidine inhibiting CYP1A2, 2C9, 2D6, and 3A4 leading to increasing theophylline concentrations).[30,51] Because of the narrow spectrum, ritonavir does not significantly affect theophylline metabolism. Table 89-2 lists moderate-major drug interactions with common allergy and asthma medications.

An understanding of the time course of pharmacokinetic interactions allows the clinician to monitor patients appropriately to avoid potential adverse consequences. Enzyme induction requires synthesis of new enzymes; thus a 3- to 4-day delay occurs for new protein synthesis before any change is seen. The peak effect depends on the half-life of the inducing drug (i.e., peak effect from rifampin with 4- to 6-hour half-life occurs sooner than from phenobarbital with 24- to 72-hour half-life). The offset is also delayed by the time it takes to eliminate the inducer and then eliminate the excess enzymes. The maximum effect depends on the dose of the inducing medication and requires a 100% increase in clearance to produce a 50% reduction in steady-state serum concentration of the coadministered medication. Enzyme induction is relatively selective; for example, tobacco smoking primarily induces CYP1A2, whereas rifampin and phenobarbital predominantly induce CYP3A4 isozymes.[30]

Enzyme inhibition is also selective, dose dependent, but primarily competitive in nature; therefore its onset is immediate, although the peak effect occurs after five half-lives of the inhibited drug.[30] The offset is shorter because the half-life of the inhibited drug decreases after elimination of the inhibitor. Although understanding the time course allows the clinician to monitor patients given interacting drugs, it is more prudent to avoid potentially serious interactions altogether.

Conclusion

Numerous factors affect the regulation and modification of the response seen with a drug, so it is remarkable that usual doses of drugs are as consistently effective as they are. The factors contributing to altered response are a reminder that drug therapy often requires individualization. With drugs that have a narrow therapeutic index, such as theophylline, individualized patient dosage should be guided by serum drug concentration monitoring.

TABLE 89-2 Major-Moderate Drug-Drug Interactions

Drug	Interaction with	Effect	Mechanism
Fluticasone	Ketoconazole, ritonavir, atazanavir, fosamprenavir, amprenavir, darunavir, nelfinavir, delavirdine, indinavir	↑ Fluticasone concentrations, reports of Cushing syndrome and secondary adrenal insufficiency	↓ Metabolism of fluticasone due to inhibition of CYP3A4 by the listed agents
Budesonide	Ketoconazole, itraconazole, ritonavir	↑ Budesonide plasma concentration, reports of Cushing syndrome	↓ Metabolism of budesonide due to inhibition of CYP3A4 by ketoconazole and itraconazole and by ritonavir
Mometasone	ketoconazole	↑ Mometasone plasma concentration	↓ Metabolism of mometasone due to inhibition of CYP3A4 ketoconazole
Montelukast	Rifampin, phenobarbital	↓ Area under curve of montelukast by 40%	↑ Metabolism montelukast due to induction of CYP2C9 and CYP3A4 by rifampin and phenobarbital
Zafirlukast	Erythromycin	↓ Zafirlukast plasma concentration by 40%	Unknown mechanism
	Theophylline	↑ Possibility of theophylline toxicity	↓ Metabolism of theophylline due to inhibition of CYP1A2, CYP2C9, CYP2D6, and CYP3A4 by zafirlukast
	Warfarin	↑ Risk of bleeding	↓ Metabolism of warfarin due to inhibition of CYP2C9 by zafirlukast
Zileuton	Theophylline	↑ Possibility of theophylline toxicity	↓ Metabolism of theophylline due to inhibition of CYP1A2 by zileuton
	Propranolol	May result in significant increase in β-adrenergic blockade	↓ Metabolism of propranolol due to inhabitation of CYP1A2 by zileuton
	Warfarin	Significant increase in prothrombin time	↓ Metabolism of R-warfarin due to inhibition of CYP1A2 by zileuton

REFERENCES

Pharmacodynamics

1. Liggett SB, Levi R, Metzger H. G-protein coupled receptors, nitric oxide, and the IgE receptor in asthma. Am J Respir Crit Care Med 1995;152:394-402.
2. Lalonde RL. Pharmacodynamics. In: Burton ME, Shaw LM, Schentag JJ, Evans WE, editors. Applied pharmacokinetics and pharmacodynamics: principles of therapeutic drug monitoring. 4th ed. Philadelphia: Lippincott Williams & Wilkins; 2006, p. 60-81.
3. Toews ML, Bylund DB. Pharmacologic principles for combination therapy. Proc Am Thorac Soc 2005;2:282-9.
4. Liggett SB. Update on current concepts of the molecular basis of β_2-adrenergic receptor signaling. J Allergy Clin Immunol 2002;110:S223-7.
5. Bakker RA, Schoonus SB, Smit MJ, Timmerman H, Leurs R. Histamine H_1-receptor activation of nuclear factor-κB: roles for G βγ- and G α(q/11)-subunits in constitutive and agonist-mediated signaling. Mol Pharmacol 2001;60:1133-42.
6. Simons FE. Advances in H_1-antihistamines. N Engl J Med 2004;351:2203-17.
7. Johnson M, Butchers PR, Coleman RA. The pharmacology of salmeterol. Life Sci 1993;52:2131-43.
8. Anderson GP. Interactions between corticosteroids and beta-adrenergic agonists in asthma disease induction, progression, and exacerbation. Am J Respir Crit Care Med 2000;161 (3 Pt 2):S188-96.
9. Jusko WJ. Pharmacokinetics and receptor-mediated pharmacodynamics of corticosteroids. Toxicology 1995;102:189-96.
10. Nelson HS. β-Adrenergic bronchodilators. N Engl J Med 1995;333:499-506.
11. Hubner M, Hochaus G, Derendorf H. Comparative pharmacology, bioavailability, pharmacokinetics, and pharmacodynamics of inhaled glucocorticosteroids. Immunol Allergy Clin North Am 2005;25:469-88.
12. Waldeck B. Enantiomers of bronchodilating β_2-adrenoceptor agonists: is there a cause for concern? J Allergy Clin Immunol 1999;103:742-8.
13. Berger WE. Levalbuterol: pharmacologic properties and use in the treatment of pediatric and adult asthma. Ann Allergy Asthma Immunol 2003;90:583-92.

Pharmaceutics

14. Fink JB. Metered-dose inhalers, dry-powder inhalers, and transitions. Respir Care 2000;45:623-35.
15. Rowe BH, Edmonds ML, Spooner CH, Diner B, Camargo CA Jr. Corticosteroid therapy for acute asthma. Respir Med 2004;98:275-84.
16. McFadden ER Jr. Acute severe asthma. Am J Respir Crit Care Med 2003;168:740-59.
17. Edwards DJ, Zarowitz BJ, Slaughter RL. Theophylline. In: Evans WE, Schentag JJ, Jusko WJ, editors. Applied pharmacokinetics: principles of therapeutic drug monitoring, 3rd ed. Vancouver: Applied Therapeutics; 1992. p. 13-38.
18. Dolovich MA. Influence of inspiratory flow rate, particle size, and airway caliber on aerosolized drug delivery to the lung. Respir Care 2000;45:597-608.
19. Ahrens R, Lux C, Bahl T, et al. Choosing the metered-dose inhaler spacer or holding chamber that matches the patient's need: evidence that the specific drug being delivered is an important consideration. J Allergy Clin Immunol 1995;96:288-94.
20. Hess DR. Nebulizers: principles and performance. Respir Care 2000;45:609-22.

Pharmacokinetic Principles

21. Evans WE. General principles of applied pharmacokinetics. In: Burton ME, Shaw LM, Schentag JJ, Evans WE, editors. Applied pharmacokinetics and pharmacodynamics: principles of therapeutic drug monitoring. 4th ed. Philadelphia: Lippincott Williams & Wilkins; 2006.
22. US Food and Drug Administration. Regulations requiring manufacturers to assess the safety and effectiveness of new drugs and biological products in pediatric patients. November 1998 (Docket No. 97N-0165).
23. Benet LZ, Kroetz DL, Sheiner LB. Pharmacokinetics. In: Hardman JG, Limbird LE, Molinoff PB, et al, editors. Goodman & Gilman's the pharmacological basis of therapeutics. 9th ed. New York: McGraw-Hill; 1996, p. 3-27.
24. Zhang Y, Benet LZ. The gut as a barrier to drug absorption: combined role of cytochrome P450 3A and P-glycoprotein. Clin Pharmacokinet 2001;40:159-68.
25. Kelly HW. Potential adverse effects of inhaled corticosteroids. J Allergy Clin Immunol 2003;112:469-78.
26. Kips JC, Pauwels RA. Long-acting inhaled β2-agonist therapy in asthma. Am J Respir Crit Care Med 2001; 164:923-32.
27. Gross NJ. Anticholinergic agents in asthma and COPD. Eur J Pharmacol 2006;533:36-9.
28. Seidenberg BC, Reiss TF. Montelukast: an anti-leukotriene treatment for asthma. In: Drazen

JM, Dahlen SE, Lee TH, editors. Five-lipoxygenase products in asthma. (Lung biology in health and disease series/120.) New York: Marcel Dekker; 1998, p. 327-46.
29. Simons FE, Simons KJ. Pharmacokinetic optimization of histamine H_1-receptor antagonist therapy. Clin Pharmacokinet 1991;21:372.
30. Kashuba ADM, Park JJ, Pershy AM, Brouwer KLR. Drug metabolism, transport, and the influence of hepatic disease. In: Burton ME, Shaw LM, Schentag JJ, Evans WE, editors. Applied pharmacokinetics and pharmacodynamics: principles of therapeutic drug monitoring. 4th ed. Philadelphia: Lippincott Williams & Wilkins; 2006, p. 121-64.
31. Scordo MG, Pengo V, Spina E, et al. Influence of CYP2C9 and CYP2C19 genetic polymorphisms on warfarin maintenance dose and metabolic clearance. Clin Pharmacol Ther 2002; 72:702-10.
32. Obase Y, Shimoda T, Kawano T, et al. Polymorphisms in the CYP1A2 gene and theophylline metabolism in patients with asthma. Clin Pharmacol Ther 2003;73:468-74.
33. Haga SB, Thummel KB, Burke W. Adding pharmacogenetics information to drug labels: lessons learned. Pharmacogenet Genomics 2006;16:847-54.

Pharmacodynamic Variability

34. Cerrina J, Ladurie ML, Labet C, et al. Comparison of human bronchial muscle responses to histamine in vivo with histamine and isoproterenol agonists in vitro. Am Rev Respir Dis 1986;134:57-61.
35. Karlsson JA, Persson CG. Influences of tracheal contraction on relaxant effects in vitro of theophylline and isoproterenol. Br J Pharmacol 1981;74:73-9.
36. Jenne JW, Shaughnessy TK, Druz WS, et al. In vivo functional antagonism between isoproterenol and bronchoconstrictants in the dog. J Appl Physiol 1987;63:812-9.
37. McWilliams BC, Menendez R, Kelly HW, et al. Effects of theophylline on inhaled methacholine and histamine in asthmatic children. Am Rev Respir Dis 1984;130:193-7.
38. Van Amsterdam RG, Meurs H, Ten Berge RE, et al. Role of phosphoinositide metabolism in human bronchial smooth muscle contraction and in functional antagonism by β-adrenoceptor agonists. Am Rev Respir Dis 1990;142:1124-8.
39. Ito K, Chung KF, Adcock IM. Update on glucocorticoid action and resistance. J Allergy Clin Immunol 2006;117:522-43.
40. Spahn JD, Leung DY, Surs W, et al. Reduced glucocorticoid binding affinity in asthma is related to ongoing allergic inflammation. Am J Respir Crit Care Med 1995;151:1709-14.
41. Weiss ST, Litonjua AA, Lange C, et al. Overview of the pharmacogenetics of asthma treatment. Pharmacogenomics J 2006;6:311-26.
42. Tantisira KG, Lasky-Su J, Harada M, et al. Genome-wide association between GLCI1 and response to glucocorticoid therapy in asthma. N Engl J Med 2011;365:1173-83.
43. Tantisira KG, Lake S, Silverman ES, et al. Corticosteroid pharmacogenetics: association of sequence variants in CRHR1 with improved lung function in asthmatics treated with inhaled corticosteroids. Hum Mol Genet 2004;13: 1353-9.
44. Pincus DJ, Humeston TR, Martin RJ. Further studies on the chronotherapy of asthma with inhaled steroids: the effect of dosage timing on drug efficacy. J Allergy Clin Immunol 1997; 100:771-4.
45. Smolensky MH, Reinberg AE, Martin RJ, et al. Clinical chronobiology and chronotherapeutics with applications to asthma. Chronobiol Int 1999;16:539-63.
46. Hendeles L, Beaty R, Ahrens R, et al. Response to inhaled albuterol during nocturnal asthma. J Allergy Clin Immunol 2004;113:1058-62.

Drug Interactions

47. Budnitz DS, Pollock DA, Weidenbach KN, et al. National surveillance of emergency department visits for outpatient adverse drug events. JAMA 2006;296:1858-66.
48. Grasela TH, Dreis MW. An evaluation of the quinolone-theophylline interaction using the Food and Drug Administration spontaneous reporting system. Arch Intern Med 1992;152: 617-21.
49. Hamilton RA, Gordon T. Incidence and cost of hospital admissions secondary to drug interactions involving theophylline. Ann Pharmacother 1992;26:1507-11.
50. Pashko S, Simons WR, Sena MM, et al. Rate of exposure to theophylline-drug interactions. Clin Ther 1994;16:1068-77.
51. Lacy CF, Armstrong LL, Goldman MP, Lance LL. Drug information handbook. 14th ed. Ohio: Lexi-Comp; 2006. p. 1762-75.

90 Pharmacogenomics of Asthma Therapies

BENJAMIN A. RABY | ELLIOT ISRAEL

CONTENTS

SUMMARY OF IMPORTANT CONCEPTS

» Pharmacogenomics is the study of how genetic differences influence the variability in patients' responses to therapy.
» Pharmacogenomic models exist for the use of β-agonists, leukotriene modifiers, inhaled corticosteroids, and theophylline in asthma.
» Pharmacogenomic information may allow clinicians to treat those who can benefit most from particular asthma medications and may prevent medication-related toxicity by targeting only those unlikely to experience adverse reactions.

Introduction

Although asthma therapies are effective in a large proportion of patients, many asthmatics fail to respond to one or more of the medications. Each of the available asthma medications is associated with adverse effects in particular individuals. Physicians use an *n*-of-one approach to assess whether asthma medications work effectively or cause adverse effects. The evolving field of pharmacogenomics holds out the promise of improving our ability to determine which patients will benefit or experience adverse effects from a particular therapy. The principles and progress of this approach to treating asthma are described in this chapter.

Definition and Background

Pharmacogenomics is the study of how the differences in an individual's genes affect the variation in responses to pharmacotherapy among individuals. Statistical studies suggest that up to 60% of the variability in response to pharmacotherapy is associated with genetic variations among individuals.[1] By using genetic information to identify the functional differences of various genes among individuals and determine the underlying mechanisms for differences in therapeutic responses, pharmacogenomics has the potential to maximize safety and efficacy of treatment.

Genetic Variations Associated with Clinical Outcomes

Pharmacogenomic studies associate variations, or polymorphisms, in the genome with patterns of response to therapy.[2] A full review of genetics is beyond the scope of this chapter, but it is important to understand the terms commonly used in the fields of genetics and pharmacogenomics. They are reviewed in Figure 90-1. A single nucleotide polymorphism (SNP) is a DNA sequence variation, or mutation, that occurs when a single nucleotide in the genome sequence is altered. SNPs can occur in coding and noncoding regions of the genome. Because the genetic code is redundant, a SNP in a coding region can be synonymous (i.e., change in the SNP that does not alter the amino acid coded for in the sequence) or nonsynonymous (i.e., change in the SNP that does alter the amino acid coded for in the sequence).

SNPs are common. They occur almost every 1000 base pairs and are polymorphisms that are stable over time. However, they are not the only type of genetic variation that occurs. Variable numbers of tandem repeats (VNTRs), or microsatellites, are another type of mutation. VNTRs are short segments of DNA that consist of multiple tandem repeats of a specific sequence of DNA bases. They may be less stable over time, and individuals may have different numbers of these segments.

In many cases, a single mutation may not be functional. Because a designated mutation likely started in an individual with a particular pattern of polymorphisms in that area of the genome and because areas that are near to one another tend to be inherited together, the mutation may be a marker for another genetic change that is responsible for the observed functional effect. The nonrandom inheritance of genetic variation in different parts of the genome (i.e., loci) is called *linkage disequilibrium* or *allelic association*. These patterns, which are

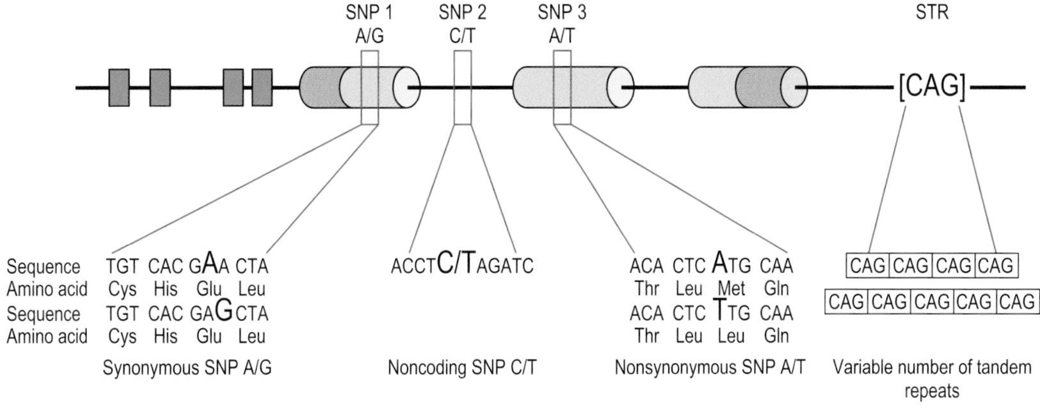

Examples of haplotype sequences

	SNP 1	SNP 2	SNP 3	STR
Hap A	A	C	A	4
Hap B	A	T	T	5
Hap C	A	C	A	5
Hap D	G	C	A	4
Hap E	G	C	A	5

Figure 90-1 Single-nucleotide polymorphisms (SNPs), copy number variations (CNVs), and haplotypes. SNPs localizing to a noncoding sequence (i.e., introns) do not alter the protein because they are not translated (i.e., SNP 2). SNPs localizing to a coding region may not produce a change in the protein sequence if the new DNA sequence does not code for a different amino acid (i.e., synonymous SNP such as SNP 1). SNPs in a coding region that do code for a different amino acid are nonsynonymous (i.e., SNP 3). Short tandem repeats (STRs) contain repetitive-sequence motifs whose number may vary between individuals (four and five repeats are shown). Haplotypes are combinations of different polymorphisms. Some haplotypes that could result from the combinations of SNPs and variation in the STRs in the single chromosome shown are listed in the table (*bottom*). A CNV consisting of a deletion of all of exon 3 and part of exon 4 is depicted. If common in the population, this variant can be seen in hemizygous form (i.e., individuals have one complete sequence and one missing exon 3, intron 3, and part of exon 4) or in homozygous form (i.e., individuals are lacking both copies of exon 3, intron 3, and part of exon 4). *(Adapted from Wechsler ME, Israel E. How pharmacogenomics will play a role in the management of asthma. Am J Respir Crit Care Med 2005;172:12-8, Copyright 2005 by the American Thoracic Society.)*

combinations of various SNPs and VNTRs on a single chromosome, are known as *haplotypes* (see Fig. 90-1), and they have been the subjects of pharmacogenomic association studies.

Another type of genetic polymorphism is *structural genetic variation,* a term that encompasses several types of large-scale genomic aberrations, including segmental rearrangements, such as translocations and inversions, and DNA copy number variations (CNVs). *Translocations* refer to the exchange of DNA sequence between two chromosomes, such as the reciprocal translocation of segments on chromosomes 9 and 22 resulting in the Philadelphia chromosome, t(9;22)(q34;q11), that causes chronic myelogenous leukemia. A *chromosomal inversion* refers to an in situ alteration in the orientation of a chromosomal sequence. CNVs are DNA segments spanning thousands to millions of bases, and the number of copies of these segments varies between individuals. Association of structural variation with rare mendelian diseases has long been known, but the importance of these DNA gains and losses in the pathogenesis of more common diseases has only recently been recognized. CNVs are common and constitute a large proportion of the total genetic variation in human populations.[3]

CNVs have not been implicated in the pharmacogenetics of asthma, likely due to the difficulty in reliably genotyping them in large cohorts. However, evidence regarding the impact of other forms of structural genetic variation suggests their importance. Tantisira and colleagues described the inhaled corticosteroid (ICS) pharmacogenetic effects of a large chromosomal inversion on chromosome 17q21.[4] The inversion spans 900 kb and includes the *CRHR1* gene, which encodes the corticotropin-releasing hormone receptor 1, a G protein–coupled receptor responsible for the downstream actions of corticotropin-releasing hormone. SNPs that serve as surrogates for the inversion were strongly associated with improvements in forced expiratory volume in 1 second (FEV_1) after ICS therapy in a cohort of adult asthmatics. Additional structural variants may have similar pharmacogenetic properties.

Pharmacogenomic Mechanisms

The field of pharmacogenomics assumes that genetic polymorphisms affect therapeutic outcomes. We usually identify three major categories of functional effects under genetic control. First, genetic variations may affect the pharmacodynamics of a therapeutic agent. They may influence the distribution, metabolism, or uptake of a medication, leading to enhanced or impaired drug clearance or inactivation of a drug. Second, a genetic variation in the drug's target, such as an altered receptor, may result in different therapeutic responses due to changes in drug binding or other phenotypic differences. Third, mutation of a gene in one pathway may lead to activation of alternative pathways that can result in idiosyncratic, unexpected effects of the drug (Table 90-1).

TABLE 90-1 **Examples of Asthma Pharmacogenomics**

Therapy	Target	Gene	Improved Outcomes
Short-acting β-agonists	β_2-Adrenergic receptor	*ADRB2*	AM PEF, FEV_1, exacerbations, rescue medication use, symptoms, bronchodilator response
Long-acting β-agonists	β_2-Adrenergic receptor	*ADRB2*	AM PEF, FEV_1, exacerbations
Leukotriene modifiers	5-Lipoxygenase	*ALOX5*	FEV_1, exacerbations
	LTC_4 synthase	*LTC4S*	FEV_1, exacerbations, exhaled nitric oxide
	LTA_4 hydrolase	*LTA4H*	FEV_1
	Multidrug resistance protein 1	*MRP1* (now called *ABCC1*)	FEV_1
Inhaled corticosteroids	T-bet	*TBX21*	Methacholine PC_{20}
	Adenylyl cyclase 9	*ADCY9*	Bronchodilator responsiveness
	Corticotropin-releasing hormone receptor 1	*CRHR1*	FEV_1
Theophylline	Theophylline degradation	*CYP1A2*	Theophylline levels

FEV_1, Forced expiratory volume in 1 second; *LTA_4*, leukotriene A_4; *LTC_4*, leukotriene C_4; *PC_{20}*, dose that induces a 20% fall in FEV_1; *PEF*, peak expiratory flow; *T-bet*, T-box expressed in T cells.

PHARMACOGENOMIC ANALYSIS

Demonstrating a pharmacogenetic effect can affect drug safety and the use of pharmacotherapy. The impetus for a specific pharmacogenomic investigation may start with the desire to define the cause of a particular response or may stem from the discovery of a gene with functional properties or associations that suggest its involvement in the therapeutic response.

The earliest pharmacogenetic studies in asthma focused on SNPs in biologically plausible candidate genes. This progressed to examination of pathways of genes (see "Pharmacogenomics of Leukotriene Modifiers"). Both approaches evolved from methods that involved a putative understanding of the mechanisms governing the action of a particular pharmacologic intervention and possible additional mechanisms related to drug delivery, metabolism, and degradation. The paradigm included several steps: defining the specific phenotypic response (e.g., FEV_1 response to therapy or asthma exacerbation); ascertaining that the given outcome or response to therapy varies within the population and is repeatable in individuals; identifying candidate polymorphisms and their variations; and ideally, testing these associations retrospectively and prospectively (Fig. 90-2).[3]

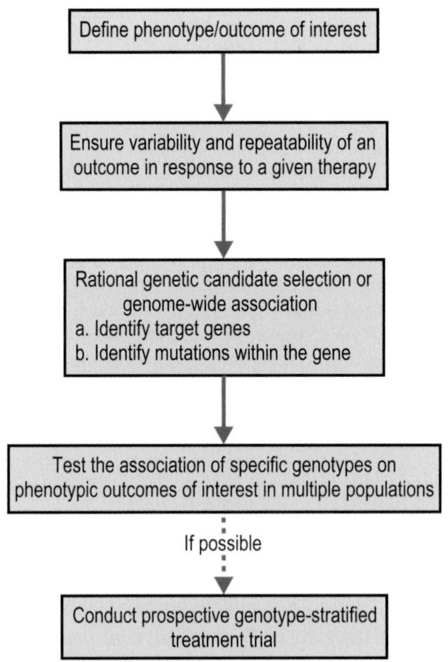

Figure 90-2 Approaches to undertaking non–genome-wide association pharmacogenomic studies. *(Adapted from Ferkol T, Israel E, Wechsler ME. Gene therapy and pharmacogenomic studies. In: Shuster D, Powers W, editors. Translational and experimental clinical research, Philadelphia: Lippincott Williams & Wilkins; 2005, p. 223-36.)*

The original paradigm has been supplemented with a nonheuristic approach that takes advantage of high-throughput genotyping platforms capable of surveying more than 500,000 variants simultaneously. These genome-wide association studies (GWASs) sample a high density of markers across the genome. They rely on the fact that, although a specific polymorphism of interest most likely will not be included in the set of polymorphisms sampled, the marker will be close enough (20 to 100 kb) to a polymorphism of interest to be in linkage disequilibrium with (i.e., travel with) the polymorphism of interest. The marker is identified as associated with the response. Due to the large number of statistical tests performed, GWASs require a very high level of associations to achieve statistical significance and require replication in multiple populations. Unlike candidate gene studies, GWASs require no prior assumptions or knowledge regarding the pharmacologic or biologic mechanisms of treatment response. Because GWASs rely on markers for chromosomal regions, follow-up studies, including detailed sequencing and fine-mapping association studies, are typically needed to define more precisely the true variants and genes underlying the observed associations. Although GWASs are designed to detect common variants, which may contribute small degrees of effect, they are usually underpowered to detect rare variants with large effects. However, the predictive utility of such rare variants and their potential relevance in clinical practice are not clear.

VARIABILITY IN ASTHMA THERAPY RESPONSES

Pharmacogenomics explains the variability in response to therapy. Does such variability occur in response to asthma therapy? Although most asthma patients derive some benefit from each of the major classes of asthma therapies, many asthmatics within a given population do not achieve full control.[5] For instance, there is significant variation in the response to β-agonists within a group of mild asthmatics exposed to the short-acting β-agonist albuterol[6] and similar differences in response to the long-acting β-agonist salmeterol.[7] Up to one third of asthmatics treated with an ICS fail to achieve good control of their asthma despite progressive increases in dose,[5] and more asthmatics may not respond to leukotriene receptor antagonists (LTRAs).[8-10] There is even more variability in populations of different ethnic backgrounds. For example, the change in FEV_1 after administration of an inhaled β-agonist bronchodilator was higher among Mexicans than Puerto Ricans, independent of asthma severity and other covariates.[11,12]

Similar heterogeneity exists for the adverse effects of asthma medications. For example, one third of patients using oral corticosteroids develop osteoporosis,[13-15] the rate of decline in bone density in response to an ICS varies,[16] and some asthmatics develop cataracts or glaucoma with ICS use.[17-20] Approximately, 3% to 5% of patients receiving 5-lipoxygenase inhibitors develop increases in liver function enzymes.[21,22] Regular long-acting β-agonist use has been associated with risk of increased morbidity in a subset of the population.[23]

Although there are several possible explanations for the distribution of these adverse effects, pharmacogenomics has an increasingly important role in understanding the heterogeneity of these responses. Several such studies have been performed. They have identified associations between a variety of loci and the response to different asthma therapies, including β-agonists, ICSs, leukotriene modifiers, and theophylline (see Table 90-1).

Pharmacogenomics of β-Agonists

The best example of the potential contribution of pharmacogenomics to treatment response in asthma comes from studies involving β-agonists. β-Agonists are the most commonly used therapy for asthma. Most asthmatics derive some benefit from these therapies on a consistent basis (i.e., repeatability), but there is a broad spectrum of response (i.e., interindividual variability) to each of these agents within populations and even more variability in populations of different ethnic backgrounds.[11] Since the 1990s, questions have been raised about whether regular exposure to β-agonists may be less effective or even produce adverse effects that increase premature mortality for a subset of patients.

Short-acting and long-acting β-agonists produce their effects by binding to the β_2-adrenergic receptor (ADRB2). Receptor binding activates adenylyl cyclase through stimulatory G proteins that activate protein kinase A, which phosphorylates several target proteins. This eventually decreases the intracellular calcium level, with resultant smooth muscle relaxation and bronchodilation. The β_2-adrenergic receptor has been extensively sequenced and found to be highly polymorphic, with more than 50 reported SNPs identified in the coding region of the gene, in the 5′ and 3′ untranslated regions, and in the adjacent genomic regions.[24,25] Studies using in vitro models found that some of these polymorphisms altered receptor function, ligand binding, and signal transduction.[26-28] For instance, β_2-adrenergic receptors containing glycine in the 16th amino acid position (Arg16Gly of ADRB2) had greater downregulation after isoproterenol exposure than receptors containing arginine. Although no association between any of these polymorphisms and a diagnosis of asthma has been established, several studies have suggested that SNPs in the gene for this receptor may significantly alter the response to short-acting and, to some extent, to long-acting β-agonists (discussed later).

SHORT-ACTING β-AGONISTS

Because of its significant minor allele frequency, one of the most commonly studied polymorphisms is that of the 16th amino acid position (Arg16Gly) of the β_2-adrenergic receptor (ADRB2). Although polymorphisms that cause amino acid changes at the 27th amino acid position are also common, associations between these variants and outcomes have been inconsistent and less studied. At the Arg16Gly locus, polymorphisms may result in arginine/glycine heterozygosity (Arg/Gly), occurring in approximately one half of whites in the United States; homozygosity for arginine (Arg/Arg), occurring in one sixth of whites and one fifth of blacks; or homozygosity for glycine (Gly/Gly), occurring in one third of whites). An early retrospective analysis of this locus in more than 250 mild asthmatics demonstrated that Arg/Arg homozygosity was associated with a decline in peak expiratory flow with regular use of the β-agonist albuterol.[29]

In another study, patients homozygous for arginine had an increased frequency of asthma exacerbations during regular treatment with albuterol compared with those receiving placebo, and they had more exacerbations than Gly/Gly individuals receiving albuterol or placebo.[30] These findings were confirmed in a genotype-stratified, prospective study in which Arg/Arg homozygotes and Gly/Gly homozygotes were screened and matched and then randomized in a double-bind, crossover study design to receive albuterol or placebo four times daily for 16 weeks.[31] To minimize β-agonist use in this study, patients used ipratropium (an inhaled anticholinergic) as their as-needed acute bronchodilator medication. The Arg/Arg homozygotes' peak expiratory flow improved when withdrawn from as-needed β-agonist use with albuterol, and the Gly/Gly patients had improved peak expiratory flow when they were treated with regular albuterol (Fig. 90-3). Similar patterns of genotype-specific effects in FEV_1, symptoms, and use of supplementary reliever medication were observed in this prospective study.[31] In

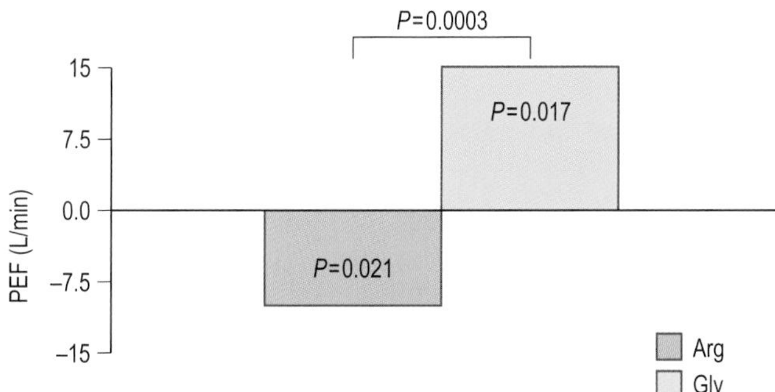

Figure 90-3 Genotype at the 16th amino acid residue of the β-adrenergic receptor affects the response to albuterol use. Arg/Arg homozygotes at Arg16Gly of ADRB2 demonstrated a reduction in peak expiratory flow (PEF) during treatment with albuterol compared with placebo. Those with the Gly/Gly phenotype had an increase in PEF during albuterol treatment compared with placebo. On the basis of these findings, bronchodilator treatments avoiding albuterol may be appropriate for patients with the Arg/Arg genotype. *(From Israel E, Chinchilli VM, Ford JG, Boushey HA, et al. Use of regularly scheduled albuterol treatment in asthma: genotype-stratified, randomised, placebo-controlled cross-over trial. Lancet 2004;364:1505-12.)*

another report, investigators revealed an association between Arg16Gly polymorphisms and airway hyperresponsiveness, particularly among nonsmokers.[32]

The Arg16Gly locus association with regular albuterol use over time has been consistent across studies, but a genotype-specific response to acute bronchodilatation with β-agonists has been inconsistent across studies. An early study examining the effects of the *ADRB2* genotype on responsiveness to β_2-agonists in children found that 60% of Arg/Arg asthmatics had a positive response to albuterol, compared with only 13% in individuals homozygous for glycine at that position.[33] A subsequent small study by Lima and colleagues found a similar association.[34] However, neither a larger study of adults[31] nor a family-based study of children found such an association.[35] Although family-based research evaluating Latinos did find an association between Arg/Arg and bronchodilator response among Puerto Ricans,[11,12] no association was observed for Mexicans, highlighting the importance of assessing genetic findings in different populations.

OTHER *ADRB2* ASSOCIATIONS AND ENVIRONMENTAL AND GENE-GENE INTERACTIONS

Several polymorphisms in the region of the β_2-adrenergic receptor gene (*ADRB2*) have pharmacogenomic associations with treatment. One study suggested an association between bronchodilator responsiveness and a synonymous SNP at nucleotide position +523 in the 3′ end of the coding region of the gene.[35] This finding suggests that additional variants, possibly in the 3′ untranslated region of the gene, may be in linkage disequilibrium with this locus and may represent the causal polymorphisms for the bronchodilator response. Another analysis suggests that the length of a poly-C repeat (−1269) in the 3′ untranslated region of the gene for the receptor may influence lung function and may be important in delineating the variation in response to β-agonists, especially in African Americans.[24]

Patterns of polymorphisms in *ADRB2* have been examined. A study of 13 SNPs in the *ADRB2* gene and its 5′ segments found that the patterns of association of the polymorphisms on the chromosome diverged significantly among different ethnic populations.[36] In this case, one of the three most common haplotypes, which contained Arg at Arg16Gly and accounted for more than three fourths of the Arg16Gly Arg alleles, was associated with a decreased response to β-agonists. In vitro, this haplotype resulted in lower production of *ADRB2*-encoded mRNA and lower receptor density compared with other haplotypes. Two family-based association studies found increased bronchodilator responsiveness to this haplotype,[12,35] but two other reports failed to identify a significant relationship between haplotype pairs and bronchodilator response.[24,37]

GENE-GENE AND ENVIRONMENTAL INTERACTIONS AT *ADRB2*

Although the *ADRB2* gene may be one of the most attractive candidate genes whose alteration may result in a modified response to β-agonists, gene-gene interactions and gene-environment interactions also need to be considered. Smoking can amplify the influence of *ADRB2* polymorphisms on the response to β-agonists.[38] Passive smoking appears to augment the downregulatory effect of arginine polymorphisms.[39]

In addition to environmental effects, some genes may affect bronchodilation itself. The products of genes in the nitrosylation pathway appear to interact with *ADRB2*-encoded proteins. *S*-nitrosoglutathione (GSNO) is an endogenous bronchodilator that can regulate proteins through nitrosylation. The enzyme GSNO reductase (GSNOR) metabolizes GSNO and reduces nitrosylation. An intronic polymorphism in GSNOR interacts with the Gly16 polymorphism of ADRB2 and reduces the response to albuterol.[40] An interaction between GSNOR and Arg16Gly of ADRB2 was identified in a study of more than 600 Puerto Rican and American families with asthma.[41]

Genes that affect the production of nitric oxide, an endogenous bronchodilator, also influence the response to β-agonists. The arginase 1 gene (*ARG1*), which influences the availability of L-arginine, a substrate for nitric oxide synthase, also may affect β-agonist responses. A study by Litonjua and colleagues suggested that polymorphisms in *ARG1* were associated with bronchodilator responses.[42] Others have identified associations between bronchodilator responses and *ARG1* and *ARG2* polymorphisms in various ethnic populations.[43,44] Although the polymorphisms identified were not identical, the findings indicate a likely role for *ARG1* variants in modulating the β-adrenergic response.

LONG-ACTING β-AGONISTS

Large, controlled, prospective studies show that long-acting β-agonists are more effective than albuterol for asthma treatment and that they further improve lung function and reduce asthma exacerbations when used with concurrent ICS treatment.[45-47] The data about whether polymorphisms in the β_2-adrenergic receptor identify patients with different responses to long-acting β-agonists are conflicting.

Similar to the associations found for asthma exacerbations and short-acting β-agonists, a study by Taylor and coworkers demonstrated a trend toward an approximately threefold increase in major asthma exacerbations in Arg/Arg patients receiving salmeterol compared with Gly/Gly individuals.[30] A suggestion that the Arg16Gly locus might be associated with a differential response to long-acting β-agonist therapy came from a retrospective analysis of two studies that demonstrated a decline in lung function in Arg/Arg patients receiving salmeterol.[7] A cross-sectional survey in Scotland that examined 546 children and young adults attending asthma clinics also found a relationship between asthma exacerbations and long-acting β-agonist use and polymorphisms at Arg16Gly, even in patients using concomitant ICS therapy.[48] In this analysis, there was an increased hazard of asthma exacerbations across all treatment steps of the British Thoracic Society asthma guidelines when comparing Arg/Arg to Gly/Gly (OR = 2.05, P = .010). This genotypic hazard was predominantly found in the salmeterol-treated Arg/Arg patients compared with Gly/Gly patients (OR = 3.40, P = .022).

Although these retrospective pharmacogenetic analyses of long-acting β-agonist use, with or without ICS use, were strikingly similar to the retrospective and prospective findings with short-acting β-agonists, an additional retrospective analysis failed to demonstrate a genotype specific difference in response to salmeterol with concurrent fluticasone therapy in Arg/Arg and Gly/Gly subjects.[49] The National Heart, Lung, and Blood Institute (NHLBI) Asthma Clinical Research Network therefore performed a prospective study to examine the effect of Arg16Gly ADRB2 polymorphisms on the response to salmeterol in the setting of moderate doses of ICSs.[50] They found that the Arg16Gly polymorphisms did not affect the peak flow response to the addition of salmeterol but did result in a differential change in methacholine reactivity between genotypes (Fig. 90-4, *A* and *B*). There was a trend toward genotype-specific effects on the peak flow response among the small number of black patients who participated in the study (see Fig. 90-4, *C*).

NON-*ADRB2* PHARMACOGENOMIC ASSOCIATIONS

The β-adrenergic receptor has been most frequently examined for associations with variations in responses to β-agonists, but polymorphisms in other genes also have been related to these variations. For example, polymorphisms in the gene for corticotropin-releasing hormone receptor 2 (*CRHR2*) have been associated with variations in the acute response to albuterol.[43] Genetic variations in the interleukin-6 (*IL6*) and IL-6 receptor (*IL6R*) genes act synergistically to modify bronchodilator responsiveness in asthma patients, and this pharmacogenetic interaction is modified by patients' genetic ancestry.[51]

OVERVIEW OF β-AGONIST PHARMACOLOGY

Although pharmacologic stimulus-response pathway for the β-agonists seems simple, occurring for the most part at a single receptor, multiple pathways likely modulate the response. *ADRB2* polymorphisms affect the response, but there also are differences between short-acting (apparent effect of Arg16Gly) and long-acting β-agonists. The influence of different polymorphisms may be affected by concomitant medication use (e.g., corticosteroids in the case of long-acting β-agonists). Variants in associated pathways may affect the response, and the response also may vary by ethnic background.

The mechanism by which specific mutations exert their effects is unclear. It has been postulated that alterations in specific amino acids result in differential upregulation, downregulation, or other remodeling of the receptor such that it functions differently in individuals harboring different genotypes. For instance, different polymorphisms may activate alternative pathways in which increased inflammation or bronchoconstriction may paradoxically result (e.g., phospholipase C activation and increased cholinergic tone).[52] Further investigation of mechanisms is warranted. A better understanding of *ADRB2*-mediated events in airway smooth muscle may lead to the design of agonists that avoid negative effects of *ADRB2* activation while enhancing muscle relaxation.

Many of these findings are being assessed by ongoing prospective, randomized, placebo-controlled trials, and it appears that pharmacogenomics will play an important role in the future use of β-agonists. Because Arg/Arg occurs in one sixth of whites and up to one fifth of blacks in the United States, the effects described previously may significantly alter recommendations for asthma pharmacotherapy for affected patients.

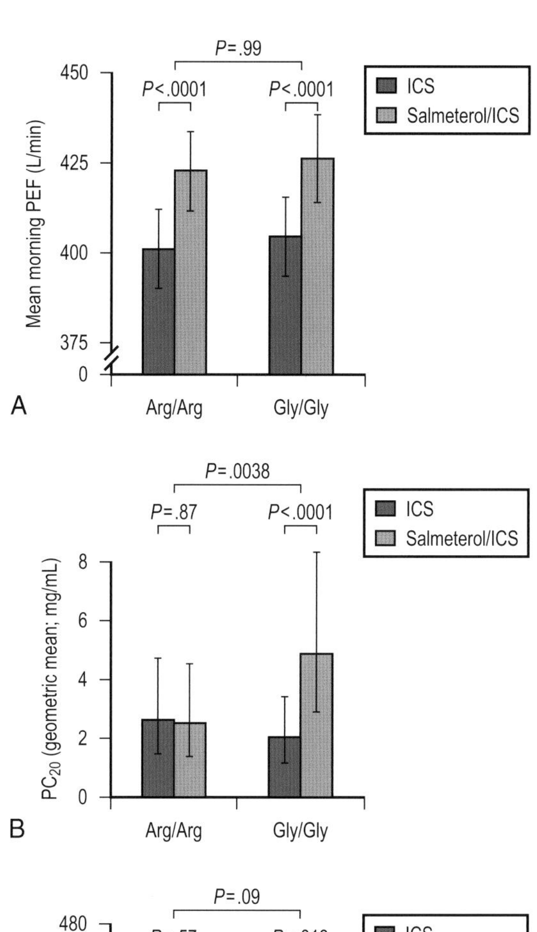

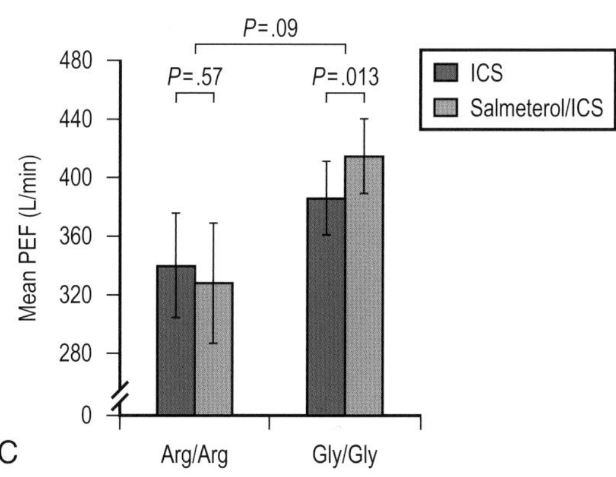

Figure 90-4 β-Adrenergic receptor genotype affects the response to salmeterol and inhaled corticosteroid (ICS) therapy. **A,** Arginine (Arg/Arg) and glycine (Gly/Gly) homozygotes at Arg16Gly of ADRB2 receiving ICS demonstrated equal improvements in forced expiratory volume in 1 second (FEV_1) when salmeterol was added to ICSs. **B,** An improvement in methacholine responsiveness occurred in Gly/Gly patients that did not occur in Arg/Arg homozygotes. **C,** There was a trend toward more improvement in peak expiratory flow (PEF) for black patients with the Gly/Gly phenotype than for those with the Arg/Arg phrnotype with the addition of salmeterol. PC_{20}, Provocative concentration of methacholine that induces a 20% decrease in FEV_1. *(Adapted from Wechsler ME, Kunselman SJ, Chinchilli VM, et al. Effect of beta(2)-adrenergic receptor polymorphism on response to long-acting beta(2) agonist in asthma (LARGE trial): a genotype-stratified, randomised, placebo-controlled, crossover trial. Lancet 2009;374:1754-64.)*

Pharmacogenomics of Leukotriene Modifiers

Leukotriene modifiers used in the treatment of asthma target the pathway of cysteinyl leukotriene formation or the cysteinyl leukotriene receptor 1 (CYSLTR1). The latter is the primary receptor that transduces the activity of these proinflammatory mediators. The biosynthesis of the cysteinyl leukotrienes has been well defined (Fig. 90-5),[53] and the enzymes involved in the synthesis of these inflammatory mediators are prime targets as potential contributors to the pharmacogenetic variability of the

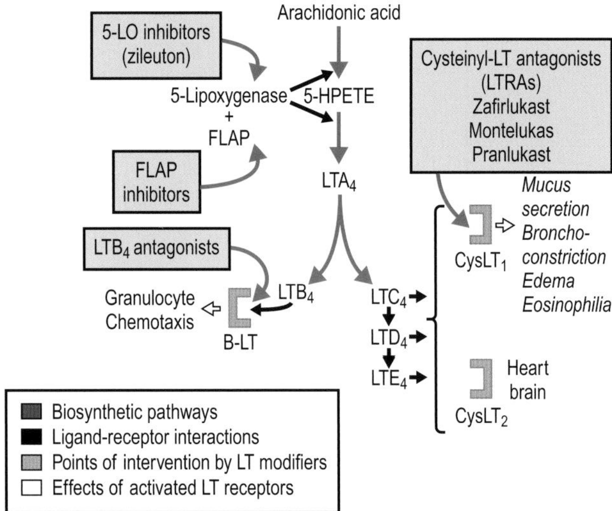

Figure 90-5 Leukotrienes are synthesized from arachidonic acid through the action of 5-lipoxygenase (5-LO) and 5-lipoxygenase activating protein (FLAP), and they play important roles in mediating airway inflammation. Leukotriene modifiers include 5-LO inhibitors and cysteinyl leukotriene antagonists. FLAP inhibitors and leukotriene B_4 (LTB_4) antagonists are being studied. *B-LT,* Leukotriene B_4 receptors 1 and 2; *CystLT*$_1$, cysteinyl leukotriene receptor 1 (CYSLTR1); *CystLT*$_2$, cysteinyl leukotriene receptor 2 (CYSLTR2); *5-HPETE,* 5-hydroperoxyeicosatetraenoic acid; *LT,* leukotriene; *LTRAs,* leukotriene receptor antagonists. *(Adapted from Deykin A, Israel E. Newer therapeutic agents for asthma. Adv Intern Med 1999;44:209-37.)*

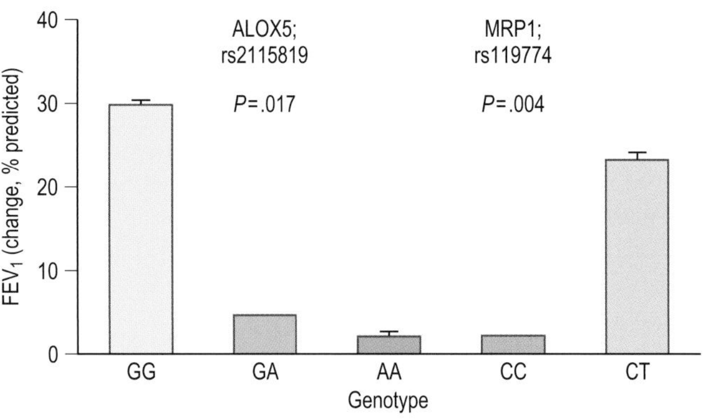

Figure 90-6 Leukotriene pathway polymorphisms in *ALOX5* and *MRP1* (now called *ABCC1*) contribute to the variability in the response to montelukast, a leukotriene receptor antagonist. *FEV*$_1$, Forced expiratory volume in 1 second. *(Adapted from Lima JJ, Zhang S, Grant A, et al. Influence of leukotriene pathway polymorphisms on response to montelukast in asthma. Am J Respir Crit Care Med 2006;173:379-85. Copyright 2006 by the American Thoracic Society.)*

treatment response to leukotriene modifiers. Two have been investigated. The first is the gene for 5-lipoxygenase (*ALOX5*), which encodes an enzyme that converts arachidonic acid into the first precursor of the cysteinyl leukotrienes. The second is the gene responsible for adding a peptide moiety to the fatty acid backbone of the leukotrienes–the leukotriene C_4 (LTC_4) synthase gene (*LTC4S*).

Studies of *ALOX5* have focused on alterations in the number of repeats in a transcription binding motif in the promoter region of the gene. Most individuals have five copies of this motif in tandem (i.e., wild-type allele). A retrospective study of the effect of a 5-lipoxygenase inhibitor (ABT-761) suggested that patients homozygous for non–wild-type alleles (i.e., possessing more or less of these repeats) had a reduced response to the inhibitor as judged by FEV_1.[54] However, less than 3% of the patients studied were homozygous for the non–wild-type allele. Consistent with this report, a study of a population that did not contain patients homozygous for the non–wild-type alleles showed no difference in bronchodilator response or bronchial hyperresponsiveness after treatment with an LTRA.[55] This finding was replicated in a study of montelukast, an LTRA, in which subjects with at least one copy of the wild-type allele had decreased exacerbations and greater improvement in FEV_1.[56]

Another study of patients treated with an LTRA suggested that the promoter repeats were associated with differences in protection from exacerbations. However, the patients who possessed at least one copy of the non–wild-type allele[57] were those who had the greatest benefit—73% fewer exacerbations than those who did not have at least one copy of the allele. The investigators also found that another SNP of this enzyme was associated with differences in rates of exacerbations in response to an LTRA. The effect of a SNP in 5-lipoxygenase was replicated in a study of zileuton, the 5-lipoxygenase inhibitor.[58] Taken together, these studies do suggest that polymorphisms of 5-lipoxygenase can affect the response to leukotriene modifiers.

Studies have consistently shown that the *LTC4S* A-444C SNP (rs730012)affects the response to leukotriene modifiers. In vitro, the C variant of the LTC_4 synthase promoter at this position is associated with enhanced expression of LTC_4 synthase in blood eosinophils[59,60] and with increased production of LTC_4 by blood eosinophils stimulated with a calcium ionophore.[61] In 23 asthmatics, treatment with the LTRA zafirlukast showed a trend toward greater improvement in lung function in those possessing at least one copy of the C variant compared with those who had no copies of this allele.[61] This same variant was associated with a 14% improvement in FEV_1 in a Japanese population in response to an LTRA compared with a 3% improvement in those not possessing the C allele ($P = .01$).[62] In children, this variant appeared to distinguish patients who had a decline in exhaled nitric oxide (a marker of airway inflammation) in response to an LTRA from those who did not.[63] In another study, those who possessed this variant, compared with those who did not, had an 80% reduction in exacerbations when treated with the LTRA, montelukast.[57] Curiously, those who possessed the variant and were treated with placebo experienced 69% fewer exacerbations, but this effect occurred only in the heterozygotes, suggesting that it might have been spurious. Taken together, these studies suggest that this promoter variant in LTC_4 synthase is associated with differential responsiveness to an LTRA.

Lima and colleagues studied the effect of leukotriene pathway polymorphismson the pharmacogenetic response to an LTRA in 61 white patients in the United States.[57] The investigators also examined SNPs and patterns of SNPs of 5-lipoxygenase; ATP-binding cassette subfamily C member 1 (ABCC1, formerly called multidrug resistance protein 1 [MRP1]), which is responsible for transporting LTC_4 into the extracellular space; and leukotriene A_4 hydrolase, which is responsible for the synthesis of the noncysteinyl leukotriene B_4 (Fig. 90-6). They observed associations between several SNPs in these genes and a variety of asthma outcomes, including improvement in FEV_1 and exacerbations.

As for ADRB2, data suggest that gene-gene interactions modulate responses to leukotriene modifiers. Polymorphisms in the genes for interleukin-13 (*IL13*), the thromboxane A_2 receptor (*TBXA2R*), and the prostaglandin D_2 receptor (*PTGDR*) have been associated with altered responses to LTRAs.[64-66]

Pharmacogenomics of Corticosteroids

ICSs are the primary medications that control asthma effectively in children and adults. However, individual responses vary. The potential to predict patient responses to corticosteroids by pharmacogenomic mechanisms holds much attraction, and a number of candidate genes and genome-wide studies have been performed.

Much of this work has been performed using the Childhood Asthma Management Program (CAMP),[67] a multicenter, randomized trial that compared regularly scheduled inhaled treatment with budesonide, nedocromil sodium, and placebo. CAMP followed 1041 children 5 to 12 years of age for 4 to 6 years. All pharmacogenetic investigations of this population have restricted themselves to the white subset (72%) of the total cohort. Candidate gene studies have identified replicable associations with inhaled glucocorticoid-responsiveness for three genes: *TBX21*, *ADCY9*, and *CRHR1* (see Table 90-1).

TBX21 encodes the transcription factor T-box expressed in T cells (T-bet), which has been implicated in asthma pathogenesis and influences naïve T lymphocyte development through induction of type 1 T helper (Th1) cells and the suppression of type 2 T helper (Th2) cells from naïve T lymphocytes. A nonsynonymous SNP was associated with a large improvement in airway hyperresponsiveness in response to corticosteroid therapy.[68] Although the minor allele frequency of this variant is less than 5%, and only five children in the treatment group possessed this allele and had the exuberant response, similar findings have been observed in independent populations of Asian decent.[69]

ADCY9 encodes adenylyl cyclase type 9, an enzyme activated by the β_2-adrenergic receptor that influences the responses to ICS therapy. An interaction was found between the nonsynonymous polymorphism at amino acid 772 and improved bronchodilator response over the 4 years of ICS treatment.[70] This finding has been reproduced in Korean populations.[71] In addition to the association of the *CRHR1* inversion with corticosteroid responsiveness, a related haplotypic combination of SNPs at this locus was associated with a twofold to threefold difference in ICS-related improvement in FEV_1 in the CAMP children and in a second adult population.[72]

Genome-wide approaches have identified functional variants that regulate the expression of the glucocorticoid-induced transcript 1 gene (*GLCCI1*) and that demonstrate consistent and reproducible ICS pharmacogenetic associations.[73] GLCCI1 is highly expressed in lung tissue, T and B lymphocytes, and natural killer cells, and it has been implicated in glucocorticoid-induced apoptosis.[74,75] *GLCCI1* gene expression is induced by glucocorticoids, and in vitro studies of lymphoblastoid B cells demonstrate a strong correlation between the degree of gene expression and clinical response to ICS. The most strongly associated functional variant is an A to G transition residing in a putative promoter sequence that is 1106 bases upstream of the *GLCCI1* translation start site (rs37973). The G allele has a

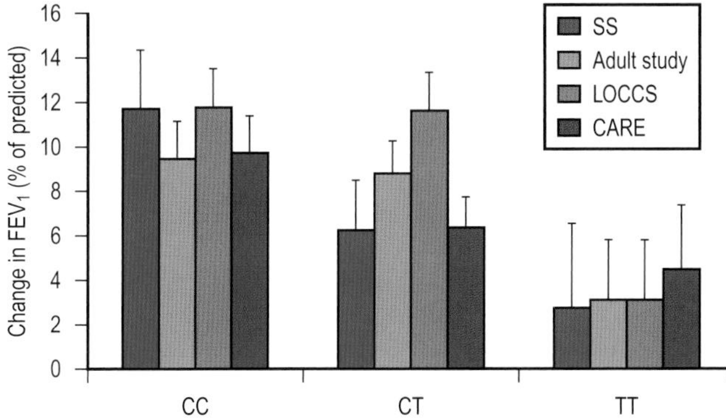

Figure 90-7 The association of *GLCCI1* (rs37972) genotypes with changes in lung function is shown as the mean (±SE) change in forced expiratory volume in 1 second (FEV_1), expressed as the percent of the predicted value after 4 to 8 weeks of therapy with inhaled corticosteroids. Results are stratified by rs37972 polymorphisms (CC, CT, and TT) that were evaluated in four studies. *Adult Study*, Study of the efficacy and tolerability of flunisolide administered once daily by AeroChamber in adults; *CARE*, childhood Asthma Research and Education Network trial; *LOCCS*, Leukotriene Modifier or Corticosteroid or Corticosteroid–Salmeterol (LOCCS) trial; *SLIC*, Salmeterol ± Inhaled Corticosteroids trial; *SOCS*, Salmeterol or Corticosteroids trial; *SS*, combined SOCS and SLIC trials. *(From Tantisira KG, Lasky-Su J, Harada M, et al. Genomewide association between GLCCI1 and response to glucocorticoid therapy in asthma. N Engl J Med 2011;365:1173-83.)*

minor allele frequency of about 40% and confers reduced *GLCCI1* gene expression relative to the more common A allele. In an analysis of four clinical trials that included CAMP subjects (combined sample size of 935), the rs37973 genotype accounted for 6.6% of the variability in response to ICS. Compared with individuals homozygous for the common AA genotype, GG homozygotes exhibited markedly reduced improvement in FEV_1 after ICS treatment (mean change: GG = 3.2% ± 1.6% versus AA = 9.4% ± 1.1%) (Fig. 90-7), and they were more than twice as likely to have a poor response to ICS therapy. Although conclusive mechanistic studies are warranted, these combined data suggest that the *GLCCI1* promoter polymorphism confers corticosteroid hyporesponsiveness by reducing *GLCCI1* gene expression and consequently attenuating glucocorticoid-induced apoptosis of airway inflammatory cells.

Gene expression profiling studies have been used to identify potential glucocorticoid pharmacogenetic candidates. A study of glucocorticoid-sensitive and glucocorticoid-resistant asthma patients from Iceland examined gene expression profiles in freshly isolated peripheral blood mononuclear cells.[76] Glucocorticoid-resistant patients did not experience improvements assessed clinically or by lung function in response to conventional therapeutic doses of glucocorticoids. Peripheral blood mononuclear cells were exposed to interleukin-1β (IL-1β) and tumor necrosis factor-α (TNF-α), and gene expression was assayed. Expression of 15 genes most accurately separated glucocorticoid responders ($n = 26$) from glucocorticoid nonresponders ($n = 18$). One of these genes, the NF-κB DNA binding subunit (*NFKB1*) predicted glucocorticoid sensitivity with an accuracy of 81% in a validation subset cohort of 79 patients. NF-κB, is a transcription factor responsible for activating the transcription of multiple cytokines, chemokines, growth factors, cellular ligands, and adhesion molecules that have been associated with asthma, and it is suppressed by corticosteroids. In addition to NF-κB, genes for signal transducer and activator of transcription 4 (*STAT4*) and interlukin-4 (*IL4*) also predicted glucocorticoid sensitivity and resistance. These findings have not been corroborated in other populations, nor have they been tested prospectively.

Woodruff and colleagues demonstrated that baseline expression of the FK506 binding protein 51 gene (*FKBP51*) in bronchial epithelium was inversely associated with corticosteroid responsiveness.[77] These findings were extended in a study of circulating peripheral blood mononuclear cells, in which dexamethasone-induced overexpression of *FKBP51* correlated with reduced improvements in lung function after oral corticosteroid use.[78] Although these studies were small (e.g., six patients studied in the latter study) and it is unclear whether a practical, inexpensive clinical test can be developed, their results suggest that *FKBP51* is a potential biomarker to predict corticosteroid responsiveness in asthma.

In summary, early studies in distinct populations have suggested that alterations in expression of or genetic polymorphisms in transcription factors associated with secondary inflammatory mediators (*NFKB1*) or T cell proliferation (*TBX21*), effector enzymes for the β_2-adrenergic receptor (*ADCY9*), or genes involved in corticosteroid pharmacodynamics (*CRHR1* and *GLCCI1*) may affect responses to corticosteroids. These preliminary studies in restricted populations require corroboration.

Pharmacogenomics of Other Asthma Therapies

Although most asthmatics are treated with β-agonists, leukotriene modifiers, or ICSs, asthma patients may also receive treatment with theophylline, omalizumab, or H_1 antihistamines. Many genetic loci have been implicated in their therapeutic pathways[79,80] (e.g., association between *FCER2* gene and IgE levels), but no studies have identified loci that predict responsiveness to any of these therapies.

A common promoter polymorphism in the *CYP1A2* gene has been associated with altered clearance of theophylline. The A allele of a G/A SNP at position −2964 of the gene was associated with decreased clearance resulting in increased serum levels in a group of 75 Japanese asthmatics. Although these findings need to be replicated, they are biologically plausible because CYP1A2 is known to degrade theophylline to 1,3-dimethyl uric acid before excretion in the urine, and poor metabolizers of theophylline have been identified. In view of theophylline's narrow therapeutic range, knowledge about the polymorphism may aid in prospective determination of a correct therapeutic dose for an individual patient.[81] As newer therapies emerge and as our understanding of the mechanisms of current therapies evolves, it is expected that additional pharmacogenomic models for these therapies will be elucidated.

Interpretation and Application of Pharmacogenomic Findings

Many of the pharmacogenomic associations detected in large populations have only small effects on the therapeutic response. However, even variations in genes that have large effects on a pharmacologic response (e.g., effects observed at the 16th position of the β-adrenergic receptor) may not produce an entirely uniform response to a therapy. Additional sources of variability can confound association studies and result in misleading associations. These sources also can introduce enough statistical noise to mask real associations. The sources of variability can be classified as simultaneous genetic interactions, host factors, and environmental effects.

Coincident genetic alterations may magnify or diminish an apparent pharmacogenomic effect. These simultaneous polymorphisms can occur within the same gene or among different genes. For example, if a combination of polymorphisms of the β-adrenergic receptor identifies patients with a diminished response to β-agonists and if these patients simultaneously possess a beneficial polymorphism in the corticosteroid pathway (e.g., corticotrophin-releasing hormone receptor 1 [CRHR1]), they may display an intermediate, rather than poor, response to a combination of long-acting β-agonists and an ICS. The overall genetic background of a specific population can further modify these interactions. Different inbred populations or ethnicities may not display the same association with a particular set of genetic markers. For example, the Arg/Arg genotype (i.e., homozygosity for arginine) at position 16 of the β-adrenergic receptor predicts the response to β-agonists in Puerto Rican but not Mexican populations.[11] Host factors such as disease severity, age, concomitant drugs, and disease cause can also affect responses. Factors such as disease severity may have their own genetic associations that are an additional genomic source of variability.

Environmental effects can modify responses. For example, studies suggest that smoking modulates the beneficial asthmatic response to ICS[82] and may alter the effects of polymorphisms of the β-adrenergic receptor.[32] A specific environmental effect may occur in a particular genetic group because of cultural differences. Because these sources of variability may confound apparent pharmacogenomic associations, it is important to reconfirm the associations, especially those without clear functional correlates, in many populations with different ethnic and genetic backgrounds.

Pharmacogenomic information may allow treatment of those who can benefit most from particular asthma medications and avoid toxicity by administering medications only to those unlikely to be susceptible because of their genetic profile. For example, if pharmacogenomics fulfills its promise, we will be able to administer corticosteroids to those least likely to experience adverse effects. Pharmacogenomics also has implications for drug development. This approach may permit the development and introduction of drugs for asthma that would have previously been abandoned due to potential toxicity in a subset of patients.

The therapeutic and detrimental genetic associations of each of the classes of commonly used asthma medications affect development of individualized therapy for asthma. Although the effects observed at position 16 of the β-adrenergic receptor may be of sufficient magnitude to affect therapy, most pharmacogenomic effects are probably of smaller magnitude or, as with 5-lipoxygenase polymorphisms, are less common. Panels of polymorphisms to ascertain relative risk-benefit ratios of particular therapeutic approaches for an individual patient are likely to be introduced as part of the tailored approach to medicine and treatments.

When will this information be ready for routine clinical use? Considering the rapid fall in the cost of simultaneous genotyping at multiple loci, it is unlikely that the technology will limit the introduction of this method. It is more likely that whole-genome sequencing (i.e., complete resequencing of all 3 billion bases) will replace genotyping in the near future due to its increasing affordability (about $5000 per genome in 2011) and its generalizability to all clinical fields. Instead, the pace of the introduction of pharmacogenomics to routine practice will be dictated by the availability of reliable predictors (validated in well-designed clinical trials) and the dissemination of this data to the general medical public. These association studies and biologically informative pharmacogenomic trials will allow us to prescribe the right drugs for the right patients.

REFERENCES

Definition and Background

1. Drazen JM, Silverman EK, Lee TH. Heterogeneity of therapeutic responses in asthma. Br Med Bull 2000;56:1054-70.

Genetic Variations Associated with Clinical Outcomes

2. Wechsler ME, Israel E. How pharmacogenomics will play a role in the management of asthma. Am J Respir Crit Care Med 2005;172:12-8.
3. Tuzun E, Sharp AJ, Bailey JA, et al. Fine-scale structural variation of the human genome. Nat Genet 2005;37:727-32.
4. Tantisira KG, Lazarus R, Litonjua AA, Klanderman B, Weiss ST. Chromosome 17: association of a large inversion polymorphism with corticosteroid response in asthma. Pharmacogenet Genomics 2008;18:733-7.

Pharmacogenomic Mechanisms

5. Bateman ED, Boushey HA, Bousquet J, et al. Can guideline-defined asthma control be achieved? The Gaining Optimal Asthma ControL study. Am J Respir Crit Care Med 2004;170:836-44.
6. Drazen JM, Israel E, Boushey HA, et al. Comparison of regularly scheduled with as-needed use of albuterol in mild asthma. N Engl J Med 1996;335:841-7.
7. Wechsler ME, Lehman E, Lazarus SC, et al. National Heart, Lung, and Blood Institute's Asthma Clinical Research Network. Beta-adrenergic receptor polymorphisms and response to salmeterol. Am J Respir Crit Care Med 2006;173:519-26.
8. Malmstrom K, Rodriguez-Gomez G, Guerra J, et al. Oral montelukast, inhaled beclomethasone, and placebo for chronic asthma. Ann Intern Med 1999;130:487-95.
9. Zeiger RS, Szefler SJ, Phillips BR, et al. Response profiles to fluticasone and montelukast in mild-to-moderate persistent childhood asthma. J Allergy Clin Immunol 2006;117:45-52.
10. Szefler SJ, Phillips BR, Martinez FD, et al. Characterization of within-subject responses to fluticasone and montelukast in childhood asthma. J Allergy Clin Immunol 2005;115:233-42.
11. Burchard EG, Avila PC, Nazario S, et al. Lower bronchodilator responsiveness in Puerto Rican than in Mexican subjects with asthma. Am J Respir Crit Care Med 2004;169:386-92.
12. Choudhry S, Ung N, Avila PC, et al. Pharmacogenetic differences in response to albuterol between Puerto Ricans and Mexicans with asthma. Am J Respir Crit Care Med 2005;171:563-70.
13. Covar RA, Leung DY, McCormick D, et al. Risk factors associated with glucocorticoid-induced adverse effects in children with severe asthma. J Allergy Clin Immunol 2000;106:651-9.
14. Wong CA, Walsh LJ, Smith CJP, et al. Inhaled corticosteroid use and bone-mineral density in patients with asthma. Lancet 2000;355:1399-403.
15. Baylink DJ. Glucocorticoid-induced osteoporosis. N Engl J Med 1983;309:306-8.
16. Israel E, Banerjee TR, Fitzmaurice GM, et al. Effects of inhaled glucocorticoids on bone density in premenopausal women. N Engl J Med 2001;345:941-7.
17. Abuekteish F, Kirkpatrick JN, Russell G. Posterior subcapsular cataract and inhaled corticosteroid therapy. Thorax 1995;50:674-6.
18. Agertoft L, Larsen FE, Pedersen S. Posterior subcapsular cataracts, bruises and hoarseness in children with asthma receiving long-term treatment with inhaled budesonide. Eur Respir J 1998;12:130-5.
19. Leone FT, Fish JE, Szefler SJ, West SL. Systematic review of the evidence regarding potential complications of inhaled corticosteroid use in asthma: collaboration of American College of Chest Physicians, American Academy of Allergy, Asthma, and Immunology, and American College of Allergy, Asthma, and Immunology. Chest 2003;124:2329-40.
20. Garbe E, LeLorier J, Boivin J-F, Suissa S. Inhaled and nasal glucocorticoids and the risks of ocular hypertension or open-angle glaucoma. JAMA 1997;277:722-7.
21. Lazarus SC, Lee T, Kemp JP, et al. Safety and clinical efficacy of zileuton in patients with chronic asthma. Am J Manag Care 1998;4:841-8.
22. Drazen JM, Israel E, O'Byrne PM. Treatment of asthma with drugs modifying the leukotriene pathway. N Engl J Med 1999;340:197-206.
23. Nelson HS, Weiss ST, Bleecker ER, Yancey SW, Dorinsky PM. The Salmeterol Multicenter Asthma Research Trial: a comparison of usual pharmacotherapy for asthma or usual pharmacotherapy plus salmeterol. Chest 2006;129:15-26.

Pharmacogenomics of β-Agonists

24. Hawkins GA, Tantisira K, Meyers DA, et al. Sequence, haplotype, and association analysis of ADRbeta2 in a multiethnic asthma case-control study. Am J Respir Crit Care Med 2006;174:1101-9.
25. Weiss ST, Litonjua AA, Lange C, et al. Overview of the pharmacogenetics of asthma treatment. Pharmacogenomics J 2006;6:311-26.
26. Green SA, Turki J, Bejarano P, Hall IP, Liggett SB. Influence of beta(2)-adrenergic receptor genotypes on signal transduction in human airway smooth muscle cells. Am J Respir Cell MolBiol 1995;13:25-33.
27. Green SA, Turki J, Hall IP, Liggett SB. Implications of genetic variability of human beta 2-adrenergic receptor structure. Pulm Pharmacol 1995;8:1-10.
28. Green SA, Cole G, Jacinto M, Innis M, Liggett SB. A polymorphism of the human beta 2-adrenergic receptor within the fourth transmembrane domain alters ligand binding and functional properties of the receptor. J Biol Chem 1993;268:23116-21.
29. Israel E, Drazen JM, Liggett SB, et al. The effect of polymorphisms of the beta2-adrenergic receptor on the response to regular use of albuterol in asthma. Am J Respir Crit Care Med 2000;162:75-80.
30. Taylor DR, Drazen JM, Herbison GP, et al. Asthma exacerbations during long term beta-agonist use: influence of beta2 adrenoceptor polymorphism. Thorax 2000;55:762-7.
31. Israel E, Chinchilli VM, Ford JG, et al. Use of regularly scheduled albuterol treatment in asthma: genotype-stratified, randomised, placebo-controlled cross-over trial. Lancet 2004;364:1505-12.
32. Litonjua AA, Silverman EK, Tantisira KG, et al. Beta 2-adrenergic receptor polymorphisms and haplotypes are associated with airways hyperresponsiveness among nonsmoking men. Chest 2004;126:66-74.
33. Martinez FD, Graves PE, Baldini M, Solomon S, Erickson R. Association between genetic polymorphisms of the beta 2-adrenoceptor and response to albuterol in children with and without a history of wheezing. J Clin Invest 1997;100:3184-8.
34. Lima JJ, Thomason DB, Mohamed MH, et al. Impact of genetic polymorphisms of the beta 2-adrenergic receptor on albuterol bronchodilator pharmacodynamics. Clin Pharmacol Ther 1999;65:519-25.
35. Silverman EK, Kwiatkowski DJ, Sylvia JS, et al. Family-based association analysis of beta2-adrenergic receptor polymorphisms in the childhood asthma management program. J Allergy Clin Immunol 2003;112:870-6.
36. Drysdale CM, McGraw DW, Stack CB, et al. Complex promoter and coding region beta 2-adrenergic receptor haplotypes alter receptor expression and predict in vivo responsiveness. Proc Natl Acad Sci U S A 2000;97:10483-8.
37. Taylor DR, Epton MJ, Kennedy MA, et al. Bronchodilator response in relation to beta2-adrenoceptor haplotype in patients with asthma. Am J Respir Crit Care Med 2005;172:700-3.
38. Zhang G, Hayden CM, Khoo SK, et al. Beta2-adrenoceptor polymorphisms and asthma phenotypes: interactions with passive smoking. Eur Respir J 2007;30:48-55.
39. Wang C, Salam MT, Islam T, et al. Effects of in utero and childhood tobacco smoke exposure and $beta_2$-adrenergic receptor genotype on childhood asthma and wheezing. Pediatrics 2008;122:e107-14.
40. Moore PE, Ryckman KK, Williams SM, et al. Genetic variants of GSNOR and ADRB2 influence response to albuterol in African-American children with severe asthma. Pediatr Pulmonol 2009;44:649-54.
41. Busse WW, Morgan WJ, Gergen PJ, et al. Randomized trial of omalizumab (anti-IgE) for asthma in inner-city children. N Engl J Med 2011;364:1005-15.
42. Litonjua AA, Lasky-Su J, Schneiter K, et al. ARG1 is a novel bronchodilator response gene: screening and replication in four asthma cohorts. Am J Respir Crit Care Med 2008;178:688-94.

43. Poon AH, Tantisira KG, Litonjua AA, et al. Association of corticotropin-releasing hormone receptor-2 genetic variants with acute bronchodilator response in asthma. Pharmacogenet Genomics 2008;18:373-82.
44. Chowdhury BA, Dal Pan G. The FDA and safe use of long-acting beta-agonists in the treatment of asthma. N Engl J Med 2010;362: 1169-71.
45. Greening AP, Ind PW, Northfield M, Shaw G. Added salmeterol versus higher-dose corticosteroid in asthma patients with symptoms on existing inhaled corticosteroid. Alen & Hanburys Limited UK Study Group. Lancet 1994; 344:219-24.
46. Taylor DR, Town GI, Herbison GP, et al. Asthma control during long-term treatment with regular inhaled salbutamol and salmeterol. Thorax 1998;53:744-52.
47. Woolcock A, Lundback B, Ringdal N, Jacques LA. Comparison of addition of salmeterol to inhaled steroids with doubling of the dose of inhaled steroids. Am J Respir Crit Care Med 1996;153:1481-8.
48. Palmer CN, Lipworth BJ, Lee S, et al. Arginine-16 β2 adrenoceptor genotype predisposes to exacerbations in young asthmatics taking regular salmeterol. Thorax 2006;61:940-4.
49. Bleecker ER, Yancey SW, Baitinger LA, et al. Salmeterol response is not affected by beta2-adrenergic receptor genotype in subjects with persistent asthma. J Allergy Clin Immunol 2006;118:809-16.
50. Wechsler ME, Kunselman SJ, Chinchilli VM, et al. Effect of beta(2)-adrenergic receptor polymorphism on response to longacting beta(2) agonist in asthma (LARGE trial): a genotype-stratified, randomised, placebo-controlled, crossover trial. Lancet 2009;374:1754-64.
51. Corvol H, De Giacomo A, Eng C, et al. Genetic ancestry modifies pharmacogenetic gene-gene interaction for asthma. Pharmacogenet Genomics 2009;19:489-96.
52. McGraw DW, Almoosa KF, Paul RJ, Kobilka BK, Liggett SB. Antithetic regulation by beta-adrenergic receptors of Gq receptor signaling via phospholipase C underlies the airway beta-agonist paradox. J Clin Invest 2003;112:619-26.

Pharmacogenomics of Leukotriene Modifiers

53. Deykin A, Israel E. Newer therapeutic agents for asthma. Adv Intern Med 1999;44:209-37.
54. Drazen JM, Yandava CN, Dube L, et al. Pharmacogenetic association between ALOX5 promoter genotype and the response to anti-asthma treatment. NatGenet 1999;22:168-70.
55. Fowler SJ, Hall IP, Wilson AM, Wheatley AP, Lipworth BJ. 5-Lipoxygenase polymorphism and in-vivo response to leukotriene receptor antagonists. Eur J Clin Pharmacol 2002;58: 187-90.
56. Telleria JJ, Blanco-Quiros A, Varillas D, et al. ALOX5 promoter genotype and response to montelukast in moderate persistent asthma. Respir Med 2008;102:857-61.
57. Lima JJ, Zhang S, Grant A, et al. Influence of leukotriene pathway polymorphisms on response to montelukast in asthma. Am J Respir Crit Care Med 2006;173:379-85.
58. Neill DR, Wong SH, Bellosi A, et al. Nuocytes represent a new innate effector leukocyte that mediates type-2 immunity. Nature 2010;464: 1367-70.
59. Sanak M, Simon HU, Szczeklik A. Leukotriene C4 synthase promoter polymorphism and risk of aspirin-induced asthma. Lancet 1997;350: 1599-600.
60. Sanak M, Pierzchalska M, Bazan-Socha S, Szczeklik A. Enhanced expression of the leukotriene C4 synthase due to overactive transcription of an allelic variant associated with aspirin-intolerant asthma. Am J Respir Cell Mol Biol 2000;23:290-6.
61. Sampson AP, Siddiqui S, Buchanan D, et al. Variant LTC(4) synthase allele modifies cysteinyl leukotriene synthesis in eosinophils and predicts clinical response to zafirlukast. Thorax 2000;55(Suppl 2):S28-31.
62. Asano K, Shiomi T, Hasegawa N, et al. Leukotriene C4 synthase gene A(-444)C polymorphism and clinical response to a CYS-LT(1) antagonist, pranlukast, in Japanese patients with moderate asthma. Pharmacogenetics 2002;12: 565-70.
63. Whelan GJ, Blake K, Kissoon N, et al. Effect of montelukast on time-course of exhaled nitric oxide in asthma: influence of LTC4 synthase A(-444)C polymorphism. Pediatr Pulmonol 2003;36:413-20.
64. Kim JH, Lee SY, Kim HB, et al. TBXA2R gene polymorphism and responsiveness to leukotriene receptor antagonist in children with asthma. Clin Exp Allergy 2008;38:51-9.
65. Kang MJ, Lee SY, Kim HB, et al. Association of IL-13 polymorphisms with leukotriene receptor antagonist drug responsiveness in Korean children with exercise-induced bronchoconstriction. Pharmacogenet Genomics 2008;18:551-8.
66. Kang MJ, Kwon JW, Kim BJ, et al. Polymorphisms of the PTGDR and LTC4S influence responsiveness to leukotriene receptor antagonists in Korean children with asthma. J Hum Genet 2011;56:284-9.

Pharmacogenomics of Corticosteroids

67. Long-term effects of budesonide or nedocromil in children with asthma. The Childhood Asthma Management Program Research Group. N Engl J Med 2000;343:1054-63.
68. Tantisira KG, Hwang ES, Raby BA, et al. TBX21: a functional variant predicts improvement in asthma with the use of inhaled corticosteroids. Proc Natl Acad Sci U S A 2004;101:18099-104.
69. Ye YM, Lee HY, Kim SH, et al. Pharmacogenetic study of the effects of NK2R G231E G>A and TBX21 H33Q C>G polymorphisms on asthma control with inhaled corticosteroid treatment. J Clin Pharm Ther 2009;34:693-701.
70. Tantisira KG, Small KM, Litonjua AA, Weiss ST, Liggett SB. Molecular properties and pharmacogenetics of a polymorphism of adenylyl cyclase type 9 in asthma: interaction between beta-agonist and corticosteroid pathways. Hum Mol Genet 2005;14:1671-7.
71. Kim SH, Ye YM, Lee HY, Sin HJ, Park HS. Combined pharmacogenetic effect of ADCY9 and ADRB2 gene polymorphisms on the bronchodilator response to inhaled combination therapy. J Clin Pharm Ther 2011;36:399-405.
72. Tantisira KG, Lake S, Silverman ES, et al. Corticosteroid pharmacogenetics: association of sequence variants in CRHR1 with improved lung function in asthmatics treated with inhaled corticosteroids. Hum Mol Genet 2004;13: 1353-9.
73. Tantisira KG, Lasky-Su J, Harada M, et al. Genomewide association between GLCCI1 and response to glucocorticoid therapy in asthma. N Engl J Med 2011;365:1173-83.
74. Chapman MS, Askew DJ, Kuscuoglu U, Miesfeld RL. Transcriptional control of steroid-regulated apoptosis in murine thymoma cells. Mol Endocrinol 1996;10:967-78.
75. Chapman MS, Qu N, Pascoe S, et al. Isolation of differentially expressed sequence tags from steroid-responsive cells using mRNA differential display. Mol Cell Endocrinol 1995;108: R1-7.
76. Hakonarson H, Bjornsdottir US, Halapi E, et al. Profiling of genes expressed in peripheral blood mononuclear cells predicts glucocorticoid sensitivity in asthma patients. Proc Natl Acad Sci U S A 2005;102:14789-94.
77. Woodruff PG, Boushey HA, Dolganov GM, et al. Genome-wide profiling identifies epithelial cell genes associated with asthma and with treatment response to corticosteroids. Proc Natl Acad Sci U S A 2007;10415858-63.
78. Chun E, Lee HS, Bang BR, et al. Dexamethasone-induced FKBP51 expression in peripheral blood mononuclear cells could play a role in predicting the response of asthmatics to treatment with corticosteroids. J Clin Immunol 2011;31: 122-7.

Pharmacogenomics of Other Asthma Therapies

79. Palmer LJ, Rye PJ, Gibson NA, et al. Association of FcepsilonR1-beta polymorphisms with asthma and associated traits in Australian asthmatic families. Clin Exp Allergy 1999;29: 1555-62.
80. Palmer LJ, Pare PD, Faux JA, et al. Fc epsilon R1-beta polymorphism and total serum IgE levels in endemically parasitized Australian aborigines. Am J Hum Genet 1997;61:182-8.
81. Obase Y, Shimoda T, Kawano T, et al. Polymorphisms in the CYP1A2 gene and theophylline metabolism in patients with asthma. Clin Pharmacol Ther 2003;73:468-74.

Interpretation and Application of Pharmacogenomic Findings

82. Chalmers GW, Macleod KJ, Little SA, et al. Influence of cigarette smoking on inhaled corticosteroid treatment in mild asthma. Thorax 2002; 57:226-30.

91 Adherence

ANDREA J. APTER | BRUCE G. BENDER | CYNTHIA S. RAND

CONTENTS

SUMMARY OF IMPORTANT CONCEPTS

» Adherence is the extent to which a person's behavior (medication regimen, diet, and lifestyle changes) corresponds with agreed recommendations from a health care provider.
» Patient nonadherence is common in all chronic diseases, including asthma.
» Self-report is not an accurate way to assess adherence.
» Nonadherence involves not only patient factors such as depression, but also adequacy of patient-provider communication, insurance coverage, and barriers to accessing the provider and prescribed medications.
» Adherence is best addressed by considering the unique and individual barriers encountered by each patient.

Introduction

Patient nonadherence to medical recommendations is common in all chronic diseases, including asthma.[1] Poor adherence likely accounts for significant morbidity and mortality associated with asthma.[2] In this chapter we define adherence; describe its measurement, barriers, and consequences; profile methods to assess it; and discuss approaches to improving or maintaining it. While many such efforts target the patient, whether the patient follows medical advice or not may be the result of multiple factors. These include the adequacy of patient-provider communication, insurance coverage, and the capability of overcoming barriers of access to the provider and the prescribed medication. Results of recent research, including evaluation of low-cost interventions targeted at the operation of medical practices or clinics, provide new insight into improving adherence.

This chapter focuses on patient adherence related to asthma and the use of inhaled corticosteroids, the treatment of choice for all but the mildest asthma. There is little research on patient adherence in other allergy/immunology-related settings, such as allergic rhinitis, urticaria, atopic dermatitis, and anaphylaxis, in part because of the difficulty in measuring adherence in these settings. For example, whether patients with food or insect allergy carry injectable epinephrine and use it appropriately has not been studied in detail. Likewise, adherence to dietary restrictions is seldom documented. There is also little research on clinician adherence to recommended practices. This chapter evaluates patient adherence and the many factors that influence it.

Definitions

Definitions of adherence have evolved in conjunction with changes in thinking about patient-physician interactions. Until fairly recently, "compliance" was the preferred term, suggesting that treatment decision making was entirely the physician's responsibility, and that the patient must obey or acquiesce.[1] In 1979, Haynes and colleagues[1] suggested that compliance could be used interchangeably with "adherence" and should be defined as "the extent to which a patient's behavior coincides with advice from professional caregivers."

Over time, emphasis has shifted from patient "obedience" to patient-physician collaboration, adequate communication, and patient satisfaction with communication. In 2003 the World Health Organization (WHO) convened a panel of experts to review the problem of nonadherence.[3] Rather than examine one chronic disease, WHO studied diseases with different characteristics that might present different barriers to adherence: communicable diseases such as tuberculosis and acquired immunodeficiency syndrome (AIDS); mental and neurologic conditions such as depression and seizure disorders; substance dependence; palliative care for cancer; and common chronic diseases such as hypertension, asthma, and diabetes. The participants concluded that adherence is "associated too closely with blame, be it of providers or patients."[3] Instead, defining adherence needs to consider the dynamic and complex changes required of patients, providers, and health systems over long periods to maintain optimal health in persons with chronic diseases.

Building on previous definitions, the WHO definition of adherence is "the extent to which a person's behavior—taking medication, following a diet, and/or executing lifestyle changes, corresponds with agreed recommendations from a health care provider."[3] This definition emphasizes *agreement* and *communication* between patient and provider and stresses a broader range of activities that should be considered beyond strict adherence to medication regimens. Adherence viewed this way may be better characterized as successful self-management.

Extent of Nonadherence with Asthma Therapies

Nonadherence with asthma therapy is widespread and a significant risk factor for morbidity. Conservative estimates indicate that almost half the prescription medications dispensed yearly are not taken as prescribed. Nonadherence can take many forms, including failing to fill the initial prescription (primary nonadherence), underuse of therapy (secondary nonadherence), and premature discontinuation of therapy. Watts and associates[4] examined *primary nonadherence* in patients with asthma by matching prescriptions written with those filled over 3 months. Approximately 70% of the prescriptions were filled, most by day 6 (91%), with over three-quarters filled on the same day as the clinic visit (76%). However, a recent study of asthmatic patients in southeastern Michigan found less than 30% of prescriptions for inhaled corticosteroids (ICS) were filled.[5] Based on fill rates, these adherence estimates represent the maximum possible levels of adherence and provide no information on the day-to-day patterns of medication use in the home.

Studies of *secondary nonadherence* suggest that long-term rates of adherence to preventive therapies (e.g., controller medications) among adult patients are low. Early studies using electronic monitoring of dispensing from metered-dose inhalers (MDIs) suggested that average adherence to asthma regimens is less than 50% of prescribed and may dip much lower.[6] Adherence appears to decline over time (Fig. 91-1),[7] and it may be better in the morning than the evening.[8] Several studies based on pharmacy database review have also suggested that persistence with a broad range of asthma therapies is poor. Sherman and coworkers[9] found that median refill adherence was 59% (95% confidence interval [CI]: 48% to 65%) for children prescribed montelukast monotherapy and 44% (90% CI: 35% to 50%) for fluticasone propionate inhaler as monotherapy. Bender and associates[10] examined refills of fluticasone/salmeterol over 12 months in over 5500 patients using records from a national pharmacy chain. On average, patients filled enough medication to cover 22.2% of days, and more than half the patients filled a 30-day prescription only once over the 1-year period.

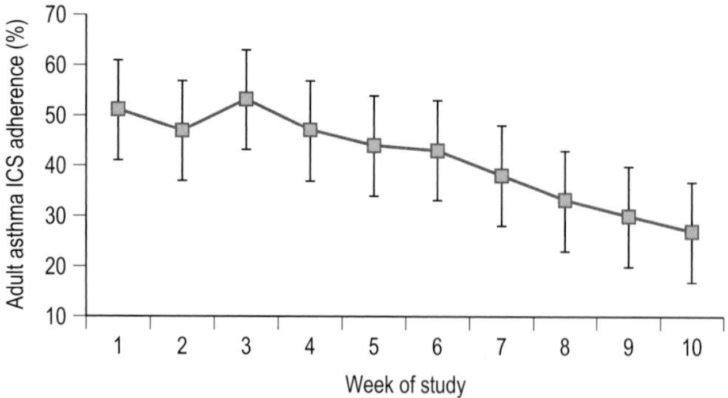

Figure 91-1 Adherence over time. Adults with moderate or severe asthma prescribed twice-daily inhaled corticosteroids were monitored with their permission. Adherence to medication regimens decreased over the observation period. *(From Onyirimba F, Apter AJ, Reisine ST, et al. Direct clinician-to-patient feedback of inhaled steroid use: its effect on adherence and asthma outcome. Ann Allergy Asthma Immunol 2003;90:411-5.)*

In a retrospective cohort study of pharmacy record–based adherence in adults with asthma enrolled in a large health maintenance organization (HMO), Williams and colleagues[2] found that overall adherence to ICS was significantly and negatively correlated with emergency department (ED) visits and number of courses and total days' supply of prescribed oral corticosteroid. This study highlights that nonadherence with asthma therapy is associated with adverse asthma outcomes. Even patients with severe, life-threatening asthma are at risk of significant nonadherence. Krishnan and coworkers[11] evaluated adherence to ICS and oral corticosteroids (OCS) after discharge in adults hospitalized for asthma exacerbations. Both ICS and OCS were measured using electronic medication monitors. Despite the provision of one-on-one asthma education and free medications on discharge, the electronically measured adherence to both corticosteroids dropped to approximately 50% within 7 days of discharge. Additionally, poor adherence to both OCS and ICS predicted significantly worse symptom control. Thus, even when asthma is severe, much medicine is not taken as prescribed, indicating significant barriers for patients.

Barriers to Adherence

Barriers can be categorized as related to the characteristics of the disease, the therapy required, the individual patient, the clinician, the practice and health system, or general societal conditions (Fig. 91-2 and Box 91-1). None of these factors is static; medications, content of patient education, access to health care, and national policy concerning access to health care all evolve rather rapidly. In addition, certain physician characteristics may result in successful interactions with some patients but lead to barriers in communication with other patients.

Barriers differ depending on the behavior required, whether appointment keeping, filling/refilling prescriptions, or abstaining from smoking. Most adherence research related to asthma examines medication taking, but other determinants of adherence, such as practice characteristics and behavior in obtaining refills, have recently been examined.

DISEASE-RELATED FACTORS

Adherence tends to be poor in patients with chronic diseases such as asthma, who may be asymptomatic for long periods and whose treatment regimen is preventive and of long duration. In addition, some asthmatic patients do not perceive airway obstruction that is measurable by other clinical parameters, such as lung examination or spirometry.[12] A patient who does not perceive symptoms is less likely to take long-term medications.[13]

THERAPY-RELATED FACTORS

Therapy-related barriers include those associated with its complexity, expense, duration, measurable or perceived success, and adverse effects. In moderate or severe asthma, the regimen is often complex and usually requires more than one inhaler and sometimes additional oral medication. Patients also must distinguish between two management regimens, one of daily preventive therapy and one for exacerbations. ICS are key components of therapy for all patients with asthma (except the mildest forms) but involve many of these therapy-related barriers. ICS are expensive and difficult to use and have an

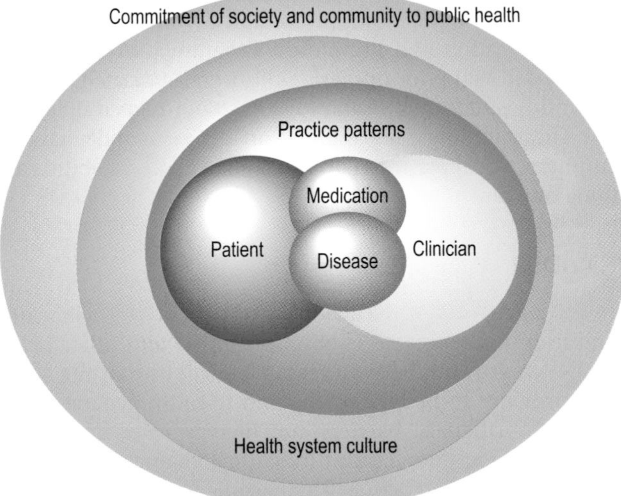

Figure 91-2 Barriers to adherence can be categorized as related to the characteristics of the disease, therapy required, individual patient, clinician, practice/health system, or general societal conditions. Characteristics of the therapy include whether the disease is chronic or acute, impacting on daily life, or life-threatening. Barriers related to the therapy include whether the medication must be taken chronically for prolonged periods and its side effects. Patient characteristics might include comorbidities and other priorities in the patient's life, such as caring for children or elderly or sick family members or maintaining a job. Clinician characteristics may include the style of interacting with the patient or ability to speak the patient's language. Examples of practice or health system characteristics that may influence adherence are the availability of evening and weekend hours and urgent care and the promptness with which providers return patient telephone calls. Societal characteristics comprise the availability of public transportation, availability of pharmacies in patient's neighborhood, and availability of health insurance regardless of ability to pay.

unpleasant taste for some patients. If the only active drug in the formulation is a corticosteroid, no immediate relief of symptoms will be experienced, and the patient may conclude that the drug does not provide any benefit. Additionally, patients may be required to take ICS indefinitely. Although ICS at low to moderate doses are relatively safe, high-dose ICS and systemic steroids have significant side effects. ICS may generate significant concern about adverse effects or possibility of addiction.[14] Patients may not distinguish the adverse effects of systemic corticosteroids from the lesser adverse effects of ICS.[14] Some of these problems may be addressed by prescribing simple, individualized regimens for patients.[15]

PATIENT FACTORS

According to the WHO, patient-related factors "represent the resources, knowledge, beliefs, perceptions, and expectations of the patient."[3] These in turn may be the products of distractions and other experiences. *Distractions* are events or factors in the patient's life that interfere with the task of managing asthma and may lead to forgetfulness or alter the perception of importance of and motivation (self-efficacy) for adherence. Personal distractions such as stresses, depression, and family conflicts can all interfere with adherence.[16] Patients living in poverty may be more prone to depression or personal stresses that can influence understanding, beliefs, and expectations. As a dramatic example, Wright and researchers[17] demonstrated that individuals exposed to community violence have an increased risk for asthma morbidity even when other demographic and socioeconomic factors are controlled. A possible link between exposure

BOX 91-1 INFLUENCES ON AND BARRIERS TO ADHERENCE BEHAVIORS*

DISEASE FACTORS

- Chronic rather than acute or limited condition
- Asymptomatic periods
- Treatment that is prophylactic rather than in response to acute symptoms
- Lack of perception of physiologic compromise (e.g., of airway obstruction)

TREATMENT FACTORS

- Cost
- Adverse effects, real or perceived
- Incomplete benefit, real or perceived
- Requirement of complex behavior (e.g., inhaler technique)
- Inconvenient treatment schedule
- Delayed benefit
- Requirement of long-term behavior

PATIENT FACTORS

- Life distractions (work, family conflicts)
- Stress, depression
- Comorbidities
- Risk versus benefit perceptions
- Limited literacy

PROVIDER FACTORS

- Ability to communicate and educate
- Ability to communicate across cultural and language differences
- Ability to assess patient's literacy and knowledge
- Ability to build trust

PRACTICE AND SYSTEM FACTORS

- Cost and copayments
- Inconvenient office hours
- Difficulty in making appointments
- Waiting times
- Fragmentation of care
- Poor accommodations for low literacy, language barriers, and cultural diversity
- Difficulties with pharmacy
- Inadequate reimbursement by health insurance
- Lack of patient and provider reminders
- Inadequate information sharing
- Poor communication: lack of prompt return of patient queries, no reminder phone calls, difficulty making appointments or scheduling tests

SOCIETY RELATED

- Lack of motivation to provide health care to all
- Transportation difficulties
- Inadequate provision of health care in schools
- Lack of community health programs
- Inability to control air quality
- Inability to control exposure to tobacco
- Unemployment
- Poverty
- Discrimination

*Behaviors include taking medication, filling refills, keeping appointments, and abstaining from smoking.

to violence and disease morbidity is the difficulty in attending to asthma self-management under these stressful conditions.

Barriers may differ according to the age of the patient. For example, elderly patients may forget medications, and polypharmacy may interfere with the taking of any one medication. For adolescents, body image, peer pressure, need for autonomy, and perceptions of invincibility all may influence their approach to adherence with medical advice.[18] Adherence in younger children is related to the ability of their caregivers to ensure medication delivery. A chaotic home life may result in impaired ability of the caregiver to deliver medication regularly to a child.[16] Maternal depression has also been shown to be a risk factor for poor adherence to medications in children.[19]

Knowledge, beliefs, perceptions, and expectations may be related not only to the patient but also to the patient's experiences in the health system. Knowledge not only is a product of a patient's ability to acquire information, but also depends on the adequacy of information presented. Knowledge of asthma and its management is necessary for adherence, but knowledge by itself is not sufficient to guarantee adherence. Patient knowledge or understanding of disease is associated with adherence in some studies.[20] However, educational programs to improve self-management skills have not always been successful.

Distrust of the medical establishment may influence health behavior of minority patients who may have experienced racism and discrimination while seeking health care, or who may perceive the medical establishment to be insensitive to their needs.[21] For example, awareness of the U.S. Public Health Service–funded Tuskegee Syphilis Study, in which African Americans who had syphilis were not treated even after penicillin became available, has generated distrust of the health care community.

Health beliefs are associated with adherence. The *perceived benefits relative to risks* of taking medications have been associated with adherence in all patient groups, including minority groups at high risk for a poor asthma outcome. Again, these perceptions may be related to trust of the health system. Poor adherence to ICS also has been associated with fears of steroid side effects and addiction.

Inadequate health literacy may lead to poor understanding of self-management instructions and inability to navigate medical systems. *Literacy* is a constellation of many skills, including the ability to read, write, and speak in English (in the United States) and to understand and use numeric concepts.[22] *Health literacy* refers to "the degree to which individuals have the capacity to obtain, process, and understand basic health information and services needed to make appropriate health decisions."[22]

The National Adult Literacy Survey reported that nearly half of all American adults have difficulty understanding and acting on health information.[23] Suboptimal health literacy is found in all patient groups, with increased prevalence among the poor, immigrants, minorities, and elderly persons, the same groups in whom asthma morbidity is excessive. In asthmatic patients, low literacy has been associated with improper use of MDIs[24] and lower asthma-related knowledge. Paasche-Orlow and associates[25] studied 73 adults hospitalized for severe asthma exacerbations and found inadequate health literacy was associated with lower asthma medication knowledge and also poor MDI technique, but not with difficulty learning or retaining instructions about their discharge regimen. These findings and the prevalence of low literacy suggest clinicians must consider providing the simplest instructions and explanations for all patients.

One aspect of literacy may be particularly important: ability to understand and use numeric concepts. A four-item questionnaire using numeric concepts adapted from the National Asthma Education and Prevention Program (NAEPP) guidelines revealed that poor numeric skills were associated with ED visits and hospitalizations and lower asthma-related quality of life.[26] These findings suggest that inadequate understanding of numeric concepts influences self-management ability and asthma outcome.

PROVIDER FACTORS

Patients' perception of the adequacy of patient-physician communication influences adherence in asthma and other health settings.[27] A growing body of research suggests that the ability of the provider to be empathetic and friendly, generate trust, account for language barriers and literacy level, and deliver education taking into account individual characteristics influences patients' adherence, self-management ability, and health outcomes.[28] With the growing diversity of patients, these skills are becoming increasingly important for practitioners.

PRACTICE AND SYSTEM FACTORS

Recent research suggests that practice and health system factors influence health outcomes, patient satisfaction, self-management, and adherence. Lowe and colleagues[29] studied primary care practices serving patients enrolled in Medicaid HMOs and found the following practice characteristics were associated with less ED use: evening hours, a lower ratio of the number of active patients per clinician hour of practice time, equipment such as nebulizers to care for exacerbations, and the absence of nurse practitioners and physicians assistants. It is reasonable to assume that these factors indirectly influence patients' ability to acquire and use appropriate medications.

Lieu and associates[28] conducted a prospective cohort study of Medicaid-insured asthmatic children and found practice-site policies that promote cultural competence (ethnically diverse or bilingual nurses and providers, cross-cultural/diversity and communication skills training available, evaluation of nurse/provider cultural competence) were associated with greater use of asthma preventive medication and more parent satisfaction with their child's care. Use of reports to clinicians (e.g., lists of patients with asthma, prompts about medication prescribing) was predictive of physician adherence to guidelines in prescribing preventive medications, better parent satisfaction, and better asthma status of the child as judged by the parent. Finally, practice polices that promoted access to medical advice, follow-up, and continuity of care all predicted higher quality of care and use of asthma medications.

Additional practice characteristics may promote patient-provider communication and empower patient self-management and thus adherence. These include appointment length, consistency of care, and the ease and effectiveness of telephone communication (e.g., provider promptness in returning calls about medical questions, ease of making an appointment, messaging for reminders/follow-up). The increasing ability of clinics and pharmacies to share information on patients' prescribed medications, refill history, and relevant medical history may improve adherence and self-management. However, confusing insurance policies regarding payment of medications doubtlessly influences adherence. Copayments for office visits (where medications are generally prescribed) vary greatly and can be so excessive, particularly for specialists, as to be a deterrent to medical follow-up. Additionally, as medication copays increase, adherence decreases.[10]

SOCIETY AND COMMUNITY FACTORS

A society's support of health and other social programs influences health outcomes. For example, society's commitment to provide broad health care coverage influences access to care and thus adherence to medical recommendations. Public assistance through Medicaid and Medicare is necessary for many patients of limited incomes to obtain medications. Some patients with limited resources are forced to choose which medications will be filled and which they can take regularly or only when disease worsens.[14] Availability of community transportation allows vulnerable patients to travel to health care facilities. Poorer communities are less likely to have school nurses and community health programs that can help children with self-management.

Measuring Adherence

The measurement of adherence, important both in clinical practice and research, typically occurs through one of two means: self-report or objective measurement. Unfortunately, patients who provide self-reported data usually overestimate their adherence. Objective measures of adherence are more accurate but are also subject to bias and are difficult to incorporate into clinical practice.

SELF-REPORT

Self-reports may be collected by interview, diaries, and questionnaires. With pediatric asthma, self-reporting refers to the combined reporting of parent and child. Self-report measures are common because they are simple, inexpensive, and generally brief. In addition, self-reporting (particularly in the clinical setting) is the best measure for collecting information about patient beliefs, risk/benefit perceptions, and experiences with medication regimens. Data from self-reporting are also useful in examining the relationship between disease exacerbation and adherence to asthma management plans.[30]

In most cases, self-reporting greatly overrepresents behavior and is an inadequate measure of adherence. When patients have completed self-reports while being monitored by other means (e.g., pill count, electronic monitoring), wide discrepancies from overreporting have been detected[6] (Fig. 91-3). Self-reports of adherence will be influenced by the setting in which the information is collected. The desire to please the physician or investigator can lead patients to exaggerate reports of adherence. Investigators continue to attempt developing a questionnaire that can accurately measure adherence in research studies, but none has established validity equal to objective adherence measures.[31] In clinical practice, physicians' and investigators' skills and sensitivity in eliciting patients' self-reports will influence the reliability and usefulness of the information they receive. Although self-reporting may not be a sufficient measure of adherence in many settings, particularly research, it is a necessary measure in all settings. When carefully collected, self-reported adherence information can provide critical information into the nature of the patients' problems with adherence.

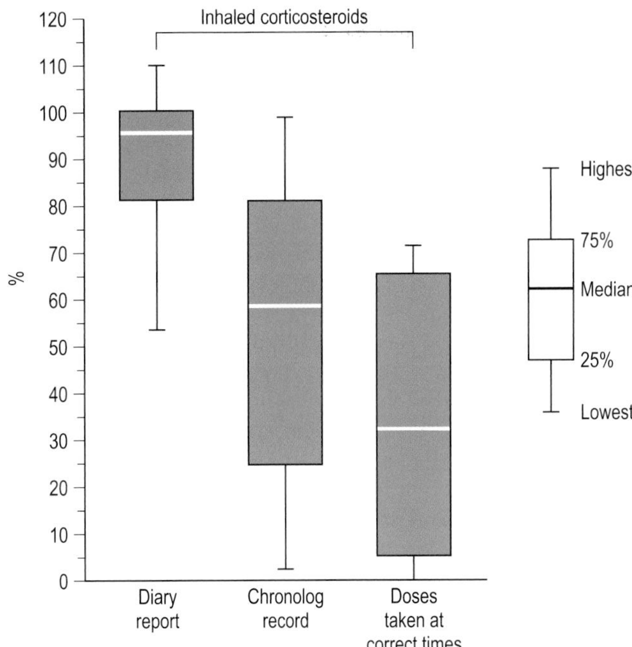

Figure 91-3 Comparison of a diary report by children and their parents of the child's inhaled corticosteroid use with data from electronic monitors. *(From Milgrom H, Bender B, Ackerson L, et al. Noncompliance and treatment failure in children with asthma. J Allergy Clin Immunol 1996;98:1051-7.)*

OBJECTIVE MEASURES

Medication adherence has been measured through biochemical assays, pill counts, pharmacy refill databases, and electronic devices that document medication events. Biochemical analysis of blood, urine, or other body fluids is an objective, accurate method of determining if a patient has recently taken a specific medication. However, these methods have several limitations. Biochemical measures can be confounded by diet or other drug use (e.g., effect of smoking on theophylline), as well as by idiosyncratic pharmacokinetic abnormalities (e.g., delayed absorption, rapid metabolism). These measures are not accurate in discerning day-to-day patterns of adherence with therapy and can be compromised if patients begin taking medications just before clinical samples are collected. Most importantly, asthma medications delivered by MDI (cromolyn, β_2-agonists, corticosteroids, or anticholinergics) are poorly absorbed and therefore cannot be measured by commercial medical laboratories.

Electronic medication monitors use microprocessors to record and store the date and time that a medication container is opened or activated. Such devices have been attached to the caps of pill bottles[32] or to MDIs to record time and date when actuation occurs.[6] These devices can confirm that the inhaler was activated or the pill bottle opened, but not that the medication was actually taken by the patient. Although they are often more accurate than other strategies to measure adherence, disadvantages of these devices include their expense, potential to malfunction, limited availability for various controller medications, and requirement of time and technical expertise from busy clinical staff.[33]

Pharmacy refill information represents a practical approach to assessing adherence and can provide a panoramic view of adherence behavior in much larger groups of patients than previously studied through clinical trials. Although not providing information about daily medication use, refill records produce epidemiologic evidence of the degree to which patients accept and obtain controller medications. Such prescription database information also introduces the concept of *persistence* (continued refills of medication over time) as a complement to the common term *adherence* (average daily medication dispensed from MDI).[10] Although the two measures are correlated, persistence typically accounts for behavior over a long period, whereas adherence is employed to typify daily behavior over periods as short as 2 weeks. Refill information has the added advantage of reflecting patient behavior in a variety of clinical practice settings rather than only a clinical trial setting.

In clinical practice, tracking of patient refills can help to determine whether patients are actually obtaining medication. Refill data are increasingly available to clinicians within HMOs and insurance databases.[34] With refill data, the treating physician can discuss options with patients not filling or refilling their prescriptions. Even the most basic refill information, consisting of the date of last refill of the prescribed controller medication, gives the provider a clear picture of which patients have abandoned therapy and therefore require attention. Given that as many as half of patients with asthma stop using their controller medications, such data represent essential information for clinicians.[10]

ESTIMATING ADHERENCE IN CLINICAL PRACTICE

Through interactions with patients, clinicians receive information that provides indirect evidence of the adequacy of adherence.[30] The following factors influence clinician insight into patient adherence:

1. A strong provider-patient relationship with trust and mutual regard is likely to allow patients to feel safe in discussing nonadherence, fear about side effects, or other barriers. A patient who admits poor adherence is providing important information that should prompt a discussion to elucidate specific barriers to adherence and how to address them.
2. *Poor disease control.* When a patient reports increased symptoms, the evaluation should include nonjudgmental questions about adherence. Permissive stems for questions (e.g., "Many patients forget to take their medications") may be helpful.
3. Erratic appointment attendance may signal that a patient also has difficulty filling and taking prescriptions.
4. Patients who cannot name or explain medications regimens, particularly the dosing intervals, are unlikely to be highly adherent. Such difficulty also may be a sign of low literacy and that communication about medications and self-management must be revised.
5. Patients with *depression* are at great risk of nonadherence to a treatment program for concomitant disease.[35] Likewise, the child of a depressed parent is less likely to receive their medication consistently.[19]
6. *Family conflict.* Families who present a picture of relative stability and emotionally close relationships tend to be more capable of administering a pediatric treatment regimen.[16] Conversely, families who present in the clinic with apparent conflict among family members, or between parents and health care provider, are likely to have difficulty with adherence.

Interventions to Improve Adherence

Because barriers to adherence can result from multiple factors, interventions to improve patient adherence need to be appropriately targeted to those factors that impede patient adherence. The implementation of these intervention strategies can occur at multiple levels (therapy, patient, provider, practice/health care system). Because poor adherence often results from multiple barriers, successful strategies to improve adherence may need to be multifactoral and multilevel.[3]

THERAPY-FOCUSED INTERVENTIONS

Because patients often report that forgetting is a key cause of nonadherence, a number of clinicians, researchers, and pharmaceutical companies have suggested that the development of simplified, once-daily asthma therapies might improve patient adherence. Nonrandomized pharmacy review–based studies in asthma do suggest some adherence advantage for once-daily versus twice-daily dosing.[36,37] Patient preference for simpler therapies may also influence adherence. However, although simplifying daily therapeutic regimens may result in decreasing the number of doses missed due to simple forgetfulness, simplified therapy is unlikely to promote adherence when a patient's nonadherence results from misunderstanding the therapy or believing therapy is no longer needed.

PATIENT-FOCUSED INTERVENTIONS

Most intervention studies to improve adherence have focused on changing patient behavior through direct education or behavioral interventions. A review of largely patient-focused adherence intervention studies indicated that the key intervention components were providing reinforcement for patients' efforts to change, providing feedback on progress, tailoring education to patients' needs and circumstances, teaching asthma self-management skills and providing access to resources, and having continuity of care (proactive).[38]

For diseases such as diabetes, cardiovascular disease, and human immunodeficiency virus (HIV) infection, many studies have examined strategies to improve adherence. In contrast, few studies have specifically focused on promoting adherence with respiratory medications. Self-management strategies for enhancing asthma medication adherence can include asthma education, self-monitoring (medication use and peak flow monitoring), MDI technique reinforcement, tailoring, and cueing. For example, Bailey and associates[39] demonstrated that appropriate asthma medication use and adherence was significantly improved among adults who participated in a six-session asthma self-management program that used such strategies as enhancing cognitive skills, increasing self-efficacy, and providing social support. More recently, in a 24-week, cluster-randomized, crossover study with 84 adults, Janson and colleagues[15] reported that an individualized asthma self-management education program improved medication adherence and markers of asthma morbidity. By study's end, participants who received the self-management intervention had threefold greater odds of more than 60% adherence and were less likely to report nighttime awakenings or use of rescue medication. Ongoing studies are also examining the benefit of combining patient self-management education with strategies designed to enhance patient motivation, such as motivational interviewing (MI). Several recent nonrandomized, pilot studies have evaluated the benefit of MI-based interventions designed to promote asthma adherence among teenagers.[40,41] Although these preliminary studies all reported significant improvements in self-reported motivation to adhere with asthma controller therapy, no controlled studies have yet been published that demonstrate that MI interventions improve patient asthma adherence behavior.

Adherence monitoring and feedback have shown promise in promoting adherence in both adults and children. In a study of adults with asthma, direct clinician-to-patient feedback of objectively measured adherence resulted in adherence above 70% in the intervention group compared with below 50% in the control group.[7] In a randomized controlled trial, a home-based adherence-monitoring and feedback intervention delivered to high-risk inner-city children and caregivers (n = 250) resulted in significant improvements in adherence to therapy with ICS (as measured by pharmacy records) and reduced asthma morbidity, although improvement was not sustained beyond 6 months.[42] In a small pediatric intervention study (n = 26), electronic monitoring and clinician feedback to parents of children with asthma resulted in improved adherence to ICS (79% versus 58%; P <.01) and improved asthma control compared with a control condition.[43]

A comprehensive review of adherence intervention studies suggested that no single intervention targeting patient behavior is effective, and that the most promising methods of improving adherence behavior are multimodal, with some combination of patient education, behavioral skills reinforcement, social support, and telephone/e-mail follow-up.[44] Patient education alone is not sufficient to ensure adherence, and the format of the educational program may be less important than the actual presentation and understanding of the information.

PROVIDER-FOCUSED INTERVENTIONS

The quality of communication between patients and their health care providers corresponds with adherence to therapy.[45] Because physicians can have a central role in patient education and motivation, improved physician-patient communication is likely to increase patient involvement and adherence to recommended therapy, as well as improve quality of care and health outcomes. Strategies to improve communication include increasing physician and patient question-asking abilities; providing an unhurried, participatory, and culturally appropriate environment; and encouraging patients to have companions accompanying them to primary care visits. Studies of physician-parent interactions in pediatric asthma suggest that strengthening physician-provided asthma education and improving communication skills are central to assisting parents of asthmatic children. Clark and coworkers[46] found that training pediatricians in communication skills led to patient-physician encounters that were of shorter duration, had an increased rate of antiinflammatory prescriptions and other guideline-based activities, decreased nonemergency physician visits, and for low-income families, decreased ED visits. Although this study did not directly measure patient adherence, the results suggest that improved patient self-management—including adherence—was responsible for the improved patient outcomes. Asthma coaches or counselors may also facilitate communication and improve patient adherence and outcomes. Results from the National Cooperative Inner City Asthma Study (NCICAS) indicated that having an asthma counselor in conjunction with physician care, an action plan, and environmental control measures improved adherence and asthma symptom control.[47]

Including patients in the therapy decision-making process is also a key component of effective provider-patient communication. In a 1-year trial of 612 adults enrolled in a managed care organization, asthma patients randomized to a shared decision-making intervention had significantly higher asthma controller adherence, as measured by pharmacy refill records (0.67 CMA versus 0.46; P <.0001), and improved measures of asthma control, including quality of life, asthma morbidity, and pulmonary function.[48]

PRACTICE AND SYSTEM-FOCUSED INTERVENTIONS

The 2003 WHO report on adherence concluded that changing adherence is not the exclusive responsibility of health care providers because they often have limited time and training to provide adherence interventions.[3] Health care systems must address nonadherence by recognizing it as a system-wide problem, allocating necessary resources, supporting clinicians efforts to change patient behavior, and facilitating improved communication both within the system (e.g., between clinics and pharmacies) and with patients (e.g., telephone contacts).

There is good reason for health care systems to concern themselves with adherence. In 2001, U.S. medical care costs were over $1.2 trillion. Almost 30% of this was paid to physicians and other health care professionals for direct services, with possibly a quarter of patients failing to follow this advice. DiMatteo[49] estimated that the cost of nonadherence to the U.S. health care system could be as high as $300 billion and concluded, "The offering of medical recommendations that are misunderstood or subsequently forgotten or ignored . . . is a waste of scarce healthcare resources and suggests a systemic problem."

However, a growing body of research suggests system-based strategies can facilitate improved adherence and disease management. Reporting on a meta-analysis of adherence interventions, Haynes and colleagues[44] concluded that simple adherence interventions, including calling patients between visits, were more cost-effective than complex interventions. Further, because no adherence intervention can cure nonadherence, the best interventions are those that can remain in place for as long as the treatment is needed.

Several asthma intervention studies have examined the value of pharmacy-based education or support to improve adherence with therapies for chronic illnesses such as asthma. For example, Clifford and associates[50] examined the value of a pharmacist-delivered telephone intervention to improve adherence using a centralized service to patients at home in England. Patients (n = 500) were eligible if they were receiving the first prescription for a new medication for a chronic condition and were 75 years or older or with asthma, stroke, cardiovascular disease, diabetes, or rheumatoid arthritis. At follow-up week 4, nonadherence was significantly lower in the intervention group compared with the control group (9% versus 16%, P = .032), as was the number of patients reporting medicine-related problems

(23% versus 34%, $P = .021$). In addition, patients receiving the intervention reported more positive beliefs about their new medicine compared with controls (5.0 versus 3.5, $P = .007$). More recently, Smith and colleagues[51] evaluated the impact of a pharmacist-delivered Asthma Self-Management Service that provided a stepwise, patient-centered intervention focused on asthma problems and goal setting. Postintervention impact included significant improvements in self-reported medication adherence, asthma control, and asthma-related quality of life.

Information technology (IT) strategies are increasingly being explored as tools for promoting patient adherence. In particular, linking a patient's electronic health record (EHR) with a patient's personal pharmacy records could enable health care providers to assess more objectively patient adherence with asthma therapies (as measured by refill patterns). Williams and associates[5] evaluated the system-level impact of providing clinicians with pharmacy-based feedback of patients' adherence with asthma therapies. In this cluster-randomized trial conducted with 2698 adult patients with asthma enrolled in a managed care health plan, intervention physicians received detailed information about how to access patients' electronic prescribing records and educational information (DVD, CD, and written format) highlighting the importance of patient adherence with asthma therapy and how to discuss adherence with patients. There were no significant differences in adherence between the intervention arm and the control arm (21.3% versus 23.3%; $P = 0.553$). Post hoc analyses, however, revealed that few physicians accessed or viewed patients' electronic adherence data. For those clinicians who did elect to view their patients' detailed adherence data, patient adherence was significantly higher (35.7%) than for clinicians who did not view adherence data ($P =.002$), suggesting that adherence information can be valuable if utilized. The trial highlighted the real-life barriers to introducing new IT-based tools into a busy practice setting and the need for practical strategies to engage clinicians in effectively using these technologies.

Interactive phone messaging systems, often called interactive voice recognition (IVR), have been used in multiple studies to collect health data, monitor patients, provide health education, and remind patients about appointments or health-screening activities.[52] IVR systems use voice-processing technology to link individuals with a computer database. Prerecorded voice files generally prompt the caller to press phone buttons to answer questions or request information. The IVR system can then retrieve appropriate health or resource information by accessing the host computer's database and provide it to the patient. With the advantages of reaching large populations at low cost with tailored health information and efficiently collecting data, use of IVR systems is a potential strategy to enhance chronic disease management. In a small, randomized, 10-week pilot study, Bender and coworkers[53] found that parent-targeted IVR calls that included reminders and core educational messages regarding therapy with ICS resulted in adherence levels that were 32% higher for intervention than control. The calls resulted in more favorable attitudes toward controller therapy as well. Vollmer and colleagues[54] evaluated the benefit of an IVR intervention designed to prompt medication refills and improve adherence to ICS over 1 year in a randomized clinical trial of adults with asthma enrolled in a large, managed care organization ($n = 8517$). In the primary outcome analysis, overall adherence increased modestly but significantly for participants in the intervention group relative to those in usual care group (Δ = 0.02; 95% CI = 0.01, 0.03), but no benefit was seem in the intervention group for asthma morbidity. However, post hoc analyses of participants receiving two or more direct IVR contacts or detailed messages found that the intervention effect was triple that observed in the primary analyses (0.06 versus 0.02), and significant differences were observed between groups in asthma control, suggesting the dose of intervention was important to outcome.

Additional promising adherence-promotion strategies, still in the evaluation phase, include the use of cell phones, MP3 players SMS/texting, e-mail, and Internet-based platforms to educate, remind, and reinforce patient adherence with asthma therapy. All these technologies offer broad outreach potential to promote adherence within the context of patients' daily lives. However, additional research is needed to determine the overall impact and sustainability of these technology-based tools in improving asthma therapy adherence and patient outcomes.

Conclusion

Poor adherence is common and contributes to morbidity associated with chronic diseases such as asthma. The extent of non-adherence is a reflection of patients' self-management but is not simply the result of patient deficiency. Rather, adherence reflects the success of overcoming dynamic and evolving barriers to self-management not only related to the medication, the disease, and the individual patient's circumstances, but also to the successful communication of health care providers with patients and the commitment of the health system and society to address barriers.

REFERENCES

Introduction

1. Haynes RB, Taylor DW, Sackett DL. Compliance in health care. Baltimore: Johns Hopkins University Press; 1979.
2. Williams LK, Pladevall M, Xi H, et al. Relationship between adherence to inhaled corticosteroids and poor outcomes among adults with asthma. J Allergy Clin Immunol 2004;114:1288-93.

Definitions

3. Sabate E. Adherence to long-term therapies: evidence for action. Noncommunicable Diseases and Mental Health Adherence to Long Term Therapies Project. Geneva: World Health Organization, 2003.

Extent of Nonadherence with Asthma Therapies

4. Watts RW, McLennan G, Bassham I, el-Saadi O. Do patients with asthma fill their prescriptions? A primary compliance study. Aust Fam Physician 1997;26(Suppl 1):S4-6.
5. Williams LK, Peterson EL, Wells K, et al. A cluster-randomized trial to provide clinicians inhaled corticosteroid adherence information for their patients with asthma. J Allergy Clin Immunol 2010;126:225-31.
6. Rand CS, Wise RA, Nides M, et al. Metered-dose inhaler adherence in a clinical trial. Am Rev Respir Dis 1992;146:1559-64.
7. Onyirimba F, Apter AJ, Reisine ST, et al. Direct clinician-to-patient feedback of inhaled steroid use: its effect on adherence and asthma outcome. Ann Allergy Asthma Immunol 2003; 90:411-5.
8. Kim C, Feldman HI, Joffe M, et al. Influences of earlier adherence and symptoms on current symptoms: a marginal structural models analysis. J Allergy Clin Immunol 2005;115:810-4.
9. Sherman J, Patel P, Hutson A, Chesrown S, Hendeles L. Adherence to oral montelukast and

inhaled fluticasone in children with persistent asthma. Pharmacotherapy 2001;21:1464-7.
10. Bender BG, Pedan A, Varasteh LT. Adherence and persistence with fluticasone propionate/salmeterol combination therapy. J Allergy Clin Immunol 2006;118:899-904.
11. Krishnan JA, Riekert KA, McCoy JV, et al. Corticosteroid use after hospital discharge among high-risk adults with asthma. Am J Respir Crit Care Med 2004;170:1281-5.

Barriers to Adherence

12. Apter AJ, Affleck G, Reisine ST, et al. Perception of airway obstruction in asthma: sequential daily analyses of symptoms, peak expiratory flow rate, and mood. J Allergy Clin Immunol 1997;99:605-12.
13. Apter AJ, ZuWallack RL, Clive J. Common measures of asthma severity lack association for describing its clinical course. J Allergy Clin Immunol 1994;94:732-7.
14. George M, Freedman TG, Norfleet AL, Feldman HI, Apter AJ. Qualitative research enhanced understanding of patients' beliefs: results of focus groups with low-income urban African American adults with asthma. J Alllergy Clin Immunol 2003;111:967-73.
15. Janson SL, McGrath KW, Covington JK, Cheng SC, Boushey HA. Individualized asthma self-management improves medication adherence and markers of asthma control. J Allergy Clin Immunol 2009;123:840-6.
16. Bender B, Milgrom H, Rand C, Ackerson L. Psychological factors associated with medication nonadherence in asthmatic children. J Asthma 1998;35:347-53.
17. Wright RJ, Mitchell H, Visness CM, et al. Community violence and asthma morbidity: the inner-city asthma study. Am J Public Health 2004;94:625-32.
18. Naimi DR, Freedman TG, Ginsburg KR, et al. Adolescents and asthma: why bother with our meds? J Allergy Clin Immunol 2009;123:1335-41.
19. Bartlett SJ, Krishnan JA, Riekert KA, et al. Maternal depressive symptoms and adherence to therapy in inner-city children with asthma. Pediatrics 2004;113:229-37.
20. Wamboldt FS, Bender BG, Rankin AE. Adolescent decision-making about use of inhaled asthma controller medication: results from focus groups with participants from a prior longitudinal study. J Asthma 2011;48:741-50.
21. US Institute of Medicine. Unequal treatment: confronting racial and ethnic disparities in health care. Washington, DC: National Academies Press; 2002.
22. Nielson-Bohlman L, Panzer A, Kindig D, editors. Health literacy: a prescription to end confusion. Washington, DC: National Academies Press; 2004.
23. US Department of Education. National assessment of adult literacy. Washington, DC: National Center for Education Statistics, Institute of Education Sciences; 2003.
24. Williams MV, Baker DW, Honig EG, Lee TM, Nowlan A. Inadequate literacy is a barrier to asthma knowledge and self-care. Chest 1998;114:1008-15.
25. Paasche-Orlow MK, Riekert KA, Bilderback A, et al. Tailored education may reduce health literacy disparities in asthma self-management. Am J Respir Crit Care Med 2005;172:980-6.
26. Apter AJ, Wang X, Bogen D, et al. Linking numeracy and asthma-related quality of life. Patient Educ Couns 2009;75:386-91.
27. Sherbourne CD, Hays RD, Ordway L, DiMatteo MR, Kravitz RL. Antecedents of adherence to medical recommendations: results from the Medical Outcomes Study. J Behav Med 1992;15:447-68.
28. Lieu TA, Finkelstein JA, Lozano P, et al. Cultural competence policies and other predictors of asthma care quality for Medicaid-insured children. Pediatrics 2004;114:e102-10.
29. Lowe RA, Localio AR, Schwarz DF, et al. Association between primary care practice characteristics and emergency department use in a Medicaid managed care organization. Med Care 2005;43:792-800.

Measuring Adherence

30. Bender BG. Screening patients for nonadherence. Female Patient 2005;30:1-4.
31. Lavsa SM, Holzworth A, Ansani NT. Selection of a validated scale for measuring medication adherence. J Am Pharm Assoc (2003) 2011;51:90-4.
32. Becker LA, Glanz K, Sobel E, et al. A randomized trial of special packaging of antihypertensive medications. J Fam Pract 1986;22:357-61.
33. Wamboldt FS, Bender BG, O'Connor SL, et al. Reliability of the model MC-311 MDI chronolog. J Allergy Clin Immunol 1999;104:53-7.
34. Grossberg R, Gross R. Use of pharmacy refill data as a measure of antiretroviral adherence. Curr HIV/AIDS Rep 2007;4:187-91.
35. DiMatteo MR, Lepper HS, Croghan TW. Depression is a risk factor for noncompliance with medical treatment: meta-analysis of the effects of anxiety and depression on patient adherence. Arch Intern Med 2000;160:2101-7.

Interventions to Improve Adherence

36. Saini SD, Schoenfeld P, Kaulback K, Dubinsky MC. Effect of medication dosing frequency on adherence in chronic diseases. Am J Manag Care 2009;15:e22-33.
37. Stoloff SW, Stempel DA, Meyer J, Stanford RH, Carranza Rosenzweig JR. Improved refill persistence with fluticasone propionate and salmeterol in a single inhaler compared with other controller therapies. J Allergy Clin Immunol 2004;113:245-51.
38. Haynes RB, Yao X, Degani A, et al. Interventions to enhance medication adherence. Cochrane Database Syst Rev 2005:CD000011.
39. Bailey WC, Richards Jr JM, Brooks CM, et al. A randomized trial to improve self-management practices of adults with asthma. Arch Intern Med 1990;150:1664-8.
40. Riekert KA, Borrelli B, Bilderback A, Rand CS. The development of a motivational interviewing intervention to promote medication adherence among inner-city, African-American adolescents with asthma. Patient Educ Couns 2011;82:117-22.
41. Halterman JS, Riekert K, Bayer A, et al. A pilot study to enhance preventive asthma care among urban adolescents with asthma. J Asthma 2011;48:523-30.
42. Otsuki M, Eakin MN, Rand CS, et al. Adherence feedback to improve asthma outcomes among inner-city children: a randomized trial. Pediatrics 2009;124:1513-21.
43. Burgess SW, Sly PD, Devadason SG. Providing feedback on adherence increases use of preventive medication by asthmatic children. J Asthma 2010;47:198-201.
44. Haynes RB, McDonald H, Garg AX, Montague P. Interventions for helping patients to follow prescriptions for medications. Cochrane Database Syst Rev 2002;(2):CD000011.
45. Zolnierek KB, Dimatteo MR. Physician communication and patient adherence to treatment: a meta-analysis. Med Care 2009;47:826-34.
46. Clark NM, Gong M, Schork MA, et al. Long-term effects of asthma education for physicians on patient satisfaction and use of health services. Eur Respir J 2000;16:15-21.
47. Evans 3rd R, Gergen PJ, Mitchell H, et al. A randomized clinical trial to reduce asthma morbidity among inner-city children: results of the National Cooperative Inner-City Asthma Study. J Pediatr 1999;135:332-8.
48. Wilson SR, Strub P, Buist AS, et al. Shared treatment decision making improves adherence and outcomes in poorly controlled asthma. Am J Respir Crit Care Med 2010;181:566-77.
49. DiMatteo MR. Variations in patients' adherence to medical recommendations: a quantitative review of 50 years of research. Med Care 2004;42:200-9.
50. Clifford S, Barber N, Elliott R, Hartley E, Horne R. Patient-centred advice is effective in improving adherence to medicines. Pharm World Sci 2006;28:165-70.
51. Smith L, Bosnic-Anticevich SZ, Mitchell B, et al. Treating asthma with a self-management model of illness behaviour in an Australian community pharmacy setting. Soc Sci Med 2007;64:1501-11.
52. Corkrey R, Parkinson L. Interactive voice response: review of studies 1989-2000. Behav Res Methods Instrum Comput 2002;34:342-53.
53. Bender BG, Apter A, Bogen DK, et al. Test of an interactive voice response intervention to improve adherence to controller medications in adults with asthma. J Am Board Fam Med 2010;23:159-65.
54. Vollmer WM, Feldstein A, Smith DH, et al. Use of health information technology to improve adherence to inhaled steroids. Am J Manag Care 2011;17(12 Spec No):SP79-87.

92

Anti-Immunoglobulin E Therapy

JEFFREY R. STOKES | THOMAS B. CASALE

CONTENTS

SUMMARY OF IMPORTANT CONCEPTS

» Omalizumab, a humanized monoclonal antibody, binds to the Fc portion (C_H3 domain) of the immunoglobulin E (IgE) molecule, resulting in decreased IgE levels.
» Omalizumab's mechanisms of action include decreased levels of circulating free IgE, expression of the IgE receptor FcεRI on critical effector cells, inflammation, and allergen-induced mediator release.
» The addition of omalizumab to standard asthma care reduced the rate of clinically significant asthma exacerbations irrespective of baseline oral corticosteroid use, concomitant treatment with other controller medications, and patient characteristics.
» In addition to moderate and severe allergic asthma, potential but unapproved clinical uses of omalizumab include seasonal and perennial allergic rhinitis with or without asthma, atopic dermatitis, food allergies, chronic urticaria (especially with autoantibodies), and as an adjuvant to allergen immunotherapy.
» Omalizumab has an excellent safety profile, but there is a small chance of allergic reactions to omalizumab, and careful observation after administration is required.

Immunoglobulin E and Immunoglobulin E Receptors

BACKGROUND

Immunoglobulin E (IgE) was originally described in 1967 by Ishizaka and colleagues.[1] The importance of IgE in atopic disorders such as asthma, allergic rhinitis, food allergies, and atopic dermatitis has since been established. Elevation of total serum IgE levels is typically found in many atopic patients, and in predisposed individuals, allergen-specific IgE is produced. IgE is then bound to the high-affinity IgE receptor, FcεRI, and subsequently expressed on the surface of several key inflammatory cells, including mast cells, basophils, and dendritic cells. Allergen binds to the Fab portion of the IgE molecule. Cross-linking of two adjacent IgE molecules on the surface of allergic effector cells initiates intracellular signaling pathways that result in the release of preformed and rapidly synthesized mediators. This type I hypersensitivity reaction is central to the pathogenesis of atopic disorders (Fig. 92-1).

Inhibition of the consequences of mast cell and basophil degranulation has been an important therapeutic goal for many years. Chronic therapy for allergic diseases has largely been limited to blocking the effects of specific mediators (e.g., leukotriene modifiers, antihistamines) or the use of corticosteroids to reduce the consequences of mediator release on the inflammatory cascade. The availability of humanized monoclonal antibodies against IgE has provided a newer therapeutic option and a tool to more closely explore the role of IgE in allergic diseases and the effects of inhibiting IgE.

Omalizumab is a humanized, monoclonal antibody that recognizes and binds to the Fc portion of the IgE molecule. Approximately 5% of omalizumab is composed of murine sequences that were engrafted onto a human immunoglobulin G (IgG1κ) framework; these Fab portions contain the antigen (IgE) binding regions of the molecule (Fig. 92-2).[2] Omalizumab binds to the heavy-chain constant C_H3 domain of the IgE molecule, which is conserved among all IgE molecules.[3] This is the same site by which IgE binds to FcεRI. The binding of omalizumab to IgE results in the formation of soluble immune complexes that are subsequently cleared by the reticuloendothelial system (i.e., mononuclear phagocyte system). Typically, omalizumab forms trimers of two omalizumab molecules per IgE antibody, but it can form other complexes (Fig. 92-3).[4] Binding of omalizumab to free IgE blocks the binding of IgE to FcεRI and the subsequent expression of IgE on the surface of allergic effector cells. Because omalizumab binds to the same site that IgE molecules use to attach to FcεRI, it cannot cross-link cell surface–expressed IgE. Therefore, because omalizumab can bind only to soluble IgE, it cannot precipitate degranulation of effector cells.[5]

IgE occurs in the serum in much smaller amounts than IgG, IgM, or IgA, and it has a half-life in the serum of only 2 days. IgE upregulates the expression of FcεRI on the surface of critical effector cells, such as basophils. This effect likely occurs through the direct interaction of IgE with FcεRIα.[6] Another IgE receptor, FcεRII [CD23], whose role is less certain, binds with much lower affinity to IgE. FcεRII appears to have opposing effects that depend on whether the molecule is expressed on the cell surface or exists free in the serum. Soluble FcεRII upregulates the production of IgE through interaction with CD21, the B cell coreceptor. Ligation of cell surface–expressed FcεRII appears to inhibit IgE production.[7]

MECHANISM OF ACTION

Administration of omalizumab results in a rapid and substantial decrease in free IgE in serum.[8] By virtue of this dramatic reduction in serum levels of free IgE, omalizumab decreases the

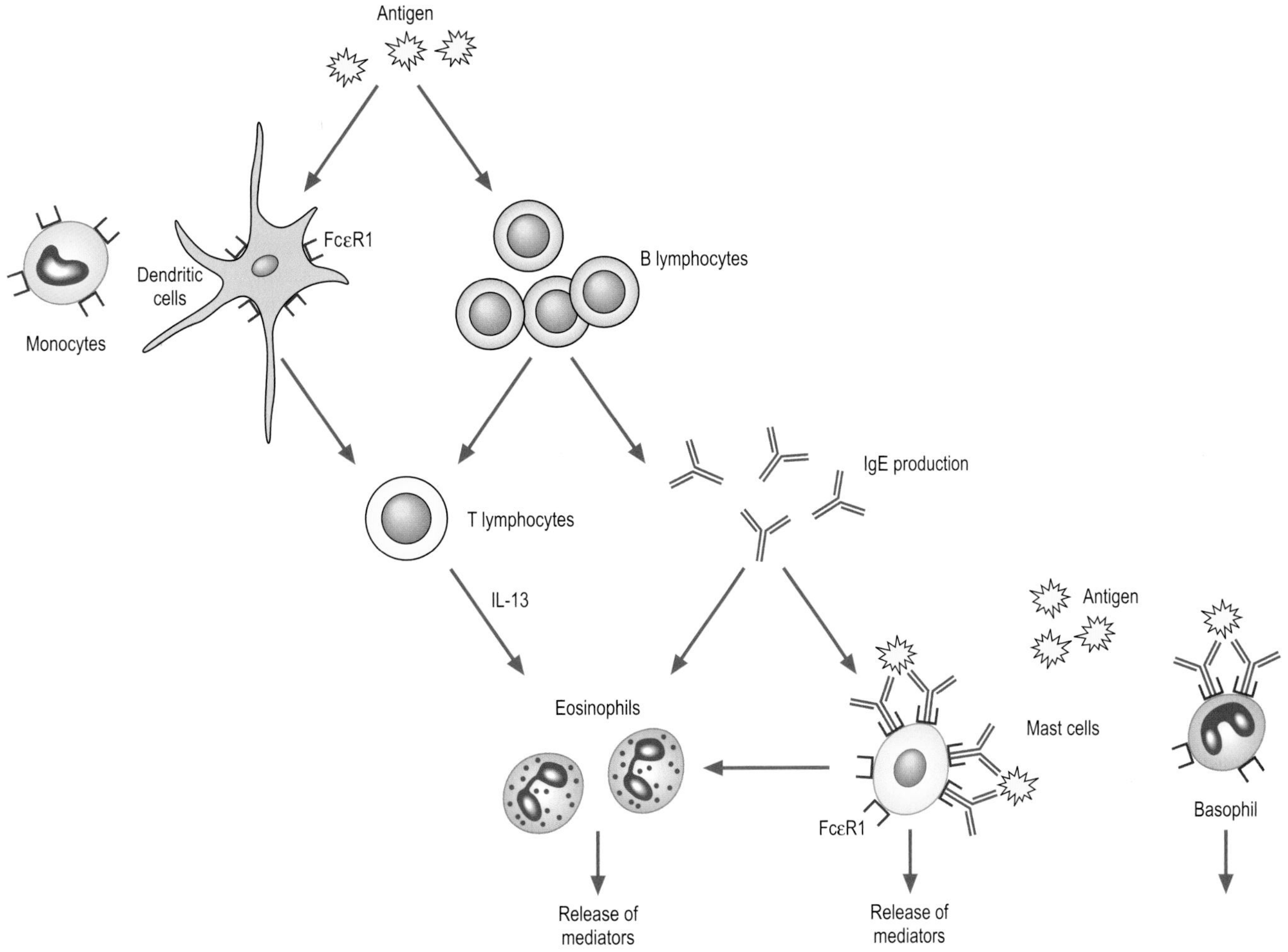

Figure 92-1 Type I hypersensitivity reaction. *FcεRI*, High-affinity IgE receptor; *IgE*, immunoglobulin E; *IL*, interleukin.

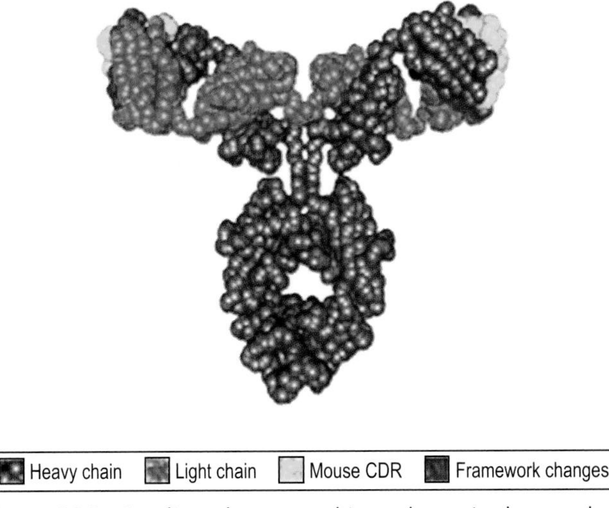

Figure 92-2 Omalizumab a recombinant humanized monoclonal antibody composed of 95% human sequence and 5% murine sequence. *CDR*, Complementarity-determining region. *(Reprinted with permission from Boushey Jr HA. Experiences with monoclonal antibody therapy for allergic asthma. J Allergy Clin Immunol 2001;108[Suppl]: S77-83.)*

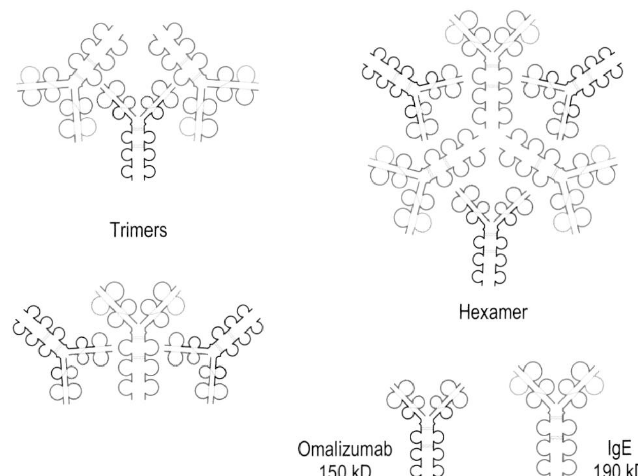

Figure 92-3 Omalizumab and immunoglobulin E (IgE) complexes. Omalizumab binds to the CH_3 domain of the IgE molecule, typically forming trimers. Hexamers are the largest complexes formed. *(Reproduced with permission from Brownell J, Casale TB. Anti-IgE therapy. Immunol Allergy Clin North Am 2004;24:551-68.)*

expression of FcεRI on several cell types.[8,9] A 99% reduction in free serum IgE levels has occurred within 2 hours after omalizumab administration. Within 3 months of therapy, human basophil responsiveness (i.e., histamine releasability) was reduced by 90%.[9] Omalizumab administration reduces allergen-induced nasal challenge responses and expression of FcεRI on basophils within 7 days.[9]

Antigen presentation by dendritic cells is facilitated by the surface expression of FcεRI.[10] Two subtypes of dendritic cells, DC1 and DC2, appear to be instrumental in the phenotypic development of T helper type 1 (Th1) cells and T helper type 2 (Th2) cells, respectively.[11] The expression of FcεRI on dendritic cells is greater in people with asthma than in nonatopic controls and correlates with serum IgE levels.[12] In ragweed-sensitive patients with seasonal allergic rhinitis treated with omalizumab, DC1 and DC2 cells showed a significant decrease in FcεRI expression as early as day 7 after initiation of treatment, which persisted through day 42. Decreased FcεRI expression correlated with a decrease in serum levels of free IgE and with decreased basophil FcεRI expression.[13] Omalizumab also reduces FcεR1 expression on monocytes.[14] These results suggest that omalizumab may have a significant effect on the sensitization phase of the allergic response by regulation of FcεRI expression on dendritic cells and monocytes.

Omalizumab's effect on cutaneous mast cell FcεRI expression appears to occur more gradually compared with basophils and dendritic cells. A small study evaluated the effect of omalizumab on intradermal allergen skin test titration and on FcεRI expression in skin biopsy samples. Omalizumab had no effect on FcεRI on day 7; however, by day 70, there was a 90% reduction in FcεRI expression in skin biopsy specimens, demonstrating a decrease in the expression of FcεRI by cutaneous mast cells.[15] Omalizumab typically has a weak and delayed effect on allergen-induced immediate skin test responses, although the inhibitory effects of omalizumab on late phase skin responses are more rapid and profound. This pattern of skin test responses makes them an unreliable surrogate biomarker for regulating and exploring dosing effects of this agent.[15,16]

MARKERS OF AIRWAY INFLAMMATION

Nitric oxide has been identified as an important noninvasive marker of airway inflammation in asthmatics. The effects of omalizumab on exhaled nitric oxide were examined in 29 children with moderate to severe allergic asthma randomized to omalizumab or placebo. The omalizumab group showed a significant reduction in exhaled nitric oxide from baseline to the end of the 52-week study period (41.9 ± 29.0 to 18.0 ± 21.8 ppb; $P = .032$) despite a substantial reduction in the dose of inhaled corticosteroids (ICS).[17]

Omalizumab treatment reduces blood eosinophil levels in patients with seasonal allergic rhinitis, correlating with reduced serum levels of free IgE.[18] Similar decreases in blood and sputum eosinophils compared with baseline values have been seen in patients with allergic asthma during omalizumab therapy.[19,20] Omalizumab treatment also has been shown to decrease B lymphocyte counts under experimental conditions. No significant differences were observed in the other lymphocyte subpopulations.[21]

Omalizumab's effects on inflammatory cells in bronchial biopsies and on sputum eosinophils have been evaluated. Forty-five patients with mild to moderate, persistent asthma with sputum eosinophilia greater than 2% were treated with omalizumab ($n = 22$) or placebo ($n = 23$) for 16 weeks. Subjects underwent sputum induction and bronchoscopy with bronchial biopsy before and after treatment. Treatment with omalizumab resulted in a significant decrease in the mean percentage of sputum eosinophils, from 6.6% to 1.7% ($P = .05$ versus placebo). This change was associated with a significant reduction in tissue eosinophils; cells positive for FcεR1; $CD3^+$, $CD4^+$, and $CD8^+$ T lymphocytes; B lymphocytes; and cells staining positive for IL-4; however, airway hyperresponsiveness to methacholine did not improve.[22] The dichotomy between omalizumab's effects on airway inflammation and on hyperresponsiveness suggests that IgE or eosinophils, or both, may not be causally linked to airway hyperresponsiveness to methacholine in mild to moderate asthma.

Thirty-five patients with moderate to severe allergic asthma were treated with omalizumab in addition to their baseline ICS, and circulating cytokines were measured. Levels of IL-13 were significantly decreased in omalizumab-treated patients compared with the placebo group; levels of IL-5 and IL-8 also declined, although not significantly. Levels of IL-6, IL-10, and soluble intercellular adhesion molecule 1 were unchanged with omalizumab therapy.[20]

Another possible mechanism of action involves the potential of omalizumab to promote mast cell apoptosis. The binding of different IgE molecules to FcεRI induces a spectrum of activation events in the absence of antigen. Highly cytokinergic IgEs induced production of cytokines and rendered mast cells resistant to apoptosis in an autocrine fashion.[23] By decreasing IgE and FcεR1 expression, omalizumab may lead to mast cell apoptosis, although this has not been demonstrated.

Omalizumab treatment induces human eosinophil apoptosis in patients with allergic asthma. After 12 weeks of therapy with omalizumab, markers of eosinophil apoptosis (i.e., immunofluorescent staining with Annexin V) were significantly increased. Fewer lymphocytes positive for granulocyte-macrophage colony-stimulating factor, IL-2, and IL-13 were evident in omalizumab-treated allergic asthma patients compared with the placebo group.[24] Figure 92-4 illustrates the mechanisms of action summarized in Box 92-1.

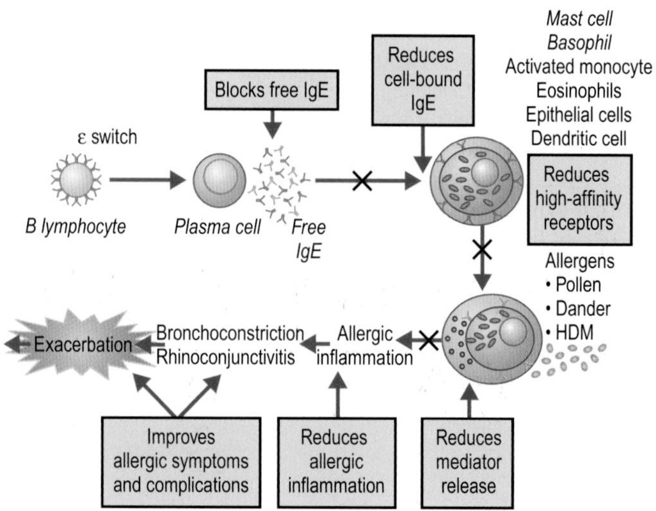

Figure 92-4 Omalizumab's mechanisms of action. *HDM*, House-dust mite; *IgE*, immunoglobulin E.

BOX 92-1 OMALIZUMAB'S MECHANISMS OF ACTION

Decreased levels of free serum immunoglobulin E
Decreased expression of FcεRI on mast cells, basophils, dendritic cells, and monocytes
Decreased fractional exhaled nitric oxide levels
Decreased levels of eosinophils in serum, sputum, and bronchial biopsies
Decreased levels of B lymphocytes
Decreased circulating levels of interleukin-13
Decreased antigen-induced mediator release from basophils and mast cells
Decreased airway inflammation

Disease-Specific Effects of Omalizumab

ASTHMA

Several studies have established the efficacy and safety of omalizumab for the treatment of patients with moderate to severe asthma. These findings led the U.S. Food and Drug Administration (FDA) to approve omalizumab for the treatment of moderate to severe, persistent allergic asthma in patients 12 years of age or older.

A phase II study examined asthma symptom scores in 317 moderate to severe allergic asthmatic patients on ICS or oral corticosteroids, or both.[25] Low-dose and high-dose intravenous treatment protocols were used: 2.5 and 5.8 μg/kg body weight per 1 ng/mL of IgE, respectively. Symptom scores improved in both groups at 12 weeks ($P = .005$ and $P = .008$, respectively). Subjects in the omalizumab treatment groups had fewer asthma exacerbations and were able to reduce or discontinue corticosteroids to a greater extent than those in the placebo group.

Three phase III trials enrolled a total of 1405 patients with moderate to severe allergic asthma.[26-28] Two trials enrolled subjects 12 years of age or older being treated with ICS.[26,28] Another trial enrolled children 6 to 12 years of age receiving ICS.[27] Omalizumab was administered subcutaneously every 2 to 4 weeks in doses ranging from 150 to 375 mg. During the initial 16 weeks, omalizumab was added to ICS at a stable dose. Subjects then underwent a steroid-reduction phase lasting 12 weeks. The primary end point in all three studies was a reduction in asthma exacerbations. Omalizumab led to a significant reduction in asthma exacerbations compared with placebo in all three studies; it also demonstrated a corticosteroid-sparing effect. Twice as many subjects in the omalizumab group successfully discontinued corticosteroids as in the placebo group. Fewer asthma symptoms, less rescue medication use, and improved quality of life scores were observed for the omalizumab-treated patients. In the adolescent and adult studies, omalizumab resulted in small but statistically significant improvements in peak expiratory flow (PEF) and forced expiratory volume in 1 second (FEV_1).[28]

The data from these three studies were later pooled to determine the effect of omalizumab on serious asthma exacerbations.[29] Significantly fewer unscheduled outpatient visits and emergency room visits were observed in the omalizumab-treated patients compared with the placebo group. Hospitalizations were also significantly reduced from 3.42 events per 100 patient-years on placebo to 0.26 on omalizumab treatment.

To examine baseline characteristics predictive of a response to omalizumab, data from 1070 adolescents and adults from two of these phase III trials were pooled.[30] Patients with features suggesting greater disease severity appeared to obtain the greatest benefit from the addition of omalizumab to the therapeutic regimen. They included patients with a history of emergency treatment of asthma in the past year, patients taking 800 μg or more of inhaled beclomethasone per day, and patients with an FEV_1 65% of the predicted value or lower. The greatest benefits were seen in patients who had two or more of these characteristics.

Of 1412 patients in phase III trials, 254 were identified as high risk (i.e., those who had ever required intubation or who had visited an emergency room, required overnight hospitalization, or received treatment in an intensive care unit during the past year). Among these high-risk patients in the corticosteroid-stable phase of the studies, those treated with omalizumab had a reduction in significant asthma exacerbation episodes by 56% and were less likely to be rehospitalized due to asthma; they also demonstrated improvements in peak flows and asthma symptoms. Omalizumab prevented exacerbations in about 17 additional patients for every 100 treated. Fifty percent of potential exacerbations were prevented by treatment with omalizumab, and 5.7 patients needed to be treated with omalizumab to maintain 1 patient free of an exacerbation.[31]

Patients with severe allergic asthma who required high-dose fluticasone (≥1000 μg/day) with or without oral corticosteroids were treated with omalizumab. At 32 weeks, the dose of ICS in the omalizumab group was significantly reduced compared with that for the placebo group (mean, 57.2% versus 43.3%; $P = .003$). Improved symptoms, less rescue medication use, and improved quality of life were also observed in the omalizumab group compared with the placebo group.[32] However, no significant reduction in exacerbations was observed in this study.

In practice, omalizumab is typically added to the therapeutic regimen for patients who remain poorly controlled despite maximal medical therapy. The addition of omalizumab to maximal conventional asthma therapy was evaluated in a 52-week trial enrolling patients with moderate to severe allergic asthma who were symptomatic despite treatment with high doses of ICS plus long-acting β_2-agonists, antileukotriene drugs, or oral steroids.[33] Compared with placebo, the omalizumab group showed a greater reduction of asthma exacerbations (60%), unscheduled physician visits, and days missed from work or school. A similar study evaluated 419 patients with severe, uncontrolled asthma despite high-dose ICS and long-acting bronchodilators.[34] Omalizumab therapy significantly reduced the rate of significant exacerbations while decreasing emergency visits by 44%. Quality of life scores, pulmonary function test results, and asthma symptom scores improved with omalizumab add-on therapy.

A study evaluated the pooled data from five double-blind trials and two open-label studies for an analysis of the effect of add-on therapy with omalizumab on asthma exacerbations in severe asthmatics.[35] A total of 4308 patients were included (2511 treated with omalizumab). Omalizumab decreased the rate of asthma exacerbations by 38% and that of emergency visits by 47%. Another study in patients with severe asthma not well controlled despite high-dose ICS and long-acting β_2-agonists found that omalizumab reduced exacerbations by 25%.[36] A review of eight clinical trials involving almost 3500 patients with asthma demonstrated that the addition of omalizumab reduced exacerbations and asthma hospitalizations for children, adolescents, and adults (risk ratio = 0.57). Omalizumab also significantly improved symptom scores, quality of life, and rescue medication use. These effects were independent of age, duration of treatment, or severity of asthma. There was no difference in adverse events or serious adverse events between the omalizumab and placebo groups.[37] Taken together, these studies suggest that omalizumab is effective as an add-on therapy in cases of severe asthma that is poorly controlled despite maximal medical therapy.

Subsequent studies have found omalizumab to be beneficial in adolescent and pediatric inner-city patients with persistent allergic asthma. Omalizumab significantly reduced the proportion of participants who had one or more exacerbations from 48.8% to 30.3% ($P < .001$).[38] This reduction was especially noticeable for seasonal exacerbations (i.e., fall and spring). In these patients, daily symptoms and daily ICS dosages were significantly reduced with omalizumab. The use of omalizumab also improved lung function, chest symptoms, and rhinoconjunctivitis symptoms compared with placebo in cat allergen–induced asthma with cat exposure.[39] Case studies found that omalizumab improved asthma control in patients with allergic asthma but baseline IgE levels of less than 17 kU/L and in a patient with no evidence of specific allergen sensitization but elevated total IgE levels.[40,41] Other data indicate that the response at 16 weeks is strongly predicts a persistent response at 32 weeks.[42] Box 92-2 provides a summary of the effects observed in patients with allergic asthma treated with omalizumab.

The cost of omalizumab is substantially higher than for other asthma medications. The cost of treatment is $4000 to $20,000 per year, depending on the dose, and the average cost is approximately $12,000 per year.[43] However, it may still be cost-effective when its use is limited to patients with severe disease, including those with frequent exacerbations, those requiring emergency care, and those requiring hospitalization. This relatively small group of patients accounts for the bulk of healthcare expenditures associated with asthma care.[44]

ALLERGIC RHINITIS

The effect of omalizumab was evaluated in 536 patients with ragweed-sensitive allergic rhinitis.[45] Patients were randomized to receive one of three omalizumab doses (50, 150, or 300 mg) or placebo. Omalizumab or placebo was administered just before the onset of the ragweed season and every 3 to 4 weeks throughout the pollen season. Subjects treated with 300 mg of omalizumab had significantly lower nasal symptoms scores, rhinitis quality of life scores, and days missed from work or school compared with the placebo group. A significant correlation was observed between reduction in serum IgE levels and improvements in nasal symptoms and rescue antihistamine use.

Another large seasonal allergic rhinitis study examined the therapeutic benefits of omalizumab in 251 birch pollen–sensitive patients with rhinitis.[46] Subjects received 300 mg of omalizumab or placebo two or three times during the birch pollen season, depending on their baseline total serum IgE values. The omalizumab-treated group showed significant improvements over the placebo group in average daily symptom scores, use of rescue antihistamines, and quality of life measures. In patients with ragweed-induced allergic rhinitis, omalizumab has been safely readministered the next year after discontinuation of the drug at the end of the previous ragweed season.[47]

Omalizumab has been shown to be effective in the treatment of perennial allergic rhinitis. A 16-week trial evaluated 289 patients with moderate to severe disease.[48] Patients were randomized to omalizumab (0.016 mg/kg/IgE [IU/mL]) or placebo every 4 weeks. Mean daily nasal severity scores and rescue antihistamine use were significantly lower in the omalizumab group than in the placebo group ($P < .001$ and $P < .005$, respectively).

The effect of omalizumab on early nasal responses to allergen challenge was investigated in two randomized, double-blind, placebo-controlled trials involving patients with allergic rhinitis.[9,49] Both studies showed significant inhibition of allergen-induced acute nasal responses, with inhibitory effects apparent within 2 weeks. Inhibition of nasal responses correlated temporally with the reduction in FcεRI on basophils, suggesting that inhibition of allergic responses by omalizumab requires reduction in FcεRI expression and serum IgE levels.[9] A significant decrease in basal levels of tumor necrosis factor-α and albumin in the nasal lavage fluid (a marker of vascular permeability) was shown in omalizumab-treated patients.[49] Box 92-3 lists the many upper airway improvements that occur with omalizumab therapy.

Allergic rhinitis and asthma frequently coexist. Poor control of rhinitis may exert a detrimental effect on asthma. The Study of Omalizumab in for Comorbid Asthma and Rhinitis (SOLAR) evaluated 405 adolescents and adults with moderate to severe asthma on stable therapy who also had persistent allergic rhinitis.[50] Patients received omalizumab or placebo for 28 weeks. Fewer asthma exacerbations were observed in the omalizumab-treated patients than placebo-treated patients (20.6% versus 30.1%). More patients in the omalizumab group demonstrated a clinically significant improvement in asthma and rhinitis quality-of-life indices (57.7% versus 40.6%). These findings suggest that omalizumab is effective in the treatment of upper and lower airway symptoms in the same patients.[50]

OMALIZUMAB PLUS IMMUNOTHERAPY

The rationale for using the combination of anti-IgE and allergen immunotherapy comes from preexisting data about the

BOX 92-2 OMALIZUMAB'S EFFECTS ON ASTHMA

Decreased exacerbations
Decreased inhaled corticosteroid doses
Decreased asthma symptoms
Decreased rescue medication use
Increased quality of life
Decreased emergency room visits
Decreased hospitalizations
Improved pulmonary functions (small effect)

BOX 92-3 OMALIZUMAB'S EFFECTS ON ALLERGIC RHINITIS

Decreased daily symptoms
Decreased rescue medication use
Increased quality of life
Decreased nasal allergen challenge responses
Decreased missed school or work days

biologic and immunologic effects of both therapies. Allergen immunotherapy has been used for 100 years for the management of allergic disorders and is the only antigen-specific immunomodulatory treatment routinely available to clinicians. The immunomodulatory effects of immunotherapy are based on several proposed mechanisms, including blunting of seasonal increases in IgE levels, increasing allergen-specific IgG levels, shifting the balance of T lymphocyte subsets away from a Th2 phenotype and toward a Th1 phenotype, and production of allergen-specific IL-10.[51] However, immunotherapy is associated with the risk of allergic reactions to the extract injections.

Omalizumab does not completely ameliorate allergic respiratory symptoms, and on discontinuation, serum IgE levels return to pretreatment levels.[45,46,52] There are no data concerning long-lasting immune tolerance as a result of anti-IgE therapy. Nonetheless, omalizumab-induced decreases in serum IgE levels and the expression of FcεRI on key immune effector cells, including basophils and dendritic cells, may lead to immunologic changes that enhance the immune tolerance to allergens delivered by immunotherapy.[8,9,13] Combining omalizumab with allergen immunotherapy improves the prospects of better clinical benefits and safety.

The addition of omalizumab to standard maintenance-dose immunotherapy was evaluated in 221 children and adolescents with sensitization to birch and grass allergens.[53] During birch season, the birch and grass immunotherapy plus omalizumab groups had symptoms decreased by 39% in the group treated with irrelevant immunotherapy (grass) and by 48% in the birch immunotherapy group compared with irrelevant immunotherapy and placebo. Similar results were seen in grass season, with irrelevant (birch) immunotherapy and omalizumab decreasing symptoms by 45%, whereas patients on grass immunotherapy and omalizumab had a reduction in symptom scores of 71% compared with irrelevant immunotherapy and placebo. When these findings were further analyzed for the grass pollen–allergic children, the groups treated with omalizumab plus immunotherapy had significantly diminished rescue medication use and number of symptomatic days compared with those using omalizumab or immunotherapy alone.[54] Combined treatment with omalizumab and grass immunotherapy was more effective than omalizumab alone.

The primary objective of a study by Casale and coworkers was to determine whether omalizumab given 9 weeks before rush immunotherapy and followed by 12 weeks of dual omalizumab and immunotherapy was more effective than rush immunotherapy followed by immunotherapy alone in ragweed-allergic patients.[55] A major secondary objective was whether omalizumab improved the safety of rush immunotherapy. Omalizumab improved the efficacy and safety of immunotherapy, and patients receiving omalizumab plus immunotherapy had fewer adverse events than those receiving immunotherapy alone. Post hoc analysis of groups receiving immunotherapy demonstrated that the addition of omalizumab resulted in a fivefold decrease in risk of anaphylaxis caused by rush immunotherapy (odds ratio = 0.17; P = .026). On an intent-to-treat basis, patients receiving omalizumab and immunotherapy showed a significant improvement in severity scores during the ragweed season compared with those receiving immunotherapy alone (0.69 versus 0.86; P = .044). In patients with persistent asthma, the use of omalizumab in conjunction with subcutaneous immunotherapy resulted in fewer systemic reactions (13.5% versus 26.2% for placebo). Omalizumab-treated patients were more likely to achieve maintenance dosing (87%, versus 72% for placebo).[56] The concurrent use of omalizumab in a few patients on venom immunotherapy demonstrated conflicting results in preventing systemic reactions caused by immunotherapy.[57,58] Omalizumab pretreatment of 11 children with cow's milk allergy has been used for oral desensitization to milk powder.[59]

Combined therapy with omalizumab and allergen immunotherapy may be an effective strategy to permit more rapid and higher doses of aeroallergen immunotherapy to be given with greater safety and efficacy to patients with allergic diseases.[55] However, there are unanswered questions: How long do you need to treat with both therapies? and Can you stop the omalizumab after reaching maintenance immunotherapy?

FOOD ALLERGY

Food allergies affect about 6% of children younger than 3 years of age and 2% of adults, with 1.5 million suffering from peanut allergy in the United States.[60] Unintended ingestion of peanut products accounts for 50 to 100 deaths each year in the United States.[60] The only treatment available is strict elimination and avoidance.

In a multicenter clinical trial, a humanized murine IgG1 monoclonal antibody against IgE (TNX-901) was evaluated in peanut-allergic patients. The double-blind, placebo-controlled, randomized trial enrolling 84 patients with proven peanut hypersensitivity evaluated three dosages of TNX-901 given every 4 weeks for 16 weeks. The mean baseline threshold of sensitivity to peanut flour was 178 to 436 mg for all the groups, which was equivalent to one-half to one and one-half peanuts ingested. At the end of 16 weeks, all treatment groups and the placebo group had a greater threshold of peanut tolerability, but only the high-dose TNX-901 group had significant improvement from the threshold dose of 178 mg (one-half peanut) to 2805 mg (almost nine peanuts). However, 25% of the patients had no improvement.

In a small study of 14 peanut-allergic patients, 44% of patients treated with omalizumab and 20% of placebo-treated patients were able to tolerate 1000 mg or greater amounts of peanut flour. The study was terminated early, and most subjects treated with omalizumab were not able to tolerate more than 1000 mg of peanut flour.[61]

ATOPIC DERMATITIS

Atopic dermatitis is a chronic inflammatory disease of the skin that affects 10% to 20% of children and 1% to 3% of adults. In the allergic form of atopic dermatitis, the total IgE serum level is elevated. A few early reports of omalizumab therapy have produced conflicting results. A small study reported three patients with severe atopic dermatitis and baseline IgE levels of 1990, 2890, and 6120 IU/mL.[62] All patients experienced significant improvement on omaluzumab (150 to 450 mg every 2 weeks for 12 weeks) as early as 2 weeks after therapy was initiated.

A study evaluated seven patients with asthma, allergic rhinitis, and atopic dermatitis. Their baseline IgE levels ranged from 262 to 2020 IU/mL.[63] Eczema symptoms were scored before therapy and after 3 and 7 months of omalizumab. Six of the seven patients had at least moderate disease before the start of

BOX 92-4 EFFECTS OF ANTI–IMMUNOGLOBULIN E THERAPY

EFFECTS ON FOOD ALLERGY

Only high-dose therapy significantly improved amount of food allergen tolerated
Minimal improvement demonstrated in small omalizumab study

EFFECTS ON ATOPIC DERMATITIS

Improved symptoms in some patients
Likely not effective for patients with extremely elevated serum immunoglobulin E levels

EFFECTS ON URTICARIA

In small case series, effective for urticaria induced by exogenous physical stimuli
Effective in small trials for chronic urticaria; possibly more effective for chronic urticaria with autoantibodies; large-scale studies under way

therapy, but only five completed 7 months of therapy as a result of problems with insurance coverage for treatment. Improvement occurred within the first 3 months of therapy. Of the five remaining patients at 7 months, three had resolution of their eczema, and two had only mild disease.[63]

In another small study, three adult patients with severe atopic dermatitis and concomitant asthma or allergic rhinitis, or both, were treated with 450 mg of omalizumab every 2 weeks.[64] After 4 months of therapy, no improvement was observed in their atopic dermatitis symptoms. A likely explanation was that the baseline values of IgE before treatment were extremely elevated (i.e., 5440, 23,000, and 24,400 IU/mL) and that omalizumab was insufficiently dosed to significantly reduce the serum IgE.[64] In these few very small trials, omalizumab improved atopic dermatitis, but the effectiveness may be limited by pretreatment IgE levels. Box 92-4 summarizes the potential effects of anti-IgE therapy on food allergy and atopic dermatitis.

URTICARIA

Several case reports and small series have detailed the utility of omalizumab in treating patients with chronic urticaria, including physical urticaria. Physical urticarias that have responded to anti-IgE therapy in one to two patient case reports include cholinergic, solar, cold-induced, delayed-pressure, dermatographic, and localized-heat urticarias.[65]

In approximately 50% of patients with chronic urticaria, the disease has an autoimmune component. The most common association is the presence of IgG antibody directed to the α-subunit of the IgE receptor, but others have IgG directed against IgE. These autoantibodies cross-link the α-subunits of the high-affinity IgE receptor or IgE bound to the cell surface, leading to degranulation of basophils and cutaneous mast cells. Because omalizumab decreases cell surface IgE levels and the number of high-affinity IgE receptors, patients with these autoantibodies are expected to have symptom improvement. In 90 symptomatic patients with chronic idiopathic urticaria despite oral antihistamines, a single dose of 300 or 600 mg of omalizumab improved hives and reduced itching. This positive effect was observed regardless of the presence or absence of autoantibodies.[66] Small samples of patients with idiopathic angioedema and chronic urticaria have demonstrated improvement and even resolution with omalizumab therapy despite refractoriness to antihistamines. Patients with the autoimmune subtype of chronic urticaria may be more responsive to the benefit of omalizumab therapy, but this should be confirmed.[67] Several phase III studies are looking at the effects of urticaria in antihistamine resistant urticaria.

OTHER ALLERGIC DISEASES

Small case reports have demonstrated the benefit of omalizumab in disease states such as allergic bronchopulmonary aspergillosis, mastocytosis, nasal polyposis or sinusitis, eosinophilic gastrointestinal diseases, latex allergy, drug allergy, and idiopathic anaphylaxis.[65]

Omalizumab Dosing

The only FDA-approved anti-IgE therapy is omalizumab (Xolair). It is supplied as a lyophilized powder in doses of 150 or 75 mg on reconstitution with sterile water for subcutaneous injection, but a liquid formulation is forthcoming. The recommended dose is 0.016 mg per kilogram of body weight per international unit of IgE every 4 weeks, and it is administered subcutaneously at 2- or 4-week intervals for adults and adolescents (i.e., ≥12 years of age) with moderate to severe perennial allergic asthma.[68] Because omalizumab is available in 75- or 150-mg vials, dosing charts are used to calculate the dose based on multiples of 75 (Table 92-1). Omalizumab doses calculated by the chart may be two times higher than the formula dosing (i.e., 0.016 mg of omalizumab/kg body weight per 1 IU/mL of free IgE).[69] It may be reasonable to base doses on the formula to achieve a decrease in total IgE approximating 90%, especially in patients who do not conform to the dosing parameters in the chart. For asthma, patients may need a trial of at least 12 weeks before clinical improvement is apparent.[43]

Omalizumab is absorbed slowly, reaching peak serum concentrations after an average of 7 to 8 days and with an average absolute bioavailability of 62%. In asthma patients, the omalizumab serum elimination half-life averaged 26 days, and apparent clearance averaging 2.4 ± 1.1 mL/kg/day.

Serum total IgE levels (i.e., bound and unbound) increase after the first dose as a result of the formation of omalizumab-IgE complexes, which have a slower elimination rate compared with that of free IgE. Total IgE levels increased with omalizumab therapy up to fivefold after 1 month and more than eight times compared with pretreatment levels after 3 months of therapy, whereas free IgE levels decreased.[70] After discontinuation of omalizumab dosing, the omalizumab-induced increase in total IgE levels and decrease in free IgE levels were reversible. Total IgE levels may take up to a year to achieve pretreatment levels after discontinuation of omalizumab.[68] Measurement of the total IgE concentration is difficult due to omalizumab-IgE complexes interfering with the accuracy of standard testing for serum IgE levels and allergen-specific IgE antibody levels.

Omalizumab is ineffective in about 40% of patients. Improvements correlate with IgE reductions, but free IgE levels in nonresponders are similar to those found in responders.[71] Possible reasons for this finding include the inexact relationship between free IgE levels and FcεR1 expression, ratios of specific IgE to total IgE that may be inordinately high for a clinically important allergen, and differences in intrinsic cellular (i.e., mast cells and basophils) sensitivity.[72]

TABLE 92-1 Omalizumab Dosing

Pretreatment Serum Immunoglobulin E Level (IU/mL)	DOSE BY BODY WEIGHT				
	30-60 kg	>60-70 kg	>70-90 kg	>90-150 kg	Frequency of Dosing
≥30-100	150	150	150	300	Every 4 weeks
>100-200	300	300	300	225	Every 2 weeks
>200-300	300	225	225	300	Every 2 weeks
>300-400	225	225	300	Not dosed	Every 2 weeks
>400-500	300	300	375	Not dosed	Every 2 weeks
>500-600	300	375	Not dosed	Not dosed	Every 2 weeks
>600-700	375	Not dosed	Not dosed	Not dosed	Every 2 weeks

Modified from Brownell J, Casale TB. Anti-IgE therapy. Immunol Allergy Clin North Am 2004;24:551-68.

Omalizumab Safety

Omalizumab has proved to be a well-tolerated medication with few adverse reactions. The most common adverse event is a local reaction at the injection site that may include burning, pruritus, hives, pain, redness, induration, swelling, warmth, and bruising. Among asthmatic patients receiving omalizumab or placebo, a local cutaneous reaction was observed in 45% and 43% of subjects, respectively. Severe local cutaneous reactions occurred in 12% of omalizumab-treated patients and 9% of the placebo group.[68] Other frequent adverse events in patients treated with omalizumab were viral infections (23%), sinusitis (16%), headaches (15%), and pharyngitis (11%). These events occurred at similar rates in omalizumab-treated patients and control patients.[68] Only 6.6% of the total adverse events were thought to be treatment related in the omalizumab group, compared with 5.6% in the placebo group. As a result of adverse events, 0.6% of omalizumab-treated patients and 1.1% of placebo-treated patients withdrew from the study.[68]

The safety of omalizumab was evaluated in more than 300 children in a randomized, double-blind, placebo-controlled study.[73] Subjects were treated for 28 weeks, followed by a 24-week open-label extension. During the double-blind, 28-week treatment period, the incidences of adverse events were similar for the omalizumab and placebo groups. Urticaria was reported in 11 patients (4.9%). With the exception of one severe case of urticaria that necessitated withdrawal from the study, all patients with urticaria had spontaneous remission or resolution with antihistamine treatment. Adverse event incidence during the open-label extension was similar to that for the omalizumab-treated group during the 28-week, double-blind phase. The study found that omalizumab was well tolerated in children and had a good safety profile.

In the original studies, 4127 patients received omalizumab; 19 (0.46%) of them developed cancer. Of the 2236 patients who received placebo, 5 (0.22%) developed cancer.[74] Of the 3726 patients who received omalizumab in controlled clinical trials, only 0.35% developed cancer. The differences between these groups were not statistically significant. All cancers were solid tumors, except for one recurrent non-Hodgkin lymphoma. It is very likely that most of these tumors were preexistent. A history of cancer was not an exclusion criterion if it occurred more than 3 months before enrollment in the initial studies. Overall, the conclusion of an independent panel of oncologists who compared the reported cancer rates for this population range was that there was no relative risk that was statistically significant for treatment with omalizumab. Nonetheless, postapproval surveillance is appropriate.

Two abstracts evaluated the possible risks of malignancy associated with omalizumab.[75,76] The first compiled data from 32 randomized, double-blind, placebo-controlled studies and assessed for incidence of primary malignancy.[75] Data collection occurred between 1994 and 2010. Studies included patients with atopic and nonatopic asthma, allergic rhinitis, atopic dermatitis, or urticaria and those receiving immunotherapy. The primary analysis identified a similar number of primary malignancies in omalizumab-treated (14 of 4254) and control patients (11 of 3178) and found no difference in the risk of malignancy for patients exposed to omalizumab compared with controls. The incidence rates per 1000 patient-years of observation were 4.14 for omalizumab-treated patients and 4.45 for the placebo group.

Evaluating Clinical Effectiveness and Long-term Safety in Patients with Moderate to Severe Asthma (EXCELS) is an ongoing epidemiologic, multicenter, prospective cohort study of approximately 5000 omalizumab-treated and 2500 non–omalizumab-treated patients recruited from a variety of practice settings in the United States.[76] Interim results compared the longer-term incidence of malignancies, including nonmelanoma skin cancers, in patients with moderate to severe, persistent asthma who have been treated with omalizumab with patients who have not been treated with omalizumab in a real-world clinical practice setting. In this interim analysis, the malignancy incidence rates were similar in the omalizumab-treated and non–omalizumab-treated cohorts. The later data suggest that omalizumab may have a better safety profile in regard to malignancy than that suggested by earlier studies.

In the clinical trials, there was no increase in type I hypersensitivity adverse events. The overall incidence of urticaria was 1.2% (39 of 3224) for the omalizumab group and 1.1% (24 of 2019) for the controls. Rare cases of acute systemic reactions occur after omalizumab treatment. These events occurred after the first and multiple doses and did not manifest until at least 60 minutes after injection. Although the mechanisms are unclear,[77] patients can be successfully desensitized to omalizumab and continue on therapy.[78] In an 18-month period during 2007 and 2008, 118 cases of anaphylaxis or multisystem allergic reactions were reported.[79] There is no evidence of any immune complex disease associated with omalizumab treatment, and among 1723 patients studied, only 1 demonstrated anti-omalizumab antibodies.

Decreasing serum IgE levels may increase the incidence or severity of helminthic infections. A 1-year clinical trial in Brazil considered this possibility in 68 patients treated with omalizumab and 69 controls receiving placebo.[80] When adjusted for study visit, baseline infection status, gender, and age, the odds ratio for helminth infection was 2.2 (95% confidence interval [CI], 0.94 to 5.15), indicating that a patient who had an infection was 0.94 to 5.15 times as likely to have received omalizumab than a patient who did not have an infection. Response to antihelminth therapy was not significantly different between treatment groups. Patients at high risk for helminthic infection should be monitored for infection while on omalizumab therapy.

Postmarketing reports of possible side effects have arisen since omalizumab was approved. One case of severe thrombocytopenia occurred. Thrombocytopenia has been added to potential adverse events associated with omalizumab, even though no causal relationship was established and routine platelet monitoring is not required. Rare (<0.1%) cases of alopecia have been reported, but no causal relation to omalizumab has been established.[68]

In response to the data on anaphylaxis resulting from omalizumab administration and placement of a black box warning by the FDA, the American Academy of Allergy, Asthma, and Immunology and the American College of Allergy, Asthma, and Immunology appointed a task force to review the data collected between June 1, 2003, and December 31, 2005.[81] A follow-up report was published in 2011 after review of data from January 1, 2006, until December 31, 2008.[82] These two reports make several recommendations for the administration of omalizumab (Box 92-5).

BOX 92-5 RECOMMENDATIONS FOR OMALIZUMAB ADMINISTRATION

Informed consent should be obtained after discussing the risks and benefits.

The patient should be educated about the signs, symptoms, and treatment of anaphylaxis.

Patients should be prescribed and educated about the proper use of an epinephrine autoinjector and advised to carry it before omalizumab administration and for the next 24 hours.

Before omalizumab administration, the patient's health is assessed, including vital signs and some measure of pulmonary function.

Patients should be observed for 2 hours after the first three injections of omalizumab. Subsequent injections require observation for 30 minutes, but the waiting period can be modified based on the physician's clinical judgment.

Conclusions

Development of a selective anti-IgE humanized monoclonal antibody represents a novel and important therapeutic option for patients with severe asthma and other allergic diseases. The data suggest that omalizumab inhibits activation of mast cells and basophils and decreases the effects of other inflammatory cells such as eosinophils through a variety of mechanisms. Omalizumab appears to be a relatively safe, well-tolerated medication, and this approach has resulted in clinical improvements, including significant reductions in exacerbations, for patients with moderate to severe allergic asthma.

The roles of omalizumab and other anti-IgE antibody strategies will continue to evolve in pediatric asthma, nonallergic asthma, food allergy, atopic dermatitis, chronic urticaria with and without autoantibodies to IgE or the high-affinity IgE receptor, allergic bronchopulmonary aspergillosis, and chronic hyperplastic sinusitis and as an adjuvant to allergen immunotherapy. A second-generation, high-affinity anti-IgE monoclonal antibody that is being evaluated for patients with moderate to severe asthma may ultimately prove to be a better IgE-blocking strategy.

REFERENCES

Immunoglobulin E and Immunoglobulin E Receptors

1. Ishizaka K, Ishizaka T, Terry WD. Antigenic structure of gamma-E globulin and reaginic antibody. J Immunol 1967;99:849-58.
2. Boushey H. Experiences with monoclonal antibody therapy for allergic asthma. J Allergy Clin Immunol 2001;108:S77-83.
3. Liu J, Lester P, Builder S, Shire SJ. Characterization of complex formation by humanized anti-E monoclonal antibody and monoclonal human IgE. Biochemistry 1995;34:10474-82.
4. Brownell J, Casale TB. Anti-IgE therapy. Immunol Allergy Clin North Am 2004;24: 551-68.
5. Easthope S, Jarvis B. Omalizumab. Drugs 2001;61:253-60.
6. MacGlashan Jr D, Lichtenstein LM, McKenzie-White J, et al. Upregulation of FcεRI on human basophils by IgE antibody is mediated by interaction of IgE with FcεRI. J Allergy Clin Immunol 1999;104:492-8.
7. Tsicopoulos A, Joseph M. The role of CD23 in allergic disease. Clin Exp Allergy 2000;30:602.
8. MacGlashan DW, Bochner BS, Adelman DC, et al. Down-regulation of FcεRI expression on human basophils during in vivo treatment of atopic patients with anti-IgE antibody. J Immunol 1997;158:1438-45.
9. Lin H, Boesel K, Griffith D, et al. Omalizumab rapidly decreases nasal allergic response and FcεRI on basophils. J Allergy Clin Immunol 2004;113:297-302.
10. Maurer D, Fiebiger E, Reininger B, et al. Fcε receptor I on dendritic cells delivers IgE-bound multivalent antigens into a cathepsin S-dependent pathway of MHC class II presentation. J Immunol 1998;161:2731-9.
11. Rissoan MC, Soumelis V, Kadowaki N, et al. Reciprocal control of T helper cell and dendritic cell differentiation. Science 1999;283:1183-6.
12. Foster B, Metcalfe DD, Prussin C. Human dendritic cell 1 and dendritic cell 2 subsets express FcεRI: correlation with serum IgE and allergic asthma. J Allergy Clin Immunol 2003;112: 1132-8.
13. Prussin C, Griffith DT, Boesel KM, et al. Omalizumab treatment downregulates dendritic cell FcεRI expression. J Allergy Clin Immunol 2003;112:1147-54.
14. Cheng YX, Foster B, Holland SM, et al. CD2 identifies a monocyte subpopulation with immunoglobulin E-dependent, high-level expression of FcεRI. Clin Exp Allergy 2006; 36:1436-45.
15. Beck LA, Marcotte GV, MacGlashan Jr D, Togias A, Saini S. Omalizumab-induced reductions in mast cell FcεRI expression and function. J Allergy Clin Immunol 2004;114: 527-30.
16. Ong YE, Menzies-Gow A, Barkans J, et al. Anti-IgE (omalizumab) inhibits late-phase reactions and inflammatory cells after repeat skin allergen challenge. J Allergy Clin Immunol 2005;116: 558-64
17. Silkoff PE, Romero FA, Gupta N, Townley RG, Milgrom H. Exhaled nitric oxide in children with asthma receiving Xolair (omalizumab), a monoclonal anti-immunoglobulin E antibody. Pediatrics 2004;113:308-12.
18. Plewako H, Arvidsson M, Petruson K, et al. The effect of omalizumab on nasal allergic

inflammation. J Allergy Clin Immunol 2002; 110:68-71.
19. Fahy JV, Fleming HE, Wong HH, et al. The effect of an anti-IgE monoclonal antibody on the early- and late-phase responses to allergen inhalation in asthmatic subjects. Am J Respir Crit Care Med 1997;155:1828-34.
20. Noga O, Hanf G, Kunkel G. Immunological changes in allergic asthma following treatment with omalizumab. Int Arch Allergy Immunol 2003;131:46-52.
21. Hanf G, Brachmann I, Kleine-Tebbe J, et al. Omalizumab decreased IgE-release and induced changes in cellular immunity in patients with allergic asthma. Allergy 2006;61:1141-4.
22. Djukanović R, Wilson SJ, Kraft M, et al. Effects of treatment with anti-immunoglobulin E antibody omalizumab on airway inflammation in allergic asthma. Am J Respir Crit Care Med 2004;170:583-93.
23. Kitaura J, Song J, Tsai M, et al. Evidence that IgE molecules mediate a spectrum of effects on mast cell survival and activation via aggregation of the FcεRI. Proc Natl Acad Sci 2003;100: 12911-6.
24. Noga O, Hanf G, Brachmann I, et al. Effect of omalizumab treatment on peripheral eosinophil and T-lymphocyte function in patients with allergic asthma. J Allergy Clin Immunol 2006;117:1493-9.

Disease-Specific Effects of Omalizumab

25. Milgrom H, Fick RB, Su JQ, et al. Treatment of allergic asthma with monoclonal anti-IgE antibody. N Engl J Med 1999;341:1966-73.
26. Busse W, Corren J, Lanier BQ, et al. Omalizumab, anti-IgE recombinant humanized monoclonal antibody, for the treatment of severe allergic asthma. J Allergy Clin Immunol 2001;108:184-90.
27. Milgrom H, Berger W, Nayak A, et al. Treatment of childhood asthma with anti-immunoglobulin E antibody (omalizumab) [editorial]. Pediatrics 2001;108:E36.
28. Solér M, Matz J, Townley R, et al. The anti-IgE antibody omalizumab reduces exacerbations and steroid requirement in allergic asthmatics. Eur Respir J 2001;18:254-61.
29. Corren J, Casale T, Deniz Y, Ashby M. Omalizumab, a recombinant humanized anti-IgE antibody, reduces asthma-related emergency room visits and hospitalizations in patients with allergic predicting response to omalizumab, and anti-IgE antibody, in patients with allergic asthma. J Allergy Clin Immunol 2003;111: 87-90.
30. Bousquet J, Wenzel S, Holgate S, et al. Predicting response to omalizumab, an anti-IgE antibody in patients with allergic asthma. Chest 2004;125:1378-86.
31. Holgate S, Bousquet J, Wenzel S, et al. Efficacy of omalizumab, an anti-immunoglobin E antibody, in patients with allergic asthma at high risk of serious asthma-related morbidity and mortality. Curr Med Res Opin 2001;17: 233-40.
32. Holgate ST, Chuchalin AG, Hebert J, et al. Efficacy and safety of a recombinant anti-immunoglobulin E antibody (omalizumab) in severe allergic asthma. Clin Exp Allergy 2004; 34:632-8.
33. Ayres JG, Higgins B, Chilvers ER, et al. Efficacy and tolerability of anti-immunoglobulin E therapy with omalizumab in patients with poorly controlled (moderate-to-severe) allergic asthma. Allergy 2004;59:701-8.
34. Humbert M, Beasley R, Ayres J, et al. Benefits of omalizumab as add-on therapy in patients with severe persistent asthma who are inadequately controlled despite best available therapy (GINA 2002 step 4 treatment): INNOVATE. Allergy 2005;60:309-16
35. Bousquet J, Cabrera P, Berkman N, et al. The effect of treatment with omalizumab, an anti-IgE antibody, on asthma exacerbations and emergency medical visits in patients with severe persistent asthma. Allergy 2005;60:302-8.
36. Hanania NA, Alpan O, Hamilos DL, et al. Omalizumab in severe allergic asthma inadequately controlled with standard therapy: a randomized trial. Ann Intern Med 2011;154:573-82.
37. Rodrigo GJ, Neffen H, Castro-Rodriguez JA. Efficacy and safety of subcutaneous omalizumab vs placebo as add-on therapy to corticosteroids for children and adults with asthma: a systematic review. Chest 2011;139:28-35.
38. Busse WW, Morgan WJ, Gergen PJ, et al. Randomized trial of omalizumab (anti-IgE) for asthma in inner-city children. N Engl J Med 2011;364:1005-15.
39. Corren J, Wood RA, Patel D, et al. Effects of omalizumab on changes in pulmonary function induced by controlled cat room challenge. J Allergy Clin Immunol 2011;127:398-405.
40. Ankerst J, Nopp A, Johansson SG, Ade'doyin J, Oman H. Xolair is effective in allergics with a low serum IgE level. Int Arch Allergy Immunol 2010;152:71-4.
41. Van den Berge M, Pauw RG, de Monchy JG, et al. Beneficial effects of treatment with anti-IgE antibodies (omalizumab) in a patient with severe asthma and negative skin-prick test results. Chest 2011;139:190-3.
42. Bousquet J, Siergiejo Z, Swiebocka E, et al. Persistency of response to omalizumab therapy in severe allergic (IgE-mediated) asthma. Allergy 2011;66:671-8.
43. Strunk RC, Bloomberg GR. Omalizumab for asthma. N Engl J Med 2006;354:2689-95.
44. Oba Y, Salzman GA. Cost-effectiveness analysis of omalizumab in adults and adolescents with moderate-to-severe allergic asthma. J Allergy Clin Immunol 2004;114:265-9.
45. Casale TB, Condemi J, LaForce C, et al. Effect of omalizumab on symptoms of seasonal allergic rhinitis. JAMA 2001;286:2956-67.
46. Adelroth E, Rak S, Haahtela T, et al. Recombinant humanized mAb-E25, an anti-IgE mAb, in birch pollen-induced seasonal allergic rhinitis. J Allergy Clin Immunol 2000;106:253-9.
47. Nayak A, Casale T, Miller SD, et al. Tolerability of retreatment with omalizumab, a recombinant humanized monoclonal anti-IgE antibody, during a second ragweed pollen season in patients with seasonal allergic rhinitis. Allergy Asthma Proc 2003;24:323-9.
48. Chervinsky P, Casale T, Townley R, et al. Omalizumab, an anti-IgE antibody, in the treatment of adults and adolescents with perennial allergic rhinitis. Ann Allergy Asthma Immunol 2003;91:160-7.
49. Hanf G, Noga O, O'Connor A, Kunkel G. Omalizumab inhibits allergen challenge-induced nasal response. Eur Respir J 2004;23:414-8.
50. Vignola AM, Humbert M, Bousquet J, et al. Efficacy and tolerability of anti-immunoglobulin E therapy with omalizumab in patients with concomitant allergic asthma and persistent allergic rhinitis: SOLAR. Allergy 2004;59:709-17.
51. Akdis M, Akdis CA. Mechanisms of allergen-specific immunotherapy. J Allergy Clin Immunol 2007;119:780-91.
52. Casale TB. Experience with monoclonal antibodies in allergic mediated disease: seasonal allergic rhinitis. J Allergy Clin Immunol 2001;108:S84-8.
53. Kuehr J, Brauburger J, Zielen S, et al. Efficacy of combination treatment with anti-IgE plus standard immunotherapy in polysensitized children and adolescents with seasonal allergic rhinitis. J Allergy Clin Immunol 2002;109:274-80.
54. Rolinck-Werninghaus C, Hamelmann E, Keil T, et al. The co-seasonal application of anti-IgE after pre-seasonal specific immunotherapy decreases ocular and nasal symptom scores and rescue medication use in grass pollen allergic children. Allergy 2004;59:973-9.
55. Casale TB, Busse WW, Kline JN, et al. Omalizumab pretreatment decreases acute reactions after rush immunotherapy for ragweed-induced seasonal allergic rhinitis. J Allergy Clin Immunol 2006;117:134-40.
56. Massanari M, Nelson H, Casale T, et al. Effect of pretreatment with omalizumab on the tolerability of specific immunotherapy in allergic asthma. J Allergy Clin Immunol 2010;125: 383-9.
57. Soriano Gomis V, Gonzalez Delgado P, Niveiro Hernandez E. Failure of omalizumab treatment after recurrent systemic reactions to bee-venom immunotherapy. J Investig Allergol Clin Immunol 2008;18:225-6.
58. Galera C, Soohun N, Zankar N, et al. Severe anaphylaxis to bee venom immunotherapy: efficacy of pretreatment and concurrent treatment with omalizumab. J Investig Allergol Clin Immunol 2009;19:225-9.
59. Nadeau KC, Schneider LC, Hoyte L, Borras I, Umetsu DT. Rapid oral desensitization in combination with omalizumab therapy in patients with cow's milk allergy. J Allergy Clin Immunol 2011;127:1622-4.
60. Leung DYM, Sampson HA, Yunginger JW, et al. Effect of anti-IgE therapy in patients with peanut allergy. N Engl J Med 2003;348:986-93.
61. Sampson HA, Leung DY, Burks AW, et al. A phase II, randomized, double blind, parallel group, placebo controlled oral food challenge trial of Xolair (omalizumab) in peanut allergy. J Allergy Clin Immunol 2011;127:1309-10.
62. Lane JE, Cheyney JM, Lane TN, Ken DE, Cohen DJ. Treatment of recalcitrant atopic dermatitis with omalizumab. J Am Acad Dermatol 2006;54:68-72.
63. Vigo PG, Girgis KR, Pfuetze BL, et al. Efficacy of Anti-IgE therapy in patients with atopic dermatitis. J Am Acad Dermatol 2006;55: 168-70.
64. Krathen RA, Hsu S. Failure of omalizumab for treatment of severe adult atopic dermatitis. J Am Acad Dermatol 2005;53:338-40.
65. Casale TB, Stokes JR. Anti-IgE therapy: clinical utility beyond asthma. J Allergy Clin Immunol 2009;123:770-1.
66. Saini S, Rosen KE, Hsieh HJ, et al. A randomized, placebo-controlled, dose-ranging study of single-dose omalizumab in patients with H1-antihistamine-refractory chronic idiopathic urticaria. J Allergy Clin Immunol 2011;128: 567-3.
67. Kaplan AP, Joseph K, Maykut RJ, Geba GP, Zeldin RK. Treatment of chronic autoimmune urticaria with omalizumab. J Allergy Clin Immunol 2008;122:569-73.

Omalizumab Dosing

68. Xolair (omalizumab). Package insert, revised. South San Francisco, CA: Genentech; 2010.

Available at http://www.gene.com/download/pdf/xolair_prescribing.pdf (accessed December 30, 2012).
69. Rambasek T, Kavuru MS. Omalizumab dosing via the recommended card versus use of the published formula. J Allergy Clin Immunol 2006;117:708-9.
70. Hamilton RG, Marcotte GV, Saini SS. Immunological methods for quantifying free and total serum IgE levels in allergy patients receiving omalizumab (Xolair) therapy. J Immunol Methods 2005;303:81-91.
71. Slavin RG, Ferioli C, Tannenbaum SJ, et al. Asthma symptom re-emergence after omalizumab withdrawal correlates well with increasing IgE and decreasing pharmacokinetic concentrations. J Allergy Clin Immunol 2009;123:107-13.
72. MacGlashan D. Therapeutic efficacy of omalizumab. J Allergy Clin Immunol 2009;23:114-5.

Omalizumab Safety

73. Berger W, Gupta N, McAlary M, Fowler-Taylor A. Evaluation of long-term safety of the anti-IgE antibody, omalizumab, in children with allergic asthma. Ann Allergy Asthma Immunol 2003;91:182-8.
74. Xolair (Omalizumab). Prescribing information and summary of product characteristics. Available at http://www.xolair.com (accessed December 13, 2012).
75. Busse W, Buhl R, Vidaurre CF, et al. Omalizumab and the risk of malignancy: results from a pooled analysis. J Allergy Clin Immunol 2012;129:983-9.
76. Miller K, Eisner M, Chou W, Rahmaoui A, Bradley M. Omalizumab and malignancy: interim results from the EXCELS study [abstract 413]. Presented at the European Respiratory Society, Amsterdam, September 27, 2011.
77. Chipps B. Systemic reaction to omalizumab. Ann Allergy Asthma Immunol 2006;97:266-7.
78. Owens G, Petrov A. Successful desensitization of three patients with hypersensitivity reactions to omalizumab. Curr Drug Saf 2011;6:339-42.
79. Lin RY, Rodriguez-Baez G, Bhargave GA. Omalizumab-associated anaphylactic reactions reported between January 2007 and June 2008. Ann Allergy Asthma Immunol 2009;103:442-5.
80. Cruz AA, Lima F, Sarinho E, et al. Safety of anti-immunoglobulin E therapy with omalizumab in allergic patients at risk of geohelminth infection. Clin Exp Allergy 2007;37:197-207.
81. Cox L, Platts-Mills TAE, Finegold I, et al. American Academy of Allergy, Asthma & Immunology/American College of Asthma, Allergy, and Immunology Joint Task Force report on omalizumab-associated anaphylaxis. J Allergy Clin Immunol 2007;120:1373-7.
82. Cox L, Lieberman P, Wallace D, Simons FE, et al. American Academy of Allergy, Asthma & Immunology/American College of Allergy Asthma & Immunology Omalizumab-Associated Anaphylaxis Joint Task Force follow-up report. J Allergy Clin Immunol 2011;128:210-2.

93

Cytokine-Specific Therapy in Asthma

CHRISTOPHER E. BRIGHTLING* | DHANANJAY DESAI | IAN D. PAVORD

CONTENTS

SUMMARY OF IMPORTANT CONCEPTS

» Cytokines and their networks are implicated in the innate and adaptive immune responses driving airway inflammation in asthma and are modulated by host-environment interactions.

» Asthma is a complex heterogeneous disease, and the paradigm of Th2 cytokine–mediated eosinophilic inflammation occurring as a consequence of allergic sensitization has been challenged and probably represents a subtype of asthma.

» There is increasing recognition of inflammatory subphenotypes driven by different cytokine networks, particularly in severe asthma.

» Cytokine networks may be specific to different clinical aspects of the condition, as well as inflammatory cell profiles.

» Cytokine-directed therapies are likely to be most effective as phenotype-specific strategies, as demonstrated by studies with anti-IL-5 and anti-IL-13.

Introduction

Asthma affects 300 million people worldwide.[1] Its prevalence is 15% to 20% in children and 5% to 10% in adults. In a majority of cases the disease can be well controlled with inhaled corticosteroid therapy, either alone or in combination with long-acting β-agonists and other therapies, in accordance with international management guidelines.[1,2] Up to 10% of asthma sufferers, however, have severe disease that remains poorly controlled despite optimal standard therapy. Severe asthma can be divided into "difficult-to-treat" and "treatment-resistant" (refractory) asthma.[1,2] The former disorder usually is a consequence of poor adherence to therapy, factors such as comorbid conditions including psychosocial factors, or persistent exposure to triggers such as smoking. People with severe asthma experience the greatest morbidity, are at greater risk for asthma-related death, and are responsible for more than 50% of health care utilization attributed to asthma.

With ongoing research, asthma, and in particular severe asthma, is increasingly recognized to be a heterogeneous condition.[3] The clinical, physiologic, and immunopathologic domains of the disease often coexist but are not necessarily related. Accordingly, elucidation of the various mechanisms that are important in the interplay between these domains can be expected to lead to the development of biomarkers and novel therapies. A good example is use of the sputum eosinophil count to more effectively target corticosteroid therapy.[4] Even with optimized corticosteroid therapy, severe asthma often remains uncontrolled; moreover, some patients suffer from unacceptable side effects of corticosteroid treatment, a scenario that is particularly likely in those who require regular oral corticosteroid therapy. A pressing need for alternatives to oral corticosteroids and for drugs that allow oral corticosteroids to be safely withdrawn is well recognized.

Anti–immunoglobulin E (IgE), available as omalizumab, has been shown to relieve symptoms, reduce the burden of systemic corticosteroids, and decrease exacerbation frequency.[5] Only 50% of people with severe asthma have atopy, however, and even in cases in which this is a major component of the disease, not all patients will respond to this agent. Therefore considerable enthusiasm has been directed at identifying new treatments for severe asthma, and the current spotlight is on cytokine-directed therapies. This chapter presents a brief overview of the role of cytokines in the biology of severe asthma and summarizes the current successes and failures of anticytokine therapies in the clinic.

Cytokines

The generic term *cytokine* was coined a few years after the discovery in the late 1960s of lymphocyte-activating factor (LAF), which proved that macrophages released a mitogenic factor that promoted T cell proliferation in the absence of other growth factors or antigens. More cytokines are being discovered as the field of immunology expands. Cytokines include the interleukins, chemokines, and growth factor families, as described in Table 93-1. This section focuses on the cytokines that have been particularly implicated in asthma and have been evaluated in therapeutic trials in humans.

CYTOKINES AND THEIR NETWORKS IN ASTHMA

The onset and course of asthma are affected by complex host-environment interactions. More than 100 studies have been published that link increased frequency or severity of asthma to cytokine gene or cytokine signaling gene polymorphisms, including interleukin (IL)-4 and its receptor IL-4RA,[6] IL-13,[7] IL-18 and IL-18R, IL-2RB, IL1RL1, IL-33, and thymic stromal

*Christopher Brightling is funded by a Wellcome Senior Clinical Fellowship.

TABLE 93-1 Cytokine Families

Superfamily	Family Members
Interleukins	IL-1 to IL-35
Chemokines	
CC subfamily	CCL1 to CCL28
CXC subfamily	CXCL1 to CXCL16
CX3C subfamily	CX3CL1
C subfamily	XCL1, XCL2
Interferons	IFN-α, IFN-β, IFN-δ, IFN-ε, IFN-γ, IFN-κ, IFN-λ, IFN-ω, IFN-τ
TNF family	TNF, TNFSF4 to TNFSF15, OX40L
PDGF family	PDGFA to PDGFD
TGF-β family	TGF-β 1-3, inhBA to inhBE, BMP-2 and -7, GDF5, AMH
NGF family	NGF, BDNF, NT-3
FGF family	FGF-1 to FGF-24
VEGF family	VEGF-A to VEGF-E
EGF family	TGF-α, NRG1 to -4, EPR

AMH, Antimüllerian hormone; *BDNF,* Brain-derived neurotrophic factor; *BMP,* bone morphogenetic protein; *EGF,* epithelial growth factor; *FGF,* fibroblast growth factor; *EPR,* epiregulin; *GDF5,* growth differentiation factor 5; *IFN,* interferon; *inh,* inhibin; *NGF,* nerve growth factor; *NRG,* neuregulin; *NT-3,* neurotrophin-3; *PDGF,* platelet-derived growth factor; *TGF,* transforming growth factor; *TNF,* tumor necrosis factor; *TNFSF,* tumor necrosis factor superfamily [protein]; *VEGF,* vascular epithelial growth factor.

lymphopoeitin (TSLP).[8] The evidence is most consistent for the IL-4/IL-13 axis, and large genome-wide association studies have in particular implicated IL-18R and IL-33. The typical symptoms of asthma and disordered airway function occur against a background of airway inflammation and remodeling. The potential interplay between Th1 and Th2 cytokine networks in asthma and their consequent cellular and functional effects are summarized in Figure 93-1.

Airway inflammation in asthma is a multicellular process involving eosinophils, $CD4^+$ T cells, mast cells, and neutrophils.[9,10] This inflammation is largely restricted to the large conducting airways in mild to moderate disease, but in severe asthma, the smaller airways often are involved.[11] A key feature of allergic asthma is the recognition of allergens and the subsequent sensitization that leads to a Th2 cytokine response. Dendritic cells in the airway epithelium and submucosa take up and process allergens and present them to T cells in association with costimulatory molecules.[12] Subsequent T cell polarization toward a Th1 or Th2 phenotype is in part under the influence of dendritic cell–derived IL-12. Increased IL-12 drives the inflammatory response toward a Th1 bias, whereas in allergic asthma the Th2 phenotype predominates. Once sensitized, T cells are able to home back to sites of allergic inflammation under the control of chemokines via activation of the receptors CCR3, CCR4, CCR7, and CCR8.[13] The Th2 cells produce Th2 cytokines (i.e., IL-3, -4, -5, -9, and -13 and granulocyte-macrophage colony-stimulating factor [GM-CSF]), a majority of which are coded for by genes on the long arm of chromosome 5. In asthma, expression of these cytokines is increased, particularly in severe disease.[14] Of note, in severe disease the inflammatory response is complex and also involves Th1 T cells. These cells secrete TNF-α and IFN-γ, among other important mediators. TNF-α expression also is increased in the airway in asthma,[15] and the TNF-α axis is upregulated as reflected by increased membrane bound TNF-α on peripheral blood monocytes.[16]

The role of the dendritic cell–T cell axis in allergic sensitization is clear, but there is increasing recognition that other cells are likely to be important in severe asthma. Mast cell numbers are increased in the airway epithelium and in the airway smooth muscle bundle.[17,18] This microlocalization with the airway smooth muscle in asthma is a consistent finding and is closely related to the degree of airway hyperresponsiveness (AHR). In the asthmatic airway, mast cells are in an activated state and are an important source of cytokines, chemokines, autocoid mediators, proteases, and histamine. These cells can be activated via both IgE and non-IgE mechanisms and have been shown to affect airway smooth muscle contractility directly and indirectly by upregulation of airway smooth muscle transforming growth factor-β (TGF-β), which in turn drives the airway smooth muscle into a more contractile phenotype via an autocrine activation.[19] Mast cells and neutrophils also are localized to the mucous glands and have been implicated in goblet cell and mucous gland hyperplasia and mucus plugging.

In severe disease, airway neutrophil numbers also are increased[20] and have been implicated in disease, but their role remains unclear. Structural cells within the airway, including epithelial cells, fibroblasts, myofibroblasts, fibrocytes, and airway smooth muscle cells, also are important sources of chemokines and growth factors and are likely to play a role in the inflammatory response. These structural cells are increased in number in severe disease and contribute to the remodeling process, which leads to progression of pathologic changes and persistent airflow obstruction.[21] The cytokines affecting particular pathophysiologic aspects of asthma are summarized in Table 93-2.

Corticosteroids are the mainstay of therapy for asthma but only attenuate the inflammatory response in patients with eosinophilic disease. In refractory asthma, this effect is inadequate to control the clinical aspects of the disease, and anticytokine therapy may be an important alternative or adjunct to standard asthma regimens. Definition and explication of the specific roles of cytokines implicated in the pathogenesis of asthma are therefore important, because the "one size fits all" approach does not necessarily apply for different asthma subphenotypes.

CYTOKINE-DIRECTED THERAPY IN ASTHMA

The complexity of the cytokine networks as described in the previous section suggests that predicting the effects of cytokine-specific therapy is likely to be difficult, in part because of substantial redundancy in biologic pathways. Much interest has focused on identifying the relative roles of key cytokines, described next. This interest has led to, and is informed by, early clinical trials of cytokine-specific therapy, summarized in Table 93-3. These studies[15,16,22-37] have been pivotal in furthering the current understanding of the role of cytokines in asthma and are beginning to present real opportunities for personalized or stratified health care.

Interleukin-2

IL-2 is a potent activator of the proliferation and function of T lymphocytes and natural killer cells. IL-2 functions as a T cell growth factor, can augment natural killer (NK) cell cytolytic activity, contributes to the development of regulatory T (Treg) cells and promotes immunoglobulin production by B cells,

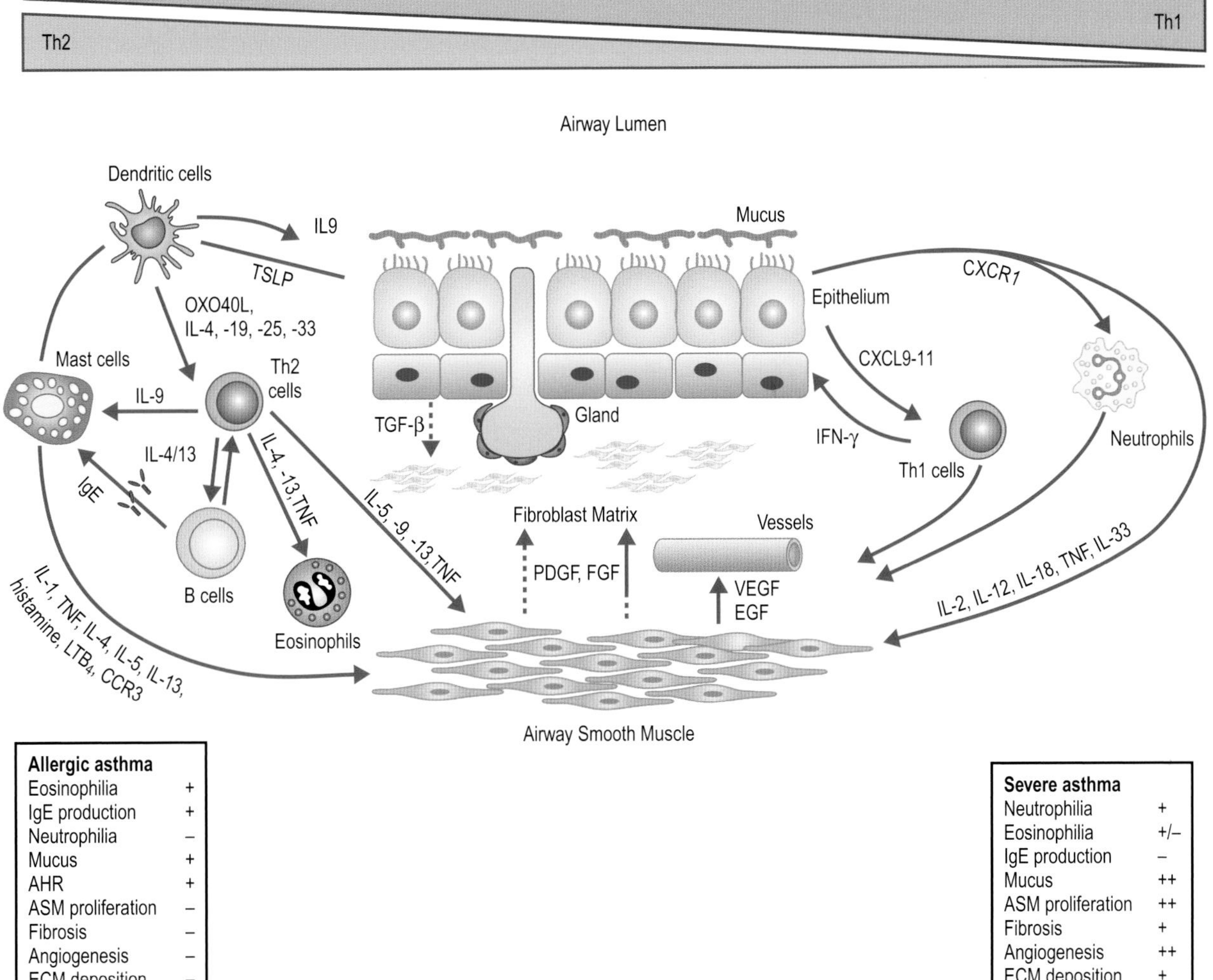

Figure 93-1 Cytokine effects on various airway components with a Th1/Th2 imbalance in mild and severe asthma. *AHR*, Airway hyperresponsiveness; *ASM*, airway smooth muscle; *ECM*, extracellular membrane; *EGF*, epidermal growth factor; *FGF*, fibroblast growth factor; *IFN*, interferon; *IgE*, immunoglobulin E; *IL*, interleukin; *LTB₄*, leukotriene B_4; *PDGF*, platelet-derived growth factor; *TGF*, transforming growth factor; *TNF*, tumor necrosis factor; *TSLP*, thymic stromal lymphopoietin; *VEGF*, vascular epithelial growth factor.

TABLE 93-2 Cytokines Associated with Pathophysiologic Features of Asthma

Feature	Interleukin(s)	Chemokine Receptor(s)	Growth Factor(s)
Airway hyperresponsiveness	IL-2, IL-4, IL-5, IL-9, IL-13, IL-18, IL-33, TNF-α	CCR7	
IgE production	IL-4, IL-9, IL-13, IL-18		
Goblet cell metaplasia	IL-4, IL-13		
Mucin hypersecretion	IL-9		EGF, TGF-β
Mastocytosis	IL-9		
Mast cell degranulation/migration	IL-9, IL-33	CCR3, CXCR1, CXCR 3, CXCR 4	
Eosinophilia	IL-4, IL-5, IL-9, IL-13, IL-17, TNF-α	CCR1, CCR3	
Neutrophilia	IL-1, IL-2, IL-18, IL-33, TNF-α, IFN-γ	CXCR1, CXCR2	
Th2 induction	IL-4, IL-5, IL-9, IL-13, IL-25, IL-33		
Airway smooth muscle hypertrophy	IL-13, IL-33	CCR7, CXCR4	TGF-α, TGF-β, PDGF, EGF
Remodeling—epithelial damage/repair	IL-5, IL-9, IL-18, IL-33		VEGF, EGFR, TGF-α
Extracellular matrix collagen deposition			TGF-β, PDGF
Subepithelial fibrosis	IL-13, IL-33	CCR7, CXCR4	TGF-β, FGF
Exacerbations	IL-4, IL-5, IL-6, IL-8, TNF-α		

EGF, Epidermal growth factor; *EGFR*, epidermal growth factor; receptor; *IgE*, immunoglobulin E; *IL*, interleukin; *TGF*, transforming growth factor; *TNF*, tumor necrosis factor; *VEGF*, vascular epithelial growth factor.

TABLE 93-3 Clinical Trials of Cytokine or Anticytokine Therapy*

Study	Study Phase	Agent	Cytokine Target	No. of Patients in Active Treatment/ Placebo Groups	Asthma Severity	Outcome
Haldar et al[22]	II	Mepolizumab	IL-5	29/32	Severe eosinophilic	Significantly reduced exacerbations
Nair et al[23]	II	Mepolizumab	IL-5	9/11	Severe eosinophilic	Reduced exacerbations and steroid-sparing
Flood-Page et al[24]	IIB	Mepolizumab	IL-5	222/119	Moderate + severe	Improved PEFR Trend toward reduced exacerbations
Flood-Page et al[25]	II	Mepolizumab	IL-5	11/13	Mild	Significant reduction in eosinophils Trend toward better PEFR
Castro et al[26]	II	Reslizumab	IL-5	53/53	Moderate + severe	Improved FEV_1, trend toward improved asthma control
Corren et al[27]	III	AMG-317	IL-4Rα	218/74	Moderate + severe	Symptomatic improvement, reduced time to exacerbations
Wenzel et al[28]	IIA	Pitrakinra	IL-4Rα	28/28	Mild	Significant attenuation of late asthmatic response Symptomatic improvement
Gauvreu et al[29]	IIB	IMA-638 and IMA-026	IL-13	28/28	Mild	Attenuation of early and late asthmatic response
Corren et al[30]	II	Lebrikizumab	IL-13	107/112	Moderate + severe	Improved lung function in high-Th2 group; no improvement in asthma control
Piper et al[31]	II	Tralokinumab	IL-13	146/48	Moderate + severe	Trend toward improved lung function, particularly in those with measurable IL-13 in sputum; no improvement in asthma control
Wenzel et al[32]	III	Golimumab	TNF-α	231/78	Severe	Unfavorable adverse effect profile
Howarth et al[15]	II	Etanercept	TNF-α	15	Severe	Improved ACQ, FEV_1; reduced AHR
Berry et al[16]	II	Etanercept	TNF-α	10/10	Moderate + severe	Improved AQLQ, FEV_1; reduced AHR
Morjaria et al[33]	II	Etanercept	TNF-α	20/19	Moderate + severe	Symptomatic improvement, reduced AHR
Holgate et al[34]	II	Etanercept	TNF-α	68/64	Moderate + severe	No benefit
Busse et al[35]	IIB	Daclizumab	IL-2Rα	88/27	Severe	Symptomatic improvement, unfavorable adverse effect profile
Oh et al[36]	II	MEDI-528	IL-9	27/9	Mild	Symptomatic improvement
Bryan et al[37]	II	Recombinant IL-12	IL-12	19/20	Mild	Reduced AHR, unfavorable adverse effect profile

AHR, Airway hyperresponsiveness; *AQLQ*, Asthma Quality of Life Questionnaire; *FEV_1*, forced expiratory volume in 1 second; *IL*, interleukin; *PEFR*, peak expiratory flow rate; *TNF*, tumor necrosis factor.
*Phase II/III only.

as well as regulating the expansion and apoptosis of activated T cells. IL-2 signals through a receptor complex consisting of IL-2–specific IL-2 receptor α (IL-2Rα) (i.e., CD25), IL-2R receptor β (IL-2Rβ), and a common γ chain (γc), which is shared by all members of this family of cytokines. The α chain of the IL-2 receptor is necessary only for high-affinity binding of the ligand and is not known to contain a signaling domain, whereas the β and γ chains are involved in transmitting the signals for IL-2–dependent cellular responses.[38] The γ_c family cytokines all signal through the JAK-STAT (Janus kinase–signal transducer and activator of transcription) pathway. IL-2, IL-7, IL-9, and IL-15 mainly activate STAT5 proteins, whereas IL-4 generally activates STAT6 and IL-21 mainly activates STAT3. This specificity may explain the differential cytokine actions. Activation of IL-2R on natural killer T (NKT) cells leads to the induction of phosphatidylinositol 3-kinase (PI3K), triggers phosphorylation of STAT3 through STAT6 and leads to the production of IFN-γ and IL-4. Phosphorylated forms of STAT3 and STAT5 can then dimerize, translocate to the nucleus, and bind DNA in the promoter region of STAT-regulated genes. Glucocorticoids exert their antiinflammatory effects by inhibiting the expression of IL-2R and JAK and also reduce STAT5 phosphorylation, thereby effectively stopping signaling, because STAT5 is unable to act on the nucleus without transcription.[39]

Among the numerous inflammatory cells present in the airways of asthmatic patients, activated lymphocytes specifically expressing IL-2R infiltrate the subepithelial tissue. Bronchoalveolar lavage (BAL) fluid obtained from patients during recovery from an exacerbation of asthma showed the presence of soluble products of T cell activation in the bronchial tree.[40] Other studies similarly showed increased levels of IL-2 and soluble IL-2R α chain in airways of patients with severe asthma.

Systemic administration of IL-2 is associated with increased AHR in murine models and an infiltration and increase in numbers of lymphocytes, eosinophils, and neutrophils in bronchial mucosa in humans. IL-2 also has direct chemoattractant activity for eosinophils, in addition to induction of IL-5 production by activated lymphocytes.

Administration of a $CD4^+$ blocking antibody to patients with asthma reduced IL-2 ($CD25^-$) lymphocytes in peripheral blood but had no significant effect on airway function assessed by the peak expiratory flow.[41] Daclizumab is a humanized monoclonal antibody that binds specifically to the CD25 subunit of the high-affinity receptor IL-2R and inhibits IL-2 binding and its biologic activity. In asthma, treatment with daclizumab was associated with a significant reduction in the mean peripheral blood eosinophil count and the serum eosinophil cationic protein level but produced no improvement in clinical outcome. A multicenter randomized, double-blind, placebo-controlled, parallel-group study in 116 patients with suboptimally controlled moderate to severe asthma failed to reach its primary end point of improved forced expiratory volume in 1 second (FEV_1). Patients in the treatment group showed an improvement in both frequency of exacerbations and time to severe exacerbation and a decrease in symptoms and rescue medication use, but only after several months of treatment. Of note, however, a number of serious adverse effects could be attributed to daclizumab, including anaphylactoid reaction, varicella-zoster meningitis, and breast cancer. The results overall do not favor further use of daclizumab in this group of patients.[42]

Interleukin-4 and Interleukin-13

IL-4 and IL-13 are the "Th2 defining" cytokines and arguably are the most important cytokines in asthma pathogenesis. Owing to structural homogeneity, their actions are broadly similar, and they are therefore considered together.

IL-4 and IL-13 are characterized by a shared receptor system—the IL-4-Rα subunit, which is a component of the heterodimeric complex common to both their cognate receptors. The IL-4 type I receptor is bound exclusively by IL-4, whereas the IL-4 type II receptor is bound by both IL-4 and IL-13; this leads to differing kinetics of signaling. In addition, the IL-13 type II receptor is exclusively bound by IL-13. The IL-4 type I receptor (IL-4Rα binds IL-4) interaction activates JAK3. IL-4 type II receptor (IL-4Rα, IL-13Rα binds IL-4/IL-13) activates tyrosine kinase 2 (TYK2) and JAK2.[43] JAKs mediate IL-4R phosphorylation, which activates STAT-6 signaling. IL-4R, under certain conditions, may even enhance IL-13 responses, and this may be relevant to the soluble IL-4 receptor's ultimate lack of efficacy in clinical trials. A negative regulatory system exists for the IL-13 pathway in form of the IL-13 decoy receptor with an IL-13Rα2 subunit, and the expression is upregulated in cells with heightened responses to IL-13.[43]

Several studies showing increased Th2 cytokine or messenger RNA (mRNA) production compared with that in normal subjects.[9,10] A bronchoscopic study in patients with moderate to severe asthma revealed that these cells also are composed to a large extent of NKT cells, which express the invariant variable region T cell receptor α chain 14–joining region 18 (V(α)14-J(α)18), which selectively recognizes the glycolipid α-galactosylceramide (α-GalCer) presented to the T cell receptor by the antigen-presenting molecule CD1d. This is a newly described subgroup of T cells with immunoregulatory function, as opposed to conventional lymphocytes.[44] The study found remarkably large numbers of NKT cells in asthmatic airways and lungs—up to 100 times the peripheral blood levels. (NKT cells constitute less than 1% of $CD4^+$ cells and less than 0.1% of mononuclear cells in peripheral blood.) This finding suggests that a subgroup of NKT cells are recruited and migrate to the lungs. IL-4 and IL-13 are thought to be key in influencing this recruitment, owing to their expression by conventional $CD4^+$ lymphocytes. Elevated IL-13 levels are similarly seen in asthmatic airways and the airway smooth muscle, and mast cells are a source of IL-4 and IL-13 as well. Some caution is required in interpretation of these findings, however, because much of the data supporting a major role for NKT cells in asthma come from mouse studies, and the bronchoscopic findings on NKT cells have not been replicated in several other studies.[45]

Most of the features of classic allergic asthma—AHR, mucin secretion, and goblet cell hyperplasia—are mediated by the activation of the STAT6 pathway. STAT6 induces the Th2 lineage in Th0 cells, is responsible for the actions of IL-4 and IL-13 and regulates chemokine production from airway smooth muscle, fibroblasts, and epithelial cells. Murine models have demonstrated the accumulation of inflammatory cells—lymphocytes, eosinophils, and neutrophils—when transgenic mice lungs expressed IL-4. AHR may be indirectly induced by activation of eosinophils and other cells, which may then act on resident airway cells to produce AHR. IL-13 itself induces AHR with eosinophilia and mucus hypersecretion; this action is independent of IL-4 actions, and neutralization with antibodies prevents these developments. Human studies also have strongly implicated a role for IL-13 in severe asthma.[14] IL-13 influences the induction of features in keeping with chronic asthma, including remodeling, airway smooth muscle hyperplasia, and subepithelial fibrosis.

Antibody therapy for IL-4/IL-13 is in advanced development, with a large number of preclinical, phase I and II trials planned or currently ongoing. The soluble, recombinant human IL-4 receptor altrakincept consists of the extracellular portion of human IL-4Rα and is nonimmunogenic. A small trial of nebulized inhaled altrakincept for 12 weeks in patients with mild to moderate asthma indicated efficacy by allowing withdrawal from treatment with inhaled corticosteroids without relapse[46]; this result was subsequently confirmed in a larger trial.[47] A phase III trial, however, failed to confirm the effectiveness of altrakincept for the treatment of asthma, although concerns were raised over the bioavailability of altrakincept in this study.

Further phase II studies are in progress using humanized IL-4–specific and IL-4Rα-blocking antibodies such as pascolizumab (SB240, 683).[48] A placebo-controlled allergen challenge study showed that an IL-4 variant, pitrakinra, administered subcutaneously or nebulized can inhibit the binding of IL-4 and IL-13 to the α-subunit of the IL-4 receptor. Pitrakinra reduced the allergen-induced late phase response and the need for rescue medication in asthmatic patients.[28] AMG-317 is a fully human monoclonal antibody to IL-4Rα that blocks both IL-4 and IL-13 pathways and was administered to mainly healthy adults and a smaller number of asthmatic adults; earlier studies established bioavailability and safety. More recently, a phase II, randomized, double-blind, placebo-controlled study of AMG-317 in 147 patients with moderate to severe asthma[27] showed a reduction in the number of exacerbations and improvement in time to exacerbation in the treatment arm. However, the study failed to meet its primary end point of improvement in ACQ.

Nevertheless, the biologic agent was well tolerated, supporting the potential for future anti–IL-4 studies.

Initial trials on animal models led to phase I and II trials of anti–IL-13 therapy. CAT-354 is a humanized IgG4 anti–IL-13 monoclonal antibody, and a phase I trial in 23 asthmatics demonstrated a good safety profile.[49] IMA-638 and IMA-026 are fully humanized IgG1 antibodies that bind to different epitopes and neutralize IL-13 bioactivity, and two double-blind, randomized, placebo-controlled, parallel-group trials were conducted in 56 patients with mild asthma.[29] The primary outcome variable was the late phase asthma reaction, and secondary outcomes were fall in FEV_1, early phase reaction, and allergen-induced shift in AHR, and sputum eosinophil count. Treatment with IMA-026 did not attenuate the asthmatic responses at day 14 or day 35. Neither antibody had an effect on allergen-induced AHR or sputum eosinophils. Some subtleties exist in the way these two monoclonal antibodies interact with IL-13. IMA-638 permits interaction of IL-13 with IL-13Rα1 or IL-13Rα2 but inhibits recruitment of IL-4Rα to the IL-13/IL-13$R\alpha_1$ complex, whereas IMA-026 competes with IL-13 interaction with IL-13$R\alpha_1$ and IL-13$R\alpha_2$.[50] The potency and efficiency of IMA-638 in effectively depleting IL-13 indicates that cell surface IL-13$R\alpha_2$ acts as an important scavenger for removal of this cytokine, with implications for the future design of IL-13 inhibitors.

Tralokinumab (CAT-354) is another anti–IL-13 antibody, and in a dose-ranging phase II study, improvement in lung function was observed in the patients on the highest dose, which was correlated with the baseline sputum IL-13 concentration[31] (Fig. 93-2). The most compelling data are with lebrikizumab.[30] A placebo-controlled trial in 219 adults with asthma showed that 12 weeks of treatment increased the FEV_1 by 5.5%. The effects were particularly evident in the subgroup with a Th2 pattern of airway inflammation as reflected by a plasma periostin levels above the median or a raised exhaled nitric oxide (eNO) concentration (Fig. 93-3). A trend for reduction in asthma exacerbations was noted, but the study was not of long-enough duration and was inadequately powered to show an effect on this outcome. Of interest, no effect on asthma symptoms was seen. Studies of both lebrikizumab and tralokinumab failed to show an effect on limiting the number of exacerbations.

Interleukin-5

IL-5 is a homodimeric glycoprotein that is produced by Th2 cells after stimulation with antigens or with allergens, and by mast cells on stimulation with allergen-IgE complex. Clusters of Th2-type cytokine genes, for IL-3, IL-4, and GM-CSF, including those encoding IL-5, have been identified on the long arm of human chromosome 5 (5q). As might be expected, significant structural similarity with the aforementioned cytokines has been confirmed. IL-5 has a two-domain configuration requiring the participation of two chains in each domain. The IL-5 receptor structure is shared by IL-2, IL-7, and GM-CSF and consists of two subunits: the high-affinity but functionally redundant α chain and a lower-affinity β chain, which induces functional activity. Receptor-ligand interaction results in activation of JAK2 by phosphorylation and via tyrosine kinase phosphorylation causes STAT1α and STAT5 activation. The phosphorylated STAT complex translocates to the cell nucleus, where it activates specific genomic sequences of DNA.

IL-5 modulates eosinophil progenitor production, maturation, activation, and survival in blood and can induce airway eosinophilia. IL-4, IL-5, IL-9, and IL-13, together with eotaxin, play critical roles in orchestrating and amplifying allergic inflammation in asthma. Available evidence indicates that the

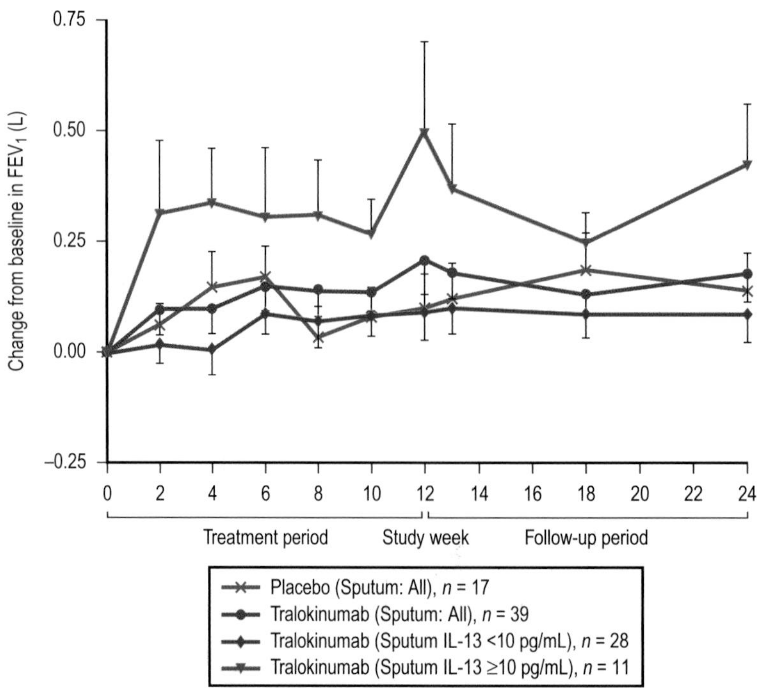

Figure 93-2 The improvement in lung function in response to anti–IL-13 (tralokinumab) was greater in those subjects with than in those without measurable sputum IL-13. Mean (SEM) change from baseline in prebronchodilator FEV_1 over time. *FEV_1*, Forced expiratory volume in 1 second; *IL-13*, interleukin-13. *(Reproduced with permission from Piper E, Brightling C, Niven R, et al. A phase II placebo-controlled study of tralokinumab in moderate-to-severe asthma. Eur Respir J 2013;41:330-8.)*

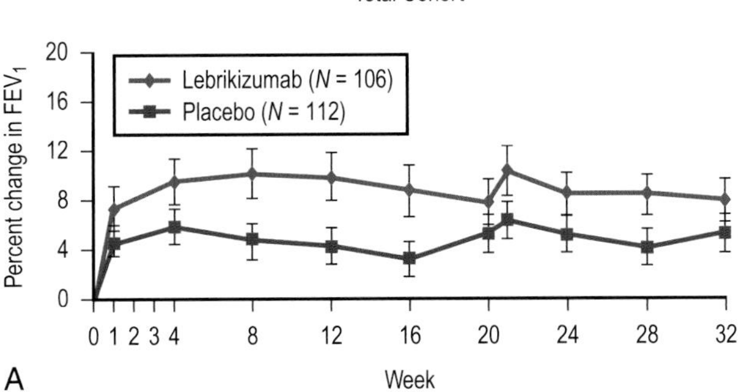

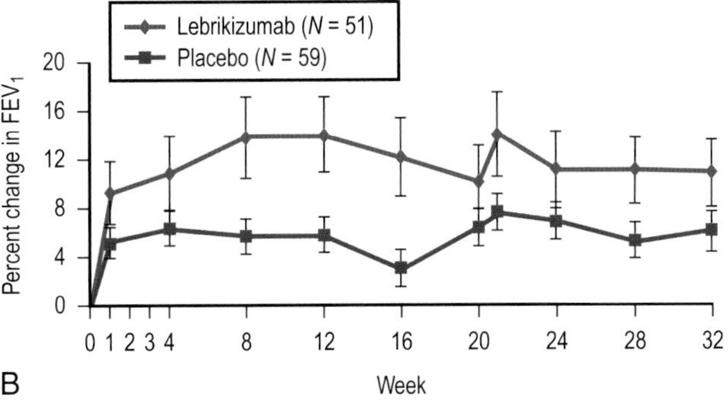

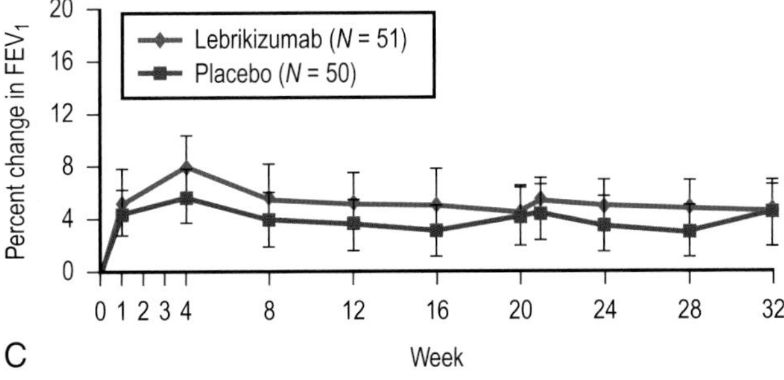

Figure 93-3 The improvement in lung function in response to anti-IL-13 (lebrikizumab) was greater in patients with than in those without high serum periostin. **A,** At week 12, the increase from baseline in FEV_1 was higher by 5.5 percentage points (95% CI, 0.8 to 10.2) in the lebrikizumab group than in the placebo group (mean [± SE] change, 9.8 ± 1.9% versus 4.3 ± 1.5%; $P = .02$). **B,** In the subgroup of patients with high periostin levels, the relative increase from baseline FEV_1 was higher by 8.2 percentage points (95% CI, 1.0 to 15.4) in the lebrikizumab group than in the placebo group (mean change, 14.0 ± 3.1% versus 5.8 ± 2.1%; $P = .03$). **C,** Among patients in the low-periostin subgroup, the relative increase from baseline FEV_1 was higher by 1.6 percentage points (95% CI, −4.5 to 7.7) in the lebrikizumab group than in the placebo group (mean change, 5.1 ± 2.4% versus 3.5 ± 2.1%; $P = .61$). *CI,* Confidence interval; *FEV_1,* forced expiratory volume in 1 second. *(Reproduced with permission from Corren J, Lemanske RF, Hanania NA, et al. Lebrikizumab treatment in adults with asthma. N Engl J Med 2011;365:1088-98.)*

eosinophil is important in cough, airway remodeling, and asthma exacerbations and is associated with worse lung function than in noneosinophilic asthma. The sputum eosinophil count has served as a useful tool to characterize asthma phenotypes, provide a biomarker for corticosteroid responsiveness, and normalize sputum eosinophilia, with consequent decreases in asthma exacerbations.[4] The major cellular sources of IL-5 are $CD4^+$ cells, mast cells, eosinophils, and basophils; more recently, invariant NKT (iNKT) cells and epithelial cells also have been discovered to be a source.

Animal models provide further insight into actions of IL-5 on AHR and its chemoattractant properties for eosinophils. Guinea pigs given inhaled recombinant IL-5 demonstrated eosinophilia and neutrophilic infiltration in BAL fluid; furthermore, on allergen challenge, sensitized animal models show AHR, which is reduced by administration of anti-IL-5 antibodies, with subsequent reduction in numbers of inflammatory cells. IL-5–deficient mice do not mount an eosinophilic response to allergic challenge, although their eosinophilia can be produced by other cytokine pathways that underpin the role of IL-5 in allergic asthma. In humans, BAL fluid and bronchial biopsy specimens from asthmatic patients show, among other mediators, increased levels of both IL-5 and mRNA, as compared with healthy volunteers. In asthmatic patients, immunostaining of bronchial mucosa after an allergen challenge showed a significant increase in both eosinophilia and IL-5 mRNA expression. A strong correlation also was found between the number of BAL fluid cells that expressed mRNA for interleukin-5, FEV_1, and bronchoconstrictor reactivity to methacholine.

Two humanized, human IL-5–specific monoclonal antibodies, Sch55700 (reslizumab CTx55700) and mepolizumab (SB-240563), and an IL-5R–specific antibody-dependent cell, cytotoxic monoclonal antibody (MEDI-563), have been developed for the treatment of asthma. In a small double-blind trial, mepolizumab resulted in a rapid dose-dependent reduction in the number of circulating and sputum eosinophils, but surprisingly, this had no effect on either the late asthmatic response or AHR.[51] A further study using mepolizumab confirmed the persistent suppression of eosinophilia in blood, bone marrow, and BAL fluid, but in airway biopsy specimens, only a 55% reduction in the number of tissue eosinophils was observed.[52] In a group of patients with severe persistent asthma, treatment with Sch-55,700 resulted in a decrease in the number of blood eosinophils, but over the course of 10 weeks it had no effect on symptoms or physiological outcomes.[53] This observation has been confirmed in a dose-ranging trial of mepolizumab in patients with severe asthma.[54] Of interest, in this study, a trend toward reduced risk of moderate to severe exacerbations, by approximately 50%, was noted in the high-dose mepolizumab arm. The study was not sufficiently powered, however, to show a difference in exacerbations.

Most recently, 61 subjects with eosinophilic refractory asthma were enrolled in a randomized, double-blind, placebo-controlled study of mepolizumab for 1 year.[22] The study differed significantly from earlier studies in that the primary outcome measure was the number of severe exacerbations per subject, and the treated population had prior evidence of a sputum eosinophilia. The study showed significant reductions in severe asthma exacerbations (2.0 mepolizumab versus 3.4 placebo) and reductions in both blood and sputum eosinophilia (Fig. 93-4). In common with previous studies, mepolizumab has no significant effect on AHR, lung function, or symptoms but did significantly reduce eosinophilic inflammation. Mepolizumab also has been shown to allow safe prednisolone withdrawal in patients with severe eosinophilic asthma[23] (Fig. 93-5). In addition to its role in asthma exacerbations, anti-IL-5 therapy also may attenuate airway remodeling, because airway wall area and immunostaining for tenascin, lumican,

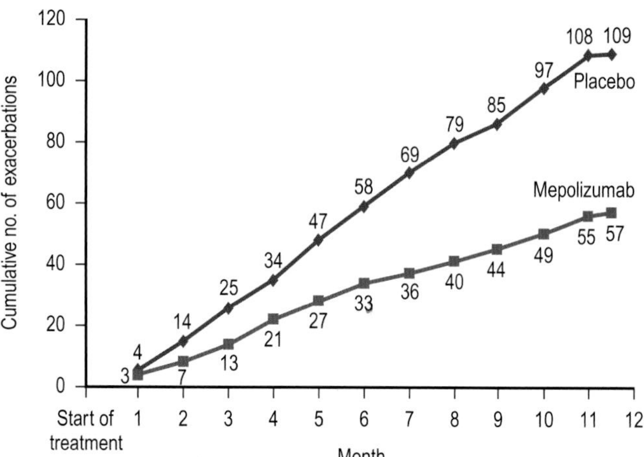

Figure 93-4 Mepolizumab therapy led to a marked reduction in severe exacerbations in patients with severe asthmatic associated with eosinophilic inflammation. The cumulative number of severe exacerbations that occurred in each study group over the course of 50 weeks is shown. The mean number of exacerbations per subject over the course of the 50-week treatment period was 2.0 in the mepolizumab group, as compared with 3.4 in the placebo group (relative risk, 0.57; 95% confidence interval, 0.32 to 0.92; $P = .02$).

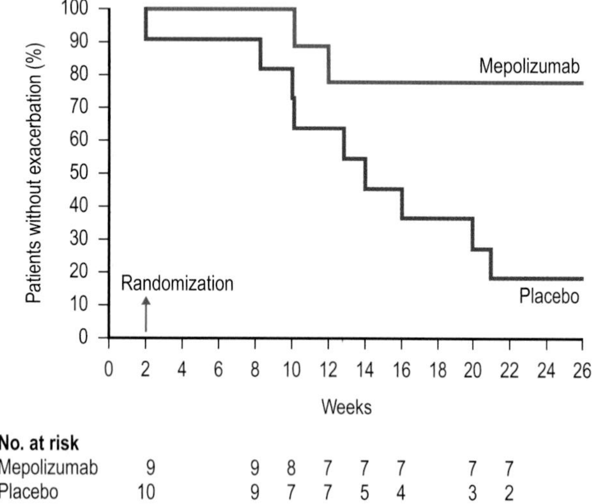

Figure 93-5 Mepolizumab therapy allowed for successful oral corticosteroid withdrawal in prednisone-dependent patients with asthma compared with placebo. The median time to exacerbation was 20 weeks in the mepolizumab group and 12 weeks in the placebo group ($P = .003$). Two asthma-related events occurred in the mepolizumab group: One patient who was withdrawn from the study because of a protocol violation had an exacerbation associated with sputum neutrophilia, and one patient was withdrawn after an adverse event; no exacerbations associated with sputum eosinophilia were reported in this group. In the placebo group, nine patients were withdrawn: Eight had exacerbations associated with sputum eosinophilia, and one patient who was withdrawn because of a protocol violation also had an exacerbation associated with sputum eosinophilia. *(Reproduced with permission from Nair P, Pizzichini MM, Kjarsgaard M, et al. Mepolizumab for prednisone-dependent asthma with sputum eosinophilia. N Engl J Med 2009;360:985-93.)*

and procollagen III in the bronchial mucosal subepithelial basal lamina was reduced.[54] Moreover, preliminary evidence showed a reduction in airway wall thickening as assessed by computed tomography (CT) after 12 months of treatment with mepolizumab.[22]

In a randomized, controlled trial in patients with eosinophilic asthma that was poorly controlled by high-dose inhaled corticosteroids, those receiving reslizumab showed significantly greater reductions in sputum eosinophils, improvement in lung function, and a trend toward greater asthma control than those in the placebo group; this benefit was especially apparent in patients with concomitant polyposis.[26] In a separate trial in patients with severe nasal polyposis, the clinical response to reslizumab was proportional to the levels of IL-5 detected in nasal lavage fluid. Both diseases are characterized by mucosal eosinophilia, and a recent small trial[54a] with mepolizumab also revealed efficacy in severe nasal polyposis.

These more recent studies have rekindled enthusiasm for anti–IL-5 in asthma and suggest that although eosinophilic inflammation and AHR are dissociated, the eosinophil does play a role in exacerbations and airway remodeling. To date, the side effect profile of anti–IL-5 has been favorable, and further studies are under way to determine the efficacy of this agent in severe asthma. Benralizumab (MEDI-563) is an anti-IL-5R humanized monoclonal antibody undergoing phase II trials in asthma, as is mepolizumab.[54b]

Interleukin-9

This Th2 cytokine drives allergic responses and has multiple effects. Interleukin-9 (IL-9) is a member of the γ chain receptor cytokine family, with other members being IL-2, IL-4, IL-7, IL-15, and IL-21. The IL-9 receptor consists of the cytokine-specific IL-9 receptor α chain (IL-9Rα) and the γ chain 1. IL-9–induced receptor activation promotes the cross-phosphorylation of Janus kinase 1 (JAK1) and JAK3. This cross-phosphorylation leads to the downstream activation of STAT1 to STAT3 and STAT5 heterodimers.[55]

IL-9 is derived from $CD4^+$ (Th9) cells, eosinophils, and mast cells. It causes T cell proliferation, increases IgE production by B cells, and increases expression of the α-subunit of IgE receptors. It uniquely promotes airway mastocytosis and mast cell progenitor development and localization to the airway. Expression of IL-9 in murine lungs increases the IgE level and causes airway inflammation, mucus hypersecretion, goblet cell hyperplasia, and epithelial cell activation, with increased AHR. Increased levels of both IL-9 and its receptor are seen in allergic asthma. IL-9 induces both IL-5 and IL-13 secretion by non–T cells and is dependent on the presence of IL-13 as a direct mediator to exert its effects. IL-9 modulates the expression of IL-5Rα in myeloid precursor cell lines and may further induce airway eosinophilia through the upregulation of IL-5 response and by enhancing IL-5–mediated maturation of eosinophil precursors. IL-9 can induce mast cell expression of several cytokines, including IL-1β, IL-5, IL-6, IL-9, IL-10, and IL-13. The IL-9–induced pathophysiologic changes described earlier can be prevented by a blocking monoclonal antibody in a mouse model; administration of intravenous anti-IL-9 antibody attenuated pulmonary eosinophilic inflammation, Th2 cytokine production (IL-4, IL-5, IL-13), and cell-specific chemokine production assayed in BAL fluid. Less information is available from human studies of IL-9. In one report, atopic asthmatics exhibited evidence of increased lymphocytes expressing IL-9 in BAL fluid.[56] Another bronchoscopy study showed that biopsied bronchial tissue from patients with atopic asthma contains an elevated number of IL-9 mRNA-positive cells in the airway compared with that in normal control subjects.

Two phase I dose-escalation studies of a humanized IL-9–specific monoclonal antibody MEDI-528 in healthy volunteers have been completed, with some hint of efficacy against the asthma-associated eosinophilia. Phase IIb trials (NCT00968669) are in progress for treating symptomatic, moderate to severe, persistent asthma.

Interleukin-12

IL-12, and also IL-23, are important for their actions in regulating the Th1/Th17 axis. Both cytokines are heterodimers sharing the IL-12 p40 ligand subunit; likewise, the IL-12 receptor IL-12Rβ chain is shared by both. Epithelial cells, dendritic cells, Langerhans cells, and mast cells are the major sources. IL-12, in conjunction with IL-18, mediates its actions partly by stimulating production of IFN-γ and induces activation and proliferation of Th and NK cells.

IL-12 directs the differentiation of naïve T cells to Th1 cells in vitro and in vivo and shifting the immune response toward cell-mediated immunity. In animal models, administration of IL-12 during sensitization suppresses allergen-induced Th2 cell responses in favor of Th1 cell development and inhibits AHR and airway eosinophilia after antigen challenge. In asthma, the production of IL-12 by whole blood cells and its expression in airway biopsy specimens is impaired; IL-12 is implicated in genome-wide association studies in asthma. Injection of recombinant human IL-12 in patients with mild asthma decreased the number of circulating blood eosinophils after allergen challenge but was associated with serious side effects attributable to the drug, and no further studies to date are planned.[37]

Tumor Necrosis Factor-α and Its Role in Severe Asthma

A number of animal model and human studies have implicated TNF-α in airway diseases including asthma, chronic obstructive pulmonary disease (COPD), and interstitial lung disease. Rheumatoid arthritis and inflammatory bowel disease are other examples of chronic disease where TNF-α has a major part to play in their pathophysiology, and treatment with anti-TNF therapy by either neutralizing antibodies or receptor blockade leads to an improvement in many indices of disease activity.

TNF-α is produced as a biologically active 26-kDa monomeric membrane bound precursor protein which is subsequently cleaved by matrix metalloproteinase (MMP) TNF-α–converting enzyme TACE to yield the 17-kDa soluble TNF-α.[57] These proteins form biologically active homotrimers that act on receptors TNFR1 and TNFR2. These receptors differ in their expression, activation, and effects. TNFR1 is activated by soluble TNF-α and is present on a variety of cells, whereas TNFR2 is activated primarily by membrane-bound TNF-α and is found mainly in cells of the immune system. The biologic effects of this receptor-ligand interaction are mediated by both receptors; however, the results of TNFR1 activation are thought to be responsible for a majority of the biologic functions of the "TNF axis." With TNFR1, the receptor binding results in intracellular signaling without internalization of the TNF-TNFR complex, leading to phosphorylation of nuclear factor of kappa light chain polypeptide gene enhancer in B cells inhibitor alpha (IκBα) and activation of protein 1. This causes activation of nuclear factor-κB (NF-κB), which interacts with DNA chromatin structure to increase the transcription of proinflammatory genes coding for cytokines such as IL6, IL-8, IL-1β, and TNF itself.

In asthma, both TNF-α protein and mRNA levels are increased in airways. The administration of inhaled recombinant TNF-α in normal subjects led to the development of AHR.[15] AHR could be caused as a direct effect of TNF-α on airway smooth muscle or indirectly mediated by the autocrine upregulation of airway smooth muscle spasmogens such as the leukotrienes LTC_4 and LTD_4. TNF-α is a chemoattractant for neutrophils, causes an airway neutrophilia and eosinophilia, increases the cytotoxic effects of eosinophils on endothelial cells, and promotes T cell recruitment. Because TNF-α is produced by various components of the airway, the role of TNF-α extends further in causing myocyte proliferation, stimulation of fibroblast growth, and maturation into myofibroblasts by promoting transforming growth factor-β (TGF-β) expression. Thus TNF-α also may have an important role in airway remodeling and promoting glucocorticoid resistance.

The first discovery that TNF-α antagonism improved lung function was reported in a retrospective study of patients who had concomitant airways disease and rheumatoid arthritis and were receiving infliximab for the latter. A significant reduction in symptoms and improvement in lung function were reported in three patients, who were able to reduce their corticosteroid use while on treatment.

In one of the first phase I studies,[58] 26 patients with mild to moderate allergic asthma received either etanercept or placebo twice weekly for 2 weeks, followed by a bronchoscopic segmental allergen challenge. TNF-α antagonism did not attenuate pulmonary eosinophilia and was not associated with a change in AHR to methacholine.

Subsequent to this initial study, enthusiasm for anti–TNF-α as a strategy for the treatment of asthma was fueled by promising efficacy in a small open-label study of 17 patients with severe asthma assigned to 12 weeks of etanercept as add-on therapy. In this report, Howarth and associates[15] noted that etanercept resulted in a significant improvement in AHR, lung function, and asthma control. These findings led to a randomized, placebo-controlled crossover study of etanercept in 10 patients with severe asthma,[16] in which improvements in asthma-related health quality and spirometry, and a reduction in AHR in the treatment arm were seen. To evaluate a similar agent, infliximab, for management of moderately severe asthma, Erin and colleagues[59] undertook a double-blinded, placebo-controlled parallel-group design study: The patients given infliximab had no significant reduction in exacerbations as compared with placebo. Another trial of etanercept in patients with severe asthma showed attenuation of AHR and symptoms but no other clinically significant parameters.[60] In a larger study of etanercept in moderate to severe asthma, no benefit was observed in terms of symptoms or lung function, although the therapy was well tolerated without serious adverse events.[34]

The largest trial thus far of anti-TNF therapy was a randomized, double-blind, placebo-controlled study of golimumab in 309 patients with severe or refractory asthma.[32] Reported findings included a small improvement in asthma quality of life scores and FEV_1 and a trend toward reduced exacerbations and time to exacerbation, but the study failed to show any meaningful improvement overall. More important, the study was stopped prematurely because of an adverse safety profile for golimumab: Up to 30% of the patients treated with this agent experienced adverse effects, reported as severe infections including pneumonia and reactivation of TB, eight malignancies, and one death reported.

In a subgroup of patients who exhibited a large acute bronchodilator response at baseline, golimumab did appear to be effective. A biologic rationale exists to support a role for TNF-α in the asthma paradigm. If TNF-α antagonism has a future as a therapeutic agent for severe asthma, clinicians will need to confirm the possibility that subgroups of patients may be identified with demonstrable efficacy without significant adverse events. In the absence of such data, current evidence does not favor the risk-benefit ratio for anti-TNF-α in severe asthma.

Interferons

Interferons are a superfamily of structurally related cytokines with immunomodulatory and antiviral properties.[61] The type I family includes IFN-α, -β, -ω, -κ, -ε, and τ; the sole member of the type II family is IFN-γ. The type III family interferons consist of IFN-λ1, IFN-λ2, and IFN-λ3, also called IL-29, IL-28A, and IL-28B, respectively. The type I and III family interferons signal through a receptor IFNαR, whereas IFN-γ signals via IFNγR. The downstream effects of receptor-ligand interaction are broadly similar to the TYK/JAK-STAT pathway activation, but the effects on asthma aspects are markedly different.

The source of secretion is predominantly host barrier defense cells, epithelial cells, dendritic cells, and T and NK cells. Interferon receptors are expressed on most cells in the body. A recent finding is that type I interferon blocked Th2 cytokine secretion through the inhibition of GATA3 during Th2 development and in fully committed Th2 cells; in addition, IFN-γ also prevented IL-4 secretion from $CD8^+$ cells, thereby abrogating the Th2 response. IFN-γ is a pleiotropic cytokine that induces and modulates an array of immune responses, but most important, it is the principal Th1 effector cytokine, with a crucial role in Th1 differentiation. IFN-γ mainly inhibits eosinophils, which are a crucial cell type in the allergic Th2 model of asthma, as evidenced when targeted disruption of the IFNγR receptor gene resulted in a prolonged airway eosinophilia in response to allergen. In addition, IFN-γ can induce AHR. In human studies, nebulized IFN-γ also has reduced the number of eosinophils in the BAL fluid of asthmatic patients.

In two different studies of IFN-γ in humans, systemic administration of recombinant agent showed a suppression of $CD4^+$ Th2 cells but increased IL-10 expression in PBMCs. Clinically, it allowed for a reduction in prednisolone dose in severe corticosteroid-dependent asthma.[62,63] Asthmatic airways are deficient in interferon production and are therefore prone to rhinovirus-induced exacerbations, and external replacement of interferon may reduce the severity of the exacerbation.[64] Currently, a randomized, double-blind, controlled trial of nebulized recombinant INF-β (Synairgen SG005) administered early in the course of a virus-induced exacerbation of asthma is under way in the United Kingdom and Australia.

OTHER POTENTIAL CYTOKINE TARGETS IN EARLY DEVELOPMENT

Interleukin-17

The IL-17 family cytokines, IL-17A to IL-17F, are linked with several autoimmune diseases such as rheumatoid arthritis, inflammatory bowel disease, and multiple sclerosis; in particular, IL-17E and IL-17F are of interest in asthma because their expression is increased in the airways of asthmatic patients, and levels have been correlated with disease severity.[65] Animal models have demonstrated that IL-17 induces inflammatory Th2 cytokines such as IL-1, IL-6, IL-21, and TNF; chemokines CXCL1 and CXCL2; inflammatory cells (eosinophils and neutrophils); and AHR. The effects may be comediated with other cytokines, as demonstrated by IL-21R–deficient mice, in which most of the Th2-mediated responses of IL-17 were reduced. IL-17F inhibitors are being studied in preclinical trials for conditions other than asthma.

Interleukin-18

IL-18 is a proinflammatory cytokine related to the IL-1 family that induces IFN-γ in activated NK cells, Th1, and $CD8^+$ cytotoxic T cells and hence was formerly called IFN-γ–inducing factor. IL-18 is implicated in many chronic inflammatory diseases, including inflammatory bowel disease and toxic shock. The IL-18R related protein complex consists of an α chain (IL-1Rrp), responsible for extracellular binding of IL-18, and a nonbinding, signal-transducing β chain (AcPL). Both chains are required for functional IL-18 signaling. IL-18 is similar to IL-6 in its ability to induce both Th responses: The Th1 action is IL-12– and IFN-γ—dependent and reduces $CD4^+$ migration, whereas the Th2 response causes reduction of airway inflammation and AHR. In addition, it can act in a Th2 fashion by inducing IL-4 and IL-13 production in T cells, NK cells, NKT cells, mast cells, and basophils.

The sources of IL-18 are $CD4^+CD8^+$ cells, macrophages, and more recently, airway epithelium. In a murine model, IL-18, with IL-12, enhanced production of IFN-γ; furthermore, this combination caused a decrease in IgE levels, prevented inflammatory cell infiltration in BAL fluid, and attenuated AHR. The other aspect of IL-18 function is to induce Th2 responses, and controversy is ongoing regarding what polarizes one response or another, and whether genetic influences play a smaller or larger role. In other work in mice, intranasal administration of an antigen and IL-18 stimulated Th1 cells to induce severe airway inflammation through IFN-γ and IL-13. In the presence of IL-3, IL-18 caused IL-18Rα expressing basophils and mast cells to release large amounts of Th2 cytokines. In human studies, serum IL-18 levels were significantly elevated during an episode of acute asthma, compared with those in patients with stable asthma or healthy control subjects and also correlated inversely with peak expiratory flow and correlated directly with soluble IL-2R (sIL-2R).[66] Interest in the potential importance of IL-18 in severe asthma also has been fueled by emerging evidence from genome-wide association studies implicating IL-18R.[8]

Interleukin-33

IL-33 is a relatively new discovery in the past decade, with ubiquitous expression of both the cytokine and its receptor in multiple organs—of importance, by bronchial epithelial cells in the lung and by many cells of the epithelial-endothelial subtype, including dendritic cells and macrophages.[67] IL-33 signaling is shared, because the heterodimeric receptor complex is made up of IL-1RAP and ST2, with downstream effects mediated by the NF-κB pathway. IL-33 can polarize naïve Th cells toward a Th2 phenotype and can induce multiple other Th1 and Th2 cytokines, chemokines, and cells in a proinflammatory manner. In murine antigen sensitization models, administration of IL-33 induced eosinophilic airway inflammation, Th2 immune deviation, and cytokine production and caused increased IgE levels; these effects were neutralized with use of a blocking antibody against IL-33 or its receptor. IL-33 is associated with mucus overproduction and goblet cell hypertrophy in the lungs, and in human studies, bronchoscopic biopsy specimens from patients with severe asthma revealed increased IL-33 expression in airway smooth muscle.[68] IL-33 also has been implicated in severe asthma in genome-wide association studies.[8]

Thymic Stromal Lymphopoietin/OX40

TSLP is released from epithelial cells after allergen exposure and activates dendritic cells, which then secrete OX40 (CD134), a key molecule that interacts with the ligand OX40L[69] to trigger the Th2 cascade and cytokine production from mast cells. In human studies, TSLP expression in airway epithelial cells is increased and, of importance, correlates with disease severity. AMG-157 is a fully human monoclonal antibody that blocks the interaction of TSLP with its receptor TSLPR, and phase I study recruitment is currently under way for atopic dermatitis, which may be extended to cover asthma. Blockade of OX40-OX40L interactions, using a neutralizing antibody specific for OX40L, inhibited the production of Th2 cytokines and TNF-α and increased antiinflammatory IL-10 production. Although human studies are lacking, it remains of potential interest.

Chemokines

Chemokines represent a large family of 8- to 15-kDa chemotactic and proinflammatory proteins expressed by many immune and nonimmune cells. They are implicated in most aspects of asthma, including AHR, mast cell degranulation, and inflammatory cell recruitment and migration, and in severe asthma by regulating remodeling and airway smooth muscle hypertrophy, among other processes. CCR3 is a potential target in eosinophilic asthma because this chemokine receptor has proved to be involved in migration of eosinophils, and in fact anti-CCR3 antibody reduced pulmonary eosinophilia in a murine model. CXCL10/CXCR3 are implicated in mast cell degranulation and may be potential targets; CXCR2 is currently under study in phase IIb studies in COPD and has shown promise, in a single exploratory phase IIa study in patients with neutrophilic asthma,[70] for modulation of neutrophilic inflammation. Whether these approaches are valuable in severe disease remains to be tested.

Summary

Asthma is a complex heterogeneous condition. The cytokine networks in asthma demonstrate that several biologic processes can result in apparently similar or distinct clinical expression, presenting a dual challenge of identifying redundancies in the system and also determining which pathway is relevant in which patient. Of importance, lessons from current cytokine-specific therapy have highlighted the need not only to consider the patient's biologic phenotype and the appropriate outcome measure but also to carefully assess the risk versus benefit of novel therapies. Emerging work on multidimensional phenotyping underpinned by the development of novel biomarkers provides the clinician with an opportunity to develop patient-specific therapy. Whether this potential is realized or is beyond our grasp will become apparent in the forthcoming decade as we move toward the goal, shared by physicians and patients alike, of personalized health care.

REFERENCES

Introduction

1. Bousquet J, Mantzouranis E, Cruz AA, et al. Uniform definition of asthma severity, control, and exacerbations: document presented for the World Health Consultation on severe asthma. J Allergy Clin Immunol 2010;126:926-38.
2. Blakey JD, Wardlaw AJ. What is severe asthma? Clin Exp Allergy 2012;42:617-24.
3. Haldar P, Pavord ID, Shaw DE, et al. Cluster analysis and clinical asthma phenotypes. Am J Respir Crit Care Med 2008;178:218-24.
4. Green RH, Brightling CE, McKenna S, et al. Asthma exacerbations and sputum eosinophil counts: a randomised controlled trial. Lancet 2002;360:1715-21.
5. Walker S, Monteil M, Phelan K, Lasserson TJ, Walters EH. Anti-IgE for chronic asthma in adults and children. Cochrane Database Syst Rev 2006;(2):CD003559.

Cytokines

6. Wenzel SE, Balzar S, Ampleford E, et al. IL4R alpha mutations are associated with asthma exacerbations and mast cell/IgE expression. Am J Respir Crit Care Med 2007;175:570-6.
7. Chen W, Ericksen MB, Levin LS, Khurana Hershey GK. Functional effect of the R110Q IL-13 genetic variant alone and in combination with IL4RA genetic variants. J Allergy Clin Immunol 2004;114:553-60.
8. Moffatt MF, Gut IG, Demenais F, et al. A large-scale, consortium-based genomewide association study of asthma. N Engl J Med 2010;363:1211-21.
9. Brightling CE, Gupta S, Gonem S, Siddiqui S. Lung damage and airway remodelling in severe asthma. Clin Exp Allergy 2012;42:638-49.
10. Holgate ST. Innate and adaptive immune responses in asthma. Nat Med 2012;18:673-83.
11. Pepe C, Foley S, Shannon J, et al. Differences in airway remodelling between subjects with severe and moderate asthma. J Allergy Clin Immunol 2005;166:544-9.
12. Hammad H, Lambrecht BN. Recent progress in the biology of airway dendritic cells and implications for understanding the regulation of asthmatic inflammation. J Allergy Clin Immunol 2006;118:331-6.
13. Thomas S, Banerji A, Medoff BD, Lilly CM, Luster AD. Multiple chemokine receptors, including CCR6 and CXCR3, regulate antigen-induced T cell homing to the human asthmatic airway. J Immunol 2007;179:1901-12.
14. Saha S, Berry M, Parker D, et al. Increased sputum and bronchial biopsy IL-13 expression in severe asthma. J Allergy Clin Immunol 2008;121:685-91.
15. Howarth PH, Babu KS, Arshad HS, et al. Tumor necrosis factor alpha as a novel therapeutic target in symptomatic corticosteroid dependent asthma. Thorax 2005;60:1012-8.
16. Berry MA, Hargadon B, Shelley M, et al. Evidence of a role of tumor necrosis factor alpha in refractory asthma. N Engl J Med 2006;354:697-708.
17. Brightling CE, Bradding P, Symon FA, et al. Mast cell infiltration of airway smooth muscle in asthma. N Engl J Med 2002;346:1699-705.
18. Siddiqui S, Mistry V, Doe C. Airway hyperresponsiveness is dissociated from airway wall structural remodeling. J Allergy Clin Immunol 2008;122:335-41.
19. Woodman L, Siddiqui S, Cruse G, et al. Mast cells promote airway smooth muscle cell differentiation via autocrine upregulation of TGF-β. J Immunol 2008;181:5001-7.
20. Wenzel S. Severe asthma in adults. Am J Respir Crit Care Med 2005;172:149-60.
21. Benayoun L, Druilhe A, Dombret MC, Aubier M, Pretolani M. Airway structural alterations selectively associated with severe asthma. Am J Respir Crit Care Med 2003;167:1360-8.
22. Haldar P, Brightling CE, Hargadon B, et al. Meoplizumab and exacerbations of eosinophilic refractory asthma. N Engl J Med 2009;360:973-84.
23. Nair P, Pizzichini MM, Kjarsgaard M, et al. Mepolizumab for prednisone-dependent asthma with sputum eosinophilia. N Engl J Med 2009;360:985-93.
24. Flood-Page PT, Menzies-Gow AN, Kay AB, Robinson DS. Eosinophil's role remains uncertain as anti-interleukin-5 only partially depletes numbers in asthmatic airway. Am J Respir Crit Care Med 2003;167:199-204.
25. Flood-Page P, Swenson C, Faiferman I, et al. A study to evaluate safety and efficacy of mepolizumab in patients with moderate persistent asthma. Am J Respir Crit Care Med 2007;176:1062-71.
26. Castro M, Mathur S, Hargreave F, et al; Res-5-0010 Study Group. Reslizumab for poorly controlled, eosinophilic asthma: a randomized, placebo-controlled study. Am J Respir Crit Care Med 2011;184:1125-32.

27. Corren J, Busse W, Meltzer EO, et al. A randomized, controlled, phase 2 study of AMG 317, an IL-4Ralpha antagonist, in patients with asthma. Am J Respir Crit Care Med 2010;181: 788-96.
28. Wenzel S, Wilbraham D, Fuller R, Getz EB, Longphre M. Effect of an interleukin-4 variant on late phase asthmatic response to allergen challenge in asthmatic patients: results of two phase 2a studies. Lancet 2007;370:1422-31.
29. Gauvreau GM, Boulet LP, Cockcroft DW, et al. The effects of IL-13 blockade on allergen-induced airway responses in mild atopic asthma. Am J Respir Crit Care Med 2011;182:1007-14.
30. Corren J, Lemanske RF, Hanania NA, et al. Lebrikizumab treatment in adults with asthma. N Engl J Med 2011;365:1088-98.
31. Piper E, Brightling C, Niven R, et al. A phase II placebo-controlled study of tralokinumab in moderate-to-severe asthma. Eur Respir J 2013; 41:330-8.
32. Wenzel S, Barnes PJ, Bleecker ER, et al. A randomized, double-blind, placebo-controlled study of tumor necrosis factor-α blockade in severe persistent asthma. Am J Respir Crit Care Med 2009;179:549-58.
33. Morjaria JB, Chauhan AJ, Babu KS, et al. The role of a soluble TNFα receptor fusion protein (etanercept) in corticosteroid refractory asthma: a double blind, randomised, placebo controlled trial. Thorax 2008;63:584-91.
34. Holgate ST, Noonan M, Chanez P, et al. Efficacy and safety of etanercept in moderate-to-severe asthma: a randomized, controlled trial. Eur Respir J 2011;37:1352-9.
35. Busse WW, Israel E, Nelson HS, et al. Daclizumab improves asthma control in patients with moderate to severe persistent asthma. Am J Respir Crit Care Med 2008;178:1002-8.
36. Oh C, Parker J, Geba G, Molfino N. Safety profile and clinical activity of multiple subcutaneous doses of MEDI-528, a humanized anti interleukin-9 monoclonal antibody in subjects with asthma. Proceedings of the European Respiratory Congress, Barcelona, 2010;39s:377. NCT00968669.
37. Bryan SA, O'Connor BJ, Matti S, et al. Effects of recombinant human interleukin-12 on eosinophils, airway hyper-responsiveness, and the late asthmatic response. Lancet 2000;356: 2149-53.
38. Rochman Y, Spolski R, Leonard WJ. New insights into the regulation of T cells by gamma(c) family cytokines. Nat Rev Immunol 2009;9:480-90.
39. Bianchi M, Meng C, Ivashkiv LB. Inhibition of IL-2-induced Jak-STAT signaling by glucocorticoids. Proc Natl Acad Sci U S A 2000;97: 9573-8.
40. Park CS, Lee SM, Uh ST, et al. Soluble interleukin 2 receptor and cellular profiles in bronchial lavage fluid from patients with bronchial asthma. J Allergy Clin Immunol 1993;91: 623-33.
41. Kon OM, Sihra BS, Compton CH, et al. Randomised, dose-ranging, placebo-controlled study of chimeric antibody to CD4 (keliximab) in chronic severe asthma. Lancet 1998;352: 1109-13.
42. Busse WW, Israel E, Nelson HS, et al; Daclizumab Asthma Study Group. Daclizumab improves asthma control in patients with moderate to severe persistent asthma: a randomized, controlled trial. Am J Respir Crit Care Med 2008;178:1002-8.
43. Brightling CE, Saha S, Hollins F. Interleukin-13: prospects for new treatments. Clin Exp Allergy 2010;40:42-9.
44. Akbari O, Faul JL, Hoyte EG, et al. CD4+ invariant T-cell-receptor+ natural killer T cells in bronchial asthma. N Engl J Med 2006;354: 1117-29.
45. Vijayanand P, Seumois G, Pickard C, et al. Invariant natural killer T cells in asthma and chronic obstructive pulmonary disease. N Engl J Med 2007;356:1410-22.
46. Borish LC, Nelson HS, Lanz MJ, et al. Interleukin-4 receptor in moderate atopic asthma. A phase I/II randomized, placebo-controlled trial. Am J Respir Crit Care Med 1999;160:1816-23.
47. Borish LC, Nelson HS, Corren J, et al. Efficacy of soluble IL-4 receptor for the treatment of adults with asthma. J Allergy Clin Immunol 2001;107:963-70.
48. Hart TK, Blackburn MN, Brigham-Burke M, et al. Preclinical efficacy and safety of pascolizumab (SB240683): a humanised anti-interleukin-4 antibody with therapeutic potential in asthma. Clin Exp Immunol 2002; 130:93-100.
49. Singh D, Kane B, Molfino NA, et al. A phase 1 study evaluating the pharmacokinetics, safety and tolerability of repeat dosing with a human IL-13 antibody (CAT-354) in subjects with asthma. BMC Pulm Med 2010;10:3.
50. Kasaian MT, Raible D, Marquette K, et al. IL-13 antibodies influence IL-13 clearance in humans by modulating scavenger activity of IL-13Rα2. J Immunol 2011;187:561-9.
51. Leckie MJ, ten Brinke A, Khan J, et al. Effects of an interleukin-5 blocking monoclonal antibody on eosinophils, airway hyper-responsiveness, and the late asthmatic response. Lancet 2000; 356:2144-8.
52. Robinson D, Hamid Q, Bentley A, et al. Activation of CD4+ T cells, increased Th2-type cytokine mRNA expression and eosinophil recruitment in bronchoalveolar lavage after allergen inhalation challenge in patients with atopic asthma. J Allergy Clin Imunol 1993;92: 313-24.
53. Kips J, O'Connor BJ, Langley SJ, et al. Effect of SCH55700, a humanized anti-human interleukin-5 antibody, in severe persistent asthma: a pilot study. Am J Respir Crit Care Med 2003;167:1655-9.
54. Flood-Page P, Menzies-Gow A, Phipps S, et al. Anti-IL-5 treatment reduces deposition of ECM proteins in the bronchial subepithelial basement membrane of mild atopic asthmatics. J Clin Invest 2003;112:1029-36.
54a. Gevaert P, Van Bruaene N, Cattaert T, et al. Mepolizumab, a humanized anti-IL5 mAb, as a treatment for severe nasal polyposis. J Allergy Clin Immunol 2011;128:989-95.
54b. Pavord ID, Korn S, Howarth P, et al. Mepolizumab for severe eosinophilic asthma (DREAM): a multicentre, double-blind placebo-controlled trial. Lancet 2012;380(9842): 651-9.
55. Noelle RJ, Nowak EC. Cellular sources and immune functions of interleukin-9. Nat Rev Immunol 2010;10:683-92.
56. Erpenbeck VJ, Hohlfeld JM, Volkmann B, et al. Segmental allergen challenge in patients with atopic asthma leads to increased IL-9 expression in bronchoalveolar lavage fluid lymphocytes. J Allergy Clin Immunol 2003;111: 1319-27.
57. Brightling C, Berry M, Amrani Y. Targeting TNF-alpha: a novel approach for asthma. J Allergy Clin Immunol 2008;121:5-10.
58. Rouhani FN, Meitin CA, Kaler M, et al. Effect of tumor necrosis factor antagonism on allergen-mediated asthmatic airway inflammation. Respir Med 2005;99:1175-82.
59. Erin EM, Leaker BR, Nicholson GC, et al. The effects of a monoclonal antibody directed against tumor necrosis factor-alpha in asthma. Am J Respir Crit Care Med 2006;174:753-62.
60. Holgate ST, Noonan M, Chanez P, et al. Efficacy and safety of etanercept in moderate-to-severe asthma: a randomised, controlled trial. Eur Respir J 2011;37:1352-9.
61. Takaoka A, Yanai H. Interferon signalling network in innate defence. Cell Microbiol 2006;6:907-22.
62. Boguniewicz M, Martin RJ, Martin D, et al. The effects of nebulized recombinant interferon-gamma in asthmatic airways. J Allergy Clin Immunol 1995;95:133-5.
63. Kroegel C, Bergmann N, Foerster M, et al. Interferon-alphacon-1 treatment of three patients with severe glucocorticoid-depedent asthma. Effect on disease control and systemic glucocorticoid dose. Respiration 2006;73: 566-70.
64. Contoli M, Message SD, Laza-Stanca V, et al. Role of deficient type III interferon-lambda production in asthma exacerbations. Nat Med 2006;12:1023-6.6.
65. Park R, Lee Y. Interleukin-17 regulation: an attractive therapeutic approach for asthma. Respir Res 2010;11:78.
66. Tanaka H, Miyazaki N, Oashi K, et al. IL-18 might reflect disease activity in mild and moderate asthma exacerbation. J Allergy Clin Immunol 2001;107:331-6.
67. Smith D. IL-33: a tissue derived cytokine pathway involved in allergic inflammation and asthma. Clin Exp Allergy 2010;40:200-8.
68. Préfontaine D, Lajoie-Kadoch S, Foley S, et al. Increased expression of IL-33 in severe asthma: evidence of expression by airway smooth muscle cells. J Immunol 2009;183:5094-103.
69. Kaur D, Brightling C. OX40/OX40 ligand in T-cell regulation and asthma. Chest 2012;141: 494-9.

Chemokines

70. Nair P, Gaga M, Zervas E, et al. Safety and efficacy of a CXCR2 antagonist in patients with severe asthma and sputum neutrophils: a randomized, placebo-controlled clinical trial. Clin Exp Allergy 2012;42:1097-103.

94 Histamine and H_1 Antihistamines

F. ESTELLE R. SIMONS | CEZMI A. AKDIS

CONTENTS

SUMMARY OF IMPORTANT CONCEPTS

» Histamine plays an important role in immune modulation and allergic inflammation through at least four histamine receptors, with HR1 and HR3 playing a pivotal role in neurotransmission.

» All four known histamine receptors exist in active and inactive forms and have constitutive activity in the absence of histamine, the agonist.

» Through HR1, histamine increases antigen-presenting capacity and Th1 priming, enhances Th1 cell proliferation and interferon-γ production, and blocks humoral immunity.

» H_1 antihistamines are functionally classified as first (old) generation and second (new) generation. PET documentation of H_1 antihistamine penetration into the human brain provides a new standard by which central nervous system H_1-receptor occupancy can be related directly to effects on CNS function.

» First (old)–generation H_1 antihistamines in standard doses may cross the blood-brain barrier, interfere with neurotransmission in the CNS, and impair alertness, learning, memory, and multitasking, with or without sedation or other adverse effects. Overdose can cause toxicity and death, and these are no longer medications of choice for allergic diseases in community settings.

» Second (new)–generation H_1 antihistamines are used in allergic rhinitis, allergic conjunctivitis, and urticaria. In standard doses, these cross the blood-brain barrier minimally; do not impair alertness, learning, memory, or multitasking; and are associated with minimal sedation. Overdose does not cause toxicity or death.

Introduction

Histamine was isolated and characterized more than 100 years ago, and medications targeting its receptors have been in clinical use for 70 years[1-5] (Fig. 94-1). Histamine plays a major role in human health and disease, exerting diverse biologic effects through four types of receptors. Knowledge about histamine metabolism, receptors, signal transduction, physiologic and pathologic effects, and complex interrelationships and crosstalk continues to increase. Histamine can influence many functions of the cells in relationship with regulation of immune response and hematopoiesis, including macrophages, dendritic cells, T lymphocytes, B lymphocytes, and endothelial cells.[6-9] These cells express histamine receptors, and some also secrete histamine, which can induce chemotaxis of mast cells and eosinophils into tissue sites and affect their maturation, activation, polarization, and effector functions, leading to chronic inflammation.[10] Importantly, mast cells and basophils are not the only cellular sources of histamine. In addition to gastric enterochromaffin-like cells, platelets, and histaminergic neurons, some cells in the immune system that do not store histamine have high histamine decarboxylase activity and are capable of producing large amounts of histamine, which is secreted immediately after synthesis.[11,12] These cells include platelets, monocytes/macrophages, dendritic cells, neutrophils, and T and B cells.[13]

Molecular Basis of Histamine Action

Histamine (2-[4-imodazole]-ethylamine) was first identified as an autocoid having potent vasoactive properties. Its smooth muscle-stimulating and vasodepressor action was demonstrated in the first experiments by Dale and Laidlaw,[14] who also found that the effects of histamine mimicked those occurring during anaphylaxis. In 1927, histamine was isolated from liver and lung tissue, followed by several other tissues, demonstrating that it is a natural constituent of the body; thus the name "histamine" was given after the Greek word for tissue, *histos.* Histamine is a low-molecular-weight amine synthesized from L-histidine exclusively by histidine decarboxylase. Histamine is produced by various cells throughout the body, including central nervous system neurons, gastric mucosa parietal cells, mast cells, basophils, and lymphocytes[1,4,15-17] (Fig. 94-2).

Histamine is involved in the regulation of many physiologic functions, including cell proliferation and differentiation, hematopoiesis, embryonic development, regeneration, and wound healing.[15,18,19] Within the central nervous system, histamine affects cognition and memory, regulation of the sleep-wake cycle, energy, and endocrine homeostasis.[20] In human pathology, histamine triggers acute symptoms because of its rapid activity on vascular endothelium and bronchial and smooth muscle cells, leading to the development of such symptoms as acute rhinitis, bronchospasm, cramping, diarrhea, and cutaneous wheal and flare responses. In addition to these effects on the immediate-type response, histamine also significantly

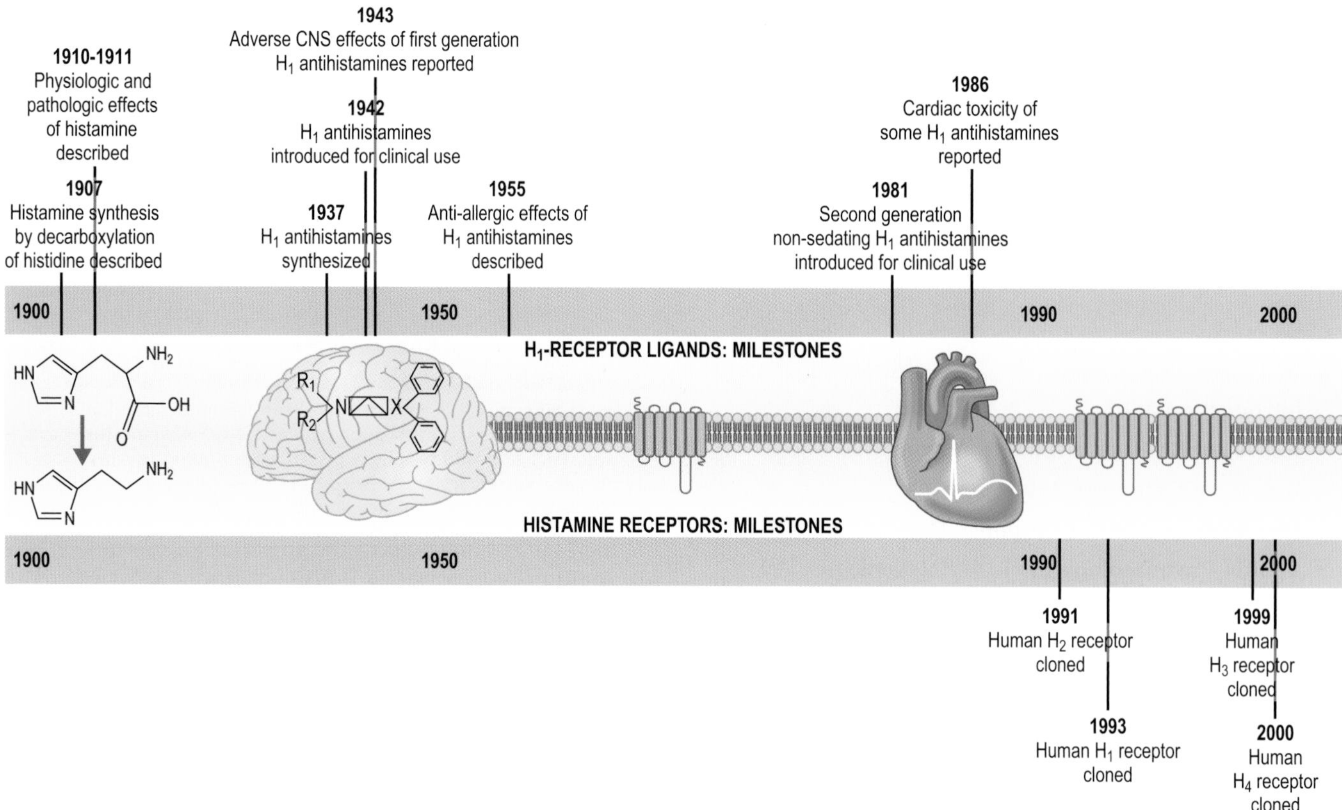

Figure 94-1 Timeline featuring historical highlights related to histamine, histamine receptors, and H_1 antihistamines. The physiologic and pathologic effects of histamine were described in 1910-1911.H_1 antihistamines were introduced for clinical use in the 1940s; for example, antergan (1942), diphenhydramine (1946), and chlorpheniramine (1949). In the 1980s, relatively nonsedating second (new)–generation H_1 antihistamines were introduced for clinical use, and histamine-containing neurons were identified in the central nervous system (*CNS*). Cloning and characterization of human histamine receptors were reported for the H_2 receptor in 1991, H_1 receptor in 1993, H_3 receptor in 1999, and H_4 receptor in 2000. *(From Simons FER, Simons KJ. Histamine and H_1-antihistamines: celebrating a century of progress; J Allergy Clin Immunol 2011;128:1139-50.)*

modulates chronic phase inflammatory events.[15-18] This chapter highlights the findings leading to a change of perspective in histamine immunobiology.

Histamine is synthesized by decarboxylation of histidine by L-histidine decarboxylase (HDC), which depends on the cofactor pyridoxal-5′-phosphate.[21] Histamine regulation is dependent on the gene of HDC enzyme, which is expressed in the cells throughout the body. The location of HDC gene is found on chromosome 2 in mice and chromosome 15 in humans, and expression is controlled by lineage-specific transcription factors. These factors interact with a promoter region consisting of a GC box, four GATA consensus sequences, a c-Myb–binding motif, and four CACC boxes.[22] Several studies have shown that the HDC transcription is regulated by various factors in gastric cancer cells (e.g., gastrin, oxidative stress, PMA) through a RAS-independent, RAF-dependent mechanism, mitogen-activated protein kinase (MAPK/ERK) and protein kinase C (PKC) pathways functioning on three overlapping cisacting gastrin response elements (GASRE 1, 2, and 3).[23] In hematopoietic cells the regulation of the HDC gene is unknown, and nuclear factor E2 (NF-E2) appears to be involved indirectly in this mechanism.[24] It is well known that the expression of HDC in basophils and mast cells results from the state of CpG methylation in the promoter region.[25] Mast cells and basophils are the major source of granule-stored histamine, where it is closely associated with the anionic proteoglycans and chondroitin-4-sulfate. Histamine is released when these cells degranulate in response to various immunologic and nonimmunologic stimuli. In addition, several myeloid and lymphoid cell types (e.g., dendritic, T cells) that do not store histamine show high HDC activity and are capable of production of high amounts of histamine.[12,26] HDC activity is modulated by cytokines, such as interleukin-1 (IL-1), IL-3, IL-12, IL-18, granulocyte-macrophage-colony-stimulating factor (GM-CSF, M-CSF, tumor necrosis factor-α (TNF-α), and calcium ionophore, in vitro.[27] HDC activity has been demonstrated in vivo in conditions such as lipopolysaccharide (LPS) stimulation, infection, inflammation, and graft rejection.[11] The generation of HDC-deficient mice provided histamine-free systems to study the role of endogenous histamine in a broad range of normal and disease processes. These mice show decreased numbers of mast cells and significantly reduced granule content, which suggests that histamine might affect the synthesis of mast cell granule proteins.[28] IgE binding to FcεRI on IL-3–dependent mouse bone marrow–derived mast cells induces the expression of HDC through a signaling pathway distinct from that during antigen-stimulated FcεRI activation.[29]

More than 97% of histamine is metabolized in two major pathways before excretion. Histamine *N*-methyltransferase metabolizes most of the histamine to *N*-methylhistamine, which is further metabolized to the primary urinary metabolite N-methyl-imidazole acetic acid by monoamine oxidase.

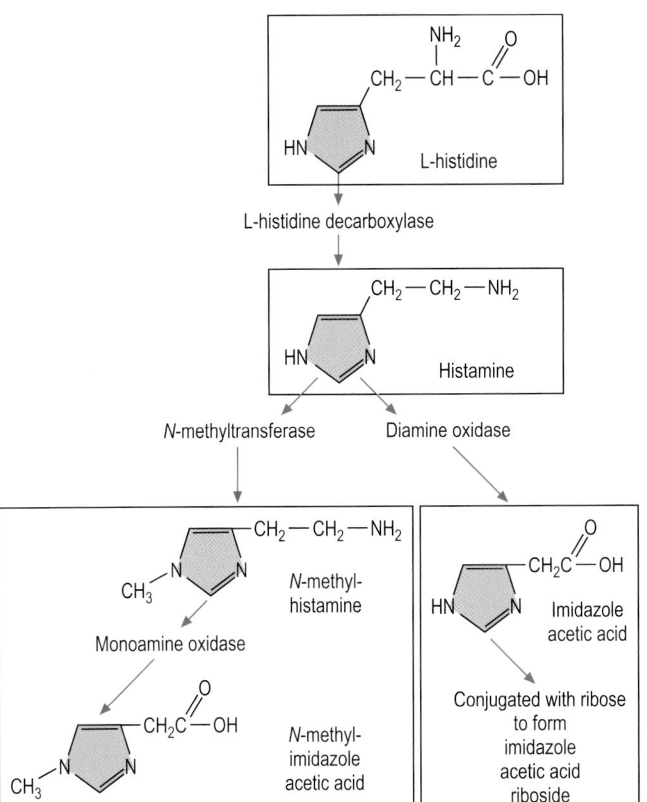

Figure 94-2 Synthesis and catabolism of histamine in humans. Histamine is a low-molecular-weight amine synthesized from L-histidine exclusively by histidine decarboxylase. Based on recovery of histamine and its metabolites in the urine during 12 hours after intradermal tests with ^{14}C histamine, 2% to 3% of histamine is excreted unchanged. Through the *N*-methyltransferase pathway in the central nervous system, small intestine mucosa, liver, and kidneys, 4% to 8% is eliminated as *N*-methylhistamine and 42% to 47% as *N*-methyl–imidazole acetic acid. Through the diamine oxidase (histaminase) pathway in the small intestine mucosa, liver, kidneys, placenta, skin, and such cells as eosinophils and neutrophils (but not in CNS), 9% to 11% is eliminated as imidazole acetic acid and 16% to 23% as imidazole acetic acid riboside.

Diamine oxidase metabolizes 15% to 30% of histamine to imidazole acetic acid. HDC is highly expressed in myeloid cells, but its function in these cells is poorly understood. Yang and associates[30] recently demonstrated that HDC-knockout mice show a high rate of colon and skin carcinogenesis, indicating key roles for HDC and histamine in myeloid cell differentiation and immature myeloid cells in early cancer development.

Histamine Receptors

The pleiotropic effects of histamine are triggered by activating one or several of histamine membrane receptors on different cells. Four subtypes of histamine receptor (HR) have been described: HR1, HR2, HR3, and HR4, or H1R to H4R (H_1 to H_4; Table 94-1).[1-3] In 1966, histamine receptors were first differentiated into HR1 and HR2.[31] In 1999 a third histamine receptor subtype was cloned and called HR3.[32] In 2000 the fourth histamine receptor subtype was named HR4.[33] All these receptors belong to the G protein–coupled receptor (GPCR) family. These heptahelical transmembrane molecules transduce extracellular signal by using G proteins and intracellular second-messenger systems.[33-35] The active and inactive states of HRs exist in equilibrium. However, it has been shown in recombinant systems that HRs can trigger downstream events in the absence of receptor occupancy by an agonist, which accounts for constitutive, spontaneous receptor activity.[36]

Histamine receptor agonists stimulate the active state in the receptor, and inverse agonists stimulate the inactive state. An agonist, with a preferential affinity for the receptor's active state, stabilizes the receptor in its active conformation, leading to continuous activation signal. An inverse agonist, with a preferential affinity for the receptor's inactive state, stabilizes the receptor in this conformation and consequently induces an inactive state, which is characterized by blocked signal transduction via the HR.[31] In reporter gene assays, constitutive HR1-mediated nuclear factor-κB (NF-κB) activation has been shown to be inhibited by many clinically used H_1 antihistamines, indicating that these agents are inverse HR1 agonists. Constitutive activity has now been shown for all four histamine receptors.[31] In addition to four membrane receptors, histamine binds to some intracellular receptors such as cytochrome P-450 (CYP) and cytochrome c, as well as high-affinity lipocalins isolated from saliva of ticks.[37] Specific activation or blockade of HRs showed that they differ in expression, signal transduction, or function and improved understanding of the role of histamine in physiology and disease mechanisms.

Histamine-releasing factor (HRF; also known as translationally controlled tumor protein [TCTP] and fortilin) has been implicated in late phase allergic reactions (LPRs) and chronic allergic inflammation.[38,39] Its overexpression in an inducible transgenic mouse model with HRF targeted to lung epithelial cells, via the Clara cells in antigen-naïve mice, yielded increases in bronchoalveolar lavage (BAL) macrophages and mRNA levels for MCP-1 in the HRF-transgenic mice compared to littermate controls. In the ovalbumin (OVA)–challenged model, HRF exacerbates the allergic, asthmatic response with increases in serum and BAL IgE, IL-4 protein, and eosinophils in transgenic mice compared to controls. Intranasally administered HRF recruits inflammatory immune cells to the lung in naïve mice in a mast cell– and Fc receptor–dependent manner. These results indicate that HRF has a proinflammatory role in asthma and skin immediate hypersensitivity that may be a therapeutic target.[38,39]

HISTAMINE RECEPTOR 1

The human $G_{q/11}$-coupled HR1 is encoded by a single exon gene located on the distal short arm of chromosome 3p25b and contains 487 amino acids. The HR1 is expressed in several cells, including airway and vascular smooth muscle cells, hepatocytes, chondrocytes, nerve cells, endothelial cells, dendritic cells, monocytes, neutrophils, T cells, and B cells.[40-42] Histamine binds to transmembrane domains 3 and 5. Activation of the HR1-coupled $G_{q/11}$ stimulates the inositol phospholipid signaling pathways, resulting in formation of inositol-1,4,5-triphosphate (IP_3) and diacylglycerol, and an increase in intracellular calcium,[43] which accounts for nitric oxide (NO) production and liberation of arachidonic acid from phospholipids. The H1R also activates phospholipase D and phospholipase A_2. HR1 has also been reported to activate the transcription factor NF-κB[44] through $G_{q/11}$ and $G_{\beta\gamma}$ on agonist binding. Constitutive activation of NF-κB occurs only through $G_{\beta\gamma}$.[43] H_1-receptor polymorphisms have been described, although it is not yet clear how

TABLE 94-1 Histamine Receptor Subtypes

Subtype	GPCR Signaling*	Expression	Representative Antihistamines	Clinical/Potential Use‡
H_1 (HR1)	G_q/G_{11} family to PLC stimulation	CNS neurons, smooth muscle cells (vascular, respiratory, GI), CVS, neutrophils, eosinophils, monocytes, macrophages, DCs, T and B cells, endothelial cells, epithelial cells	Chlorpheniramine, diphenhydramine, hydroxyzine, cetirizine, desloratadine, fexofenadine, levocetirizine, loratadine, and 40 others	Allergic rhinitis, allergic conjunctivitis, urticaria, and many other allergic and nonallergic diseases, including CNS diseases
H_2 (HR2)	G_s family to adenylate cyclase stimulation and increase in cAMP	Gastric parietal cells, smooth muscle, CNS, CVS, neutrophils, eosinophils, monocytes, macrophages, DCs, T and B cells, endothelial cells, epithelial cells	Cimetidine, ranitidine, famotidine, nizatadine	Peptic ulcer disease, gastroesophageal reflux disease
H_3 (HR3)	$G_{i/o}$ family to adenylate cyclase inhibition and decrease in cAMP	CNS and peripheral neurons,† CVS, lungs, monocytes, eosinophils, endothelial cells	No agents approved for use to date; those in clinical trials have included JNJ 39220675 and PF-03654746 for allergic rhinitis	Potentially useful in allergic rhinitis and neurologic disorders, including Alzheimer disease, attention-deficit hyperactivity disorder, schizophrenia, epilepsy, narcolepsy, and neuropathic pain; also in obesity
H_4 (HR4)	$G_{i/o}$ family to adenylate cyclase inhibition and decrease in cAMP	Neutrophils, eosinophils, monocytes, DCs, Langerhans cells, T cells, basophils, mast cells, fibroblasts, bone marrow, endocrine cells, CNS	No agents approved for use to date; those in clinical trials have included JNJ 7777120 for allergic rhinitis and pruritus and UR 65380 and UR 63825 for pruritus	Potentially useful in allergic rhinitis, atopic dermatitis, asthma, and in other chronic inflammatory and autoimmune disorders

cAMP, Cyclic adenosine monophosphate; *CNS,* central nervous system; *CREB,* cAMP response element–binding; *CVS,* cardiovascular system; *DAG,* 1,2-diacylglycerol; *DCs,* dendritic cells; *EPAC,* exchange protein directly activated by cAMP; *GI,* gastrointestinal; *GPCR,* G protein–coupled receptor; *IP_3,* inositol-1,4,5-triphosphate; *PIP2,* phosphatidylinositol-4,5-biphosphate; *PKA,* protein kinase A; *PKC,* protein kinase C; *PLC,* phospholipase C.

*The primary signaling mechanism is shown. Additional intracellular signals at the H_1 receptor include PLC, DAG, IP_3, PIP2, PKC, and intracellular calcium. Additional intracellular signals at the H_2 receptor include PKA, CREB, and EPAC. At the H_3 and H_4 receptors, stimulation of calcium mobilization from intracellular stores constitutes an important signal.

†The H_3 receptor is a presynaptic autoreceptor on histaminergic neurons in the CNS and on non-histamine-containing neurons in the CNS and peripheral nervous system. H_3 regulates levels of a variety of neurotransmitters,including norepinephrine, acetylcholine, serotonin, and dopamine.

‡Issues in the development of H_3 and H_4 antihistamines include nondisclosure of ligand structure, instability of some synthesized ligands, different outcomes in different species, and adverse events in some clinical trials. Nevertheless, H_3 and H_4 antihistamines should eventually prove effective and safe in the treatment of allergic disorders, not only in patients with allergic rhinitis, but also in those with atopic dermatitis/and asthma.

they influence the clinical response to H_1 antihistamines.[45] Activation of HR1 results in airway and vascular smooth muscle contraction. The contractile responses to HR1 stimulation initially involve mobilization of calcium (Ca^{2+}) from intracellular stores such as inositol phospholipids hydrolysis.[41] HR1 stimulation causes various cellular responses in vascular endothelial cells, including changes in vascular permeability as a result of cell contraction, synthesis of prostacyclin and platelet-activating factor, release of von Willebrand factor, and in NO release.[15,46]

Thus HR1 mediates many pathologic processes, including allergenic rhinitis, atopic dermatitis, conjunctivitis, urticaria, asthma, and anaphylaxis.[3,47] The receptors also mediate bronchoconstriction and enhanced vascular permeability in the lung.[40,46] Targeted disruption of the HR1 gene in mice impairs neurologic functions such as memory, learning, locomotion, and nociception, and in aggressive behavior. Immunologic abnormalities have also been described in HR1-deleted mice, with impairment of both T and B cell responses.[8,48] Potential mechanisms of HR1 antagonists for a general immune suppressive effect were tested in mice infected with *Listeria monocytogenes* and in a human trial.[49] Clemastine and desloratadine strongly reduced innate responses to *L. monocytogenes* in mice comparable to dexamethasone. The immune suppression, characterized by inhibition of the MAPK-extracellular signal–regulated signaling pathway, led to an overall impaired innate immunity with reduced TNF-α and IL-6 production. In addition, one intravenous dose of clemastine reduced the TNF-α secretion potential of peripheral blood macrophages and monocytes in a double-blind placebo-controlled (DBPC) clinical trial.[49] This inhibition could be exploited to find applications in the treatment of inflammatory diseases.

HISTAMINE RECEPTOR 2

In humans the intronless gene encoding HR2 is located on chromosome 5. The human HR2 is a protein of 359 amino acids coupled to both adenylate cyclase and phosphoinositide second-messenger systems by separate guanosine triphosphate (GTP)–dependent mechanisms, including $G_{\alpha s}$. Similar to that demonstrated for HR1, histamine binds to transmembrane (TM) domains 3 (aspartate) and TM 5 (threonine and aspartate). The short third intracellular loop and the long C-terminal tail are features of the HR2 subtype.[50] Similar to HR1, HR2 is expressed in various cell types. Studies in different species and several human cells demonstrated that inhibition of characteristic features of the cells by primarily cyclic adenosine monophosphate (cAMP) formation dominates in HR2-dependent effects of histamine. Receptor binding stimulates activation of FOS (formerly c-Fos), JUN (c-Jun), protein kinase C (PKC), and p70S6 kinase.[15,41] These cAMP-independent effects might depend on the level of receptor expression or subtle differences between clonal cell lines. Effects of H_2 receptors can inhibit a variety of functions within the immune system. H_2 receptors negatively regulate the release of histamine on basophils and mast cells.[51] The inhibition of antibody synthesis, T cell proliferation, cell-mediated cytolysis, and cytokine production are evidence of H_2 receptors on lymphocytes.[18] Rapid upregulation of HR2 has been reported within the first 6 hours of the buildup phase of venom immunotherapy (VIT).[52] HR2 strongly suppressed FcεRI-induced activation and mediator release of basophils, including histamine and sulfidoleukotrienes, as well as cytokine production in vitro. Data suggest that HR2-mediated basophil suppression might contribute to early protective mechanisms during the buildup phase of VIT.[52]

HISTAMINE RECEPTOR 3

Human HR3 is encoded by a gene that consists of four exons on chromosome 20 and has been cloned.[32] More than one HR3 subtype has been suggested.[53] HR3 has initially been identified in the central and peripheral nervous system as presynaptic receptors controlling the release of histamine and other neurotransmitters (dopamine, serotonin, noradrenaline, GABA, and acetylcholine). HR3 signal transduction involves $G_{i/o}$ of G proteins leading to inhibition of cAMP and accumulation of Ca^{2+} and activation of the MAPK pathway. R-α-methylhistamine and imetit are agonists, and thioperamide and clobenpropit are HR3 antagonists. HR3 is mainly involved in brain functions and mast cells, via H_3 receptors.[54] HR3 is involved in cognition, sleep-wake cylce, homeostatic regulation, and inflammation and is presynaptically located as an autoreceptor controlling the synthesis and release of histamine.[55] H_3-autoreceptor activation stimulates a negative feedback mechanism to reduce central histaminergic activity.[56] The control of mast cells by histamine acting on HR3 involves neuropeptide-containing nerves might be related to a local neuron–mast cell feedback loop controlling neurogenic inflammation.[54] Dysregulation of this feedback loop may lead to excessive inflammatory responses, suggesting a novel therapeutic approach by using H_3 agonists.

HISTAMINE RECEPTOR 4

Human HR4 is encoded by a gene containing three exons and separated by two large introns located in chromosome 18q11.2. HR4 has 37% to 43% homology to HR3 (58% in TM region). HR4 is functionally coupled to $G_{i/o}$, which inhibits cAMP formation as does HR3.[35] H_4 activation leads to an inhibition of adenylyl cyclase and downstream of cAMP-responsive elements (CREs) as well as activation of MAPK and phospholipase C with Ca^{2+} mobilization. HR4 shows high expression in bone marrow and peripheral blood hematopoietic cells (neutrophils, eosinophils, T cells) and moderate expression in spleen, thymus, lung, small intestine, colon, and heart.[35] Both basophils and mast cells express H_4 messenger RNA.[57] Related to high homology between the two receptors, presently available HR3 agonists and antagonists are also recognized by HR4.[42] However, clobenpropit, an H_3 antagonist, exerts agonistic activity on H_4. Relatively little is known about the biologic function of HR4. It seems to be involved in immune regulatory functions, including chemotaxis and cytokine secretion. Presumably, HR4 plays an important role in autoimmune disorders, allergic conditions, and nociceptive responses. Early results in animal models suggest that H_4 antagonists may be helpful in treating conditions in which H_1 antagonists are not clinically effective.[58] Selective H_4 antagonists (e.g., JNJ7777120) show a potential role in treatment of inflammation in humans.[58]

The H_1 antagonists doxepin, cinnarizine, and promethazine are reported to exhibit high affinity binding to the H_4 receptor.[59] HRs form dimers, and even oligomers, which allow cooperation between HRs and other GPCRs. The affinity of histamine binding to different histamine receptors varies significantly, with K_i values ranging from 5 to 10 nM for the H_3 and H_4 receptors to 2 to 10 μM for the H_1 and H_2 receptors. Thus the effects of histamine on receptor stimulation can be complex.

NONCONVENTIONAL BINDING SITES OF HISTAMINE

Histamine can affect cell function by binding to nonclassic binding sites that include cytochrome P-450 (CYP) and histamine transporters. Histamine's binding to CYP suggested a second messenger role for intracellular histamine via this binding site. This hypothesis was based mainly on a finding that N, N diethyl-2-(4-(phenylmethyl) phenoxyethanamine (DPPE), an arylalkylamine analog of tamoxifen, inhibits binding of histamine to CYP.[60] The effect of DPPE on histamine binding depends on activity of the CYP enzymes; CYP2E1 and CYP3A are upregulated in HDC-deficient mice.[61] Vesicular monoamine histamine transporter 2 (VMAT2) had been cloned from rat and human brain. The gene expression of VMAT2 can be modulated via cytokines, either positively (TGF-β) or negatively (IL-1 and TNF-α).[62] The bone marrow–derived mast cells from HDC-deleted mice are completely devoid of endogenous histamine but can take it up from histamine-supplemented medium and store it in their secretory granules.

Histamine in Immune Response Regulation

ANTIGEN-PRESENTING CELLS

The first step in allergen-specific immune response development is sensitization with stimulation and clonal expansion of specific T and B cells by allergens/antigens, autoantigens, superantigens, and infectious agents and production of specific antibodies[63,64] (Fig. 94-3).

Dendritic cells (DCs) are often located near various histamine sources, such as connective tissue mast cells, and are potent antigen-presenting cells (APCs) and cytokine-producing cells. Therefore histamine may effectively influence the immune response through DCs. These professional APCs mature from monocytic and lymphoid precursors and acquire DC1 and DC2 phenotypes, which in turn facilitate development of helper T type 1 (Th1) and type 2 (Th2) cells, respectively. Endogenous histamine is actively synthesized during cytokine-induced DC differentiation, which acts in autocrine and paracrine fashion

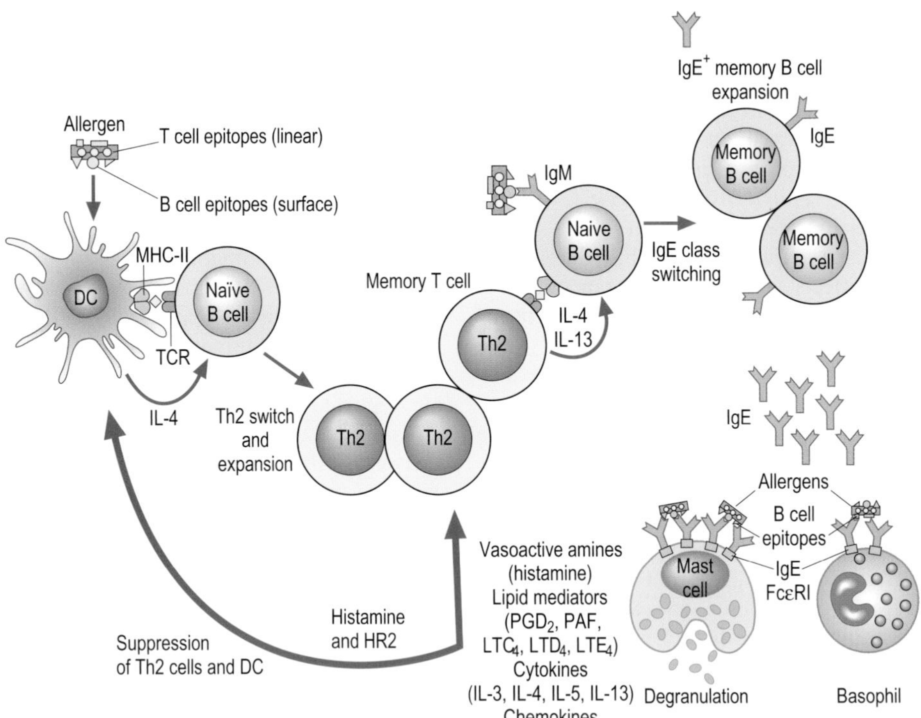

Figure 94-3 Immunologic events during the sensitization phase against allergens. After antigen presentation by dendritic cells (*DC*) in the presence of low-dose innate immune response–stimulating substances, Th2 cells develop from naïve T cells and show clonal expansion (*TCR*, T cell receptor). Th2 cell interaction with naïve B cells lead to immunoglobulin class switch to IgE and expansion of allergen-specific memory B cells. IgE produced by plasma cells sensitizes mast cells and basophils by binding to surface FcεRI. The cross-linking of mast cell and basophil surface FcεRI-bound IgE by B cell epitopes of allergens leads to the release of vasoactive amines (e.g., histamine), lipid mediators such as prostaglandin D_2 (*PGD_2*), platelet-activating factor (*PAF*), and leukotrienes LTC_4, LTD_4, and LTE_4, as well as cytokines and chemokines, and to immediate symptoms of allergic disease (type I hypersensitivity), including pruritus, wheal and flare, nasal conjunctival discharge, angioedema, systemic anaphylaxis, and bronchoconstriction. *(From Jutel M, Watanabe T, Adkis M, Blaser K, Adkis CA. Immune regulation by histamine. Curr Opin Immunol 2002;14:735-40.)*

and modifies DC markers.[26] Histamine actively participates in the function and activity of DC precursors as well as their immature and mature forms (see Fig. 94-3). Immature and mature DCs express all four HRs; however, their levels of expression has not yet been compared. In the differentiation process of DC1 from monocytes, HR1 and HR3 act as positive stimulants to increase antigen presentation capacity and proinflammatory cytokine production and Th1 priming activity. In contrast, HR2 acts as a suppressive molecule for antigen presentation capacity by enhancing IL-10 production and inducing IL-10–producing T cells or Th2 cells.

In monocytes stimulated with Toll-like receptor (TLR)–triggering bacterial products, histamine inhibits the production of proinflammatory IL-1-like activity, TNF-α, IL-12, and IL-18, but enhances IL-10 secretion through HR2 stimulation.[65,66] Histamine also downregulates CD14 expression via H_2 receptors on human monocytes. The inhibitory effect of histamine via H_2 receptor appears through the regulation of intercellular adhesion molecule 1 (ICAM-1) and B7.1 expression, leading to the reduction of innate immune response stimulated by LPS.[66]

Histamine induces intracellular Ca^{2+} flux, actin polymerization, and chemotaxis in immature DCs due to stimulation of HR1 and HR3 subtypes. Maturation of DCs results in loss of these responses. In maturing DCs, however, histamine, in a dose-dependent fashion, enhances intracellular cAMP levels and stimulates IL-10 secretion while inhibiting production of IL-12 via HR2.[67] Interestingly, although human monocyte-derived DCs have both histamine H_1 and H_2 receptors and can induce CD86 expression by histamine, human epidermal Langerhans cells express neither H_1 nor H_2 receptors.[68] Inflammatory DCs express a functionally active HR4, which on stimulation leads to downregulation of CCL2 and IL-12. This might have implications for the treatment of atopic dermatitis.[69]

T CELLS AND ANTIBODY ISOTYPES

Histamine has been shown to intervene in the Th1, Th2, regulatory T (Treg) cell balance and consequently antibody formation. Differential patterns of histamine receptor expression on Th1 and Th2 cells determine reciprocal T cell responses after histamine stimulation[7] (Fig. 94-4). Th1 cells show predominant, but not exclusive, expression of HR1, whereas Th2 cells show increased expression of HR2. Histamine enhances Th1-type responses by triggering the HR1, whereas both Th1- and Th2-type responses are negatively regulated by HR2 from activation of different biochemical intracellular signals.[7] In mice, deletion of HR1 results in suppression of interferon-γ (IFN-γ) and dominant secretion of Th2 cytokines (IL-4, IL-13). HR2-deleted mice show upregulation of both Th1 and Th2 cytokines. *Bphs*, a non–major histocompatibility complex–linked gene involved in the susceptibility to many autoimmune diseases, has been identified as HR1 gene in mice. HR1-deleted mice show delayed disease onset and decreased disease severity when immunized to develop experimental allergic encephalomyelitis.[70] Also, histamine stimulation induces IL-10 secretion through HR2.[71] Increased IL-10 production in both DCs and

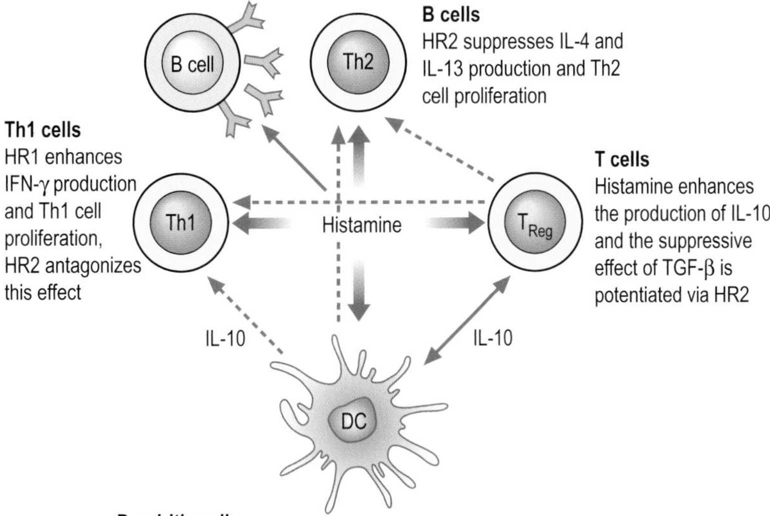

Figure 94-4 Regulation of the immune system through histamine receptors (HRs). In lymphatic organs and subepithelial tissues of allergic inflammation, histamine regulates monocytes, dendritic cells (DCs), T cells, and B cells. Monocytes and DCs express all known HRs. HR1 and HR3 induce proinflammatory activity and increased antigen-presenting cell (APC) capacity, whereas HR2 plays a suppressive role on monocytes and monocyte-derived DCs. Helper T type 1 (*Th1*) cells show predominant, but not exclusive, expression of HR1, whereas Th2 cells show upregulation of HR2. Histamine induces increased proliferation and interferon-γ (*IFN-γ*) production in Th1 cells. Th2 cells express predominant HR2, which acts as the negative regulator of proliferation, IL-4 and IL-13 production. Histamine enhances Th1-type responses by triggering the HR1, whereas both Th1- and Th2-type responses are negatively regulated by HR2, showing an essential role for immune regulation for this receptor. These distinct effects may suggest roles of HR1 and HR2 on T cells for autoimmunity and peripheral tolerance, respectively. Histamine also modulates antibody production. Histamine directly effects B cell antibody production as a costimulatory receptor on B cells. HR1 predominantly expressed on Th1 cells may block humoral immune responses by enhancing Th1-type cytokine IFN-γ. In contrast, HR2 enhances humoral immune responses. Allergen-specific IgE production is differentially regulated in HR1- and HR2-deficient mice. HR1-deleted mice show increased allergen-specific IgE production, whereas HR2-deleted mice show suppressed IgE production. *TGF*, Transforming growth factor. *(From Jutel M, Watanabe T, Adkis M, Blaser K, Adkis CA. Immune regulation by histamine. Curr Opin Immunol 2002;14:735-40.)*

T cells may account for an important regulatory mechanism in the control of inflammatory functions through histamine. Various cytokines regulate the production of histamine and its receptor expression. IL-3 and GM-CSF enhance histamine release from basophils, while stem cell factor (SCF) accomplishes this action for mast cells.[15] In addition, IL-3 stimulation significantly increases HR1 expression on Th1, but not on Th2 cells.[7]

In mice, histamine enhances anti-IgM–induced proliferation of B cells, which is abolished in HR1-deleted mice. In HR1-deleted mice, antibody production against a T cell–independent antigen, TNP-Ficoll, is decreased,[48] suggesting an important role of HR1 signaling in responses triggered from B cell receptors. Antibody responses to T cell–dependent antigens (e.g., OVA) show a different pattern.[48] HR1-deleted mice produced high OVA-specific IgG1 and IgE compared with wild-type mice. In contrast, HR2-deleted mice showed decreased serum levels of OVA-specific IgE compared with wild-type mice and HR1-deficient mice. Although T cells of H2R-deficient mice secreted increased IL-4 and IL-13, OVA-specific IgE was suppressed in the presence of highly increased IFN-γ. Thus HR1 and the related Th1 response may play a dominant role in the suppression of humoral immune response.

Peripheral T cell tolerance characterized by immune deviation to regulatory/suppressor T cells represents a key event in the control of specific immune responses during allergen-specific immunotherapy[72] (Fig. 94-5). Although, multiple suppressor factors, including contact dependent or independent mechanisms, might be involved, IL-10 and transforming growth factor β (TGF-β) predominantly produced by allergen-specific T cells play an essential role.[72,73] High-dose bee venom exposure in beekeepers by natural bee stings represents a model to understand mechanisms of T cell tolerance to allergens in healthy individuals. Continuous exposure of nonallergic beekeepers to high doses of bee venom antigens induces diminished T cell–related cutaneous late phase swelling to bee stings in parallel with suppressed allergen-specific T cell proliferation and Th1 and Th2 cytokine secretion.[74] After multiple bee stings, venom antigen-specific Th1 and Th2 cells show a clonal switch toward IL-10–secreting type 1 Treg (Tr1) cells. T cell regulation continues as long as antigen exposure persists and returns to initial levels within 2 to 3 months after bee stings stop. HR2, upregulated on specific Th2 cells, displays a dual effect by directly suppressing allergen-stimulated T cells and increasing IL-10 production. Thus, rapid clonal switch to and expansion of IL-10–producing Tr1 cells and the HR2-related effects represent

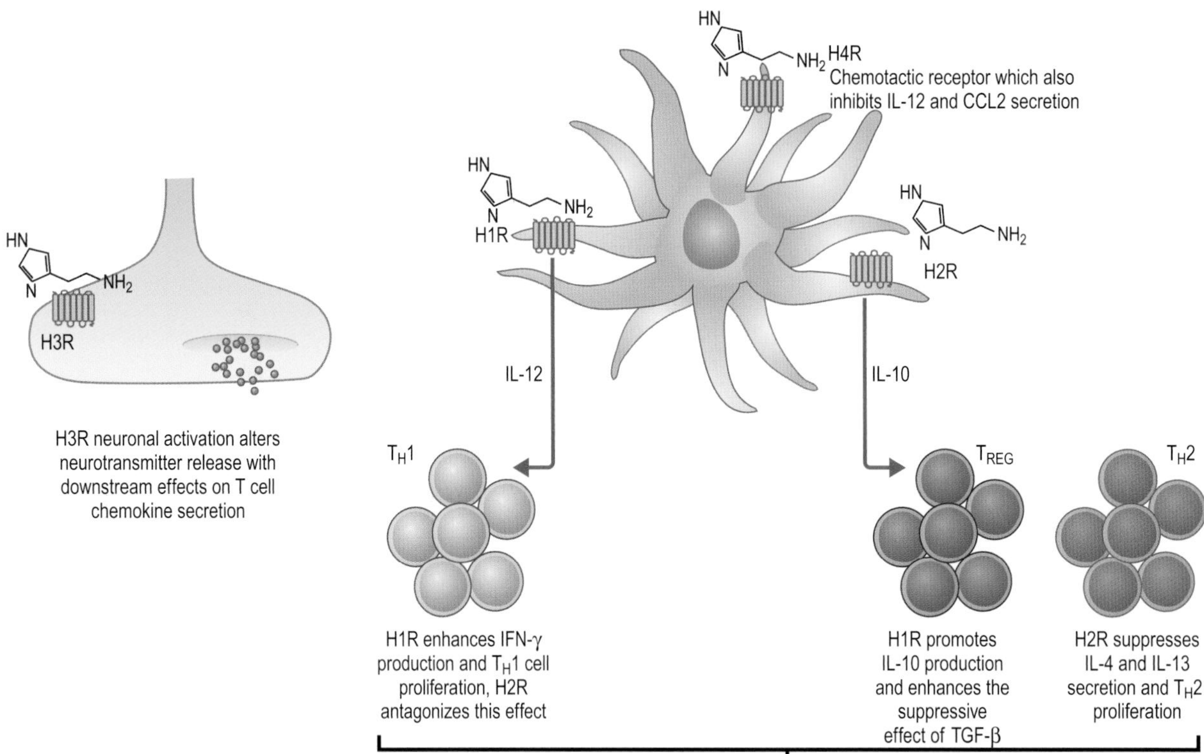

Figure 94-5 Induction and regulation of immune tolerance to allergens by histamine. Histamine released during allergen-specific immunotherapy plays a suppressive role on monocytes and monocyte-derived dendritic cells (DCs) through H2R (HR2). Th2 cells express predominantly HR2, which acts as the negative regulator of proliferation, and suppression of IL-4 and IL-13 production, suggesting a role for HR2 on T cells for peripheral tolerance. Histamine also modulates antibody production by directly effecting B cell antibody production as a costimulatory receptor on B cells and enhances humoral immune responses through HR2. *(From O'Mahony L, Akdis M, Akdis CA. Regulation of the immune response and inflammation by histamine and histamine receptors. J Allergy Clin Immunol 2011;128:1153-62.)*

essential mechanisms in immune tolerance to high dose of allergens in nonallergic individuals.[74] Apparently, histamine interferes with the peripheral tolerance induced during specific immunotherapy (SIT) in several pathways. Histamine induces the production of IL-10 by DCs.[67] In addition, histamine induces IL-10 production by Th2 cells.[71,74,75] Furthermore, histamine enhances the suppressive activity of TGF-β on T cells.[76] All three of these effects are mediated through HR2, which is relatively highly expressed on Th2 cells and suppresses IL-4 and IL-13 production and T cell proliferation. Apparently, these recent findings suggest that HR2 may represent an essential receptor that participates in peripheral tolerance or active suppression of inflammatory/immune responses. In the murine model, HR4 stimulation enriches for a Foxp3$^+$ Treg cell with potent suppressive activity for proliferation.[77]

A DBPC trial analyzed the long-term protection from honeybee stings by terfenadine premedication during rush immunotherapy with honeybee venom.[78] After an average 3 years of treatment, 41 patients were stung by a honeybee. Surprisingly, none of the 20 patients given HR_1 antihistamine premedication had a systemic allergic reaction to the reexposure by either a field sting or a sting challenge, whereas 6 of 21 given placebo did. This highly significant difference suggests that H_1 antihistamine premedication during the initial dose-increase phase may have enhanced the long-term efficacy of immunotherapy. Expression of HR1 on T lymphocytes is strongly reduced during ultrarush immunotherapy, which may lead to a dominant expression and function of tolerance-inducing HR2. This indicates a positive role of histamine in immune regulation during SIT.[79] In a recent DBPC prospective study, the effect of treatment with L-cetirizine during ultrarush venom immunotherapy was investigated. Patients treated with L-cetirizine produced significantly more IFN-γ. IL-10 production was induced in both groups but only significantly in L-cetirizine group. Decreased HR1/HR2 expression ratio, indicating H_2 signal dominance after 21 days, was observed in the placebo group.[80]

Selective H_2 antagonists have attracted interest because of their potential immune response–modifying activity.[81] Most data suggest that cimetidine has a stimulatory effect on the immune system, possibly by blocking the receptors on subsets of T lymphocytes and inhibiting HR2-induced immune suppression. Cimetidine has also been used successfully to restore immune functions in patients with malignant disorders, hypogammaglobulinemia, and AIDS-related complexes. On the other hand, H_2 agonists such as dimaprit significantly reduce disease severity in mice with experimental allergic encephalomyelitis.[82]

Clinical Pharmacology of H_1 Antihistamines

More than 45 H_1 antihistamines are available worldwide, representing the largest class of medications used in the treatment of allergic diseases. Since the previous edition of this textbook,[1] new H_1 antihistamines include bilastine and rupatadine for oral administration[83-86] and bepotastine and alcaftadine for ophthalmic application.[87-89] New clinically relevant information is available about the molecular basis of action, clinical pharmacology, efficacy, and safety of H_1 antihistamines in the treatment of allergic diseases.[2,83-89]

Histamine receptors are heptahelical transmembrane molecules that transduce extracellular signals by way of G proteins to intracellular second-messenger systems. These receptors have *constitutive activity,* defined as the ability to trigger downstream events, even in the absence of ligand binding. Their active and inactive states exist in equilibrium. At rest, the inactive state isomerizes with the active state, and vice versa[2,4,10,41] (Fig. 94-6).

The low H_1-receptor selectivity of first (old)–generation H_1 antihistamines has been attributed to direct interaction with tryptophan 428[6,48], a highly conserved key residue in GPCR activation. In contrast, second (new)–generation H_1 antihistamines interact with lysine 191[5,39], and/or lysine 179[ECL2], a residue in GPCR activation that confers high selectivity.[9] H_1-deleted mice have neurologic abnormalities, including aggressive behavior and impaired vigilance, learning, memory, and locomotion, in addition to immunologic and metabolic abnormalities.[48]

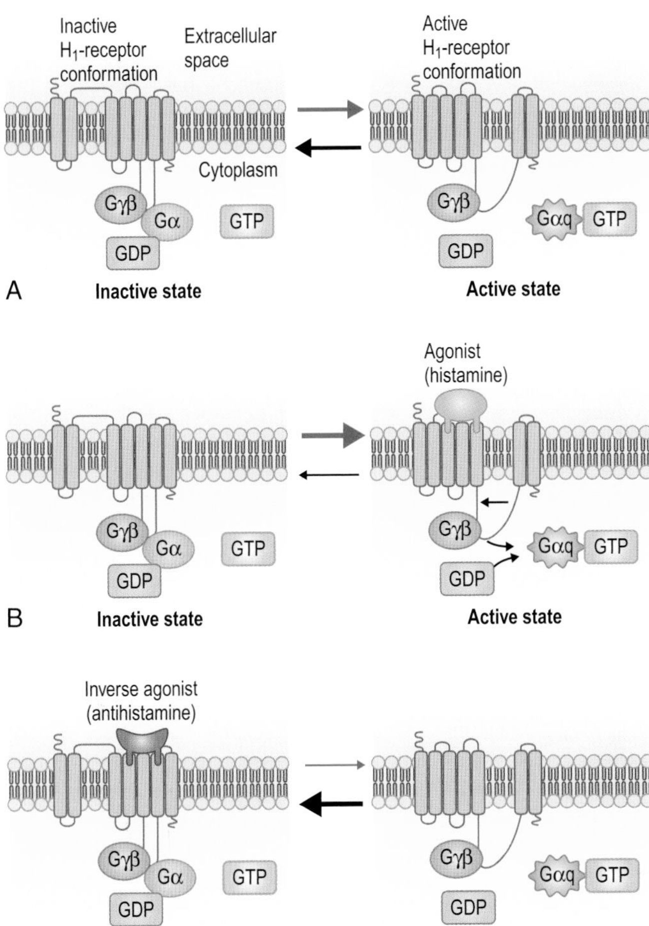

Figure 94-6 Molecular basis of action of histamine and antihistamines. **A,** The inactive state of histamine H_1 receptor is in equilibrium with the active state. **B,** The agonist, histamine, has preferential affinity for the active state, stabilizes the receptor in this conformation, and shifts the equilibrium toward the active state. **C,** An H_1 antihistamine (inverse agonist) has preferential affinity for the inactive state, stabilizes the receptor in this conformation, and shifts the equilibrium toward the inactive state. *GDP,* Guanosine diphosphate; *GTP,* guanosine triphosphate. *(From Simons FER, Simons KJ. Histamine and H_1 antihistamines: celebrating a century of progress; J Allergy Clin Immunol 2011;128:1139-50.)*

STRUCTURE AND CLASSIFCATION

The chemical structures of representative H_1 antihistamines are shown in Figure 94-7. The presence of multiple aromatic or heterocyclic rings and alkyl substituents in first (old)–generation H_1 antihistamines results in lipophilicity. Along with other properties, such as relatively low molecular weight, positive electrostatic charge, and for many of these H_1 antihistamines, *lack of recognition* by the P-glycoprotein efflux transporter enhances brain penetration.[1,90-92]

Historically, H_1 antihistamines have been categorized into six groups: ethanolamines, ethylene diamines, alkylamines, piperazines, piperidines, and phenothiazines (Table 94-2).[1-3] This traditional classification system now has limited clinical relevance, because H_1 antihistamines *within* each group (e.g., the large piperazine group) differ considerably in H_1 activity and adverse effects.[1]

First (old)–generation H_1 antihistamines have poor specificity for the H_1 receptor, as noted previously. To varying degrees, they inhibit transmission at muscarinic cholinergic receptors, α-adrenergic receptors, and 5-hydroxytryptamine (5-HT, serotonin) receptors. In high concentrations, diphenhydramine and dimethindene also have local anesthetic activity. In contrast, second (new)–generation H_1 antihistamines are highly specific for the H_1 receptor and have little or no affinity for muscarinic cholinergic, α-adrenergic, or serotonin receptors.[1,2,4]

PHARMACOKINETICS: CONCENTRATION VERSUS TIME

Using gas-liquid chromatography (GLC), high-performance liquid chromatography (HPLC), and HPLC with tandem mass spectrometry (MS/MS) assays and immunoassays, after usual doses, H_1 antihistamine concentrations can be detected in picogram to nanogram amounts in plasma, urine, and tissue, facilitating pharmacokinetic studies. After overdose, H_1 antihistamine concentrations can be detected in milligram amounts, facilitating forensic studies.[1,93-100]

Pharmacokinetic Studies

Pharmacokinetic studies provide clinically relevant information on bioavailability (rate and extent of H_1 antihistamine absorption), volume of distribution, protein binding, elimination half-life, clearance, and interactions with other drugs, foods, or herbal products. The pharmacokinetics of the first (old)–generation H_1 antihistamines have not been optimally investigated in healthy adults or in vulnerable patients, such as children, elderly persons, patients with hepatic or renal dysfunction, or in drug interaction studies (Table 94-3).[1,2] In contrast, the pharmacokinetics of all the second (new)–generation H_1 antihistamines have been studied in healthy young adults, with most also studied in children, elderly persons, patients with hepatic or renal impairment, and those concomitantly ingesting drugs, foods, or herbal products that potentially interfere with H_1 antihistamine elimination.[1,2,4,94-100]

After oral administration, H_1 antihistamines are typically well absorbed. Peak plasma concentrations are reached within 0.7 to 2.6 hours after administration to fasting individuals

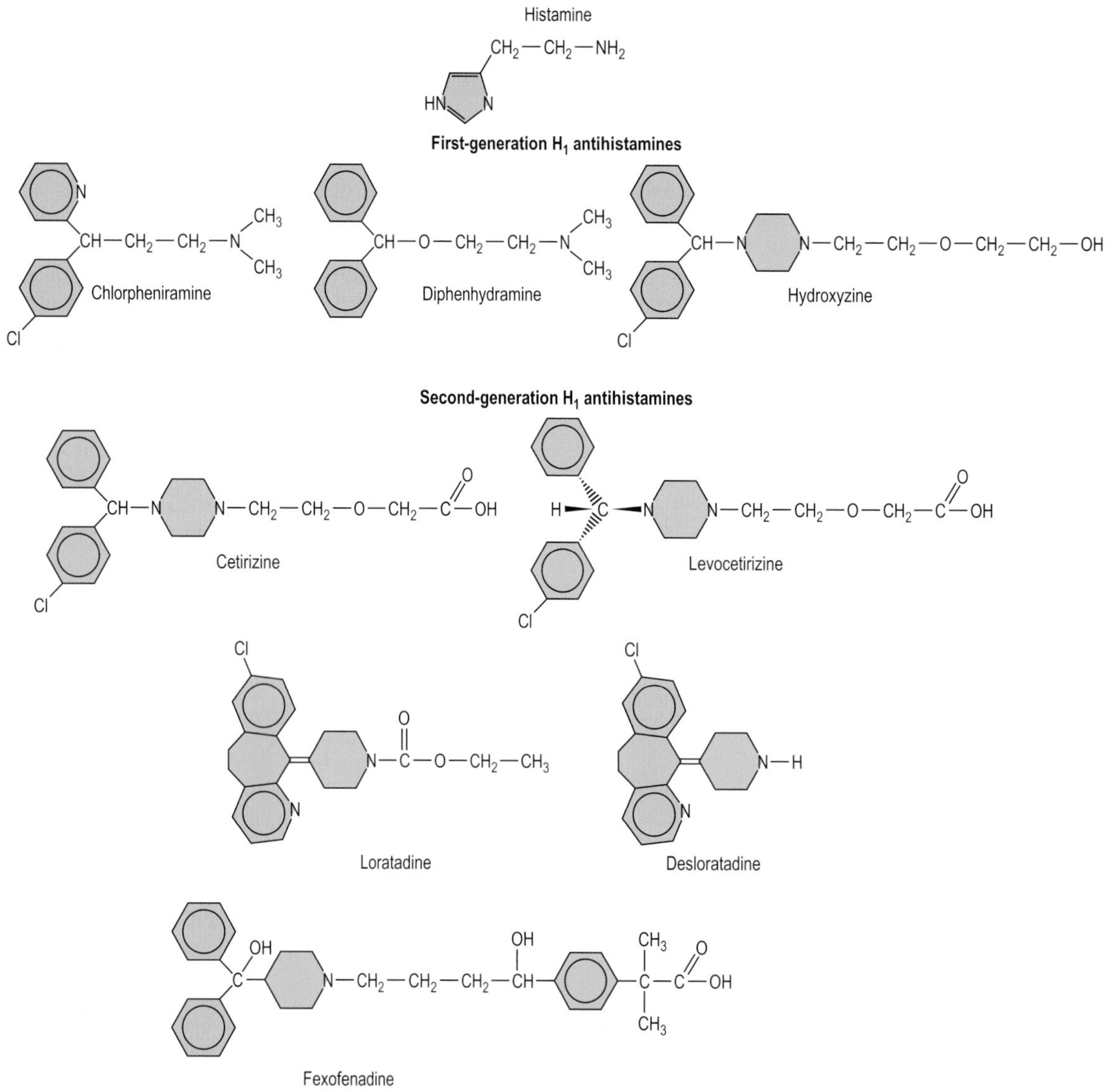

Histamine

First-generation H_1 antihistamines

Chlorpheniramine

Diphenhydramine

Hydroxyzine

Second-generation H_1 antihistamines

Cetirizine

Levocetirizine

Loratadine

Desloratadine

Fexofenadine

Figure 94-7 Chemical structures of representative H_1 antihistamines: first (old)-generation and second (new)-generation. Many H_1 antihistamines are structurally similar to each other; for example, cetirizine is a metabolite of hydroxyzine; levocetirizine is an enantiomer of cetirizine; desloratadine is a metabolite of loratadine; and fexofenadine is a metabolite of terfenadine (not shown; no longer approved for use or used in the United States and most other countries). Also, the availability of different H_1 antihistamines and different formulations of the same H_1 antihistamine varies from country to country; for example, azelastine, ketotifen, and olopatadine, available in topical, intranasal, and ophthalmic formulations in the United States, are also available in oral formulations in some countries.

(see Table 94-3). Bioavailability is influenced by several types of drug transporters, including ATP-binding cassette (ABC transporters) such as organic anion transport protein (OATP) and P-glycoprotein expression on the luminal surfaces of intestinal endothelial cells. Fexofenadine is a well-studied example of an H_1 antihistamine that is dependent on transport proteins for absorption and elimination. P-glycoprotein *inducers* such as grapefruit juice, rifampin, and St. John's wort have the potential to decrease fexofenadine absorption. P-glycoprotein *inhibitors* such as erythromycin and ketoconazole have the potential to increase fexofenadine absorption.[98,99] However, fexofenadine is a substrate of the P-glycoprotein efflux transporter in the blood-brain barrier, which prevents its penetration into the central nervous system and contributes to its favorable therapeutic index. Fexofenadine is also an organic acid that binds to aluminum/magnesium-containing antacids; therefore administration within 15 minutes of ingestion of these agents should be avoided to prevent a clinically relevant decrease in absorption.[94-100]

Pharmocokinetic values for H_1 antihistamine volume of distribution are proportionality factors between plasma concentrations and the dose administered, rather than actual volumes. These values vary from 0.33 L/kg for levocetirizine and 0.5 L/kg for cetirizine to more than 100 L/kg for loratadine. H_1 antihistamine plasma protein binding also varies considerably, from 60% for fexofenadine to more than 95% for cetirizine, levocetirizine, and desloratadine. Elimination half-life values range from 2 hours for acrivastine to 27 hours for desloratadine[94-100] (see Table 94-3).

Some second (new)–generation H_1 antihistamines are excreted largely unchanged in the urine and feces. For example, more than 50% of a cetirizine dose is eliminated unchanged

TABLE 94-2 H_1 Antihistamines: Chemical and Functional Classification

CHEMICAL CLASS	FUNCTIONAL CLASS	
	First (Old) Generation	Second (New) Generation
Alkylamines	Brompheniramine, chlorpheniramine, dexchlorpheniramine, dimethindene,† pheniramine, triprolidine*	Acrivastine*
Piperazines	Buclizine, cyclizine, hydroxyzine,* meclizine, oxatomide†	**Cetirizine,* levocetirizine***
Piperidines	Azatadine, cyproheptadine, diphenylpyraline, ketotifen	Astemizole,† bepotastine, bilastine,† **desloratadine,*** ebastine,† **fexofenadine,*** levocabastine, **loratadine,*** mizolastine,† rupatadine,*† terfenadine,*† alcaftadine
Ethanolamines	Carbinoxamine, clemastine, dimenhydrinate, diphenhydramine, doxylamine, phenyltoloxamine†	—
Ethylenediamines	Antazoline, pyrilamine, tripelennamine	—
Phenothiazines	Methdilazine, promethazine	—
Other	Doxepin‡	Azelastine, emedastine, epinastine, olopatadine

*Some of the H_1 antihistamines listed are related to each other; for example, acrivastine is a derivative of triprolidine; cetirizine is a metabolite of hydroxyzine; levocetirizine is an enantiomer of cetirizine; and desloratadine is a metabolite both of loratadine and rupatadine. Of the H_1 antihistamines currently approved for use in the United States, cetirizine, levocetirizine, desloratadine, fexofenadine, and loratadine are the most thoroughly investigated in randomized controlled trials and other prospective studies.
†In the United States, these H_1 antihistamines either are not yet approved or have never been approved. Regulatory approval was withdrawn for astemizole and terfenadine in the 1990s.
‡Doxepin is classified as both an H_1 antihistamine and a tricyclic antidepressant. It has potent H_1- and H_2-antihistaminic properties and inhibits reuptake of serotonin and norepinephrine.

in the urine, more than 85% of a levocetirizine dose is eliminated unchanged in the urine, and more than 80% of a fexofenadine dose is eliminated unchanged in the feces after biliary excretion[94-100] (see Table 94-3).

Phenotypic polymorphism has been observed in the metabolism of some H_1 antihistamines. Some individuals, for example, have decreased ability to form 3-hydroxy-desloratadine, the major metabolite of desloratadine, although the increased exposure to desloratadine in these poor metabolizers does not affect the safety and tolerability profiles of desloratadine.[96]

Drug–drug interaction studies are of practical clinical relevance for all of the first (old)–generation H_1 antihistamines as well as for second (new)–generation H_1 antihistamines such as desloratadine and loratadine, which are extensively metabolized in the hepatic CYP450 system. Metabolism of the first (old)–generation H_1 antihistamines is potentially decreased by CYP inhibitors such as erythromycin, azithromycin, and other macrolide antibiotics or ketoconazole and other imidazole antifungals. Plasma and tissue concentrations of unmetabolized H_1 antihistamines may increase and potentially lead to toxicity. Loratadine (as well as desloratadine and rupatadine) are also metabolized through the alternative CYP2D6 pathway, which greatly reduces potential increases in serum concentrations and potential toxicity. In vitro screening systems are now used to predict in vivo metabolic drug–drug interactions, and to prescreen H_1 antihistamine candidate drugs for future development.[1,95,99]

Population Pharmacokinetics

Population pharmacokinetic data can be obtained during phase II and III clinical trials of H_1 antihistamines involving large numbers of patients with allergic rhinitis or urticaria. In such studies, plasma antihistamine concentrations are measured in the intermittent blood samples taken for hematology and chemistry tests,[100] and the intervals between H_1 antihistamine dosing and blood samples are precisely documented. In these studies the influence on H_1 antihistamine pharmacokinetics from clinical and biologic covariates such as H_1 antihistamine dosage form, allergic disease, age, gender, ethnicity, and body mass can be examined. Theoretically, the influence of hepatic and renal function on pharmacokinetics and assessment of drug–drug interactions can also be investigated. However, patients with impaired hepatic or renal function and those taking other systemic medications with the potential for drug–drug interactions are typically excluded from phase II and III clinical trials.[1,2,4]

PHARMACODYNAMICS: CONCENTRATION VERSUS EFFECT

The pharmacodynamics of H_1 antihistamines can be studied objectively using the allergic rhinoconjunctivitis model and the cutaneous wheal and flare model.

Allergic Rhinoconjunctivitis Model

H_1 antihistamines prevent and suppress the response to histamine, allergen, and other agents in the nasal and conjunctival mucosa and can be tested in patients with allergic rhinitis or allergic conjunctivitis who are challenged intranasally or conjunctivally, respectively, with these agents. Experimental models involve pretreatment of a patient with an H_1 antihistamine followed by allergen challenge in that patient, pretreatment of a group of patients followed by natural allergen challenge of the group in an outdoor setting such as a park, or group challenge with high doses of allergen in an indoor environmental exposure unit. These experimental models can be used to investigate H_1 antihistamine onset of action, peak effect, and duration of action.[84,87,88,101,102]

Cutaneous Wheal and Flare Model

Objective information about the onset, intensity, and offset of H_1 antihistamine activity is often obtained by measuring the

TABLE 94-3 H_1 Antihistamines: Pharmacokinetics and Pharmacodynamics in Healthy Adults

Medication	Time to Maximum Plasma Concentration (t_{max}, hr) after Single Dose	Terminal Elimination Half-life ($t_{1/2}$, hr)	Clinically Relevant Drug–Drug Interactions*	Onset of Action (hr)†	Duration of Action (hr)
ORALLY ADMINISTERED H_1 ANTIHISTAMINES					
FIRST (OLD) GENERATION					
Chlorpheniramine‡	2.8 ±0.8	27.9 ±8.7	Possible	3	24
Diphenhydramine‡	1.7 ±1.0	9.2 ±2.5	Possible	2	12
Doxepin‡	2	13-17	Possible	n/a	n/a
Hydroxyzine‡	2.1 ±0.4	20.0 ±4.1	Possible	2	24
SECOND (NEW) GENERATION					
Bilastine	1.2	14.5	Unlikely	2	24
Cetirizine	1.0 ±0.5	6.5-10	Unlikely	0.7	≥24
Desloratadine	1-3	27	Unlikely	2-2.6	≥24
Fexofenadine*	1-3	11-15	Unlikely	1-3	24
Levocetirizine	0.8 ±0.5	7 ±1.5	Unlikely	0.7	>24
Loratadine (metabolite: descarboethoxyloratadine)	1.2 ±0.3 (1.5 ±0.7)	7.8 ±4.2 (24 ±9.8)	Unlikely	2	24
Rupatadine	0.75-1.0	6 (4.3-14.3)	Unlikely	2	24
NASAL/OPHTHALMIC H_1 ANTIHISTAMINE FORMULATIONS§					
Alcaftadine (ophthalmic)	0.25	8-12	No	0.05	24
Azelastine (metabolite: desmethylazelastine, nasal and ophthalmic)	5.3 ±1.6 (20.5)	22-27.6 (54 ±15)	No	0.5	12
Bepotastine (ophthalmic)	1.3	2.5	No	0.25	12-24
Emedastine (ophthalmic)	1.4 ±0.5	7	No	0.25	12
Epinastine (ophthalmic)	2	6.5	No	0.1	12
Ketotifen (ophthalmic)	2-4	20-22	No	0.25	12
Levocabastine (ophthalmic)	1-2	35-40	No	0.25	12
Olopatadine (nasal and ophthalmic)	0.5-2	8-12	No	0.25	12-24

Results are expressed as mean ± standard deviation, unless otherwise indicated. *n/a,* Information not available or incomplete.

*Clinically relevant drug–drug interactions are unlikely with most of the second (new)–generation H_1 antihistamines. Clinically relevant drug–food interactions have been well studied for fexofenadine. Naringin, a flavonoid in grapefruit juice, and hesperidin, a flavonoid in orange juice, reduce the oral bioavailability of fexofenadine through inhibition of OATP-1A2. This interaction can be avoided by waiting 4 hours between juice consumption and fexofenadine dosing.

†For oral H_1 antihistamines, onset and duration of action are based on wheal and flare studies. For nasal and ophthalmic H_1 antihistamine formulations, onset and duration of action are based on standard adult doses, such as 1 or 2 sprays in each nostril or 1 drop in each eye, as determined in nasal and conjunctival challenge studies, respectively.

‡Six or 7 decades ago, when many of the first (old)–generation H_1 antihistamines were introduced, regulatory agencies did not require pharmacokinetic and pharmacodynamic studies for any medication. Although subsequently these studies were performed for some H_1 antihistamines, empiric dosage regimens persist. For example, manufacturers' recommended diphenhydramine dose for allergic rhinitis is 25 to 50 mg every 4 to 6 hours, yet the diphenhydramine dose for insomnia is 25 to 50 mg at bedtime. Despite the long terminal elimination half-life values identified for some of the medications, traditionally they are still dosed several times daily. For example, doxepin, which has an elimination half-life of 13 to 17 hours, is given in doses of up to 25 to 50 mg three times daily for chronic spontaneous urticaria, yet a considerably lower dose of doxepin, 3 mg or 6 mg once daily at bedtime, is FDA-approved for insomnia. Chlorpheniramine has an elimination half-life longer than 24 hours; yet traditionally it is either given several times daily or in an extended-release formulation.

§For nasal and ophthalmic H_1 antihistamines, t_{max}, $t_{1/2}$, and drug–drug interaction information are based on serum levels obtained after *oral* administration. After topical applications, serum levels are too low to permit calculation of pharmacokinetic parameters; most of these medications cause minimal systemic effects, including skin test suppression.

suppression of the histamine-induced or (less often) the allergen-induced wheal and flare response (Fig. 94-8). In some studies, plasma and skin H_1 antihistamine concentrations have been measured concomitantly[83,85,86,94-97,104-106] (Fig. 94-9). H_1 antihistamines decrease the size of the wheal directly by acting on endothelial cells to decrease postcapillary venule permeability and leakage of plasma protein. They decrease the size of the flare indirectly by blocking the histamine-induced axon reflex. Using a standardized wheal and flare bioassay, dose-response curves can be identified for each H_1 antihistamine (see Fig. 94-8), and significant differences in onset, amount, and duration of activity among H_1 antihistamines can be consistently identified (see Fig. 94-9). For some H_1 antihistamines such as cetirizine, fexofenadine, and levocetirizine (Fig. 94-10), wheal and flare suppression in humans has been shown to correlate with H_1-receptor occupancy by free (unbound) H_1 antihistamine.[1,2,4,104-108]

Onset of Action and Peak Action

The pharmacodynamics of H_1 antihistamines are medication and dose dependent. For second (new)–generation H_1 antihistamines, peak plasma concentrations (C_{max}) in target organs such as the skin are achieved rapidly after oral administration (see Figs. 94-8 and 94-9). After a single oral dose, significant suppression of the histamine-induced wheal and flare begins within 1 hour (bilastine, cetirizine, levocetirizine) to 2 hours

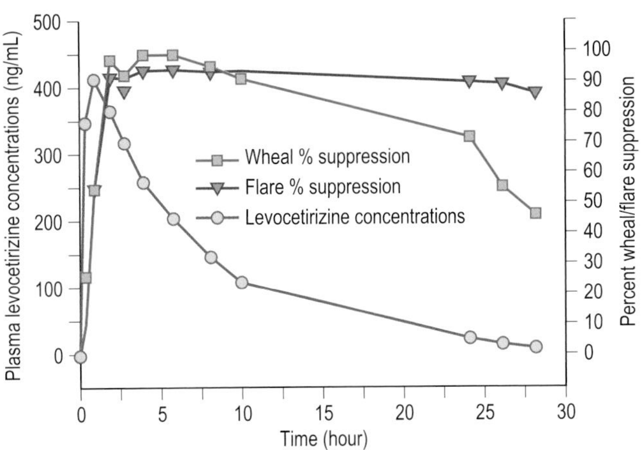

Figure 94-8 Levocetirizine plasma concentrations and effect on the wheals and flares (erythema) produced by skin prick tests with histamine phosphate 1 mg/mL. Mean plasma levocetirizine concentrations (**A**) and mean wheal and flare percent suppression (**B**) are plotted against time before and after ingestion of levocetirizine 5 mg by children age 6 to 11 years. Compared with predose values, wheals were significantly suppressed from 1 to 28 hours, inclusive, and flares were also significantly suppressed from 1 to 28 hours, inclusive (data not shown). *(From Simons FER, Simons KJ. Levocetirizine: pharmacokinetics and pharmacodynamics in children age 6 to 11 years. J Allergy Clin Immunol 2005;116:355-61.)*

(loratadine, desloratadine) of H_1 antihistamine ingestion, and peak suppression occurs at 5 to 8 hours.[83,94-97,103-106]

Duration of Action and Residual Action

The duration of action of a single dose of an H_1 antihistamine, assessed objectively from suppression of the histamine- or allergen-induced wheals and flares in the skin, or subjectively by suppression of nasal symptoms after allergen challenge, is more prolonged than might be expected from elimination half-life values. This persistent effect is associated with high tissue/plasma concentration ratios of H_1 antihistamines such as cetirizine or fexofenadine[106] (see Fig. 94-9). For other H_1 antihistamines such as desloratadine or loratadine, it is likely associated with the presence of active metabolites, although these have not been directly measured in human tissue.

The duration of action of most second (new)–generation H_1 antihistamines is at least 24 hours, facilitating once-daily dosing (see Table 94-3). For some of these medications, it may be even longer in elderly persons and in patients with hepatic or renal dysfunction, necessitating a reduced dose or dose frequency. Some topically administered H_1 antihistamines such as azelastine and levocabastine have long elimination half-life values but still need to be administered every 12 hours because of medication washout by continuous bathing of the nasal mucosa and conjunctivae with secretions and tears.

After discontinuing a second (new)–generation H_1 antihistamine taken regularly for 1 or more weeks, residual suppression of skin test reactivity to histamine and allergens varies with the H_1 antihistamine, lasting 1 day after loratadine or desloratadine, 2 days after fexofenadine, and 3 to 4 days after cetirizine or levocetirizine.[1,4]

Peripheral H_1 Activity during Regular Administration

No loss of H_1 antihistamine effects during regular daily administration has been found in rigorously controlled, double-blind studies of up to 12 weeks' duration that monitor skin wheal and flare suppression or in long-term clinical studies monitoring symptom suppression in allergic rhinitis or urticaria. The apparent subsensitivity to some first (old)–generation H_1 antihistamines described decades ago may have resulted from their weak, inconsistent pharmacologic effects or lack of compliance because of adverse effects.

Clinical Relevance of Wheal and Flare Studies

Significant, clinically relevant differences among H_1 antihistamines can be clearly shown in 10 to 20 participants in clinical pharmacology studies using objective outcomes in the wheal and flare model.[83,85,95,103,105,106] Wheal and flare suppression has direct clinical relevance for patients with urticaria. For some H_1 antihistamines (e.g., cetirizine, fexofenadine, levocetirizine), wheal and flare suppression also correlates with relief of allergic rhinitis symptoms. For others, however, such as loratadine and desloratadine, there is poor correlation with relief of rhinitis symptoms. This may involve dosing issues; in the wheal and flare model, desloratadine 10 mg and levocetirizine 1.25 mg provide equivalent suppression for 4 hours after dosing, although manufacturers' recommended dose for allergic rhinitis treatment is desloratadine 5 mg or levocetirizine 5 mg daily.[104] Significant, clinically relevant differences in efficacy among H_1 antihistamines or among different doses of the same H_1 antihistamine are difficult to demonstrate in randomized controlled trials (RCTs) in allergic rhinitis, with hundreds of participants in each treatment group and the main outcomes being subjective symptom scores and quality-of-life scores.

Allergic Rhinitis

H_1 antihistamines are medications of initial choice in allergic rhinitis[109] (Fig. 94-11).

Histamine plays an important role in the pathophysiology of allergic rhinitis, especially in the early allergic response.[43] Acting at H_1 receptors, histamine causes sneezing and itching of the nose and potentially the palate, throat, and ears through sensory nerve stimulation. It contributes to rhinorrhea through parasympathetic reflex stimulation of glandular secretions, and to both rhinorrhea and congestion through vasodilation and increased permeability of postcapillary venules. It also plays a role in the late allergic response; in the recruitment, adherence, and activation of epithelial cells, eosinophils, basophils, mast cells, T cells, and Langerhans cells; and in the upregulation of the expression and mobilization of cell adhesion molecules. H_1 antihistamines downregulate allergic inflammation mainly through the H_1 receptor[1,2] (Fig. 94-12).

It has been proposed that the traditional classification of allergic rhinitis into "seasonal" and "perennial" disease should be changed to "intermittent" and "persistent." However, the traditional classification is used here because to date, it has defined the inclusion criteria in most RCTs of H_1 antihistamines in allergic rhinitis.[109] Few RCTs of *first (old)–generation* H_1 antihistamines in seasonal or perennial allergic rhinitis have been conducted, and where performed, few of them meet current standards. Optimal masking in clinical trials of these H_1 antihistamines is difficult to achieve because of sedation and other adverse effects that often occur.[91] The evidence base for their use in allergic rhinitis is therefore small, and recommendations for dose and dose frequency remain largely empiric.[1,4,91]

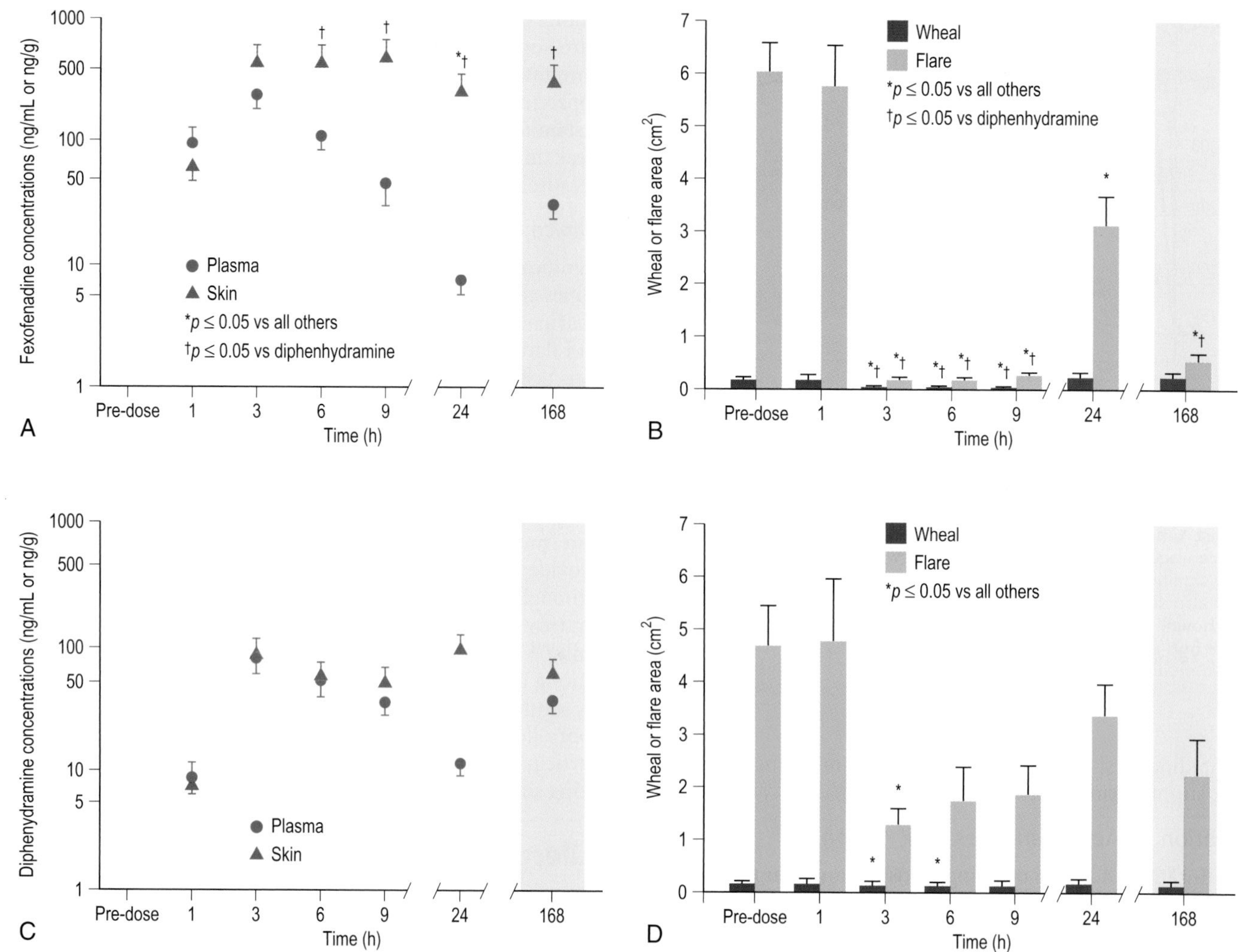

Figure 94-9 Correlation of skin and plasma H_1 antihistamine concentrations during multidose administration. In a randomized, double-blind, multiple-dose, parallel-group study, fexofenadine 120 mg/day or diphenhydramine 50 mg/day was administered for 1 week. At predose baseline and 1, 3, 6, 9, and 24 hours after the initial H_1 antihistamine dose, skin and plasma antihistamine concentrations were monitored, and wheal and flare areas were measured after epicutaneous tests with histamine phosphate 1 mg/mL. Subsequently, on each of 6 consecutive days, participants took their H_1 antihistamine dose at 9 PM. All the tests were repeated at 168 hours (i.e., at steady-state, depicted in *shaded area*), exactly 12 hours after the seventh and last dose. The values shown are mean ± SEM. Fexofenadine (**A** and **B**) achieved significantly higher concentrations in the skin and significantly greater wheal and flare suppression than did diphenhydramine (**C** and **D**). Predose, plasma concentrations of both H_1 antihistamines were zero. *(From Simons FER, Silver NA, Gu X, et al. Skin concentrations of H_1-receptor antagonists. J Allergy Clin Immunol 2001;107:526-30.)*

In contrast, in both seasonal and perennial allergic rhinitis, there is a solid evidence base for the use of orally administered *second (new)–generation* H_1 antihistamines such as bilastine, cetirizine, desloratadine, fexofenadine, loratadine, levocetizirine, and rupatadine, as well as for nasal H_1 antihistamine formulations such as azelastine and olopatadine and ophthalmic formulations such as alcaftadine and bepotastine. Efficacy has been well documented in hundreds of randomized DBPC parallel-group clinical trials involving thousands of participants. Additional studies are still needed in children and elderly persons.[110-132]

Traditional "diary card" studies in seasonal allergic rhinitis involve self-report of symptoms and quality of life during the pollen season. Typically, regular H_1 antihistamine treatment begins before peak pollination and is continued for the duration of the season. The duration of clinical trials in perennial allergic rhinitis is usually 4 to 8 weeks, although some studies have lasted 26 to 52 weeks. In seasonal allergic rhinitis and perennial allergic rhinitis studies, participants demonstrate a predefined pretreatment level of self-recorded nasal symptoms (e.g., itch, sneezing, rhinorrhea) and nonnasal symptoms (e.g., itchy watery eyes; itchy throat, palate, or ears; cough). Such studies document sensitization to the allergens likely to be encountered. In seasonal allergic rhinitis studies, daily allergen exposure (e.g., pollen counts) is monitored. In addition to subjective self-assessment of rhinitis symptoms used to evaluate efficacy, objective measurements such as measurement of nasal peak inspiratory flow have been incorporated into some clinical trials.[110-121]

Most studies of H_1 antihistamines have involved regular daily administration, which is associated with a significant decrease in symptoms and nasal mucosal inflammation compared with "as needed," "on demand," or "on-again, off-again" use.[115,116]

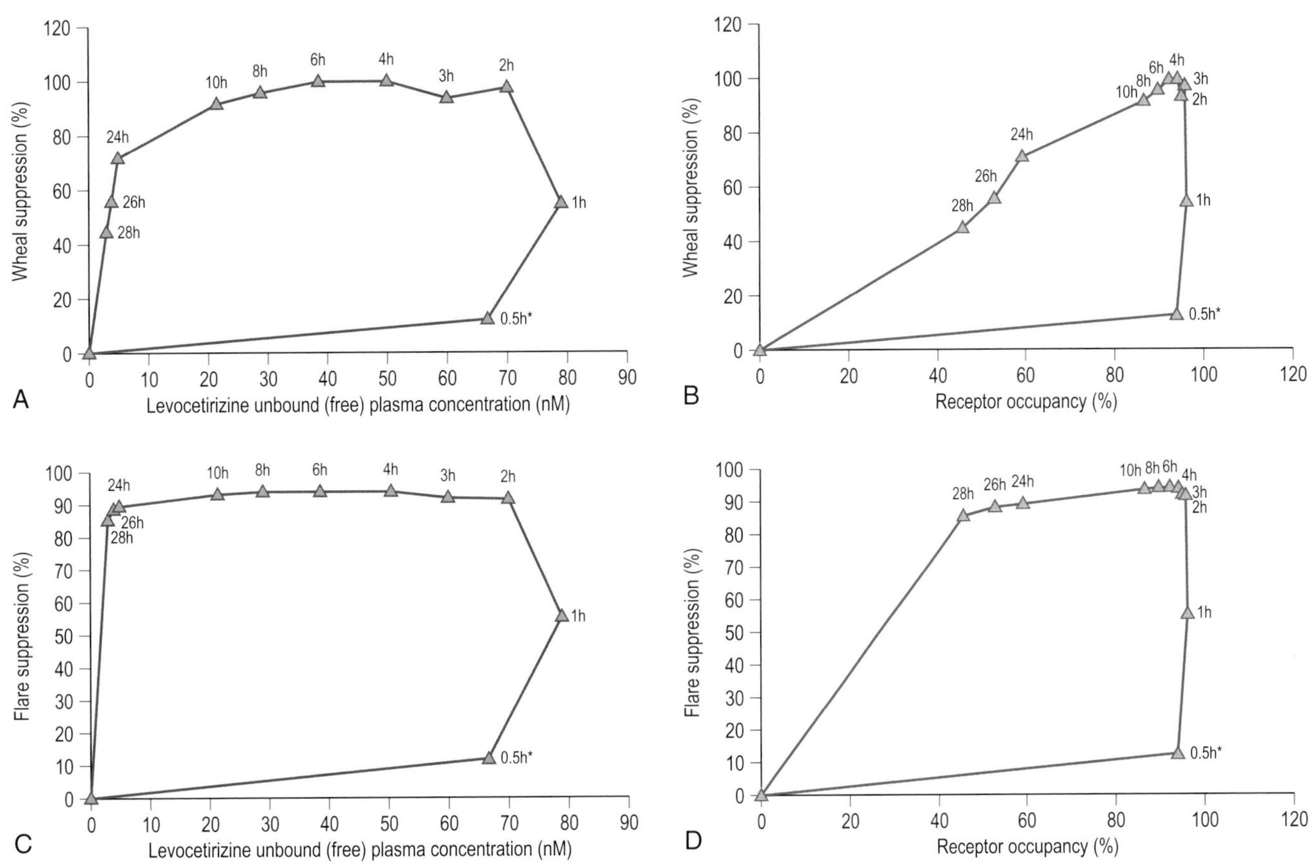

Figure 94-10 H_1 antihistamines and H_1-receptor occupancy. **A**, Percent suppression of the histamine-induced wheal versus levocetirizine unbound (free) plasma concentrations. **B**, Percent suppression of the histamine-induced wheal versus percent levocetirizine H_1-receptor occupancy. **C**, Percent suppression of the histamine-induced flare versus levocetirizine unbound (free) plasma concentrations. **D**, Percent suppression of the histamine-induced flare versus percent levocetirizine H_1-receptor occupancy. Receptor occupancy kinetics are a better representation of the time course of H_1 antihistamine pharmacodynamics than plasma pharmacokinetics. *(From Simons KJ, Benedetti MS, Simons FE, Gillard M, Baltes E. Relevance of H_1-receptor occupancy to H_1 antihistamine dosing in children. J Allergy Clin Immunol 2007;119:1551-4.)*

PRACTICAL ISSUES

The H_1 antihistamines reduce symptoms in allergic rhinitis and improve quality of life significantly. They relieve nasal itching, sneezing, and rhinorrhea to a greater extent than placebo and are also effective for relieving itching of the palate, throat, and ears. Overall, a 50% to 70% reduction in symptoms is typically documented, versus a 30% to 40% reduction after placebo. The dose-response curve for symptom relief from H_1 antihistamines is relatively flat.[110-118]

Small, inconsistent but statistically significant differences in efficacy among oral H_1 antihistamines have been demonstrated in a few allergic rhinitis studies. When all RCTs are reviewed, however, no H_1 antihistamine emerges with an overall superior efficacy profile that is clinically relevant. Selection of an H_1 antihistamine for allergic rhinitis treatment should therefore be based first on safety and considerations such as convenience of dose regimen and patient preference.[119-121]

In some studies, oral H_1 antihistamines have had a small, statistically significant decongestant effect that may or may not be clinically relevant.[119] Some H_1 antihistamines are therefore marketed in fixed-dose combination with a decongestant such as pseudoephedrine to improve relief of nasal congestion and overall efficacy.[122] Concomitant administration of an H_1 antihistamine and an H_3 antihistamine might be useful in prevention of nasal congestion and other allergic rhinitis symptoms.[123] Although second (new)–generation H_1 antihistamines are more efficacious than montelukast or cromolyn, all three of these classes of medication are less efficacious than nasal glucocorticoids. Nonresponders to H_1 antihistamines who are adherent to treatment thus should be considered candidates for nasal glucocorticoid treatment.[109-114,124,125]

Now that relatively inexpensive generic second (new)–generation H_1 antihistamines such as cetirizine and loratadine are available, additional comprehensive cost-effectiveness studies of H_1 antihistamines in allergic rhinitis are needed. In such studies the indirect costs incurred from adverse effects of first (old)–generation H_1 antihistamines need to be considered.[126] Pharmacoeconomic evaluations of allergic rhinitis should include comparisons of patients with severe versus mild chronic upper airway disease.[127]

Nasal H_1 antihistamine formulations have a more rapid onset of action than oral H_1 antihistamine formulations, for example, 15 minutes for intranasal azelastine versus 150 minutes for oral desloratadine.[128-130] In patients with seasonal allergic rhinitis, intranasal H_1 antihistamines are reported to be as

Conditions Currently Treated with H_1 Antihistamines

Strong evidence base for second (new)-generation H_1 antihistamine use	Weak evidence base for H_1 antihistamine use	Weak evidence base for first (old)-generation H_1 antihistamine use in CNS and vestibular disorders
√ Allergic rhinitis	Atopic dermatitis	Insomnia
√ Allergic conjunctivitis	Asthma	Conscious sedation
√ Urticaria	Anaphylaxis	Perioperative sedation
	Nonallergic angioedema	Analgesia
	Upper respiratory tract infections (colds)	Anxiety
	Otitis media	Serotonin syndrome
	Sinusitis	Akathisia
	Nasal polyps	Migraine
	Nonspecific cough	Motion sickness
	Nonallergic, nonspecific itching	Vertigo

Figure 94-11 Science versus reality: evidence-based use of H_1 antihistamines in allergic diseases and other disorders. On the basis of well-designed randomized controlled trials and meta-analyses of such trials, the evidence base for the efficacy and safety of second (new)–generation H_1 antihistamines is strong in patients with allergic rhinitis, allergic conjunctivitis, and urticaria (category of evidence I, strength of recommendation A), but not in those with atopic dermatitis and other diseases (category of evidence II to IV, strength of recommendation B, C, or D, depending on the disease). The evidence base for the efficacy and safety of first (old)–generation H_1 antihistamines remains weak in patients with allergic rhinitis, allergic conjunctivitis, urticaria, atopic dermatitis, and other diseases, including central nervous sytem (*CNS*) and vestibular disorders (category of evidence II to IV, strength of recommendation B, C, or D, depending on the disease). The potential adverse effects of these first (old)–generation H_1 antihistamines remain a concern. *(From Simons FER, Simons KJ. Histamine and H_1-antihistamines: celebrating a century of progress; J Allergy Clin Immunol 2011;128:1139-50.)*

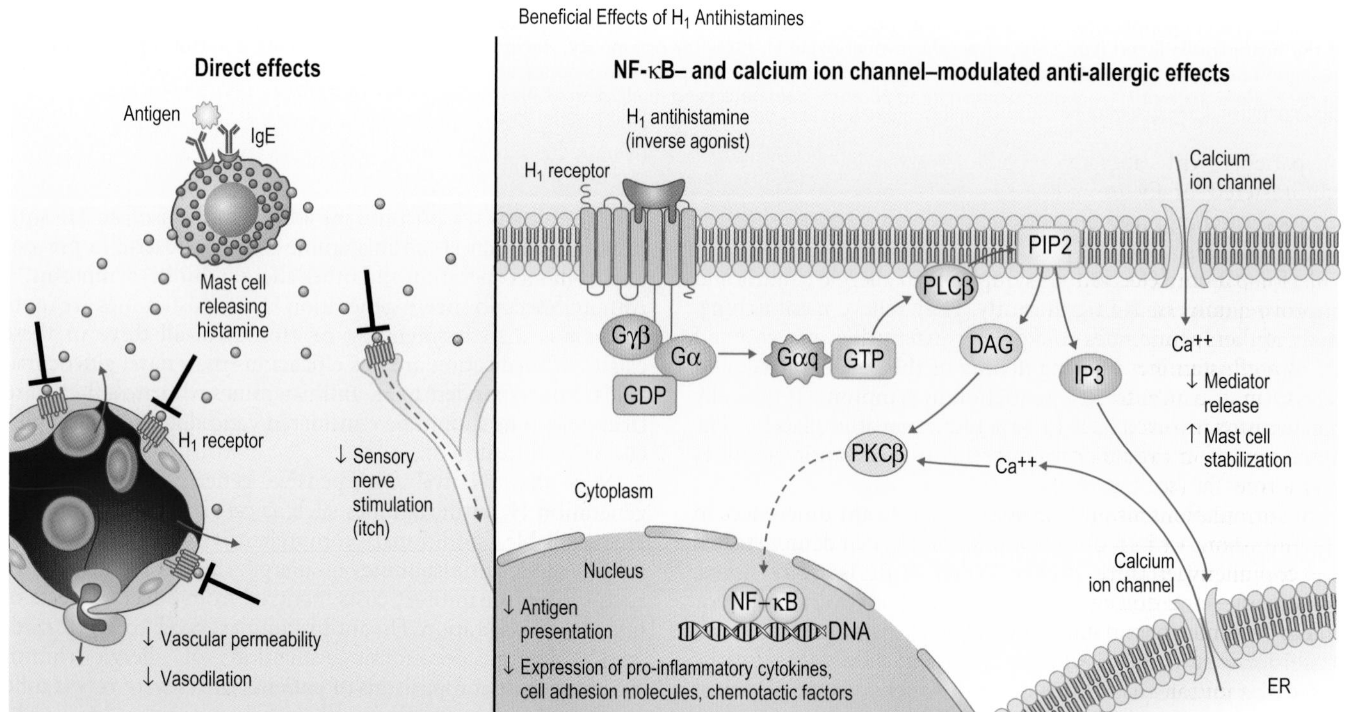

Figure 94-12 Mechanisms underlying beneficial effects of H_1 antihistamines. In addition to acting directly to interfere with histamine action at H_1 receptors on sensory neurons and small blood vessels, mainly postcapillary venules, H_1 antihistamines also downregulate allergic inflammation indirectly through nuclear factor-κB and through calcium ion channels. *DAG,* 1,2-Diacylglycerol; *ER,* endoplasmic reticulum; *GDP,* guanosine diphosphate; *GTP,* guanosine triphosphate; *IP3,* inositol 1,4,5-triphosphate; *PIP2,* phosphatidylinositol-4,5-bisphosphate; *PKC,* protein kinase C; *PLC,* phospholipase C. *(From Simons FER, Simons KJ. Histamine and H_1-antihistamines: celebrating a century of progress; J Allergy Clin Immunol 2011;128:1139-50.)*

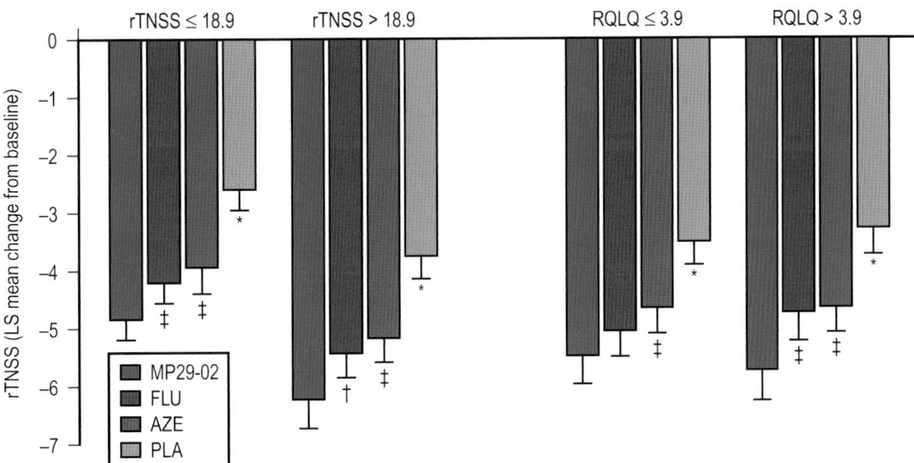

Figure 94-13 Nasal H_1 antihistamine combined with nasal glucocorticoid for allergic rhinitis treatment. Effect of azelastine and fluticasone in combination (MP29-02) versus fluticasone propionate (FLU), azelastine (AZE), and placebo (PLA) on the reflective total nasal symptom scores (rTNSSs) (morning plus evening) by severity in patients with seasonal allergic rhinitis (SAR). Data are presented as least squares (*LS*) mean change from baseline for the meta-analysis. **P* ≤.001 versus all active treatment. Patients with moderate-to-severe SAR (rTNSS >18.9 and Rhinitis Quality of Life Questionnaire [RQLQ] >3.9) had the best response to treatment. *(From Carr W, Bernstein J, Lieberman P, et al. A novel intranasal therapy of azelastine with fluticasone for the treatment of allergic rhinitis; J Allergy Clin Immunol 2012;129:1282-9).*

efficacious as (or more efficacious than) oral H_1 antihistamines, particularly for relief of nasal congestion. They improve symptoms in patients who are unresponsive to oral H_1 antihistamines and in those with vasomotor rhinitis.[130] Patient preference should be considered when recommending a nasal versus an oral H_1 antihistamine.[131] Nasal azelastine combined with nasal fluticasone in a single–nasal spray delivery device provides a significantly greater improvement of symptoms, including congestion, than either medication alone[132] (Fig. 94-13).

Allergic Conjunctivitis

In patients with allergic conjunctivitis, H_1 antihistamines administered orally or applied directly to the conjunctivae relieve the itching, erythema, tearing, and edema that characterize the early response to allergens.[87-89,109,133-137] Standardized criteria for patient selection and quantifiable primary outcomes are not yet universally incorporated into randomized controlled trials of therapeutic interventions in allergic conjunctivitis.[134]

H_1 antihistamines inhibit mast cell activation and histamine release in a concentration-dependent manner. Although the mechanisms involved have not yet been delineated fully, downregulation of intracellular calcium ion accumulation seems to play a role[43,138] (see Fig. 94-12). Most ophthalmic H_1 antihistamine formulations also function as mast cell stabilizers because H_1 antihistamines in high concentrations are applied directly to the conjunctivae; these high concentrations are difficult to achieve after oral dosing.[87-89,138]

Ophthalmic formulations have a rapid onset of action of 3 to 15 minutes.[133-137] Some are reported to treat nasal symptoms in addition to conjunctival symptoms. In patients with allergic conjunctivitis,[89] H_1 antihistamines have a more favorable benefit/risk ratio than all other classes of medications, including nonsteroidal antiinflammatory drugs (NSAIDs), decongestants, and glucocorticoids,[109] although the new ophthalmic glucocorticoid loteprednol might prove to be an exception to this.[139]

Urticaria

Histamine, acting through H_1-receptors, is the main mediator of pruritus in acute and chronic urticaria. Along with proteases, tachykinins, eicosanoids, prostanoids, neuropeptides such as substance P, and other vasoactive substances, it leads to increased vascular permeability, vasodilation, and wheals and flares that blanch under pressure.[104,109] In chronic urticaria, skin tissue fluid histamine concentrations are increased in urticarial lesions and in uninvolved skin. The presence of urticarial lesions correlates with increased histamine releasing activity by autoantibodies. Clinical tolerance to histamine is reduced in individuals with chronic urticaria. In localized urticarial lesions induced by cold challenge or other relevant stimulus, plasma histamine concentrations are not increased; however, histamine concentrations in venous blood draining the site increase transiently, peaking at 2 to 5 minutes, and declining to baseline within 30 minutes.[1]

In urticaria, H_1 antihistamines provide symptomatic relief of itching, and reduce the number, size, and duration of flares (erythema). Relief may be incomplete because additional vasoactive mediators contribute to the vasodilation, vascular permeability, and extravasation.[1,4,140]

In *acute* urticaria, defined as hives lasting less than 6 weeks, the evidence base for the use of either first (old)–generation or second (new)–generation H_1 antihistamines remains small. In young atopic children, a planned secondary outcome was H_1 antihistamine efficacy in intermittent acute urticaria in two large randomized DBPC trials, each 18 months in duration; cetirizine[142] and levocetirizine[143] were significantly more effective than placebo in preventing and reducing urticarial lesions.

In *chronic* urticaria, defined as hives lasting 6 weeks or more, the evidence base for the use of first (old)–generation antihistamines remains surprisingly small by current standards. H_1 antihistamines such as chlorpheniramine, diphenhydramine, doxepin, and hydroxyzine remain in use for urticaria treatment despite the absence of randomized DBPC trials to confirm their

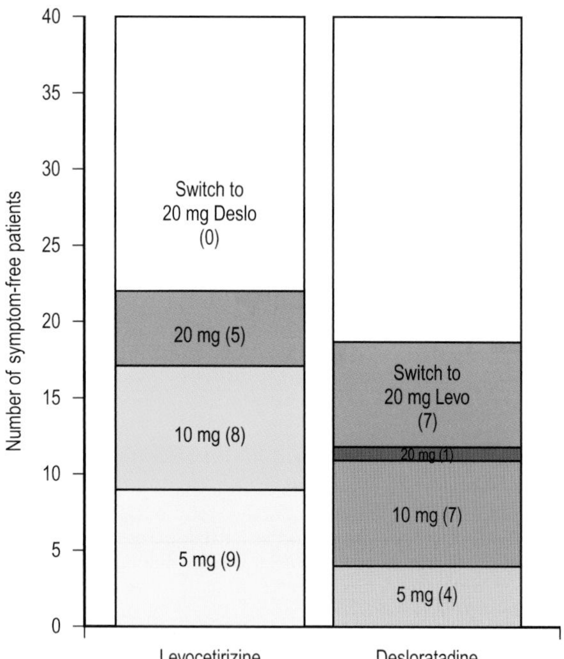

Figure 94-14 Effectiveness of levocetirizine and desloratadine in up to 4 times conventional doses in difficult-to-treat urticaria. The number of patients whose symptoms were relieved by levocetirizine (Levo) and desloratadine (Deslo) during the 4 weeks of the study are shown. The numbers in parentheses refer to the number of patients who were symptom free on 5 mg (week 1), 10 mg (week 2), 20 mg (week 3), or after switching from one drug to the other (week 4). *(From Staevska M, Popov TA, Kralimarkova T, et al. The effectiveness of levocetirizine and desloratadine in up to 4 times conventional doses in difficult-to-treat urticaria. J Allergy Clin Immunol 2010;125:676-82.)*

efficacy and safety. Moreover, some are given three or four times daily despite their long elimination half-life values associated with prolonged wheal and flare suppression in pharmacokinetic studies (see Table 94-3).

In contrast, randomized DBPC trials constitute a strong evidence base for use of second (new)-generation H_1 antihistamines such as bilastine, cetirizine, desloratadine, fexofenadine, levocetirizine, loratadine, and rupatadine in chronic urticaria (Fig. 94-14). In these trials, they have been given on a regular basis rather than on an as-needed or on-again, off-again basis, which is less effective.[144] In RCTs, second (new)–generation H_1 antihistamines are as effective as first (old)–generation H_1 antihistamines and also are less impairing and sedating.[145,146]

Some treatment regimens involving H_1 antihistamines remain in use for chronic urticaria despite no scientific rationale or prospective randomized DBPC trials to support their use. These include sequential administration of two different second (new)–generation H_1 antihistamines on the same day or administration of a second (new) generation in the morning and a first (old) generation at bedtime, sometimes leading to an "antihistamine hangover" the next morning.[1,4,91]

Although many patients respond to usual doses of a second (new)–generation H_1 antihistamine, even more respond to increasing the daily dose of some of these medications up to fourfold. In a randomized DBPC trial, 13 of 40 patients became symptom free with 5 mg of levocetirizine, but 28 of the 40 patients became symptom free receiving 10 or 20 mg of levocetirizine, without experiencing adverse effects from the higher dose. Additionally, in objective tests in patients with acquired cold urticaria, high-dose desloratadine (20 mg) or rupatadine (20 mg) decreased wheal volume and increased the threshold for cold provocation significantly, compared with usual doses. Treatment guidelines for chronic urticaria now recommend second (new)–generation H_1 antihistamines as the medications of choice, starting with usual doses and increasing the doses up to fourfold as needed to provide relief.[147-153] However, this approach is not universally recommended[154] and is not effective in all patients.[155] Chronic urticaria is not well studied in children, and strategies to improve this situation are being developed.[156]

Guidelines recommend different approaches to treatment of severe chronic urticaria refractory to second (new)–generation H_1 antihistamines.[141] Based on evidence from RCTs,[140] it can be helpful to add omalizumab,[157] cyclosporine, or dapsone. A recent Cochrane review found that addition of an H_2 antihistamine to an H_1 antihistamine for treatment of chronic urticaria did not significantly enhance relief.[158] The evidence base for the efficacy of sulfasalazine, hydroxychloroquine, mycophenolate, and oral tacrolimus in chronic urticaria is weak. Exacerbations of hives can be treated with a brief 3- to 7-day course of a glucocorticoid, but long-term glucocorticoid treatment should be avoided. Patients with urticaria taking cyclosporine, dapsone, sulfasalazine, hydroxychloroquine, mycophenolate, or oral tacrolimus need regular monitoring and dose adjustments when indicated to avoid potentially severe adverse effects.[140]

Other Diseases and Uses

FIRST (OLD)– AND SECOND (NEW)–GENERATION H_1 ANTIHISTAMINES

Medications of Choice[78,80,159]

A small RCT supports H_1 antihistamine use to prevent and relieve itching and flushing in mastocytosis.[160] Similarly, small RCTs support the use of H_1 antihistamines such as cetirizine, ebastine, levocetirizine, and rupatadine for prevention and relief of the itching, redness, and swelling of early and late allergic reactions to mosquito bites.[161,162] Small RCTs also support pretreatment with an H_1 antihistamine to reduce adverse effects and modulate allergen-specific immune responses during subcutaneous immunotherapy with stinging insect venoms.[162]

Not Medications of First Choice

Largely on the basis of tradition, H_1 antihistamines remain in widespread use for many diseases despite a weak evidence base for drug efficacy and safety and not being supported by RCTs that meet current standards (see Fig. 94-11).

Atopic Dermatitis. In some patients with atopic dermatitis, histamine concentrations are elevated in the skin and plasma. Histamine acts as a pruritogen through H_4 receptors as well as H_1 receptors and through cytokines (e.g., IL-31), neuropeptides, proteases, and eicosanoids. Relief of itching in atopic dermatitis is therefore typically incomplete after H_1 antihistamine use. Moreover, the evidence that these medications have significant topical glucocorticoid-sparing effects in dermatitis is not convincing.[163] No high-quality randomized DBPC trials of H_1 antihistamines confirm their overall efficacy in atopic dermatitis. Regardless, some physicians still recommend first (old)–generation H_1 antihistamines because of their sedative effects.

This is a concern, particularly in infants and young children, in whom adverse effects are well documented not only after usual doses but also when higher doses or extra doses are given due to lack of efficacy.[163-165]

Asthma. The role of histamine and of H_1 antihistamines in asthma has been extensively reviewed.[1,4] H_1 antihistamine treatment for asthma has evolved through several phases, with initial enthusiasm for first (old)–generation H_1 antihistamines fading quickly. Later, they were thought to be contraindicated in asthma because of their anticholinergic effects and potential drying and inspissation of secretions. Recent RCTs suggest that, although they are not medications of first choice for asthma, second (new)–generation H_1 antihistamines provide indirect benefit in patients with concomitant seasonal asthma and allergic rhinitis and are safe for use.[110,166,167]

In an 18-month study in very young children with atopic dermatitis and house-dust mite or grass sensitization at risk for development of asthma, regular administration of cetirizine was reported to delay asthma onset. However, this observation was not confirmed with levocetirizine.[1,4]

Anaphylaxis. A Cochrane review of 2070 H_1 antihistamine studies identified no RCTs that provided satisfactory evidence for use of this class of medications in anaphylaxis. The onset of action of oral H_1 antihistamines is slow, ranging from 0.7 to 2.6 hours. Although they decrease itch and hives, H_1 antihistamines do not prevent or relieve laryngeal edema, lower respiratory tract obstruction, hypotension, or shock and are not lifesaving. First (old)–generation H_1 antihistamines such as diphenhydramine potentially impair recognition of anaphylaxis symptoms. Improvement in anaphylaxis attributed to H_1 antihistamine treatment may reflect spontaneous improvement from endogenous production of epinephrine, endothelin, angiotensin II, and other agents. Epinephrine (adrenaline) is the lifesaving medication of choice for initial use.[168]

First (old)–generation H_1 antihistamines (diphenhydramine, chlorpheniramine) are available in parenteral formulations for intravenous injection and remain in use in hospital settings for relief of itching and generalized hives in patients with anaphylaxis. The sedation that typically accompanies their use might be relevant in emergency department settings from which patients are discharged within hours of treatment.

In a randomized trial in young patients with food challenge-associated acute allergic reactions confined to the skin, cetirizine (0.25 mg/kg) had a similar onset of action compared with diphenhydramine (1 mg/kg), as well as similar efficacy, longer duration of action, and reduced sedation profile. Similar numbers of children in each treatment group received epinephrine and glucocorticoid treatment.[169]

Prevention of Allergic Reactions. In a variety of protocols an H_1 antihistamine in combination with other medications, such as an H_2 antihistamine and a glucocorticoid, is recommended for prophylaxis of anaphylaxis triggered by agents such as radiocontrast media, volume expanders, plasma exchange transfusion, fluorescein, morphine, protamine, and other drugs. With a few exceptions,[170] the protocols in use are based on clinical experience rather than RCTs.[1,4]

Nonallergic Angioedema. In the absence of itching or urticaria, angioedema is typically nonallergic, not mediated by histamine, and not prevented or relieved by H_1 antihistamines. The recommended pharmacologic treatment of hereditary angioedema type I, II, and III attacks includes C1-esterase inhibitor concentrates, ecallantide, or icatibant.[171] Treatment of nonallergic angioedema associated with angiotensin-converting enzyme (ACE) inhibitor use involves substitution of another medication if possible. Treatment of malignancy-associated nonallergic angioedema focuses on definitive treatment of the malignancy.

Weak Efficacy and Off-label Uses

H_1 antihistamines are used to treat symptoms of upper respiratory tract infections, acute otitis media, otitis media with effusion, sinusitis, nasal polyps, and acute and chronic nonspecific cough. However, their efficacy and safety have not been confirmed in high-quality RCTs in patients with these conditions.[172-178]

First (old)–generation H_1 antihistamines are also used to relieve nonspecific itching and to relieve intractable itching in patients with polycythemia vera or those with hepatic disease or renal disease in which pruritis is not histamine-mediated.[179] Lack of H_1 antihistamine efficacy, leading to updosing and potential adverse effects, is a concern in these clinical situations.

In addition, H_1 antihistamines are used "off label" in many other diseases, including neurofibromatosis, eosinophilic gastroenteritis, eosinophilic fasciitis, interstitial cystitis, aphthous ulceration, lichen nitidus, rheumatoid arthritis, scleroderma, myotonic congenita, and chronic fatigue syndrome. In most of these diseases, claims of H_1 antihistamine efficacy are anecdotal and are not supported by randomized controlled trials: either such trials have not been performed, or they have been performed with negative results.

Interestingly, in malaria, RCTs do support the concomitant use of the first (old)–generation H_1 antihistamine chlorpheniramine with the antimalarial chloroquine or amodiaquine. Chlorpheniramine plays a cost-effective role by acting as a CYP inhibitor and increasing plasma levels of the antimalarial to reverse drug resistance.[180]

FIRST (OLD)–GENERATION H_1 ANTIHISTAMINES

Insomia and Other Central Nervous System Symptoms. First (old)–generation H_1 antihistamines have a comparable sedative effect to that of triazolam or ethanol. These drugs decrease the time elapsed before falling asleep but also may distort sleep architecture and cause rebound insomnia. Diphenhydramine, doxepin, doxylamine, and pyrilamine are the most frequently used medications in the world for the treatment of insomnia and are effective when given in low doses, such as 25 mg of diphenhydramine or 3 or 6 mg of doxepin once daily at bedtime. RCTs of first (old)–generation H_1 antihistamine use in insomnia and other central nervous system (CNS) diseases are being conducted.[1,4,181]

Sedation. Although not drugs of choice, first (old)–generation H_1 antihistamines such as diphenhydramine, hydroxyzine, and promethazine are still prescribed, often in combination with other medications, for patients needing conscious sedation, perioperative sedation, and analgesia.[182]

Nausea. Dimenhydrinate, diphenhydramine, and promethazine are used for prevention and treatment of nausea and vomiting during the postoperative period and after chemotherapy.[183] Doxylamine is used to decrease nausea and vomiting in pregnancy.[1,4,184]

Movement Disorders. Diphenhydramine or cyproheptadine is still used to decrease rigidity and increase voluntary movement in some patients with dystonia and akathisia, including those who develop extrapyramidal reactions during treatment with antipsychotic drugs. Cyproheptadine is still used to treat serotonin syndrome and also for relief of sweating during treatment with selective serotonin reuptake inhibitors (SSRIs).

Anxiety. Hydroxyzine is still used as an inexpensive treatment for anxiety disorders.[1,4,185]

Vertigo and Motion Sickness. First (old)–generation H_1 antihistamines, including cinnarizine, dimenhydrinate, diphenhydramine, meclizine, and promethazine, are among the limited therapeutic options available for the prevention and treatment of vertigo and motion sickness. They block the signal sent through the histaminergic nervous system from the vestibular nucleus to the vomiting center in the medulla. Their impairing and sedating effects are widely recognized, and first (old)–generation H_1 antihistamines are contraindicated for use by pilots and others in safety-critical jobs that require a continuous high level of alertness. Second (new)–generation H_1 antihistamines do not prevent motion sickness.[1,4,186]

Adverse Effects

The risk of adverse effects from an H_1 antihistamine is fundamentally associated with its chemical structure and functional classification. First (old)–generation H_1 antihistamines are more likely to cause known H_1 antihistamine adverse effects than second (new)–generation H_1 antihistamines.[1,4,187] First (old)–generation H_1 antihistamines have been marketed to the medical profession and general public as safe medications since the 1940s and 1950s, despite extensive documentation of their adverse effects and toxicity during this period (Fig. 94-15 and Table 94-4). Even in standard doses, all these medications may cause adverse effects in the central nervous system and elsewhere.[1,4,91,92,187] After accidental or intentional overdose, all first (old)–generation H_1 antihistamines may cause serious toxicity and, in the absence of supportive treatment, death.[187] Some antihistamines (e.g., diphenhydramine) are documented drugs of abuse.[188] First (old)–generation H_1 antihistamines are not selective for the H_1 receptor (see Fig. 94-15). Their antimuscarinic anticholinergic effects include mydriasis, dry eyes, dry mouth, constipation, and urinary hesitancy and retention; antiserotonin effects include increased appetite and weight gain; and anti-α-adrenergic effects include dizziness and orthostatic hypotension.[189-191] These first-generation H_1 antihistamines have also been implicated in impairing the innate immune response to bacterial infection, although this is more likely attributable to coadministered H_2 antihistamines.[192,193]

CENTRAL NERVOUS SYSTEM

Histamine plays an important role in neurotransmission in the CNS.[194,195] It is produced in neurons with cell bodies located in the tuberomamillary nucleus of the posterior hypothalamus that send their axons throughout the histaminergic nervous system in the cerebrum, cerebellum, posterior pituitary, and spinal cord. Histamine has natural anticonvulsant activity and contributes to regulation of vigilance (alertness), cognition and learning, memory, and the circadian sleep-wake cycle, as well as to energy and endocrine homeostasis. First (old)–generation H_1 antihistamines cross the blood-brain barrier (BBB) and interfere with neurotransmission in the histaminergic system.[1,4,91,92,196-209]

First (Old)–Generation H_1 Antihistamines

Use of positron emission tomography (PET) to document H_1 antihistamine penetration into the human brain provides objective criteria by which occupancy of H_1 receptors can be directly related to effects on CNS function[92,196-200] (Fig. 94-16). PET studies with ^{11}C-doxepin as the positron-emitting ligand (positive control) confirm that in standard or even low doses,

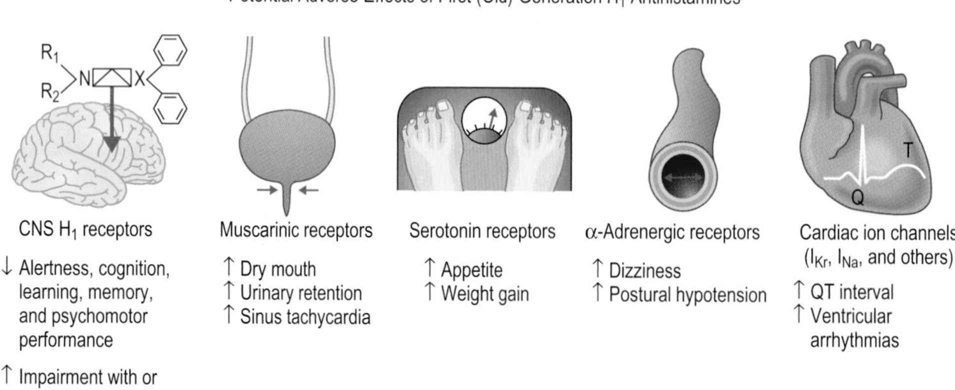

Figure 94-15 Mechanisms associated with potential adverse H_1 antihistamine effects. First (old)–generation H_1 antihistamines cross the blood-brain barrier and occupy central nervous sytem *(CNS)* H_1 receptors, as documented by means of positron emission tomography. High H_1-receptor occupancy correlates directly with impairment of CNS function, with or without accompanying sedation. These medications also may cause adverse effects through other mechanisms, such as their antimuscarinic and antiserotonin effects. I_{Kr}, Rapid component of the delayed outward rectifying potassium channel; I_{Na}, rapid component of the inward rectifying sodium channel. *(From Simons FER, Simons KJ. Histamine and H_1-antihistamines: celebrating a century of progress. J Allergy Clin Immunol 2011;128:1139-50.)*

TABLE 94-4 H_1 Antihistamines: Potential Adverse Effects

Mechanism	First (Old) Generation*,†	Second (New) Generation†,‡
CENTRAL NERVOUS SYSTEM (CNS) EFFECTS		
Inhibition of neurotransmitter effect of histamine at CNS H_1 receptors	After standard doses, there is potential impairment of alertness, cognition, learning, memory, and performance (especially of complex sensorimotor tasks), with or without drowsiness, somnolence, fatigue, or sedation. Other potential CNS adverse effects include headache, dizziness, confusion, agitation, behavioral changes (children), and less often, dystonia, dyskinesia, and hallucinations.	Minimal or no adverse effects reported with bilastine 10 mg, cetirizine 5 mg, desloratadine 5 mg, fexofenadine 120 mg or 240 mg (standard doses), fexofenadine 360 mg (off-label dose), levocetirizine 5 mg, loratadine 10 mg, or rupatadine 10 mg. Except for fexofenadine, at higher doses these H_1 antihistamines might cause dose-related CNS effects in some adults with some allergic diseases.
CARDIAC EFFECTS		
Antimuscarinic effects, anti-α-adrenergic effects, and blockade of cardiac ion currents (I_{Kr}, I_{Na}, I_{to}, I_{Ki}, and I_{Ks})	Dose-related sinus tachycardia; reflex tachycardia, prolonged atrial refractive period, and supraventricular arrhythmias potentially occur. Prolongation of the QTc interval and ventricular arrhythmias reported after standard doses but more likely after overdose (see Toxicity after Overdose).	Concerns are minimal in countries where regulatory agencies scrutinize second (new)–generation H_1 antihistamines for potential cardiac toxicity and do not approve them for use if identified.
OTHER POTENTIAL ADVERSE EFFECTS		
Blockade of muscarinic, serotonin, and α-adrenergic receptors Unknown mechanisms§	After standard doses: potential anti-muscarinic effects include mydriasis (dilation of pupils), blurred vision, dry eyes, dry mouth, urinary retention/hesitancy, constipation, erectile dysfunction, and memory deficits; these H_1 antihistamines are contraindicated in patients with glaucoma or prostatic hypertrophy. Antiserotonin effects include appetite stimulation and weight gain, especially with cyproheptadine and ketotifen. Anti-α-adrenergic effects include peripheral vasodilation, orthostatic hypotension, and dizziness.	None
TOXICITY AFTER OVERDOSE		
Multiple nechanisms	In adults, potential CNS effects include extreme drowsiness, confusion, delirium, coma, and respiratory depression. In infants and young children, paradoxic excitation, irritability, hyperactivity, insomnia, hallucinations, and seizures can precede coma and respiratory depression. Prolongation of QTc interval and ventricular arrhythmias reported after overdose of cyproheptadine, diphenhydramine, doxepin, hydroxyzine, promethazine, and others. Adverse CNS effects typically predominate over adverse cardiac effects. In untreated patients, death can occur within hours.	Up to 30-fold overdoses of cetirizine, fexofenadine, and loratadine have not been causally associated with serious adverse events or fatality.
DRUG ABUSE		
Through H_1 receptors and other CNS receptors	Euphoria, hallucinations, and "getting high" are reported for cyclizine, diphenhydramine, dimenhydrinate, and others.	None reported

I_{Kr}, Rapid component of the delayed outward rectifying potassium current; I_{Na}, rapid component of the inward rectifying sodium current; I_{to}, transient outward potassium current; I_{Ki}, inward rectifying current; I_{Ks}, slow component of the delayed rectifying potassium current.

*Information about adverse effects and toxicity of first (old)–generation H_1 antihistamines is based largely on descriptions in case reports and case series since the 1940s. For example, promethazine is no longer recommended because it may cause sedation and respiratory depression/arrest and by the intravenous route, vascular irritation, local necrosis, and gangrene. Applied topically to the skin, diphenhydramine or doxepin may cause contact dermatitis, and when applied to abraded or thin skin, may also cause systemic adverse effects and rarely, death.

†Nasal and ophthalmic formulations of H_1 antihistamines are minimally absorbed and seldom cause systemic adverse effects. Some are associated with a transient bitter or unpleasant taste sensation. Ophthalmic H_1 antihistamines can cause stinging or burning on application. These H_1 antihistamines should be applied at least 10 minutes before contact lens insertion because the preservative benzalkonium chloride 0.01% in the formulations can cloud the lenses.

‡Information about relative lack of adverse effects from second (new)–generation H_1 antihistamines is from prospective randomized placebo-controlled trials in patients with allergic rhinitis or chronic urticaria and from occasional case reports of overdose with remarkable absence of toxicity.

§Both first (old)–generation and second (new)–generation H_1 antihistamines are reported to cause rare adverse effects for which the mechanisms are incompletely understood. These include agranulocytosis, fever, urticaria, anaphylaxis, hepatic enzyme elevation/hepatitis, fixed-drug eruptions, and photosensitivity. Rhabdomyolysis has been reported after overdose with diphenhydramine and doxylamine.

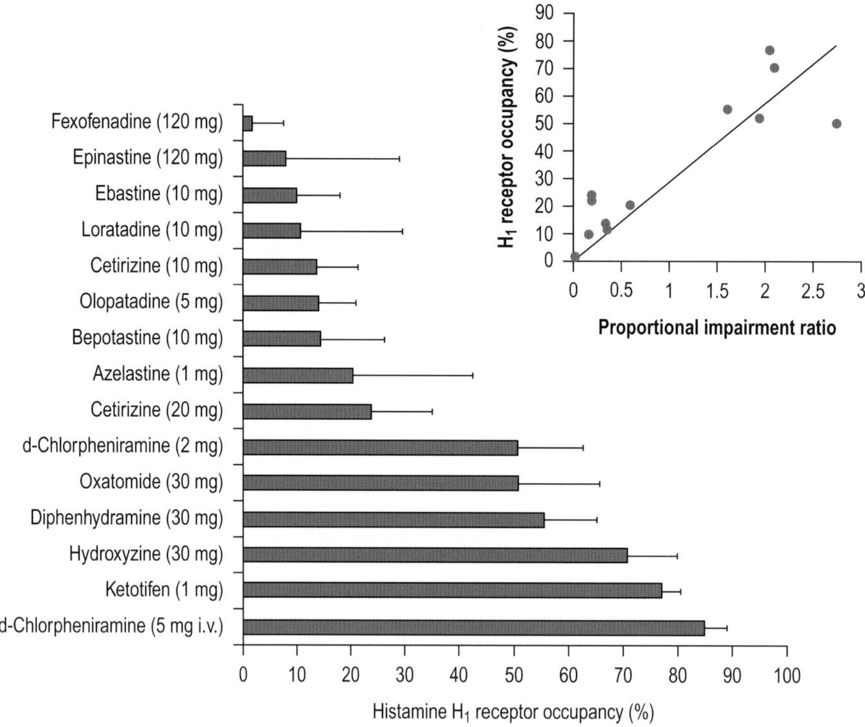

Figure 94-16 The sedative effects of H_1 antihistamines is proportional to their CNS H_1 receptor occupancy, which varies considerably among drugs in this class. H_1 receptor occupancy also varies with dose and route of administration. First-generation H_1 antihistamines such as chlorpheniramine, diphenhydramine, hydroxyzine, ketotifen, and oxatomide have the highest CNS H_1 receptor occupancy. *(From Yanai K, Zhang D, Tashiro M, et al. Positron emission tomography evaluation of sedative properties of antihistamines. Expert Opin Drug Saf 2011;10:613-22.)*

first (old)–generation H_1 antihistamines cross the BBB and occupy greater than 50% to 70% of the H_1 receptors located on the presynaptic membranes of histaminergic neurons throughout the CNS, especially in the frontal cortex, temporal cortex, hippocampus, and pons. High H_1-receptor occupancy is associated with decreased histaminergic neurotransmission and impaired CNS function on objective testing, with or without associated sedation, drowsiness, fatigue, or somnolence.[201]

Impairment can be documented in the absence of CNS symptoms, regardless of the patient population studied, the test used, the first-generation H_1 antihistamine given, or the dose given. Even in low doses such as 2 mg of chlorpheniramine 2 mg or diphenhydramine 25 mg, old H_1 antihistamines potentially impair alertness, cognition, learning, and rapid response/waking memory, especially during multitasking and performance of complex sensorimotor tasks, including divided-attention, critical tracking, and attention-switch tasks such as objectively monitored car driving.[201-207]

The likelihood of CNS adverse effects is high; after ingestion of a first-generation H_1 antihistamine in randomized double-blind crossover studies, only six participants are needed to demonstrate significant differences between an old H_1 antihistamine versus placebo or versus a new H_1 antihistamine[202] (Fig. 94-17). This contrasts with the hundreds of participants per treatment group typically required in clinical trials to demonstrate clinical efficacy versus placebo, as in allergic rhinitis. Few studies involve objective tests of CNS function in children or elderly patients, and the results are more variable in the studies in these age groups.[1,4]

The CNS adverse effects of the first (old)–generation H_1 antihistamines are underestimated by health care professionals and by patients. As with ethanol and other CNS-active chemicals and medications, impairment is often subclinical and occurs long before drowsiness is perceived. The warnings contained in the package insert for these medications (e.g., may cause drowsiness; avoid activities requiring mental alertness) are critically important in this high-technology era, in which mental alertness is required for most activities of daily life. Impaired performance on school examinations, loss of productivity in the workplace, and on-the-job injuries are attributed to first (old)–generation H_1 antihistamines. These medications are implicated as a cause of civil (i.e., noncommercial, nonmilitary) aviation accidents and fatalities, and traffic accidents and fatalities, based on documentation of elevated levels of H_1 antihistamine (e.g., chlorpheniramine) in postmortem blood and tissue samples. In some jurisdictions, motorists faulted for causing traffic fatalities can be fined or imprisoned if they have taken a first (old)–generation H_1 antihistamine. For obvious reasons, commercial and military aircraft pilots are prohibited from using these medications before or during flights.[201-206]

The adverse CNS effects of first-generation H_1 antihistamines are potentially exacerbated by concurrently ingested ethanol, benzodiazepines, and other CNS-active chemicals. Driving performance has been reported to be worse after diphenhydramine ingestion than after alcohol ingestion sufficient to produce blood alcohol levels of 0.1%.[207]

Some physicians recommend giving the old H_1 antihistamine only at bedtime so that somnolence will occur during the night. When taken at bedtime, however, these H_1 antihistamines increase the latency to onset of rapid eye movement sleep and reduce the duration of rapid eye movement sleep.[91,92,196] As noted in the previous section on Urticaria, the morning after,

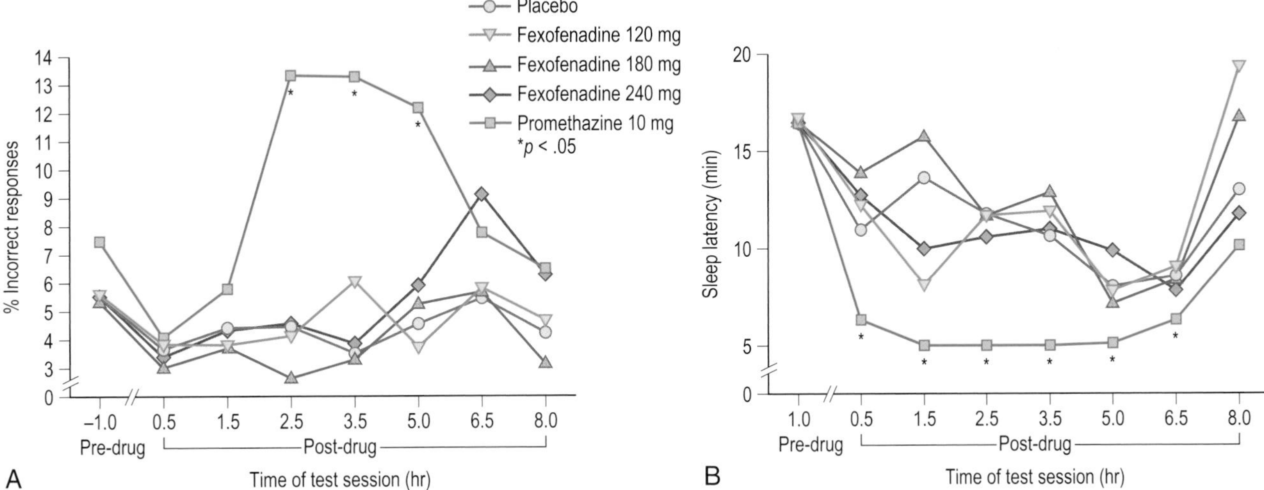

Figure 94-17 Central nervous system effects of first (old)–generation versus second (new)–generation H_1 antihistamines. First (old)–generation promethazine impairs psychomotor performance and increases sedation; second (new)–generation fexofenadine does not. In a single-dose DBPC crossover study in six participants, psychomotor performance tests included visual vigilance (**A**) and multiple sleep latency tests (**B**). Compared with fexofenadine (120, 180, and 240 mg) or placebo, promethazine (10 mg) significantly impaired vigilance at 2.5 to 5 hours and increased the likelihood of falling asleep, as assessed by electroencephalograms in the multiple sleep latency tests between 1.5 and 3.5 hours after administration. In contrast, at all test times, the effect of fexofenadine (120, 180, and 240 mg) did not differ from placebo on any test. *(Modified from data in Nicholson AN, Stone BM, Turner C, Mills SL. Antihistamines and aircrew: usefulness of fexofenadine. Aviat Space Environ Med 2000;71:2-6.)*

in patients who have CNS residual effects such as impairment with or without sedation (antihistamine hangover), PET documents residual H_1-receptor occupancy.[200] Other physicians advise regular daytime use to develop tolerance to the adverse CNS effects; however, on objective testing, tolerance may or may not be confirmed. First (old)–generation H_1 antihistamines are available in fixed-dose combination with a decongestant to counteract the sedative effects of the antihistamine, although the sedative effects typically predominate.

Second (New)–Generation H_1 Antihistamines

By definition, second-generation H_1 antihistamines do not cross the BBB readily.[92] These drugs are relatively free from adverse effects in standard doses and free from toxicity and fatality in overdose (see Table 94-4). Fexofenadine is least likely to cross the BBB; in PET studies, even in a high, off-label dose of 360 mg, it occupies CNS receptors minimally and does not impair cognitive function or cause sedation.[202,207] By definition, all the new H_1 antihistamines impair CNS function significantly less than their predecessors,[210] and in standard doses can be coadministered with alcohol, lorazepam, and other CNS-active chemicals without exacerbation of the impairment or sedation associated with these agents.[211] Some, however, such as cetirizine, loratadine, and rupatadine, may have CNS activity at higher doses.[198]

Regulatory agencies do not require screening of second (new)–generation H_1 antihistamines for potential CNS adverse effects. Information about the CNS safety of these medications can be obtained from pharmacokinetic studies performed in healthy adults, elderly patients, and those with impaired renal or hepatic function; from reported adverse events in clinical trials; and from phase IV prescription event-monitoring studies in clinical practice.[212]

Nasal and Ophthalmic H_1 Antihistamines

Nasal and ophthalmic formulations of H_1 antihistamines are minimally absorbed through the nasal mucosa or conjunctivae, respectively. After application to the nasal mucosa or the conjunctivae, first (old)–generation H_1 antihistamines (e.g., ketotifen) are significantly less sedating than after administration in oral formulations, where available for comparison.[91]

CARDIAC EFFECTS

H_1 antihistamines are among many medications that potentially prolong the QTc interval and lead to cardiac arrhythmias, including polymorphic ventricular tachycardia, with torsades de pointes, ventricular fibrillation, and even death.[46,213] Cardiac toxicity from H_1 antihistamines is not an HR1 effect but rather is caused by blockade of cardiac ion currents, such as the rapid component of the delayed outward rectifying potassium channel (I_{Kr}) or the rapid component of the inward rectifying sodium channel (I_{Na})[213] (see Table 94-4).

In overdose, first (old)–generation H_1 antihistamines potentially cause cardiac effects such as prolongation of the QTc interval, atrial and ventricular arrhythmias and may cause torsades de pointes.[214-216]

Several years after the second (new)–generation H_1 antihistamines astemizole and terfenadine were introduced for clinical use, sporadic reports linked their administration with occurrence of torsades de pointes and other potentially fatal ventricular arrhythmias. Subsequently, in most countries, regulatory approval was withdrawn for these medications. During the past 2 decades, regulatory agencies have mandated extensive testing for potential cardiac toxicity of second (new)–generation H_1 antihistamines. This scrutiny begins during the preclinical and early clinical studies of each H_1 antihistamine and continues through phase II, III, and IV studies, including long-term pharmacovigilance.[46,213]

Second (new)–generation H_1 antihistamines such as bilastine, cetirizine, desloratadine, fexofenadine, levocetirizine, loratadine, and rupatadine have been extensively investigated for potential cardiac toxicity, which has not been detected even when therapeutic doses are greatly exceeded. Lack of cardiac toxicity has also been confirmed in thousands of patients by using drug prescription event monitoring in postmarketing surveillance studies. In the rare clinical reports where cardiac toxicity has been attributed to one of these medications, causality has been deemed unlikely.[1,4,217-219]

OVERDOSE TOXICITY AND FATALITY[220-226]

Toxicity and fatality after overdose of first (old)–generation H_1 antihistamines were reported soon after these medications were introduced for clinical use 70 years ago[187] and still lead to tens of thousands of phone calls to poison control centers and emergency department visits in the United States every year. Evidence-based guidelines detail triage and management of diphenhydramine poisoning in adults and children[220,221] (see Table 94-4).

First (old)–generation H_1 antihistamines such as brompheniramine, chlorpheniramine, cyproheptadine, dimenhydrinate, diphenhydramine, and doxylamine remain widely available without prescription and are used in suicide attempts. Palatable liquid formulations have been implicated in homicides of infants and young children. After accidental or intentional overdose in infants and young children, paradoxic excitation with irritability, hyperalertness, hallucinations, and seizures typically precedes drowsiness, confusion, delirium, coma, and respiratory depression. In patients of all ages, prominent features of overdose include anticholinergic effects such as dryness of the mucous membranes, fever, flushed face, pupillary dilation, urinary retention, decreased gastrointestinal motility, hypotension, and tachycardia.[187,220-226] In patients with thin or abraded epidermis, topical H_1 antihistamines such as diphenhydramine or promethazine can produce toxic effects.[187,224]

After H_1 antihistamine overdose, monitoring of vital signs, including continuous electrocardiographic monitoring, should be instituted, and CNS function should be monitored. Supportive measures should be implemented promptly when needed. Rarely, hemodialysis is effective in facilitating H_1 antihistamine elimination.[223] In patients who have overdosed on a first (old)–generation H_1 antihistamine such as diphenhydramine, although CNS signs usually predominate, dose-dependent cardiac toxicity, including increased QTc interval and torsades de pointes, can occur.[213-216] If the QTc interval is prolonged, the patient should be monitored until it normalizes. If torsades de pointes develops, cardioversion and pacing should be instituted. In patients with H_1 antihistamine-induced cardiac toxicity, some antiarrhythmics are contraindicated because they also potentiate the QTc interval further.[1,213]

In contrast, intentional or accidental overdose of second (new)–generation H_1 antihistamines has not been reported to cause toxicity or fatality. A 6-year-old child who ingested 300 mg of loratadine and a 13-month-old child who ingested 180 mg of cetirizine developed only minimal symptoms.[4,91]

VULNERABLE PATIENTS

Many first (old)–generation H_1 antihistamines remain in widespread use in vulnerable patients with impaired hepatic or renal function, elderly people, pregnant women, infants, and children, in whom their unfavorable benefit/risk ratio has been well documented[1,4,223-241] (Table 94-5). The brain is a sensitive target in old age and elderly people are vulnerable to adverse effects from any CNS-active chemical, including first (old)–generation H_1 antihistamines. In hospitalized elderly patients, diphenhydramine administration has been associated with an increased risk of cognitive decline, delirium, inattention, disorganized speech, altered consciousness, and need for urinary catheter placement.[228-230]

During pregnancy, H_1 antihistamines are used for symptomatic treatment of rhinitis and urticaria, and as noted previously, the first (old)–generation H_1 antihistamine doxylamine is used to prevent nausea and vomiting. All H_1 antihistamines cross the placenta. Their relative risk with regard to causing teratogenicity when taken in the first trimester is briefly reviewed in Table 94-5. Practical information about the safety of H_1 antihistamine use in pregnancy based on prospective controlled observational studies is summarized (and updated regularly) at the Motherisk Program (http://www.motherisk.org/women/index.jsp) and the Pregnancy Healthline.[231-233] Pregnant women who receive large therapeutic doses or take an overdose of a first (old)–generation H_1 antihistamine (e.g., diphenhydramine) can experience oxytocin-like effects and uterine contractions as well as other symptoms and signs of toxicity. Maternal ingestion of a first (old)–generation H_1 antihistamine before parturition can lead to irritability, tremulousness, seizures, and respiratory depression in the neonate. H_1 antihistamines are excreted in small amounts (less than 0.1% of a maternal dose) in breast milk. Nursing infants whose mothers have ingested first-generation H_1 antihistamines can experience irritability or drowsiness. In contrast, after maternal ingestion of second (new)–generation H_1 antihistamines, neonates and nursing infants have not been reported to develop symptoms.[1,4]

Adverse effects, toxicity, and fatalities from first (old)–generation H_1 antihistamines such as diphenhydramine in infants and children have been reported since the 1940s and 1950s.[187] In this population, few short-term and no long-term RCTs of efficacy and safety of old H_1 medications are available. Most publications relate to their adverse effects. First-generation drugs are widely used off-label in atopic dermatitis, cough, colds, and otitis media, despite lack of evidence for their efficacy and safety in these disorders. They are often given in mixtures containing decongestants, analgesics, and other drugs. In some countries, regulatory agencies have mandated that many of these medications be withdrawn from the market or relabeled as "not safe for use in children less than 6 years of age."[223-226,234,235] In contrast, second (new)–generation H_1 antihistamines such as cetirizine, desloratadine, levocetirizine, and loratadine have been relatively well studied in the pediatric population, including a short-term RCT of cetirizine in infants age 6 to 11 months.[237] In randomized DBPC studies in atopic children age 1 to 3 years, no long-term effects on behavioral, cognitive, or psychomotor development have been found after cetirizine or levocetirizine administration daily for 18 months.[238-240] A 12-month RCT of loratadine in young children documented no safety concerns[241] (see Table 94-5).

Summary and Future Directions

The cells involved in the regulation of immune responses and hematopoiesis express histamine receptors and also secrete histamine. Histamine can selectively recruit the major effector cells into tissue sites and affect their maturation, activation, polarization, and other functions, leading to chronic inflammation. Histamine also regulates dendritic cells, T cells, and B cells,

TABLE 94-5 H_1 Antihistamines: Potential Adverse Effects in Vulnerable Patients

Population	First (Old)–Generation H_1 Antihistamines	Second (New)–Generation H_1 Antihistamines
Patients with impaired hepatic or renal function	Few prospective studies are available. In these patients, including those receiving hemodialysis, use of standard doses may be associated with adverse effects, including central nervous system (CNS) effects (e.g., impaired cognitive function, drowsiness).	Clinical pharmacology (absorption, distribution, metabolism, elimination) of most medications has been studied prospectively in these patients; specific instructions for reduction in dose or dose frequency are provided where relevant.
Elderly people	Few randomized controlled trials of first (old)–generation H_1 antihistamines are available. Elderly patients often use these drugs, which may impair cognition and memory and cause inattention, disorganized speech, falls, incontinence, sedation, altered consciousness, and delirium.	Clinical pharmacology of most medications has been studied prospectively in elderly patients; specific instructions for reduction in dose or dose frequency are provided where relevant.
Pregnant and lactating women*	With regard to teratogenicity, these drugs are classified as FDA Pregnancy Category B (chlorpheniramine, diphenhydramine) or C (hydroxyzine, ketotifen). In nursing infants, these drugs potentially cause irritability or drowsiness.	With regard to teratogenicity, these medications are classified as FDA Pregnancy Category B (alcaftadine, cetirizine, emedastine, loratadine) or C (azelastine, bepotastine, desloratadine, epinastine, fexofenadine, levocetirizine, olopatadine). No adverse CNS effects reported in nursing infants.
Neonates	When given to the mother immediately before parturition, these medications potentially cause irritability, seizures, drowsiness, and respiratory depression in the neonate.	No CNS adverse effects reported in neonates.
Infants and young children	These drugs are often assumed to be effective and safe in infants and children with allergies, coughs, and colds, either alone or in a mixture with other medications, but are often associated with adverse effects and occasionally with fatalities.† Since 2006, regulatory agencies in the U.S. and other countries have mandated that more than 1500 pediatric oral allergy, cough, and cold formulations containing first (old)–generation H_1 antihistamines be withdrawn from the market or relabeled as "not safe for use in children less than 6 years."	Long-term safety of cetirizine, desloratadine, fexofenadine, levocetirizine, and loratadine has been confirmed in young children.

*No medications, including H_1 antihistamines, are classified as Pregnancy Category A (no risk) by the U.S. Food and Drug Administration (FDA). The Pregnancy Category B designation means that medications are not teratogenic in animals and are therefore thought to be relatively low risk in humans. Pregnancy Category C designates "teratogenicity in animals/adequate information about use in human pregnancies not yet available/should therefore be used during pregnancy only if the expected benefits to the mother exceed the unknown risks to the fetus."

†First (old)–generation H_1 antihistamines, particularly the phenothiazine class, have been associated with sudden infant death syndrome and apparent life-threatening events, although causality has never been proved.

related antibody isotype responses, and through HR2, it positively interferes with the peripheral antigen tolerance induced by Treg cells. The diverse effects of histamine on immune regulation are caused by differential expression and regulation of four types of histamine receptors and their distinct intracellular signals. In addition, differences in affinity of these receptors for histamine are decisive for the biologic effects of histamine and drugs that target histamine receptors.

At H_1 receptors, the molecular mechanisms of action of histamine and H_1 antihistamines involve inverse agonism. Second (new)–generation H_1 antihistamines are preferred to first (old)–generation H_1 antihistamines in the treatment of allergic rhinitis, allergic conjunctivitis, and urticaria because the new H_1 antihistamines have been investigated extensively with regard to clinical pharmacology, efficacy, and safety. They are significantly less likely to impair CNS function or cause sedation or other adverse effects. The second-generation drugs are not causally linked with fatalities after overdose. Important advances include introduction of high (up to fourfold) doses of some second (new)–generation H_1 antihistamines for effective and safe chronic urticaria treatment and nasal and ophthalmic formulations with rapid onset of action (minutes) for allergic rhinitis and conjunctivitis. Using PET to study H_1 antihistamine penetration in the human brain, CNS H_1-receptor occupancy can now be directly related to CNS functional effects. Oral first (old)–generation H_1 antihistamines are contraindicated in anyone who requires alertness and ability to learn, remember, and perform complex tasks. Despite safety concerns, the old H_1 antihistamines remain in use for insomnia and other CNS disorders as well asfor motion sickness and other vestibular disorders.

Further research is needed into the molecular mechanisms of action of H_1 antihistamines as inverse agonists and the molecular basis of their specificity for the H_1 receptor. Additional clinical pharmacology studies and high-quality RCTs of H_1 antihistamine efficacy and safety are needed, especially comparative studies of different second (new)–generation H_1 antihistamines in allergic rhinitis, allergic conjunctivitis, chronic urticaria, and prevention of allergic reactions, and additional RCTs in infants, children, and the elderly. Further comparative PET studies of old and new H_1 antihistamines need to correlate BBB penetration and CNS H_1-receptor occupancy as well as CNS functional effects. Ongoing prospective observational studies of the safety of second (new)–generation H_1 antihistamines are required in pregnancy.[58,123]

Regarding other HR antihistamines, the H_3 antihistamines lead to an increase in norepinephrine and might have an advantageous decongestant effect in patients with allergic rhinitis, administered with or without H_1 antihistamines. The H_4 antihistamines might play an important role in the downregulation of inflammation in patients with allergic rhinitis, administered with or without H_1 antihistamines, in patients with atopic dermatitis, asthma, and other chronic inflammatory diseases. Accelerated investigation of H_3 antihistamines and H_4 antihistamines in allergic diseases is needed.[242-250]

Acknowledgments

The authors thank Dr. Mübeccel Akdis, Dr. Marek Jutel, and Dr. Keith J. Simons for insightful discussions and long-term collaboration. They also acknowledge the assistance of Lori McNiven.

REFERENCES

Introduction

1. Simons FER, Akdis CA. Histamine and H_1-antihistamines. In: Adkinson NF Jr, Bochner BS, Busse WW, et al, editors. Middleton's allergy: principles and practice. 7th ed. St Louis: Mosby; 2009. p. 1517-47.
2. Simons FER, Simons KJ. Histamine and H_1-antihistamines: celebrating a century of progress. J Allergy Clin Immunol 2011;128:1139-50.
3. O'Mahony L, Akdis M, Akdis CA. Regulation of the immune response and inflammation by histamine and histamine receptors. J Allergy Clin Immunol 2011;128:1153-62.
4. Simons FER. Advances in H_1-antihistamines. N Engl J Med 2004;351:2203-17.
5. Jutel M, Blaser K, Akdis CA. Histamine receptors in immune regulation and allergen-specific immunotherapy. Immunol Allergy Clin North Am 2006;26:249-59.
6. Akdis CA, Simons FER. Histamine receptors are hot in immunopharmacology. Eur J Pharmacol 2006;533:69-76.
7. Jutel M, Watanabe T, Klunker S, et al. Histamine regulates T-cell and antibody responses by differential expression of H1 and H2 receptors. Nature 2001;413:420-5.
8. Banu Y, Watanabe T. Augmentation of antigen receptor-mediated responses by histamine H_1 receptor signaling. J Exp Med 1999;189:673-82.
9. Shimamura T, Shiroishi M, Weyand S, et al. Structure of the human histamine H_1 receptor complex with doxepin. Nature 2011;475:65-70.
10. Nijmeijer S, Leurs R, Vischer HF. Constitutive activity of the histamine H(1) receptor. Methods Enzymol 2010;484:127-47.
11. Dy M, Lebel B, Kamoun P, Hamburger J. Histamine production during the anti-allograft response: demonstration of a new lymphokine enhancing histamine synthesis. J Exp Med 1981;153:293-309.
12. Kubo Y, Nakano K. Regulation of histamine synthesis in mouse $CD4^+$ and $CD8^+$ T lymphocytes. Inflamm Res 1999;48:149-53.
13. Radvany Z, Darvas Z, Kerekes K, et al. H_1 histamine receptor antagonist inhibits constitutive growth of Jurkat T cells and antigen-specific proliferation of ovalbumin-specific murine T cells. Semin Cancer Biol 2000;10:41-5.

Molecular Basis of Histamine Action

14. Dale HH, Laidlaw PP. The physiological action of beta-iminazolylethylamine. J Physiol 1910;41:318-44.
15. Dy M, Schneider E. Histamine-cytokine connection in immunity and hematopoiesis. Cytokine Growth Factor Rev 2004;15:393-410.
16. Schneider E, Rolli-Derkinderen M, Arock M, Dy M. Trends in histamine research: new functions during immune responses and hematopoiesis. Trends Immunol 2002;23:255-63.
17. MacGlashan D Jr. Histamine: a mediator of inflammation. J Allergy Clin Immunol 2003;112:S53-9.
18. Jutel M, Watanabe T, Akdis M, Blaser K, Akdis CA. Immune regulation by histamine. Curr Opin Immunol 2002;14:735-40.
19. Akdis CA, Blaser K. Histamine in the immune regulation of allergic inflammation. J Allergy Clin Immunol 2003;112:15-22.
20. Higuchi M, Yanai K, Okamura N, et al. Histamine H(1) receptors in patients with Alzheimer's disease assessed by positron emission tomography. Neuroscience 2000;99:721-9.
21. Endo Y. Simultaneous induction of histidine and ornithine decarboxylases and changes in their product amines following the injection of *Escherichia coli* lipopolysaccharide into mice. Biochem Pharmacol 1982;31:1643-7.
22. Nakagawa S, Okaya Y, Yatsunami K, et al. Identification of multiple regulatory elements of human L-histidine decarboxylase gene. J Biochem 1997;121:935-40.
23. Hocker M, Henihan RJ, Rosewicz S, et al. Gastrin and phorbol 12-myristate 13-acetate regulate the human histidine decarboxylase promoter through Raf-dependent activation of extracellular signal-regulated kinase-related signaling pathways in gastric cancer cells. J Biol Chem 1997;272:27015-24.
24. Ohtsu H, Kuramasu A, Suzuki S, et al. Histidine decarboxylase expression in mouse mast cell line P815 is induced by mouse peritoneal cavity incubation. J Biol Chem 1996;271:28439-44.
25. Kuramasu A, Saito H, Suzuki S, Watanabe T, Ohtsu H. Mast cell–/basophil-specific transcriptional regulation of human L-histidine decarboxylase gene by CpG methylation in the promoter region. J Biol Chem 1998;273:31607-14.
26. Szeberenyi JB, Pallinger E, Zsinko M, et al. Inhibition of effects of endogenously synthesized histamine disturbs in vitro human dendritic cell differentiation. Immunol Lett 2001;76:175-82.
27. Yoshimoto T, Tsutsui H, Tominaga K, et al. IL-18, although antiallergic when administered with IL-12, stimulates IL-4 and histamine release by basophils. Proc Natl Acad Sci USA 1999;96:13962-6.
28. Ohtsu H, Tanaka S, Terui T, et al. Mice lacking histidine decarboxylase exhibit abnormal mast cells. FEBS Lett 2001;502:53-6.
29. Tanaka S, Takasu Y, Mikura S, Satoh N, Ichikawa A. Antigen-independent induction of histamine synthesis by immunoglobulin E in mouse bone marrow–derived mast cells. J Exp Med 2002;196:229-35.
30. Yang XD, Ai W, Asfaha S, et al. Histamine deficiency promotes inflammation-associated carcinogenesis through reduced myeloid maturation and accumulation of $CD11b^+Ly6G^+$ immature myeloid cells. Nat Med 2011;17:87-95.

Histamine Receptors

31. Ash AS, Schild HO. Receptors mediating some actions of histamine. Br J Pharmacol Chemother 1966;27:427-39; Br J Pharmacol 1997;120(Suppl. 4):302-14 (reprint).
32. Lovenberg TW, Roland BL, Wilson SJ, et al. Cloning and functional expression of the human histamine H_3 receptor. Mol Pharmacol 1999;55:1101-7.
33. Oda T, Morikawa N, Saito Y, Masuho Y, Matsumoto S. Molecular cloning and characterization of a novel type of histamine receptor preferentially expressed in leukocytes. J Biol Chem 2000;275:36781-6.
34. Le Coniat M, Traiffort E, Ruat M, Arrang JM, Berger R. Chromosomal localization of the human histamine H_1-receptor gene. Hum Genet 1994;94:186-8.
35. Nakamura T, Itadani H, Hidaka Y, Ohta M, Tanaka K. Molecular cloning and characterization of a new human histamine receptor, HH4R. Biochem Biophys Res Commun 2000;279:615-20.
36. Milligan G, Bond RA, Lee M. Inverse agonism: pharmacological curiosity or potential therapeutic strategy? Trends Pharmacol Sci 1995;16:10-3.
37. Paesen GC, Adams PL, Harlos K, Nuttall PA, Stuart DI. Tick histamine-binding proteins: isolation, cloning, and three-dimensional structure. Mol Cell 1999;3:661-71.
38. Yeh YC, Xie L, Langdon JM, et al. The effects of overexpression of histamine releasing factor (HRF) in a transgenic mouse model. PLoS One 2010;5:e11077.
39. Kashiwakura J, Ando T, Matsumoto K, et al. Histamine-releasing factor has a proinflammatory role in mouse models of asthma and allergy. J Clin Invest 2012;122:218-28.
40. Togias A. H_1-receptors: localization and role in airway physiology and in immune functions. J Allergy Clin Immunol 2003;112:S60-8.
41. Leurs R, Smit MJ, Timmerman H. Molecular and pharmacological aspects of histamine receptors. Pharmacol Ther 1995;66:413-63.
42. Smit MJ, Hoffmann M, Timmerman H, Leurs R. Molecular properties and signalling pathways of the histamine H_1 receptor. Clin Exp Allergy 1999;29(Suppl 3):19-28.
43. Bakker RA, Schoonus SB, Smit MJ, Timmerman H, Leurs R. Histamine H_1-receptor activation of nuclear factor-τB: roles for Gβτ and $G\alpha_{q/11}$ subunits in constitutive and agonist-mediated signaling. Mol Pharmacol 2001;60:1133-42.
44. Aoki Y, Qiu D, Zhao GH, Kao PN. Leukotriene B4 mediates histamine induction of NF-κB and IL-8 in human bronchial epithelial cells. Am J Physiol 1998;274:L1030-9.
45. Hall IP. Pharmacogenetics of asthma. Eur Respir J 2000;15:449-51.
46. Leurs R, Church MK, Taglialatela M. H_1-antihistamines: inverse agonism, anti-inflammatory actions and cardiac effects. Clin Exp Allergy 2002;32:489-98.
47. Vanbervliet B, Akdis M, Vocanson M, et al. Histamine receptor H_1 signaling on dendritic cells plays a key role in the IFN-γ/IL-17 balance in T cell–mediated skin inflammation. J Allergy Clin Immunol 2011;127:943-53.e1-10.

48. Yanai K, Son LZ, Endou M, Sakurai E, Watanabe T. Targeting disruption of histamine H_1 receptors in mice: behavioral and neurochemical characterization. Life Sci 1998;62:1607-10.
49. Johansen P, Weiss A, Bunter A, et al. Clemastine causes immune suppression through inhibition of extracellular signal-regulated kinase-dependent proinflammatory cytokines. J Allergy Clin Immunol 2011;128:1286-94.
50. Del Valle J, Gantz I. Novel insights into histamine H_2 receptor biology. Am J Physiol 1997; 273:G987-96.
51. Plaut M, Liu MC, Conrad DH, et al. Histamine release from human basophils is induced by IgE-dependent factor(s) derived from human lung macrophages and an Fc epsilon receptor-positive human B cell line. Trans Assoc Am Physicians 1985;98:305-12.
52. Novak N, Mete N, Bussmann C, et al. Early suppression of basophil activation during allergen-specific immunotherapy by histamine receptor 2. J Allergy Clin Immunol 2012;130: 1153-8.
53. Drutel G, Peitsaro N, Karlstedt K, et al. Identification of rat H_3 receptor isoforms with different brain expression and signaling properties. Mol Pharmacol 2001;59:1-8.
54. Dimitriadou V, Rouleau A, Dam Trung Tuong M, et al. Functional relationship between mast cells and C-sensitive nerve fibres evidenced by histamine H_3-receptor modulation in rat lung and spleen. Clin Sci (Lond) 1994;87:151-63.
55. Leurs R, Bakker RA, Timmerman H, de Esch IJP. The histamine H_3 receptor: from gene cloning to H_3 receptor drugs. Nat Rev Drug Discov 2005;4:107-20.
56. Teuscher C, Subramanian M, Noubade R, et al. Central histamine H_3 receptor signaling negatively regulates susceptibility to autoimmune inflammatory disease of the CNS. Proc Natl Acad Sci USA 2007;104:10146-51.
57. Zhu Y, Michalovich D, Wu H, et al. Cloning, expression, and pharmacological characterization of a novel human histamine receptor. Mol Pharmacol 2001;59:434-41.
58. Thurmond RL, Gelfand EW, Dunford PJ. The role of histamine H_1 and H_4 receptors in allergic inflammation: the search for new antihistamines. Nat Rev Drug Discov 2008;7:41-53.
59. Nguyen T, Shapiro DA, George SR, et al. Discovery of a novel member of the histamine receptor family. Mol Pharmacol 2001;59: 427-33.
60. Brandes LJ, Queen GM, LaBella FS. Displacement of histamine from liver cells and cell components by ligands for cytochromes P450. J Cell Biochem 2002;85:820-4.
61. Tamasi V, Fulop AK, Hegyi K, Monostory K, Falus A. Upregulation of CYP2e1 and CYP3a activities in histamine-deficient histidine decarboxylase gene targeted mice. Cell Biol Int 2003;27:1011-5.
62. Kazumori H, Ishihara S, Rumi MAK, et al. Transforming growth factor-alpha directly augments histidine decarboxylase and vesicular monoamine transporter 2 production in rat enterochromaffin-like cells. Am J Physiol Gastrointest Liver Physiol 2004;286:G508-14.

Histamine in Immune Response Regulation

63. Akdis M, Simon HU, Weigl L, et al. Skin homing (cutaneous lymphocyte-associated antigen-positive) $CD8_+$ T cells respond to superantigen and contribute to eosinophilia and IgE production in atopic dermatitis. J Immunol 1999;163:466-75.
64. Abernathy-Carver KJ, Sampson HA, Picker LJ, Leung DY. Milk-induced eczema is associated with the expansion of T cells expressing cutaneous lymphocyte antigen. J Clin Invest 1995; 95:913-8.
65. Takahashi HK, Iwagaki H, Mori S, et al. Histamine inhibits lipopolysaccharide-induced interleukin (IL)-18 production in human monocytes. Clin Immunol 2004;112:30-4.
66. Morichika T, Takahashi HK, Iwagaki H, et al. Histamine inhibits lipopolysaccharide-induced tumor necrosis factor-alpha production in an intercellular adhesion molecule-1- and B7.1-dependent manner. J Pharmacol Exp Ther 2003;304:624-33.
67. Mazzoni A, Young HA, Spitzer JH, Visintin A, Segal DM. Histamine regulates cytokine production in maturing dendritic cells, resulting in altered T cell polarization. J Clin Invest 2001;108:1865-73.
68. Ohtani T, Aiba S, Mizuashi M, et al. H_1 and H_2 histamine receptors are absent on Langerhans cells and present on dermal dendritic cells. J Invest Dermatol 2003;121:1073-9.
69. Dijkstra D, Stark H, Chazot PL, et al. Human inflammatory dendritic epidermal cells express a functional histamine H_4 receptor. J Invest Dermatol 2008;128:1696-703.
70. Hellings PW, Vandenberghe P, Kasran A, et al. Blockade of CTLA-4 enhances allergic sensitization and eosinophilic airway inflammation in genetically predisposed mice. Eur J Immunol 2002;32:585-94.
71. Osna N, Elliott K, Khan MM. Regulation of interleukin-10 secretion by histamine in TH2 cells and splenocytes. Int Immunopharmacol 2001;1:85-96.
72. Akdis CA, Blesken T, Akdis M, Wuthrich B, Blaser K. Role of interleukin 10 in specific immunotherapy. J Clin Invest 1998;102: 98-106.
73. Jutel M, Akdis M, Budak F, et al. IL-10 and TGF-β cooperate in the regulatory T cell response to mucosal allergens in normal immunity and specific immunotherapy. Eur J Immunol 2003;33:1205-14.
74. Meiler F, Zumkehr J, Klunker S, et al. In vivo switch to IL-10-secreting T regulatory cells in high dose allergen exposure. J Exp Med 2008;205:2887-98.
75. Simon T, Gogolák P, Kis-Tóth K, et al. Histamine modulates multiple functional activities of monocyte-derived dendritic cell subsets via histamine receptor 2. Int Immunol 2012;24: 107-16.
76. Kunzmann S, Mantel PY, Wohlfahrt JG, et al. Histamine enhances TGF-β1-mediated suppression of Th2 responses. FASEB J 2003; 17:1089-95.
77. Morgan RK, McAllister B, Cross L, et al. Histamine 4 receptor activation induces recruitment of $FoxP3^+$ T cells and inhibits allergic asthma in a murine model. J Immunol 2007; 178:8081-9.
78. Muller U, Hari Y, Berchtold E. Premedication with antihistamines may enhance efficacy of specific-allergen immunotherapy. J Allergy Clin Immunol 2001;107:81-6.
79. Jutel M, Zak-Nejmark T, Wrzyszcz M. Histamine receptor expression on peripheral blood $CD4_+$ lymphocytes is influenced by ultra-rush bee venom immunotherapy. Allergy 1997;52 (Suppl. 37):88.
80. Muller UR, Jutel M, Reimers A, et al. Clinical and immunologic effects of H_1 antihistamine preventive medication during honeybee venom immunotherapy. J Allergy Clin Immunol 2008; 122:1001-7.
81. Gifford RR, Schmidtke JR. Cimetidine-induced augmentation of human lymphocyte blastogenesis: comparison with levamisole in mitogen stimulation. Surg Forum 1979;30: 113-5.
82. Emerson MR, Orentas DM, Lynch SG, LeVine SM. Activation of histamine H_2 receptors ameliorates experimental allergic encephalomyelitis. NeuroReport 2002;13:1407-10.

Clinical Pharmacology of H_1 Antihistamines

83. Church MK. Comparative inhibition by bilastine and cetirizine of histamine-induced wheal and flare responses in humans. Inflamm Res 2011;60:1107-12.
84. Horak F, Zieglmayer P, Zieglmayer R, Lemell P. The effects of bilastine compared with cetirizine, fexofenadine, and placebo on allergen-induced nasal and ocular symptoms in patients exposed to aeroallergen in the Vienna Challenge Chamber. Inflamm Res 2010;59:391-8.
85. Church MK. Efficacy and tolerability of rupatadine at four times the recommended dose against histamine- and platelet-activating factor-induced flare responses and ex vivo platelet aggregation in healthy males. Br J Dermatol 2010;163:1330-2.
86. Pena J, Carbo ML, Solans A, et al. Antihistaminic effects of rupatadine and PKPD modelling. Eur J Drug Metab Pharmacokinet 2008; 33:107-16.
87. Bohets H, McGowan C, Mannens G, et al. Clinical pharmacology of alcaftadine, a novel antihistamine for the prevention of allergic conjunctivitis. J Ocul Pharmacol Ther 2011; 27:187-95.
88. Abelson MB, Torkildsen GL, Williams JI, et al. Time to onset and duration of action of the antihistamine bepotastine besilate ophthalmic solutions 1.0% and 1.5% in allergic conjunctivitis: a phase III, single-center, prospective, randomized, double-masked, placebo-controlled, conjunctival allergen challenge assessment in adults and children. Clin Ther 2009;31:1908-21.
89. Torkildsen GL, Williams JI, Gow JA, et al. Bepotastine besilate ophthalmic solution for the relief of nonocular symptoms provoked by conjunctival allergen challenge. Ann Allergy Asthma Immunol 2010;105:57-64.
90. Chen C, Hanson E, Watson JW, Lee JS. P-glycoprotein limits the brain penetration of nonsedating but not sedating H_1-antagonists. Drug Metab Dispos 2003;31:312-8.
91. Church MK, Maurer M, Simons FER, et al. Risk of first-generation H_1-antihistamines: a GA(2)LEN position paper. Allergy 2010;65: 459-66.
92. Yanai K, Zhang D, Tashiro M, et al. Positron emission tomography evaluation of sedative properties of antihistamines. Expert Opin Drug Saf 2011;10:613-22.
93. Rodrigues WC, Castro C, Catbagan P, Moore C, Wang G. Immunoassay screening of diphenhydramine (Benadryl) in urine and blood using a newly developed assay. J Anal Toxicol 2012;36:123-9.
94. Church MK, Gillard M, Sargentini-Maier ML, et al. From pharmacokinetics to therapeutics. Drug Metab Rev 2009;41:455-74.
95. Simons FER, Simons KJ. Levocetirizine: pharmacokinetics and pharmacodynamics in children age 6 to 11 years. J Allergy Clin Immunol 2005;116:355-61.

96. Devillier P, Roche N, Faisy C. Clinical pharmacokinetics and pharmacodynamics of desloratadine, fexofenadine and levocetirizine: a comparative review. Clin Pharmacokinet 2008; 47:217-30.
97. Phan H, Moeller ML, Nahata MC. Treatment of allergic rhinitis in infants and children: efficacy and safety of second-generation antihistamines and the leukotriene receptor antagonist montelukast. Drugs 2009;69:2541-76.
98. Bailey DG. Fruit juice inhibition of uptake transport: a new type of food-drug interaction. Br J Clin Pharmacol 2010;70:645-55.
99. Shon JH, Yoon YR, Hong WS, et al. Effect of itraconazole on the pharmacokinetics and pharmacodynamics of fexofenadine in relation to the MDR1 genetic polymorphism. Clin Pharmacol Ther 2005;78:191-201.
100. Gupta SK, Kantesaria B, Banfield C, Wang Z. Desloratadine dose selection in children aged 6 months to 2 years: comparison of population pharmacokinetics between children and adults. Br J Clin Pharmacol 2007;64:174-84.
101. Day JH, Ellis AK, Rafeiro E, Ratz JD, Briscoe MP. Experimental models for the evaluation of treatment of allergic rhinitis. Ann Allergy Asthma Immunol 2006;96:263-77.
102. Hyo S, Fujieda S, Kawada R, Kitazawa S, Takenaka H. The efficacy of short-term administration of 3 antihistamines vs. placebo under natural exposure to Japanese cedar pollen. Ann Allergy Asthma Immunol 2005; 94:457-64.
103. Jones DH, Romero FA, Casale TB. Time-dependent inhibition of histamine-induced cutaneous responses by oral and intramuscular diphenhydramine and oral fexofenadine. Ann Allergy Asthma Immunol 2008;100:452-6.
104. Church MK, Maurer M. H_1-antihistamines and urticaria: how can we predict the best drug for our patient? Clin Exp Allergy 2012;42: 1423-9.
105. Frossard N, Strolin-Benedetti M, Purohit A, Pauli G. Inhibition of allergen-induced wheal and flare reactions by levocetirizine and desloratadine. Br J Clin Pharmacol 2008;65:172-9.
106. Simons FER, Silver NA, Gu X, Simons KJ. Skin concentrations of H_1-receptor antagonists. J Allergy Clin Immunol 2001;107: 526-30.
107. Gillman S, Gillard M, Strolin Benedetti M. The concept of receptor occupancy to predict clinical efficacy: a comparison of second-generation H_1 antihistamines. Allergy Asthma Proc 2009; 30:366-76.
108. Simons KJ, Strolin-Benedetti M, Simons FER, Gillard M, Baltes E. Relevance of H_1-receptor occupancy to antihistamine dosing in children. J Allergy Clin Immunol 2007;119:1551-4.

Allergic Rhinitis

109. Drugs for allergic disorders. Treat Guidel Med Lett 2010;8:9-18.
110. Brozek JL, Bousquet J, Baena-Cagnani CE, et al. Allergic rhinitis and its impact on asthma (ARIA) guidelines: 2010 revision. J Allergy Clin Immunol 2010;126:466-76.
111. Scadding GK, Durham SR, Mirakian R, et al. BSACI guidelines for the management of allergic and non-allergic rhinitis. Clin Exp Allergy 2008;38:19-42.
112. Wallace DV, Dykewicz MS, Bernstein DI, et al. The diagnosis and management of rhinitis: an updated practice parameter. J Allergy Clin Immunol 2008;122:S1-84.
113. Hoyte FCL, Katial RK. Antihistamine therapy in allergic rhinitis. Immunol Allergy Clin North Am 2011;31:509-43.
114. Bousquet J, Bachert C, Canonica GW, et al. Efficacy of desloratadine in persistent allergic rhinitis: A GA[2]LEN study. Int Arch Allergy Immunol 2010;153:395-402.
115. Canonica GW, Fumagalli F, Guerra L, et al. Levocetirizine in persistent allergic rhinitis: continuous or on-demand use? A pilot study. Curr Med Res Opin 2008;24:2829-39.
116. Laekeman G, Simoens S, Buffels J, et al. Continuous versus on-demand pharmacotherapy of allergic rhinitis: evidence and practice. Respir Med 2010;104:615-25.
117. Mosges R, Konig V, Koberlein J. The effectiveness of levocetirizine in comparison with loratadine in treatment of allergic rhinitis: a meta-analysis. Allergol Int 2011;60:541-6.
118. Bachert C, Bousquet J, Canonica GW, et al. Levocetirizine improves quality of life and reduces costs in long-term management of persistent allergic rhinitis. J Allergy Clin Immunol 2004;114:838-44.
119. Bachert C. A review of the efficacy of desloratadine, fexofenadine, and levocetirizine in the treatment of nasal congestion in patients with allergic rhinitis. Clin Ther 2009;31: 921-44.
120. Fantin S, Maspero J, Bisbal C, et al. A 12-week placebo-controlled study of rupatadine 10 mg once daily compared with cetirizine 10 mg once daily, in the treatment of persistent allergic rhinitis. Allergy 2008;63:924-31.
121. Bousquet J, Ansotegui I, Canonica CW, et al. Establishing the place in therapy of bilastine in the treatment of allergic rhinitis according to ARIA: evidence review. Curr Med Res Opin 2012;28:131-39.
122. Grubbe RE, Lumry WR, Anolik R. Efficacy and safety of desloratadine/pseudoephedrine combination vs. its components in seasonal allergic rhinitis. J Investig Allergol Clin Immunol 2009;19:117-24.
123. Stokes JR, Romero FA Jr, Allan RJ, et al. The effects of an H_3 receptor antagonist (PF-03654746) with fexofenadine on reducing allergic rhinitis symptoms. J Allergy Clin Immunol 2012;129:409-12.
124. Benninger M, Farrar JR, Blaiss M, et al. Evaluating approved medications to treat allergic rhinitis in the United States: an evidence-based review of efficacy for nasal symptoms by class. Ann Allergy Asthma Immunol 2010;104: 13-29.
125. Greiner AN, Meltzer EO. Overview of the treatment of allergic rhinitis and nonallergic rhinopathy. Proc Am Thorac Soc 2011;8:121-31.
126. Hay JW, Kaliner MA. Costs of second-generation antihistamines in the treatment of allergic rhinitis: U.S. perspective. Curr Med Res Opin 2009;25:1421-31.
127. Bousquet J, Bachert C, Canonica GW, et al. Unmet needs in severe chronic upper airway disease (SCUAD). J Allergy Clin Immunol 2009;124:428-33.
128. Kaliner MA, Berger WE, Ratner PH, Siegel CJ. The efficacy of intranasal antihistamines in the treatment of allergic rhinitis. Ann Allergy Asthma Immunol 2011;106:S6-11.
129. Shah SR, Nayak A, Ratner P, et al. Effects of olopatadine hydrochloride nasal spray 0.6% in the treatment of seasonal allergic rhinitis: a phase III, multicenter, randomized, double-blind, active- and placebo-controlled study in adolescents and adults. Clin Ther 2009;31: 99-107.
130. Lieberman P, Meltzer EO, LaForce CF, Darter AL, Tort MJ. Two-week comparison study of olopatadine hydrochloride nasal spray 0.6% versus azelastine hydrochloride nasal spray 0.1% in patients with vasomotor rhinitis. Allergy Asthma Proc 2011;32:151-8.
131. Hellings PW, Dobbels F, Denhaerynck K, et al. Explorative study on patient's perceived knowledge level, expectations, preferences, and fear of side effects for treatment for allergic rhinitis. Clin Transl Allergy 2012;2:9.
132. Carr W, Bernstein J, Lieberman P, et al. A novel intranasal therapy of azelastine with fluticasone for the treatment of allergic rhinitis. J Allergy Clin Immunol 2012;129:1282-9.

Allergic Conjunctivitis

133. Bielory L, Friedlaender MH. Allergic conjunctivitis. Immunol Allergy Clin North Am 2008; 28:43-58.
134. Mantelli F, Lambiase A, Bonini S, Bonini S. Clinical trials in allergic conjunctivitis: a systematic review. Allergy 2011;66:919-24.
135. Greiner JV, Edwards-Swanson K, Ingerman A. Evaluation of alcaftadine 0.25% ophthalmic solution in acute allergic conjunctivitis at 15 minutes and 16 hours after instillation versus placebo and olopatadine 0.1%. Clin Ophthalmol 2011;5:87-93.
136. Torkildsen G, Shedden A. The safety and efficacy of alcaftadine 0.25% ophthalmic solution for the prevention of itching associated with allergic conjunctivitis. Curr Med Res Opin 2011;27:623-31.
137. Mahvan TD, Buckley WA, Hornecker JR. Alcaftadine for the prevention of itching associated with allergic conjunctivitis. Ann Pharmacother 2012;46:1025-32.
138. Lambiase A, Micera A, Bonini S. Multiple action agents and the eye: do they really stabilize mast cells? Curr Opin Allergy Clin Immunol 2009;9:454-65.
139. Gong L, Sun X, Qu J, et al. Loteprednol etabonate suspension 0.2% administered qid compared with olopatadine solution 0.1% administered bid in the treatment of seasonal allergic conjunctivitis: a multicenter, randomized, investigator-masked, parallel group study in Chinese patients. Clin Ther 2012;34: 1259-72.

Urticaria

140. Zuberbier T, Asero R, Bindslev-Jensen C, et al. EAACI/GA(2)LEN/EDF/WAO guideline: management of urticaria. Allergy 2009;64:1427-43.
141. Ortonne JP. Chronic urticaria: a comparison of management guidelines. Expert Opin Pharmacother 2011;12:2683-93.
142. Simons FER, on behalf of the Early Treatment of the Atopic Child (ETAC) Study Group. Prevention of acute urticaria in young children with atopic dermatitis. J Allergy Clin Immunol 2001;107:703-6.
143. Simons FER, for the Early Prevention of Asthma in Atopic Children Study Group. H_1-antihistamine treatment in young atopic children: effect on urticaria. Ann Allergy Asthma Immunol 2007;99:261-6.
144. Weller K, Ardelean E, Scholz E, et al. Can on-demand non-sedating antihistamines improve urticaria symptoms? A double-blind, randomized, single-dose study. Acta Derm Venereol 2013;93:168-74.

145. Potter PC, Kapp A, Maurer M, et al. Comparison of the efficacy of levocetirizine 5 mg and desloratadine 5 mg in chronic idiopathic urticaria patients. Allergy 2009;64:596-604.
146. Zuberbier T, Oanta A, Bogacka E, et al. Comparison of the efficacy and safety of bilastine 20 mg vs. levocetirizine 5 mg for the treatment of chronic idiopathic urticaria: a multi-centre, double-blind, randomized, placebo-controlled study. Allergy 2010;65:516-28.
147. Gimenez-Arnau A, Izquierdo I, Maurer M. The use of a responder analysis to identify clinically meaningful differences in chronic urticaria patients following placebo-controlled treatment with rupatadine 10 and 20 mg. J Eur Acad Dermatol Venereol 2009;23:1088-91.
148. Staevska M, Popov TA, Kralimarkova T, et al. The effectiveness of levocetirizine and desloratadine in up to 4 times conventional doses in difficult-to-treat urticaria. J Allergy Clin Immunol 2010;125:676-82.
149. Zuberbier T. Pharmacological rationale for the treatment of chronic urticaria with second-generation non-sedating antihistamines at higher-than-standard doses. J Eur Acad Dermatol Venereol 2012;26:9-18.
150. Weller K, Ziege C, Staubach P, et al. H_1-antihistamine up-dosing in chronic spontaneous urticaria: patients' perspective of effectiveness and side effects: a retrospective survey study. PLoS One 2011;6:e23931.
151. Siebenhaar F, Degener F, Zuberbier T, Martus P, Maurer M. High-dose desloratadine decreases wheal volume and improves cold provocation thresholds compared with standard-dose treatment in patients with acquired cold urticaria: a randomized, placebo-controlled, crossover study. J Allergy Clin Immunol 2009;123:672-9.
152. Metz M, Scholz E, Ferran M, et al. Rupatadine and its effects on symptom control, stimulation time, and temperature thresholds in patients with acquired cold urticaria. Ann Allergy Asthma Immunol 2010;104:86-92.
153. Magerl M, Pisarevskaja D, Staubach P, et al. Critical temperature threshold measurement for cold urticaria: a randomized controlled trial of H_1-antihistamine dose escalation. Br J Dermatol 2012;166:1095-9.
154. Kavosh ER, Khan DA. Second-generation H_1-antihistamines in chronic urticaria: an evidence-based review. Am J Clin Dermatol 2011;12:361-76.
155. Maurer M, Weller K, Bindslev-Jensen C, Gimenez-Arnau A, Bousquet PJ, Bousquet J, et al. Unmet clinical needs in chronic spontaneous urticaria: a GA(2)LEN task force report. Allergy 2011;66:317-30.
156. Church MK, Weller K, Stock P, Maurer M. Chronic spontaneous urticaria in children: itching for insight. Pediatr Allergy Immunol 2011;22:1-8.
157. Saini S, Rosen KE, Hsieh HJ, et al. A randomized, placebo-controlled, dose-ranging study of single-dose omalizumab in patients with H_1-antihistamine-refractory chronic idiopathic urticaria. J Allergy Clin Immunol 2011;128:567-73.
158. Fedorowicz Z, van Zuuren EJ, Hu N. Histamine H_2-receptor antagonists for urticaria. Cochrane Database Syst Rev 2012;(3):CD008596.

Other Diseases and Uses

159. Arock M, Valent P. Pathogenesis, classification and treatment of mastocytosis: state of the art in 2010 and future perspectives. Expert Rev Hematol 2010;3:497-516.
160. Siebenhaar F, Fortsch A, Krause K, et al. Rupatadine improves quality of life in mastocytosis: a randomized, double-blind, placebo-controlled trial. Allergy 2013 (in press), DOI: 10.1111/all.12159.
161. Karppinen A, Brummer-Korvenkontio H, Petman L, et al. Levocetirizine for treatment of immediate and delayed mosquito bite reactions. Acta Derm Venereol Stockh 2006;86:329-31.
162. Muller UR, Jutel M, Reimers A, et al. Clinical and immunologic effects of H_1-antihistamine preventive medication during honeybee venom immunotherapy. J Allergy Clin Immunol 2008;122:1001-7.
163. Buddenkotte J, Maurer M, Steinhoff M. Histamine and antihistamines in atopic dermatitis. Adv Exp Med Biol 2010;709:73-80.
164. Diepgen TL. Long term treatment with cetirizine of infants with atopic dermatitis: a multi-country, double-blind, randomized, placebo-controlled trial (the ETAC trial) over 18 months. ETAC Study Group. Pediatr Allergy Immunol 2002;13:278-86.
165. Apfelbacher CJ, Ebert I, Scheidt R, Diepgen TL, Weisshar E. H_1-antihistamines for eczema. Cochrane Database Syst Rev 2009;(2):CD007770.
166. Dunford PJ, Holgate ST. The role of histamine in asthma. Adv Exp Med Biol 2010;709:53-66.
167. Bachert C, Maspero J. Efficacy of second-generation antihistamines in patients with allergic rhinitis and comorbid asthma. J Asthma 2011;48:965-73.
168. Sheikh A, Ten Broek V, Brown SGA, Simons FER. H_1-antihistamines for the treatment of anaphylaxis: Cochrane systematic review. Allergy 2007;62:830-7.
169. Park JH, Godbold JH, Chung D, et al. Comparison of cetirizine and diphenhydramine in the treatment of acute food-induced allergic reactions. J Allergy Clin Immunol 2011;128:1127-8.
170. De Silva HA, Pathmeswaran A, Ranasinha CD, et al. Low-dose adrenaline, promethazine, and hydrocortisone in the prevention of acute adverse reactions to antivenom following snakebite: a randomised, double-blind, placebo-controlled trial. PLoS Med 2011;8:e1000435.
171. Cicardi M, Bork K, Caballero T, et al. Evidence-based recommendations for the therapeutic management of angioedema owing to hereditary C1 inhibitor deficiency: consensus report of an International Working Group. Allergy 2012;67:147-57.
172. De Sutter AIM, van Driel ML, Kumar AA, Lesslar O, Skrt A. Oral antihistamine-decongestant-analgesic combinations for the common cold. Cochrane Database Syst Rev 2012;(2):CD004976.
173. Coleman C, Moore M. Decongestants and antihistamines for acute otitis media in children. Cochrane Database Syst Rev 2008;(3):CD001727.
174. Griffin G, Flynn CA. Antihistamines and/or decongestants for otitis media with effusion (OME) in children. Cochrane Database Syst Rev 2011;(9):CD003423.
175. Meltzer EO, Hamilos DL. Rhinosinusitis diagnosis and management for the clinician: a synopsis of recent consensus guidelines. Mayo Clin Proc 2011;86:427-43.
176. Shaikh N, Wald ER, Pi M. Decongestants, antihistamines and nasal irrigation for acute sinusitis in children. Cochrane Database Syst Rev 2012;(9):CD007909.
177. Smith SM, Schroeder K, Fahey T. Over-the-counter (OTC) medications for acute cough in children and adults in ambulatory settings. Cochrane Database Syst Rev 2012;(8):CD001831.
178. Chang AB, Peake J, McElrea MS. Antihistamines for prolonged non-specific cough in children. Cochrane Database Syst Rev 2010;(2):CD005604.
179. Greaves MW. Pathogenesis and treatment of pruritus. Curr Allergy Asthma Rep 2010;10:236-42.
180. Egan TJ, Kaschula CH. Strategies to reverse drug resistance in malaria. Curr Opin Infect Dis 2007;20:598-604.
181. Krystal AD, Durrence HH, Scharf M, et al. Efficacy and safety of doxepin 1 mg and 3 mg in a 12-week sleep laboratory and outpatient trial of elderly subjects with chronic primary insomnia. Sleep 2010;33:1553-61.
182. Roach CL, Husain N, Zabinsky J, Welch E, Garg R. Moderate sedation for echocardiography of preschoolers. Pediatr Cardiol 2010;31:469-73.
183. Lu CW, Jean WH, Wu CC, Shieh JS, Lin TY. Antiemetic efficacy of metoclopramide and diphenhydramine added to patient-controlled morphine analgesia: a randomised controlled trial. Eur J Anaesthesiol 2010;27:1052-7.
184. Niebyl JR. Clinical practice. Nausea and vomiting in pregnancy. N Engl J Med 2010;363:1544-50.
185. Guaiana G, Barbui C, Cipriani A. Hydroxyzine for generalised anxiety disorder. Cochrane Database Syst Rev 2010;(12):CD006815.
186. Golding JF, Gresty MA. Motion sickness. Curr Opin Neurol 2005;18:29-34.

Adverse Effects

187. Wyngaarden JB, Seevers MH. The toxic effects of antihistaminic drugs. JAMA 1951;145:277-82.
188. Thomas A, Nallur DG, Jones N, Deslandes PN. Diphenhydramine abuse and detoxification: a brief review and case report. J Psychopharmacol 2009;23:101-5.
189. Tanaka T, Takasu A, Yoshino A, et al. Diphenhydramine overdose mimicking serotonin syndrome. Psychiatry Clin Neurosci 2011;65:534.
190. Ratliff JC, Barber JA, Palmese LB, Reutenauer EL, Tek C. Association of prescription H_1 antihistamine use with obesity: results from the National Health and Nutrition Examination Survey. Obesity (Silver Spring) 2010;18:2398-400.
191. Shi SJ, Platts SH, Ziegler MG, Meck JV. Effects of promethazine and midodrine on orthostatic tolerance. Aviat Space Environ Med 2011;82:9-12.
192. St Peter SD, Sharp SW, Ostlie DJ. Influence of histamine receptor antagonists on the outcome of perforated appendicitis: analysis from a prospective trial. Arch Surg 2010;145:143-6.
193. Metz M, Doyle E, Bindslev-Jensen C, et al. Effects of antihistamines on innate immune responses to severe bacterial infection in mice. Int Arch Allergy Immunol 2011;155:355-60.
194. Thakkar MM. Histamine in the regulation of wakefulness. Sleep Med Rev 2011;15:65-74.
195. Haas HL, Sergeeva OA, Selbach O. Histamine in the nervous system. Physiol Rev 2008;88:1183-241.

196. Yanai K, Rogala B, Chugh K, Paraskakis E, Pampura AN, Boev R. Safety considerations in the management of allergic diseases: focus on antihistamines. Curr Med Res Opin 2012;28:623-42.
197. Kubo N, Senda M, Ohsumi Y, et al. Brain histamine H_1 receptor occupancy of loratadine measured by positron emission topography: comparison of H_1 receptor occupancy and proportional impairment ratio. Hum Psychopharmacol 2011;26:133-9.
198. Tashiro M, Kato M, Miyake M, et al. Dose dependency of brain histamine H(1) receptor occupancy following oral administration of cetirizine hydrochloride measured using PET with [11C]doxepin. Hum Psychopharmacol 2009;24:540-8.
199. Tashiro M, Duan X, Kato M, et al. Brain histamine H_1 receptor occupancy of orally administered antihistamines, bepotastine and diphenhydramine, measured by PET with 11C-doxepin. Br J Clin Pharmacol 2008;65:811-21.
200. Zhang D, Tashiro M, Shibuya K, et al. Next-day residual sedative effect after nighttime administration of an over-the-counter antihistamine sleep aid, diphenhydramine, measured by positron emission tomography. J Clin Psychopharmacol 2010;30:694-701.
201. McDonald K, Trick L, Boyle J. Sedation and antihistamines: an update—review of inter-drug differences using proportional impairment ratios. Hum Psychopharmacol 2008;23:555-70.
202. Nicholson AN, Stone BM, Turner C, Mills SL. Antihistamines and aircrew: usefulness of fexofenadine. Aviat Space Environ Med 2000;71:2-6.
203. Walker S, Khan-Wasti S, Fletcher M, et al. Seasonal allergic rhinitis is associated with a detrimental effect on examination performance in United Kingdom teenagers: case-control study. J Allergy Clin Immunol 2007;120:381-7.
204. Officer J. Trends in drug use of Scottish drivers arrested under Section 4 of the Road Traffic Act: a 10 year review. Sci Justice 2009;49:237-41.
205. Zhuo X, Cang Y, Yan H, Bu J, Shen B. The prevalence of drugs in motor vehicle accidents and traffic violations in Shanghai and neighboring cities. Accid Anal Prev 2010;42:2179-84.
206. Canfield DV, Dubowski KM, Chaturvedi AK, Whinnery JE. Drugs and alcohol found in civil aviation accident pilot fatalities from 2004-2008. Aviat Space Environ Med 2012;83:764-70.
207. Weiler JM, Bloomfield JR, Woodworth GG, et al. Effects of fexofenadine, diphenhydramine, and alcohol on driving performance: a randomized, placebo-controlled trial in the Iowa driving simulator. Ann Intern Med 2000;132:354-63.
208. Conen S, Theunissen EL, Vermeeren A, Ramaekers JG. Short-term effects of morning versus evening dose of hydroxyzine 50 mg on cognition in healthy volunteers. J Clin Psychopharmacol 2011;31:294-301.
209. Katayose Y, Aritake S, Kitamura S, et al. Carry-over effect on next-day sleepiness and psychomotor performance of nighttime administered antihistaminic drugs: a randomized controlled trial. Hum Psychopharmacol 2012;27:428-36.
210. Tzanetos DB, Fahrenholz JM, Scott T, Buchholz K. Comparison of the sedating effects of levocetirizine and cetirizine: a randomized, double-blind, placebo-controlled trial. Ann Allergy Asthma Immunol 2011;107:517-22.
211. Garcia-Gea C, Ballester MR, Martinez J, et al. Rupatadine does not potentiate the CNS depressant effects of lorazepam: randomized, double-blind, crossover, repeated dose, placebo-controlled study. Br J Clin Pharmacol 2010;69:663-74.
212. Layton D, Osborne V, Gilchrist A, Shakir SAW. Examining the utilization and tolerability of the non-sedating antihistamine levocetirizine in England using prescription-event monitoring data. Drug Saf 2011;34:1177-89.
213. Woosley RL. Cardiac actions of antihistamines. Annu Rev Pharmacol Toxicol 1996;36:233-52.
214. Nia AM, Fuhr U, Gassanov N, Erdmann E, Er F. Torsades de pointes tachycardia induced by common cold compound medication containing chlorpheniramine. Eur J Clin Pharmacol 2010;66:1173-5.
215. Park S-J, Kim K-S, Kim E-J. Blockade of HERG K^+ channel by an antihistamine drug brompheniramine requires the channel binding within the S6 residue Y652 and F656. J Appl Toxicol 2008;28:104-11.
216. Jo SH, Hong HK, Chong SH, Lee HS, Choe H. H_1 antihistamine drug promethazine directly blocks hERG K^+ channel. Pharmacol Res 2009;60:429-37.
217. Hulhoven R, Rosillon D, Letiexhe M, et al. Levocetirizine does not prolong the QT/QTc interval in healthy subjects: results from a thorough QT study. Eur J Clin Pharmacol 2007;63:1011-7.
218. Tyl B, Kabbaj M, Azzam S, et al. Lack of significant effect of bilastine administered at therapeutic and supratherapeutic doses and concomitantly with ketoconazole on ventricular repolarization: results of a thorough QT study (TQTS) with QT-concentration analysis. J Clin Pharmacol 2012;52:893-903.
219. Donado E, Izquierdo I, Perez I, et al. No cardiac effects of therapeutic and supratherapeutic doses of rupatadine: results from a 'thorough QT/QTc study' performed according to ICH guidelines. Br J Clin Pharmacol 2010;69:401-10.
220. Scharman EJ, Erdman AR, Wax PM, et al. Diphenhydramine and dimenhydrinate poisoning: an evidence-based consensus guideline for out-of-hospital management. Clin Toxicol (Phila) 2006;44:205-23.
221. Bebarta VS, Blair HW, Morgan DL, Maddry J, Borys DJ. Validation of the American Association of Poison Control Centers out of hospital guideline for pediatric diphenhydramine ingestions. Clin Toxicol (Phila) 2010;48:559-62.
222. Kim HJ, Oh SH, Youn CS, et al. The associative factors of delayed-onset rhabdomyolysis in patients with doxylamine overdose. Am J Emerg Med 2011;29:903-7.
223. McKeown NJ, West PL, Hendrickson RG, Horowitz BZ. Survival after diphenhydramine ingestion with hemodialysis in a toddler. J Med Toxicol 2011;7:147-50.
224. Turner JW. Death of a child from topical diphenhydramine. Am J Forensic Med Pathol 2009;30:380-1.
225. Rimsza ME, Newberry S. Unexpected infant deaths associated with use of cough and cold medications. Pediatrics 2008;122:e318-22.
226. Dart RC, Paul IM, Bond GR, et al. Pediatric fatalities associated with over the counter (nonprescription) cough and cold medications. Ann Emerg Med 2009;53:411-7.
227. Kurella Tamura M, Larive B, Unruh ML, et al. Prevalence and correlates of cognitive impairment in hemodialysis patients: the Frequent Hemodialysis Network trials. Clin J Am Soc Nephrol 2010;5:1429-38.
228. Meurer WJ, Potti TA, Kerber KA, et al. Potentially inappropriate medication utilization in the emergency department visits by older adults: analysis from a nationally representative sample. Acad Emerg Med 2010;17:231-7.
229. Chang CM, Chen MJ, Tsai CY, et al. Medical conditions and medications as risk factors of falls in the inpatient older people: a case-control study. Int J Geriatr Psychiatry 2011;26:602-7.
230. McEvoy LK, Smith ME, Fordyce M, Gevins A. Characterizing impaired functional alertness from diphenhydramine in the elderly with performance and neurophysiologic measures. Sleep 2006;29:957-66.
231. Weber-Schoendorfer C, Schaefer C. The safety of cetirizine during pregnancy: a prospective observational cohort study. Reprod Toxicol 2008;26:19-23.
232. Schwarz EB, Moretti ME, Nayak S, Koren G. Risk of hypospadias in offspring of women using loratadine during pregnancy: a systematic review and meta-analysis. Drug Saf 2008;31:775-88.
233. So M, Bozzo P, Inoue M, Einarson A. Safety of antihistamines during pregnancy and lactation. Can Fam Physician 2010;56:427-9.
234. Vassilev ZP, Kabadi S, Villa R. Safety and efficacy of over-the-counter cough and cold medicines for use in children. Expert Opin Drug Saf 2010;9:233-42.
235. Shehab N, Schaefer MK, Kegler SR, Budnitz DS. Adverse events from cough and cold medications after a market withdrawal of products labeled for infants. Pediatrics 2010;126:1100-7.
236. Ostroff C, Lee CE, McMeekin J. Unapproved prescription cough, cold, and allergy drug products: recent U.S. Food and Drug Administration regulatory action on unapproved cough, cold, and allergy medications. Chest 2011;140:295-300.
237. Simons FER, Silas P, Portnoy JM, et al. Safety of cetirizine in infants 6 to 11 months of age: a randomized double-blind placebo-controlled trial. J Allergy Clin Immunol 2003;111:1244-8.
238. Simons FER, on behalf of the ETAC Study Group. Prospective, long-term safety evaluation of the H_1-receptor antagonist cetirizine in very young children with atopic dermatitis. J Allergy Clin Immunol 1999;104:433-40.
239. Simons FER, on behalf of the Early Prevention of Asthma in Atopic Children (EPAAC) Study Group. Safety of levocetirizine treatment in young atopic children: an 18-month study. Pediatr Allergy Immunol 2007;18:535-42.
240. Stevenson J, Cornah D, Evrard P, et al. Long-term evaluation of the impact of the H_1-receptor antagonist cetirizine on the behavioral, cognitive and psychomotor development of very young children with atopic dermatitis. Pediatr Res 2002;52:251-7.
241. Grimfeld A, Holgate ST, Canonica GW, et al. Prophylactic management of children at risk for recurrent upper respiratory infections: the Preventia I Study. Clin Exp Allergy 2004;34:1665-72.

Summary and Future Directions

242. Leurs R, Vischer HF, Wijtmans M, de Esch IJP. En route to new blockbuster antihistamines:

surveying the offspring of the expanding histamine receptor family. Trends Pharmacol Sci 2011;32:250-7.

243. Beaton G, Moree WJ. The expanding role of H_1 antihistamines: a patent survey of selective and dual activity compounds 2005-2010. Expert Opin Ther Pat 2010;20:1197-218.

244. Yu F, Bonaventure P, Thurmond RL. The future antihistamines: histamine H_3 and H_4 receptor ligands. Adv Exp Med Biol 2010;709: 125-40.

245. Lazewska D, Kiec-Kononowicz K. Recent advances in histamine H_3 receptor antagonists/inverse agonists. Expert Opin Ther Pat 2010; 20:1147-69.

246. Romero FA Jr, Allan RJ, Phillips PG, et al. The effects of an H_3 receptor antagonist in a nasal allergen challenge model. J Allergy Clin Immunol 2010;125:AB191.

247. Huang JF, Thurmond RL. The new biology of histamine receptors. Curr Allergy Asthma Rep 2008;8:21-7.

248. Cowden JM, Riley JP, Ma JY, Thurmond RL, Dunford PJ. Histamine H_4 receptor antagonism diminishes existing airway inflammation and dysfunction via modulation of Th2 cytokines. Respir Res 2010;11:86.

249. Walter M, Kottke T, Stark H. The histamine H_4 receptor: targeting inflammatory disorders. Eur J Pharmacol 2011;668:1-5.

250. Zampeli E, Tiligada E. The role of histamine H_4 receptor in immune and inflammatory disorders. Br J Pharmacol 2009;157:24-33.

Inhaled β_2-Agonists

PAUL M. O'BYRNE | MALCOLM R. SEARS

Withdrawn

CONTENTS

SUMMARY OF IMPORTANT CONCEPTS

» Inhaled short-acting β_2-agonists (SABAs) are the most widely used asthma medications for symptom relief.
» Regular use of potent SABAs as monotherapy for asthma leads to worsening of asthma control, and their overuse increases asthma-related mortality.
» Long-acting β_2-agonist (LABA) monotherapy for asthma also increases the risks of asthma-related hospitalization and death.
» When β_2-agonists are used together with an inhaled corticosteroid (ICS), particularly in a single inhaler, the combination improves asthma control and reduces asthma exacerbation risk.
» Use of ICS-LABA combinations containing the LABA formoterol for both maintenance and rescue treatment reduces the risk of severe asthma exacerbations compared with treatment approaches that use inhaled β_2-agonist alone as rescue treatment, irrespective of the baseline ICS or ICS-LABA combination selected for maintenance therapy.

Introduction

Inhaled β_2-agonists are the most widely used medications for the treatment of asthma, because they rapidly reverse bronchoconstriction. Treatment guidelines recommend use of these agents for the relief of asthma symptoms.[1,2] They also are used to prevent bronchoconstriction in situations recognized by the patient as likely to precipitate the condition (most commonly in association with exercise), owing to their ability to act as functional antagonists.

Inhaled β_2-agonists are now classified as *short-acting* (SABAs), with a rapid onset of effect in the airways but a relatively short duration of action (3 to 4 hours); *long-acting* (LABAs), with a 12- to 24-hour duration of activity; or *ultra-long-acting* (ultra-LABAs), with a duration of activity of at least 24 hours.

Historical Background

It was recognized in the mid 1940s that the catecholamine epinephrine, when delivered by inhalation, provided relief from bronchoconstriction in asthmatic patients.[3] The first synthetic inhaled catecholamine to be used for the treatment of asthma was isoprenaline, with initial reports of beneficial effects published in 1948.[4] The modern β_2-agonists were developed after it was recognized that catecholamines such as epinephrine exerted their effects via distinct α- and β-receptors.[5] Subsequently, Lands and colleagues[6] characterized the β-adrenoceptors into β_1- and β_2-subtypes, leading to efforts to develop selective agonists for the β_2-receptor in the lungs. β_2-Agonist selectivity was improved by modifying the structure of catecholamines; other modifications extended the duration of action after inhalation. The commonly available SABAs, such as albuterol[7] (also called salbutamol) and terbutaline,[8] were the result of this initial pharmacologic effort.

Several decades later, selective β_2-agonists with longer durations of action were developed (LABAs). The initial members of this class were salmeterol and formoterol. Salmeterol was developed from salbutamol, modified to attach the drug molecule near the β_2-receptor by extending its aliphatic side-chain.[9] By contrast, formoterol initially was developed as an oral β_2-agonist by Japanese medicinal chemists, and its long duration of activity when inhaled was discovered serendipitously.[10] Although it is most likely that the binding of albuterol, terbutaline, and formoterol is similar to that of epinephrine to the β_2-receptor, the nature of salmeterol binding remains controversial. The main difference between the two LABA drugs is that salmeterol is intrinsically long-acting, whereas the duration of action of formoterol is critically dependent on its route of administration. Finally, LABAs with very long duration of effect (more than 24 hours), such as indacaterol, have been developed (ultra-LABAs).[11,12]

Pharmacology of β_2-Agonists

Important considerations with regard to the pharmacologic properties of β_2-agonists are their selectivity, potency, and efficacy. *Selectivity* reflects the ratios of binding affinities to receptors (β_2- versus β_1-receptors) in in vitro assays. All currently available inhaled β_2-agonists have excellent selectivity for β_2- versus β_1-receptor–mediated effects. *Potency* is the molar concentration of drug required to produce a half-maximal effect. *Efficacy* is the degree of effect observed compared with the maximal possible effect in a system. Full agonists produce a full response, whereas partial agonists provide a lesser response. However, the efficacy of a drug depends on the system in which it is tested; if receptors are abundant and well-coupled, partial agonists may appear to be full agonists. Isoprenaline is the classic full agonist on the β-receptor, whereas albuterol is a partial agonist on human airway smooth muscle in vitro; however, the bronchodilator activity of albuterol in humans is not distinguishable from that of isoproterenol. Terbutaline and formoterol are almost full agonists, whereas salmeterol is a partial agonist on human airway smooth muscle.

β_2-Receptor Structure and Activation

BASIC CONCEPTS

The β_2-receptor is a member of the family of seven-transmembrane G protein–coupled receptors and, in 1987, was the first receptor to be cloned.[13] The receptor is composed of a single amino acid chain that forms seven α-helix coils, localized to the cell membrane and connected by intracellular and extracellular loops. A ligand-binding pocket, open to the extracellular space, is formed when the seven α-helices of the receptor cluster together in a loose ring. The ligand-binding pocket involves an aspartate residue (Asp113) on transmembrane ring (TM) 3, and several critical serines (Ser 203, Ser 204, and Ser 207) on TM5. Signaling is promoted by interactions with Asn 293 (TM6), Ile 169 (TM4), Val 117 (TM3), and Phe 290 (TM6). The binding of synthetic β_2-agonists closely follows but does not exactly mimic the binding conformation of epinephrine.

SIGNAL TRANSDUCTION

A small fraction of the β_2-receptor population is in an active signaling state at rest. When activated by β_2-agonists, the receptor's G protein trimer, called Gs, disassociates into a Ga subunit and a β/γ dimer (Fig. 95-1). Ga binds to and activates adenylyl cyclase, causing increased cAMP, which in turn activates protein kinases A (PKA) and G (PKG). PKA phosphorylates myosin light chain kinase, which is ineffective in sustaining active tone in airway smooth muscle, and therefore, the tissue relaxes. Rho kinases, which are needed for contraction, also are targeted. The β_2-receptor also activates some transduction pathways, such as the sodium-hydrogen exchanger regulatory protein, without involving Gs protein, and also couples directly to potassium channels linked to relaxation of airway smooth muscle.

The β_2-receptor also is phosphorylated by G protein receptor kinases, which facilitate binding of β-arrestins that desensitize the receptor by uncoupling it from Gs, and promote receptor internalization. Once internalized, the receptor may be recycled after enzymatic dephosphorylation or may be destroyed in lysosomes.

As shown by both in vitro and in vivo evidence, receptors that evoke contraction, mediated by Gi and Gq G protein–coupled receptors (such as cysteinyl leukotriene receptors or muscarinic M_3 receptors), antagonize β_2-receptor responses. This causes the β_2-agonist concentration-response curves for relaxation to shift to the right and move downward, demonstrating that the drugs lose potency and efficacy. This loss of efficacy probably is very important in uncontrolled asthma,

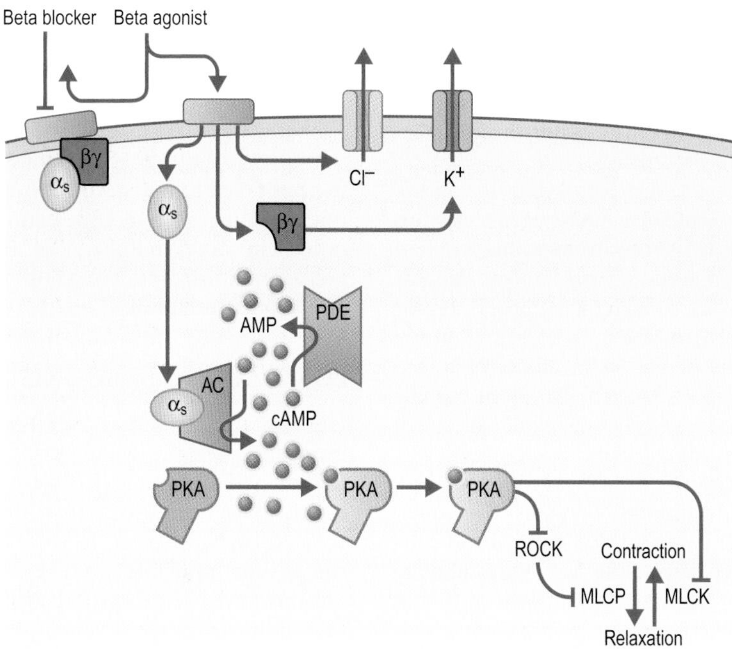

Figure 95-1 Intracellular signaling after activation of the β_2-receptor by a β_2-agonist. When activated by β_2-agonists, the receptor's G protein trimer, called Gs, disassociates into a Ga subunit and a β/γ dimer. Ga binds to and activates adenylyl cyclase, causing increased cyclic adenosine monophosphate (*cAMP*), which in turn activates protein kinase A (*PKA*). PKA phosphorylates myosin light chain kinase (*MLCK*), which is ineffective in sustaining active tone in airway smooth muscle, so that the tissue relaxes. Rho kinases (*ROCK*), which are needed for contraction, also are targeted. The β_2-receptor also activates some transduction pathways, such as the sodium-hydrogen exchanger regulatory protein, without involving Gs protein, and also couples directly to potassium channels linked to relaxation of airway smooth muscle. *MLCP*, Myosin light chain phosphatase; *PDE*, phosphodiesterase.

characterized by high levels of contractile agonists in the airways. In addition, inflammatory mediators, such as interleukin-1β and tumor necrosis factor-α, which have been implicated in severe asthma, can uncouple the β_2-receptor from its transduction pathways.

Efficacy of Inhaled β_2-Agonists

SHORT-ACTING β_2-AGONISTS

All asthma treatment guidelines recommend rapid-onset inhaled β_2-agonists for the relief of airflow obstruction.[1,2] Inhaled SABAs are the most widely used, acting rapidly (within 5 to 10 minutes) to reverse airflow obstruction. If the airflow obstruction is not severe, low doses of inhaled SABAs usually can fully reverse it; however, when airflow obstruction is severe, even high doses of inhaled SABAs usually are not fully effective. As described earlier, activation of the β_2-receptor can decouple it from its transduction pathways, with the potential for loss of responsiveness with repeated use of SABAs. By contrast, very little evidence supports loss of effect in bronchodilator responses. Thus, even with regular use of a β_2-agonist over 1 year, the magnitude of bronchodilation can be maintained,[14] probably because the intracellular mechanisms that result in bronchodilation require activation of only a relatively small fraction of the available β_2-receptors on an airway smooth muscle to evoke a maximal response.

Another recommended use of SABAs results from their ability to act as functional antagonists to protect against bronchoconstrictor stimuli. This counteracting effect can be demonstrated with any agonist that causes bronchoconstriction, including inhaled methacholine, histamine, and the cysteinyl leukotrienes. The most clinically relevant stimulus, however, is exercise.[15] The effect is rapid in onset and can provide greater than 80% protection[16] (Fig. 95-2). Regular use of β_2-agonists, however, results in tolerance to this protective effect,[17] suggesting that, in contrast with the mechanisms of bronchodilation, the bronchoprotective effects of β_2-agonists require a large fraction of available β_2-receptors to be activated.

Although inhaled β_2-agonists are very effective in alleviating asthma symptoms in the short term, use of these agents also has been associated with worsening asthma control and an increased risk of asthma-related death in some circumstances. Regular inhaled SABA use formerly was considered appropriate for asthma management,[18] apparently on the basis of a single study of regular versus as-needed use of the SABA albuterol[19]: In a crossover trial, 18 patients received albuterol 200 μg or matching placebo four times daily for 1 week. During regular albuterol treatment, fewer rescue doses of albuterol were used, and evening and bedtime peak expiratory flow measurements were higher than with placebo. Accordingly, regular β_2-agonist therapy was deemed to provide better asthma control and subsequently was widely promoted, despite the fact that total daily dose of albuterol was actually substantially higher, and that the improved peak flow rates were measured shortly after use of albuterol. By contrast, a year-long randomized, placebo-controlled crossover trial using a more potent SABA, fenoterol, demonstrated worsened asthma control with regular four-times-daily SABA compared with use only as needed.[20] As a consequence of these findings, coupled with the recognition that asthma is predominantly an inflammatory airway disease, necessitating antiinflammatory medication as part of regular

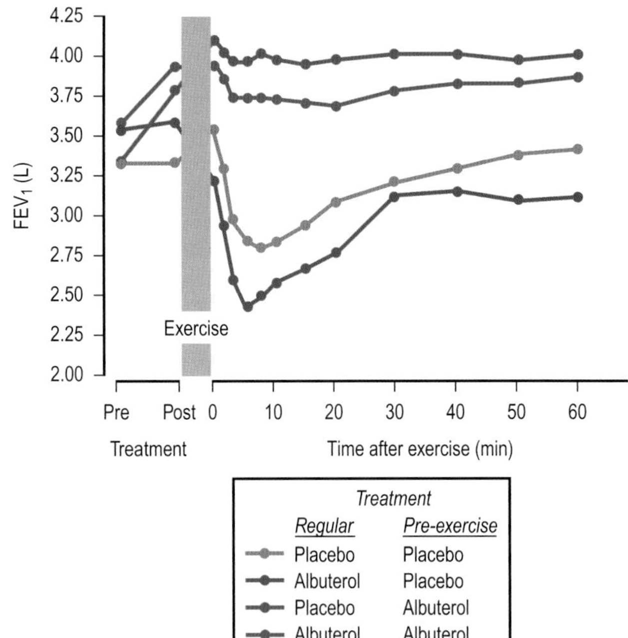

Figure 95-2 Effects of regular treatment with an inhaled short-acting β_2-agonist (SABA), albuterol, or placebo four times daily, as well as treatment immediately before exercise, on exercise-induced bronchoconstriction. The fall in forced expiratory volume at 1 second (FEV_1) after exercise, after regular placebo treatment and pretreatment with placebo immediately before exercise, is depicted by the *orange curve*. Regular treatment with albuterol and pretreatment with placebo before exercise significantly increased the maximal exercise-induced fall in FEV_1 (*purple curve*). Regular treatment with placebo and pretreatment with albuterol before exercise provided the best protection (*green curve*); a protocol of regular treatment with albuterol and use of albuterol before exercise was significantly less effective (*blue curve*). *(Redrawn from Inman MD, O'Byrne PM. The effect of regular inhaled albuterol on exercise-induced bronchoconstriction. Am J Respir Crit Care Med 1996;153:65-69.)*

therapy for patients with persisting symptoms, regular SABA use has fallen into disfavor. It is now recognized that SABAs do not have any inherent antiinflammatory activity in asthma and indeed, in some circumstances, may increase early and late allergic asthmatic responses[21] and in fact promote eosinophilic airway inflammation.[22]

LONG-ACTING β_2-AGONISTS

LABAs were introduced for asthma treatment in 1990 and over time have become widely used in both asthma and chronic obstructive pulmonary disease (COPD). In both diseases, LABAs have been used either for monotherapy or added to an inhaled corticosteroid (ICS). Both salmeterol and formoterol, the LABAs available for chronic maintenance treatment in asthma, have been shown in large randomized, controlled trials in asthma to provide better clinical outcomes (symptom control, improved lung function, and reduced exacerbations) when added to an ICS than those achieved by doubling the dose of ICS.[23] These findings initially were interpreted as indicating that LABAs had antiinflammatory activity. Most researchers, however, now regard LABAs as providing stability of airway function and increased asthma control, accounting for their "steroid-sparing" properties in asthma. Formoterol has a rapid onset of bronchodilation and is approved for the acute relief of airflow obstruction in many countries, unlike salmeterol, for which onset to peak bronchodilation takes significantly longer than with formoterol.[24]

The use of LABAs for the treatment of asthma is now recommended only in combination with ICS, ideally in a single inhaler.[1,2] Such ICS-LABA combinations provide better asthma control than high doses of ICS alone in patients whose asthma is not well controlled on lower ICS doses[25] and also reduce asthma exacerbations. The effect was first demonstrated in the Formoterol and Corticosteroids Establishing Therapy (FACET) study,[14] in which the most substantial impact on reducing mild and severe exacerbations in asthma was observed in the group of patients given both increased ICS and formoterol. This benefit has been consistently reproduced in other studies.[26] Most asthma treatment guidelines now recommend use of low-dose ICS-LABA combinations as the preferred treatment if ICS monotherapy is not providing optimal asthma control.[1,2] If asthma control remains suboptimal, higher doses of ICS-LABA combinations are recommended.

The mechanisms by which ICS-LABA combinations provide superior overall asthma control over that achieved with ICS alone are not well understood. LABAs stimulate the glucocorticoid receptor and promote its translocation to the nucleus, increasing corticosteroid-mediated gene transcription,[27] whereas corticosteroids increase the transcription of the β_2-receptor gene in the lung.[28] Suggestions that LABAs possess intrinsic antiinflammatory properties have been debated, but a recent systematic review of the effects of LABAs on a wide range of inflammatory indices (induced cell counts; markers of cell activation in sputum, bronchoalveolar lavage fluid, bronchial biopsy specimens, and serum; and exhaled nitric oxide) concluded that LABA therapy was neither antiinflammatory nor proinflammatory.[29]

Safety of Inhaled β_2-Agonists Alone and with Inhaled Corticosteroids

SHORT-ACTING β_2-AGONISTS

Questions regarding the safety of SABAs in asthma go back to a report in 1948 of increased mortality associated with use of nebulized epinephrine,[30] a very nonselective β-agonist, with effects on β_1-receptors on the myocardium. Concern became more widespread in the 1960s when England and Wales, Australia, and New Zealand experienced an increase in asthma mortality among young people, associated in time with introduction of a high-dose formulation of another nonselective β-agonist, isoprenaline.[31] A further epidemic of asthma mortality occurred in New Zealand from 1976 through the 1980s. Case-control studies suggested a relationship to prescription of fenoterol,[32] a more potent and slightly longer-acting beta agonist than albuterol. These concerns were increased by the findings of a randomized placebo-controlled clinical trial which demonstrated that regular use of fenoterol could increase asthma severity despite concomitant use of ICS.[20] Asthma mortality in New Zealand decreased abruptly when fenoterol was severely restricted, just as mortality in the United Kingdom, Australia, and New Zealand had decreased in the late 1960s when use of high-dose isoprenaline was discouraged. An accompanying substantial reduction in morbidity, as reflected in hospital admissions for severe asthma, with restriction of fenoterol suggested the epidemic was more likely to be mediated through increased asthma severity rather than through cardiac adverse effects. SABAs are no longer recommended for regular use in asthma[1,2] but remain the mainstay of rescue therapy, and these short-acting agents are the most widely used inhaled medication for asthma.

LONG-ACTING β_2-AGONISTS USED FOR MONOTHERAPY

After the launch of salmeterol in the United Kingdom, Castle and associates[33] conducted a large randomized, controlled trial comparing twice-daily salmeterol with albuterol four times daily in subjects considered to require regular β_2-agonist therapy. Although exacerbations did not differ, and study discontinuations decreased with salmeterol treatment, a disconcerting, albeit nonsignificant, threefold increase was observed in the risk of death in the salmeterol treatment group. The study authors considered lack of adequate ICS a likely contributor to many of the 14 deaths.

Because of these concerning but inconclusive findings, a large study of salmeterol versus placebo added to usual therapy was conducted in the United States, powered on death as the primary outcome.[34] The study was terminated prematurely, in part because of preliminary findings of a higher proportion of deaths and serious adverse events with salmeterol. The odds ratio (OR) for respiratory-related deaths was 2.16, and for asthma-related deaths it was 4.37. African Americans in this study appeared to be at higher risk, and the question arose regarding the possible impact of β-receptor genotype, because the prevalence of Arg-Arg at position 16 is higher in African Americans. This apparent increased risk, however, largely reflected the higher baseline risk of death in this population group, because the actual mortality rates in the study in African Americans and whites were similarly increased, being about fourfold and threefold higher, respectively, than those expected in relation to their age- and race-matched populations. ICS use was not recorded throughout the study, but at baseline, only 38% of African Americans and 49% of whites used ICS. Post hoc analysis showed that deaths were dominantly among patients not prescribed ICS at baseline; among those not using ICS at baseline, 9 deaths occurred in the salmeterol arm and none in the placebo arm, whereas among those using ICS at baseline, no difference was seen in the risk of death (4 versus 3 deaths).

The concern that inflammation might increase because of insufficient ICS while concomitant LABA use maintained apparent control of asthma was highlighted by a study evaluating the use of salmeterol with reduced ICS doses. This study demonstrated that salmeterol can mask the clinical effects of inflammation by controlling symptoms and maintaining stable lung function as the sputum eosinophil count increases during steroid reduction.[35]

The results of the large U.S. study of salmeterol reported by Nelson and colleagues led the Food and Drug Administration (FDA) to impose a "black box" warning on all products containing salmeterol or formoterol, both as monotherapy and in combination with ICS. This action, and the safety concerns leading to it, resulted in a number of meta-analyses examining safety of LABA therapy in asthma. Salpeter and colleagues[36] assessed the effect of LABAs on severe asthma exacerbations requiring hospitalization, life-threatening asthma attacks, and asthma-related deaths in adults and children. Randomized, placebo-controlled asthma trials of LABAs with duration of more than 3 months were included, but those without placebo control groups were excluded. The OR for asthma-related deaths for LABA compared with placebo was 3.5 (95% confidence interval [CI], 1.3 to 9.3). Major criticisms of this meta-analysis were that some 80% of the subjects included were participants in the single study of Nelson and colleagues,[34] exclusion of pivotal studies on the addition of LABAs to ICS because these studies did not have a placebo-controlled arm, and the lack of verification of concomitant use of ICS during therapy with LABAs. Ernst and colleagues compared the analysis of Salpeter and associates with those reported in previous Cochrane reviews and took the contrary view that LABA used with ICS was safe.[37]

Safety data relating to formoterol exposure in clinical trials were examined by Sears and colleagues[38]: The rates of asthma-related death were 0.34 per 1000 patient-years among subjects randomized to receive formoterol (92% using ICS) and 0.22 per 1000 patient-years among those not receiving formoterol (83% using ICS) (RR, 1.57). The rate of asthma-related serious adverse events (SAEs), more than 90% of which were hospitalizations, was significantly lower among formoterol-randomized patients. No increase in asthma-related SAEs was observed with increased daily doses of formoterol; rather, a significant trend in the opposite direction was evident. The investigators concluded that despite the very large sample size (with review of data on more than 68,000 patients), the power was insufficient to conclude no increased mortality with formoterol, but that asthma-related SAEs were significantly reduced with formoterol.

INHALED CORTICOSTEROID–LONG-ACTING β_2-AGONIST COMBINATIONS

A meta-analysis of all studies in which formoterol or salmeterol was used with concomitant ICS was completed by Jaeschke and co-workers.[39] On the basis of data from 62 studies with more than 29,000 participants, these workers concluded that in patients with asthma using ICS, LABA use did not increase the risk of asthma-related hospitalizations (Table 95-1). The OR for all-cause mortality was 1.26 (95% CI, 0.58-2.74), reflecting 14 and 8 deaths in the LABA treatment and control groups, respectively. The 3 reported asthma-related deaths and 2 asthma-related nonfatal intubations (all in LABA groups, with no more than one event per study) were too few to establish the effect of LABA on these outcomes.

In addition, Bateman and associates[40] reported data from 20,966 participants in 66 studies involving use of ICS with or without salmeterol. Only one death and one intubation were reported, both in patients using salmeterol with ICS, with no difference in hospitalizations.

Rodrigo and colleagues[23] examined asthma exacerbations requiring systemic corticosteroids or hospitalization, life-threatening exacerbations, and asthma-related deaths in LABA trials. Asthma-related deaths were increased with LABA, but ICS provided a protective effect. LABA with ICS was equivalent to ICS in rate of life-threatening exacerbations and asthma-related deaths, and the combination significantly reduced exacerbations (OR, 0.73; 95% CI, 0.67 to 0.79) and hospitalizations (O.R, 0.58; 95% CI, 0.45 to 0.74).

Salpeter and associates[41] subsequently published quite different results derived from a further meta-analysis of these existing data, reporting not only that use of LABA with or without ICS was associated with a twofold risk of death and need for intubation (OR, 2.10; 95% CI, 1.37 to 3.22) but also that concomitant ICS use further increased that risk (OR, 3.65; 95% CI ,1.39 to 9.55). Even more surprising, this meta-analysis reported that use of an LABA with ICS as an integral part of the study intervention carried an even higher risk of deaths and intubations (OR, 8.19; 95% CI, 1.10 to 61.18). Critical appraisal of these reported outcomes suggests confounding by ICS dose. In the 12 trials in which asthma-related deaths and intubations occurred, 5 of the protocols did not require concomitant ICS (use ranged from 0% to 67%). ICS doses are not provided in 3 of the remaining 7 trials, providing no assurance that equal ICS doses were used in each arm; in one trial, ICS plus LABA was compared with higher-dose ICS only, and the remaining 3 studies used two doses of ICS in the LABA and/or non-LABA arms. For a true assessment of safety of LABA, equal doses of ICS are required in each treatment arm with and without LABA, to ensure that any difference in safety signals reflect the addition of LABA.

A substantive independent meta-analysis involving 110 trials and 60,954 subjects was conducted as part of the FDA evaluation of the safety of LABAs, in which the risk difference (RD) was calculated for LABA versus non-LABA.[42] The RD for the composite outcomes of asthma-related death, intubation, and hospitalization for patients receiving LABA without mandatory randomized ICS was significantly increased, at 3.63 per 1000 (95% CI, 1.51 to 5.75), whereas among patients receiving LABA *with* mandatory ICS, the RD was not increased, at 0.25 per 1000 (95% CI, 1.69 to 2.18). Furthermore, 43 of 44 deaths and intubations in LABA-exposed patients occurred in trials that did not mandate the use of ICS, compared with 1 death in all trials with mandatory ICS. Despite these reassuring data on safety of LABAs when used with ICS, the black box warning remains on all LABA products in the United States. The FDA has provided guidelines suggesting that whenever possible, LABAs should be withdrawn when asthma becomes controlled.[43] In clinical trials, however, asthma control apparently worsened on withdrawal of LABA when this β_2-agonist had been used to gain control, resulting in a requirement for higher ICS doses.[44] Most recently, the FDA has required the four pharmaceutical companies marketing LABAs in the United States to each undertake a large randomized controlled study (involving some 50,000 patients in all) comparing LABA plus ICS with the identical dose of the same ICS to determine whether there is any safety signal.[45]

Use of Inhaled Corticosteroid–Long-Acting β_2-Agonists as Single-Inhaler Maintenance and Reliever Therapy

As an interesting hypothesis, use of a combination inhaler containing both an ICS and an LABA for relief as well as for regular maintenance therapy was postulated to be advantageous compared with use of an inhaled β_2-agonist (SABA or LABA) alone for relief on a background of maintenance therapy with the same ICS-LABA. This hypothesis implied that the additional ICS delivered when the combination was used to relieve symptoms would provide additional antiinflammatory benefit, reducing the risk for the severe asthma exacerbations known to be associated with worsening airway inflammation.

TABLE 95-1 **Effects of Treatment with Long-Acting β2-Agonists on Total Mortality among Patients Using Inhaled Corticosteroids (ICS), with Forest Plot***

Study or Subgroup†	Treatment Events	Treatment Total	Control Events	Control Total	Weight	Odds Ratio: M-H, Random (95% CI)
40.7.1 FORMOTEROL—ICS DOSES SIMILAR IN BOTH GROUPS						
Pauwels, 1997	1	426	0	427	5.9%	3.01 (0.12-74.20)
O'Byrne, 2001	1	869	0	862	5.9%	2.98 (0.12-73.24)
Zetterstrom, 2001	1	238	0	124	5.8%	1.57 (0.06-38.89)
Buhl, 2003	1	352	0	171	5.9%	1.46 (0.06-30.12)
Jenkins, 2006	1	341	0	115	5.8%	1.02 (0.04-25.15)
Subtotal (95% CI)		3603		2626	29.3%	1.84 (0.44-7.72)
TOTAL EVENTS	5		0			
Heterogeneity: tau-square = 0.00; chi-square = 0.34, df = 4 (P = 0.99); I^2 = 0%						
Test for overall effect: Z = 0.83 (P = 0.40)						
40.7.2 FORMOTEROL—ICS DOSE HIGHER IN CONTROL GROUP						
Scicchitano, 2004	1	947	2	943	10.4%	0.50 (0.05-5.49)
O'Byrne, 2005	2	1592	1	818	10.4%	1.03 (0.09-11.35)
Subtotal (95% CI)		3385		2615	20.8%	0.71 (0.13-3.91)
TOTAL EVENTS	3		3			
Heterogeneity: tau-square = 0.00; chi-square = 0.18, df = 1 (P = 0.68); I^2 = 0%						
Test for overall effect: Z = 0.39 (P = 0.70)						
40.7.3 SALMETEROL—ICS DOSES SIMILAR IN BOTH GROUPS						
van Noord, 2001	1	337	0	172	5.9%	1.54 (0.06-37.95)
Bateman, 2004	3	1709	2	1707	18.8%	1.50 (0.25-8.98)
Strand, 2004	0	78	1	72	5.8%	0.30 (0.01-7.57)
SAS40068	0	262	1	270	5.9%	0.34 (0.01-8.44)
Subtotal (95% CI)		4326		3819	36.3%	0.92 (0.25-3.33)
TOTAL EVENTS	4		4			
Heterogeneity: tau-square = 0.00; chi-square = 1.21, df = 3 (P = 0.75); I^2 = 0%						
Test for overall effect: Z = 0.13 (P = 0.90)						
40.7.4 SALMETEROL—ICS DOSE HIGHER IN CONTROL GROUP						
Baraniuk, 1999	1	118	1	232	7.8%	1.97 (0.12-31.85)
Ind, 2003	1	173	0	329	5.9%	5.73 (0.23-141.41)
Subtotal (95% CI)		4273		4510	13.6%	3.12 (0.38-25.49)
TOTAL EVENTS	2		1			
Heterogeneity: tau-square = 0.00; chi-square = 0.24, df = 1 (P = 0.62); I^2 = 0%						
Test for overall effect: Z = 1.06 (P = 0.29)						
SUMMARY						
TOTAL (95% CI)		15,587		13,570	100.0%	1.26 (0.58-2.74)
TOTAL EVENTS	14		8			
Heterogeneity: tau-square = 0.00; chi-square = 3.61, df = 12 (P = 0.99); I^2 = 0%						
Test for overall effect: Z = 0.59 (P = 0.56)						

Odds Ratio: M-H, Random (95% CI)

0.01 0.1 1 10 100

Favors treatment Favors control

Reproduced with permission from Jaeschke R, O'Byrne PM, Mejza F, et al. The safety of long-acting beta-agonists among patients with asthma using inhaled corticosteroids: systematic review and metaanalysis. Am J Respir Crit Care Med 2008;178:1009-16.

CI, Confidence interval; *df*, degrees of freedom; I^2, index of inconsistency given as percent of total variation across studies as a result of heterogeneity; *M-H*, Mantel-Haenszel method; *tau-square*, estimate of between-study variance; *Z*, effect size.

*No significant increase was demonstrated in patients treated with ICS–long-acting β2-agonist combinations.

†Only studies with at least one event are included.

This hypothesis was evaluated using a combination inhaler containing formoterol and budesonide. Formoterol has a rapid onset of bronchodilator action (within the first minute), and its pharmacologic characteristics demonstrate a dose-response effect whereby increasing doses provides additional bronchodilation. Several large studies have consistently demonstrated specific benefits of the combination of budesonide and formoterol for both maintenance and symptom relief—namely, decreased frequency of severe exacerbations requiring medication intervention; reduction in need for oral steroids, in reliever medication use, and in night-time symptoms including awakenings; and improved lung function—compared with maintenance budesonide-formoterol (or a fourfold higher dose of budesonide) with SABA for relief[46,47] (see Table 95-1). The benefits were seen in both children and adults with moderate to severe asthma not controlled on moderate doses of ICS (some also on LABAs) at randomization, all of whom had a previous history of severe asthma exacerbations. The benefit of another ICS-LABA combination, beclomethasone and formoterol, for reliever therapy has been shown in a population of patients with milder asthma.[48]

The mechanism by which the combination of ICS plus an LABA containing formoterol reduces the risk of severe asthma exacerbations is not yet explained. Asthma exacerbations generally develop over a period of 5 to 7 days before the problem is recognized and treatment is initiated, during which patients experience deteriorating symptoms and lung function. This timing suggests that there is an opportunity to intervene early with an increase in ICS dose for symptom relief over several days before the exacerbation becomes severe enough to necessitate medical intervention. Of note, however, studies that have doubled the maintenance dose of ICS well into the course of an exacerbation have failed to show the anticipated benefits. These interventions usually have been in response to a fixed increase in symptoms and decline in lung function (as dictated by study protocol), which is likely to be too late for the increased dose of ICS to provide benefit. It is plausible—but not yet proved—that using a combination of ICS and formoterol for maintenance and reliever therapy more effectively combats the worsening inflammation, because ICS is always delivered when the combination is used to relieve the increase in symptoms much earlier in the development of an exacerbation.

Conclusions

Inhaled β_2-agonists are a mainstay of asthma treatment. SABAs remain the most widely used asthma medications for relieving symptoms and preventing bronchoconstriction (bronchoprotection). Tolerance to the bronchoprotective benefit of inhaled β_2-agonists occurs with their regular use. In addition, regular use of potent SABAs as monotherapy in asthma leads to worsening of asthma control, and their overuse increases the likelihood of asthma-related death. LABA monotherapy also increases the risk of asthma-related hospitalization and mortality rates; however, when used together, particularly in a single inhaler, the ICS-LABA combination improves asthma control, reduces asthma exacerbation risk, and allows effective maintenance at a lower overall dose of ICS. As demonstrated by substantial evidence that patients with asthma use beta agonists in preference to ICSs when these drugs are provided in separate inhalers, the practical recommendation is that LABAs should be provided as a component of combination products in a single inhaler in which every dose of LABA is accompanied by ICS.

In patients with a history of severe asthma exacerbations, use of ICS-LABA combinations that contain formoterol for both maintenance and rescue treatment reduces the risk of severe exacerbations more than do treatment approaches that use an inhaled β_2-agonist alone for rescue treatment, irrespective of the baseline ICS or ICS-LABA selected for maintenance therapy.

REFERENCES

Introduction

1. Expert Panel Report 3 (EPR-3): Guidelines for the Diagnosis and Management of Asthma-Summary Report 2007. J Allergy Clin Immunol 2007;120:S94-138.
2. Bateman ED, Hurd SS, Barnes PJ, et al. Global strategy for asthma management and prevention: GINA executive summary. Eur Respir J 2008;31:143-78.

Historical Background

3. Hartmann MM. Ethyl-nor-epinephrine by inhalation for bronchial asthma; a comparison with epinephrine. J Allergy 1946;106-11.
4. Lowell FC, Curry JJ, Schiller IW. A clinical and experimental study of Isuprel in spontaneous and induced asthma. N Engl J Med 1948;239: 45-51.
5. Alquist RP. A study of the adrenotropic receptors. Am J Physiol 1948;153:586-600.
6. Lands AM, Luduena FP, Buzzo HJ. Differentiation of receptors responsive to isoproterenol. Life Sci 1967;6:2241-9.
7. Cullum VA, Farmer JB, Jack D, Levy GP. Salbutamol: a new, selective beta-adrenoceptive receptor stimulant. Br J Pharmacol 1969;35:141-51.
8. Hedstrand U. The effect of a new sympathomimetic beta-receptor stimulating drug (terbutaline) on the pulmonary mechanics in bronchial asthma. Scand J Respir Dis 1970;51:188-94.
9. Johnson M. The pharmacology of salmeterol. Lung 1990;168(Suppl):115-9.
10. Ullman A, Bergendal A, Linden A, et al. Onset of action and duration of effect of formoterol and salmeterol compared to salbutamol in isolated guinea pig trachea with or without epithelium. Allergy 1992;47:384-7.
11. Beeh KM, Derom E, Kanniess F, et al. Indacaterol, a novel inhaled beta2-agonist, provides sustained 24-h bronchodilation in asthma. Eur Respir J 2007;29:871-8.
12. O'Byrne PM, van der Linde J, Cockcroft DW, et al. Prolonged bronchoprotection against inhaled methacholine by inhaled BI 1744, a long-acting beta(2)-agonist, in patients with mild asthma. J Allergy Clin Immunol 2009;124: 1217-21.

β_2-Receptor Structure and Activation

13. Chung FZ, Lentes KU, Gocayne J, et al. Cloning and sequence analysis of the human brain beta-adrenergic receptor. Evolutionary relationship to rodent and avian beta-receptors and porcine muscarinic receptors. FEBS Lett 1987;211: 200-6.

Efficacy of Inhaled β_2-Agonists

14. Pauwels RA, Lofdahl CG, Postma DS, et al. Effect of inhaled formoterol and budesonide on exacerbations of asthma. Formoterol and Corticosteroids Establishing Therapy (FACET) International Study Group. N Engl J Med 1997; 337:1405-11.
15. Anderson SD, Seale JP, Rozea P, et al. Inhaled and oral salbutamol in exercise-induced asthma. Am Rev Respir Dis 1976;114:493-500.
16. Inman MD, OByrne PM. The effect of regular inhaled albuterol on exercise-induced bronchoconstriction. Am J Respir Crit Care Med 1996; 153:65-9.
17. Ramage L, Lipworth BJ, Ingram CG, Cree IA, Dhillon DP. Reduced protection against exercise induced bronchoconstriction after chronic dosing with salmeterol. Respir Med 1994;88: 363-8.
18. Rebuck AS, Chapman KR. Asthma: 2. Trends in pharmacologic therapy. CMAJ 1987;136:483-8.
19. Shepherd GL, Hetzel MR, Clark TJ. Regular versus symptomatic aerosol bronchodilator treatment of asthma. Br J Dis Chest 1981;75: 215-7.
20. Sears MR, Taylor DR, Print CG, et al. Regular inhaled beta-agonist treatment in bronchial asthma. Lancet 1990;336:1391-6.
21. Cockcroft DW, O'Byrne PM, Swystun VA, Bhagat R. Regular use of inhaled albuterol and the allergen-induced late asthmatic response. J Allergy Clin Immunol 1995;96:44-9.
22. Gauvreau GM, Jordana M, Watson RM, Cockroft DW, OByrne PM. Effect of regular inhaled albuterol on allergen-induced late responses and sputum eosinophils in asthmatic subjects. Am J Respir Crit Care Med 1997;156: 1738-45.
23. Greening AP, Ind PW, Northfield M, Shaw G. Added salmeterol versus higher-dose corticosteroid in asthma patients with symptoms on existing inhaled corticosteroid. Lancet 1994;344: 219-24.
24. Palmqvist M, Ibsen T, Mellen A, Lotvall J. Comparison of the relative efficacy of formoterol and salmeterol in asthmatic patients. Am J Respir Crit Care Med 1999;160:244-9.
25. O'Byrne PM, Naya IP, Kallen A, Postma DS, Barnes PJ. Increasing doses of inhaled corticosteroids compared to adding long-acting inhaled β2-agonists in achieving asthma control. Chest 2008;134:1192-9.
26. O'Byrne PM, Barnes PJ, Rodriguez-Roisin R, et al. Low dose inhaled budesonide and formoterol in mild persistent asthma: the OPTIMA randomized trial. Am J Respir Crit Care Med 2001;164:1392-7.
27. Roth M, Johnson PR, Rudiger JJ, et al. Interaction between glucocorticoids and beta2 agonists on bronchial airway smooth muscle cells through synchronised cellular signalling. Lancet 2002;360:1293-9.
28. Cheng JB, Goldfien A, Ballard PL, Roberts JM. Glucocorticoids increase pulmonary beta-adrenergic receptors in fetal rabbit. Endocrinology 1980;107:1646-8.
29. Sindi A, Todd DC, Nair P. Antiinflammatory effects of long-acting beta2-agonists in patients with asthma: a systematic review and metaanalysis. Chest 2009;136:145-54.

Safety of β_2-Agonists Alone and with Inhaled Corticosteroids

30. Benson RL, Perlman F. Clinical effects of epinephrine by inhalation. J Allergy 1948;19: 129-40.

31. Speizer FE, Doll R, Heaf P, Strang LB. Investigation into use of drugs preceding death from asthma. BMJ 1968;1:339-43.
32. Grainger J, Woodman K, Pearce N, et al. Prescribed fenoterol and death from asthma in New Zealand, 1981-7: a further case-control study. Thorax 1991;46:105-11.
33. Castle W, Fuller R, Hall J, Palmer J. Serevent nationwide surveillance study: comparison of salmeterol with salbutamol in asthmatic patients who require regular bronchodilator treatment. BMJ 1993;306:1034-7.
34. Nelson HS, Weiss ST, Bleecker ER, Yancey SW, Dorinsky PM. The Salmeterol Multicenter Asthma Research Trial: a comparison of usual pharmacotherapy for asthma or usual pharmacotherapy plus salmeterol. Chest 2006;129:15-26.
35. McIvor RA, Pizzichini E, Turner MO, et al. Potential masking effects of salmeterol on airway inflammation in asthma. Am J Respir Crit Care Med 1998;158:924-30.
36. Salpeter SR, Buckley NS, Ormiston TM, Salpeter EE. Meta-analysis: effect of long-acting beta-agonists on severe asthma exacerbations and asthma-related deaths. Ann Intern Med 2006;144:904-12.
37. Ernst P, McIvor A, Ducharme FM, et al. Safety and effectiveness of long-acting inhaled beta-agonist bronchodilators when taken with inhaled corticosteroids. Ann Intern Med 2006;145:692-4.
38. Sears MR, Ottosson A, Radner F, Suissa S. Long-acting beta-agonists: a review of formoterol safety data from asthma clinical trials. Eur Respir J 2009;33:21-32.
39. Jaeschke R, O'Byrne PM, Mejza F, et al. The safety of long-acting beta-agonists among patients with asthma using inhaled corticosteroids: systematic review and metaanalysis. Am J Respir Crit Care Med 2008;178:1009-16.
40. Bateman E, Nelson H, Bousquet J, et al. Meta-analysis: effects of adding salmeterol to inhaled corticosteroids on serious asthma-related events. Ann Intern Med 2008;149:33-42.
41. Salpeter SR, Wall AJ, Buckley NS. Long-acting beta-agonists with and without inhaled corticosteroids and catastrophic asthma events. Am J Med 2010;123:322-8.
42. Levenson M. Long-acting beta-agonists and adverse asthma events meta-analysis. Statistical briefing package for joint meeting of the Pulmonary-Allergy Drugs Advisory Committee, Drug Safety and Risk Management Advisory Committee, and Pediatric Advisory Committee, U.S. Food and Drug Administration, Bethesda, Md. December 10-11, 2008.
43. Chowdhury BA, Dal PG. The FDA and safe use of long-acting beta-agonists in the treatment of asthma. N Engl J Med 2010;362:1169-71.
44. Reddel HK, Gibson PG, Peters MJ, et al. Down-titration from high-dose combination therapy in asthma: removal of long-acting beta(2)-agonist. Respir Med 2010;104:1110-20.
45. Chowdhury BA, Seymour SM, Levenson MS. Assessing the safety of adding LABAs to inhaled corticosteroids for treating asthma. N Engl J Med 2011;364:2473-5.

Use of Inhaled Corticosteroid–Long-Acting β_2-Agonist Combinations as Single-Inhaler Maintenance and Reliever Therapy

46. Rabe KF, Atienza T, Magyar P, et al. Effect of budesonide in combination with formoterol for reliever therapy in asthma exacerbations: a randomised controlled, double-blind study. Lancet 2006;368:744-53.
47. O'Byrne PM, Bisgaard H, Godard PP, et al. Budesonide/formoterol combination therapy as both maintenance and reliever medication in asthma. Am J Respir Crit Care Med 2005;171:129-36.
48. Papi A, Canonica GW, Maestrelli P, et al. Rescue use of beclomethasone and albuterol in a single inhaler for mild asthma. N Engl J Med 2007;356:2040-52.

96

Theophylline and Phosphodiesterase Inhibitors

C.P. PAGE | DOMENICO SPINA

CONTENTS

SUMMARY OF IMPORTANT CONCEPTS

» Oral theophylline is now third-line therapy for respiratory disease because of its narrow therapeutic window and propensity for drug-drug interactions.
» Lower-than-conventional doses of theophylline considered to be bronchodilating have antiinflammatory actions relevant to treatment of respiratory disease.
» The molecular mechanisms of action of theophylline are not well understood, but targets may include nonselective inhibition of phosphodiesterase (PDE), phosphoinositide 3-kinase, and increased activity of certain histone deacetylases.
» Several selective PDE inhibitors have been identified to improve the therapeutic window of theophylline, but only the PDE4 inhibitor roflumilast is currently registered as a medicine and approved for exacerbations in patients with severe chronic obstructive pulmonary disease.
» Oral roflumilast is dose limited because of side effects, and therefore novel inhalant PDE inhibitors are under investigation, including combination treatments that provide bronchodilator and antiinflammatory activity (PDE3/4 inhibitors) or greater antiinflammatory activity (PDE4/7).
» Studies are ongoing to ascertain whether histone deacetylase is a viable target for novel drugs in treatment of respiratory disease.

Introduction

Theophylline has been in clinical use for more than a century, although in regular use for the treatment of respiratory disease only the last 50 years. In 1886, Henry Hyde Salter described the efficacious use of strong coffee taken on an empty stomach as a treatment for asthma.[1] The principal agent in coffee producing the bronchodilator effect observed is the methylxanthine *caffeine*. Theophylline has a similar chemical structure to caffeine (Fig. 96-1). In 1937 it was administered intravenously for the treatment of acute asthma, and in 1940 theophylline was first used orally in combination with ephedrine. Many studies now describe the effects of theophylline in the treatment of both asthma[2,3] and chronic obstructive pulmonary disease (COPD).[4]

Theophylline is presently used in various slow-release formulations to overcome rapid metabolism and maintain constant plasma levels. Over the last decade, however, the number of prescriptions for theophylline has declined as newer medications are introduced to treat respiratory disease, and mainly because of concerns about the narrow therapeutic window of theophylline, typically classified as 10 to 20 μg/mL in plasma.[2,3] An understanding of the molecular mechanism by which theophylline exerts its antiinflammatory activity might lead to the development of novel and safer antiinflammatory agents.

This chapter discusses the mechanism of action, dosage, side effects, and indications for theophylline. Also, because one of the molecular mechanisms of action proposed for theophylline is inhibition of phosphodiesterases, the selective phosphodiesterase inhibitors are also summarized.

Mechanism of Action

BRONCHODILATION

Theophylline has traditionally been classified as a bronchodilator drug; concentrations greater than 9 to 18 μg/mL are required to induce a 50% reversal of contraction of isolated bronchial preparations in vitro obtained from otherwise healthy subjects or from individuals who died as a result of severe asthma.[5] Despite these high concentrations required to produce relaxation in vitro, clinical studies have shown that bronchodilation in asthmatic patients can be achieved after intravenous administration of theophylline associated with plasma levels of about 10 μg/mL.[6] This beneficial action associated with theophylline could result from a direct relaxation of airway smooth muscle, although the concentration required to inhibit phosphodiesterases is one to two orders of magnitude greater than that achievable in plasma. Theophylline is also an antagonist for adenosine receptors, although the potency of this drug for adenosine A_1 and A_{2B} receptors is modest, with affinity (K_i) values of about 2 μg/mL for theophylline at both receptors (Table 96-1).

The bronchodilator action of theophylline may result from antagonism of adenosine receptors, although another xanthine, enprophylline, was as effective as theophylline, while the plasma levels were below the K_i value for enprophylline against the human, cloned A_1 adenosine receptor.[6] This receptor is expressed on airway smooth muscle from subjects with asthma.[7] Theophylline or enprophylline might block the stimulatory effect of endogenously released adenosine on mast cell A_{2B} receptors, with a subsequent downstream effect of reversing baseline airway constriction. However, neither xanthine has a

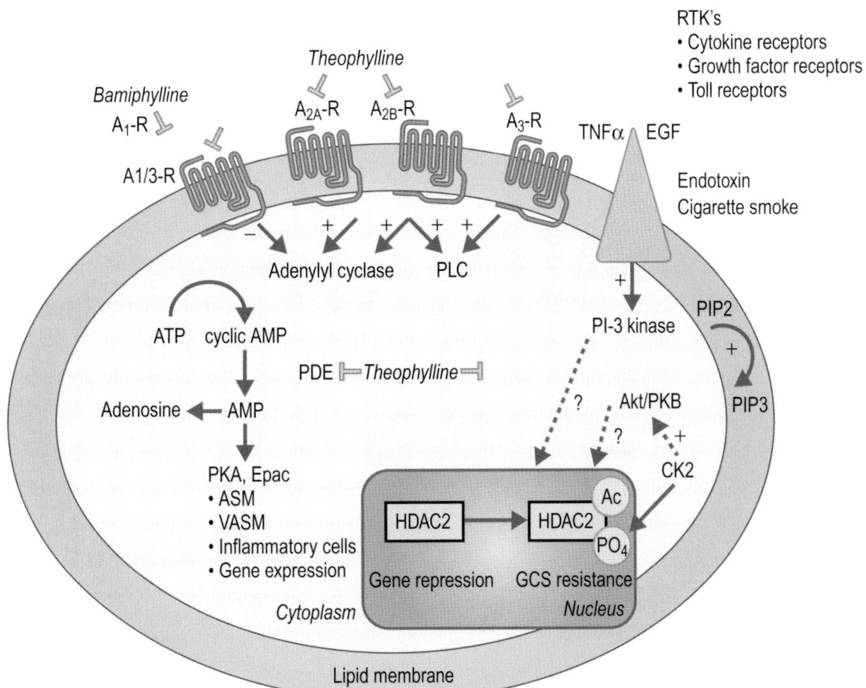

Figure 96-1 Diagrammatic representation showing the potential targets that could explain the beneficial action of theophylline. Theophylline is a relatively weak adenosine receptor antagonist, although targeting adenosine A_1 receptors might explain some of its beneficial actions. Xanthines such as bamiphylline are more potent antagonists at this receptor. Paradoxically, inhibition of adenosine A_{2A} receptor signaling could worsen inflammation, but current evidence supports that theophylline is predominantly antiinflammatory. Theophylline inhibits phosphodiesterase *(PDE)*, and the selective PDE4 inhibitor roflumilast is used to treat severe COPD. Mixed inhibitors such as RPL554 could provide both bronchodilator (PDE3) and antiinflammatory (PDE4) activity.* A third mechanism involves inhibition of phosphoinositide 3-kinase *(PI-3 kinase)* and reduction in histone deacetylase 2 *(HDAC2)* activity. PI-3 kinase (δ and γ isoforms) in certain circumstances contributes to cell recruitment to the airways. However, the δ isoform promotes steroid resistance, particularly in asthmatic smokers and COPD patients. The molecular mechanism might involve the acetylation and phosphorylation of HDAC2 by Akt/PKB (downstream of PI-3 kinase) and CK2-dependent pathways. Low doses of theophylline (0.18-1.8 μg/mL) are thought to restore glucocorticosteroid sensitivity in these subjects after inhibition of PI-3 kinase (δ isoform). *Akt/PKB,* Akt/protein kinase B; *AMP,* adenosine monophosphate; *ASM,* airway smooth muscle; *ATP,* adenosine triphosphate; *CK2,* casein kinase 2; *EGF,* epidermal growth factor; *Epac,* exchange protein directly activated by cyclic AMP; *GCS,* glucocorticosteroid; *PIP2,* phosphoinositidyl (4,5)-bisphosphate; *PIP3,* phosphoinositidyl (3,4,5)-triphosphate; *PKA,* protein kinase A; *PLC,* phospholipase C; *RTKs,* receptor tyrosine kinases; *TNF-α,* tumor necrosis factor alpha; *VASM,* vascular smooth muscle. (**Data from Boswell-Smith V, Spina D, Oxford AW, et al. The pharmacology of two novel long-acting phosphodiesterase 3/4 inhibitors, RPL554 [9,10-dimethoxy-2(2,4,6-trimethylphenylimino)-3-(n-carbamoyl-2-aminoethyl)-3,4,6,7-tetrahydro-2H-pyrimido[6,1-a]isoquinolin-4-one] and RPL565 [6,7-dihydro-2-(2,6-diisopropylphenoxy)-9,10-dimethoxy-4H-pyrimido[6,1-a]i soquinolin-4-one]. J Pharmacol Exp Ther 2006;318:840-8.*)

demonstrable effect against acute allergen-induced bronchospasm (see next section), thereby ruling out a major role for adenosine A_{2B} receptors in regulating airway caliber or influencing mast cell degranulation in humans. Furthermore, theophylline at clinically effective doses does not inhibit allergen-induced release of mast cell–derived mediators recovered from bronchoalveolar lavage fluid.[8] Another possibility is that theophylline might impair afferent neuronal activity, thereby reducing airway caliber indirectly[9] and the increased respiratory drive associated with lung disease.[4]

ANTIINFLAMMATORY ACTIONS

The allergen-induced late asthmatic response is often associated with the recruitment of inflammatory cells to the airways, including activated eosinophils, which can be significantly reduced after 4 to 6 weeks of treatment with theophylline.[10,11] Importantly, this antiinflammatory effect occurred at plasma levels of theophylline below 10 μg/mL. Not only was the number, but also the activation status of eosinophils reduced after theophylline therapy, as evidenced by a reduction in the number of cells expressing EG2, a marker used to indicate that cells were actively secreting eosinophil-derived cationic protein.[10] A significant reduction in the number of eosinophils in the airways of stable, mildly asthmatic patients was observed at plasma levels of theophylline (6 μg/mL) that was insufficient to alter pulmonary lung mechanics.[11] Similarly, after nasal allergen challenge, the late phase response and the accumulation/activation of eosinophils in the nose was also significantly attenuated in allergic rhinitis patients after chronic treatment with theophylline.[12]

Regular theophylline treatment has also produced antiinflammatory activity in patients with natural exacerbations of their asthma, in the form of nocturnal asthma. Theophylline treatment significantly improved the overnight deterioration in lung function associated with nocturnal asthma compared with placebo treatment,[13] a finding consistent with previous studies of theophylline for asthma.[14] Chronic treatment with theophylline also protected individuals from nocturnal falls in baseline forced expiratory volume in 1 second (FEV_1) and was associated with a reduction in the number of neutrophils migrating into the airways of these subjects.[13] The magnitude of inhibition of neutrophil recruitment to the airways was correlated with plasma concentrations of theophylline (12 to 24 μg/mL).

TABLE 96-1 Examples of Xanthines and Drug Targets

Name	Structure	Known Drug Targets*
Theophylline	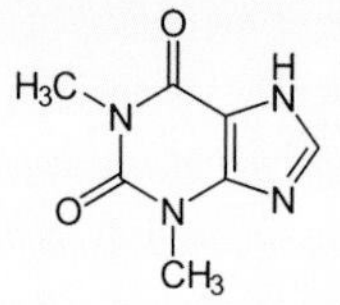	A_1 receptor (6.8 μM) A_{2A} receptor (2 μM) A_{2B} receptor (9/10/74 μM) A_3 receptor (22 μM) PDE3 (98 μM) PDE4 (150 μM) PI-3 kinase (100 μM)
Enprophylline	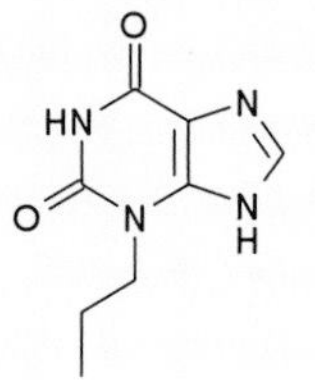	A1 receptor (42/156 μM) A_{2A} receptor (32/81 μM) A_{2B} receptor (5/10/20 μM) A_3 receptor (65/93 μM) PDE1, 2, 3, 4, 5 (>100 μM)
Doxophylline	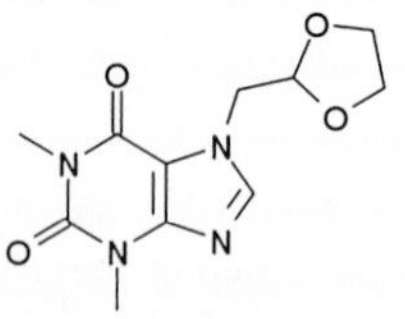	A_1 receptor (>100 μM) A_2 receptor (>100 μM)
Bamiphylline	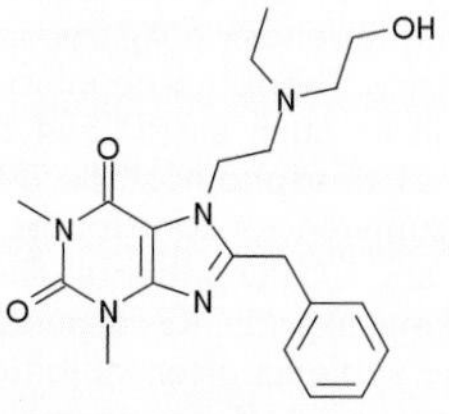	$A_1 > A_2$ (562 times)

*Values represent affinity constants and inhibitory potency for xanthines against adenosine receptors and phosphodiesterase (*PDE*)/phosphoinositide (*PI*) 3-kinase, respectively. The therapeutic window for theophylline is about 10 to 20 μg/mL, which is equivalent to 50 to 100 μM.

Moreover, the ability of these neutrophils to release leukotriene B_4 (LTB_4) stimulated with a calcium ionophore in culture ex vivo was suppressed in these patients. This indicated that theophylline could inhibit not only the migration of cells to the airways, but also their ability to be activated once recruited to the lung. This is consistent with an antiinflammatory action of theophylline (Table 96-2) and supports earlier work that regular treatment with theophylline can reduce neutrophil activation.[15] In contrast, withdrawing theophylline from asthma patients who were taking glucocorticosteroids resulted in a significant deterioration of their disease, with a concomitant rise in the number of $CD4^+$ and $CD8^+$ T lymphocytes in bronchial biopsies.[16] The antiinflammatory effects of theophylline have also been documented in patients with COPD. Various indices of inflammation were significantly reduced, including sputum number of neutrophils (40%), interleukin-8 (IL-8; 24%), and myeloperoxidase (31%), at plasma levels of theophylline between 9 and 11 μg/mL.[17]

Studies in pediatric asthma have shown that the effect of theophylline is comparable to low doses of glucocorticosteroids.[18] This observation is of particular interest given that theophylline is an orally active drug shown to have a better compliance rate than inhaled medications. Given the low cost

TABLE 96-2 Experimental Findings Showing Antiinflammatory Property of Xanthines and Phosphodiesterase 4 (PDE4) Inhibitors in Human Cells

Cell Type	Theophylline	PDE4 Inhibitors
T lymphocytes	Migration through endothelium Promote IL-10 production Tolerance induction Increase T suppressor cell function Inhibit graft rejection in vitro and in vivo	Suppress proliferation Suppress cytokine release
Eosinophils	Reduce survival	Decrease ROS and LTC_4 production
Neutrophils	Reduced superoxide generation, LTB_4 release, and chemotaxis	Reduce IL-8 and LTB_4 production Reduce chemotaxis Reduce elastase and MMP-9 release
Mast cells	Reduce mediator release	Decrease mediator release
Monocytes	Inhibition of TNF-α release Inhibition of IL-12 release Promoted IL-10 production	Decrease TNF-α production Increase IL-10 production
Macrophages	Inhibition of TNF-α release	Decrease TNF-α production Increase IL-10 production
Vascular endothelium	Inhibition of adhesion molecule expression	Decrease adhesion molecule expression and lymphocyte transmigration
Fibroblasts	Inhibition of collagen mRNA expression and proliferation	

Data from Page CP, Spina D. Phosphodiesterase inhibitors in the treatment of inflammatory diseases. Handb Exp Pharmacol 2011;204:391-414; and Spina D, Landells LJ, Page CP. The role of phosphodiesterase enzymes in allergy and asthma. Adv Pharmacol 1998;44:33-89.

IL, Interleukin; *LT*, leukotriene; *MMP*, matrix metalloproteinase; *ROS*, reactive oxygen species; *TNF-α*, tumor necrosis factor alpha.

of theophylline relative to other antiasthma medications, and that it is still one of the few oral drugs available for asthma therapy, the evidence that theophylline is antiinflammatory and immunomodulatory at lower-than-conventional plasma levels suggest it should have a greater role in the treatment of asthma.

MOLECULAR MECHANISMS

Adenosine Receptor Antagonism

Theophylline and enprophylline are antagonists of adenosine receptors with affinities against the human, cloned adenosine A_1, A_{2B}, and A_3 receptors in the micromolar range, levels that can be achieved clinically[6] (see Table 96-1). It has been argued that the similarity in clinical effectiveness between theophylline and enprophylline against the early and late phase asthmatic response[18a] and against histamine but not adenosine-induced bronchoconstriction,[6] suggested that adenosine receptor antagonism could not account for the bronchoprotective action exhibited by the xanthines. Also, both theophylline and enprophylline inhibited mediator secretion from human lung mast cells by acting as a selective adenosine A_{2B} receptor antagonist and with affinities in the order of 1.8 μg/mL.[19] Patients with asthma are very sensitive to inhaled adenosine, an effect that is blocked by theophylline and enprophylline. Both drugs have an equivalent inhibitory effect on allergen-induced late response,[19] although theophylline was more effective in causing bronchoprotection against inhaled adenosine at plasma levels that caused a similar degree of bronchodilation.[6] Therefore, it is unlikely that the effect of xanthines in asthma is through antagonism of A_{2B} receptors.

Other studies have revealed that isolated bronchial airways from asthmatic patients[20] and passively sensitized human bronchial tissue[21] contract in response to adenosine through an A_1-receptor–dependent mechanism. This is consistent with the increased expression of these receptors in epithelium and airway smooth muscle in biopsies obtained from mildly asthmatic subjects.[22] In support of A_1-receptor antagonism as a mechanism of action of xanthines are the clinical observations that bamiphylline, used in Europe for the treatment of respiratory disease, is 562 times more potent at adenosine A_1 versus A_2 receptors. On the other hand, another clinically effective xanthine, doxophylline, appears to lack adenosine receptor antagonism (see Table 96-1).

Phosphodiesterase Inhibition

Theophylline has long been recognized as a nonselective phosphodiesterase (PDE) inhibitor, and this molecular action may contribute to the effectiveness of theophylline clinically as well as account for many of the side effects of xanthines.[23] However, it is now recognized that an ever-growing family of PDE enzymes, most of which are not sensitive to inhibition by theophylline at plasma levels, can be safely achieved clinically. Nonetheless, the pharmaceutical industry has expended considerable effort in developing selective PDE inhibitors because of the modest clinical effectiveness of theophylline and its narrow therapeutic window.

Currently, the focus is in developing PDE4 inhibitors that target inflammatory cells and PDE3 inhibitors that primarily target airway smooth muscle, based on the assumption that the plasma concentration of theophylline required to achieve 50% inhibition (IC_{50}) of these enzymes only occur above 18 μg/mL and is only a relatively poor inhibitor. PDE4 has been found in many inflammatory cells thought to participate in respiratory diseases (e.g., asthma, COPD), and inhibition of this enzyme can suppress cell function (see Table 96-2). Such observations have underpinned the development of *roflumilast,* a potent and selective PDE4 inhibitor, now marketed in the European Union (EU) for treatment of exacerbations in patients with severe COPD. However, although it has proved effective in the treatment of patients with asthma,[24] roflumilast has not yet been approved for this indication (see later).

Phosphodiesterases comprise at least 11 gene families, metabolize the second messengers, cyclic adenosine monophosphate (cAMP) and cyclic guanosine monophosphate (cGMP), thereby finely controlling their intracellular levels. Also of relevance to respiratory diseases is the presence of PDE3 in airway and vascular smooth muscle. In homogenates of human bronchus, PDE3, PDE4, and PDE5 are present in equal abundance, and theophylline inhibited cAMP PDE activity by about 40% at a plasma levels equivalent to 18 μg/mL and at this concentration, caused relaxation of spontaneously contracted human bronchial tissue 60% below baseline tone.[25] This is consistent with clinical data showing a 10% improvement in baseline FEV_1 with plasma levels of theophylline at about 12 μg/mL in atopic asthmatic patients[6] and suggests selective PDE3 inhibitors could provide a novel class of bronchodilator.

OTHER INTRACELLULAR TARGETS

Phosphoinositide 3-Kinase

Phosphoinositide 3-kinase (PI-3 kinase) belongs to a family of lipid kinase enzymes of which there are four classes (IA, IB, II and III) based on their in vitro substrate specificities, and there activation by various receptors (e.g., cytokine, growth hormone, Toll, G-protein coupled). Class IA and IB kinases phosphorylate phosphatidylinositol,(4,5) bisphosphate (PtdIns[4,5]) P2 in the 3 position to give rise to PtdIns(3,4,5) P3, which triggers a cascade of intracellular events involved in metabolism, cell survival, migration, growth, and proliferation that are characteristics of such diseases as cancer and inflammation. As an example, the generation of PtdIns(3,4,5)-triphosphate (PIP3) leads to the translocation of Akt/protein kinase B (PKB) and subsequent binding by virtue of the plekstrin homology (PH) domain of PIP3 on the inner leaflet of cell membranes. A similar interaction between 3′-phosphoinositide–dependent kinase-1 (PDK1) results in the phosphorylation and subsequent activation of Akt/PKB. A downstream target of Akt/PKB of relevance to airway inflammatory disease is inhibitory protein I-κB kinase, which subsequently phosphorylates nuclear factor (NF)-κB, a proinflammatory transcription factor.[26] Inactivation of either the δ or γ isoform of PI-3 kinase did not affect airways inflammation in mice exposed to cigarette smoke,[27] although these enzymes appeared to contribute to the inflammatory response in other models.[28]

Theophylline inhibits the enzyme activity of human recombinant PI-3 kinase with an IC_{50} value of 75, 300, and 800 μM for the class IA heterodimers p85α/p110δ, p85α/p110α, and p85α/p110β, respectively, and 800 μM for the class IB monomeric p110γ PI-3 kinase. The IC_{50} value against PI-3 δ isoform would be achieved with plasma levels of theophylline between 10 and 20 μg/mL. These studies also showed that xanthines can interfere with the lipid kinase activity of this enzyme, with a clear structure-activity relationship among xanthines, and interestingly, enprophylline did not inhibit lipid kinase activity at a concentration of 1 mM.[29]

As mentioned previously, one consequence of the activation of PI-3 kinase is the formation of PIP3, resulting in the translocation of Akt/PKB to the cell membrane and subsequent phosphorylation of Akt/PKB on threonine-308 and serine-473 by PDK1 and PDK2, respectively. Theophylline inhibited insulin-induced phosphorylation of Akt/PKB in rat soleus muscle and CHO cells with an IC_{50} value of 100 and 500 μM, respectively, showing that natively expressed PI-3 kinase can be inhibited by theophylline.[29] Whether these effects of theophylline on PI-3 kinase contribute to the drug's beneficial effect remains to be established clinically.

Histone Deacetylases

A significant improvement in a number of clinical variables was observed in subjects with poorly controlled asthma taking existing glucocorticosteroid therapy after concomitant treatment with theophylline, compared with increasing the dose of glucocorticosteroid[30] at plasma levels of theophylline not sufficient to induce bronchodilation. In contrast, withdrawing theophylline from asthmatic patients taking glucocorticosteroids resulted in a significant deterioration of their disease together with a concomitant rise in the number of $CD4^+$ and $CD8^+$ T lymphocytes in bronchial biopsies.[16,31] These results suggest that theophylline may offer additional benefit to glucocorticosteroids, as previously suggested by other clinical studies using different protocols.[16,31,32]

A novel mechanism was proposed that might explain the apparent beneficial effect of theophylline in patients with severe asthma taking glucocorticosteroids, as well as the relative ineffectiveness of glucocorticosteroids in COPD treatment involving the activation of a family of nuclear proteins regulating gene transcription.[33] At a molecular level, the rate of gene transcription can be controlled by transcriptional coactivators (e.g., p300, CBP), which link transcription factors to RNA–polymerase II complex through protein-protein interactions. Both p300 and CBP possess intrinsic histone acetyltransferase (HAT) activity, resulting in the acetylation of lysine on the N-terminal regions of histone. This leads to a neutralization of positive charge, resulting in the remodeling of chromatin and unwinding of DNA and a more favorable environment for transcription factors to bind in order to regulate gene transcription.

Conversely, gene transcription can be silenced by a family of proteins called histone deacetylases (HDACs), which deacetylate lysine residues in chromatin, thereby silencing gene transcription.[34] Theophylline and enprophylline at concentrations between 1 and 10 μM increased the activity of HDAC, whereas concentrations above this value inhibited the activity of this enzyme.[33] A functional consequence of these low doses of theophylline was a suppression of IL-8 release when administered with low concentrations of dexamethasone. This may explain the clinical observations of the deterioration in asthma symptoms after removal of theophylline from patients taking glucocorticosteroids.[33] It is proposed that theophylline might act as an allosteric activator of HDAC or might inhibit the activity of a kinase that phosphorylated HDAC and thereby restore glucocorticosteroid sensitivity. Adenosine receptor antagonism and inhibition of cAMP metabolism did not account for the ability of theophylline to increase HDAC activity.[33] Further studies showed that the ability of theophylline to restore glucocorticosteroid sensitivity was dependent on the activation of the p110δ isoform of PI-3 kinase.[27,35] It appears that the inhibitory activity of theophylline is increased by 65-fold in cells exposed to oxidant stress, which would explain why low concentrations of theophylline, both in vitro and in vivo, can augment HDAC2 activity.[35]

It is proposed that oxidant stress activates PI-3 kinase (e.g., Akt/PKB, both cell membrane–localizing proteins), which leads to the subsequent phosphorylation of HDAC2, located in the nucleus, although the precise molecular details have yet to be established. For example, Akt/PKB has been shown to translocate to the nucleus and promote phosphorylation of p300, with subsequent increased gene transcription of the intercellular adhesion protein ICAM-1 in response to tumor necrosis factor alpha (TNF-α),[36] although it is unclear whether Akt can phosphorylate HDAC2. The only kinase currently known to phosphorylate HDAC2 is casein-dependent kinase II (CK2), which during oxidant stress promotes loss of deacetylase activity and reduces transrepression, loss of HDAC2 protein, and steroid resistance.[37]

Dosages and Routes of Administration

Theophylline is rapidly and completely absorbed when administered as a capsule or solution but is delayed when given as a coated tablet, although absorption is nonetheless complete. Absorption may be delayed when taken with a meal or when administered in the evening. There is some degree of variability between the absorption of theophylline from different formulations manufactured for slow release (Table 96-3).[2,3,38]

Dosing is usually commenced at 10 mg/kg for children older than 6 months and adults, to a maximum of 300 mg/day and subsequently increased by 13 to 16 mg/kg/day (maximum 450

TABLE 96-3 Examples of Theophylline Formulations and Absorption Characteristics

Formulation	Doses (mg)	Comments
Slo-bid Gyrocap*‡	50-300 mg	C_{max} ~ 5-9 hours every 12 hours. For children, can be swallowed whole or with granules sprinkled on food. Rapid and complete absorption in the absence or presence of food.
Slo-Phyllin†‡	60-250 mg	C_{max} ~ 4-8 hours every 12 hours. For children, can be swallowed whole or with granules sprinkled on food. Rapid and complete absorption in the absence or presence of food.
Theo-24*‡	100-400 mg	C_{max} ~ 6-14 hours every 24 hours. Absorption is variable in the morning, after meals, or in the evening.
Theo-Dur*	100, 200, 300 mg	C_{max} ~ 4-10 hours every 12 hours. Tablets (100, 300 mg) are scored. Complete absorption in the absence or presence of food.
Uni-Dur*	400, 600 mg	C_{max} ~ 8-12 hours; once-daily evening dose. Complete absorption in the absence or presence of food.
Uniphyl*	200, 400 mg	C_{max} ~ 8-12 hours every 12 hours. Incomplete absorption after overnight fast; more complete when taken after food.
Uniphyllin Continuous†	200, 300, 400 mg	Some evidence of delay in absorption with food in children.
Nuelin SA†	175, 250 mg	C_{max} ~ 4-8 hours every 12 hours.
Phyllocontin Continuous†	225 mg	Aminophylline hydrate: C_{max} ~ 4-8 hours. Taken twice daily, to two tablets twice daily after 1 week.

Data from Hendeles L, Massanari M, Weinberger M. Update on the pharmacodynamics and pharmacokinetics of theophylline. Chest 1985;88(Suppl. 2):103S-11S; Weinberger M, Hendeles L. Theophylline in asthma. N Engl J Med 1996;334:1380-8; and Weinberger M, Hendeles L, Wong L. Relationship of formulation and dosing interval to fluctuation of serum theophylline concentration in children with chronic asthma. J Pediatr 1981;99:145-52.

C_{max}, Maximum drug concentration.

*Marketed in United States.

†Marketed in United Kingdom.

‡Indicates delivery by capsule; otherwise, tablet form.

TABLE 96-4 **Examples of Drug-Drug Interactions with Theophylline**

Drug/Class	Nature of Interaction	Effect on Theophylline
Alcohol (large dose)		Reduced plasma clearance
Allopurinol (high dose)		Reduced plasma clearance
Antibacterials		
Fluoroquinolones		
Ciprofloxacin Norfloxacin Enoxacin	Inhibition of CYP1A2	Reduced plasma clearance
Macrolides		
Clarithromycin Erythromycin Troleandomycin	Inhibition of CYP3A and uptake into hepatocytes	Reduced plasma clearance
Antidepressants		
Fluvoxamine St John's wort	Inhibition of CYP1A2	Reduced plasma clearance (halve dose of theophylline)
Antiviral: Ritonavir	Inducer of CYP1A2	Increased plasma clearance
Barbiturate: Phenobarbital	Inducer of CYP1A2	Increased plasma clearance
Calcium channel blocker: Verapamil	Substrate of CYP1A2	Reduced plasma clearance
Oral contraceptive: Estrogen	Substrate of CYP1A2	Reduced plasma clearance
Miscellaneous		
Disulfiram	Inhibitor for CYP2E1	Reduced plasma clearance (affects hydroxylation pathway)
Cimetidine	Inhibitor for CYP1A2	Reduced plasma clearance
Interferon-α	Decrease CYP1A2 expression	Reduced plasma clearance
Methotrexate, mexiletine, propafenone, pentoxifylline, propranolol, tacrine, thiabendazole, ticlopidine	Substrate for CYP1A2	Reduced plasma clearance
Zileuton	Inhibitor for CYP1A2 5-lipoxygenase inhibitor	Reduced plasma clearance
Aminoglutethimide, carbamazepine, phenytoin, primidone, rifampicin, sulfinpyrazone	Inducers of CYP1A2	Increased plasma clearance
Tobacco	Inducer of CYP1A2	Increased plasma clearance
β-Adrenergic agonists		Increased risk of hypokalemia with theophylline
Benzodiazepines		Theophylline reduces the effects of these drugs.
Lithium carbonate, erythromycin, phenytoin		Theophylline increases excretion of these drugs.
Corticosteroids Diuretics		Increased risk of hypokalemia with theophylline
Ephedrine		Avoid use with theophylline, particularly in children.

Data from Hendeles L, Massanari M, Weinberger M. Update on the pharmacodynamics and pharmacokinetics of theophylline. Chest 1985;88 (Suppl. 2):103S-11S; Weinberger M, Hendeles L. N Engl J Med 1996;334:1380-8; and http://medicine.iupui.edu/flowchart/table.html.

to 600 mg/kg). If the dose achieves plasma concentrations less than 10 μg/mL, the dose is increased by 25%. The dose is maintained if plasma levels of 10 to 15 μg/mL are achieved and the patient tolerates the dose. A dose reduction of 10% should be considered if plasma levels of 15 to 20 μg/mL are observed, and if plasma levels of 20 to 25 μg/mL and greater than 25 μg/mL are observed, the next dose and next 2 doses should be withheld, respectively, and treatment resumed on the next-lower dose increment.[2,3,38]

Theophylline rapidly distributes into nonadipose tissue and body water (volume of distribution [Vd] approximately 0.5 L/kg), and this value can increase in patients who have liver disease, elderly patients, and those with factors that alter albumin binding (40% plasma protein binding). Theophylline is metabolized extensively in the liver (up to 70%), where it undergoes N-demethylation to 1- and 3-methylxanthine through cytochrome P-450 (CYP) 1A2 and 8-hydroxylation by CYP2E1.[3] The metabolism of theophylline is influenced by environmental factors (e.g., CYP1A2 activity is increased by cigarette smoking), hepatic disease, genetic factors, and important drug-drug interactions, which increase, decrease, or interfere with CYP1A2 activity (Table 96-4).[2,3]

The elimination half-life of theophylline is approximately 8 hours in adults and 4 hours in children, and 10% is excreted unchanged by the kidney in adults. Theophylline does cross the placenta, but there have been no reports of teratogenicity in the neonate when theophylline is administered during the first trimester. However, if the dose is not adjusted during pregnancy, potentially harmful plasma levels can be achieved, particularly as the clearance of theophylline during the third trimester is delayed (pregnancy category C). Furthermore, the accumulation of the metabolite *caffeine* in the neonate, particularly in the first 6 months of life, means that is advisable to monitor the neonate for signs of theophylline toxicity.[2,3,38]

Major Side Effects

The major side effects associated with theophylline occur when plasma concentration rises above 20 μg/mL, which include gastrointestinal (GI) side effects such as nausea, vomiting, and diarrhea. Other side effects occurring above this level include insomnia, irritability, and headache. At concentrations greater than 30 μg/mL the potential for cardiac arrhythmia (probably via A_1-receptor antagonism), hypotension, hypokalemia, and hyperglycemia (PDE3 inhibition) are more likely. Seizures, brain damage, and death occur at levels greater than 40 μg/mL. The side effects associated with high plasma levels of theophylline are only likely to be achieved after rapid intravenous administration and are unlikely to occur after oral ingestion with proper monitoring. The propensity for these side effects is exacerbated in elderly patients with comorbidities, those with impaired renal and liver function or cardiac failure, and patients taking other medications that could cause drug-drug interactions, particularly if chronic overdosing occurs. Consequently, monitoring of plasma levels is important, particularly during pregnancy, when neonatal levels of theophylline can achieve toxic levels because of reduced clearance, as described earlier.

The numerous side effects associated with theophylline, drug-drug interactions, and the requirement for plasma monitoring limit the utility of theophylline, although its demonstrable antiinflammatory effect in asthma and COPD at doses below the therapeutic window and its ease of administration can justify its use.[2,3]

Indications and Contraindications

Reviews of randomized controlled clinical trials (RCTs) investigating the effectiveness of theophylline in patients with asthma[39] and with COPD[40] have concluded that this drug has modest clinical effectiveness. Theophylline can improve lung function and reduce exacerbations in patients with mild to moderate asthma taking inhaled glucocorticosteroids or in whom asthma is poorly controlled with glucocorticosteroids, although these effects are relatively modest.[39]

A Cochrane report concluded that theophylline was as effective as long acting β_2-adrenoceptor agonists in the control of nocturnal asthma in adolescents and adults with persistent asthma.[41] An earlier report concluded that although some evidence suggests that theophylline has beneficial actions in terms of reducing symptoms and the need for rescue medication in children with mild to moderate asthma, it was less effective than inhaled glucocorticosteroids.[42] One potential problem in treating children with theophylline is the possibility of a deterioration in cognitive and behavioral scores, but no significant changes were found.[42] Oral versus inhaled treatment is clearly advantageous in the pediatric asthmatic population, and some evidence indicates that theophylline may be beneficial as add-on therapy in children with severe asthma not controlled with inhaled glucocorticosteroids, although large RCTs are required to address this issue.

Randomized clinical trials have highlighted that long-term treatment with theophylline for patients with COPD significantly improved lung function (0 to 120 mL), reduced exacerbations (by 50%), and diminished worsening of symptoms (12 vs. 4 days without symptoms), although no study has investigated whether theophylline can reduce the decline in lung function and mortality and improve quality of life. However, it was concluded that the utility of theophylline is compromised by numerous side effects (e.g., risk of nausea about sevenfold greater than with placebo) even within its normal therapeutic window (e.g., headache, irritability, arrhythmia, seizures).[40] The risk of these adverse effects is clearly an issue for COPD patients, who tend to be older with systemic comorbidities and who may be prescribed other medications leading to drug-drug interactions (see Table 96-4), and the need for monitoring plasma levels makes this treatment far from ideal.

Selective Phosphodiesterase Inhibitors

MECHANISM OF ACTION

The development of selective PDE4 inhibitors for use in the treatment of respiratory diseases is based in part on the understanding of the role of intracellular cyclic AMP in the regulation of inflammatory cell function.[43] There are 11 isoenzymes (PDE1 to PDE11) within the PDE superfamily, and each isoenzyme has different tissue distribution and biochemical properties, enabling targeted therapy with potentially fewer side effects than theophylline. Particular interest is in targeting the PDE4 isoenzyme, which is expressed in inflammatory cells (e.g., neutrophils, macrophages, lymphocytes, eosinophils) and structural cells (e.g., fibroblasts, epithelium, sensory nerves, airway smooth muscle cells) within the lung.[43] The presence of the PDE4 isoenzyme in many of the cell types implicated in asthma and COPD has made it a promising target for disease-modifying therapy, given the strong relationship among chronic airway inflammation, structural remodeling, and changes in lung function (e.g., nonreversible decline in lung function in COPD[44]). Numerous studies have documented the ability of PDE4 inhibitors to attenuate many aspects of inflammatory cell function relevant to respiratory disease (see Fig. 96-1 and Table 96-2).

Thus, it is not surprising that PDE4 inhibitors attenuate various characteristics of respiratory diseases, including recruitment of inflammatory cells to the lung, bronchial hyperresponsiveness (BHR), and airway edema when administered into preclinical "asthma" models. This is exemplified by the most clinically advanced PDE4 inhibitor, roflumilast, which suppresses various aspects of the allergic inflammatory response in asthma models and neutrophil activation and recruitment in COPD models.[43,45]

Although PDE4 inhibitors exhibit antiinflammatory activity, they do not exhibit significant bronchodilator activity. Thus, oral administration of roflumilast (500 μg) had no significant effect on the acute bronchoconstriction following allergen challenge,[46] which is consistent with the suggestion that PDE3 rather than PDE4 is the important isoenzyme regulating airway smooth muscle tone in asthmatic patients.[47] It also suggests that targeting PDE4 alone may not be sufficient to inhibit mast cell degranulation.[48] The effect of PDE4 inhibitors on cellular recruitment to the airways has recently been reported in COPD with another PDE4 inhibitor, cilomilast, and after 10-week treatment, a significant reduction in the number of $CD8^+$ T lymphocytes, macrophages, and neutrophils was observed in bronchial biopsies.[49] These studies show that PDE4 inhibitors have the potential to reduce not only the traffic of cells to inflammatory sites, but also their activity.

A number of clinical studies have now shown the ability of roflumilast to improve lung function in patients with asthma[24] and with COPD,[50,51] which is unlikely to be caused by bronchodilation, because these drugs have only modest effects on airway smooth muscle function.[43] Another explanation for the beneficial effect of PDE4 inhibitors in patients with asthma might include suppression of BHR secondary to a reduction of airway inflammation.

DOSAGES AND ROUTES OF ADMINISTRATION

Roflumilast is currently available to be prescribed only as a once-daily treatment (500 μg) for patients with severe COPD. Roflumilast is rapidly metabolized to the N-oxide, which has similar pharmacology to the parent compound. Roflumilast is rapidly and completely absorbed following a single oral dose, with a minor delay when ingested with a high-fat diet, although the pharmacokinetics of the N-oxide is not affected.[52] Both roflumilast and the N-oxide have high plasma protein binding. Roflumilast is metabolized in the liver to the N-oxide by CYP4A3 and CYP1A2; consequently, a number of drug-drug interactions have been investigated[52] (Table 96-5). However, none of these interactions appears to alter the pharmacodynamics of roflumilast. The parent compound and N-oxide are excreted in the urine with a half-life of 17 and 30 hours, respectively, the N-oxide metabolite contributing to the drug's once-daily activity.

TABLE 96-5 Examples of Drug-Drug Interactions with Roflumilast

Drug/Class	Nature of Interaction	Effect on Roflumilast
ANTIBACTERIALS		
Erythromycin	Inhibition of CYP3A4	Increased plasma levels (adjustment not required)
Rifampicin	Inducer of CYP4A4	Reduced plasma levels (dose adjustment may be required)
Enoxacin	Inhibition of CYP1A2	Increased plasma levels (adjustment not required)
Antifungal: Ketoconazole	Inhibition of CYP3A4	Increased plasma levels (adjustment not required)
Anxiolytic: Midazolam	Substrate for CYP3A4	Roflumilast did not interfere with plasma levels for midazolam.
Antidepressant: Fluvoxamine	Inhibitor of CYP1A2, CYP2C19, CYP2D6, and CYP3A4	Increased plasma levels (adjustment may be required)
Cigarette smoke	Inducer of CYP1A2	Reduced plasma levels (but no adjustment necessary)
Digoxin	P-glycoprotein transporter	No adjustment necessary
Antacids	Possible effects on absorption	No difference

Data from Lahu G, Nassr N, Huennemeyer A. Pharmacokinetic evaluation of roflumilast. Expert Opin Drug Metab Toxicol 2011;7: 1577-91.

MAJOR SIDE EFFECTS

The most common adverse effects reported by COPD patients receiving PDE inhibitors included central adverse events (nausea, headache, insomnia), GI side effects (diarrhea), and (modest) weight loss.[50,51] Adverse events mostly became evident during the first 4 to 12 weeks and although usually subsiding with continued treatment, these events caused an increased patient withdrawal in the roflumilast arms. In addition, no clinically relevant cardiac toxicity was reported.[50,51] The potential to cause nausea and emesis is based on the localization of PDE4B and PDE4D isoforms in the area postrema in humans.[53] This region of the brainstem is not completely behind the blood-brain barrier, and thus inhibition of these enzymes can lead to elevations in cAMP within area postrema neurons, which can trigger an emetogenic response. One way to minimize the nausea and vomiting in susceptible patients is to dose every other day until tolerance develops.

In all four registration trials for roflumilast, weight loss was reported, with a mean of 2.1 kg, mostly occurring in the first 6 months of the trial,[50] and with a similar mean weight loss of 1.9 kg.[51] The largest absolute weight loss was seen in patients with a body mass index (BMI) greater than 30. If this weight loss is ascribed primarily to fat loss, it remains to be established how this relates to the systemic antiinflammatory potential of roflumilast. In the COPD safety-pooled analysis, including more than 12,000 COPD patients from several RCT trials (797 patients receiving roflumilast, 250 μg; 5766 taking roflumilast, 500 μg; 5491 receiving placebo), three suicides were reported, all receiving roflumilast treatment (one at 250 μg; two at 500 μg).[54] Despite relatively small numbers and possible preexisting depression among these patients, these findings obviously require close monitoring.

INDICATIONS AND CONTRAINDICATIONS

The clinical benefits of roflumilast have been confirmed in four RCTs in patients with moderate to severe COPD.[50,51] Two of these studies evaluated the effect of roflumilast versus placebo in patients already treated with regular salmeterol (M2-127 study) or tiotropium (M2-128 study) therapy.[51] In both trials, roflumilast was associated with consistent and sustained improvement in both the prebronchodilator and postbronchodilator FEV_1. In the salmeterol combination the mean increase in prebronchodilator FEV_1 versus placebo was 49 mL; in the tiotropium combination the mean increase was 80 mL ($P < .0001$). Patients receiving roflumilast tended to have fewer exacerbations, and the dropout rate was greater in the roflumilast arm, with significantly more withdrawals in the salmeterol-roflumilast arm ($P = .0019$). The most frequently reported roflumilast-related side effects were nausea, diarrhea, and mild weight loss (mean 1.8 and 2 kg).[51]

In two other clinical trials (M2-124 and M2-125) an identical study design was used, including the recruitment of chronic smokers or ex-smokers (≥20 pack-years) with symptomatic, (very) severe COPD characterized by chronic cough, sputum production, and exacerbations.[50] In both studies, patients received either roflumilast or placebo for 52 weeks, concomitantly with their existing COPD medication after a 4 week placebo run-in period. There was a mean increase in prebronchodilator FEV_1 of 48 mL ($P < .0001$) and a significant decrease in both moderate and severe exacerbations of 17% in the roflumilast versus placebo group ($P < .0003$). The improvement in lung function and reduction in exacerbations were independent of concomitant use of long-acting β_2-agonists or short-acting muscarinic antagonists, or prior inhaled corticosteroid use or smoking behavior. The mortality from COPD was similar in both treatment arms in both studies (2% to 3%).

The mechanism of improvement in lung function, exacerbation rates, and quality of life scores cannot be attributed to a direct bronchodilating action of this drug class, as we have previously discussed for cilomilast. It is more likely that these beneficial actions are secondary to an antiinflammatory activity of roflumilast (see Table 96-2), although the reduction in proinflammatory cell numbers found in two other studies was modest.

Summary

Theophylline has been used in the treatment of respiratory disease for nearly a century, but its precise mechanism of action remains to be established. Theophylline is a bronchodilator, but its antiinflammatory activity has gained increasing acceptance. However, the antiinflammatory effectiveness is modest compared with the "gold standard," glucocorticosteroids, for the treatment of asthma. Theophylline has found a niche as add-on therapy in patients with severe asthma. In patients with COPD the bronchodilator action of theophylline is accepted, although it remains to be established whether this drug is antiinflammatory in this disease, with some evidence that theophylline might facilitate glucocorticosteroid activity in COPD patients. However, theophylline has significant potential for side effects, and drug-drug interactions require monitoring of plasma levels, a disadvantage for oral treatment. Mechanistic studies have revealed potential drug targets, and PDE4 is a target successfully exploited with roflumilast treatment of COPD. Other targets may offer novel therapeutic agents for future treatment of asthma and COPD.

REFERENCES

Introduction

1. Persson CGA, Pauwels R. Pharmacology of antiasthma xanthines. In: Page CP, Barnes PJ, editors. Pharmacology of asthma. Berlin: Springer-Verlag; 1991, p. 207-25.
2. Hendeles L, Massanari M, Weinberger M. Update on the pharmacodynamics and pharmacokinetics of theophylline. Chest 1985;88 (Suppl. 2):103S-11S.
3. Weinberger M, Hendeles L. Theophylline in asthma. N Engl J Med 1996;334:1380-8.
4. Ashutosh K, Sedat M, Fragale-Jackson J. Effects of theophylline on respiratory drive in patients with chronic obstructive pulmonary disease. J Clin Pharmacol 1997;37:1100-7.

Mechanism of Action

5. Goldie RG, Spina D, Henry PJ, Lulich KM, Paterson JW. In vitro responsiveness of human asthmatic bronchus to carbachol, histamine, beta-adrenoceptor agonists and theophylline. Br J Clin Pharmacol 1986;22:669-76.
6. Clarke H, Cushley MJ, Persson CG, Holgate ST. The protective effects of intravenous theophylline and enprofylline against histamine- and adenosine 5′-monophosphate-provoked bronchoconstriction: implications for the mechanisms of action of xanthine derivatives in asthma. Pulm Pharmacol 1989;2:147-54.
7. Brown RA, Clarke GW, Ledbetter CL, et al. Elevated expression of adenosine A_1 receptor in bronchial biopsy specimens from asthmatic subjects. Eur Respir J 2008;31:311-9.
8. Jaffar ZH, Sullivan P, Page CP, Costello J. Low-dose theophylline modulates T-lymphocyte activation in allergen-challenged asthmatics. Eur Respir J 1996;9:456-62.
9. Barlinski J, Lockhart A, Frossard N. Modulation by theophylline and enprofylline of the excitatory non-cholinergic transmission in guinea-pig bronchi. Eur Respir J 1992;5:1201-5.
10. Sullivan P, Bekir S, Jaffar Z, et al. Anti-inflammatory effects of low-dose oral theophylline in atopic asthma]. Lancet 1994;343(8904):1006-8; erratum 343(8911):1512.
11. Lim S, Tomita K, Caramori G, et al. Low-dose theophylline reduces eosinophilic inflammation but not exhaled nitric oxide in mild asthma. Am J Respir Crit Care Med 2001;164:273-6.
12. Aubier M, Neukirch C, Maachi M, et al. Effect of slow-release theophylline on nasal antigen challenge in subjects with allergic rhinitis. Eur Respir J 1998;11:1105-10.
13. Kraft M, Torvik JA, Trudeau JB, Wenzel SE, Martin RJ. Theophylline: potential antiinflammatory effects in nocturnal asthma. J Allergy Clin Immunol 1996;97:1242-6.
14. D'Alonzo GE, Smolensky MH, Feldman S, et al. Twenty-four hour lung function in adult patients with asthma: chronoptimized theophylline therapy once-daily dosing in the evening versus conventional twice-daily dosing. Am Rev Respir Dis 1990;142:84-90.
15. Nielson CP, Crowley JJ, Morgan ME, Vestal RE. Polymorphonuclear leukocyte inhibition by therapeutic concentrations of theophylline is mediated by cyclic-3′,5′-adenosine monophosphate. Am Rev Respir Dis 1988;137:25-30.
16. Kidney J, Dominguez M, Taylor PM, et al. Immunomodulation by theophylline in asthma: demonstration by withdrawal of therapy. Am J Respir Crit Care Med 1995;151:1907-14.
17. Culpitt SV, de Matos C, Russell RE, et al. Effect of theophylline on induced sputum inflammatory indices and neutrophil chemotaxis in chronic obstructive pulmonary disease. Am J Respir Crit Care Med 2002;165:1371-6.
18. Tinkelman DG, Reed CE, Nelson HS, Offord KP. Aerosol beclomethasone dipropionate compared with theophylline as primary treatment of chronic, mild to moderately severe asthma in children. Pediatrics 1993;92:64-77.
18a. Pauwels R, van Renterghem D, van der Straeten M, Johannesson N, Persson CG. The effect of theophylline and enprofylline on allergen-induced bronchoconstriction. J Allergy Clin Immunol 1985;76:583-90.
19. Feoktistov I, Biaggioni I. Adenosine A_{2b} receptors evoke interleukin-8 secretion in human mast cells: an enprofylline-sensitive mechanism with implications for asthma. J Clin Invest 1995;96:1979-86.
20. Bjorck T, Gustafsson LE, Dahlen SE. Isolated bronchi from asthmatics are hyperresponsive to adenosine, which apparently acts indirectly by liberation of leukotrienes and histamine. Am Rev Respir Dis 1992;145:1087-91.
21. Calzetta L, Spina D, Cazzola M, et al. Pharmacological characterization of adenosine receptors on isolated human bronchi. Am J Respir Cell Mol Biol 2011;45:1222-31.
22. Brown RA, Clarke GW, Ledbetter CL, et al. Elevated expression of adenosine A1 receptor in bronchial biopsy specimens from asthmatic subjects. Eur Respir J. 2008;31:311-9.
23. Nicholson CD, Challiss RA, Shahid M. Differential modulation of tissue function and therapeutic potential of selective inhibitors of cyclic nucleotide phosphodiesterase isoenzymes. Trends Pharmacol Sci 1991;12:19-27.
24. Lipworth BJ. Phosphodiesterase-4 inhibitors for asthma and chronic obstructive pulmonary disease. Lancet 2005;365(9454):167-75.
25. Rabe KF, Magnussen H, Dent G. Theophylline and selective PDE inhibitors as bronchodilators and smooth muscle relaxants. Eur Respir J 1995;8:637-42.
26. Wymann MP, Zvelebil M, Laffargue M. Phosphoinositide 3-kinase signalling: which way to target? Trends Pharmacol Sci 2003;24:366-76.
27. Marwick JA, Caramori G, Stevenson CS, et al. Inhibition of PI3Kδ restores glucocorticoid function in smoking-induced airway inflammation in mice. Am J Respir Crit Care Med 2009;179:542-8.
28. Hirsch E, Katanaev VL, Garlanda C, et al. Central role for G protein–coupled phosphoinositide 3-kinase gamma in inflammation. Science 2000;287(5455):1049-53.
29. Foukas LC, Daniele N, Ktori C, et al. Direct effects of caffeine and theophylline on p110δ and other phosphoinositide 3-kinases. Differential effects on lipid kinase and protein kinase activities. J Biol Chem 2002;277:37124-30.
30. Evans DJ, Taylor DA, Zetterstrom O, et al. A comparison of low-dose inhaled budesonide

plus theophylline and high-dose inhaled budesonide for moderate asthma. N Engl J Med 1997;337:1412-8.
31. Brenner M, Berkowitz R, Marshall N, Strunk RC. Need for theophylline in severe steroid-requiring asthmatics. Clin Allergy 1988;18: 143-50.
32. Ukena D, Harnest U, Sakalauskas R, et al. Comparison of addition of theophylline to inhaled steroid with doubling of the dose of inhaled steroid in asthma. Eur Respir J 1997;10:2754-60.
33. Ito K, Lim S, Caramori G, et al. A molecular mechanism of action of theophylline: induction of histone deacetylase activity to decrease inflammatory gene expression. Proc Natl Acad Sci USA 2002;99:8921-6.
34. Shakespear MR, Halili MA, Irvine KM, Fairlie DP, Sweet MJ. Histone deacetylases as regulators of inflammation and immunity. Trends Immunol 2011;32:335-43.
35. To Y, Ito K, Kizawa Y, et al. Targeting phosphoinositide-3-kinase-delta with theophylline reverses corticosteroid insensitivity in chronic obstructive pulmonary disease. Am J Respir Crit Care Med 2010;182:897-904.
36. Huang WC, Chen CC. Akt phosphorylation of p300 at Ser-1834 is essential for its histone acetyltransferase and transcriptional activity. Mol Cell Biol 2005;25:6592-602.
37. Adenuga D, Rahman I. Protein kinase CK2-mediated phosphorylation of HDAC2 regulates co-repressor formation, deacetylase activity and acetylation of HDAC2 by cigarette smoke and aldehydes. Arch Biochem Biophys 2010;498: 62-73.

Dosages and Routes of Administration

38. Weinberger M, Hendeles L, Wong L. Relationship of formulation and dosing interval to fluctuation of serum theophylline concentration in children with chronic asthma. J Pediatr 1981;99:145-52.

Indications and Contraindications

39. Dennis RJ, Solarte I. Asthma in adults. Clin Evid (Online) 2011;(07):1512-72.
40. McIvor RA, Tunks M, Todd DC. COPD. Clin Evid (Online) 2011;(06):1502-602.
41. Tee AK, Koh MS, Gibson PG, et al. Long-acting β_2-agonists versus theophylline for maintenance treatment of asthma. Cochrane Database Syst Rev 2007;(3):CD001281.
42. Seddon P, Bara A, Ducharme FM, Lasserson TJ. Oral xanthines as maintenance treatment for asthma in children. Cochrane Database Syst Rev 2006;(1):CD002885.

Selective Phosphodiesterase Inhibitors

43. Page CP, Spina D. Phosphodiesterase inhibitors in the treatment of inflammatory diseases. Handb Exp Pharmacol 2011;204:391-414.
44. Vestbo J, Prescott E, Lange P. Association of chronic mucus hypersecretion with FEV_1 decline and chronic obstructive pulmonary disease morbidity. Copenhagen City Heart Study Group. Am J Respir Crit Care Med 1996;153:1530-5.
45. Spina D, Landells LJ, Page CP. The role of phosphodiesterase enzymes in allergy and asthma. Adv Pharmacol 1998;44:33-89.
46. Nell H, Louw C, Leichtl S, et al. Acute anti-inflammatory effect of the novel phosphodiesterase 4 inhibitor roflumilast on allergen challenge in asthmatics after a single dose. Am J Respir Crit Care Med 2000;161:A200.
47. Rabe KF, Tenor H, Dent G, et al. Phosphodiesterase isozymes modulating inherent tone in human airways: identification and characterization. Am J Physiol 1993;264(5 Pt 1): L458-64.
48. Schmidt DT, Watson N, Dent G, et al. The effect of selective and non-selective phosphodiesterase inhibitors on allergen- and leukotriene C(4)-induced contractions in passively sensitized human airways. Br J Pharmacol 2000;131: 1607-18.
49. Gamble E, Pavord ID, Vignola AM, et al. Cilomilast reduces CD8+ T-lymphocytes and macrophages in patients with chronic obstructive pulmonary disease (COPD): a double-blind placebo-controlled, parallel-group quantitiative study of bronchial biopsies. Eur Respir J 2001; 17:P2238.
50. Calverley PM, Rabe KF, Goehring UM, et al. Roflumilast in symptomatic chronic obstructive pulmonary disease: two randomised clinical trials. Lancet 2009;374(9691):685-94.
51. Fabbri LM, Calverley PM, Izquierdo-Alonso JL, et al. Roflumilast in moderate-to-severe chronic obstructive pulmonary disease treated with long-acting bronchodilators: two randomised clinical trials. Lancet 2009;374(9691):695-703.
52. Lahu G, Nassr N, Huennemeyer A. Pharmacokinetic evaluation of roflumilast. Expert Opin Drug Metab Toxicol 2011;7:1577-91.
53. Mori F, Pérez-Torres S, De Caro R, et al. The human area postrema and other nuclei related to the emetic reflex express cAMP phosphodiesterases 4B and 4D. J Chem Neuroanat 2010; 40:36-42.
54. US Food and Drug Administration. Available at: www.fda.gov/downloads/advisorycommittees/committeesmeetingmaterials/drugs/pulmonary-allergydrugsadvisorycommittee/UCM207377.pdf.

97 Anticholinergic Therapies

STEPHEN P. PETERS | MARK S. DYKEWICZ

CONTENTS

SUMMARY OF IMPORTANT CONCEPTS

» Cholinergic mechanisms have the potential to play an important role in the pathogenesis of asthma and chronic obstructive pulmonary disease (COPD) through many mechanisms, such as increasing bronchial hyperresponsiveness, causing and modulating airway constriction, and acting through the numerous muscarinic receptors on airway structural and inflammatory cells.
» The short-acting anticholinergic agent ipratropium bromide, often used in combination with a short-acting β-agonist, provides relief in patients with COPD.
» Except in the acute setting, the short-acting anticholinergic agent ipratropium bromide provides minimal benefit in asthma, although it has been successfully used as a substitute for albuterol in some clinical trials.
» In patients with COPD, the long-acting anticholinergic agent tiotropium bromide has improved pulmonary function, dyspnea, health status, exercise tolerance, exacerbations of COPD, and hospitalizations.
» Although the most comprehensive clinical trial (i.e., Understanding Potential Long-term Impacts on Function with Tiotropium [UPLIFT] study) did not show that tiotropium could alter the natural history of COPD by decreasing the rate of decline of forced expiratory volume in 1 second (FEV_1) over time, subgroup analyses suggested possible benefits for younger patients and patients with milder disease.
» Although there is some disagreement on the issue of safety, anticholinergic agents are considered to have an acceptable risk-benefit profile for patients with COPD.
» Initial clinical trials suggest that tiotropium may be an effective controller when used in conjunction with inhaled corticosteroids in patients with asthma.
» Data suggest that tiotropium can improve asthma control when added to an inhaled corticosteroid plus a long-acting β-agonist combination and that it can reduce asthma exacerbations.
» The long-term safety of anticholinergic agents and their effect on exacerbations have not been established in patients with asthma.
» In rhinitis, intranasal ipratropium reduces local mucus production and is an effective treatment for rhinorrhea.

Introduction

Cholinergic mechanisms, especially those involving muscarinic nerves and receptors, can affect several key elements central to obstructive lung disease, such as asthma and chronic obstructive pulmonary disease (COPD). First, patients with asthma and COPD often have an exaggerated response to a variety of stimuli, a condition called *airway* or *bronchial hyperresponsiveness*. The most commonly used agent to evaluate this response, methacholine, produces bronchoconstriction by activating cholinergic receptors. Second, episodic bronchoconstriction produced by a wide variety of stimuli, which is a hallmark of asthma and often found in COPD, can similarly be induced by activating cholinergic mechanisms. An imbalance between the opposing bronchodilating (i.e., sympathetic) and bronchoconstriction (i.e., parasympathetic) elements of the nervous system has been postulated as one mechanism by which an asthmatic state can be achieved. Third, muscarinic receptors are present on neurons and on a number of structural and immunologic elements thought to be important in asthma and perhaps in COPD pathogenesis, including airway smooth muscle, epithelial cells, mucous glands, mast cells, eosinophils, macrophages, and neutrophils.

Agents that antagonize these effects have the potential to produce pronounced benefits for patients with obstructive lung diseases, but until recently, the use of anticholinergic medications had been viewed as standard treatment for COPD but not asthma. For decades, anticholinergic agents were known to reduce acute bronchospasm in patients with asthma, but recent studies have suggested that they also can help to maintain asthma control. Anticholinergic agents have a defined role for treatment in some subsets of patients with rhinitis.

Airway Cholinergic Hyperresponsiveness

Airway (bronchial) hyperresponsiveness to a wide variety of stimuli is a characteristic feature of asthma.[1] As stated in the 2007 report of the National Asthma Education and Prevention Program, "Asthma is a complex disorder characterized by variable and recurring symptoms, airflow obstruction, bronchial hyperresponsiveness, and an underlying inflammation."[2] Although natural, pharmacologic, or other triggers can cause bronchoconstriction and can be used to diagnose bronchial hyperresponsiveness,[3] challenge tests have most frequently been performed using methacholine, histamine, or exercise[4-6] (see Chapter 64).

Airway hyperresponsiveness is not unique to asthma. It occurs in some individuals with COPD, allergic rhinitis, bronchiectasis, cystic fibrosis, and even in normal individuals.[1,7] Bronchial hyperresponsiveness was once considered an almost universal finding in asthma,[8] and exceptions were worthy of case reports,[9] but later observations have suggested that as many as 27% of patients with physician-diagnosed asthma have a negative response to methacholine testing,[10] and the reported sensitivity of the test is 77%.[11] Approximately 60% of the individuals studied by McGrath and Fahy[10] had symptoms characteristic of asthma (e.g., cough, dyspnea, chest tightness, wheeze), and 39% reported emergency department visits for these symptoms. Whether these observations suggest a shift in the pathogenic mechanisms responsible for the clinical condition we describe as asthma is not clear. However, methacholine hyperreactivity remains a hallmark of asthma.

Cholinergic Nervous System as a Target for Anticholinergic Agents

The innervations of the lung are complex. Alterations in the adrenergic (sympathetic), cholinergic (parasympathetic), and nonadrenergic/noncholinergic portions of the nervous system and the neural mediators that are the effectors of these systems appear to be altered in the lungs of patients with asthma[12,13] and COPD. Although there are differences between asthma and COPD in the relative magnitude of these alterations, obstructive lung diseases, especially asthma, typically are associated with β-adrenergic hyporesponsiveness (promoting bronchospasm), α-adrenergic hyporesponsiveness, and cholinergic hyperresponsiveness (promoting bronchospasm). The importance of these neurogenic mechanisms compared with inflammatory and immunologic mechanisms in the pathogenesis of asthma has long been debated and often underappreciated.[14,15] For example, the National Asthma Education and Prevention Program (NAEPP) 2007 guidelines (Section 2, Definition, Pathophysiology, and Pathogenesis of Asthma and Natural History of Asthma) present a thorough discussion of airway histology, remodeling, and the role of inflammatory and immunologic cells and mechanisms, but it does not mention the importance of neural mechanisms or their interactions with inflammatory mechanisms.[2]

PARASYMPATHETIC NERVES SUPPLYING LUNG AIRWAYS

Parasympathetic nerve impulses originate in the medulla, travel in the vagus nerves, and then course through their smaller branches that relay through the cardiac plexus to supply the lower trachea and bronchi. Preganglionic nerves release the cholinergic neurotransmitter acetylcholine and supply clusters of postganglionic cell bodies located in parallel chains along smooth muscle of the trachea and bronchi.[16] Stimulated postganglionic fibers from these cell bodies directly innervate smooth muscle and glands. Cholinergic postganglionic fibers do not extend beyond the terminal bronchi,[17] consistent with the absence of functional changes in respiratory bronchioles or alveoli with vagal stimulation.[18] Consequently, parasympathetic nerves are not thought to have a significant effect on smaller airways in obstructive lung disease, although this does not preclude acetylcholine-mediated effects on smaller airways through nonneuronal mechanisms.

NICOTINIC AND MUSCARINIC RECEPTORS

Although the principal source of acetylcholine in the lungs is its release from preganglionic cholinergic nerves, acetylcholine may also be produced from other cells in the airway such as epithelial cells, particularly in response to inflammatory stimuli. Acetylcholine acts on two types of receptors: muscarinic and nicotinic. Neurotransmission through parasympathetic ganglia is principally mediated by nicotinic receptors on postganglionic nerves that produce a fast excitatory postsynaptic potential. This fast potential can be positively and negatively modulated by postganglionic muscarinic receptors, and muscarinic receptors on other lung tissues can have other important effects.

Muscarinic receptors, through altered expression and function, are thought to play a greater role than nicotinic receptors in the pathogenesis of obstructive lung disease, which provides the underlying pharmacologic rationale for using antimuscarinic receptor agents in treatment. Muscarinic receptors are concentrated in smooth muscle and are proximate to submucosal glands of the airways. They have the highest density in the proximal airways and hilum, which corresponds to where there is greatest parasympathetic innervation of the lungs.[19]

MUSCARINIC RECEPTOR SUBTYPES IN THE LUNG

Five muscarinic receptor subtypes (M_1 through M_5), all of which are inhibited by atropine, have been identified and reviewed by Fryer and Jacoby.[20] M_1, M_2, and M_3 are the principal receptors in the airways. Different subtypes are located on different airway structures (Fig. 97-1), and their activation can lead to different downstream effects. The M_1, M_3, and M_5 receptors have a stimulatory cholinergic effect on target tissue and cells, whereas M_2 receptors can be inhibitory or stimulatory, depending on their location, and M_4 receptors are inhibitory.

M_1 receptors are principally postganglionic, where their stimulation promotes ganglionic transmission primarily mediated by nicotinic receptors. M_1 receptors are also present on smooth muscle, where their stimulation can augment cholinergic reflex bronchoconstriction, but they are thought to have a less important role than other subtypes of muscarinic receptors.

At parasympathetic ganglia, prejunctional M_2 receptors provide negative presynaptic feedback to inhibit acetylcholine release to modulate cholinergic responses. Blocking prejunctional M_2 receptors with pharmacologic agents can increase acetylcholine release, with the potential to increase cholinergically mediated bronchoconstriction.[21] However, through inhibition of adenylate cyclase, postjunctional M_2 receptors limit β-adrenoceptor–mediated relaxation,[22] and postjunctional M_2 stimulation may indirectly contribute to smooth muscle contraction, a clinical effect that is opposite to the stimulation of prejunctional M_2 receptors. M_2 receptors are the most highly expressed muscarinic receptors on airway smooth muscle, but they are less clinically important than M_3 receptors.[19,23]

M_3 receptors on smooth muscle elicit mucus secretion, and compared with other muscarinic receptors, have a greater effect

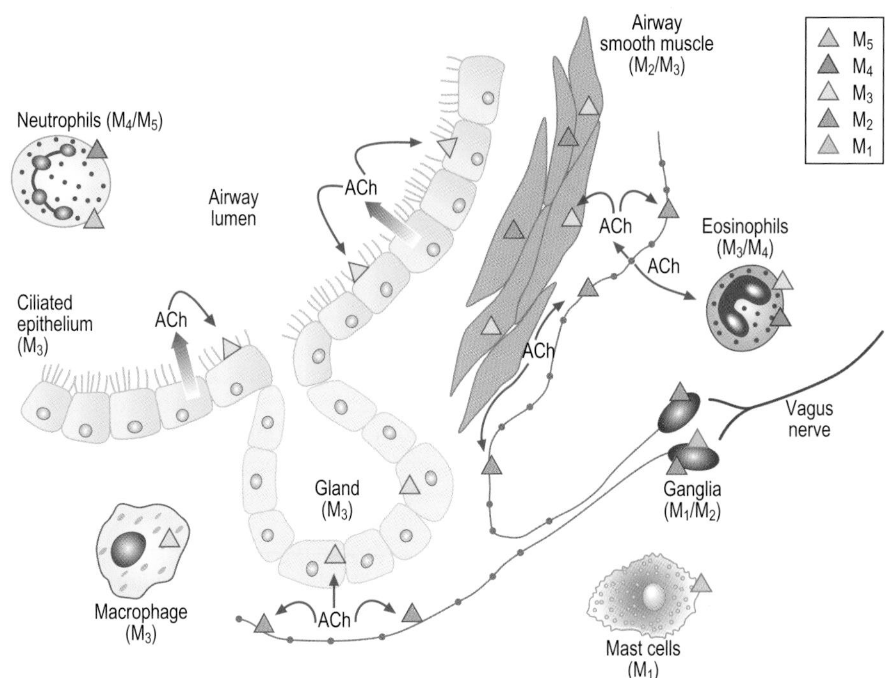

Figure 97-1 Muscarinic receptor subtypes found in the lung and on inflammatory cells. *Ach*, Acetylcholine. *(From Fryer AD, Jacoby DB. Cholinergic mechanisms and anticholinergic therapy in respiratory diseases. In: Adkinson NF Jr, Bochner BS, Busse WW, et al., editors. Middleton's allergy: principles and practice, 7th ed. Philadelphia: Mosby; 2009, p. 1603-18.)*

in promoting cholinergically mediated bronchoconstriction, which is the principal basis for use of M_3 receptor antagonists in obstructive lung disease. M_3 receptors are also present on epithelium, glands, macrophages, eosinophils, and possibly neutrophils. M_4 receptors are present on neutrophils and eosinophils, whereas M_5 receptors are present on neutrophils and lymphocytes.[21,24-26]

MUSCARINIC RECEPTOR EFFECTS ON AIRWAY SMOOTH MUSCLE TONE

In humans and animals, some degree of resting bronchomotor tone occurs because of tonic vagal nerve release of acetylcholine adjacent to airway smooth muscle.[27] Although airway smooth muscle expresses M_2 and M_3 receptors in approximately a 4:1 ratio,[28] M_3 receptors have a greater role in bronchial smooth muscle contraction. Consistent with this concept are the airway effects of selective antagonists of different muscarinic receptor subtypes[29-31] and the absence of vagal and methacholine-induced bronchoconstriction in M_3-knockout but not M_2-knockout mice.[32] Pharmacologically, antagonism of M_3 receptors is considered the most important mechanism for a bronchodilator effect from anticholinergic agents.

MUSCARINIC RECEPTOR EFFECTS ON MUCUS HYPERSECRETION

In asthma and COPD, mucus hypersecretion is a characteristic feature that contributes to airway obstruction and airflow limitation.[33] Mucus production in the central airways is under cholinergic control.[34,35] Although goblet cells can produce mucus in response to muscarinic receptor stimulation,[34] airway submucosal glands are the primary source of cholinergically mediated mucus production. Submucosal glands are innervated and express M_1 and M_3 receptors in approximately a 1:2 ratio.[36,37] M_3 receptors are the principal receptor subtype that mediates mucus secretion, whereas M_1 and M_3 receptors likely mediate electrolyte and water secretion.[38,39]

MUSCARINIC RECEPTOR EFFECTS ON INFLAMMATION

Functional muscarinic receptors are expressed on most inflammatory cells, including lymphocytes (M_1), mast cells (M_1), eosinophils (M_3 and M_4), macrophages (M_3), and neutrophils (M_4, M_5, and possibly M_3) (see Fig. 97-1). There is evidence that through activation of muscarinic receptors on inflammatory cells and production of acetylcholine from nonneuronal sources, various inflammatory processes are promoted, including lymphocyte proliferation and activation, cytokine release, cytotoxicity, and eosinophilic chemotactic activity.[25,26,40-44] Bronchial epithelial cells respond to acetylcholine by release of eosinophil, monocyte, and neutrophil chemotactic activity and granulocyte-macrophage colony-stimulating factor (GM-CSF).[43-45] Because bronchial epithelial cells can also express nonneuronal acetylcholine,[46] epithelial acetylcholine may initiate inflammatory responses.[47] Overall, these data indicate that acetylcholine can influence inflammatory processes through paracrine and autocrine mechanisms,[48,49] and they provide a possible rationale for the antiinflammatory effect of antimuscarinic agents in the airways.

MUSCARINIC RECEPTOR REGULATION OF AIRWAY REMODELING

Although airway remodeling is different in asthma and COPD, there is evidence that cholinergic mechanisms may play a significant role in airway smooth muscle remodeling, mucous gland hypertrophy, and goblet cell hyperplasia.[48,50,51] Proliferation of primary cultured human lung fibroblasts is promoted through stimulation of muscarinic receptors, and it correlates best with a role for M_2 receptors.[52] Although stimulation of muscarinic receptors alone does not induce airway smooth muscle proliferation, there is evidence that muscarinic receptor stimulation can increase the mitogenic response of myocytes to platelet-derived growth factor (PDGF), apparently an effect mediated through M_3 receptors.[53,54]

DYSREGULATION OF MUSCARINIC RECEPTORS IN ASTHMA

In asthma, increased acetylcholine release and increased cholinergic hyperreactivity have been proposed as a consequence of abnormal muscarinic receptor expression by means of an increase in M_1 and M_3 receptors or dysfunction of M_2 receptors, although current evidence does not suggest that ganglionic muscarinic M_1 receptor expression is altered.[48,55] In patients with asthma, viral infections can induce $CD8^+$ T lymphocytes that cause M_2 receptor dysfunction and result in enhanced cholinergic activation in the airway.[56-58] Airway inflammation can impact cholinergic effects on the airway. For example, eosinophilic major basic protein (MBP) has been shown to be an allosteric inhibitor of M_2 receptors, with consequent loss of autoinhibition of acetylcholine release and the potential for enhancement of vagally mediated bronchoconstriction.[59-61]

Pharmacology of Anticholinergic Agents

OVERVIEW

As competitive inhibitors of muscarinic receptors, anticholinergic agents used in the treatment of obstructive lung disease have pharmacologic action that decreases intracellular levels of cyclic guanosine monophosphate (cGMP), with a consequent decrease of tonic cholinergic activity and promotion of bronchodilation. Considering the stimulatory effect of M_1 and M_3 receptors and the overall inhibitory effect of M_2 receptors, the optimal pharmacologic profile for anticholinergic agents in obstructive lung disease is antagonism of M_1 and M_3 receptors with minimal affinity for M_2 receptors.[21,62]

Historically, the anticholinergic agent atropine was a standard treatment for asthma before the introduction of adrenergic agents and methylxanthines. As a tertiary amine, atropine is systemically absorbed even when administered locally to the airways, and it lost favor because of its significant anticholinergic adverse effects, including decreased pulmonary mucociliary clearance, urinary retention, and increased intraocular pressure.[63]

Ipratropium bromide and tiotropium bromide, the principal quaternary amine anticholinergic agents used as inhaled treatments for respiratory disease, have relatively little absorption through respiratory mucosa, do not penetrate the blood-brain barrier, and usually avoid the systemic adverse effects associated with atropine. When used at approved doses in pulmonary airways, ipratropium and tiotropium do not significantly alter mucociliary clearance or respiratory secretions. These drugs compete with acetylcholine at muscarinic receptors on airway smooth muscle, which decreases the intracellular concentration of cGMP and inhibits tonic cholinergic activity. Bronchodilation from these drugs is principally a local, site-specific effect.

IPRATROPIUM BROMIDE

Ipratropium bromide is a nonselective antagonist of M_1, M_2, and M_3 receptors. Although ipratropium produces a net bronchodilatory effect, blockade of M_2 receptors allows further release of presynaptic acetylcholine, and it may antagonize the bronchodilatory effect of blocking M_3, a possible basis for reports of paradoxical bronchoconstriction.[64] Ipratropium bromide has a half-life of elimination of 1.6 hours after inhalation, and it is partially metabolized by ester hydrolysis to inactive products. Table 97-1 lists muscarinic receptor antagonists and their properties.[65]

TIOTROPIUM BROMIDE

Tiotropium is different from other anticholinergic agents in its relative selectivity and higher affinity for muscarinic receptor subtypes. Tiotropium has a 6- to 20-fold higher affinity for muscarinic receptors than ipratropium.[21] Although it binds to M_2 and M_3 receptors with approximately equal affinity, it dissociates from M_3 receptors approximately 10 times more slowly

TABLE 97-1 Muscarinic Receptor Antagonists and Their Properties

Muscarinic Receptor Antagonists	Affinity at M_3 Receptors (pK_i)*	$M_3 > M_2$ Affinity	Half-Life at M_3 Receptors (h)
Atropine	9.68[66]	None[66]	3.5[70]
Ipratropium	9.58[66]	None[66]	3.2[71]
Tiotropium	11.02[66]	Functional selectivity[21]	34.7[21]
Glycopyrrolate	10.04[66]	3-5 times more selective[23]	3.7[23]
Aclidinium	10.74[66]	Functional selectivity[69]	29[69]
OrM3	9.38[67]	120 times more selective[67]	14.2[67]
CHF 5407	9.23[68]	Functional selectivity[68]	–32[68]

Reproduced with permission from Moulton BC, Fryer AD. Muscarinic receptor antagonists, from folklore to pharmacology; finding drugs that actually work in asthma and COPD. Br J Pharmacol 2011;163:44-52.

CHF 5407, Selective muscarinic M_3 receptor antagonist; *OrM3*, oral M-selective anticholinergic agent.

*The pK_i (–log dissociation constant) was determined in heterologous competition experiments against [*N*-methyl-^{3}H]scopolamine methyl chloride.

than from M_2 receptors and approximately 100 times more slowly from M_1 and M_3 receptors than ipratropium.[20,72] This kinetic selectivity for M_3 receptors results in a functionally more selective antagonist action for M_3 muscarinic receptor subtypes that is the basis for its clinical effectiveness. The half-life of the tiotropium–M_3 receptor complex is approximately 35 hours, compared with 0.3 hour for the ipratropium–M_3 receptor complex. These characteristics result in a long duration of action and permit once-daily dosing. The most common adverse event is a dry mouth, which occur in approximately 10% to 15% of patients.[72-74]

OTHER LONG-ACTING ANTICHOLINERGIC AGENTS AND MUSCARINIC ANTAGONISTS

Muscarinic antagonists that have been under development include glycopyrrolate, aclidinium bromide, OrM3, and CHF 5407.[65] Glycopyrrolate has been used clinically to mitigate the cholinergic side effects of bradycardia and increased secretions that can be associated with invasive procedures such as bronchoscopy, but it may be useful in obstructive lung diseases when administered by inhalation,[75,76] Aclidinium has an advantage over tiotropium of being rapidly metabolized in plasma. OrM3, an oral M_3-selective anticholinergic agent, appears to have less activity with more side effects that ipratropium. CHF 5407 is a potent and long-acting antagonist of M_3 receptors with a significantly shorter half-life at M_2 receptors than tiotropium.[65] Whether any of these agents will be approved for the treatment of COPD must be determined by ongoing research.

Anticholinergic Agents in Obstructive Lung Diseases

SHORT-ACTING ANTICHOLINERGIC AGENTS IN CHRONIC OBSTRUCTIVE PULMONARY DISEASE

In stable COPD, ipratropium bromide has been reported to produce an increase in FEV_1 that is as great as or sometimes greater than that achieved with a short-acting β-agonist (SABA).[77-80] There is no tachyphylaxis with prolonged use. The duration of bronchodilation due to ipratropium can persist for up to 8 hours after administration, longer than a SABA.[81] Some evidence suggests that spirometric measurements of FEV_1 and forced vital capacity (FVC) may not be the best measures of the therapeutic response in COPD. Perhaps of more importance is the demonstration that short-acting anticholinergic agents acutely decrease functional residual capacity and residual volume and increase inspiratory capacity, consistent with a reduction in hyperinflation that is commonly observed in COPD.[63,82] Fixed-dose combinations of ipratropium and a SABA produce greater peak increases in FEV_1 than monotherapy with either agent.[83]

A meta-analysis of 11 long-term (at least 4 weeks' duration) studies of COPD treatment compared ipratropium monotherapy, ipratropium in combination with SABAs, and β-agonist monotherapy.[80] Lung function after bronchodilator use was greater with combination therapy or with ipratropium monotherapy than with SABA monotherapy. Small benefits in favor of ipratropium monotherapy were found for health-related quality of life and a reduction in requirement for oral corticosteroids. Although there was no benefit for combination therapy in subjective improvements in health-related quality of life, there was a reduction in the requirement for oral corticosteroids.

In COPD exacerbations, FEV_1 improvement at 90 minutes showed no significant difference between SABA monotherapy, ipratropium monotherapy, or combination treatment.[84-87] Evaluation after 24 hours showed similar results.[87] Treatment guidelines nonetheless state that for an acute exacerbation of COPD, SABAs, with or without short-acting anticholinergic agents, are usually the preferred bronchodilators for treatment.[88]

SHORT-ACTING ANTICHOLINERGIC AGENTS IN ASTHMA

Clinical trials have examined anticholinergic agents, mainly ipratropium bromide, for acute bronchodilation when used alone or in combination with short- or intermediate-acting $β_2$-adrenergic agents in asthma in nonemergent settings. A meta-analysis that reviewed these data found that these agents, when used alone, had a small effect on asthma symptoms (i.e., daytime dyspnea −0.09 and 95% confidence interval [CI], −0.14 to −0.04 in three studies with 59 patients) and lung function (i.e., increase in morning peak expiratory flow [PEF] of 14.38 L/min and 95% CI, 7.69 to 21.08 in three studies with 59 patients), but these changes were thought to have minimal clinical significance.[89] When used in combination with a $β_2$-agonist, as is commonly done in clinical practice, there was no indication that they produced improvements in symptoms or lung function above those obtained with a $β_2$-agonist alone.[89] However, ipratropium bromide was an effective reliever medication in asthmatic subjects in clinical trials in which the confounding effect of "as needed" albuterol rescue was minimized (i.e., trials studying the pharmacogenetics of short- and long-acting β-adrenergic agonists).[90,91]

Results of another meta-analysis found that when anticholinergic agents were used in combination with $β_2$-agonists in *acute asthma*, they produced an improvement in lung function and in rates of hospitalization for children and adults.[92] For children and adolescents, the relative risk for hospitalization was 0.73 (95% CI, 0.63 to 0.85; P = .0001), and it was 0.68 (95% CI, 0.53 to 0.86; P = .002) for adults (Fig. 97-2).[92]

Tiotropium for Treating Chronic Obstructive Pulmonary Disease

GENERAL OBSERVATIONS

In patients with COPD, tiotropium can improve pulmonary function, dyspnea, health status, exercise tolerance, exacerbations of COPD, and hospitalizations.[74,93-95] The most frequent adverse event is a dry mouth, which occurs in approximately 10% to 15% of patients.[72-74]

Tiotropium has been compared with other treatment strategies to prevent exacerbations of COPD. In a year-long trial enrolling 7376 patients with moderate or severe COPD (FEV_1 of 1.41 L, 49% of predicted) in which tiotropium was compared with salmeterol, tiotropium increased the time to the first exacerbation (187 versus 145 days) and the time to the first severe exacerbation (hazard ratio = 0.72; 95% CI, 0.61 to 0.85; P < .001), and it reduced the annual number of moderate or severe exacerbations (0.64 versus 0.72; rate ratio = 0.89; 95% CI, 0.83 to 0.96; P = .002) and the annual number of severe exacerbations (0.09 versus 0.13; rate ratio = 0.73; 95% CI, 0.66 to 0.82;

$P < .001$).[96] A 2-year study of 1323 patients with slightly more severe COPD (FEV_1 of 1.12 L, 39% of predicted) found no difference in the exacerbation rates produced by use of tiotropium versus salmeterol plus fluticasone propionate.[97] Small benefits in probability of withdrawal from the study and health status (measured with the St. George's Respiratory Questionnaire) favored salmeterol plus fluticasone, and an unexpected difference in deaths, an outcome for which the trial was not powered, also favored the combination of salmeterol and fluticasone.

UPLIFT STUDY OF TIOTROPIUM IN CHRONIC OBSTRUCTIVE PULMONARY DISEASE

Current therapies for COPD provide symptom relief only. They do not change the natural history of the disease, such as the rate of loss of lung function over time or the mortality rate. The possibility of affecting these end points was raised by the results of the meta-analysis by Barr and colleagues,[95] which showed that patients receiving tiotropium had a 30 mL/yr slower decline inFEV_1 than patients treated with placebo. An ambitious 4-year trial of tiotropium in COPD, the Understanding Potential Long-term Impacts on Function with Tiotropium (UPLIFT) trial, studied the long-term effects of this agent on the coprimary end points of rate of decline in the mean FEV_1 value before and after bronchodilation and on the secondary outcomes of FVC, responses to the St. George's Respiratory Questionnaire, and mortality.[98] In this trial of 5993 patients, with an average age of 65 years and a mean FEV_1 of 1.32 L (48% of predicted), 2987 were randomly assigned to tiotropium and 3006 were assigned to placebo while continuing all other

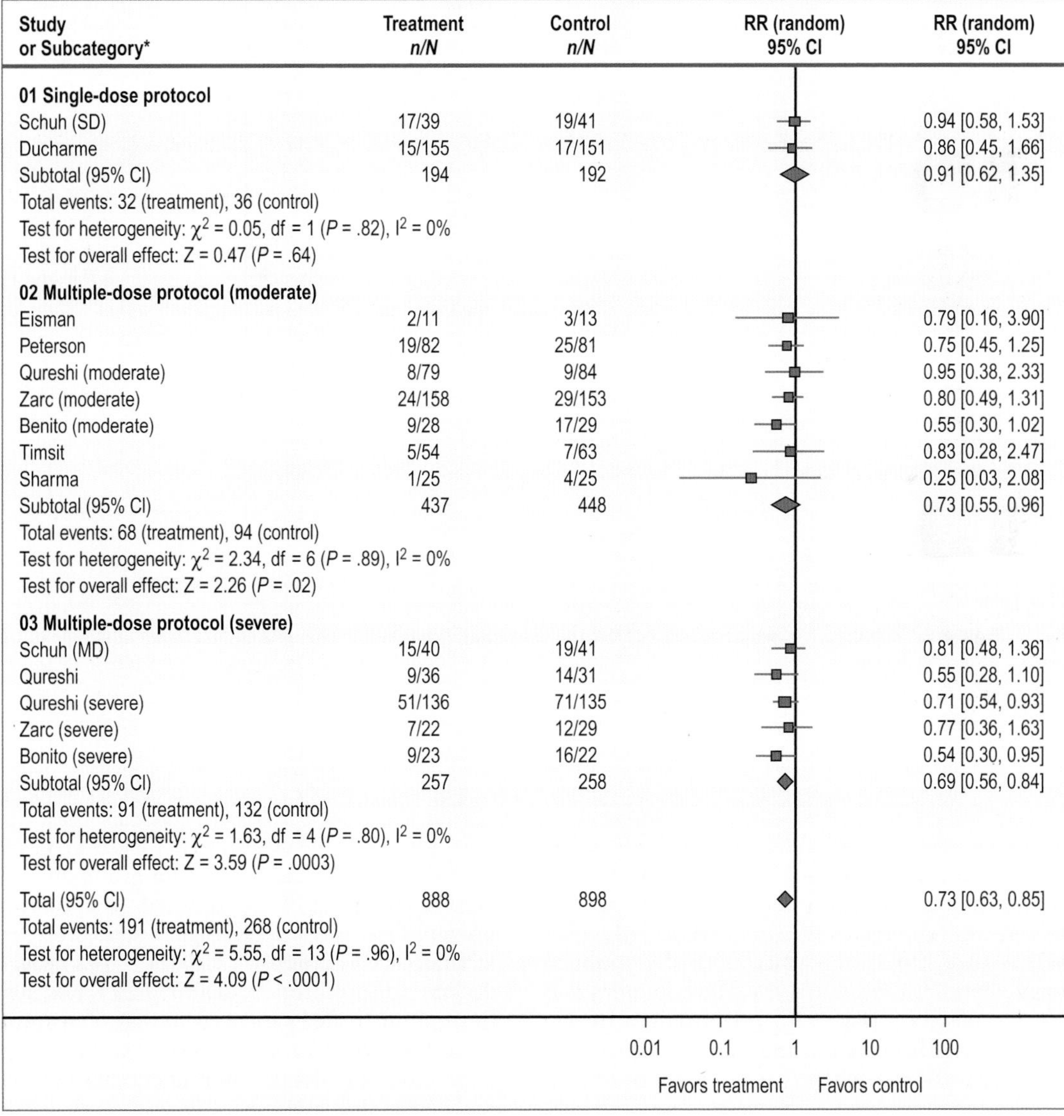

Figure 97-2 Hospitalization rates for children (**A**) and adults (**B**, see next page) with asthma are shown for the addition of anticholinergic agents to β_2-agonists (Treatment) and for β_2-agonists used alone (Control). *CI*, Confidence interval; *RR*, relative risk. *Complete sources for these studies are listed in the source article for this figure. *(From Rodrigo GJ, Castro-Rodríguez JA. Anticholinergics in the treatment of children and adults with acute asthma: a systematic review with meta-analysis. Thorax 2005;60:740-6.)*

Continued

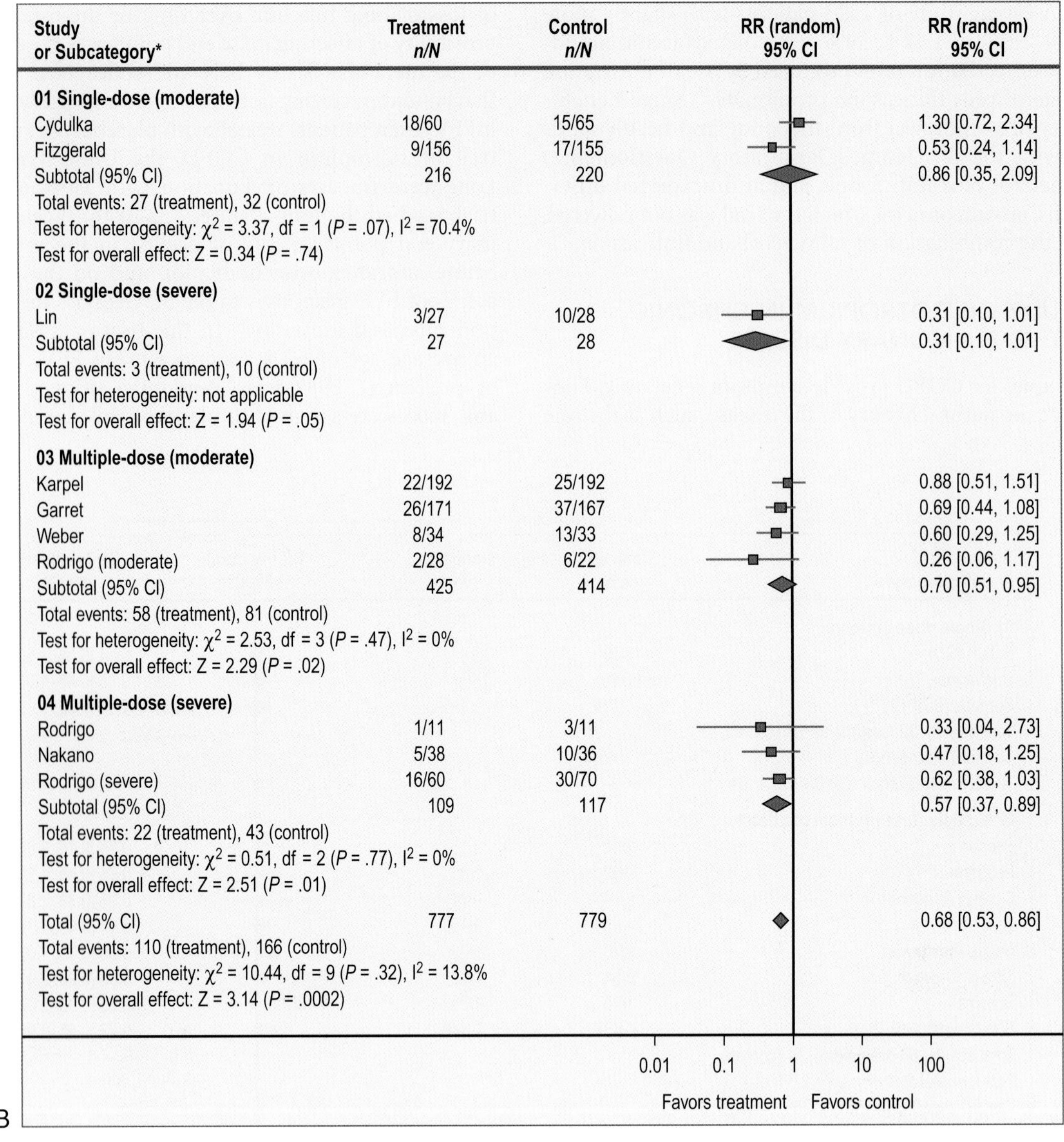

Figure 97-2 cont'd *Complete sources for these studies are listed in the source article for this figure.

respiratory treatments except anticholinergic agents. There was no difference in the rate of decline of FEV_1 values for patients who took tiotropium compared with those who took placebo among the patients who completed the study (38 ± 1 mL/yr for tiotropium versus 40 ± 1 mL/yr for placebo) or discontinued the study drug prematurely (55 ± 4 mL/yr for tiotropium versus 57 ± 4 mL/yr for placebo) (Fig. 97-3). Tiotropium-treated patients showed positive benefits for lung function, quality of life, and COPD exacerbations. Whether there might have been a small decrease in the mortality rate between the two groups, which favored tiotropium, depends on the type of analysis performed.[98-100]

In a subsequent analyses of the 810 UPLIFT patients who were treated *only* with tiotropium (403 patients) or placebo (407 patients), the rate of decline in FEV_1 was slower in the tiotropium group (postbronchodilator FEV_1 rate of decline of 42 ± 4 mL/yr for the tiotropium group and 53 ± 4 mL/yr for the placebo group; $P = .026$), and at 48 months, the morning predose FEV_1 was 134 mL higher in the tiotropium group than in the placebo group ($P < .001$).[101] A similar smaller rate of decline in postbronchodilator FEV_1 was also observed in tiotropium-treated patients who were 50 years of age or younger (38 mL/yr for tiotropium versus 58 mL/yr for placebo; $P = .01$)[102] and in patients with milder, stage II COPD according to the Global Initiative for Chronic Obstructive Lung Disease (GOLD) classification (postbronchodilator FEV_1 rate of decline of 43 ± 2 mL/yr for tiotropium versus 49 mL ± 2 mL/year for placebo; $P = .024$).[103]

Additional publications reported subgroup analyses of men and women who received similar beneficial effects.[104] They

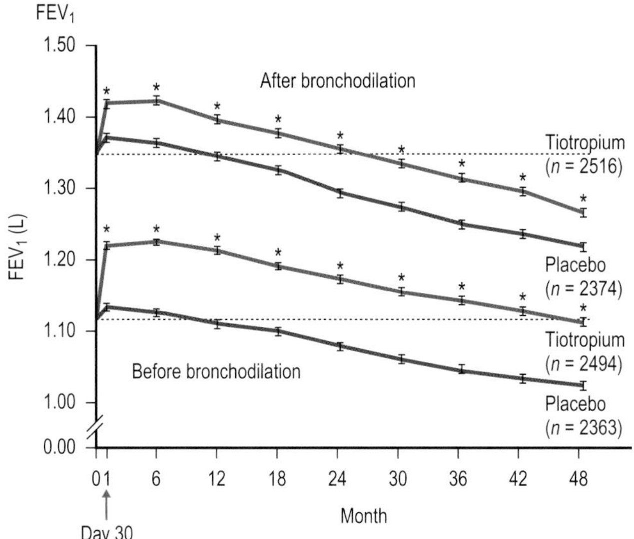

Figure 97-3 Decline in forced expiratory volume in 1 second (FEV_1) values documented before and after bronchodilation in the 4-year Understanding Potential Long-term Impacts on Function with Tiotropium (UPLIFT) study. *(From Tashkin DP, Celli B, Senn S, et al; UPLIFT Study Investigators. A 4-year trial of tiotropium in chronic obstructive pulmonary disease. N Engl J Med 2008;359:1543-54.)*

also described the characteristic of patients who discontinue study participation early, a potentially more vulnerable population.[105]

TRIPLE COMBINATION THERAPY FOR CHRONIC OBSTRUCTIVE PULMONARY DISEASE

The literature describing positive benefits for patients with COPD treated with the anticholinergic agent tiotropium is rich and convincing. However, these data were derived primarily from a comparison of tiotropium with placebo or one other comparator. It is important to know whether a long-acting anticholinergic agent can provide additional benefit when added to the combination therapy of an inhaled corticosteroid (ICS) plus a long-acting β-agonist (LABA) and to determine which set of COPD end points to use for outcome assessment. Several trials,[106-108] including the meta-analysis performed by Rodrigo and colleagues,[109] suggest that the addition of tiotropium to ICS/LABA results in improvements in several important end points, including lung function, quality of life, symptoms, rescue bronchodilator use, and perhaps hospitalization rates, but it does not appear to have a significant beneficial effect on exacerbations of COPD. Although there is guarded enthusiasm for this approach to treating diseases of the airways, these results are based on limited data, and additional studies addressing these questions are needed.[110]

SAFETY CONCERNS FOR ANTICHOLINERGIC AGENTS IN PATIENTS WITH CHRONIC OBSTRUCTIVE PULMONARY DISEASE

A meta-analysis of 17 randomized, controlled trials for anticholinergic agents, including ipratropium and tiotropium, found an increased risk of major cardiovascular events (i.e., stroke; myocardial infarction; cardiovascular deaths, including sudden death) among COPD patients treated with inhaled anticholinergics (relative risk [RR] = 1.58; 95% CI, 1.21 to 2.06; $P < .001$).[111] However, the UPLIFT trial found no increase in mortality rates or cardiovascular events.[98] A clinical trial safety database for tiotropium that enrolled 19,545 patients (10,846 on tiotropium, 8699 on placebo) from 30 trials found a significant reduction in the risk of all-cause mortality, cardiovascular mortality, and cardiovascular events.[112] These data were subsequently reviewed by the U.S. Food and Drug Administration (FDA), which concluded that there was no apparent increased risk of mortality when using tiotropium with the HandiHaler device and bemoaned the "urgent calls to take immediate regulatory action without acknowledgment of potential pitfalls in the interpretation of data from meta-analyses and pooled analyses, such as those encountered in the tiotropium evaluation."[113] However, a subsequent meta-analysis of trials of COPD patients using a tiotropium mist inhaler (Respimat), which exposes patients to higher doses of the drug than does the powder formulation (HandiHaler), found a 52% increased risk of mortality associated with the mist inhaler.[114] These observations are troubling, and they contributed to the 2010 recommendation of the U.K. Medicines and Healthcare Regulatory Agency that tiotropium Respimat should be used with caution in patients with known cardiac rhythm disorders and the 2011 FDA decision not to approve tiotropium Respimat on the basis of available data. A large, controlled study is directly comparing the mortality rates of COPD patients receiving tiotropium using these delivery devices.

Tiotropium for Treating Asthma

INITIAL CLINICAL OBSERVATIONS

Before the results of the current asthma clinical trials were reported, observations in the literature suggested that tiotropium bromide could be an effective asthma controller. Kapoor and coworkers[115] found tiotropium to be a corticosteroid-sparing drug in a case report of a patient who required oral corticosteroids to control his disease (Table 97-2). Iwamoto and colleagues[116] reported the effect of 4 weeks of open-label tiotropium treatment of 17 patients with severe persistent asthma after characterizing their airway inflammatory characteristics in induced sputum. Their findings suggest that tiotropium had greater benefit in patients with a noneosinophilic airway phenotype and produced equivalent outcomes for nonsmokers and smokers. The usefulness of tiotropium in patients with concomitant COPD and asthma was confirmed in a double-blind, randomized, placebo-controlled, parallel-design trial of 472 patients in which inclusion criteria included a diagnosis of both diseases, age of 40 years or older, smoking history of more than 10 pack-years, and 1 or more years of ICS use.[117] Tiotropium was superior to placebo in terms of spirometric measures (FEV_1 and FVC area under the curve [AUC] from 0 to 6 hours and morning predose FEV_1 and FVC) and rescue β-agonist use.

Park and colleagues[118] studied 138 patients with severe asthma who were treated with open-label tiotropium for at least 12 weeks. They classified 46 of the 138 patients as *responders* based on an improvement in FEV_1 of at least 15% (or 200 mL) for at least 8 successive weeks. Analysis showed that an Arg16Gly substitution in the *ADRB2* gene in a minor allele

TABLE 97-2 Selected Studies Examining the Effect of Tiotropium in Patients with Asthma

Study	Population	Study Design	N	Findings	Comments
Kapoor et al, 2009[115]	GINA step 4,[123] severe and persistent asthma; oral corticosteroid-requiring asthma patient	Case report, open label TIO: 18 μg by HandiHaler	1	TIO demonstrated to be corticosteroid sparing	
Iwamoto et al, 2008[116]	GINA step 4,[123] severe and persistent asthma; nonsmokers and smokers	Open label, 4-wk treatment period with TIO	17	TIO appeared to work better in patients with noneosinophilic phenotype and was equally effective in nonsmokers and smokers	Induced sputum used to examine sputum eosinophils and neutrophils
Magnussen et al, 2008[117]	Diagnosis of COPD (≥40 yr old, >10 pack-year smoking) and asthma, on ICS ≥1 yr; other medications allowed except anticholinergic agents	DBR PC parallel group, 2-wk run-in, then 12-wk treatment (a) TIO: 18 μg by HandiHaler (b) Placebo	472	TIO superior to placebo for FEV_1, FVC, and rescue β-agonist use	
Park et al, 2009[118]	GINA step 4,[124] severe and persistent asthma; all received high-dose ICS plus LABA	Open label, at least 12-wk treatment TIO: 18 μg by HandiHaler	138	46 (33%) of 138 responders to TIO: improvement in FEV_1 by ≥ 15% (or 200 mL) for at least 8 successive weeks	Arg16Gly in *ADRB2* (in a minor allele [Arg]–dominant model) significantly associated with response to tiotropium
Peters et al (TALC), 2010[119]	GINA step 3,[124] moderate persistent asthma; inadequately controlled on low-dose ICS (beclomethasone, 80 μg bid)	DBR crossover, 4-wk run-in, then 14-wk treatment (a) Double ICS dose (b) TIO: 18 μg by HandiHaler (c) Salmeterol: 50 μg bid	210	TIO superior to double ICS dose for AM PEF, PM PEF, asthma-control days, symptoms, ACQ, pre-BD FEV_1, post-BD FEV_1; noninferior to salmeterol for AM PEF, PM PEF, asthma-control days, symptoms, ACQ; superior for pre-BD FEV_1, post-BD FEV_1	Insufficient power to assess asthma exacerbations and long-term safety
Bateman et al, 2011[120]	GINA step 3,[123] moderate and persistent asthma; inadequately controlled on ICS (400-1000 μg of budesonide equivalent), in B16-Arg/Arg genotype	DBR PC parallel group, 4-wk run-in with salmeterol, then 16-wk treatment (a) TIO: 5 μg in evening by Respimat (b) Salmeterol: 50 μg bid by MDI (c) Placebo	388	TIO noninferior to salmeterol, superior to placebo for AM PEF and other lung functions; TIO and salmeterol numerically superior to placebo for symptoms	Insufficient power to assess asthma exacerbations and long-term safety
Kerstjens et al, 2011[121]	GINA step 4,[124] severe and persistent asthma; uncontrolled on high-dose ICS plus LABA	DBR PC crossover, 8-wk treatment (a) TIO: 5 μg by Respimat (b) TIO: 10 μg by Respimat (c) Placebo	100	Both doses of TIO add-on superior for peak and trough FEV_1, PEF; no difference in asthma-related health status or symptoms	Dry mouth more common with TIO 10-μg dose
Kerstjens et al, 2012[122]	GINA step 4,[124] severe and persistent asthma; uncontrolled on high-dose ICS plus LABA	Two replicate, DBR PC parallel group trials, 48-wk treatment (a) TIO: 5 μg by Respimat (b) Placebo	912 total (459 in trial 1 and 453 in trial 2)	Mean change in FEV_1 was 86 ± 34 mL (SE) in trial 1 and 154 ± 32 mL (SE) in trial 2; risk reduction for severe asthma exacerbations was 21% ($P = .03$)	Only allergic rhinitis occurred more commonly in the tiotropium group; asthma events and insomnia were more common in placebo group

ACQ, Asthma Control Questionnaire; *BD*, bronchodilator; *COPD*, chronic obstructive pulmonary disease; *DBR*, double-blind, randomized; *FEV_1*: forced expiratory volume in 1 second; *FVC*, forced vital capacity; *GINA*, Global Initiative for Asthma study; *ICS*, inhaled corticosteroids; *LABA*, long-acting β2-agonist (bronchodilator); *MDI*, metered-dose inhaler; *N*, patient population; *PC*, placebo-controlled; *PEF*, peak expiratory flow; *SE*, standard error; *TALC:* Tiotropium Bromide as an Alternative to Increased Inhaled Corticosteroid in Patients Inadequately Controlled on a Lower Dose of Inhaled Corticosteroids trial; *TIO*, tiotropium.

(Arg)–dominant model was significantly associated with a greater response to tiotropium.

CONTROLLED TRIALS

Several published clinical trials have provided encouraging results for the use of tiotropium as add-on therapy in patients with asthma inadequately controlled with ICS alone or in combination with an LABA.

The National Heart, Lung, and Blood Institute–funded Asthma Clinical Research Network (ACRN) has reported on the effect of adding tiotropium (18 μg/day by HandiHaler) or salmeterol (50 μg twice daily) versus doubling the dose of the ICS (from 80 μg of beclomethasone HFA twice daily to 160 μg twice daily) in patients with asthma inadequately controlled on low-dose ICS alone.[118] The *T*iotropium Bromide as an *A*lternative to Increased Inhaled Glucocorticoid in Patients Inadequately Controlled on a *L*ower Dose of Inhaled *C*orticosteroids (TALC) trial tested two hypotheses: whether tiotropium plus low-dose ICS would be superior to the doubled dose of ICS and whether tiotropium and low-dose ICS would be noninferior to salmeterol plus low-dose ICS. The trial randomized 210 participants in a double-blind, randomized, triple-dummy, crossover design that included 14-week treatment periods and 2-week run-out, run-in periods between periods of active treatment. The use of tiotropium resulted in a superior primary outcome compared with doubling the dose of an inhaled glucocorticoid. Assessment by measuring the morning peak expiratory flow (PEF) found a mean difference of 25.8 L/min ($P < .001$) and superiority in most secondary outcomes, including evening PEF, with a difference of 35.3 L/min ($P < .001$); the proportion of asthma-control days, with a difference of 0.079 ($P = .01$); the FEV_1 before bronchodilation, with a difference of 0.10 L ($P = .004$); and daily symptom scores, with a difference of −0.11 points ($P < .001$).[119] Figure 97-4 shows data for morning PEF, evening PEF, prebronchodilator FEV_1, and asthma-control days for the three treatment regimens. The addition of tiotropium was also noninferior to the addition of salmeterol for all assessed outcomes, and it increased the prebronchodilator FEV_1 more than did salmeterol, with a difference of 0.11 L ($P = .003$).[119]

Two additional studies reported positive results for tiotropium add-on therapy in patients with inadequately controlled asthma.[120,121] Bateman and colleagues[120] reported the results of treating 388 patients homozygous for the Arg/Arg variant at the 16th amino acid coding position of the β_2-adrenergic receptor gene *(ADRB2)*, whose asthma had been inadequately controlled by ICS, with placebo, salmeterol or tiotropium (5 μg by Respimat). The changes in weekly PEF from the last week of the run-in period (on salmeterol) to the last week of treatment (on tiotropium, salmeterol, or placebo), for which the primary end point was the change in PEF, were −3.9 ± 4.87 L/min ($n = 128$) for tiotropium and −3.2 ± 4.64 L/min ($n = 134$) for salmeterol,

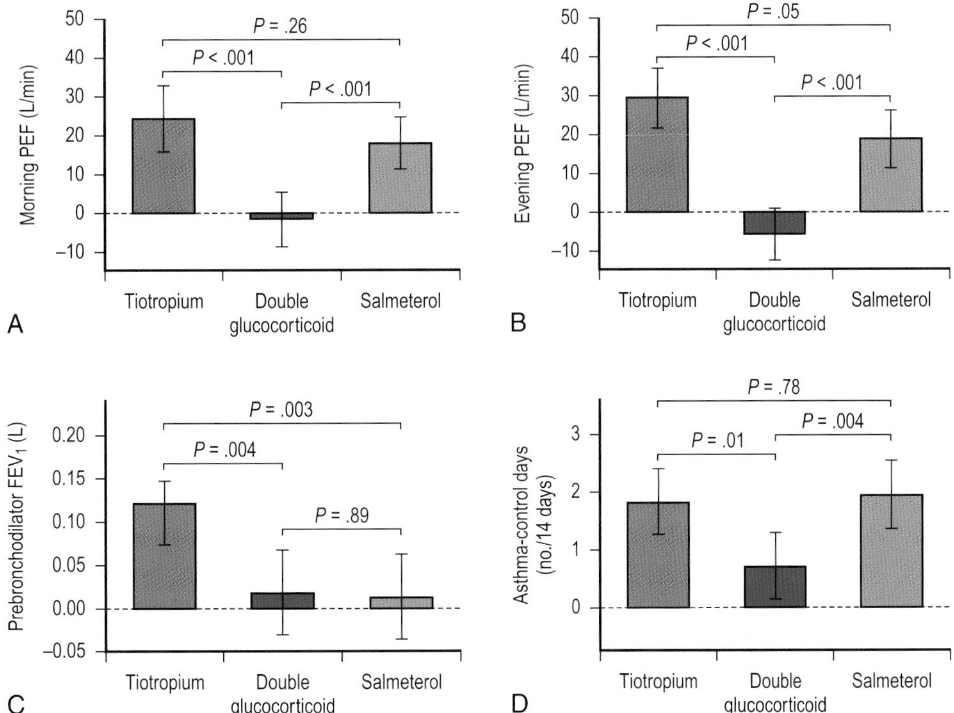

Figure 97-4 Comparison of the efficacy of tiotropium plus low-dose or double-dose inhaled corticosteroid (ICS) and salmeterol plus low-dose ICS in the TALC asthma trial. Shown in the graphs are the mean differences among patients receiving tiotropium, double glucocorticoid, or salmeterol doses with respect to the morning peak expiratory flow (PEF) **(A)**, the evening PEF **(B)**, the prebronchodilator forced expiratory volume in 1 second (FEV_1) **(C)**, and the proportion of asthma-control days per 14-day period **(D)**. The *I bars* indicate 95% confidence intervals. *TALC*, Tiotropium Bromide as an Alternative to Increased Inhaled Corticosteroid in Patients Inadequately Controlled on a Lower Dose of Inhaled Corticosteroids trial. *(From Peters SP, Kunselman SJ, Icitovic N, et al; National Heart, Lung, and Blood Institute Asthma Clinical Research Network. Tiotropium bromide step-up therapy for adults with uncontrolled asthma. N Engl J Med 2010;363:1715-26.)*

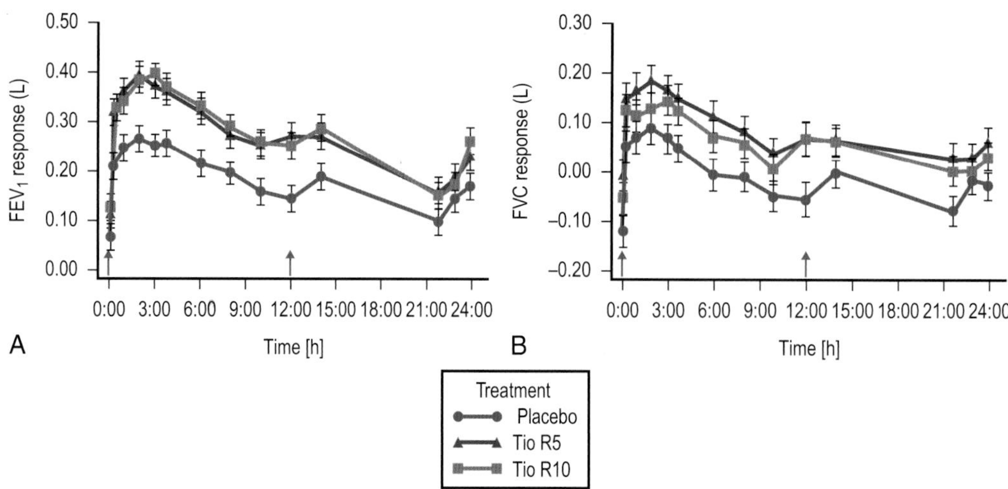

Figure 97-5 Effects of adding tiotropium (5 or 10 μg daily) administered through the Respimat inhaler with placebo as add-on therapy in patients with uncontrolled, severe asthma despite maintenance treatment with a high-dose inhaled corticosteroid plus a long-acting β_2-agonist. *FEV_1*, Forced expiratory volume in 1 second; *FVC*, forced vital capacity; *R10*, 10-μg dose; *R5*, 5-μg dose. *(From Kerstjens HA, Disse B, Schröder-Babo W, et al. Tiotropium improves lung function in patients with severe uncontrolled asthma: a randomized controlled trial. J Allergy Clin Immunol 2011;128:308-14.)*

and these results were superior to placebo (−24.6 ± 4.84 L/min; $n = 125$; $P < .05$). Using this end point, tiotropium was noninferior to salmeterol. Tiotropium was also superior to placebo in terms of FEV_1, FVC, and activity limitation.

Kerstjens and colleagues[121] reported the results of treating 107 patients with severe asthma that was inadequately controlled on high-dose ICS plus LABA (100 of whom completed all treatment periods) with placebo or with 5 or 10 μg/day of tiotropium by Respimat for 8-week periods in a randomized, double-blind, crossover study. The peak FEV_1 value was significantly higher with 5 μg (difference of 139 mL; 95% CI, 96 to 181 mL) and 10 μg (difference of 170 mL; 95% CI, 128 to 213 mL) of tiotropium than with placebo (both $P < .0001$), as was the trough FEV_1 at the end of the dosing interval (5 μg: 86 mL [95% CI, 41 to 132 mL]; 10 μg: 113 mL [95% CI, 67 to 159 mL]; both $P < .0004$). Data for the 67 patients who underwent 24-hour monitoring of spirometry are presented in Figure 97-5. Only the adverse effect of dry mouth was more common in the 10-μg tiotropium treatment period.

Kerstjens and coworkers[122] reported the results of treating 912 patients with severe asthma who were inadequately controlled (i.e., Asthma Control Questionnaire [ACQ]-7 score ≥1.5) on high-dose ICS (≥800 μg of budesonide or equivalent) plus LABA in two companion trials (459 in trial 1 and 453 in trial 2) with 5 μg/day of tiotropium by Respimat or with placebo for 48 weeks (Fig. 97-6). At 24 weeks, the mean (±SE) change in the peak FEV_1 from baseline was greater with tiotropium than with placebo in the two trials: a difference of 86 ± 34 mL in trial 1 ($P = .01$) and 154 ± 32 mL in trial 2 (P < .001). The predose (i.e., trough) FEV_1 also improved in trials 1 and 2 with tiotropium compared with placebo: a difference of 88 ± 31 mL ($P = .01$) and 111 ± 30 mL ($P < .001$), respectively. The addition of tiotropium increased the time to the first severe exacerbation (282 versus 226 days), with an overall reduction of 21% in the risk of a severe exacerbation (hazard ratio = 0.79; $P = .03$).[122] Most adverse events were similar in the two groups, with only allergic rhinitis occurring more commonly in the tiotropium group, and asthma events and insomnia more common in the placebo group.

Anticholinergic Agents for Treating Rhinitis

Nasal provocation with methacholine causes rhinorrhea in normal subjects and in patients with allergic and nonallergic rhinitis, a response that can be blocked by atropine and ipratropium bromide. Studies indicate that M_1 and M_3 muscarinic receptor subtypes regulate mucous glycoprotein secretion from human nasal mucosa, but that the M_3 receptor has the predominant role.[125] Although oral anticholinergic agents such as methscopolamine are sometimes used as adjunctive treatments for rhinitis, they have the disadvantage of causing atropine-like systemic side effects. Nasal ipratropium bromide reduces rhinorrhea caused by allergic rhinitis, nonallergic rhinitis, and viral respiratory infections (e.g., common cold).[126] Ipratropium bromide has no adverse effect on physiologic nasal functions (e.g., sense of smell, ciliary beat frequency, mucociliary clearance) and is associated with a low incidence of epistaxis and nasal dryness. Concomitant use of ipratropium bromide and intranasal corticosteroids has an additive effect in controlling rhinorrhea.[126]

Summary

Asthma and COPD have cholinergic hyperactivity that can cause bronchospasm and may contribute to inflammatory and airway remodeling processes. The use of anticholinergic agents as bronchodilators is well established for the treatment of COPD, and the data suggest a role for these drugs in the treatment of asthma. We are on the verge of adding a new class of drugs that can be used to improve asthma control. The extent to which different groups of patients with asthma respond to different classes of long-acting bronchodilator drugs, such as long-acting β-agonists or long-acting cholinergic and muscarinic antagonists, has yet to be determined. Appropriate use of these novel agents has the potential to advance the goal of tailoring treatment strategies for patients with asthma. Anticholinergic agents also have a well-recognized role in the treatment of rhinorrhea of rhinitis or the common cold.

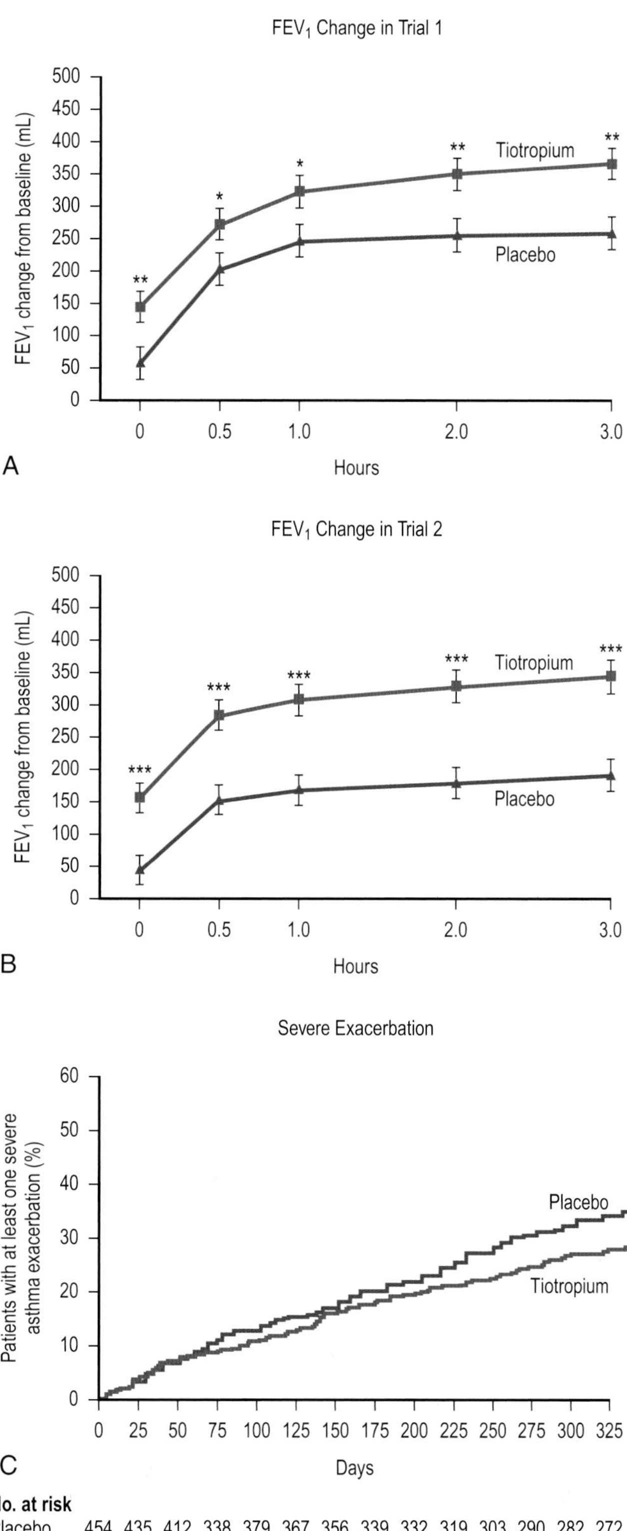

Figure 97-6 Effects of tiotropium or placebo (both delivered by mist inhaler once daily for 48 weeks) on lung function and asthma exacerbations in patients whose disease was uncontrolled on an inhaled corticosteroid plus a long-acting β_2-agonist. **A** and **B,** Lung function data were collected from two companion trials. At 24 weeks, the mean change in the peak forced expiratory volume in 1 second (FEV_1) from baseline was greater with tiotropium than with placebo in both trials. **C,** Data from the two trials were combined to examine asthma exacerbations, and showed that addition of tiotropium increased the time to the first severe exacerbation and provided modest, sustained bronchodilation. *, $P < 0.05$; **, $P < 0.01$; ***, $P < 0.001$. *(From Kerstjens HA, Engel M, Dahl R, et al. Tiotropium in asthma poorly controlled with standard combination therapy. N Engl J Med 2012;367:1198-207.)*

REFERENCES

Airway Cholinergic Hyperresponsiveness

1. Boushey HA, Holtzman MJ, Sheller JR, Nadel JA. Bronchial hyperreactivity. Am Rev Respir Dis 1980;121:389-413.
2. National Asthma Education and Prevention Program. Expert panel report 3 (EPR3): guidelines for the diagnosis and management of asthma. NIH publication no. 08-4051. Bethesda, MD: National Institutes of Health, National Heart, Lung, and Blood Institute, 2007. Available at www.nhlbi.nih.gov/guidelines/asthma/asthgdln.htm (accessed February 18, 2013).
3. Cockcroft DW. Airways hyperresponsiveness: therapeutic implications. Ann Allergy 1987; 405-14.
4. Cockcroft DW, Killian DN, Mellon JJ, Hargreave FE. Bronchial reactivity to inhaled histamine: a method and clinical survey. Clin Allergy 1977;7:235-43.
5. Hargreave FE, Ryan G, Thomson NC, et al. Bronchial responsiveness to histamine or methacholine in asthma: measurement and clinical significance. J Allergy Clin Immunol 1981;68:347-55.
6. Guidelines for methacholine and exercise challenge testing—1999: official statement of the American Thoracic Society. Am J Respir Crit Care Med 2000;161:309-29.
7. Fish JE, Shaver JR, Peters SP. Airway hyperresponsiveness in asthma: is it unique? Chest 1995;107:S154-6.
8. Bleecker ER. Airways reactivity and asthma: significance and treatment. J Allergy Clin Immunol 1985;75:21-4.
9. Stanescu DC, Frans A. Bronchial asthma without increased airway reactivity. Eur J Respir Dis 1982;63:5-12.
10. McGrath KW, Fahy JV. Negative methacholine challenge tests in subjects who report physician-diagnosed asthma. Clin Exp Allergy 2010;41:46-51.
11. Sumino K, Sugar EA, Irvin CG, et al. American Lung Association Asthma Clinical Research Centers. Methacholine challenge test: diagnostic characteristics in asthmatic patients receiving controller medications. J Allergy Clin Immunol 2012;130:69-75.

Cholinergic Nervous System as a Target for Anticholinergic Agents

12. O'Byrne PM, Inman MD. New considerations about measuring airway hyperresponsiveness. J Asthma 2000;37:293-302.
13. Undem BJ, Carr MJ. The role of nerves in asthma. Curr Allergy Asthma Rep 2002;2:159-65.
14. Barnes PJ. Pathogenesis of asthma: a review. J Royal Soc Med 1983;76:580-6.
15. Lemanske RF Jr, Kaliner MA. Autonomic nervous system abnormalities and asthma. Am Rev Respir Dis 1990;141:S157-61.
16. Baker DG, McDonald DM, Basbaum CB, et al. The architecture of nerves and ganglia of the ferret trachea as revealed by acetylcholinesterase histochemistry. J Comp Neurol 1986;246:513-26.
17. Richardson J. Nerve supply to the lungs. Am Rev Respir Dis 1979;119:785-802.
18. Nadel JA, Cabezas A, Austin JHM. In vivo roentrographic examination of parasympathetic innervation of small airways: use of tantalum and fine focal spot X-ray tube. Invest Radiol 1971;6:9-17.
19. Barnes PJ. Muscarinic receptor subtypes in airways. Eur Respir J 1993;6:328-31.
20. Fryer AD, Jacoby DB. Cholinergic mechanisms and anticholinergic therapy in respiratory diseases. In: Adkinson NF Jr, Bochner BS, Busse WW, et al, editors. Middleton's allergy: principles and practice, 7th ed. Philadelphia: Mosby; 2009, p. 1603-18.
21. Disse B, Reichl R, Speck G, et al. Ba 679 BR, a novel long-acting anticholinergic bronchodilator. Life Sci 1993;52:537-44.
22. Fernandes LB, Fryer AD, Hirshman CA. M2 muscarinic receptors inhibit isoproterenol-induced relaxation of canine airway smooth muscle. J Pharmacol Exp Ther 1992;262:119-26.
23. Haddad E-B, Landry Y, Gies J-P. Muscarinic receptor subtypes in guinea-pig airways. Am J Physiol 1991;261:L327-33.
24. Witek TJ Jr. The fate of inhaled drugs: the pharmacokinetics and pharmacodynamics of drugs administered by aerosol. Respir Care 2000;45:826-30.
25. Fujii T, Yamada S, Watanabe Y, et al. Induction of choline acetyltransferase mRNA in human mononuclear leukocytes stimulated by phytohemagglutinin, a T-cell activator. J Neuroimmunol 1998;82:101-7.
26. Fujii T, Watanabe Y, Inoue T, Kawashima K. Upregulation of mRNA encoding the M5 muscarinic acetylcholine receptor in human T- and B-lymphocytes during immunological responses. Neurochem Res 2003;28:423-9.
27. Barnes PJ. Anticholinergics. In: Celli BR, editor. Pharmacotherapy in chronic obstructive pulmonary disease. New York: Marcel Dekker; 2004.
28. Roffel AF, Elzinga CR, Van Amsterdam RG, De Zeeuw RA, Zaagsma J. Muscarinic M2 receptors in bovine tracheal smooth muscle: discrepancies between binding and function. Eur J Pharmacol 1988;153:73-82.
29. Ten Berge RE, Roffel AF, Zaagsma J. The interaction of selective and non-selective antagonists with pre- and postjunctional muscarinic receptor subtypes in the guinea pig trachea. Eur J Pharmacol 1993;233:279-84.
30. van Nieuwstadt RA, Henricks PA, Hajer R, et al. Characterization of muscarinic receptors in equine tracheal smooth muscle in vitro. Vet Q 1997;19:54-7.
31. Roffel AF, Elzinga CR, Zaagsma J. Muscarinic M3 receptors mediate contraction of human central and peripheral airway smooth muscle. Pulm Pharmacol 1990;3:47-51.
32. Fisher JT, Vincent SG, Gomeza J, Yamada M, Wess J. Loss of vagally mediated bradycardia and bronchoconstriction in mice lacking M2 or M3 muscarinic acetylcholine receptors. FASEB J 2004;18:711-3.
33. Jeffery PK. Remodeling and inflammation of bronchi in asthma and chronic obstructive pulmonary disease. Proc Am Thorac Soc 2004;1:176-83.
34. Rogers DF. Motor control of airway goblet cells and glands. Respir Physiol 2001;125:129-44.
35. Rogers DF. Airway mucus hypersecretion in asthma: an undervalued pathology? Curr Opin Pharmacol 2004;4:241-50.
36. Laitinen A, Partanen M, Hervonen A, Laitinen LA. Electron microscopic study on the innervation of the human lower respiratory tract: evidence of adrenergic nerves. Eur J Respir Dis 1985;67:209-15.
37. Mak JC, Barnes PJ. Autoradiographic visualization of muscarinic receptor subtypes in human and guinea pig lung. Am Rev Respir Dis 1990;141:1559-68.
38. Ramnarine SI, Haddad EB, Khawaja AM, Mak JC, Rogers DF. On muscarinic control of neurogenic mucus secretion in ferret trachea. J Physiol 1996;494:577-86.
39. Ishihara H, Shimura S, Satoh M, et al. Muscarinic receptor subtypes in feline tracheal submucosal gland secretion. Am J Physiol 1992; 262:L223-8.
40. Strom TB, Deisseroth A, Morganroth J, Carpenter CB, Merrill JP. Alteration of the cytotoxic action of sensitized lymphocytes by cholinergic agents and activators of adenylate cyclase. Proc Natl Acad Sci U S A 1972;69:2995-9.
41. Profita M, Giorgi RD, Sala A, et al. Muscarinic receptors, leukotriene B4 production and neutrophilic inflammation in COPD patients. Allergy 2005;60:1361-9.
42. Sato E, Koyama S, Okubo Y, Kubo K, Sekiguchi M. Acetylcholine stimulates alveolar macrophages to release inflammatory cell chemotactic activity. Am J Physiol 1998;274:L970-9.
43. Koyama S, Rennard SI, Robbins RA. Acetylcholine stimulates bronchial epithelial cells to release neutrophil and monocyte chemotactic activity. Am J Physiol 1992;262:L466-71.
44. Koyama S, Sato E, Nomura H, et al. Acetylcholine and substance P stimulate bronchial epithelial cells to release eosinophil chemotactic activity. J Appl Physiol 1998;84:1528-34.
45. Klapproth H, Racke K, Wessler I. Acetylcholine and nicotine stimulate the release of granulocyte-macrophage colony stimulating factor from cultured human bronchial epithelial cells. Naunyn Schmiedebergs Arch Pharmacol 1998;357:472-5.
46. Proskocil BJ, Sekhon HS, Jia Y, et al. Acetylcholine is an autocrine or paracrine hormone synthesized and secreted by airway bronchial epithelial cells. Endocrinology 2004;145:2498-506.
47. Gosens R, Zaagsma J, Meurs H, Halayko AJ. Muscarinic receptor signaling in the pathophysiology of asthma and COPD. Respir Res 2006;7:73-8.
48. Verhein KC, Fryer AD, Jacoby DB. Neural control of airway inflammation. Curr Allergy Asthma Rep 2009;9:484-90.
49. Kawashima K, Fujii T. Extraneuronal cholinergic system in lymphocytes. Pharmacol Ther 2000;86:29-48.
50. Gosens R, Zaagsma J, Grootte Bromhaar M, Nelemans A, Meurs H. Acetylcholine: a novel regulator of airway smooth muscle remodelling? Eur J Pharmacol 2004;500:193-201.
51. Halayko AJ, Tran T, Ji SY, Yamasaki A, Gosens R. Airway smooth muscle phenotype and function: interaction with current asthma therapies. Curr Drug Targets 2006;7:525-40.
52. Matthiesen S, Bahulayan A, Kempkens S, et al. Muscarinic receptors mediate stimulation of human lung fibroblast proliferation. Am J Respir Cell Mol Biol 2006;35:621-7.
53. Krymskaya VP, Orsini MJ, Eszterhas AJ, et al. Mechanisms of proliferation synergy by receptor tyrosine kinase and G protein-coupled

receptor activation in human airway smooth muscle. Am J Respir Cell Mol Biol 2000;23: 546-54.
54. Gosens R, Nelemans SA, Grootte Bromhaar MM, et al. Muscarinic M3-receptors mediate cholinergic synergism of mitogenesis in airway smooth muscle. Am J Respir Cell Mol Biol 2003;28:257-62.
55. Ayala LE, Ahmed T. Is there loss of protective muscarinic receptor mechanism in asthma? Chest 1989;96:1285-91.
56. Fryer AD, Jacoby DB. Parainfluenza virus infection damages inhibitory M2 muscarinic receptors on pulmonary parasympathetic nerves in the guinea-pig. Br J Pharmacol 1991;102:267-71.
57. Fryer AD, Jacoby DB. Effect of inflammatory cell mediators on M2 muscarinic receptors in the lungs. Life Sci 1993;52:529-36.
58. Adamko DJ, Fryer AD, Bochner BS, Jacoby DB. CD8+ T lymphocytes in viral hyperreactivity and M2 muscarinic receptor dysfunction. Am J Respir Crit Care Med 2003;167:550-6.
59. Evans CM, Fryer AD, Jacoby DB, Gleich GJ, Costello RW. Pretreatment with antibody to eosinophil major basic protein prevents hyperresponsiveness by protecting neuronal M2 muscarinic receptors in antigen-challenged guinea pigs. J Clin Invest 1997;100:2254-62.
60. Jacoby DB, Gleich GJ, Fryer A. Human eosinophil major basic protein is an endogenous allosteric antagonist at the inhibitory muscarinic M2 receptor. J Clin Invest 1993;91:1314-8.
61. Jacoby DB, Costello R, Fryer AD. Eosinophil recruitment to the airway nerves. J Allergy Clin Immunol 2001;107:211-8.

Pharmacology of Anticholinergic Agents

62. Restrepo RD. Use of inhaled anticholinergic agents in obstructive airway disease. Respir Care 2007;52:833-51.
63. Gross NJ, Skorodin MS. Anticholinergic, antimuscarinic bronchodilators. Am Rev Respir Dis 1984;129:856-70.
64. van Bever HP, Desager KN. Paradoxical bronchoconstriction in wheezing infants after nebulized ipratropium bromide. BMJ 1990;300: 397-8.
65. Moulton BC, Fryer AD. Muscarinic receptor antagonists, from folklore to pharmacology: finding drugs that actually work in asthma and COPD. Br J Pharmacol 2011;163:44-52.
66. Casarosa P, Bouyssou T, Germeyer S, et al. Preclinical evaluation of long-acting muscarinic antagonists: comparison of tiotropium and investigational drugs. J Pharmacol Exp Ther 2009;330:660-8.
67. Lu S, Parekh DD, Kuznetsova O, et al. An oral selective M3 cholinergic receptor antagonist in COPD. Eur Respir J 2006;28:772-80.
68. Patacchini R, Bergamaschi M, Harrison S, et al. In vitro pharmacological profile of CHF 5407, a potent, long-acting and selective muscarinic M3 receptor antagonist. Eur Respir J 2007;30: s25-6.
69. Gavaldà A, Miralpeix M, Ramos I, et al. Characterization of aclidinium bromide, a novel inhaled muscarinic antagonist, with long duration of action and a favorable pharmacological profile. J Pharmacol Exp Ther 2009;331: 740-51.
70. Goodman LS, Gilman A, Brunton LL, Lazo JS, Parker KL. Goodman and Gilman's the pharmacological basis of therapeutics. 11th ed. New York: McGraw-Hill; 2006.
71. Pakes GE, Brogden RN, Heel RC, Speight TM, Avery GS. Ipratropium bromide: a review of its pharmacological properties and therapeutic efficacy in asthma and chronic bronchitis. Drugs 1980;20:237-66.
72. Barnes PJ. Tiotropium bromide. Expert Opin Investig Drugs 2001;10:733-40.
73. Littner MR, Ilowite JS, Tashkin DP, et al. Long-acting bronchodilation with once-daily dosing of tiotropium (Spiriva) in stable chronic obstructive pulmonary disease. Am J Respir Crit Care Med 2000;161:1136-42.
74. Casaburi R, Mahler DA, Jones PW, et al. A long-term evaluation of once-daily inhaled tiotropium in chronic obstructive pulmonary disease. Eur Respir J 2002;19:217-24.
75. Haddad EB, Patel H, Keeling JE, et al. Pharmacological characterization of the muscarinic receptor antagonist, glycopyrrolate, in human and guinea-pig airways. Br J Pharmacol 1999; 127:413-20.
76. Hansel TT, Neighbour H, Erin EM, et al. Glycopyrrolate causes prolonged bronchoprotection and bronchodilatation in patients with asthma. Chest 2005;128:1974-9.

Anticholinergic Agents in Obstructive Lung Diseases

77. Gross N, Tashkin D, Miller R, et al. Inhalation by nebulization of albuterol-ipratropium combination (Dey combination) is superior to either agent alone in the treatment of chronic obstructive pulmonary disease. Dey Combination Solution Study Group. Respiration 1998; 65:354-62.
78. Lefcoe NM, Toogood JH, Blennerhassett G, Baskerville J, Paterson NA. The addition of an aerosol anticholinergic to an oral beta-agonist plus theophylline in asthma and bronchitis: a double-blind single dose study. Chest 1982;82: 300-5.
79. Tashkin DP, Ashutosh K, Bleecker ER. Comparison of the anticholinergic bronchodilator ipratropium bromide with metaproterenol in chronic obstructive pulmonary disease: a 90-day multi-center study. Am J Med 1986; 81:81-90.
80. Appleton S, Jones T, Poole P, et al. Ipratropium bromide versus short acting β2 agonists for stable chronic obstructive pulmonary disease. Cochrane Database Syst Rev 2006;(2): CD001387.
81. COMBIVENT Inhalation Aerosol Study Group. In chronic obstructive pulmonary disease, a combination of ipratropium and albuterol is more effective than either agent alone: an 85-day multicenter trial. Chest 1994; 105:1411-9.
82. Gross NJ, Skorodin MS. Role of the parasympathetic system in airway obstruction due to emphysema. N Engl J Med 1984;311:421-5.
83. Gross NJ. Ipratropium bromide. N Engl J Med 1988;319:486-94.
84. Backman R, Hellstrom PE. Fenoterol and ipratropium in respiratory treatment of patients with chronic bronchitis. Curr Ther Res Clin Exper 1985;38:135-40.
85. Karpel JP, Pesin J, Greenberg D, Gentry E. A comparison of the effects of ipratropium bromide and metaproterenol sulfate in acute exacerbations of COPD. Chest 1990;98:835-9.
86. Lloberes P, Ramis L, Montserrat JM, et al. Effect of three different bronchodilators during an exacerbation of chronic obstructive pulmonary disease. Eur Respir J 1988;1:536-9.
87. McCrory DC, Brown CD. Anti-cholinergic bronchodilators versus β2-sympathomimetic agents for acute exacerbations of chronic obstructive pulmonary disease. Cochrane Database Syst Rev 2002;(4):CD003900.
88. Global Initiative for Chronic Obstructive Lung Disease. Global strategy for the diagnosis, management and prevention of chronic obstructive pulmonary diseases, revised 2011. Available at www.goldcopd.org (accessed February 18, 2013).
89. Westby M, Benson M, Gibson P. Anticholinergic agents for chronic asthma in adults. Cochrane Database Syst Rev 2004;(3): CD003269.
90. Israel E, Chinchilli VM, Ford JG, et al; National Heart, Lung, and Blood Institute's Asthma Clinical Research Network. Use of regularly scheduled albuterol treatment in asthma: genotype-stratified, randomised, placebo-controlled cross-over trial. Lancet 2004;364: 1505-12.
91. Wechsler ME, Kunselman SJ, Chinchilli VM, et al; National Heart, Lung and Blood Institute's Asthma Clinical Research Network. Effect of beta2-adrenergic receptor polymorphism on response to longacting beta2 agonist in asthma (LARGE trial): a genotype-stratified, randomised, placebo-controlled, crossover trial. Lancet 2009;374:1754-64.
92. Rodrigo GJ, Plaza V, Castro-Rodríguez JA. Comparison of three combined pharmacological approaches with tiotropium monotherapy in stable moderate to severe COPD: a systematic review. Pulm Pharmacol Ther 2012;25: 40-7.

Tiotropium for Treating Chronic Obstructive Pulmonary Disease

93. O'Donnell DE, Flüge T, Gerken F, et al. Effects of tiotropium on lung hyperinflation, dyspnoea and exercise tolerance in COPD. Eur Respir J 2004;23:832-40.
94. Niewoehner DE, Rice K, Cote C, et al. Prevention of exacerbations of chronic obstructive pulmonary disease with tiotropium, a once-daily inhaled anticholinergic bronchodilator: a randomized trial. Ann Intern Med 2005;143: 317-26.
95. Barr RG, Bourbeau J, Camargo CA, Ram FS. Tiotropium for stable chronic obstructive pulmonary disease: a meta-analysis. Thorax 2006;61:854-62.
96. Vogelmeier C, Hederer B, Glaab T, et al; POET-COPD Investigators. Tiotropium versus salmeterol for the prevention of exacerbations of COPD. N Engl J Med 2011;364:1093-103.
97. Wedzicha JA, Calverley PM, Seemungal TA, et al; INSPIRE Investigators. The prevention of chronic obstructive pulmonary disease exacerbations by salmeterol/fluticasone propionate or tiotropium bromide. Am J Respir Crit Care Med 2008;177:19-26.
98. Tashkin DP, Celli B, Senn S, et al; UPLIFT Study Investigators. A 4-year trial of tiotropium in chronic obstructive pulmonary disease. N Engl J Med 2008;359:1543-54.
99. Celli B, Decramer M, Kesten S, et al; UPLIFT Study Investigators. Mortality in the 4-year trial of tiotropium (UPLIFT) in patients with chronic obstructive pulmonary disease. Am J Respir Crit Care Med 2009; 180:948-55.
100. McGarvey LP, Magder S, Burkhart D, et al. Cause-specific mortality adjudication in the

UPLIFT COPD trial: findings and recommendations. Respir Med 2012;106:515-21.
101. Troosters T, Celli B, Lystig T, et al; UPLIFT Investigators. Tiotropium as a first maintenance drug in COPD: secondary analysis of the UPLIFT trial. Eur Respir J 2010;36:65-73.
102. Morice AH, Celli B, Kesten S, et al. COPD in young patients: a pre-specified analysis of the four-year trial of tiotropium (UPLIFT). Respir Med 2010;104:1659-67.
103. Decramer M, Celli B, Kesten S, et al; UPLIFT investigators. Effect of tiotropium on outcomes in patients with moderate chronic obstructive pulmonary disease (UPLIFT): a prespecified subgroup analysis of a randomised controlled trial. Lancet 2009;374:1171-8.
104. Tashkin D, Celli B, Kesten S, Lystig T, Decramer M. Effect of tiotropium in men and women with COPD: results of the 4-year UPLIFT trial. Respir Med 2010;104:1495-504.
105. Decramer M, Molenberghs G, Liu D, et al; UPLIFT investigators. Premature discontinuation during the UPLIFT study. Respir Med 2011;105:1523-30.
106. Aaron SD, Vandemheen KL, Fergusson D, et al; Canadian Thoracic Society/Canadian Respiratory Clinical Research Consortium. Tiotropium in combination with placebo, salmeterol, or fluticasone/salmeterol for treatment of chronic obstructive pulmonary disease: a randomized trial. Ann Intern Med 2007;146:545-55.
107. Singh D, Brooks J, Hagan G, Cahn A, O'Connor BJ. Superiority of "triple" therapy with salmeterol/fluticasone propionate and tiotropium bromide versus individual components in moderate to severe COPD. Thorax 2008;63:592-8.
108. Hanania NA, Crater GD, Morris AN, et al. Benefits of adding fluticasone propionate/salmeterol to tiotropium in moderate to severe COPD. Respir Med 2012;106:91-101.
109. Rodrigo GJ, Castro-Rodriguez JA. Anticholinergics in the treatment of children and adults with acute asthma: a systematic review with meta-analysis. Thorax 2005;60:740-6.
110. Barnes PJ. Triple inhalers for obstructive airways disease: will they be useful? Expert Rev Respir Med 2011;5:297-300.
111. Singh S, Loke YK, Furberg CD. Inhaled anticholinergics and risk of major adverse cardiovascular events in patients with chronic obstructive pulmonary disease: a systematic review and meta-analysis. JAMA 2008;300:1439-50.
112. Celli B, Decramer M, Leimer I, et al. Cardiovascular safety of tiotropium in patients with COPD. Chest 2010;137:20-30.
113. Michele TM, Pinheiro S, Iyasu S. The safety of tiotropium: the FDA's conclusions. N Engl J Med 2010;363:1097-9.
114. Singh S, Loke YK, Enright PL, Furberg CD. Mortality associated with tiotropium mist inhaler in patients with chronic obstructive pulmonary disease: systematic review and meta-analysis of randomised controlled trials. BMJ 2011;342:d3215.

Tiotropium for Treating Asthma

115. Kapoor AS, Olsen SR, O'Hara C, Puttagunta L, Vethanayagam D. The efficacy of tiotropium as a steroid-sparing agent in severe asthma. Can Respir J 2009;16:99-101.
116. Iwamoto H, Yokoyama A, Shiota N, et al. Tiotropium bromide is effective for severe asthma with noneosinophilic phenotype. Eur Respir J 2008;31:1379-80.
117. Magnussen H, Bugnas B, van Noord J, et al. Improvements with tiotropium in COPD patients with concomitant asthma. Respir Med 2008;102:50-6.
118. Park HW, Yang MS, Park CS, et al. Additive role of tiotropium in severe asthmatics and Arg-16Gly in ADRB2 as a potential marker to predict response. Allergy 2009;64:778-83.
119. Peters SP, Kunselman SJ, Icitovic N, et al; National Heart, Lung, and Blood Institute Asthma Clinical Research Network. Tiotropium bromide step-up therapy for adults with uncontrolled asthma. N Engl J Med 2010;363:1715-26.
120. Bateman ED, Kornmann O, Schmidt P, et al. Tiotropium is noninferior to salmeterol in maintaining improved lung function in B16-Arg/Arg patients with asthma. J Allergy Clin Immunol 2011;128:315-22.
121. Kerstjens HA, Disse B, Schröder-Babo W, et al. Tiotropium improves lung function in patients with severe uncontrolled asthma: a randomized controlled trial. J Allergy Clin Immunol 2011;128:308-14.
122. Kerstjens HA, Engel M, Dahl R, et al. Tiotropium in asthma poorly controlled with standard combination therapy. N Engl J Med 2012;367:1198-207.
123. Grossman J, Banov C, Boggs P, et al. Use of ipratropium bromide nasal spray in chronic treatment of nonallergic perennial rhinitis, alone and in combination with other perennial rhinitis medications. J Allergy Clin Immunol 1995;95:1123-7.
124. Global Strategy for Asthma Management and Prevention, Global Initiative for Asthma (GINA). Available at: http://www.ginasthma.org (accessed February 18, 2013).

Anticholinergic Agents for Treating Rhinitis

125. Mullol J, Baraniuk JN, Logun C, et al. M1 and M3 muscarinic antagonists inhibit human nasal glandular secretion in vitro. J Appl Physiol 1992;73:2069-73.
126. Wallace DV, Dykewicz MS, et al, and The Joint Force on Practice Parameters, representing the AAAAI, ACAAI, JCAAI. The diagnosis and management of rhinitis: an updated practice parameter. J Allergy Clin Immunol 2008;122:S1-84.

98

The Chromones: Cromolyn Sodium and Nedocromil Sodium

ALAN M. EDWARDS | STEPHEN T. HOLGATE

Withdrawn

CONTENTS

SUMMARY OF IMPORTANT CONCEPTS

» The chromones, cromolyn sodium and nedocromil sodium, were developed from the naturally occurring chromone khellin, an extract of the plant *Ammi visnaga.*

» The primary mode of action of the chromones is as stabilizers of mast cells. They also modulate sensory nerve activity and can reduce severity of skin itch.

» The chromones act directly on the mucosal surface involved in allergic disease. They are poorly absorbed, not metabolized, and excreted unchanged and have low toxicity and few adverse effects.

» Efficacy of cromolyn and nedocromil depends on the efficiency of distribution on the surface affected: bronchial mucosa, nasal mucosa, conjunctivae, or gut mucosa.

» The effect of cromolyn and nedocromil on mast cells depends on dose and route of administration to the relevant mast cells.

» Dose frequency of the chromones should be increased if symptoms worsen.

Introduction

Cromolyn sodium and nedocromil sodium, members of the chromone group of chemical compounds, were discovered in 1965 and 1979, respectively. These compounds are used in the treatment of allergic diseases, including: allergic asthma, seasonal and perennial allergic rhinitis, allergic conjunctivitis, vernal keratoconjunctivitis, food allergy, atopic dermatitis, and systemic mastocytosis. The chromones are chemically and pharmacologically distinct from other drugs used in the treatment of allergic disease.

HISTORY AND BACKGROUND

The first chromone used in allergic disease was *khellin*, purified from an extract of the plant *Ammi visnaga* (Fig. 98-1). Following a trial showing the efficacy of khellin in asthma,[1] new chromones based on the khellin molecule were synthesized at Benger's Research Laboratories (Cheshire, UK) and screened for potential bronchodilator and antianaphylactic activities. For antianaphylaxis, a modification of the Herxheimer guinea pig model was used. Guinea pigs sensitized to egg albumin were challenged with a bronchial aerosol of ovalbumin. New compounds were tested for their ability to prevent the release of histamine and slow-releasing substance of anaphylaxis (SRS-A), now known as the *leukotrienes.*

Figure 98-2 shows the chemical structure of two early chromones. K18 was synthesized from khellin itself; GR4 was a newly synthesized compound. In animal models, both compounds were shown to prevent the release of histamine and SRS-A and to have anti–SRS-A activity, but no antihistamine properties.

In the late 1950s the UK research team was joined by Dr. Roger E.C. Altounyan, who induced asthmatic attacks in himself by inhaling antigens to which he was sensitive. He then measured the degree of protection against the ensuing bronchoconstriction provided by the prechallenge administration of new compounds. One of the first compounds tested was K18, which had been shown to have strong antileukotriene properties. In these experiments it was given with and without an antihistamine.[2] K18 was also given to 25 asthmatic patients as continuous therapy for several months during 1957 and was therefore the first antileukotriene drug to be used in the treatment of asthma. Remarkably, Altounyan tested more than 300 compounds on himself over 8 years. Almost complete protection was provided by the compound K84 (Fig. 98-2). However, repeat experiments failed, and it was eventually realized that the initial success had been caused by an impurity resulting from two K84 molecules joining at the 5-position during the synthesis to form a bischromone; thus cromolyn sodium was born.

Another compound, GR4, was the first drug to be tested using bronchial antigen challenge in asthmatic patients in a controlled trial. Although GR4 was never developed, it was the starting point when work on new monochromones began in the 1970s. From this developmental work, nedocromil sodium emerged.

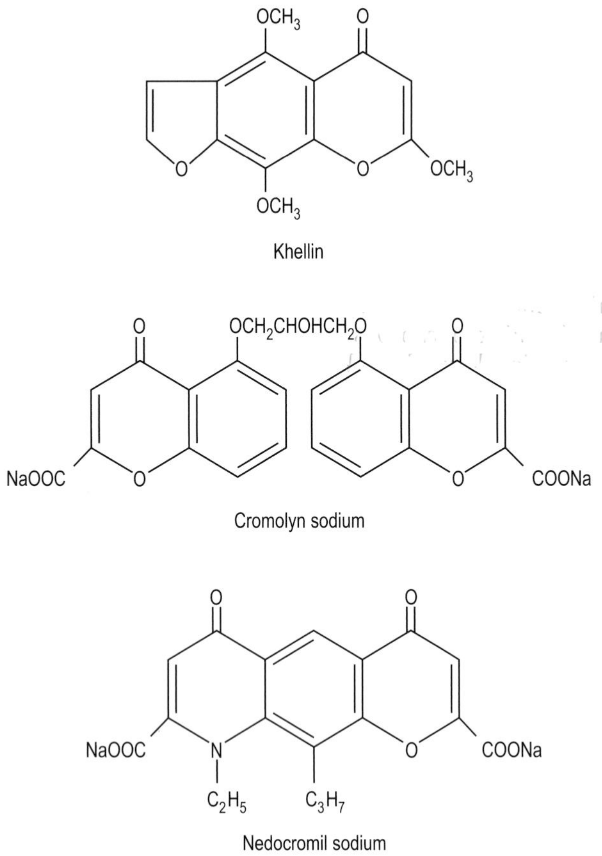

Khellin

Cromolyn sodium

Nedocromil sodium

Figure 98-1 Structures of khellin, cromolyn sodium, and nedocromil sodium.

K18

GR4

K84

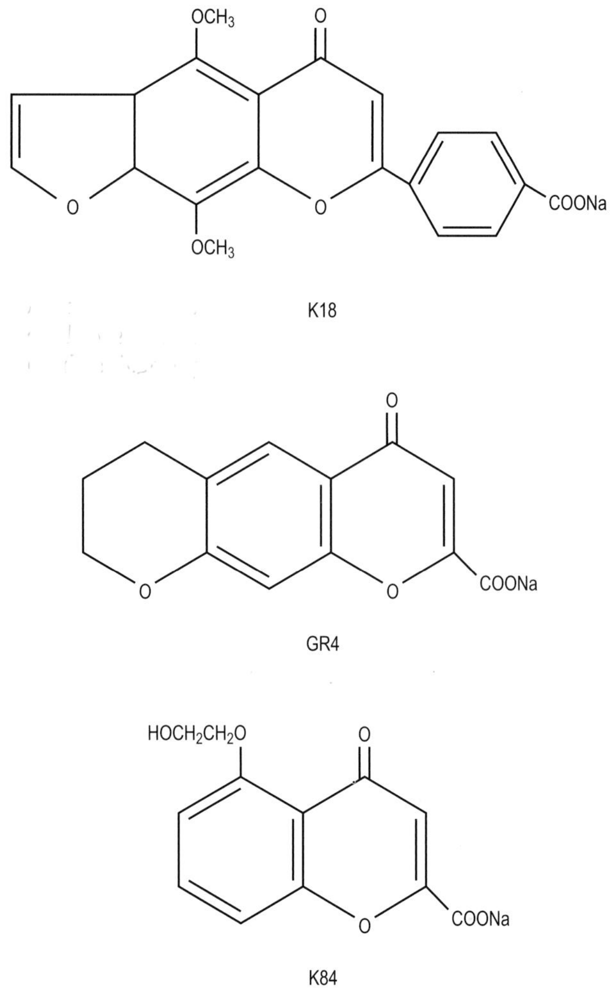

Figure 98-2 Structures of early chromones: K18, GR4, and K84.

CHALLENGE STUDIES

Single doses of cromolyn sodium and nedocromil sodium, when inhaled, have been shown to protect against a wide variety of stimuli, including antigen (early and late reactions)[3] (Fig. 98-3), physical challenges (exercise, fog, cold air), chemical challenges (adenosine, hypertonic saline, mannitol, sulpyrine), and neuronal challenges (sulfur dioxide, sodium metabisulfite, bradykinin, substance P, neurokinin A). Nedocromil prevented the increase in histamine in bronchoalveolar lavage (BAL) specimens after segmental allergen challenge in asthmatic subjects.

Inhalation of mannitol causes bronchoconstriction in asthmatic patients, but not in healthy individuals. Pretreatment with cromolyn sodium reduces the degree of bronchoconstriction and the increase in urinary 9α,11β-prostaglandin F_2 (PGF_2) that occurs with this challenge; 9α,11β-PGF_2 is a metabolite of mast cell–derived PGD_2.[4]

Mechanism of Action

The chromones have been shown to have three pharmacologic activities potentially useful in clinical medicine, as mast cell stabilizers, inhibitors of sensory nerve activity, and inhibitors of immunoglobulin E (IgE) production.

MAST CELL STABILIZATION

Cromolyn sodium was the first drug used in clinical medicine shown to prevent the antigen-induced release of histamine and leukotrienes from passively sensitized human lung.[5] The release

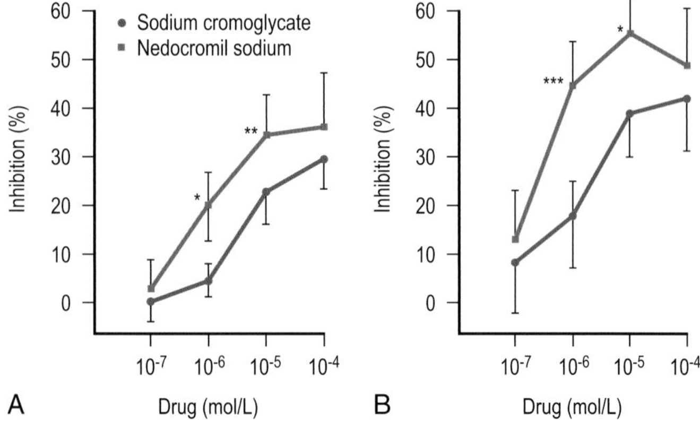

Figure 98-3 Effect of sodium cromoglycate (●) and nedocromil sodium (■) on immunologically induced histamine release from, **A**, dispersed human lung mast cells, and, **B**, human lavage mast cells. In each experiment a single pool of cells was used to construct parallel dose inhibition curves for the two drugs. Values are means and standard errors (SE) for eight (**A**) or five (**B**) experiments. The control, immunologically induced release of histamine, was 24.8% (±4.9%) (**A**) and 21.6% (±4.9%) (**B**) of the respective totals. **P* < .05; ***P* < .01, *** *P* < .001 (paired *t* test). *(Reproduced from Leung KB, Flint KC, Brostoff J, et al. Effects of sodium cromoglycate and nedocromil sodium on histamine secretion from human lung mast cells. Thorax 1988;43:756-61.)*

of these mediators was accompanied by alterations in mast cells,[6] and these were prevented by pretreatment with cromolyn along with the reduction of mediator release.

Many experiments examining the effects of chromones on mast cell activity followed, showing that these effects depend on the animal species and tissues from which the mast cells are derived, the challenge used, and the mediators released.[7-12]

In experiments examining the release of histamine and PGD_2 from mast cells derived from human skin, lung, tonsils, adenoids, and intestine challenged with anti-IgE, both cromolyn sodium and nedocromil sodium inhibited histamine release from lung, tonsillar, adenoidal, and intestinal mast cells.[7] Nedocromil was more effective than cromolyn against histamine release from lung, tonsillar, and adenoidal mast cells. Cromolyn was more effective on intestinal mast cells. Both compounds showed tachyphylaxis on the effects on lung and tonsillar mast cells but not in intestinal mast cells. Of importance, neither compound had any inhibitory effect on allergen-induced mediator release of skin (connective tissue) mast cells. When human skin is exposed to ultraviolet B irradiation, the inflammatory cytokine tumor necrosis factor alpha (TNF-α) is released, and skin mast cells are the source of this cytokine. Cromolyn sodium inhibits the release of TNF-α in these experiments.[13] Human lung mast cells release a number of proinflammatory cytokines, including interleukin-4 (IL-4), IL-5, IL-8, Il-13, and TNF-α, that contribute to the inflammatory response in asthma. Cromolyn significantly reduces the amount of TNF-α and IL-5 released from sensitized human lung specimens challenged with *Dermatophagoides* antigen.[14] Exposure of healthy volunteers to the inhalation of dust in a swine confinement building results in an intense inflammatory reaction in the lower and upper airways. In these individuals, cromolyn sodium reduces the increase in neutrophils, myeloperoxidase, soluble intercellular adhesion molecule 1 (ICAM-1), IL-6, and TNF-α in BAL and nasal lavage fluid.[15]

Atmospheric pollution with diesel exhaust particles plays an important role in the establishment of airway inflammation in asthmatic persons. Diesel exhaust particles instilled into the trachea of hamsters results in airway inflammation, as shown by an increase in inflammatory cells in BAL fluid and plasma histamine. These inflammatory changes are prevented by pretreatment with cromolyn sodium.[16] Pollutant gases such as nitrogen dioxide and sulfur dioxide increase airway reactivity in asthmatic patients and are potent activators of bronchial epithelial cells, resulting in the release of cytokines. In vitro studies have shown that nedocromil sodium reduces the release of TNF-α, IL-8, and soluble ICAM-1 from cultured human bronchial epithelial cells exposed to 50 parts per billion (ppb) of ozone.[17]

Differential effects of cromolyn and nedocromil on mast cells depend on the source of the mast cells and the challenge used. BAL specimens obtained from macaque monkeys infected with the nematode *Ascaris suum* contain large numbers of mast cells. When challenged with antigen, these cells release histamine, leukotriene C_4 (LTC_4), and PGD_2. This release is inhibited by nedocromil sodium but not by cromolyn sodium.[18] Both compounds inhibited the release of histamine from human lung mast cells challenged with anti–human IgE, but were more active against cells obtained by BAL versus those derived from dispersed human lung tissue (see Fig. 98-3).[9] This has clinical relevance, implying that when inhaled, optimal dose of the drugs should be directed into the smaller airways and alveoli.

EFFECTS ON SENSORY NERVES

Although unlikely to be involved in the initiation of inflammation in asthma, neurogenic mechanisms probably amplify the inflammatory response through the release of tachykinins (proinflammatory neuropeptides) from sensory nerves, which contribute to the symptoms of asthma (e.g., cough, wheeze, chest tightness). Cromolyn sodium inhibits substance P–induced microvascular leakage in the rat trachea, substance P–induced edema in rat paw skin, and substance P–induced and neurokinin B–induced edema in human skin. Cromolyn and nedocromil inhibit bronchoconstriction induced by irritants such as sulfur dioxide and bradykinin. These effects likely result from inhibition of neural reflex mechanisms in the airways. This conclusion is supported by evidence that cromolyn sodium blocks both myelinated and nonmyelinated C-fiber transmission in canine airways.[19]

Itch is a feature of many skin diseases. The transmission of itch sensation to the brain is the function of dense nerve networks in the skin and unmyelinated C-neurons, which are histamine sensitive. Cromolyn sodium reduces the severity of the itch induced in human skin with intradermal allergen, codeine, and histamine, as a result of inhibition of sensory nerve activation.[20]

INHIBITION OF IGE PRODUCTION

Cromolyn sodium and nedocromil sodium inhibit production of IgE expression of mature epsilon (ε) transcripts, inhibited IgE synthesis, and inhibited IgE release from purified B cells that were stimulated with IL-4 and B cell–activating agents such as T cells, monoclonal antibody (mAb) to B cell antigen, CD40, and hydrocortisone. The drug inhibited the Sμ to Sε switch/recombination mechanism in response to B cell–activating stimuli in IL-4–treated cells and had no effect on the induction of ε germline transcripts induced by IL-4 alone[21] (Fig. 98-4).

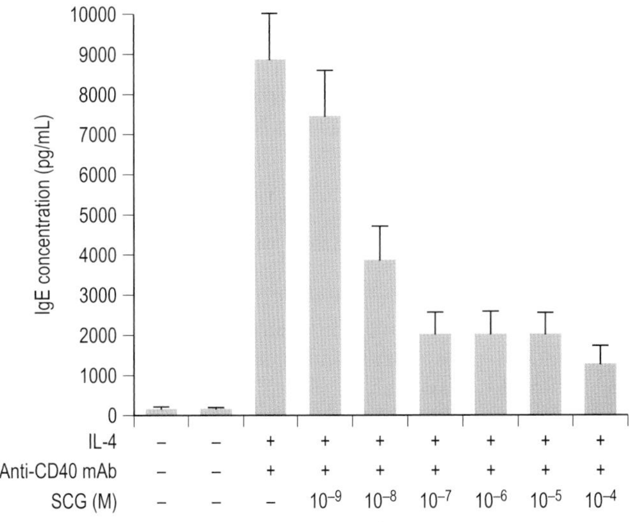

Figure 98-4 Effect of cromolyn sodium on IgE production by T cell–depleted, B cell–enriched populations of cells (10^6 cells/mL) in the presence of IL-4 (50 U/mL) and anti-CD40 monoclonal antibody (5 μg/mL). Results represent mean ± SE net synthesis IgE (pg/mL) of five experiments. *(Reproduced from Loh RK, Jabara HH, Geha RS. Disodium cromoglycate inhibits Sμ→Sε deletional switch recombination and IgE synthesis in human B cells. J Exp Med 1994;180:663-71.)*

Inhaled cromolyn sodium reduced the levels of house-dust mite (HDM)–specific IgE in asthmatic patients showing the best clinical response to the treatment.[22] In this study, adult patients were treated in a double-blind manner for 4 weeks with either 40 mg four times daily of inhaled cromolyn ($n = 19$) or placebo ($n = 17$). BAL was carried out before treatment and at the end of treatment. Cromolyn-treated subjects were divided into responders ($n = 14$) or nonresponders ($n = 5$) based on their diary card symptom scores during the 28-day period. Similarly, the placebo-treated patients were divided into spontaneous improvers ($n = 6$) and spontaneous nonimprovers ($n = 11$). The cromolyn-treated responders demonstrated a significant reduction in HDM-specific IgE ($P = .025$) between the first and second lavage. The other groups showed no change.

Experimental Pharmacology

Electrophysiologic studies on rat peritoneal mast cells have demonstrated that degranulation depends on a sustained elevation of intracellular calcium after a transient inositol triphosphate (IP_3)–induced increase in calcium caused by the release of calcium from intracellular stores. The sustained phase of increased calcium is mediated by influx through a small-conductance, highly specific calcium ion (Ca^{2+}) channel that can be activated by intracellular application of IP_3 and that requires membrane hyperpolarization to support the influx. A small-conductance chloride ion (Cl^-) channel has been observed in rat peritoneal mast cells activated by secretagogues and by intracellular application of cyclic 3′,5′-adenosine monophosphate (cAMP) and high Ca^{2+} concentration; this channel can provide the negative membrane potential or hyperpolarization necessary to maintain calcium influx and its sustained elevation, leading to degranulation. The calcium current activated by this mechanism is described as *calcium release–activated calcium* (I_{CRAC}) because it is likely to be responsible for the refilling of depleted intracellular calcium stores.

Incubation of mast cells with cromolyn sodium abolishes or inhibits Ca^{2+} channel activation that follows cross-linking of membrane-bound IgE by antigen. Further studies have shown that cromolyn inhibits uptake of radioactive calcium into purified rat mast cells after stimulation with compound 48/80 and antigen, although it is now considered unlikely that this effect is caused by a direct blocking action on Ca^{2+} channels. However, the ability of cromolyn to block an "intermediate-conductance" Cl^- channel in rat mucosal mast cells correlates with its inhibitory effect on antigen-induced mediator secretion, which may be a consequence of lowering intracellular calcium levels indirectly.

The ability of both chromones to impair a cell volume–dependent Cl^- current may be related to the findings showing drug-induced phosphorylation of a 78-kilodalton protein in rat peritoneal mast cells.[23] The 78-kD protein undergoes phosphorylation after 30 to 60 seconds and may be related to events associated with termination of mediator release. Thus, cromolyn sodium and nedocromil sodium may be imitating a natural cellular inhibitory process, which may also explain the lack of toxicity with these agents. The 78-kD protein has been identified as *moesin*,[24] a member of the band 4.1 (ERM) superfamily of proteins. The ability of moesin to interact with the cytoskeleton of cells may be the link between the inhibitory effects of cromolyn and nedocromil on cell activation and secretion, with inhibition of cell swelling–induced chloride currents.

The G protein–coupled receptor 35 (GPR35) expressed in a variety of tissues and cells, including human mast cells and GPR35 mRNA, is upregulated on challenge with anti-IgE antibodies. Using calcium flux and inositol phosphate accumulation assays, both chromones were potent GPR35 agonists, with greater potency on human versus rat or mouse GPR35 (Fig. 98-5).[25] These data suggest that GPR35 is the chromone receptor present on mast cells. GPR35 was first identified from human genomic DNA, corresponding to a polypeptide located on chromosome 2.[26] Expression of GPR35 is reported to be predominantly in the gastrointestinal tract and immune tissues,[27] suggesting potential roles in immunomodulation and allergic inflammation. The loop diuretic drugs bumetanide and furosemide are GPR35 agonists, and the receptor is expressed in human skin.[28] Both loop diuretics and nedocromil sodium inhibit histamine-induced flare and itch responses, suggesting that GPR35 may play an important role in skin cell biology.[29]

Cromolyn sodium is often used to demonstrate that a specific pathologic process is mast cell dependent. Using cromolyn to block mast cell effects has shown that mast cells have a central role in experimental intestinal permeability and oral antigen sensitization and thus an important role in food allergy.[30] Cromolyn has also been used to demonstrate that the tissue remodeling, increase in blood vessel density, and increase in submesothelial matrix thickness induced by peritoneal dialysis in rats is caused by mast cell activation.[31]

METABOLISM

Studies in animals and humans show that cromolyn and nedocromil are not metabolized and are excreted unchanged in the bile and urine. The plasma clearance rates and tissue distribution are similar in all species, with differences only in the relative proportions of biliary and urinary excretion. Because both chromones are poorly and reversibly bound to plasma protein, the incidence of drug interactions is very low.

Pharmacokinetics

The pharmacokinetics of the chromones has mainly been studied following intravenous infusion and inhalation. There have been limited studies after oral use and topical application to the skin, but no studies after use in the nose or the eye. Both cromolyn and nedocromil are disodium salts of strong acids, and the pharmacokinetic principles are similar.

CROMOLYN SODIUM

The pharmacokinetics of cromolyn sodium were established in four healthy volunteers after slow intravenous (IV) infusion and inhalation.[32] After IV infusion the drug is cleared rapidly from the plasma (mean clearance rate, 7.9 ± 0.9 mL/min^{-1}/kg^{-1}). This is caused by extremely rapid excretion, the mean half-life calculated from k_{10} being 13.5 minutes; 91% of the total urinary excretion ($43.8 \pm 4.1\%$ of dose) occurred within 90 minutes of cessation of the infusion. Inhalation pharmacokinetics was studied after administration of a single 20-mg dose administered using a dry powder inhaler (DPI, Spinhaler). Mean ± standard error (SE) peak plasma levels of 46 ± 7 ng/mL^{-1} were

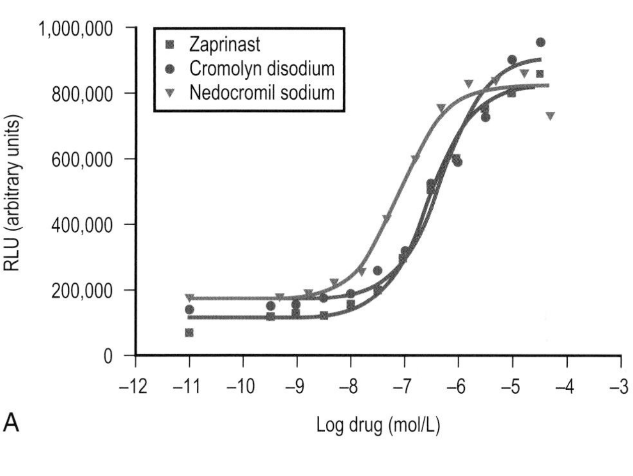

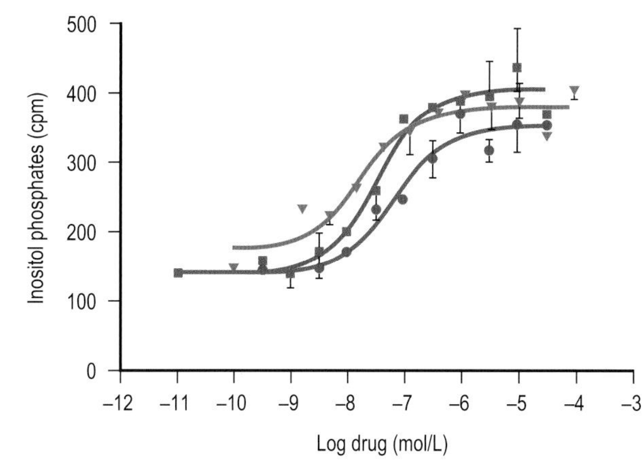

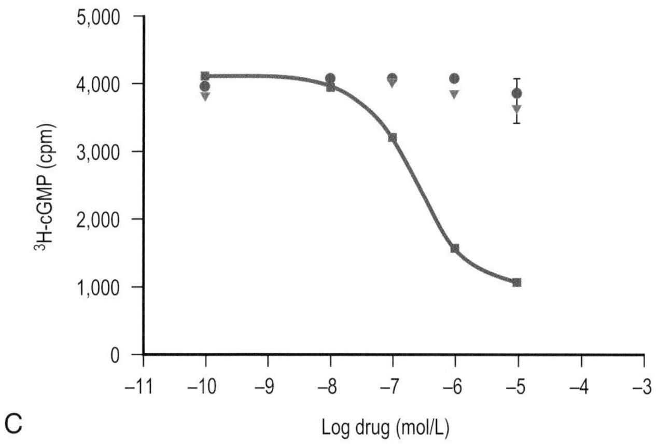

Figure 98-5 **A,** Cromolyn disodium and nedocromil sodium promote intracellular Ca^{2+} flux in human GPR35-transfected cells. Chinese hamster ovary cells were transiently transfected with human GPR35, Gq_u5 and the photoprotein aequorin. Agonists were added at the indicated concentrations, and increases in intracellular Ca^{2+} were measured by the amount of light emitted from the cells by the photochemical reaction between aequorin and coelenterazine F. *RLU,* Relative light units. **B,** Cromolyn disodium and nedocromil sodium promote inositol phosphate turnover in human GPR35-transfected cells. HEK293 cells were transiently transfected with human GPR35 and Gq05. Cells were prelabeled with ^{3}H-inositol overnight. **C,** Cromolyn disodium and nedocromil sodium do not inhibit phosphodiesterase 5 (PDE5). Compounds were added at the indicated concentrations to a purified preparation of PDE5. Zaprinast, a cGMP-specific PDE inhibitor, was an unsuccessful precursor to the PDE5 inhibitors. *cGMP,* Cyclic guanosine monophosphate; *cpm,* counts per minute.

reached after 5 minutes, with an inhalation plasma half-life of 91 minutes. Interpreting the results of the IV and inhalation pharmacokinetics, it was concluded that after inhalation, two absorption rates are observed, a fast absorption rate constant with a mean value of 0.54 min^{-1} and a slower rate constant with a mean value of 0.0097 min^{-1}. Also, after inhalation the drug is deposited in varying amounts in at least two sites with different absorption rates. Drug deposited in the alveoli and smaller bronchi may be absorbed rapidly, whereas that deposited higher in the larger airways may be absorbed more slowly. This has important implications for the efficacy of the drug on the basis of its primary mode of action being as a mast cell stabilizer and recent work outlining the distribution of mast cells in the bronchial tree in asthma.[33]

Support for these conclusions comes from a study combining distribution and efficacy. Using a radiolabeled 1-mg metered-dose inhaler (MDI) and a large-volume spacer (≈700 mL), Laube and colleagues[34] showed that the proportion of radiolabel delivered to the lung increased from 8.6% to 11.8% if the inhalation rate from the spacer was reduced from about 70 L/min to 30 L/min. This also increased the protection against allergen challenge, the amount of drug delivered to the peripheral versus the central areas of the lung, and the homogeneity of distribution within the lung field.

The pharmacokinetic profile using the Spinhaler is variable and depends on inhalation technique, with particular reference to inhalation rate. Higher inhalation rates provide greater peak plasma levels at the rapid absorption site, indicating better distribution to the peripheral airways. Forced expiratory maneuvers also result in a secondary peak.

When the drug is inhaled as an aqueous solution, administered using a powered nebulizer, the pharmacokinetic profile and the amount absorbed vary according to the tonicity of the solution and whether a β_2-agonist bronchodilator is added. In a study of healthy adult volunteers, a 1% aqueous solution containing 20 mg of drug, peak plasma levels, which occurred 5 to 10 minutes after administration, were 8.8 ± 6.2 ng/mL^{-1} using 2 mL of the aqueous solution alone, 17.2 ± 16.3 ng/mL^{-1} when 5 mL of isotonic saline was added, and 24.5 ± 11.9 ng/mL^{-1} when 5 mL isotonic saline and 0.3 mL procaterol (β_2-agonist) were added.[35] The early peak drug levels show the amount of drug reaching the smaller airways, so these results suggest that when using nebulizer solution, the solution should be isotonic and a small dose of a β_2-agonist added. This should improve efficacy.

When administered using a 1-mg/puff or 5-mg/puff MDI, the optimal amount reaching the lungs is achieved using a large (750-mL) spacer.

NEDOCROMIL SODIUM

Nedocromil sodium has also been studied in healthy volunteers and asthmatic patients. When inhaled at about 30 L/min from an MDI alone, 7.5% ± 2.9% of the nominal dose is delivered to the lung. In vitro measurements of particle sizes suggest that this can be improved by the use of a large-volume spacer. Its pharmacokinetic profile is similar to cromolyn sodium.

ORAL ADMINISTRATION

After oral administration, approximately 0.8% (range 0.6% to 1.0%) of the chromone dose is absorbed.[36]

Dosages and Routes of Administration

ASTHMA

Cromolyn Sodium

In the early development of cromolyn sodium, it was considered necessary to provide continuous protection against inhaled allergens. To provide adequate protection (50% or greater) for at least 6 hours, an inhaled unit dose of 20 mg was required.

Capsules containing 20 mg of cromolyn sodium for inhalation using the E-haler (Eclipse) or other inhalers are available in some countries. For children over 5 years and for adults, inhaled powder from capsules is preferred. The starting dose should be 1 capsule four times daily, which can be reduced to 1 capsule twice daily once improvement has been achieved. In some asthmatic patients, 1 capsule daily is adequate for maintenance treatment. However, increasing the dose frequency to four times daily is required if exacerbations occur.

Metered-dose aerosols delivering 1 or 5 mg per actuation are manufactured, with the 1-mg dose used in the United States and Japan and the 5-mg size in Canada, Australia, and Europe. No evidence indicates that the two dose sizes differ in efficacy, and both have been shown to be effective in absolute terms. The delivered dose of the two products is likely much closer than the nominal dose, and with the 5-mg MDI, the use of a large-volume (750-mL) spacer increases the delivered dose by 28.2% to 87.3%. Similarly, with the 1-mg MDI, the dose to the lung increases when used with a large-volume spacer. If MDIs are used, they should be used with a large-volume spacer. The starting-dose frequency should be four times daily, which can be reduced to twice daily when asthma has been controlled.

Cromolyn sodium is available as a 1% aqueous solution in most countries and as an isotonic solution in Japan, which has been shown to achieve higher blood levels, which are increased further by adding a short-acting β_2-agonist. For children less than 5 years, the starting-dose frequency should be four times daily in severe cases, which can be reduced to twice daily in moderate cases and after asthma has been controlled.

For efficient lung deposition to the smaller airways, particularly in children, inhaled drug particles should be less than 3.3 μm in size. In the case of cromolyn sodium, because of its hygroscopicity (moisture retention), drug particles tend to grow in the inspired air. A study investigating drug delivery using an MDI, a DPI, an existing nebulizer, and a nebulizer under development showed that the *amount* of drug of particle size less than 3.3 μm was 0.14, 1.6, 4.4, and 9.4 μg, respectively.[37] These are important considerations with respect to the potential clinical efficacy of cromolyn in patients with asthma.

Nedocromil Sodium

Only one formulation of nedocromil sodium exists, a 2-mg/actuation MDI. Most trials have been conducted using a dose of either 2 inhalations × 2 mg twice daily or 2 × 2 mg four times daily. In a trial in severe, steroid-dependent asthmatic patients, when nedocromil was added to inhaled steroids, using both dosage regimens, Wells and associates[38] showed no overall difference between the two doses in symptom control and peak flow changes, but those receiving the higher nedocromil dose of 16 mg daily required fewer emergency courses of oral corticosteroids.[39]

A long-term trial in children using a dose of 8 mg twice daily (no spacer) failed to show a clear drug effect, apart from a reduction in urgent care visits and courses of prednisone. In a trial using 4 mg three times daily through a spacer, however, there were significant differences with placebo for all the primary outcome measures. Because the use of a spacer increases the effective delivered dose by 19.8% to 52.3% depending on the spacer used, a spacer should always be used in children and possibly in adults as well. For children, a starting dose of nedocromil sodium should be 2 inhalations × 2 mg three or four times daily using a spacer, which may be reduced to twice daily once asthma has improved. For adults, starting dose should be 2 × 2 mg four times daily, with a possible reduction to 2 × 2 mg twice daily when the asthma has improved.

Chromones versus Corticosteroids

Chromones and corticosteroids are both used in the treatment of allergic diseases, but with differences in their mode of action. The chromones are effective in blocking the acute reaction to allergic challenge; corticosteroids are not. Both block the allergen-induced late asthmatic reaction. Single doses of chromones will prevent exercise-induced asthma and other acute challenges; corticosteroids will not. The number of comparative trials of these two drug classes in asthma patients implies that both can be used in similar circumstances. Such trials assume that all patients with asthma have a common underlying mechanism potentially responsive to the two types of drug. There is substantial evidence, however, that asthma involves more than one type of inflammation; some asthmatic patients are atopic, whereas others are not. Also, different types of asthma exist; some patients have recurrent episodes or reversible wheezy breathlessness, whereas others progress into a chronic state of airway obstruction with exacerbations.

Many of the early trials of inhaled cromolyn sodium in asthma were conducted in patients who were inadequately controlled with oral corticosteroids. Adding cromolyn to existing treatment provided significantly better control of the asthma and in many cases allowed the oral corticosteroid dose to be reduced without loss of benefit.[40,41] In some individuals, inhaled corticosteroids do not adequately control asthma. The addition of nedocromil sodium to such patients provides better asthma control. In the treatment of vernal keratoconjunctivitis, cromolyn and nedocromil eyedrops are used in conjunction with corticosteroid eyedrops and allow a reduced use of the latter. In a trial of cromolyn skin lotion in atopic dermatitis, the addition of cromolyn resulted in an improvement in the severity of the atopic dermatitis and a significant reduction in the use of topical corticosteroids.

In their report on the first 100 patients treated with inhaled cromolyn sodium, Altounyan and Howell[42] noted that the therapeutic effects of cromolyn and corticosteroids are not wholly interchangeable. They concluded that at least two processes might coexist in asthma, one mainly responsive to cromolyn and the other to corticosteroids. These principles hold true today and are reflected in the use of the two classes of drugs in asthma, vernal keratoconjunctivitis, and atopic dermatitis; these two drug classes are complementary and not competitive.

ALLERGIC EYE DISEASE

Cromolyn Sodium Ophthalmic Solution (Opticrom)

Adults: 1 or 2 drops in each eye four to six times daily at regular intervals.

Children (4 years and older): 1 or 2 drops in each eye four to six times daily at regular intervals.

One drop of ophthalmic solution contains approximately 1.6 mg of cromolyn sodium.

Nedocromil Sodium Ophthalmic Solution

The recommended dosage of nedocromil solution is 1 or 2 drops in each eye twice daily.

ALLERGIC RHINITIS

Intranasal Cromolyn Sodium

Adults: 1 spray (5.2 mg) in each nostril three or four times daily.

Children (2 years and older): 1 spray (5.2 mg) in each nostril three or four times daily.

When necessary, intranasal cromolyn may be used up to six times daily in both adults and children.

Oral Cromolyn Sodium (Gastrocrom)

Adults and adolescents (13 years and older): 2 ampules four times daily, taken one-half hour before meals and at bedtime.

Children (2 to 12 years): 1 ampule four times daily, taken one-half hour before meals and at bedtime.

If satisfactory control of symptoms is not achieved within 2 to 3 weeks, the dosage of oral cromolyn may be increased but should not exceed 40 mg/kg/day.

Major Side Effects

Extensive safety evaluation studies in a range of species by various routes of administration and different durations of dosing at many multiples of the clinical doses have shown cromolyn sodium[43] and nedocromil sodium[44] to possess a very low order of toxicity. Both compounds show almost no systemic pharmacologic activity, with no effect on normal host defense mechanisms, no teratogenic effects, and no influence on the incidence of neoplasia. A summary of human safety considerations showed that nedocromil has an excellent safety profile and is well-tolerated, and adverse effects are generally mild. Clinical experience with cromolyn suggests that adverse reactions are rare events.

Tables 98-1, 98-2, and 98-3 list the side effects associated with inhaled, intranasal, and oral cromolyn sodium, respectively, along with their incidence. Box 98-1 lists ophthalmic cromolyn side effects, and Boxes 98-2 and 98-3 list side effects of inhaled and ophthalmic nedocromil.

Use in Pregnancy

Cromolyn sodium has been assigned to pregnancy category B by the U.S. Food and Drug Administration (FDA). Animal studies using doses up to 338 times the normal human dose have revealed no evidence of teratogenicity. There are no controlled data in human pregnancies, but available information suggests that cromolyn use in human pregnancy is not associated with fetal toxicity or teratogenicity. Cromolyn is only recommended for use during pregnancy when benefit outweighs risk. Evaluation of 296 women treated with cromolyn throughout pregnancy revealed four newborns with congenital malformations (1.35%), which is lower than the expected rate. The malformations included club foot, harelip, nonfused septum, and patent ductus arteriosus.

TABLE 98-1 Inhaled Cromolyn Sodium: Side Effects and Incidence

Side Effect	Incidence	Comments
Transient cough	1 in 5 patients	Treatment or discontinuation of drug rarely required
Mild wheezing	1 in 25 patients	Treatment or discontinuation of drug rarely required
Laryngeal edema, swollen parotid gland, angioedema, bronchospasm, joint swelling/pain, dizziness, dysuria, urinary frequency, nausea, cough, wheezing, headache, nasal congestion, rash, urticaria, lacrimation	<1 in 10,000 patients	Attributed to cromolyn sodium, based on recurrence after readministration
Anaphylaxis, nephrosis, periarteritic vasculitis, pericarditis, peripheral neuritis, pulmonary infiltrates with eosinophilia, polymyositis, exfoliative dermatitis, hemoptysis, anemia, myalgia, hoarseness, photodermatitis, vertigo	<1 in 100,000 patients	Uncertain whether attributable to drug

TABLE 98-2 Intranasal Cromolyn Sodium: Side Effects and Incidence

Side Effect	Incidence
Sneezing	1 in 10 patients
Nasal stinging	1 in 20 patients
Nasal burning	<1 in 25 patients
Nasal irritation	<1 in 40 patients
Headaches, bad taste	1 in 50 patients
Epistaxis, postnasal drip, rash	<1 in 100 patients
Anaphylaxis	One patient in clinical trials

TABLE 98-3 Oral Cromolyn Sodium: Side effects and Incidence

Side Effect	Incidence
Headache, diarrhea	4 in 87 patients
Pruritus, nausea, myalgia	3 in 87 patients
Abdominal pain, rash, irritability	2 in 87 patients
Malaise	One report

BOX 98-1 OPHTHALMIC CROMOLYN SODIUM: SIDE EFFECTS

Transient ocular stinging or burning on instillation
Conjunctival injection; watery eyes; itchy eyes; dryness around the eye; puffy eyes; eye irritation; styes
Immediate hypersensitivity reported rarely, including dyspnea, edema, and rash

BOX 98-2 INHALED NEDOCROMIL: SIDE EFFECTS

Unpleasant taste, headache
Cough, fatigue
Nausea, vomiting, dyspepsia
Diarrhea, abdominal pain
Conjunctivitis
Pharyngitis, rhinitis, upper respiratory infection

BOX 98-3 OPHTHALMIC NEDOCROMIL: SIDE EFFECTS

Unpleasant taste, headache
Ocular burning, irritation, stinging
Nasal congestion, rhinitis
Conjunctivitis, eye redness, photophobia
Asthma

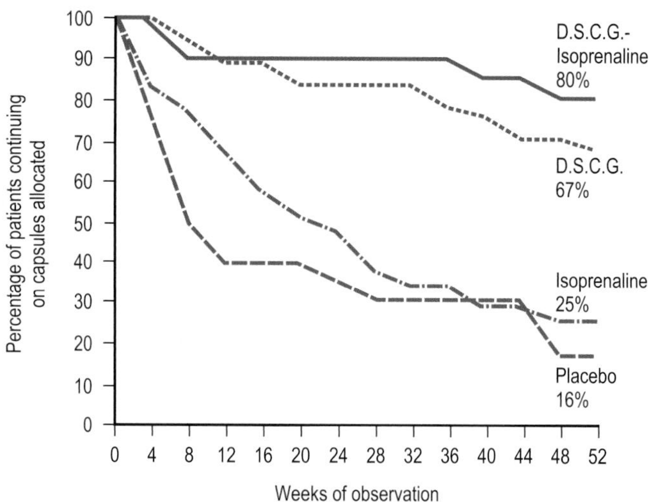

Figure 98-6 Percentage of patients remaining in trial, whose progress was satisfactory, and who completed at least 36 weeks in the trial. Comparison of cromolyn sodium (disodium cromoglycate, D.S.C.G.) + isoproterenol (Isoprenaline), D.S.C.G. alone, isoproterenol alone, and placebo. *(Reproduced from Brompton Hospital–Medical Research Council (MRC) collaborative trial. Long-term study of disodium cromoglycate in treatment of severe extrinsic or intrinsic bronchial asthma in adults. BMJ 1972;4[5837]:383-8.)*

Nedocromil sodium has also been assigned to pregnancy category B by the FDA. Animal studies using doses of 100 mg/kg/day subcutaneously have not revealed evidence of adverse fetal outcome. There are no controlled data in human pregnancy. Nedocromil is only recommended for use during pregnancy when benefit outweighs risk.

Indications

ASTHMA

Both chromones are indicated for the management of patients with asthma.

Adults

Cromolyn Sodium. The first controlled trial of cromolyn sodium was conducted in adult patients with severe, corticosteroid-dependent, allergic asthma. The trial compared cromolyn plus isoproterenol with isoproterenol alone. All variables favored the combination.[45] The isoproterenol combination possibly provides better distribution of cromolyn to the alveoli and smaller airways, where the mast cells involved in severe asthma predominate. The definitive trials that established efficacy in adult asthmatic patients were organized by the United Kingdom Medical Research Council (UK MRC) Tuberculosis and Chest Diseases Unit,[46] the New Zealand Medical Research Council (NZ MRC) Clinical Trials Committee,[47] and the American Academy of Allergy (AAA) Drug Committee.[48]

The UK MRC trial (114 patients) compared cromolyn sodium plus isoproterenol, cromolyn alone, isoproterenol alone, and placebo during a 12-month treatment period using a parallel group design, in symptomatic patients not receiving corticosteroids.[46] The starting dose was 20 mg four times daily delivered by inhalation from a capsule. After 8 weeks, half the patients in each treatment group reduced the dose at weekly intervals, initially to 1 capsule three times daily, then twice daily, and finally to 1 capsule daily. This dose was then maintained for 1 year, but could be increased if symptoms recurred. The end point was treatment failure, when patients were withdrawn from the trial. At the end of 12 months, 73% of patients treated with cromolyn + isoproterenol remained under good control, compared with 62% of those taking cromolyn alone, 31% of those treated with isoproterenol alone and 19% of the placebo group (Fig. 98-6). No difference was evident between the patients receiving the full or the reducing dosage.

The NZ MRC trial involved a comparison of cromolyn sodium alone with placebo, in 117 patients with moderately severe asthma.[47] Half the patients were taking regular oral corticosteroids. Pulmonary function tests, forced expiratory volume in the first second (FEV_1; $P < 0.001$), and vital capacity (VC; $P < 0.01$) were significantly improved after cromolyn compared to placebo. Significant differences in symptom improvement also favored cromolyn.

The AAA trial in 252 individuals compared 20 mg of cromolyn sodium alone inhaled from a capsule four times daily with placebo, using a crossover design and treatment period of 8 weeks.[48] A carryover effect was observed in asthmatic patients receiving cromolyn as the first treatment. A significant treatment effect was observed with symptom scores, use of concomitant treatments, physician evaluation, and patient preference.

Pressurized MDI formulations of cromolyn sodium delivering 1 mg and 5 mg per actuation were introduced in the 1980s. Efficacy of the 1-mg MDI was established by transferring patients controlled on 20-mg Spincaps to the 1-mg MDI without loss of clinical control.[49] Trials using a hydrofluoroalkane-driven formulation for the 1-mg MDI of cromolyn sodium versus the original chlorofluorocarbon-driven MDI have confirmed the efficacy of this dosage form. In a trial comparing 8 mg/day of cromolyn sodium, 16 mg/day of nedocromil sodium, and placebo, both chromones were shown to be significantly better than placebo, but with no difference between the two active treatments.[50]

A multicenter comparative trial of nebulized isotonic cromolyn sodium and normal saline in 251 adults with severe persistent asthma showed a significant improvement in the primary end point, the peak expiratory flow (PEF) measured each morning, in the atopic individuals but not in the nonatopic individuals.[51]

Nedocromil Sodium. Nedocromil has a similar clinical profile to cromolyn sodium. Trials in adults have used dosage regimens of 2 inhalations × 2 mg twice daily or 2 × 2 mg four times daily. An overview analysis of all double-blind, placebo-controlled clinical trials, both published and unpublished, involving 4723 patients at 127 trial centers showed that nedocromil sodium is significantly better than placebo in regard to all variables, including daytime and nighttime asthma symptoms, cough, daily mean PEF, FEV_1, rescue bronchodilator use, and patient satisfaction. Optimal effects were seen in patients currently using bronchodilators alone as treatment. Corticosteroid-sparing effect was demonstrated by a 50% reduction in inhaled corticosteroid usage, when nedocromil was added without loss of effect. Added benefit was demonstrated in patients inadequately controlled using inhaled corticosteroid treatment, when the drug was added.[52]

Children

Cromolyn Sodium. Cromolyn is an effective treatment in children with asthma, particularly in those 5 years and older. In a placebo-controlled trial in the United States, using inhaled 20-mg capsules of 276 asthmatic patients age 5 to 18 years, all the outcome measures were significantly in favor of cromolyn.[53] It is effective when delivered as a nebulized solution in children, with moderate to severe intractable asthma, treated with either the combination of cromolyn plus salbutamol, or cromolyn alone or salbutamol alone, the combination was significantly better than either component administered alone.[54] Trials in children younger than 5 years, in whom the diagnosis of asthma is less secure and the dose delivered variable, have used either nebulizer solution or metered-dose aerosols with and without spacers. Under these conditions, demonstration of clear efficacy is less certain.

A retrospective study showed that if treatment with cromolyn sodium in children is started within 3 years of the onset of asthma (early intervention) compared with children in whom it is started after 6 years (late intervention), the outcomes, as determined by overall severity of asthma, emergency department visits, and hospitalizations, are significantly better in the early intervention group.[55]

Nedocromil Sodium. Nedocromil is effective in childhood asthma. In a placebo-controlled trial of 209 asthmatic children age 6 to 17 years, total symptom scores were reduced by 50% in the nedocromil group, which was significantly better than the placebo group.[56] A similar improvement in symptoms was shown in a trial of 79 children with a recent acute asthma attack, often triggered by a viral infection and requiring acute corticosteroid treatment. Differences between nedocromil sodium and placebo in the changes from baseline were significantly in favor of nedocromil for all variables (daytime and nighttime asthma symptoms, morning and evening PEF, use of rescue bronchodilators).

Cromolyn/Nedocromil Comparison Trials

Cromolyn sodium and nedocromil sodium are the only chromones currently available, but few studies have compared the two drugs in asthma. In two trials using a three-way comparison between the two drugs and placebo, nedocromil was administered at a dose of 4 mg four times daily and cromolyn sodium at 2 mg four times daily.[57,58] Both drugs were significantly better than placebo in both trials, and the few differences between the two drugs are not considered clinically relevant. As often occurs with more than one drug in a particular class, individuals may respond to one drug in the class, but not to another.

ALLERGIC EYE DISEASES

Cromolyn sodium ophthalmic solution (Opticrom) is indicated in the treatment of vernal keratoconjunctivitis, vernal conjunctivitis, and vernal keratitis.

Nedocromil ophthalmic solution is indicated for the treatment of itching associated with allergic conjunctivitis.

An overview of the ophthalmic use of cromolyn sodium concluded that it is effective in relieving the subjective symptoms and clinical signs of allergic rhinitis, acute allergic conjunctivitis, chronic allergic conjunctivitis, vernal keratoconjunctivitis, and giant papillary conjunctivitis.[59] Evidence indicates that nedocromil sodium is more efficacious than cromolyn sodium in vernal conjunctivitis.

The drugs can also be useful in the relief of acute eye symptoms. Cromolyn sodium eyedrops, when administered to one eye after symptoms of redness, itching, swelling, and tearing had been induced by the instillation of either grass or birch pollen in sensitive individuals, resulted in a significant reduction in these symptoms compared with placebo drops in the other eye at 2, 10, and 30 minutes after allergen challenge.[60]

The mechanisms of these effects have been examined in a group comparative trial of nedocromil sodium, levocabastine, and placebo eyedrops administered for 2 weeks before challenge with ryegrass extract.[61] Compared with the placebo-treated group, nedocromil reduced total symptom scores, particularly of itching, hyperemia, and lacrimation. In addition, nedocromil reduced tear concentrations of histamine and PGD_2 and in bulbar biopsies reduced the number of 3H4-positive mast cells.

ALLERGIC RHINITIS

Cromolyn sodium nasal spray is used to prevent and relieve nasal symptoms of hay fever and other nasal allergies (runny/itchy nose, sneezing, allergic stuffy nose). There is a full review of the use of cromolyn sodium in the management of chronic rhinitis.[62]

Food Allergy (Not an FDA-Approved Indication)

Oral cromolyn sodium is useful in the management of food allergy. Doses of 100 to 800 mg taken as a single dose 15 to 30 minutes before the food to which the individual is sensitive will either prevent or reduce the severity of the symptoms produced by ingesting the food. This treatment is *not* recommended for prevention of anaphylaxis to food. In a series of food challenges in individuals who developed either a lower respiratory tract reaction or a skin reaction after eating egg, immune complexes containing IgE and IgG could be detected in the serum of subjects who became symptomatic after challenge. Serum levels of ovalbumin rose to peak levels at 3 hours after challenge, falling to prechallenge levels after 24 hours. Both the development of the immune complexes and the rise in absorbed ovalbumin were prevented or reduced by pretreatment with 2 doses of 500 mg of oral cromolyn taken 2 hours and ½ hour before challenge. Oral cromolyn sodium prevents the increased absorption of undigested protein in sensitized patients and in the production of immune complexes.[63]

Systemic Mastocytosis

Systemic mastocytosis is a group of disorders characterized by a pathologic increase in mast cells. Oral cromolyn sodium can be useful in the management, particularly in patients with gastrointestinal (GI) symptoms. A dose of 400 mg/day in adults had a significant effect on both GI and non-GI symptoms compared with placebo.[64] Doses of 400 mg or 800 mg daily showed a significant effect on GI symptoms and a nonsignificant effect on non-GI symptoms.[65] In an infant with diffuse cutaneous mastocytosis, the combination of oral cromolyn with the dose maintained at 25 mg/kg/day with topical 4% cutaneous emulsion applied twice daily has been shown to be beneficial, with reduction in serum tryptase levels.[66] In a patient with severe bone pain and fatigue caused by systemic mastocytosis, adequate symptom control required both inhaled and oral cromolyn administration.

Allergic Skin Disease (Not an FDA-Approved Indication)

Cromolyn sodium has been used in a number of different topical skin preparations for the treatment of atopic dermatitis. A 4% cutaneous emulsion reduced the severity of itch and flare induced by intradermal histamine in atopic subjects and was beneficial in children with atopic skin dermatitis.[67]

Summary

The major recent change is that the chromones (cromolyn sodium and nedocromil sodium) are no longer recommended as a treatment for asthma in the 2010 Global Initiative for Asthma Care (GINA). The withdrawal of recommendation in children under 5 years of age is based on one clinical trial and a Cochrane review showing insufficient evidence of clinical efficacy over placebo, both of which have been criticized. In adults and older children, although mentioned, the chromones are not recommended in the key guidelines.

The primary mode of action of the chromones is as mast cell stabilizers, so it is important to deliver an adequate dose of the compound to the mast cells causing the disease pathology. In patients with asthma, this requires good distribution of the drug throughout the bronchial tree and particularly to the peripheral airways. This could be achieved previously with the 20-mg capsules if the powder inhaler was used correctly and the capsules contained a mixture of cromolyn sodium and isoproterenol. To achieve this with currently available products, metered-dose aerosols are used with large-volume spacers and nebulizer solution made isotonic by mixing with normal saline and adding a small dose of a short-acting bronchodilator. Both cromolyn and nedocromil are still recommended for ophthalmic use, with cromolyn also delivered intranasally and orally.

Over the past 10 years, more than 500 articles on cromolyn sodium have been recorded by the U.S. National Library of Medicine in the MedLine database. Many are scientific experiments in which the ability of the compound to stabilize mast cells is used to demonstrate that mast cells are involved in a pathologic process under investigation. These conditions include human thyroid cancer, insulin-induced lipoatrophy, acute pancreatitis, apoptosis in sepsis, hypoxic pulmonary hypertension, pruritus in renal failure, diet-induced obesity, cardiac arrhythmia, acute inflammatory pain, itching, intestinal permeability, ischemic cerebral injury, dystrophin-deficient muscle fibers, and sickle cell anemia.

REFERENCES

Introduction

1. Anrep GV, Barsoum GS, Kenawy MR, et al. Therapeutic uses of khellin. Lancet 1947;249(6542):557-8.
2. Edwards AM, Howell JB. The chromones: history, chemistry and clinical development. A tribute to the work of Dr. R. E. C. Altounyan. Clin Exp Allergy 2000;30:756-74.
3. Pepys J, Hargreave FE, Chan M, et al. Inhibitory effects of disodium cromoglycate on allergen-inhalation tests. Lancet 1968;2:134-7.
4. Brannan JD, Gukliksson M, Anderson SD, et al. Inhibition of mast cell PGD_2 release protects against mannitol-induced airway narrowing. Eur Respir J 2006;27:944-50.

Mechanism of Action

5. Sheard P, Blair AM. Disodium cromoglycate: activity in three in vitro models of the immediate hypersensitivity reaction in lung. Int Arch Allergy Appl Immunol 1970;38:217-24.
6. Parish WE. Release of histamine and slow-reacting substance with mast cell changes after challenge of human lung sensitized passively with reagin in vitro. Nature 1967;215:738-9.
7. Okayama Y, Benyon RC, Rees PH, et al. Inhibition profiles of sodium cromoglycate and nedocromil sodium on mediator release from mast cells of human skin, lung, tonsil, adenoid and intestine. Clin Exp Allergy 1992;22:401-9.
8. Pearce FL, Ali H, Barrett KE, et al. Functional characteristics of mucosal and connective tissue mast cells of man, the rat, and other animals. Int Arch Allergy Appl Immunol 1985;77:274-6
9. Leung KB, Flint KC, Brostoff J, et al. Effects of sodium cromoglycate and nedocromil sodium on histamine secretion from human lung mast cells. Thorax 1988;43:756-61.
10. Bissonnette EY, Enciso JA, Befus AD. Inhibition of tumour necrosis factor-alpha (TNF-α) release from mast cells by the anti-inflammatory drugs, sodium cromoglycate and nedocromil sodium. Clin Exp Immunol 1995:102:78-84.
11. Okuda M, Ohnishi M, Ohtsuka H. The effects of cromolyn sodium on nasal mast cells. Ann Allergy 1988;55:721-3.
12. Esposito P, Gheorghe D, Kandere K, et al. Acute stress increases permeability of the blood-brain barrier through activation of mast cells. Brain Res 2001;888;117-27.
13. Walsh LJ. Ultraviolet B irradiation of skin induces mast cell degranulation and release of tumour necrosis factor-alpha. Immunol Cell Biol 1995;73:226-33.
14. Matsuo N, Shimoda T, Matsuse H, et al. Effects of sodium cromoglycate on cytokine production following antigen stimulation of a passively sensitized human lung model. Ann Allergy Asthma Immunol 2000;84:72-8.
15. Larsson K, Larsson BM, Sandstrom T, et al. Sodium cromoglycate attenuates pulmonary inflammation without influencing bronchial responsiveness in healthy subjects exposed to organic dust. Clin Exp Allergy 2001;31:1356-68.
16. Nemmar A, Hoet PH, Vermylen J, et al. Pharmacological stabilization of mast cells abrogates late thrombotic events induced by diesel exhaust particles in hamsters. 1. Circulation 2004;110:1670-7.
17. Rusznak C, Devalia JL, Sapsford RJ, et al. Ozone-induced mediator release from human

bronchial epithelial cells in vitro and the influence of nedocromil sodium. Eur Respir J 1996;9: 2298-305.
18. Wells E, Jackson CG, Harper ST, et al. Characterization of primate bronchoalveolar mast cells. II. Inhibition of histamine, LTC_4, and PGD_2 release from primate bronchoalveolar mast cells and a comparison with rat peritoneal mast cells. J Immunol 1986;137:3941-5.
19. Dixon M, Jackson DM, Richards IM. The action of sodium cromoglycate on "C" fibre endings in the dog lung. Br J Pharmacol 1980; 70:11-3.
20. Viera dos Santos R, Mageri M, Martus P, et al. Topical sodium cromoglicate relieves allergen- and histamine-induced dermal pruritus. Br J Dermatol 2010;162:674-6.
21. Loh RK, Jabara HH, Geha RS. Disodium cromoglycate inhibits $S\mu \rightarrow S\varepsilon$ deletional switch recombination and IgE synthesis in human B cells. J Exp Med 1994;180:663-71.
22. Diaz P, Galleguillos FR, Gonzalez MC, et al. Bronchoalveolar lavage in asthma: the effect of disodium cromoglycate (cromolyn) on leukocyte counts, immunoglobulins, and complement. J Allergy Clin Immunol 1984;74:41-8.

Experimental Pharmacology

23. Theoharides TC, Sieghart W, Greengard P, et al. Antiallergic drug cromolyn may inhibit histamine secretion by regulating phosphorylation of a mast cell protein. Science 1980;207:80-2.
24. Wang L, Corriea I, Pang X, et al. Rat moesin: cloning, phosphorylation and localisation in mast cells. FASEB J 1995;9:2P-803.
25. Yang Y, Lu JY-L, Wu X, et al. G-protein-coupled receptor 35 is a target of the asthma drugs cromolyn disodium and nedocromil sodium. Pharmacol 2010;86:1-5.
26. O'Dowd BF, Nguyen T, Marchese A, et al. Discovery of three novel G-protein-coupled receptor genes. Genomics 1998;47:310-3.
27. Wang J, Simonavicius N, Wu X, et al. Kynurenic acid as a ligand for orphan G protein–coupled receptor GPR35. J Biol Chem 2006;281: 22021-8.
28. Yang Y, Fu A, Wu X, et al. GPR35 is a target of the loop diuretic drugs bumetanide and furosemide. Pharmacology 2012;89:13-7.
29. Willis EF, Clough GF, Church MK. Investigation into the mechanisms by which nedocromil sodium, furosemide and bumetanide inhibit the histamine-induced itch and flare response in human skin in vivo. Clin Exp Allergy 2004;34: 450-5.
30. Forbes EE, Groschwitz K, Abonia JP, et al. IL-9-and mast cell–mediated intestinal permeability predisposes to oral antigen hypersensitivity. J Exp Med 2008;205:897-913.
31. Zareie M, Fabbrini P, Hekking LHP, et al. Novel role for mast cells in omental tissue remodeling and cell recruitment in experimental peritoneal dialysis. J Am Soc Nephrol 2006; 17:3447-57.

Pharmacokinetics

32. Neale MG, Brown K, Hodder RW, et al. The pharmacokinetics of sodium cromoglycate in man after intravenous and inhalation administration. Br J Clin Pharmacol 1986;22:373-82.
33. Balzar S, Fajt ML, Comhair SAA, et al. Mast cell phenotype, location, and activation in severe asthma. Am J Respir Crit Care Med 2011;183: 299-309.
34. Laube BL, Edwards AM, Dalby RN, et al. The efficacy of slow versus faster inhalation of cromolyn sodium in protecting against allergen challenge in patients with asthma. J Allergy Clin Immunol 1998;101:475-83.
35. Kato Y, Muraki K, Fujitaka M, et al. Plasma concentrations of disodium cromoglycate after various inhalation methods in healthy subjects. Br J Clin Pharmacol 1999;48:154-7.
36. Walker SR, Evans ME, Richards AJ, et al. The fate of [^{14}C]disodium cromoglycate in man. J Pharm Pharmacol 1972;24:525-31.

Dosages and Routes of Administration

37. Keller M, Hug M, Schuschnig U, et al. Importance of the inhaler system and relative humidity on the fine particle dose (FPD) of disodium cromoglicate (DSCG). Respir Drug Deliv Eur 2007;1:307-10.
38. Wells A, Drennan C, Holst P, et al. Comparison of nedocromil sodium at two dosage frequencies with placebo in the management of chronic asthma. Respir Med 1992;86:311-16.
39. Edwards AM, Patel B. Inhaled nedocromil sodium in the management of asthma. Respir Med 1993;87:238-9.
40. Campbell AH, Tandon MK. A trial of disodium cromoglycate in older asthmatics. Med J Aust 1969;535-7.
41. Engström I, Krapelien S. The corticosteroid sparing effect of disodium cromoglicate in children and adolescents with bronchial asthma. Acta Allergol 1971;26:90-100.
42. Altounyan RE, Howell JB. Treatment of asthma with disodium cromoglycate (FPL 670, "Intal"). Respiration 1969;26(Suppl):131-40.

Major Side Effects

43. Cox JS, Beach JE, Blair AM, et al. Disodium cromoglycate (Intal). Adv Drug Res 1970;5:115-96.
44. Clark B. General pharmacology, pharmacokinetics, and toxicology of nedocromil sodium. J Allergy Clin Immunol 1993;92:200-2.

Indications

45. Howell JBL, Altounyan REC. A double-blind trial of disodium cromoglycate in the treatment of allergic bronchial asthma. Lancet 1967;290 (7515):539-42.
46. Brompton Hospital–Medical Research Council (MRC) collaborative trial. Long-term study of disodium cromoglycate in treatment of severe extrinsic or intrinsic bronchial asthma in adults. BMJ 1972;4(5837):383-8.
47. Gebbie T, Harris EA, O'Donnell TV, et al. Multicentre, short-term therapeutic trial of disodium cromoglycate, with and without prednisone, in adults with asthma. BMJ 1972;4:576-80.
48. Bernstein IL, Siegel SC, Brandon ML, et al. A controlled study of cromolyn sodium sponsored by the Drug Committee of the American Academy of Allergy. J Allergy Clin Immunol 1972;50:235-45.
49. Blumenthal MN, Selcow J, Spector S, et al. A multicenter evaluation of the clinical benefits of cromolyn sodium aerosol by metered-dose inhaler in the treatment of asthma. J Allergy Clin Immunol 1988;81:681-7.
50. Schwartz HJ, Blumenthal M, Brady R, et al. A comparative study of the clinical efficacy of nedocromil sodium and placebo: how does cromolyn sodium compare as an active control treatment? Chest 1996;109:945-52.
51. Sano Y, Adachi M, Kiuchi T, et al. Effects of nebulized sodium cromoglycate on adult patients with severe refractory asthma. Respir Med 2006;100:420-33.
52. Edwards AM, Stevens MT. The clinical efficacy of inhaled nedocromil sodium (Tilade) in the treatment of asthma. Eur Respir J 1993;6: 35-41.
53. Berman BA, Fenton MM, Girsch LS, et al. Cromolyn sodium in the treatment of children with severe, perennial asthma. Pediatrics 1975;55: 621-9.
54. Furusho K, Nishikawa K, Sasaki S, et al. The combination of nebulized sodium cromoglycate and salbutamol in the treatment of moderate-to-severe asthma in children. Pediatr Allergy Immunol 2002;13:209-16.
55. Yoshihara S, Kanno N, Yamada Y, et al. Effects of early intervention with inhaled sodium cromoglycate in childhood asthma. Lung 2006;184: 63-72.
56. Armenio L, Baldini G, Bardare M, et al. Double-blind, placebo-controlled study of nedocromil sodium in asthma. Arch Dis Child 1993;68: 193-7.
57. Nathan RA, Minkwitz MC, Bonuccelli CM. Two first-line therapies in the treatment of mild asthma: use of peak flow variability as a predictor of effectiveness. Ann Allergy Asthma Immunol 1999;82:497-503.
58. Lal S, Dorrow PD, Venho KK, et al. Nedocromil sodium is more effective than cromolyn sodium for the treatment of chronic reversible obstructive airway disease. Chest 1993;104:438-47
59. Sorkin EM, Ward A. Ocular sodium cromoglycate: an overview of its therapeutic efficacy in allergic eye disease. Drugs 1986;31:131-48.
60. Montan P, Zetterstrom O, Eliasson E, et al. Topical sodium cromoglycate (Opticrom) relieves ongoing symptoms of allergic conjunctivitis within 2 minutes. Allergy 1994;49:637-40.
61. Ahluwalia P, Anderson DF, Wilson SJ, et al. Nedocromil sodium and levocabastine reduce the symptoms of conjunctival allergen challenge by different mechanisms. J Allergy Clin Immunol 2001;108:449-54.
62. Simons FE, Simons KJ. Optimum pharmacological management of chronic rhinitis. Drugs 1989;38:313-31.
63. Carini C, Brostoff J, Wraith DG. IgE complexes in food allergy. Ann Allergy 1987;59:110-17.
64. Soter NA, Austen KF, Wasserman SI. Oral disodium cromoglycate in the treatment of systemic mastocytosis. N Engl J Med 1979;301: 465-69.
65. Horan RF, Sheffer AL, Austen KF. Cromolyn sodium in the management of systemic mastocytosis. J Allergy Clin Immunol 1990;85:852-5.
66. Edwards AM, Čapková Š. Oral and topical sodium cromoglicate in the treatment of diffuse cutaneous mastocytosis in an infant. BMJ Case Rep 2011. doi:10.1136/bcr.02.2011.3910.
67. Stainer R, Matthews S, Arshad SH, et al. Efficacy and acceptability of a new topical skin lotion of sodium cromoglicate (Altoderm) in atopic dermatitis in children aged 2-12 years: a double-blind, randomized, placebo-controlled trial. Br J Dermatol 2005;152:334-41.

99

Glucocorticosteroids

IAN M. ADCOCK | KIAN FAN CHUNG

CONTENTS

SUMMARY OF IMPORTANT CONCEPTS

» Glucocorticosteroids are the most effective antiinflammatory drugs and act through a nuclear receptor–dependent process to attenuate the allergic and nonallergic cascade in asthma.
» Glucocorticosteroids target the expression of most inflammatory mediators, including cytokines, chemokines, growth factors, and their receptors, as well as enzymes involved in arachidonic acid and nitric oxide metabolism.
» Topical glucocorticosteroids act locally at the site of application with reduced systemic side effects, high receptor-binding affinity, and rapid metabolism and elimination from the systemic circulation.
» The glucocorticosteroid receptor exists in many isoforms expressed differentially in disease and may exert distinct functional effects.
» Whether switching off inflammatory gene expression or enhancing antiinflammatory gene expression, the glucocorticosteroid receptor acts through a chromatin-dependent process involving changes in histone acetylation.
» Glucocorticosteroids enhance many aspects of the immune response, including epithelial barrier function and production of antimicrobial peptides, attenuating their immunosuppressive actions.

Introduction

Glucocorticosteroids (GCs) are endogenous hormones produced from the adrenal cortex. Cortisol secretion increases in response to physical stress (illness, trauma, surgery, temperature extremes) and psychological stress.[1] More than a simple marker of stress levels, however, cortisol is important for the correct functioning of most cells and tissues. GCs are potent suppressors of the immune and inflammatory systems that are activated in the normal response to exogenous stimuli/challenges and therefore are highly effective therapeutic agents.[2]

Since the groundbreaking work of Hench, Kendall, and Reichstein[3] and the discovery of cortisol, its use in rheumatoid arthritis and inflammatory skin disease, and the advent of safe inhaled steroids, corticosteroids have become the mainstay of antiinflammatory therapy in asthma. Synthetic GCs are the most effective antiinflammatory drugs currently used.[4] This chapter discusses the general pharmacologic aspects of GCs, their mechanism of antiinflammatory action, and possible mechanisms for their limited effectiveness in severe, treatment-refractory asthma.

Circulating cortisol levels display a diurnal variation, with the highest levels seen early in the morning (about 8 AM) and lowest levels just after midnight.[1] Diurnal variation in inflammatory and immune function is also evident in the physiology and pathology of asthma. This diurnal variation in cortisol release is under control of local and central "clocks." The nuclear receptor REV-ERBα is critical is regulating the circadian clock and the cellular response to inflammation. In human macrophages, administration of a synthetic REV-ERB ligand or genetic knockdown of REV-ERBα expression modulates the expression and release of interleukin-6 (IL-6). Thus the timing and duration of drug dosing may have profound consequences for the efficacy and safety of GCs because of the molecular clock. For example, mimicking this pulsatile cortisol release or giving a GC at the correct time is done to reduce the detrimental side effects of exogenous GCs while enhancing their antiinflammatory properties.[5,6]

Chemical Structure

Glucocorticosteroids are 21-carbon steroid hormones composed of four rings[7] (Fig. 99-1). The basic structure of the A-ring is a 1α,2β-half-chair, whatever the substitutions, whereas rings B and C are semirigid chairs with minimal structural influence by substituent groups. In contrast, the shape of the D-ring is highly dependent on both the nature and the environment of the substituent groups. Modern GCs such as prednisolone, prednisone, methylprednisolone, and dexamethasone are based on the cortisol (hydrocortisone) structure with modification to enhance the antiinflammatory effects. Such modifications include insertion of a C=C double bond at C1,C2 and the introduction of 6α-fluoro, 6α-methyl, 9α-fluoro, or further substitutions with α-hydroxyl, α-methyl, or β-methyl at the 16 position, as in dexamethasone.[7] The insertion of the C=C double bond has the additional benefit of reducing binding to the mineralocorticoid receptor (nuclear receptor subfamily 3, group C, member 2; NR3C2), as does the addition of a 16-methyl group to the D-ring, as evidenced by dexamethasone. Lipophilic substituents such as 16α- and 17α-acetals, 17α-esters, and

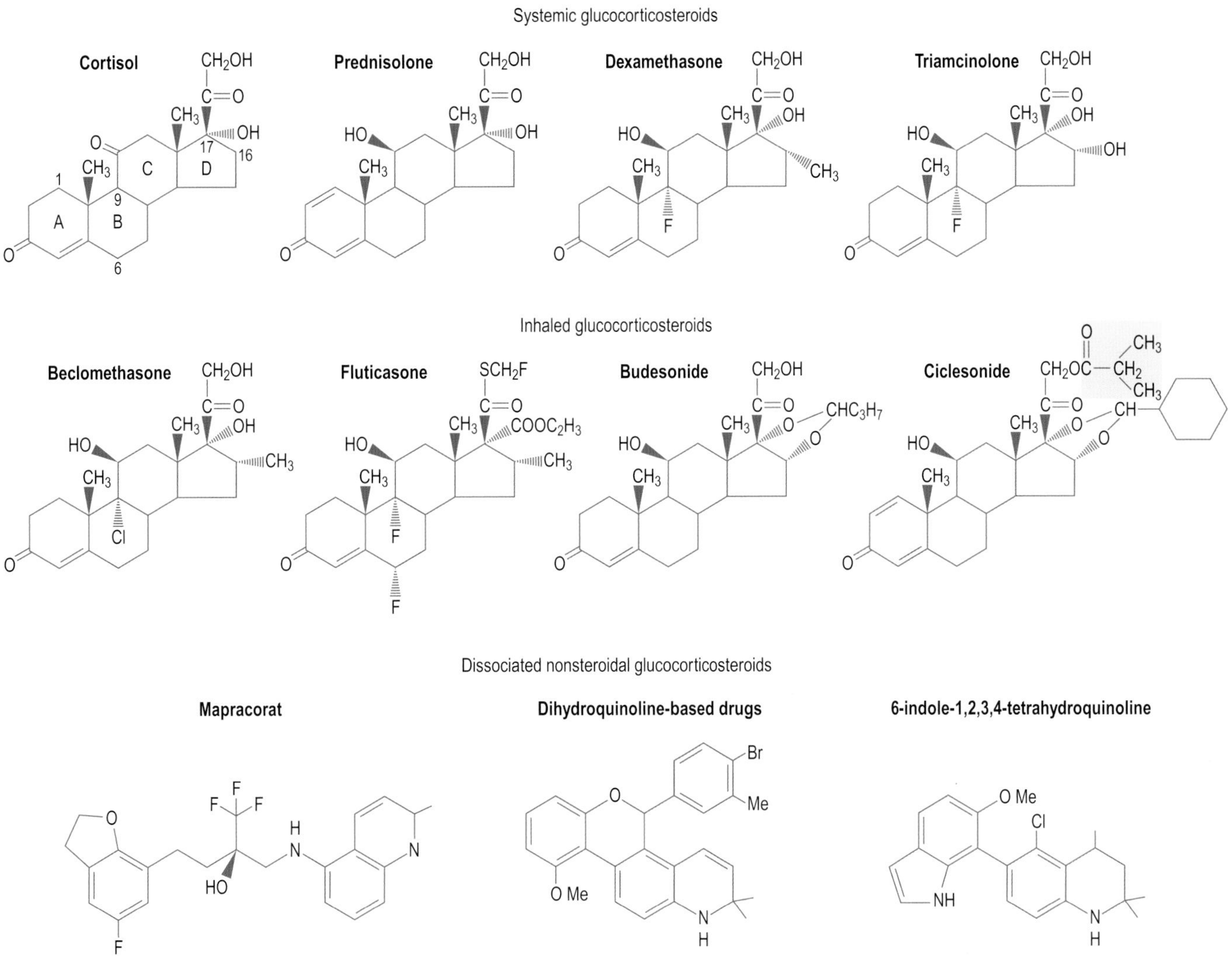

Figure 99-1 Structural modifications of cortisol that produce the clinically used systemic glucocorticosteroids (GCs) prednisolone, methylprednisolone, dexamethasone and triamcinolone and the inhaled GCs beclomethasone, flunisolide, mometasone, fluticasone propionate, fluticasone furoate, fluticasone, budesonide, and ciclesonide (the cleaved ester is shaded). The structures of some novel dissociated nonsteroidal GCs are also shown.

21α-esters attached to the D-ring enhance glucocorticosteroid receptor (nuclear receptor subfamily 3, group C, member 1; NR3C1; GR) binding affinity. Cortisol and other agents prolong local topical deposition and enhance hepatic metabolism in this receptor, as exemplified by the structures of budesonide and fluticasone, two of the most common topical GCs[8] (Fig. 99-1). The 11-ketone group on some GCs (e.g., cortisone, prednisone) must be converted to an 11-hydroxyl group to enable GC activity, whereas cleavage of 16α or 17α groups after absorption can dramatically reduce systemic effects.[8]

The glucocorticosteroid receptor (GR) ligand-binding domain has been crystallized in the presence of a number of ligands and indicates that the ligand-binding cleft has a pocket that lies beneath the C17 residue of the steroid backbone.[9] GR binding characteristics such as affinity, duration, and side effect profile are believed to be regulated by the degree of occupancy of this pocket on the floor of the binding cleft. Computational drug discovery has used this knowledge to produce steroidal and nonsteroidal GR agonists called selective glucocorticosteroid receptor agonists (SEGRA). SEGRAs fill the GR ligand cleft spatially and have many classic GR activities, but can avoid the side effects associated with the steroid backbone, such as association with other nuclear hormone receptors[10] (Fig. 99-1). However, the exact structural and lipophilic requirements that will optimize GC pharmacokinetics, tissue retention, and longevity of action remain to be established, and improved drugs are still likely to be synthesized. The use of a nonsteroidal backbone has additional benefits in that it has proved difficult to remove the cross–nuclear receptor binding of ligands with a traditional steroidal backbone.[11]

Pharmacokinetics

Synthetic GCs are easily absorbed after oral, subcutaneous, intravenous, or topical administration largely because their lipophilic nature allows prolonged retention in the airways[12] (Fig. 99-2). The pharmacokinetics for most synthetic GR ligands has been well described. Generally, plasma concentrations of GCs vary greatly (up to tenfold) after oral administration of the same dose to normal volunteers and patients;[13] the reasons

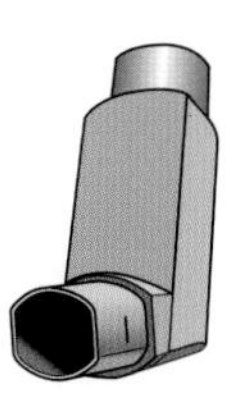
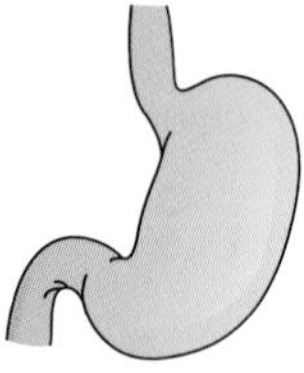
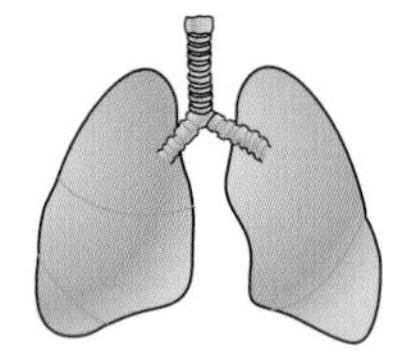
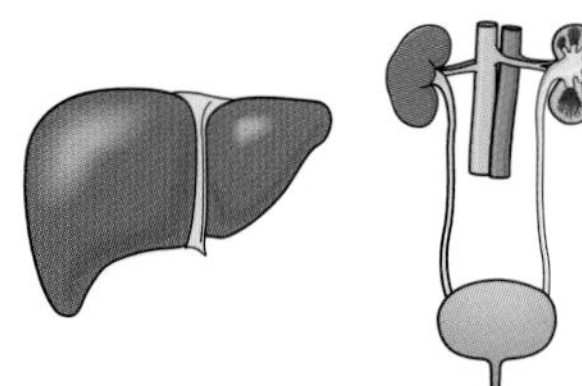

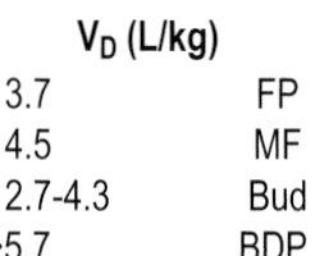

Figure 99-2 Factors affecting local and systemic effects of inhaled corticosteroids (*ICS*)/glucocorticosteroids: fluticasone propoionate (FP), mometasone furoate (*MF*), budesonide (*Bud*), and beclomethasone dipropionate (*BDP*).

TABLE 99-1 Relative Potencies of Common Glucocorticosteroids

Drug	Potency Relative (Hydrocortisone)	Equivalent Dose*	Duration of Action (hr)†
ORAL DRUGS			
Hydrocortisone	1	20 mg	8-12
Cortisone	0.8	25 mg	8-12
Prednisolone	4	5 mg	12-36
Prednisone	4	5 mg	12-36
6α-Methylprednisolone	5	4 mg	12-36
Triamcinolone	5	4 mg	12-36
Dexamethasone	25	0.75 mg	36-72
Betamethasone	25	0.75 mg	36-72
INHALED DRUGS			
Budesonide	3750	400 μg	1.5-2.8
Fluticasone	7200	200 μg	3.1-14
Mometasone	8800	200/400 μg	4.5
des-Ciclesonide	4800	320 μg	0.7-7
Beclomethasone (BDP/BMP)	2100/5400	400 μg	0.5/2.7

BDP, Beclomethasone dipropionate; *BMP*, beclomethasone monopropionate.
*Equivalence to hydrocortisone for oral drugs (milligrams) and to BDP for inhaled drugs (micrograms).
†Biologic half-life (hours).

remain unclear, except where functional genetic variants occur. Depot preparations are also available for subcutaneous injection to allow sustained release into the circulation.[14] However, most patients with asthma, allergic rhinitis, and dermatologic conditions are treated with topical GCs, with oral preparations limited to patients with more severe disease because of the risk of adverse side-effects.[14,15]

Initial attempts to use hydrocortisone or dexamethasone as topical inhaled corticosteroids (ICS) were minimally effective because of their rapid absorption and highly systemic bioavailability through the airways and gastrointestinal (GI) tract. However, modern ICS have high receptor affinity, are retained in the airways, and are rapidly metabolized after absorption from the GI tract (Table 99-1). The relative safety profile of these ICS is evidenced by their use in increasing doses to treat more severe asthma or exacerbations.[16] There is a fourfold lower effect on the hypothalamic-pituitary-adrenal (HPA) axis with ICS than with oral GCs, for the same degree of antiasthma efficacy,[17] although the use of increasing doses of ICS produces the same spectrum of side effects as seen with oral corticosteroids.[18] Currently, 10% to 20% of drug is delivered to the lungs from a metered-dose inhaler (MDI) or dry powder inhaler

(DPI), whereas greater than 50% of the drug is deposited in the mouth and pharynx and swallowed, available for GI absorption (Fig. 99-2).

Some GCs (budesonide, flunisolide, triamcinolone) have a plasma half-life of less than 2 hours, and others (BDP/BMP, fluticasone, mometasone) greater than 5 hours, whereas their biologic effects have a half-life ranging from 18 to 36 hours.[13] The pharmacokinetic properties of topical drugs depend on a combination of tissue deposition and targeting, receptor binding, volume of distribution, tissue retention, and lipid conjugation. An inhaled drug with a good therapeutic index possesses low oral bioavailability, small particle size, rapid metabolism, high clearance, high plasma protein binding, and low systemic half-life. Furthermore, an ideal compound is inactive at sites distal to the target organ.[12]

The systemic activity of topical GCs can be blunted by reducing GI bioavailability and prolonging tissue residency.[13] In asthma, changing the inhaler device can decrease oral delivery and GI availability of the same drug, as well as increase lung deposition by altering the particle size (e.g., MDI versus DPI).[13,19] In one study a similar bronchodilator response was obtained with one-twelfth the dose of salbutamol (albuterol) by using 3-μm particles rather than the dispersed size of particles emitted from a standard inhaler.[19] Similar effects will likely be seen with monodispersed particle sizes of GCs. Prolonged lung retention can be achieved by increasing lipophilicity, as with fluticasone propionate and mometasone, or by forming soluble intracellular esters, as with budesonide and ciclesonide.[12]

Lipophilicity generally correlates well with absorption characteristics. For example, fluticasone propionate has high lipophilicity and binding affinity for the GR, resulting in a high volume of distribution and long plasma half-life. However, the systemic side effects of fluticasone that arise from systemic absorption are limited because of its almost complete first-pass metabolism in the liver and, with enteric delivery, low absorption from the GI tract. In general for topical GCs, treatment efficacy and side-effects are directly related to tissue dose. This may also vary depending on disease severity for fluticasone propionate but apparently not for budesonide.[12] The pharmacokinetic profile of topical GCs varies with the drug, the delivery mechanism, and patient profile.[12]

METABOLISM AND EXCRETION

More than 90% of circulating cortisol is bound to plasma proteins and either to high-affinity, low-capacity steroid-binding globulin transcortin or to low-affinity, high-capacity serum albumin.[14,15] For example, the transcortin binding of dexamethasone is only 0.1% that of prednisolone. GCs undergo a common metabolic fate in that the 4,5 double bond and 3-ketone groups are reduced, resulting in an inactive compound.[14,15] This subsequently forms a glucoronide by conjugation, creating readily excreted, highly water-soluble compounds.[14,15] Alternately, the 2-position in the A-ring is hydroxylated. 11β-Hydroxysteroid dehydrogenase 2 (HSD2) converts the 11-hydroxyl group to a ketone group, thereby removing GC activity.[20] This process is reversible by HSD1.[20] These metabolic processes are generally very efficient, and more than 98% of cortisol is metabolized before being excreted into the urine (see Fig. 99-2).

Hepatic enzymes such as the cytochrome P-450 (CYP)–dependent mixed-function oxidases (MFOs) and glucuronyl transferases (and other conjugating enzymes) are important in steroid metabolism. Therefore, diseases and drugs that affect liver function can impact steroid half-life. Thus, barbiturates, diphenylhydantoin, and ephedrine—all agents that induce liver MFOs—shorten steroid half-life by increasing their metabolism.[14,15] In contrast, troleandomycin (TAO) prolongs the plasma half-life and function of methylprednisolone (but not prednisolone) by preventing its metabolic breakdown.[14,15] However, the clinical utility of TAO is limited by its hepatotoxicity.[14,15]

Local metabolism of endogenous cortisol at tissue sites has been found to regulate GC action. For example, inhibition of HSD2, which catalyzes the conversion of hydrocortisone to inactive cortisone by glycyrrhetinic acid (found in licorice), leads to enhanced steroid effects in the skin and possibly the lungs.[20] Two further examples of local metabolism are the conversion of beclomethasone dipropionate (BDP) to beclomethasone 17α-monopropionate (BMP), which has high-affinity for GR, and the reversible fatty acid conjugation of budesonide, triamcinolone, and cortisol, which results in prolonged retention and longer-lasting antiinflammatory action.[21] The active metabolite of ciclesonide, des-ciclesonide, which is produced by removal of the isobutyryl group at C21, can also undergo esterification in airway tissue.[22] Thus, individual variation in the local metabolism of an inhaled GC may alter the drug's efficacy and may account in part for variability in individual patient responses.

Side Effects

The recognition that GCs protected an organism from the harmful effects of stress and dampened inflammation and immune responses to infection led to their development as antiinflammatory therapies.[3] More recent work suggests that GCs may be important in activating components of the innate immune response, thereby increasing resistance to some infections.[15,23] GCs regulate the formation of glucose as well as carbohydrates, lipids, and proteins. GCs also control water and electrolyte homeostasis, and their effects impact all the major organ systems. [18] However, prolonged GC use is the greatest risk factor for adverse effects. Although all currently available topical GCs have some systemic effects, these are considerably less than seen with oral GCs (Table 99-2). Duration of use, dosage, dosing regimen, and specific drug used all affect the occurrence and severity of side effects, depending somewhat on patient variability.[18]

The side effects of topical GCs include glaucoma, cataracts, tissue atrophy, and reduced wound healing. At high doses there is an increased risk of infection, adrenal suppression, and osteoporosis. The growth retardation seen with oral GCs does not appear to be a problem with modern topical GCs, although growth velocity may be reduced on initiation of therapy.[24,25]

The most common adverse effects associated with use of oral GCs are skin and muscle atrophy, delayed wound healing and increased risk of infection, osteoporosis and bone necrosis, glaucoma and cataracts, behavioral changes, hypertension, peptic ulcers and GI bleeding, and diabetes.[18] Striae (stretch marks) induced by GC therapy results from major tissue atrophy and is permanent, whereas striae from early skin atrophy are reversible.[18]

These side effects often occur concomitantly, as seen in patients with Cushing syndrome: hypertension, diabetes mellitus, abdominal striae, fatigue, depression, moodiness, buffalo

TABLE 99-2 **Tissue/Organ-specific Side Effects of Topical and Systemic Corticosteroids**

Tissue/Organ	Effects
Skeleton and muscle	Muscle atrophy/myopathy Osteoporosis Bone necrosis
Skin	Atrophy, striae, distention Delayed wound healing Steroid acne, perioral dermatitis Erythema, telangiectasia, petechia, hypertrichosis
Endocrine system (metabolism, electrolytes)	Cushing syndrome Diabetes mellitus Adrenal atrophy Growth retardation Hypogonadism, delayed puberty Increased sodium retention and potassium excretion
Eye	Glaucoma Cataract
Immune system	Increased risk of infection Reactivation of latent viruses
Central nervous system	Disturbances in mood, behavior, memory, and cognition "Steroid psychosis," steroid dependence Cerebral atrophy
Gastrointestinal (GI) tract	Peptic ulcer GI bleeding Pancreatitis
Cardiovascular system	Hypertension Dyslipidemia Thrombosis Vasculitis

hump, and moon face.[1,18] Women with Cushing syndrome also have irregular menstrual periods and facial hair, and men have decreased libido. Therefore the risk/benefit ratio (or therapeutic index) is crucial in patients with severe asthma and allergy taking regular high-dose GCs. This issue has led to the search for novel agents with similar antiinflammatory capacity as GCs but reduced side effects.

Acute administration of GCs can produce central nervous system (CNS) effects, including suppression of the HPA axis and dramatic mood swings and occasionally frank psychosis.[26] The mood swings disappear on treatment cessation. Further, chronic oral GC therapy results in high circulating levels of GCs and a long-lasting inhibition of corticotropin (ACTH) secretion and atrophy of the anterior pituitary gland. Rapid GC withdrawal can have serious consequences.[27]

Although transrepression (see later) by GR is likely the major cause of the antiinflammatory effects of corticosteroids, a single mechanism does not as readily explain the major drivers for steroid side effects.[18] For example, transactivation drives diabetes and glaucoma, HPA suppression results from transrepression, and osteoporosis mechanisms are unclear but probably require both gene induction and gene repression.[18] Despite this uncertainty over the mechanisms involved in the generation of side-effects, there has been a search for GCs that can dissociate the ability of GR to transrepress without significant transactivation capabilities, to reduce the risk of systemic side effects. As noted earlier, several SEGRAs recently showed both steroidal and nonsteroidal backbones, with good dissociative properties in the skin for some.[10,18] Whether these drugs are dissociated in the lung and can reduce systemic side effects needs to be demonstrated in asthmatic patients (see Fig. 99-1).

The development of ciclesonide as an ICS for asthma took an alternative approach to reducing side effects. The active form des-ciclesonide is produced after cleavage by lung-specific esterases. Suppression of serum cortisol levels was greatly reduced with ciclesonide compared with an equipotent dose of beclomethasone dipropionate.[28]

Targeting other inflammatory pathways using kinase inhibitors may result in corticosteroid-sparing effects in addition to the antiinflammatory actions. Such combinations may become particularly important in exacerbations of disease where the need for short-term pulse therapy may overcome issues with potential side effects of kinase inhibition.[29,30]

EFFECTS ON ASTHMATIC INFLAMMATION

Most cases of asthma are accompanied by atopy and characterized by an inflammatory response within the airways involving mast cell activation, eosinophil influx, and increased numbers of activated type 2 helper T (Th2) cells.[31] However, this single mechanistic view of asthma has been modified with the realization that subsets of asthmatic patients may even reflect different diseases,[32,33] and in particular that inflammatory phenotypes may define the response to GCs.[32,34]

GCs are the most successful antiinflammatory treatment used in asthma because they target all the cells implicated in asthmatic inflammation (Fig. 99-3). The routine use of ICS to prevent airway inflammation in combination with relievers (e.g., β_2-agonists to help airway smooth muscle relax after contraction) is effective in treating symptoms, reducing exacerbations, and improving lung function and has greatly improved asthma control and quality of life in most patients.[35] Unfortunately, a minority of asthmatic patients show refractoriness to GC treatment.[36,37] The burden of costs (economic, morbidity/mortality) of these GC-refractory patients is much greater than that of GC-sensitive patients with nonsevere asthma.[36]

The GC-refractory nature of the inflammatory response is not confined to a subset of asthmatic patient and is also seen in most chronic inflammatory diseases.[37] The inflammatory patterns found in refractory asthma may also contribute to relative GC insensitivity, because drivers of specific disease subphenotypes may themselves be GC refractory. Better understanding of GC regulation of inflammation and the processes that prevent GC effectiveness in some patients will result in novel therapeutic agents or combinations to treat patients with severe asthma.[37]

EFFECTS ON INFLAMMATORY CELLS

Glucocorticosteroids given orally or intravenously cause an acute (4 to 6 hours) 80% reduction in circulating leukocytes, particularly basophils, eosinophils, and monocytes,[14] but an increase in neutrophils. In addition, the T cell/B cell ratio alters because of a greater effect on T cells.[14] In contrast, levels of cytotoxic $CD8^+$ and natural killer (NK) cells are not affected by acute GC administration; these changes revert back to baseline 24 to 48 hours after a single administration.[14]

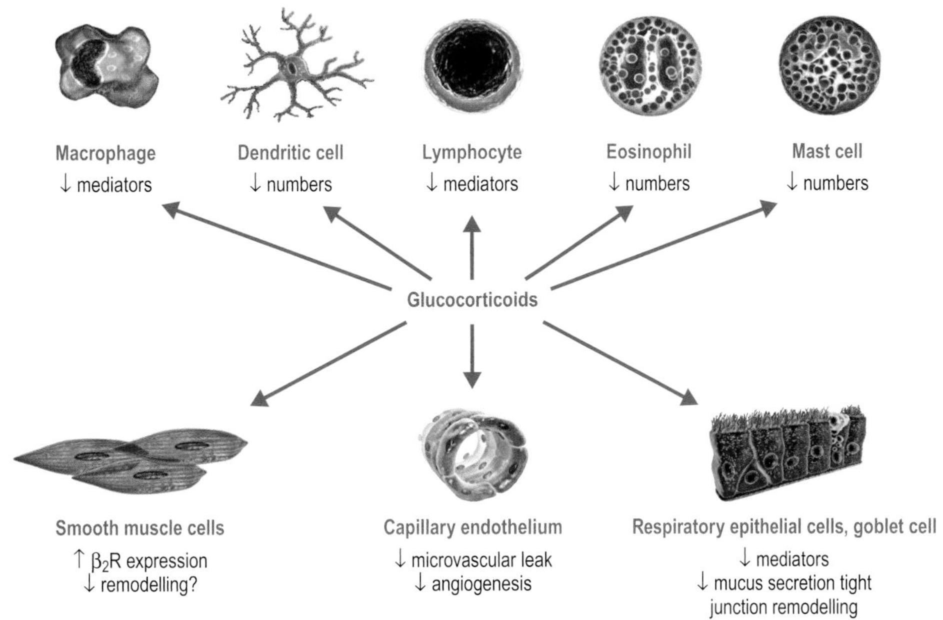

Figure 99-3 Effects of glucocorticosteroids (GCs) on inflammation in asthma. GCs have effects on many inflammatory aspects of infiltrating and resident inflammatory cells to suppress inflammation. The activity (T lymphocytes, macrophages) and number of infiltrating cells (eosinophils, T lymphocytes, macrophages, basophils, mast cells, dendritic cells) are decreased by GCs. GCs also have a suppressive effect on resident tissue cells and can reduce mediator release and adhesion molecule expression on epithelial and endothelial cells, microvascular leak from blood vessels, angiogenesis, and both the numbers of mucus glands and the release of mucus from these glands.

Eosinophils

Although a major eosinophilopoietic factor, interleukin-5 (IL-5) is not the only driver of eosinophil production; factors such as IL-3 and granulocyte-macrophage colony-stimulating factor (GM-CSF) are also important.[38] This probably underlies the initial disappointing effects of anti–IL-5 therapies in asthma.[39] However, more recent clinical trials indicate that a subset of severely asthmatic patients with eosinophilia despite high-dose ICS or oral steroids respond to the anti–IL-5 monoclonal antibody mepolizumab with respect to exacerbation rate, but not lung function or other asthma outcome measures.[40-42] Although promising, whether mepolizumab will be GC sparing in patients with severe asthma is unknown at present. GCs prevent eosinophil migration to the lung and the increase in blood eosinophil progenitors after antigen challenge.[43] In addition, intranasal GCs attenuate the seasonal rise in circulating eosinophil numbers associated with allergic rhinitis.[38] These data suggest that topical GCs modulate bone marrow actions directly or indirectly.[38]

GCs induce eosinophil apoptosis in vitro either in the absence or in the presence of survival factors such as IL-3, IL-5, and GM-CSF.[38] GCs also repress the expression of eosinophil survival factors from lymphocytes, which is enhanced after allergen challenge and in chronic allergic diseases.[38] The regulation of eosinophil apoptosis by survival factors and GCs is reciprocal in that steroid-induced eosinophil apoptosis is reversed by addition of survival factors.[38] GC-induced eosinophil apoptosis is linked to caspase-3 activation rather than effects on Bcl-family member proteins.[43] Importantly, GCs do not modulate eosinophil chemotaxis, adhesion, or degranulation to any extent.[38] Despite the lack of other potential mechanisms for eosinophil removal from the airways by GCs, apoptotic eosinophils have proved difficult to visualize after corticosteroid treatment in vivo.[43]

Neutrophils

Glucocorticosteroids have the opposite effect on neutrophils as on eosinophils, increasing peripheral blood neutrophil numbers. Proposed mechanisms include decreased cell migration from blood, increased neutrophil survival, and increased bone marrow production. In rabbits, GC-induced granulocytosis is primarily caused by a movement of polymorphonuclear leukocytes (PMNs) into the circulating pool from the marginated pool, with only a minor contribution made by the release of PMNs from the bone marrow. However, since GCs have little effect on circulating neutrophil numbers in patients with bone marrow dysfunction, this may be more important. Of note is also the opposite effect of GCs on neutrophil and eosinophil apoptosis, with GCs prolonging neutrophil survival in contrast to inducing eosinophil cell death.[44,45]

Lymphocytes

Total blood lymphocyte numbers are reduced in asthmatic patients who receive oral GCs. GCs inhibit lymphocyte activation and inflammatory mediator expression through a variety of mechanisms and induce lymphocyte apoptosis.[46] GC effects on lymphocyte cell survival are context dependent but can involve actions on mitochondrial proteins and early apoptotic events.[47] This may be caused by GC effects on mitochondrial metabolite and protein transporter, resulting in changes in mitochondrial membrane properties.[47] Alternatively, the GR can modulate mitochondrial oxidative stress and function more directly. GRs are localized to the mitochondria and can regulate expression from the mitochondrial genome through DNA binding sites in mitochondrial oxidative phosphorylation genes, mitochondrial transcription factors A, B1, and B2, and mitochondrial ribosomal RNA.[48] In addition to the nuclear transcription of mitochondrial genes, this can result in altered cell function.[48] Furthermore, thioredoxin (Trx2) is a mitochondrial antioxidant that helps regulate both GR and nuclear factor-κB (NF-κB) function by direct protein-protein interaction.[48] Cofilin-1, which regulates mitochondrial function, is abnormally expressed in CD4$^+$ lymphocytes in severe asthma.[49]

In contrast to the pronounced effects seen on T cells, GC therapy has little effect on B cell IgE production because they do not affect B cell proliferation or differentiation.[14] However, large doses of GCs may produce a small increase in IgG and IgM release.[14] This is in contrast to the ability of GCs to inhibit the seasonal increase in IgE levels seen in patients with rhinitis.[14] Delayed-type hypersensitivity (DTH) reactions (e.g., tuberculin test) are Th1 mediated and blocked by GCs in vivo because of effects on lymphocyte migration and proliferation.[14] The ability of GCs to prevent lymphocyte cytotoxicity is at least partly mediated by downregulation of granzyme B expression.[14] In allergic diseases, GCs are effective inhibitors of Th2 functions, including proliferation, survival, and cytokine/chemokine expression.[46] However, the relative importance of GC-induced suppression of lymphocyte cytokine expression versus suppression of lymphocyte accumulation or proliferation is unclear.[46]

GCs can also modulate the immune response in allergic asthma through effects on CD4$^+$CD25$^+$ Foxp3$^+$ regulatory T cells (Tregs).[14,50] The expression of IL-10 from human mononuclear cells is enhanced by GCs. Alone or with vitamin D_3, GCs can enhance expression of transcription factor Foxp3, inducing formation and activation of Treg cells.[50] The effects of GCs on Th17 and NK cells are not well established, although IL-17 can attenuate GC function in murine models of asthma[51] and in primary human epithelial cells.[52]

Monocytes, Macrophages, and Dendritic Cells

Monocyte and alveolar macrophage numbers are increased in the airways of asthmatic patients and express both high-affinity (FcεRI) and low-affinity (FcεRII, CD23) IgE receptors.[53] GCs have many effects on macrophage/monocye function, terminal differentiation, and activation status.[54] GCs reduce the expression of macrophage-derived proinflammatory cytokines such as IL-1, tumor necrosis factor-α (TNF-α), and IL-6.[54] The number of blood monocytes and their expression of low-affinity IgE receptors are reduced by in vivo therapy with GCs.[14] GCs also greatly reduce the numbers of major histocompatibility complex (MHC) class II (Ia)–positive cells residing in airway tissues.[14] GCs inhibit the inducible release of enzymes such as plasminogen activator, elastase, and collagenase, but not of the constitutively released lysozyme, suggesting that enzyme induction rather than release is the target of GC function.[14] Intracellular killing of *Nocardia, Listeria,* and *Salmonella* is reduced by GCs in vitro despite macrophage phagocytosis being relatively resistant to GCs.[14]

Dendritic cells (DCs) are major drivers of the adaptive immune response and key cells in mediating allergic inflammation.[55] DCs can sense the airway environment and are activated in asthma in response to allergic and noxious stimuli, leading to the release of TNF-α, IL-17A, and IL-5 and subsequent neutrophilia.[55] DCs also respond to the release of innate immune mediators from bronchial epithelial cells.[55] IL-1α and IL-1β are also released from bronchial epithelial cells after microbial and environmental stimulation of the NLRP3 inflammasome and are often present in Th17-driven inflammatory disease.[56] Indeed, elevated levels of IL-1β, IL-17, and the acute-phase protein serum amyloid A (SAA) are present in patients with severe allergic asthma.

Migration of DCs to local lymphoid collections is regulated by GCs, probably through modulation of cell surface CCR7 expression.[55] In addition, GCs prevent the release of Th1- and Th2-polarizing cytokines such as IL-4, IL-12, IL-13, thymic stromal lymphopoietin (TSLP), and interferon-γ (IFN-γ) from DCs, inhibiting development of both Th1 and Th2 cells.[14,57] IL-10 release from DCs is important for Treg development and likely is increased by upregulation of GC-induced leucine zipper (GILZ) expression.[55]

Asthmatic patients receiving GCs have reduced numbers of HLA-DR$^+$ cells in their airways,[55] probably because of induced cell death.[55] In vitro experiments using human monocyte–derived macrophages showed that GCs stimulate the phagocytosis of apoptotic eosinophils and neutrophils[58] and enhance monocyte differentiation into phagocytic macrophages.[14] Overall, although reducing the number of activated macrophages and DCs, steroids probably counter this by increasing their phagocytic activity.

Mast Cells

Many studies have demonstrated that topical and oral GCs can reduce bronchoalveolar lavage (BAL) and biopsy mast cell numbers.[14,59] However, up to 1 month of intranasal GC therapy had no effect on nasal biopsy mast cell numbers.[14,59] In contrast, 7 days of budesonide treatment reduced nasal mucosal biopsy histamine levels, indicating that GCs may affect mast cell mediator release in vivo.[14,59] However, topical GCs were able to reduce the numbers of mast cells localized adjacent to the nasal epithelium, probably indirectly through release of mast cell–directed chemokines such as eotaxin (CCL11), monocyte chemoattractant protein 4 (MCP-4, CCL13), and regulated on activation, normal T cell expressed and secreted (RANTES, CCL5) from epithelial cells.[59] Prolonged treatment with topical high-dose, highly potent GCs for 6 weeks, however, may reduce mast cell numbers in the skin through cell toxicity, requiring up to 4 months to return to baseline levels.[14,59] This effect may underpin the benefits seen with GC pulse therapy in patients with urticaria pigmentosa (mastocytosis).[14,59] Topical GCs are also able to reduce the large increase in nasal mucosal mast cells seen in patients with seasonal rhinitis during allergen season.[59] GCs also modulate human mast cell maturation and IgE receptor expression.[59]

Human mast cells obtained from the lung or skin do not reduce histamine or leukotriene release in response to GCs in vitro.[14,59] However, GCs can inhibit the stimulated release of macrophage inflammatory protein 1α (MIP-1α, CCL3), MCP-1 (CCL2), IL-5, IL-8–CXCL8, IL-13, and GM-CSF from human cord blood mast cells[59] and can enhance GILZ expression.[59] However, overall, GCs are unable to prevent the acute release of mediators from human lung mast cells, which likely accounts for the failure of topical and oral GCs to suppress the early asthmatic response Clinically, patients receiving systemic steroids still have positive skin-prick tests.[14,59]

Basophils

Basophils are major sources of IL-4 and IL-13 and are found in high numbers in the airways of asthmatic patients and after allergen challenge.[14] GCs have similar effects on specific subsets of basophils as on eosinophils because of induction of apoptosis,[14] and this is prevented by basophil growth factors such as IL-3.[14,60] In addition, GCs cause basophils to be sequestered in specific vascular beds.[60] GCs also have an indirect effect on basophil survival by repressing IL-3 production.[60] Basophil degranulation and release of histamine and leukotrienes are also GC sensitive.[14] However, this effect depends on the stimulus used, because IgE-dependent mediator release is inhibited, but not ionophore-, phorbal ester–, or formyl-methionyl-leucyl-phenylalanine (fMLP)–dependent mediator release.[14,60] ICS therapy in patients with asthma substantially reduces blood basophilia but noticeably, not histamine release.[14] In contrast, prolonged treatment with oral GCs has no effect on number of blood basophils, which are still able to release histamine in response to IgE stimulation.[14] GC treatment reduces basophil release of IL-4 and IL-13 in vitro, and prednisone treatment in vivo reduces airway basophilia and IL-4 expression induced by allergen challenge.[60]

Sparing Innate Immune Responses

Although GCs inhibit most inflammatory responses in the airways, it is increasingly evident that some innate immune responses are not reduced, or may even be enhanced, by GCs.[15,23] Such innate responses include increased production and survival of neutrophils, increased macrophage phagocytosis, and improved epithelial survival.[15,23] In addition, expression of innate immune genes such as Toll-like receptors (TLRs), complement, pentraxins, collectins, SAA, and other host defense genes are either enhanced or not repressed by GCs.[15,23] The mechanisms for these effects are not clear but involve in part the transcription factor C/EBPβ and the MAPK pathways.[23]

EFFECTS ON CELL RECRUITMENT TO THE AIRWAYS

The recruitment of inflammatory cells into the airways from blood depends on the expression of cell adhesion molecules (CAMs) expressed on endothelial cells and on the release of chemokines from airway resident cells (e.g., epithelium).[61,62] Expression of most CAMs is under control of NF-κB activation induced by proinflammatory mediators (e.g., IL-1, TNF-α) and thus should be GC responsive,[61,62] but evidence is minimal. GCs had no effect on CAM expression induced by cutaneous challenge with tuberculin[61,62] or endotoxin.[14] In addition, prednisone did not modulate the expression of allergen-induced intercellular adhesion molecule 1 (ICAM-1) or E-selectin in asthmatic airways despite GCs downregulating the levels of soluble E-selectin in BAL fluid.[61,62] This may reflect the importance of alternative sources of E-selectin expression. In contrast, expression of vascular cell adhesion molecule 1 (VCAM-1, CD106) and the numbers of VCAM-1–positive cells was reduced in nasal polyps and asthma biopsies after GC treatment, linked to reduction in eosinophilia and indirect actions of GCs on inflammatory mediator expression.[61,62] Further, transendothelial migration of eosinophils is not inhibited by GCs,[14] suggesting that the reduced airway eosinophilia may also be indirect through a reduction in chemokine or chemokine receptor expression. GCs are effective in suppressing the expression of most chemokines involved in recruitment of key asthma inflammatory cells into the airway, including macrophage-derived chemokine (MDC, CCL22), thymus and activation-regulated chemokine (TARC, CCL17), I-309 (CCL1), MCP-4 (CCL13), CCL5, stromal cell–derived factor 1α (SDF-1α, CXCL12), eotaxins 1 to 3 (CCL11, 24, 26), MIP-3α–CCL20, and CCR3 ligands such as CXCL8, IFN-γ–induced protein (IP-10, CXCL10), and fractalkine (CX3CL1).[4,31]

EFFECTS ON AIRWAY EPITHELIAL CELLS

In addition to their physical barrier function, airway epithelial cells play a key role in defense of the airways against environmental stimuli. In response to these stimuli, airway epithelial cells regulate the initiation and flares in disease by producing numerous inflammatory mediators, including lipid mediators, oxygen radicals, innate host defense molecules, cytokines, and chemokines, along with fibrogenic and growth-stimulating factors.[31] Most inflammatory mediators are induced by the proinflammatory transcription factors NF-κB and activator protein 1 (AP-1).[31]

GCs suppress the expression and release of a host of inflammatory cytokines (e.g., IL-1, IL-6, IL-11, GM-CSF, TNF-α), chemokines (CXCL8, CXCL12, CXCL10, growth-regulated oncogene-α [GRO-α, CXCL1], GRO-γ [CXCL3], CCL2, CCL13; CCL11, 24, 26; CCL17, CCL22, CCL5), and growth factors (e.g., TGF-β, PDGF, bFGF [FGF2], IGF-1) from epithelial cells in vitro and in vivo.[31] This suppression is likely through an effect on NF-κB, which is reduced in vivo by ICS in some studies.[57] As a result, there are marked effects on the downstream actions involving recruitment and activation of infiltrating inflammatory cells (DCs, Th2, eosinophils, basophils) and the function of structural cells (e.g., fibroblasts, airway smooth muscle cells).[4]

Also, GCs modulate the expression of specific CAMs (e.g., VCAM-1) on airway epithelial cells, modulating their interaction with the basement membrane and basal cells and with adjacent cells that form functional permeability barriers and prevent neutrophil and eosinophil migration into the airway lumen of the airway.[4,31] Epithelial mucus production[63] and fluid flux across the epithelium[31,61,62] are also regulated by GCs. GC actions on mucus production and secretion appear to target NF-κB by recruiting corepressors (see later), whereas the effect on transepithelial electrical resistance requires remodeling of tight junctions.[61,62] In the latter process, zonula occludens-1 (ZO-1) expression is induced and, along with β-catenin and F-actin, recruited to the junctional region.

GCs enhance the expression of surfactant protein B (SP-B) and SP-C to reduce airway surface tension.[15] This may be important in preventing neonatal respiratory distress syndrome, although this remains controversial.[64] The expression of the important host defense collectins SP-A and SP-D are also induced in airway epithelial cells by GCs.[15]

Airway Smooth Muscle Cells

In addition to contractile properties, airway smooth muscle (ASM) cells also have the major synthetic capacity to generate and release key proinflammatory cytokines, chemokines, and growth factors.[65] ASM cells also contribute to asthma pathophysiology by demonstrating increased proliferation and hypertrophy that correlate with asthma severity.[65] GCs can attenuate ASM cell proliferation, depending on the cellular growth matrix,[65,66] and also can downregulate the expression of inflammatory mediators.[65,66] However, the responsiveness of ASM cells to GCs in culture appears to reflect that of the disease;

cells from patients with severe asthma are less responsive to GCs than cells from patients with nonsevere asthma.[67] The regulation of some inflammatory genes (e.g., GRO-α) by dexamethasone involves the rapid induction of dual MAPK phosphatase 1 (MKP-1) and subsequent modulation of mitogen-activated protein kinases MAPK14 (P38α) and JUN N-terminal (JNK).[29]

EFFECT ON AIRWAY VASCULATURE

Numerous inflammatory mediators, including histamine, bradykinin, prostaglandins, leukotriene B_4 (LTB_4), complement (C5a), fMLP, arachidonic acid metabolites, and cytokines modulate epithelial barrier function.[31] The effects of GCs on these processes are not well described, however, although GCs can prevent the release of cyclooxygenase (COX) enzyme products and their metabolites and nitric oxide (NO) release.[4] This may explain the skin blanching seen in the McKenzie test.[4] Patients with severe steroid-refractory asthma have reduced steroid-induced skin blanching.[57] GCs also reduce microvascular leak in the airways of patients with asthma, although whether this is a direct effect on endothelial cells (increased tight junctions and ZO-1 expression) or an indirect effect on suppression of inflammatory mediator expression is unclear.[14]

Asthmatic patients express higher levels of vascular endothelial growth factor (VEGF) and VEGF receptors linked to increased angiogenesis by vessels with a larger cross-sectional area.[68] The number of blood vessels was reduced in asthmatic patients taking ICS or combined fluticasone/salmeterol therapy.[68] These effects likely are a result of GCs inhibiting VEGF expression.[68]

TISSUE REPAIR

Short-term treatment with steroids has minimal effect on wound healing and tissue repair. However, wound healing is delayed and more complications arise in patients receiving long-term GC therapy. The mechanisms for these effects probably relate to cell recruitment, activation, and proliferation as well as actions on fibrosis and repair processes. The role of GCs in modulating angiogenic and angiostatic chemokines in tissue repair is unclear, although steroids can inhibit both fibroblast growth and cytokine release. The wound repair response in differentiated epithelial cells is greatly inhibited by GCs.[18,69]

CROSSTALK BETWEEN ADRENERGIC SYSTEM AND GLUCOCORTICOSTEROIDS

Prolonged β_2-adrenoceptor (β_2-AR) stimulation by an agonist results in downregulation of β_2-AR expression.[70] GCs can counteract this effect and enhance β_2-AR mRNA expression through binding to specific sites in the promoter region.[4] The desensitization seen with β_2-AR ligands depends on single-nucleotide polymorphisms (SNPs) within the receptor-coding region.[71] Thus asthmatic patients, particularly African Americans, with the B16Arg/Arg allele are at greater risk of exacerbation and death when treated with a long-acting β_2-agonist (LABA) as monotherapy.[71]

Activation of the β_2-AR by LABAs can also impinge on GR function.[72] LABAs such as salmeterol and formoterol can enhance several aspects of GC function in different cell types,[71] believed to result from priming of GR by protein kinase A (PKA)–mediated events, which can result in enhanced GR nuclear translocation.[72] This is also seen in vivo in asthmatic patients in whom the combination of low-dose fluticasone with salmeterol is as effective as high-dose fluticasone in inducing sputum cell GR nuclear import.[73] The complementary effects of LABAs on ASM function and GCs on inflammation are also likely to be important in underlying the clinical efficacy of these combination drugs.[72]

Arachidonic Acid Metabolites

A number of arachidonic acid (AA) products, including prostaglandins, thromboxanes, prostacyclin, monohydroxyeicosatetraenoic acids (HETEs), diHETEs, lipoxins, and LTB_4 and the sulfidopeptide leukotrienes (LTC_4, LTD_4, LTE_4) are important in inflammation. GCs can block the formation of AA metabolites in many cell types via suppression of phospholipase A_2 (PLA_2), and COX-2 expression, with subsequent effects on the induction of chemokine and cytokine receptors and their ligands.[74,75] Dexamethasone, along with the proresolving omega-3 polyunsaturated fatty acid (PUFA)–derived mediators, including resolvin E1 (RvE1)[4] and protectin D1 (PD1),[76] regulate the function of inflammatory (CD11b-low) macrophages in vivo.[77] This is achieved by resetting the level at which ingestion of apoptotic leukocytes act to convert macrophages into CD11b-low macrophages and thereby enhance the termination of the acute inflammatory response.

Inflammatory Gene Expression

Most inflammatory genes are regulated by the actions of proinflammatory transcription factors such as NF-κB.[78,79] However, the degree of inflammatory gene expression induced by NF-κB may be regulated by the coordinated activation of other proinflammatory transcription factors (e.g., STATs, AP-1) and activation of distinct intracellular signaling pathways (e.g., MAPK14). These transcription factors and signaling pathways may modulate NF-κB function by protein-protein interaction or by modulation of NF-κB signaling from induction of posttranslational modifications (PTMs) of NF-κB, affecting NF-κB–induced inflammatory gene transcription.[78,79]

NUCLEAR FACTOR-κB INFLAMMATORY PATHWAY

The NF-κB pathway is one of the major signaling pathways activated in inflammatory cells and a master regulator of the expression of inflammatory mediators, including cytokines, chemokines, growth factors, and proteases. It is also involved in the innate and adaptive immune system. NF-κB comprises homodimers or heterodimers of members of two protein families: the REL family (RELA/P65, c-REL, and RELB) and the NF-κB family (P100 and P105). The NF-κB family of proteins is cleaved after PTMs by proteolysis to enable formation of active DNA-binding proteins (e.g., P100 to P52, P105 to P50). in contrast to P100 and P105, REL proteins contain a C-terminal transcription activation domain (TAD) that enables gene transcription. The NF-κB family members P52 and P50 must therefore associate with a REL family member to induce gene transcription.[78,79]

The classic form of NF-κB contains a heterodimer of P50 and P65 that interacts with a specific 9– to 10–base pair (bp) site in the promoter region of κB-responsive genes known as a κB response element. This sequence is variable, enabling the expression of diverse subsets of inflammatory genes in a cell-specific and stimulus-specific manner. NF-κB is found as an inactive complex in the cytoplasm of most cells and is activated through a classical (canonical) or alternative (noncanonical) pathway. These two pathways, alone or together, are activated by specific stimuli to target the expression of distinct spectrums of inflammatory genes.[78,79]

CLASSICAL NF-κB PATHWAY

In nonstimulated cells, NF-κB heterodimer (P65/RELA and P50 subunits) resides in the cytoplasm in an inactive state, bound by the inhibitory IκBα protein. Cell activation by binding of an inflammatory stimulus or even allergen to its cell surface receptor (e.g., TNFR, IL1R, or TLRs to respective receptor) results in activation of the myeloid differentiation primary response gene 88 (MYD88)–dependent pathway, leading to NF-κB activation. Ligand binding results in receptor dimerization and enables the receptor to initiate a phosphorylation cascade that eventually leads to TAK1 (TGF-β–activated kinase 1 or MAP3K7) activating the IKK complex.[78,79]

The IκB kinase (IKK) complex contains three subunits, IKKα, IKKβ, and the regulatory molecule IKKγ/NEMO. The IKK complex phosphorylates IκBα (on SER32 and SER36), which is targeted for ubiquination and degradation by the E3 ubiquitin-ligase (E3RS IκB) and the 26S proteasome, respectively.[78,79] The degradation of IκBα allows the translocation of NF-κB P65/P50 dimer into the nucleus, where it binds to promoter regions of inflammatory genes and forms a complex containing transcriptional coactivators such as P300, cyclic adenosine monophosphate (cAMP) response element binding protein (CBP), P300/CBP-associated protein (PCAF), and TATA-binding protein (TBP)–associated factor 2 (ATF-2).[80,81]

REGULATION BY CHROMATIN AND HISTONE MODIFICATIONS

Deoxyribonucleic acid is packaged within the nucleus by the formation of nucleosomes, wrapping 146 bp around a histone octomer (two each of histones 2A, 2B, 3, and 4).[82,83] The linker histone H1 stabilizes the chromatin structure by binding to DNA between nucleosomes, and H1 loss from this complex is therefore essential for upregulating gene expression.[84] All histones, including H1, undergo PTMs linked to modulation of gene expression.[82,83] Histone acetylation and methylation are the most extensively studied modifications and are deposited on histones by the action of specific enzymes to form marks or tags. These tags allow "readers" of these marks to recruit chromatin-remodeling engines such as switch/sucrose nonfermentable (SWI/SNF), resulting in changes in chromatin structure. This is an active ATP-dependent process that results in the open chromatin structure associated with active gene transcription or the closed, repressive chromatin state linked to a lack of active transcription. For example, an acetylated lysine residue forms a bromodomain that is read by many enzymes and transcription-regulating factors, resulting in upregulation of gene expression. Histone methylation is slightly more complex; the functional outcome depends on the target residue. For example, H3 lysine 4 trimethylation (H3K4me3) is associated with active gene expression and is most often found at the transcriptional start site, whereas H3K9 and H3K27 methylation tags are associated with gene repression. Similar to histone acetylation, these methyl tags are reversible and are removed by an active demethylation process. Thus, alterations in histone methyltransferase (HMT) and histone demethylase (HDM) activity modulate gene expression profiles.[82,83]

BROMODOMAIN-CONTAINING PROTEINS

Transcriptional coactivator molecules have intrinsic histone acetyltransferase (HAT) activity and subsequently acetylate core histones.[80,81] This results in disruption of electrostatic attraction between histones and DNA, producing a looser structure, and tags histones for subsequent recruitment of other regulatory factors previously spatially prevented from joining the transactivation complex.[4,85] This process often involves looping out of the DNA to contact gene promoters and enhancers associated with multiple genes either locally, such as at the Th2 locus on chromosome 5, or even on other chromosomes.[86] The resultant effect on gene expression is context dependent.

The acetylated lysine tag left by HAT activation can be read by bromodomain-containing proteins. Proteins such as BRD4 are involved in many aspects of gene expression, including initiation complex formation, mRNA elongation, and cell proliferation.[87,88] Removal of this acetylation tag by histone deacetylases (HDACs) can reverse or block gene expression.[4] Bromodomain mimics are small, peptidelike molecules that sit in the bromodomain pocket and prevent BRD4 from binding to acetylated lysine residues that have shown marked, specific suppression of inflammatory gene expression in human and murine macrophages and in animal models of sepsis and cancer.[88] The use of these bromodomain mimics confirms the key role of histone acetylation in the expression of key inflammatory genes, although their role in models of allergic asthma has yet to be established. Other histone modifications include phosphorylation and ubiquitination.

FEEDBACK REGULATION OF NF-κB PATHWAY

Nuclear factor-κB controls the expression of many genes involved in inflammation and regulation of the immune response. Therefore, its biologic activity requires tight regulation to maintain a cellular/tissue homeostasis. This balance is achieved through several negative regulatory mechanisms. During transcription, NF-κB also transcribes its negative regulatory proteins IκBα and A20. The newly synthesized IκBα can shuttle the P65:P50 heterodimer back into the nucleus or bind to NF-κB within the cytoplasm. A20 is an ubiquitin-modifying enzyme directly induced by NF-κB. A20 deubiquitinates the IKK complex, resulting in its destabilization, preventing phosphorylation and degradation of IκBα. PTMs of P65 can have profound effects on NF-κB function. Several lysine sites on P65 have been identified as acetylated by CBP/P300 acetyltransferase (e.g., lysines 123, 218, 221, 310, 314, and 315). CBP/P300-interacting transactivator-2 (CITED2) protein has been shown to inhibit P65 acetylation and interaction with CBP/P300 acetyltransferase, leading to reduced DNA-binding affinity.[78,79]

Mechanisms of Corticosteroid Action

GLUCOCORTICOSTEROIDS RECEPTORS

Oral and topical GCs pass rapidly through the cell membrane by passive diffusion into the cytoplasm. Within the cytoplasm,

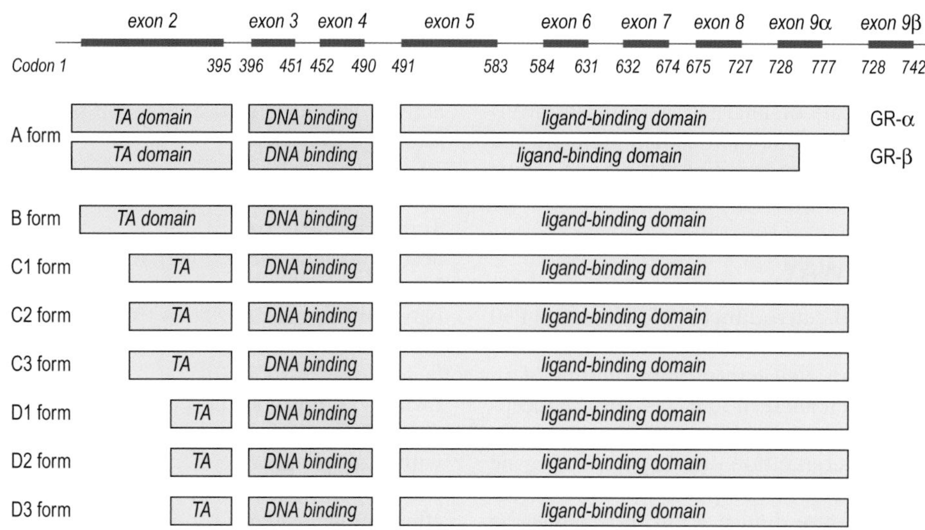

Figure 99-4 Modular structure of the glucocorticosteroid receptor (GR). The coding region of GR results from splicing together of exons 2 to 9 of the GR gene. The GR-β isoform of GR results from the use of the short 9β exon, which removes the ligand-binding domain (LBD) seen in GR-α. The modular design of GR enables distinct regions of the protein to function in isolation as LBDs, DNA-binding domain, and transactivating domain (TA domain). N-terminal truncated forms of GR (labeled *A* to *D*) are produced by alternative use of ATG sites in exon 2. These have different functions (e.g., than the GR-αA form).

GCs bind to and activate their receptor (GR, NR3C1) through interaction with the specific receptor ligand-binding domain (LBD).[87] GR, as with all nuclear hormone receptors, is divided into distinct functional modules: an LBD, a nuclear translocation domain (NTD), and transactivation domains (AF1, AF2). The latter enables GR to associate with transcriptional coactivators or repressors.[87]

The primary form of GR is GR-α, although other forms exist[89] (Fig. 99-4). GR-α is expressed in all resident and infiltrating cells within the airways and lungs, which accounts for the ability of GCs to affect the recruitment and activation of most inflammatory cells, as well as the effectiveness of ICS in controlling symptoms and allergic asthmatic inflammation.[90] The expression of GR-α may vary between cell types, but the number of GR molecules that must be activated in each cell to induce a full functional response may not be limiting; even when GR-α expression is reduced by up to 70%, this is not enough to prevent effective antiinflammatory responses.[91] Specifically, in a smoking model of acute inflammation, there is a rapid loss of total GR within the murine lung associated with a loss of budesonide sensitivity.[91] Overexpression of a PI3Kδ-active site mutant that retains the PI3Kδ structure without enzymic activity in these mice does not affect the numbers of inflammatory cells or mediators in the lung in response to cigarette smoke or GR-α expression levels, but does restore budesonide responsiveness.

Posttranslational Modifications and GR Function

Newly synthesised GR is phosphorylated at three sites—SER203, SER211, and SER226—but these phosphate groups are removed once within the multisubunit complex. Ligand binding, which results in heat shock protein 90 (HSP90) dissociation, allows kinases to again interact with GR, which becomes phosphorylated. GR phosphorylation status can alter GR function; for example, phosphorylation of SER211 correlates with ligand binding, nuclear translocation, and transactivation.[92] Human GR is rapidly phosphorylated on S211 and S226 in response to dexamethasone, and maximal GR-mediated transcriptional activation of GILZ and mouse mammary tumor virus (MMTV) transcription requires phosphorylation at one or more serine residues (from S203, S211, and S226).[93] GR phosphorylation at these sites has no effect on GR half-life but alters the ability of DNA-bound GR associating with transcriptional cofactors such as GR-interacting protein-1 (GRIP-1).[93] The extent of S226 and S211 GR phosphorylation, GR half-life, and transcriptional response depends on the precise ligand used to stimulate the cell.[94] GR phosphorylation and half-life correlated with ligand-induced transactivation and transrepression, whereby S211 phosphorylation is required for maximal transactivation, but not transrepression efficacy, and S226 phosphorylation was linked to maximal transcription efficacy.[94] Correct GR phosphorylation is essential for optimal GR function because when GR is phosphorylated at S226, but not S226 and S221 together as seen with dexamethasone stimulation, this results in the formation of an inactive GR transactivation complex.[95]

As with other nuclear hormone receptors,[96] GR is an acetylated protein, and ligand binding induces GR acetylation on K494 and K495.[97] Acetylation of GR affects its ability to interact with P65, and removal of these tags is important for the suppression of subsets of inflammatory genes.[97]

GR also undergoes sumoylation, in which small ubiquitin-like modifier (SUMO) proteins are attached to and detached from other proteins in cells to alter their function. Sumoylation affects GR transactivation potential, particularly at promoters with multiple GREs.[98] Sumoylation is increased in the presence of high levels of oxidative stress, whereas low levels of oxidative stress can remove sumoylate conjugates.[99] This may have implications for GR function under conditions of altered oxidative stress.

Glucocorticosteroid Receptor Isoforms

There are N- or C-terminally truncated forms of GR that have distinct activities and may modulate GC activity in treatment-refractory diseases[89,100] (see Fig. 99-4). GR-β, the most well studied of these alternatively spliced isoforms, possesses a divergent truncated C terminus, resulting in an inability to bind correctly to conventional GCs or activate gene expression,[101] although it does act as a dominant negative modulator of GR-α.[102] A specific ligand for GR-β has been reported as the glucocorticosteroid antagonist RU-486.[102] Some patients with treatment-refractory asthma have enhanced expression of GR-β,[102] possibly in response to high levels of proinflammatory cytokines, including TNF-α and IL-1, IL-2, and IL-4.[102] However, the precise role of GR-β in regulating GC function in these steroid-refractory patients remains controversial, because its relative expression level compared to GR-α may not be high enough to allow suppression of GR-α actions.[102]

GR mutations can cause global GC insensitivity.[103] Patients with hypercortisolism without cushingoid features are described as having glucocorticosteroid insensitivity syndrome and exhibit a resetting of the HPA axis associated with elevated plasma cortisol levels.[103] This rare disease was first described in 1976 and to date only 20 kindreds exists, with only occasional additional reports of cases caused by GR mutations.[103] The clinical spectrum ranges from completely asymptomatic patients to those with severe symptoms; most patients diagnosed to date, often during other studies, were asymptomatic, with only biochemical changes apparent.[103] These mutations occur across GRs and tend to exhibit a partial loss of GR function resulting from reduced GR number, ligand binding, stability, nuclear translocation, and cofactor association.[103] For example, GR nuclear translocation is reduced with the I559N mutant, resulting in attenuation of GRE-mediated gene transduction.[103] Other mutations such as N363S, however, are linked to increased GR function.[103]

Peripheral blood mononuclear cells (PBMCs) from healthy subjects treated with GCs indicate that almost 25% exhibit some form of resistance to dexamethasone.[104] Therefore a proportion of the population may have reduced GC sensitivity even without disease.[104] Furthermore, alterations in specific genes such as the P50 component of NF-κB and the GR chaperone protein FKBP51 have been proposed to play a role in class switch recombination (CSR), but this link is still unproved.[104]

Glucocorticosteroid Receptor Nuclear Translocation

Nucelocytoplasmic shuttling of GR occurs through the nuclear pore complex (NPC) and is a dynamic process regulated by nuclear import and export receptors in a sequential manner.[105] The mechanisms that govern GR nucleocytoplasmic shuttling are unclear, but GR contains two nuclear localization signals, NLS1 and NLS2. (An NLS is an amino acid sequence that tags a protein for import into the cell nucleus by nuclear transport and typically consists of one or more short sequences of positively charged lysines or arginines exposed on the protein surface.) NLS1 is located within the DNA-binding domain and is responsible for rapid GR nuclear translocation (4 to 6 minutes). NLS2 is located in the LBD and mediates relatively slower GR nuclear translocation (45 minutes to 1 hour).[106] The rates of hormone-induced nuclear localization of both the full-length receptor and the NLS2-fusion proteins were similar.[106] Several nuclear importin receptors, such as importins 7, 8, 13, and α/β heterodimer, interact with the GR.[107] For example, immunoprecipitation of S-methionine–labeled fragments of GR in reticulocyte lysate indicates that importin-7 binds to both NLS1 and NLS2.[107] It is unclear whether these different importins act in combination or individually to facilitate GR nuclear translocation.

TABLE 99-3 Induction and Inhibition by Glucocorticosteroids (GCs) on Expression of Proinflammatory and Antiinflammatory Gene Classes

Induced by GCs	Inhibited by GCs
Soluble interleukin receptors	Interleukins
Membrane functional proteins	Chemokines
Membrane regulatory proteins	Metalloproteinases and other proteinases
Intracellular regulatory proteins	Enzymes involved in synthesis of prostanoids, inflammatory peptides, and nitric oxide
Interleukin-10	

Similarly, nuclear export of proteins is also regulated by the RAN–guanosine triphosphatases (GTPases) system. A nuclear export signal (NES) located on the cargo protein is recognized by exportins. Exportin-1 (CSR-1) is best characterized and is inhibited by leptomycin B (LMB). LMB inhibits GR nuclear export, leading to enhanced, unliganded, and hormone-treated GR nuclear localization.[106] However, this has not been confirmed in other studies proposing the importance of nuclear export receptors such as calreticulin (CRT). CRT binds GR at a unique 15–amino acid sequence localized between the two zinc fingers of the DNA-binding site under the control of intracellular calcium levels.[108] Data to date are unable to clarify whether GR usses specific importins and exportins in a cell-specific manner.

Once within the nucleus, GR has two major roles. First, GR can bind to DNA as a dimer at specific glucocorticosteroid response elements (GREs), stimulating antiinflammatory gene expression (transactivation). Second, the GR monomer can tether to DNA-bound proinflammatory transcription factors, bringing transcriptional regulator proteins close to the activated transcriptional complexes and generally suppressing inflammatory gene expression[87] (Table 99-3). The major targets for tethering are redox-sensitive inflammatory transcription factors such as NF-κB. These factors are implicated in the regulation of many, if not most, inflammatory and immune genes.[57]

GENE INDUCTION BY CORTICOSTEROIDS

Activated GR binds to an imperfect palindrome of two hexamers separated by a 3-bp linker AGAACA*nnn*TGTTCT (GRE)[109] (Fig. 99-5). Each half of the hexamer within the GRE provides sites for GR interaction.[110] Most of the bases are highly variable, with little or no effect on GR function and only a few invariant bases critical for GR DNA binding.[110] However, even a single base-pair change in a GRE may affect the GR-GRE conformation and subsequent transcriptional activity.[110] Similar results are seen with other transcription factors, such as NF-κB.[111] In contrast to other transcription factors whose GREs are located just upstream of the transcription start site (TSS), only 17% of GREs are found close to a TSS.[110] In addition, the localization of GREs differs with respect to the TSS, depending on whether the gene is activated (closer to TSS) or repressed by GR.[112]

Interestingly, GRE flanking regions are able to bind many other transcription factors (e.g., AP-1, ETS, SP1, C/EBP, HNF2), which are conserved across cells and species in a gene-specific manner. This suggests that each GRE acts as a composite element that also provides potential combination regulation/

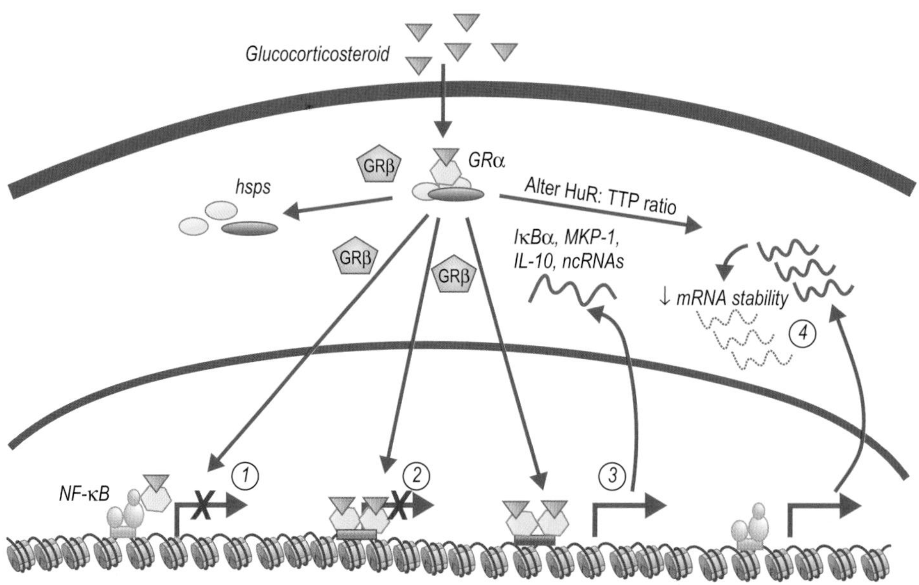

Figure 99-5 Mechanisms of glucocorticosteroid receptor (GR) action. The glucocorticosteroid ligand can freely migrate across the plasma membrane, where it associates with the cytoplasmic GR. This results in activation of the GR and dissociation from its chaperone complex, which contains the heat shock proteins (*hsps*) HSP90 and HSP51. The activated GR translocates to the nucleus, where it can bind as a monomer either directly or indirectly with the transcription factor nuclear factor-κB (*NF-κB*), preventing it from switching on inflammatory gene expression (*1*). This involves a change in local histone acetylation status and chromatin remodeling. Second, the GR dimer can bind to a glucocorticosteroid response element that overlaps the DNA binding site for a proinflammatory transcription factor or the start site of transcription, to prevent inflammatory gene expression impairing formation of an active transcriptional complex (*2*). Third, the GR dimer can induce the expression of antiinflammatory genes such as the NF-κB inhibitor *IκBα*, mitogen-activated protein kinase phosphatase 1 (*MKP-1*), *IL-10*, or the production of distinct subsets of noncoding (nc) RNA (*3*). Fourth, corticosteroids can increase the levels of cell ribonucleases and mRNA-destabilizing proteins such as *HuR* and tristetraprolin (*TTP*), thereby reducing *mRNA* levels (*4*). The increased expression of the *GRβ* isoform found in some patients with glucocorticosteroid-insensitive severe asthma can act as a dominant negative regulator of *GRα*.

modulation of specific genes by the presence of these factors along with the activated GR.[110] For example, even if activated GR is found within a complex at a specific gene, it may be functionless without the correct profile of composite factors, transcriptional cofactors, or DNA accessibility to create the correct transcriptional environment.[4,113] Just as different GC ligands have subtle differences on GR function, the specific DNA sequence at and around each GRE could act as an allosteric GR ligand that modifies GR function in a gene-specific and cell/tissue-specific manner.[110]

DNA BINDING

The classic model of GR binding to a GRE, recruiting cofactors such as chromatin-remodeling enzymes, and causing local unwinding of chromatin structure,[4,113] has recently been reevaluated in light of a series of experiments using a combination of chromatin immunoprecipitation-deep sequencing (ChIP-seq), live-cell imaging and photobleaching of GR binding to repeated GRE sequences, and mathematical modeling.[114,115] Standard ChIP analysis suggests that transcription factors remain associated with GREs for long periods because of saturable binding to the GRE, during which changes in local histone modification status and chromatin remodeling occur, allowing gene expression to occur. However, evidence now suggests that GR bound GREs only for seconds before leaving and being replaced by a distinct GR.[115] Binding of GR to GREs is not saturable, and indeed, binding of a single GR to a specific GRE can enhance loading of another GR at this site, a process called assisted loading. In this process the initial rapid on-off binding of an activated GR to a GRE evokes an ATP-dependent remodeling that is generally reversed before stoichastic binding of another GR occurs. However, if the remodeling is still present when the second GR arrives at the GRE site, it will meet a chromatin structure more amenable to GR-GRE binding, enhancing its subsequent transcriptional effect.[115] These data emphasize the importance of a coordinated order of recruitment to access the full genomic information available.[115]

The requirement for activated GR to bind to both GREs and to tether to other transcription factors at open chromatin that is accessible before hormone treatment suggested that some factors, presumably transcription factors, were critical to maintenance of these regulated domains, probably in a tissue-dependent manner.[115] Combining DNase I accessibility and chromatin immunoprecipitation with high-throughput sequencing identified AP-1 as a major partner for productive GR-chromatin interactions. AP-1 is critical for GR-regulated transcription and recruitment to jointly occupied regulatory elements, illustrating an extensive AP-1–GR interaction network. Importantly, the maintenance of baseline chromatin accessibility facilitates GR recruitment and is dependent on AP-1 binding. Thus, distinct transcription factors, particularly AP-1 in murine mammary epithelial cells, occupy sites close to GREs and prime chromatin, allowing binding of inducible factors such as activated GR by assisted loading.[114,115]

Rapid exchange of GR at a GRE requires chaperone and proteasome activity.[116] The protein kinase CDK2 controls H1 phosphorylation, chromatin remodeling, and transcription from the mouse mammary tumor virus (MMTV) promoter. Using photobleaching of live cells, inhibition of CDK2 by

Roscovitine resulted in slower GR exchange at the MMTV, resulting in more GR being tightly associated with MMTV. This was associated with reduced GR-mediated transactivation and changes in H1 phosphorylation.[116] This suggests that chromatin remodeling is important in the rapid exchange of GR at MMTV.

Methylation by DNA at the core GRE can interfere with the maintenance of locally accessible chromatin required for GR-GRE binding. The classic GRE itself does not contain cytosine-phosphate-guanine (CpG) oligonucleotides, but nucleotide substitutions are able to create CpG sites within key sites in the GRE hexamer to regulate GR-GRE binding. In contrast, CpG formation within the spacer region or outside the core 15-mer did not affect DNA binding. CpG density is greater at open, preprogrammed chromatin elements, whereas the sites that undergo de novo remodeling on GR activation have a characteristically low CpG density and lack the capacity for regulation by DNA methylation. Interestingly, exposure to GCs and binding of activated GR to specific de novo sites (e.g., Suox-GRE) results in rapid loss (5 minutes) of CpG methylation at selected sites through an active demethylation process. These results introduce the concept of DNA methylation as an essential component of the complex regulatory processes that control gene expression by nuclear receptors.[117]

More recently, a novel type of repressive function of GR has been described whereby GR binds to a palindromic sequencing consisting of two inverted repeats (IRs) separated by a single base pair (IR1 nGRE).[118] These sequences are implicated in the control of over 1000 human genes.[118] Further, GR-mediated downregulation of MUC5AC gene expression in primary human bronchial epithelial cells is controlled by two distinct GREs within the MUC5AC promoter, GRE3 and GRE5.[63] HDAC2 was recruited to the GR-GRE complex on DNA in a temporal manner, as determined by ChIP analysis and thereby reduced MUC5AC expression.

GENE REPRESSION BY CORTICOSTEROIDS

In contrast to its role in activating antiinflammatory genes via DNA binding, GR also plays an important role in the repression of proinflammatory genes. The mechanisms involved in this process involve direct inhibition of transcriptional complex activation by binding across the TSS of some genes or by preventing DNA binding of proinflammatory transcription factors at composite elements or indirectly through tethering to transcription factors such as DNA-bound NF-κB[87] (Fig. 99-5). The interaction between GR and NF-κB is mutually antagonistic, and NF-κB activation can therefore repress GR function.[97] Increased NF-κB activation at the nuclear localization and expression level is associated with severe asthma.[57]

The mutually antagonistic interaction between GR and NF-κB is regulated at least in part by the acetylation status of GR.[97] GR deacetylation is catalyzed by the enzyme HDAC2, which is rapidly recruited to the activated GR, allowing GR to interact with P65.[97] GR-associated corepressor activity can also reduce P65-induced local histone deacetylation and chromatin remodeling, allowing suppression of subsets of inflammatory genes. HDAC2-mediated GR deacetylation does not affect GR nuclear translocation, DNA binding, or transactivation.[97] HDAC2 expression or activity linked to enhanced HAT activity has been shown to be reduced in severely asthmatic patients, particularly children.[119] Interestingly, GR-β has been reported to reduce HDAC2 expression in human BAL macrophages.[120]

During NF-κB–induced proinflammatory gene activation, the local chromatin structure is modified by HATs, allowing sequential recruitment of bromodomain complexes, which in turn induce chromatin remodeling, RNA polymerase-2 recruitment, and gene expression.[81] Loss of a specific HDAC may therefore lead to changes in the histone acetylation at the promoter regions of inflammatory genes, resulting in either altered transcription factor DNA accessibility or association with bromodomain-containing transcription cofactors, modulating gene expression.[87] GR-mediated repression of the proopiomelanocortin (POMC) gene requires the ATPase-dependent chromatin remodeling enzyme BRG1 and the recruitment of HDAC2. Recruitment of HDAC2 by GR resulted in deacetylation of histones around the POMC promoter. Also, 50% of corticosteroid-resistant human and dog corticotroph pituitary adenomas, a characteristic of Cushing disease, are deficient in the nuclear expression of BRG1 or HDAC2. This suggests that a relative insufficiency of BRG1 or HDAC2 would induce GC insensitivity.[121]

Remodeling of the POMC promoter by BRG1 is an essential requirement for RNA polymerase-2 initiation and reinitiation[121] a process that coincides with alterations in the phosphorylation status of RNA polymerase-2 C-terminal domain (CTD) phosphorylation. Dexamethasone attenuates TNF-α/NF-κB–induced CTD S2 phosphorylation at the CXCL8 promoter,[122] through prevention of the association of the SER2 CTD kinase P-TEFb.[123] This indicates a potential role for GR in blocking BRD4-mediated transcription, possibly acting in a functionally similar manner to BRD4 mimics. Biladeau and colleagues[121] demonstrated that reduced HDAC2 expression results in attenuation of BRG1 function, with failure to remove the CTD S2 phosphotag and stalling of RNA polymerase 2 on the promoters of steroid-responsive genes.

Other Transcriptional Corepressors

There are 18 HDACs belonging to four major classes,[82] and other HDACs in addition to HDAC2 have been implicated in the modulation of GR function. However, the precise role for each enzyme in lung disease requires further investigation. HDAC6 expression is increased in chronic obstructive pulmonary disease (COPD) and has been reported to reverse acetylation of HSP90, the GR chaperone. This affects the release and maturation of activated from the HSP90/GR complex and subsequent GR nuclear translocation.[124] HDAC1 has also been implicated in GR function, as described earlier in relation to GR-GRE retention time,[125] but is also involved in dexamethasone-induced repression of Th2 cytokines via recruitment to the GR-GATA3 complex located on the promoters of Th2 genes.[126] HDAC3 can also modulate GR functions: HDAC3 complexes with silencing mediator for retinoid and thyroid receptors (SMRT) and nuclear receptor corepressor (N-CoR) to obtain full activity and is recruited to GR repressing its transactivation function by the action of the chaperone protein BCL2-associated athanogene 1M (Bag-1M).[127] Recently, SIRT1, a member of the sirtuin family of deacetylases, was reported to act as a major repressor of dexamethasone-induced uncoupling protein-3 (UCP3) expression through deacetylation of the *UCP3* promoter. This effect is indirect through impairing the association of P300 with GR.[128] Histone methyltransferases have also been reported to play a role in GR function.[129]

STAT PROTEINS

Glucocorticosteroid receptors can also interact with the signal transducer and activator of transcription (STAT) family of transcription factors, including STATs 1, 3, and 5, to modulate gene expression.[130] STAT-family members activate a host of inflammatory and acute phase genes under the control of distinct inflammatory stimuli.[131] For example, STAT3 is activated by interferons (IFNs), IL-5, and IL-6 as well as growth factors (e.g., EGF).[131] IL-6 has been increasingly recognized as an important factor in the inflammatory cascade; for example, targeting this cytokine has been a clinically effective strategy in rheumatoid arthritis.[131] IL-6 expression is increased in asthma and thought to be important in asthma pathophysiology,[132] particularly since mast cell–epithelial cell interactions enhance IL-6 expression.[132] IL-6 may be even more important in severe asthma, where sputum IL-6 levels were positively correlated with the Asthma Control Questionnaire and inversely related to forced expiratory volume in 1 second (FEV_1).[132] IL-6 expression is also linked to exacerbations because exposure of human epithelial cells to virus leads to enhanced IL-6 expression.[133] A genome-wide association study in asthmatic patients of European descent reported an association between an IL-6R SNP (rs4129267) and asthma susceptibility.[132] The rs4129267 is in linkage disequilibrium with the IL-6R coding SNP rs2228145, which encodes for the N358A mutation. The minor C allele of rs2228145 was associated with a lower percent FEV_1 predicted, forced vital capacity (FVC), and provocative concentration (PC_{20}) in patients from the Severe Asthma Research Program (SARP) and Collaborative Study on the Genetics of Asthma (CSGA) cohorts.[134] Furthermore, an increased serum level of soluble IL-6R was associated with reduced lung function.[134]

The interaction between activated GR and STAT3 is complex and drives distinct patterns of gene expression.[130] GR tethering to DNA-bound STAT3 results in transcriptional repression of STAT3-activated genes without the loss of STAT3 or P300 DNA binding or the recruitment of the corepressor proteins SMRT and NCoR. These GR-STAT3 repressive sites are linked to the proximity of key inflammatory transcription factors such as AP-1, CREB, forkhead box (FOX), and SP-1, all associated with asthma.[36,66]

In contrast, STAT3 tethering to DNA-bound activated GR results in a synergistic upregulation of gene expression. A similar synergistic enhancement of gene expression is also seen when GR and STAT3 interact through composite or neighboring response elements.[130] DNA binding of both STAT3 and GR occurs predominantly at preset open or regulatory chromatin tagged by an H3K4me1 mark, and neither GR nor STAT3 acts as a pioneer factor.

REGULATION OF MESSENGER RNA STABILITY

The stability of proinflammatory gene mRNAs that contain adenylate-uridylate–rich elements (AREs) within their 3′ untranslated regions are also regulated by GCs[135] (Fig. 99-5). Tristetrapolin (TTP) and other ARE-binding proteins, which promote mRNA decay, and Hu antigen R (HuR) family members, which are associated with mRNA stability, interact with AREs to form messenger ribonucleoprotein complexes.[135] The activity of MAPK14 modulates HuR binding to AREs[135] and evidence suggests that the levels of HuR and TTP are dexamethasone dependent.[135] Dexamethasone therefore can attenuate the levels of COX-2, CCL11, and other ARE-containing inflammatory gene mRNAs through modulation of the MAPK14–MKP-1 axis. However, this is likely to be important for only a subset of inflammatory genes in specific cell types,[135] including airway epithelial cells.[136]

Noncoding MicroRNAs

Less than 2% of the human genome encodes proteins, but a large percentage of genome is transcribed and not translated into functional proteins.[137,138] These noncoding RNAs (ncRNAs) include microRNAs (miRNAs) that are now known to modulate the expression of most cellular pathways through effects on mRNA degradation and translation, depending upon the degree of homology between the specific miRNA and the target mRNA. GR expression is regulated by a number of miRNAs, and in turn GR can modulate the expression miRNAs (Fig. 99-5). In primary rat thymocytes, dexamethasone can induce apoptosis in part through modulating global miRNA expression through downregulation of the key miRNA-processing enzymes Dicer, Drosha, and DGCR8/Pasha.[138] However, dexamethasone has more specific effects on miRNA expression in other cell types.

GR expression and activity (e.g., induction of GILZ expression) is reduced in human neuronal cells by miR-18 and miR-124a.[138] A similar role is seen for miR-18 in the brain of rats.[138] Abnormal expression of miR-18 and miR-124 may be a cause of relative steroid insensitivity in severe asthma.[138] MiR-124 was shown to specifically downregulate GR-α expression, but not GR-β, in human blood lymphocytes.[139] In sepsis patients, hydrocorticosone induced a threefold increase in mi-R124 expression, resulting in downregulation of GR-α expression and a relative steroid insensitivity.[139]

Although the expression of these microRNAs in severe asthma has not been reported, their expression in bronchial epithelial cells from patients with mild asthma is reduced.[140] The expression of nine microRNAs is significantly altered in bronchial epithelial cells of mildly asthmatic patients after 8 weeks of treatment with budesonide (200 μg twice daily).[140] These include four miRNAs that were downregulated (miR-2146, 663a, 1275, 92b-5p) and five upregulated (let-7c, miR-24-3p, 34a-5p, 34b-5p, 34c-5p). Interestingly, miR-34 family members upregulated by budesonide in vivo were downregulated by 14 days of treatment with IL-13 (10 ng/mL) in human bronchial epithelial cells.[140] In contrast, Jardim and colleagues[141] reported that 66 miRNAs were differentially expressed in bronchial epithelial cells of normal and asthmatic subjects. There was minimal overlap in miRNA expression (e.g., miR-18 and miR-92b) in the data sets, which may reflect different severity and treatments in the asthma groups studied.

MicroRNA-145, miR-21, and let-7b regulate abnormal inflammation and airway structural cell function in asthma.[138] In BALB/c mice sensitized and challenged with house-dust mite, inhibition of miR-145 prevented eosinophilia, mucus secretion, and airway hyperresponsiveness (AHR) to the same extent as dexamethasone.[138] Similar antiinflammatory effects were seen with inhibitors of miR-126.[138]

The majority of noncoding RNAs are defined as long ncRNAs (lncRNAs; more than 200 nucleotides), and this class is the least well understood. Long ncRNAs were originally thought to be transcriptional "noise," but it is now clear that they have specific functions, often relating to their conserved secondary structure.[142] More than 3000 novel lncRNAs have been described,[142] and two have opposing effects on GR function. Steroid receptor

RNA activator (SRA) was the first lncRNA to be described in 1999 and is part of the steroid receptor coactivator 1 (SRC-1)/SRC-2 complex. Its structure contains five stem loops that allow the complex to enhance the transcriptional activity of liganded GR.[143] In contrast, growth arrest–specific 5 (GAS-5) can act as a decoy GRE and binds to the DNA-binding site of active GR.[144]

Steroid-refractory Asthma

The failure of inhaled corticosteroids or even oral GCs to suppress inflammation is seen in some patients with severe asthma. These patients present a major health care problem and account for a large percentage of the overall costs for asthma worldwide.[145] These patients should not be confused with those who either do not take their antiinflammatory medication or do not have access to the correct treatments.[145] The inability of corticosteroids to function effectively in refractory asthma has been linked to abnormalities at each stage of GR activation: expression, ligand binding, nuclear translocation, and binding to the GRE[36,37,87,104] (Fig. 99-6).

BIOMARKERS OF STEROID RESPONSIVENESS

Transcriptomic analysis of airway cells is transforming our views on the molecular classification of allergic asthma and monitoring drug responses.[34] For example, microarray analysis

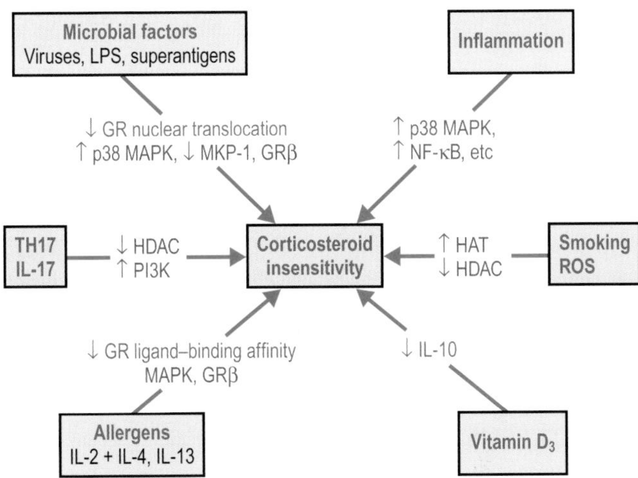

Figure 99-6 Mechanisms implicated in glucocorticosteroid (GC) insensitivity in severe asthma. Infection, oxidative stress (directly or indirectly from cigarette smoking), allergen exposure (leading to Th2 cytokine expression), inflammation (e.g., *IL-17* production from *Th17* and other cells), and a lack of *vitamin D_3* can modulate GC function and are important in patients with severe GC-refractory asthma. These factors affect most aspects of glucocorticosteroid receptor (*GR*) function, such as ligand binding, nuclear translocation, and modulation of gene expression. These effects are mediated through actions on key regulatory pathways, including enhanced (*p38*) mitogen-activated protein kinase (*MAPK*) and reduced MAPK phosphatase-1 (*MKP-1*) activity, increased nuclear factor-κB (*NF-κB*) function, elevated phosphatidylinositol 3-kinase (*PI3K*) function, or reduced *IL-10* expression. The production of IL-10 by GR can be improved by vitamin D_3 supplementation in some patients. A change in histone deacetylase (*HDAC*) and histone acetyltransferase (*HAT*) activity also occurs in some patients. Many of these factors also alter the expression of the dominant negative isoform of GRα, *GRβ*. Drugs that target these abnormal processes or signaling pathways may prove of benefit in patients with severe asthma. *LPS*, Lipopolysaccharide; *ROS*, reactive oxygen species.

of epithelial cells from asthmatic patients has confirmed the presence of distinct subsets of mild/moderate asthma and identified a gene profile in bronchial epithelial cells that predicts drug responsiveness: a high-Th2 phenotype that indicates a GC-responsive asthma group of patients.[146] However, the high-Th2 signature is variable[147] and has also been linked to markers of airway remodeling.[146] High periostin levels, a key part of the Th2 signature, is released from epithelial cells stimulated with IL-13, also distinguishing patients with severe asthma who responded to anti–IL-13 therapy.[148]

When GC enters the cytoplasm, it must bind to GR to enable the release and nuclear translocation of active GR from the inactive chaperone complex.[87] Exposure of T lymphocytes to high levels of cytokines such as IL-2, IL-4, and IL-13 reduced GR affinity. Importantly, these cytokines are expressed at higher levels in a subtype of therapy-refractory asthma patients.[57,102] Overexpression of these cytokines in the airways of severely asthmatic patients may therefore be responsible for localized resistance to GC action and has been associated with an increase in the expression of GR-β[102] and with changes in GR phosphorylation status.[92] For example, IL-2, IL-4, and IL-13 can induce GR phosphorylation under the control of the MAPK14 pathway.[29,149]

The precise mechanisms by which enhanced activation or increased expression of p38 MAPK in the airways of refractory asthma is unclear.[82] but P38 MAPK (MAPK14) inhibitors were able to restore GC sensitivity in peripheral blood cells and BAL macrophages from patients with severe asthma which failed to respond to exogenous GCs.[29,150] For example, the ability of dexamethasone to suppress LPS-induced CCL2, CCL3, CCL5, TNFα, IL-1β, CXCL8, IFNγ, IL-6, IL-10, and GM-CSF release from PBMCs, BAL macrophages and ASM cells of severe treatment refractory asthmatics is compromised in relation to that seen in patients with nonsevere asthma. This has been associated with both enhancement of p38 MAPK activity and alterations in nuclear HDAC and HAT activities. In the latter case, whilst the reduced HDAC activity correlated directly with steroid insensitivity the reduction in HAT activity related to corticosteroid use.[104] Similar results have been reported in children where severity of disease was measured by bronchial hyperresponsiveness.[104]

The expression and activity of MAPK14 is elevated in these patients without directly modulating the expression of inflammatory cytokines released from these cells.[29,150] This data indicates that a combination of MAPK14 inhibitor with an ICS, but neither alone, may be of clinical benefit. Intriguingly, Goleva and colleagues[150] have shown that IFN-γ mimics the effects of MAPK inhibition by restoring GR function. Another mechanism by which MAPK14 may regulate CS sensitivity in human T-cells has also been described. In T-cells, MAPK14-mediated activation of GATA3 can also regulate GR nuclear import.[105]

Phosphorylation of GR on S134 is induced by a number of proinflammatory insults in a P38 MAPK (MAPK14)–dependent manner and significantly alters dexamethasone-dependent genome-wide transcriptional responses and cell functions. S134 phosphorylation enhanced the ability of DNA-bound GR to associate with the adapter protein 14-3-3ζ. Since 14-3-3 proteins have a highly rigid structure, this induces a conformational change in the GR complex, resulting in downregulation of GR responses.[151]

MAPK phosphatase 1 (MKP-1) is responsible for the dephosphorylation and inactivation of MAPK14 and JNK MAPK.

Patients with severe asthma have impaired induction of MKP-1, which results in inappropriate overexpression of MAPK14, compared to patients with nonsevere asthma.[119] A feedback loop involves GR, MAPK14, and MKP-1 in that MKP-1 is a steroid-inducible gene.[119] MKP-1 induction by dexamethasone is unique in that it is driven by GR monomers acting at three GRE-half site motif.[152] MKP-1 expression is also regulated by microRNAs, including miR-110, and its overexpression leads to prolonged MAPK14 and JNK activation. MicroRNA-110 induction is stimulated by many TLR ligands, and in lipopolysaccharide (LPS)–stimulated macrophages, this enhanced expression is blocked by dexamethasone, providing an additional mechanism for steroids and MAPK14 crosstalk.[153] The activity of MAPK14 is enhanced by P300-mediated acetylation to a greater extent than seen with changes in phosphorylation,[154] suggesting that enhanced HAT activity or reduced HDAC activity increases MAPK14 activity.

The precise stimulus to which a cell is exposed can modify the pathways that regulate relative GC refractoriness. Thus, other MAPK inhibitors, particularly those directed against MEK/ERK, have been shown to restore GR function in cells from patients with refractory asthma.[57] Furthermore, cyclin-dependent kinase (CDK), glycogen synthase kinase-3, and JNKs can also target GR phosphorylation or phosphorylation of GR-associated cofactors.[37,82]

Phosphorylation of GR is reversible, under the control of several protein phosphatases, including PP1, PP2A, and PP5, which impact several aspects of GR function. For example, PP5-induced changes in GR phosphorylation modulate expression of subsets of GR-inducible genes in different cell types.[87] PP5 is part of the HSP90/GR complex, and estrogen-induced changes in PP5 expression in breast cancer cells results in GR dephosphorylation and reduced functional responses. Inhibition of PP2A by okadaic acid reduced corticosteroid sensitivity at the level of GR nuclear translocation and was associated with increased GR phosphorylation in U937 monocytic cells. The induction of relative steroid insensitivity induced by IL-2/IL-4 was associated with reduced PP2A expression/activity and was mimicked by PP2A siRNA. In addition, PP2A expression in PBMCs from subjects with severe asthma was reduced compared with that in nonsevere asthma and linked to elevated PP2A Y307 phosphorylation and negatively correlated with GR S226 phosphorylation.[155] Further evidence is needed to confirm whether changes in phosphatase activity occur in primary cells from patients with severe steroid-insensitive asthma.

There is often a divergent response to GCs between $CD4^+$ and $CD8^+$ T cells, resulting in lingering populations of $CD8^+$ cells despite systemic GC treatment.[157] Although the mechanisms of GC actions are the same in both cell types, alternate effects of GC on histone H4 acteylation have been attributed to deficient HAT activity, specifically of ATF2, in the $CD8^+$ cells, resulting in reduced gene silencing.[156] This may account for the differential patterns of gene and microRNA expression seen on peripheral blood $CD8^+$ T cells in patients with severe asthma compared to those with nonsevere asthma.[157] There was a specific reduction in miR-28-5p expression in $CD8^+$ T cells and a reduction of both miR-146a and miR-146b in $CD4^+$ and $CD8^+$ T cells in severe asthma.

Interleukin-17 and Th17 Cells

Neutrophillic asthma, a subset of corticosteroid-refractory asthma, is associated with the enhanced presence of IL-17 and Th17 cells.[52] Th17 cells represent a distinct population of $CD4^+$ T helper cells characterized by IL-17, IL-22, and IL-6 expression under the control of the transcription factor RORγt. The expression of key CXCR2 chemokines, including CXCL1, CXCL6, and CXCL8, along with the neutrophil survival factors GM-CSF and G-CSF, are greatly elevated in airway epithelial cells in response to IL-17. Structural cells also respond to IL-17 by enhancing the production of profibrotic cytokines and extracellular matrix proteins.[159] The expression of inflammatory mediators by viral-stimulated or TNF-α–stimulated epithelial cells is also enhanced by IL-17 exposure.[158] In an ovalbumin challenge model of asthma, the transfer of polarized Th17 cells resulted in a neutrophilic inflammatory response and AHR to metacholine, which was dexamethasone insensitive.[51] IL-17 inhibitory effects on corticosteroid responsiveness have been recapitulated in primary human bronchial epithelial cells.[52] IL-17A pretreatment of cells significantly attenuated the ability of budesonide to inhibit TNF-α–induced CXCL8 production. The mechanism of IL-17A–induced GC insensitivity involved PI3K, reduced HDAC2 expression, and HDAC2 overexpression. These data indicate that IL-17 and Th17 cells may play a major role in severe asthma, and several groups have analyzed IL-17 expression in biologic samples from patients with severe refractory asthma.

Interleukin-17 levels are elevated in sputum and serum from patients with severe asthma, and sputum IL-17 levels correlate with sputum neutrophilia.[52] Furthermore, IL-17 levels, along with IL-9, CCL2, and CCL5 levels, are one of the dominant variables for severely asthmatic patients with intermittent airflow obstruction, as determined by principal component analysis.[159] This supports the results that indicate that serum IL-17 levels greater than 20 pg/mL are an independent risk factor for severe asthma.

The major cellular site of IL-17 expression is still unclear. Although infiltrating cells as the predominant site of IL-17A expression in severe asthma was not confirmed, increased IL-17F expression in the epithelium was confirmed in patients with severe asthma. In addition, evidence was limited at best that the numbers of IL-17A–positive and IL-17F–positive cells correlated with neutrophilic inflammation, although submucosal eosinophils correlated with IL-17F–positive cells.[52]

ASTHMA EXACERBATIONS AND STEROID SENSITIVITY

Viral infections are associated with up to 80% of asthma exacerbations in children and adults. Rhinovirus (RV) is the most frequently identified virus in natural asthma exacerbations and can exacerbate asthma symptoms in a human experimental model. RV infection worsens the inflammation observed in both the upper and the lower airway of asthmatic patients. This heightened postinfection inflammatory response remains despite antiinflammatory treatment. Several studies show that high doses of inhaled or systemic GCs are ineffective in treating or preventing virus-induced acute asthma exacerbations, particularly in children.[160] Viral infection produces similar steroid-refractory inflammation in experimental models of asthmatic exacerbations; neither inhaled corticosteroid[161] nor oral prednisolone[162] prevents the worsening of airway inflammation or improves clinical symptoms. In addition, cytokine production in nasal lavage during experimental RV infection of asthmatic patients is not affected by budesonide.[160] The mechanisms making corticosteroid treatment ineffective against viral infections are unclear, although steroid-insensitive respiratory syncytial virus (RSV) infection is replication dependent and NF-κB independent. In these studies, RSV infection of primary human airway epithelial cells prevented the maximal induction of the GR-inducible genes GILZ, FK506-binding protein (FKBP),[51] and MKP-1 at the level of preventing GR DNA binding.[163]

Principal component analysis indicated that IFN-γ was one of the dominant variables for chronic persistent obstruction in severe asthma.[159] Viral infection results in the elevated expression of IFN-γ and IFN-γ–inducible genes. The presence of inflammatory mediators such as TNF-α along with IFN-γ can induce relative GC insensitivity despite the same genes being steroid sensitive when induced by other stimuli.[164] The transcription factor interferon regulatory factor (IRF) is activated by IFN-γ, and its overexpression in human ASM cells leads to attenuation of GR function, possibly caused by competition for limiting amounts of the transcriptional coregulator GRIP-1.[165] GRIP-1 forms a coactivating complex with phosphorylated GR that enables induction of several antiinflammatory genes as well as the repression of inflammatory genes. GRIP-1/IRF-1 interaction is associated with the production of RANTES and CD38 as well as other inflammatory genes. IRF-1 is able to pull GRIP-1 from the GR complex and prevent full GR function; conversely, overexpression of GRIP-1 restores steroid responsiveness in TNF-α/IFN-γ–stimulated cells. These results suggest that GR function depends on relative GRIP-1 levels and may regulate steroid insensitivity in patients with severe asthma.[165] GRIP-1 expression in severe asthma needs to be determined.

Role of Superantigen

Intrinsic and extrinsic asthma have similar pathologic features, and IgE synthesis has been found in the airways of patients with intrinsic asthma despite negative skin-prick tests and low serum-specific IgE. Microbial superantigens, particularly staphylococcal enterotoxins, are probably more important in amplifying inflammation in intrinsic asthma than driving asthma itself. Colonization of airway epithelial cells by staphylococci and other superantigen-producing microbes leads to the local production of specific IgE as well as polyclonal IgE. Specific IgE antibodies against staphylococcal enterotoxins are present in patients with severe asthma and are able to sensitize mast cells and DCs, activate mast cells, and induce clonal expansion of T cells and suppression of Treg cells.[166]

The presence of antinuclear antigens (ANAs) in severely asthmatic patients was associated with severe exacerbations and high ICS intake (annual decline in FEV_1 greater than 100 mL in one small study)[167] as well as death. Autoantibodies against α-enolase protein have also been associated with severe asthma, particularly in female patients with late-onset severe asthma. These antibodies were IgG1 in nature, which may be implicated in complement activation in these patients.

Staphylococcal enterotoxin B can drive neutrophilic inflammation in severe asthma by stimulating Th17 cells.[168] Staphylococcal superantigens may also inhibit the immunosuppressive activity of Treg cells and may therefore amplify the activity of Th2 cells and $CD8^+$ cells.[169] Superantigens can induce corticosteroid resistance by activating the ERK/MAPK pathway either through increasing expression of GR-β or by affecting GR-α phosphorylation status. In either case, CS responsiveness was restored by coincubation with a selective ERK inhibitor.[170] In addition, activation of DCs obtained from patients with systemic lupus erythematosus (SLE) through TLR7 and TLR9 can reduce the ability of dexamethasone to attenuate NF-κB activation and DC death and subsequent attenuation of IFN-α levels.[171]

Regulatory T Cells and Vitamin D_3

Glucocorticosteroids induce the antiinflammatory gene *IL-10*, particularly in Treg cells, thereby inhibiting cytokine secretion by allergen-specific Th2 cells.[87] The ability of dexamethasone to induce IL-10 by these cells is impaired in some patients with severe steroid-refractory asthma.[165] Vitamin D_3 (calcitriol) was able to increase the secretion of IL-10 from Treg cells isolated from steroid-refractory patients up to levels seen in cells from patients with nonsevere asthma after dexamethasone therapy alone.[50] Furthermore, treatment of three patients with severe steroid-refractory asthma with vitamin D_3 supplementation restored the T cell IL-10 response to dexamethasone, suggesting this might be a useful therapeutic approach. Therefore, low dietary intake of vitamin D or lack of sunlight might contribute to reduced GC responses in inflammatory disease.

Children with severe therapy-resistant asthma have reduced serum levels of vitamin D compared with children with mild asthma and controls, which correlated with percent FEV_1 predicted.[172] There was also a positive correlation with asthma control scores (ACT test) and an inverse correlation with exacerbations and ICS use.[173] An inverse relationship was also seen between serum vitamin D_3 levels and both ASM mass and bronchodilator reversibility, indicating that vitamin D_3 supplementation may be useful in pediatric patients with severe therapy-resistant asthma.[173] The mechanisms underlying this process in vivo include increasing the frequency of both Tregs and upregulating the expression of CD200 on peripheral blood human $CD4^+$ T cells, a cell surface immunoglobulin-like molecule expressed by immune cells that dampens inflammatory cell activity.[50]

Reactive Oxygen Species

Oxidative stress levels are higher in patients with refractory asthma than in those with nonsevere asthma and controls. Oxidative stresses such as hydrogen peroxide (H_2O_2) have been shown to reduce GR translocation in primary human airway fibroblasts.[173] This suggests that in addition to enhancing the inflammatory response in severe asthma, oxidative stress may also modulate corticosteroid action in both patients with severe treatment-refractory asthma and in smoking asthmatic patients. Antioxidants should therefore be of benefit in these patients by enhancing GR nuclear translocation.[36,37] This may be one mechanism by which the combination of ICS and LABA significantly enhances GR nuclear translocation above that seen with ICS alone both in vitro and in vivo.[73]

Activator protein 1 is a redox-sensitive transcription factor whose expression and activity are increased in PBMCs from patients with severe steroid-refractory asthma compared to those from nonsevere asthmatics.[174] AP-1 is generally found as a FOS/JUN heterodimer[170] and is involved in the regulation of the expression of many asthma-relevant inflammatory genes, including *IL-5*, *GM-CSF*, and *TNF-α*, through the JNK-MAPK pathway.[173] As with NF-κB, AP-1 forms a mutually repressive complex with GR and has been implicated in corticosteroid resistance.[87] JNK activity is higher and FOS expression is greater in PBMCs and bronchial biopsies from patients with corticosteroid-resistant asthma.[57] Furthermore, there is no reduction in JNK activity or JUN expression in PBMCs and biopsies from patients with corticosteroid-resistant asthma after high doses of oral GCs.[164]

The induction of nitric oxide synthase (NOS) and subsequently increased exhaled NO levels seen in severe asthma[175] may be a consequence of enhanced ROS production.[173] NO reacts with critical SH groups on GR, which leads to nitrosylation of both GR and GR-associated cofactors, resulting in reduced ligand binding and affinity. However, this may be selective because enhancing GR nitrosylaton using the NO-donating steroid NCX-1080 enhances GR function. Conversion of NO to peroxinitrate in smoking asthmatic patients may also result in even greater steroid insensitivity because of the more profound oxidant effects of peroxynitrite.[173] Increased formation of peroxynitrite results in nitration of specific tyrosine residues on HDAC2, resulting in its rapid inactivation (Y146), ubiquitination, and degradation (Y253).[176] In addition, C262 and C274 S-nitrosylation of HDAC2 has been shown to affect its association with chromatin and may also contribute to reduced GR function.[177]

However, reduced HDAC2 expression or activity is not seen in all patients with therapy-refractory asthma, possibly reflecting the heterogeneity of severe asthma phenotype.[33] HDAC2 has been shown to be important in GR-mediated repression of inflammatory genes such as *GM-CSF* and *CXCL8*,.[97] and its expression and activity are decreased in smokers with asthma, some severely asthmatic patients, COPD patients,[179] and those with cystic fibrosis,[179] all steroid refractory. In addition, a negative correlation exists between the repressive effect of dexamethasone on cytokine production and total HDAC activity in alveolar macrophages from smokers and nonsmokers.[82]

Although overexpression of HDAC2 (but not HDAC1) enhances dexamethasone responsiveness toward suppressing LPS-induced GM-CSF release in primary macrophages from COPD patients,[97] similar experiments have not been performed in cells from patients with severe corticosteroid-refractory asthma. Recent evidence suggests a link between GR-β and HDAC2 in patients with severe steroid-insensitive asthma.[120] Thus, increased GR-β expression selectively reduces HDAC2 and can prevent GR-α–induced enhancement of HDAC2 promoter reporter gene activity in a concentration-dependent manner. Treatment options for the restoration of HDAC2 may include the bronchodilator theophylline, which has been used in vitro to restore HDAC2 activity in cells[179] and in COPD patients.[180] Generic theophylline can help restore GC sensitivity at least in smoking asthmatic patients.[178,181]

Other related pathways are also activated by oxidative stress, including the phosphatidylinositol 3-kinase-δ (PI3Kδ) pathway, which also leads to the inactivation of HDAC2 via an effect of HDAC2 phosphorylation. Pharmacologic and genetic inhibition of PI3Kδ, but not PI3Kγ, restored dexamethasone functions in animal models and ex vivo studies under conditions where steroids alone were ineffective.[91,182]

CLINICAL IMPLICATIONS

In the future, unbiased cluster analysis of large, complex datasets from patients with severe treatment-refractory asthma will likely reveal key pathways involved in the inflammatory profile observed in these patients that may indicate novel therapeutic targets.[183] The subset of asthmatic patients whose smoking habit drives disease severity and GC insensitivity should be encouraged to quit smoking, thereby reducing their oxidant load.[173] Currently, evidence shows that subsets of patients with severe treatment-insensitive disease will respond to specific antiinflammatory agents, including anti–IL-5,[40,41] anti–IL-13,[148] and JAK/STAT inhibitors.[184] However, many of these new, single-mediator approaches, such as anti–TNF-α have not proved successful in clinical trials in severe asthma as hoped compared with their efficacy in other chronic inflammatory diseases, such as rheumatoid arthritis.[36,185]

In these patients an alternative strategy is to restore the ability of steroids to suppress the inflammatory response that has been rendered defective (see Fig. 99-6). The results of experiments conducted in vitro, ex vivo, and in vivo implicate several inflammatory mediators and signaling pathways in driving the molecular defects in GR activation associated with severe treatment-refractory asthma (Table 99-4). Activation or overexpression of many of these mediators and pathways results in enzyme-mediated PTMs of GR or GR-associated proteins. These processes therefore make attractive targets to enable enhancement or restoration of steroid sensitivity in these patients. Thus the presence of high levels of IL-2 and IL-4, oxidative stress, and various infectious agents that activate MAPK and PI3K pathways (e.g., modulate GR function) could be reduced by using anticytokine approaches or small-molecule inhibitors. An additional benefit may be further direct suppression of some aspects of the inflammatory response by the drug alone in the absence of ICS. Clinical trials examining the benefit of ICS along with a MAPK14 inhibitor, for example, may produce enhanced antiinflammatory effects and clinical benefit with reduced side effects from both drugs, although actions on feedback pathways that divert the inflammatory drive to other signaling pathways slow the development of these compounds.[30] Anti–IL-2 has clinical efficacy in patients with severe inflammatory bowel disease despite ongoing high-dose steroid treatment.[104] Placebo-controlled studies in patients with severe asthma may therefore be warranted.

It is essential to develop noninvasive biomarkers for aberrant pathway activation and for discerning which components of the GR activation cascade are abnormal so that future treatments can be tailored to address these specific issues. For example, periostin may be used as a biomarker for patients with severe refractory asthma who may be responsive to anti–IL-13.[148] FK501-binding protein is another potential biomarker for GC responsiveness.[186]

Infection, whether bacterial or viral, may also affect GC responsiveness.[163] Thus, LPS levels are considerably higher in BAL fluid of patients with severe steroid-insensitive asthma than in steroid-sensitive asthmatic patients, and prolonged exposure to LPS can induce relative dexamethasone insensitivity in human monocytes.[187] In addition, exposure to superantigen can induce a relative steroid insensitivity in human T cells.[170] This effect requires the presence of antigen-presenting cells and is mediated through ERK-induced GR phosphorylation and loss of GR nuclear translocation. Rhinovirus infection can also attenuate GR nuclear translocation and suppression of inflammatory cytokine release from primary human epithelial cells in an NF-κB–dependent manner.[188] These data suggest that antiinfective agents may also be beneficial in patients with severe disease.

There is increasing evidence for an autoimmune component in asthma,[189] which may be important in relation to steroid

TABLE 99-4 Mediators and Pathways in Glucocorticosteroid Receptor (GR) Function

Mediators/Pathways	References
MEDIATORS	
Infection/Toll-like receptor (TLR) agonists	Bellattato et al,[189] 2003; Goleva et al,[188] 2008; Guiducci et al,[172] 2010; Hinzey et al,[164] 2011; Li et al,[171] 2004
Interleukin-2 (IL-2), IL-4	Ito et al,[57] 2006; Kam et al,[a] 1993; Kino et al,[102] 2009
Interferon-γ (IFN-γ)	Bhandare et al,[166] 2010; Goleva et al,[151] 2009; Tliba et al,[b] 2008; Tudhope et al,[c] 2007
Oxidative stress	Okamoto et al,[d] 1999; Kirkham and Rahman,[e] 2006
Vitamin D_3	Xystrakis et al,[f] 2006; Gupta et al,[173] 2011
SIGNALING PATHWAYS	
Cyclin-dependent kinase 1 (CDK1)	Adcock and Barnes,[74] 2008; Luecke and Yamamoto,[123] 2005
GSK3β	Adcock and Barnes,[74] 2008; Roth and Black,[g] 2006
Interferon regulatory factor 1 (IRF-1)	Bhandare et al,[166] 2010
Histone deacetylase 2 (HDAC2)	Adcock et al,[82] 2006; Aoyagi and Archer,[h] 2005; Bhavsar et al,[i] 2008; Hew et al,[j] 2006; Ito et al,[k,97] 2005, 2006; Kovacs et al,[124] 2005; Li et al,[81,120] 2007, 2010; Marwick et al,[91] 2009; Nott et al,[178] 2008; Osoata et al,[177] 2009; Su et al,[l] 2009; To et al,[183] 2010; Wang et al,[m,n] 2008, 2009; Zylstra et al,[o] 2011
Mitogen-activated protein kinase (MAPK) pathways (p38, JNK, ERK/MEK)	Bhavsar et al,[29] 2009; D'Elia et al,[p] 2010; Goleva et al,[151] 2009; Loke et al,[q] 2006; Kent et al,[r] 2009; Maneechotesuwan et al,[105] 2009
Phosphatases PP1, PP2A, PP5	Beck et al,[87] 2009; Zhang et al,[s] 2009
Phosphatidylinositol 3-kinase (PI3K)	Marwick et al,[91] 2009; To et al,[183] 2010; Zylstra et al,[o] 2011
Redox-sensitive transcription factors (e.g., NF-κB)	Ito et al, 2006;[57,97] Leung et al,[111] 2004; Loke et al,[q] 2006; Roth and Black,[g] 2006

ERK, Extracellular signal–regulated kinase; *GSK,* glycogen synthase kinase; *JNK,* JUN N-terminal kinase; *MEK,* mitogen-activated protein kinase/extracellular signal–regulated kinase kinase; *NF-κB,* nuclear factor-κB; *PP,* protein phosphatase.

[a]Kam JC, Szefler SJ, Surs W, et al. Combination IL-2 and IL-4 reduces glucocorticoid receptor–binding affinity and T cell response to glucocorticoids. J Immunol 1993;151:3460; [b]Tliba OG, Damera A, Banerjee SGu, et al. Cytokines induce an early steroid resistance in airway smooth muscle cells: novel role of interferon regulatory factor-1. Am J Respir Cell Mol Biol 2008;38:463-72; [c]Tudhope SJ, Catley MC, Fenwick PS, et al. The role of IkappaB kinase 2, but not activation of NF-kappaB, in the release of CXCR3 ligands from IFN-gamma-stimulated human bronchial epithelial cells. J Immunol 2007;179:6237-45; [d]Okamoto KH, Tanaka H, Ogawa Y, et al. Redox-dependent regulation of nuclear import of the glucocorticoid receptor. J Biol Chem 1999;274:10363-71; [e]Kirkham P, Rahman I. Oxidative stress in asthma and COPD: antioxidants as a therapeutic strategy. Pharmacol Ther 2006;111:476-94; [f]Xystrakis E, Kusumakar S, Boxwell S, et al. Reversing the defective induction of IL-10-secreting regulatory T cells in in glucocorticoid-resistant asthma patients. J Clin Invest 2006;116:146-55; [g]Roth M, Black JL. Transcription factors in asthma: are transcription factors a new target for asthma therapy? Curr Drug Targets 2006;7:589-95; [h]Aoyagi S, Archer TK. Modulating molecular chaperone Hsp90 functions through reversible acetylation. Trends Cell Biol 2005;15:565-7; [i]Bhavsar P, Hew M, Khorasani N, et al. Relative corticosteroid insensitivity of alveolar macrophages in severe asthma compared to non-severe asthma. Thorax 2008;63:784-90; [j]Hew M, Bhavsar P, Torrego A, et al. Relative corticosteroid insensitivity of peripheral blood mononuclear cells in severe asthma. Am J Respir Crit Care Med 2006;174:134-41; [k]Ito K, Ito M, Elliott WM, et al. Decreased histone deacetylase activity in chronic obstructive pulmonary disease. N Engl J Med 2005;352:1967-76; [l]Su RC, Becker AB, Kozyrskyj AL, Hayglass KT. Altered epigenetic regulation and increasing severity of bronchial hyperresponsiveness in atopic asthmatic children. J Allergy Clin Immunol 2009;124:1116-8; [m]Wang ZC, Zang JA, Rosenfeld DE, et al. Combinatorial patterns of histone acetylations and methylations in the human genome. Nat Genet 2008;40:897-903; [n]Wang ZC, Zang K, Cui DE, et al. Genome-wide mapping of HATs and HDACs reveals distinct functions in active and inactive genes. Cell 2009;138:1019-31; [o]Ziljstra JG, ten Hacken NH, Hoffmann RF, Van Oosterhout AJ, Heijink IH. IL-17A induces glucocorticoid insensitivity in human bronchial epithelial cells. Eur Respir J 2012;39:439-45; [p]D'Elia M, Patenaude J, Dupras C, Bernier J. T cells from burn-injured mice demonstrate a loss of sensitivity to glucocorticoids. Am J Physiol Endocrinol Metab 2010;299:E299-E307; [q]Loke TK, Mallett KH, Ratoff J, et al. Systemic glucocorticoid reduces bronchial mucosal activation of activator protein 1 components in glucocorticoid-sensitive but not glucocorticoid-resistant asthmatic patients. J Allergy Clin Immunol 2006;118:368-75; [r]Kent LM, Smyth LJ, Plumb J, et al. Inhibition of lipopolysaccharide-stimulated chronic obstructive pulmonary disease macrophage inflammatory gene expression by dexamethasone and the p38 mitogen-activated protein kinase inhibitor N-cyano-N'-(2-{[8-(2,6-difluorophenyl)-4-(4-fluoro-2-methylphenyl)-7-oxo-7,8-dihy dropyrido[2,3-d] pyrimidin-2-yl]amino}ethyl)guanidine (SB706504). J Pharmacol Exp Ther 2009,328:458-68; [s]Zhang Y, Leung DY, Nordeen SK, Goleva E. Estrogen inhibits glucocorticoid action via protein phosphatase 5 (PP5)-mediated glucocorticoid receptor dephosphorylation. J Biol Chem 2009;284:24542-52.

responsiveness, because many autoimmune diseases such as systemic lupus erythematosus (SLE) are relatively steroid insensitive.[171] Stimulation of TLR7 and TLR9 on DCs by self DNA can attenuate the ability of steroids to suppress NF-κB–mediated IFN-α production in vitro and in vivo, and blockade of these receptors may improve GC function.

Summary

Although GCs remain the optimal treatment for asthmatic patients, a significant subpopulation still does not benefit from GC effects. This apparently heterogeneous population does not respond to GCs for various reasons; genetic factors, behavior, and environmental risk appear to play a role. Better understanding of the molecular mechanisms of GC-refractory asthma should identify new targets (kinases, inflammatory mediators) for inhibition to restore responsiveness in at least in some of these patients. Epigenetics is involved in many areas of GC function and perhaps in the development of allergy and asthma, offering better understanding and treatment or even cure for these theoretically preventable environmental diseases.

Acknowledgment

Research in the authors' laboratories is supported by the EU (IMI), MRC (UK), Wellcome Trust, BBSRC, NERC, NIH, and by Asthma UK. The authors have no conflicts of interest. IMA and KFC are principal investigators in the MRC/Asthma UK Centre for Asthma and Allergic Mechanisms and are supported by the NIHR Respiratory Disease Biomedical Research Unit at the Royal Brompton and Harefield NHS Foundation Trust and Imperial College London.

REFERENCES

Introduction

1. Magiakou MA, Chrousos GP. Cushing's syndrome in children and adolescents: current diagnostic and therapeutic strategies. J Endocrinol.Invest 2002;25:181-94.
2. Barnes PJ, Adcock IM. How do corticosteroids work in asthma? Ann Intern Med 2003;139:359-70.
3. Raju TN. The Nobel chronicles. Edward Calvin Kendall (1886-1972); Philip Showalter Hench (1896-1965); and Tadeus Reichstein (1897-996). Lancet 1950:1999;353:1370.
4. Barnes PJ. How corticosteroids control inflammation. Quintiles Prize Lecture 2005. Br J Pharmacol 2006;148:245-54.
5. Gibbs JE, Blaikley J, Beesley S, et al. The nuclear receptor REV-ERBα mediates circadian regulation of innate immunity through selective regulation of inflammatory cytokines. Proc Natl Acad Sci USA 2012;109:582-7.
6. Farrow SN, Solari R, Willson TM. The importance of chronobiology to drug discovery. Expert Opin Drug Discov 2012;7:535-41.

Chemical Structure

7. Johnson M. Pharmacodynamics and pharmacokinetics of inhaled glucocorticoids. J Allergy Clin Immunol 1996;97:169-76.
8. Hochhaus G, Druzgala P, Hochhaus R, Huang MJ, Bodor N. Glucocorticoid activity and structure activity relationships in a series of some novel 17α-ether-substituted steroids: influence of 17α-substituents. Drug Des Discov 1991;8:117-25.
9. Bledsoe RK, Montana VG, Stanley TB, et al. Crystal structure of the glucocorticoid receptor ligand binding domain reveals a novel mode of receptor dimerization and coactivator recognition. Cell 2002;110:93-105.
10. Schacke H, Berger M, Rehwinkel H, Asadullah K. Selective glucocorticoid receptor agonists (SEGRAs): novel ligands with an improved therapeutic index. Mol Cell Endocrinol 2007;275:109-17.
11. Uings IJ, Farrow SN. A pharmacological approach to enhancing the therapeutic index of corticosteroids in airway inflammatory disease. Curr Opin Pharmacol 2005;5:221-6.

Pharmacokinetics

12. O'Connor D, Adams WP, Chen ML, et al. Role of pharmacokinetics in establishing bioequivalence for orally inhaled drug products: workshop summary report. J.Aerosol Med Pulm Drug Deliv 2011;24:119-35.
13. Winkler J, Hochhaus G, Derendorf H. How the lung handles drugs: pharmacokinetics and pharmacodynamics of inhaled corticosteroids. Proc Am Thorac Soc 2004;1:356-63.
14. Umland SP, Schleimer RP, Johnston SL. Review of the molecular and cellular mechanisms of action of glucocorticoids for use in asthma. Pulm Pharmacol Ther 2002;15:35-50.
15. Schleimer RP. Glucocorticoids suppress inflammation but spare innate immune responses in airway epithelium. Proc Am Thorac Soc 2004;1:222-30.
16. Barnes PJ. Corticosteroids: the drugs to beat. Eur J Pharmacol 2006;533:2-14.
17. Shaw RJ. Inhaled corticosteroids for adult asthma: impact of formulation and delivery device on relative pharmacokinetics, efficacy and safety. Respir Med 1999;93:149-60.
18. Schacke H, Docke WD, Asadullah K. Mechanisms involved in the side effects of glucocorticoids. Pharmacol Ther 2002;96:23-43.
19. Usmani OS, Biddiscombe MF, Barnes PJ. Regional lung deposition and bronchodilator response as a function of β_2-agonist particle size. Am J Respir Crit Care Med 2005;172:1497-504.
20. Pretorius E, Wallner B, Marx J. Cortisol resistance in conditions such as asthma and the involvement of 11β-HSD-2: a hypothesis. Horm Metab Res 2006;38:368-76.
21. Edsbacker S, Brattsand R. Budesonide fatty-acid esterification: a novel mechanism prolonging binding to airway tissue—review of available data. Ann Allergy Asthma Immunol 2002;88:609-16.
22. Derendorf H. Pharmacokinetic and pharmacodynamic properties of inhaled ciclesonide. J Clin.Pharmacol 2007;47:782-9.

Side Effects

23. Zhang N, Truong-Tran QA, Tancowny B, Harris KE, Schleimer RP. Glucocorticoids enhance or spare innate immunity: effects in airway epithelium are mediated by CCAAT/enhancer binding proteins. J Immunol 2007;179:578-89.
24. Barnes PJ. Inhaled glucocorticoids for asthma. N Engl J Med 1995;332:868-75.
25. Barnes PJ, Pedersen S, Busse WW. Efficacy and safety of inhaled corticosteroids: new developments. Am J Respir Crit Care Med 1998;157(3 Pt 2):S1-53.
26. Sirois F. Steroid psychosis: a review. Gen Hosp Psych 2003;25:27-33.
27. Fietta P, Fietta P, Delsante G. Central nervous system effects of natural and synthetic glucocorticoids. Psychiatry Clin Neurosci 2009;63:613-22.
28. Kanniess F, Richter K, Bohme S, Jorres RA, Magnussen H. Effect of inhaled ciclesonide on airway responsiveness to inhaled AMP, the composition of induced sputum and exhaled nitric oxide in patients with mild asthma. Pulm Pharmacol Ther 2001;14:141-7.
29. Bhavsar P, Khorasani N, Hew M, Johnson M, Chung KF. Effect of p38 MAPK inhibition on corticosteroid suppression of cytokine release in severe asthma. Eur Respir J 2010;35:750-6.
30. Chung KF. p38 mitogen-activated protein kinase pathways in asthma and COPD. Chest 2011;139:1470-9.
31. Holgate ST, Arshad HS, Roberts GC, et al. A new look at the pathogenesis of asthma. Clin Sci Lond 2010;118:439-50.
32. Haldar P, Pavord ID, Shaw DE, et al. Cluster analysis and clinical asthma phenotypes. Am J Respir Crit Care Med 2008;178:218-24.
33. Moore WC, Meyers DA, Wenzel SE, et al. Identification of asthma phenotypes using cluster analysis in the Severe Asthma Research Program. Am J Respir Crit Care Med 2010;181:315-23.
34. Woodruff PG, Boushey HA, Dolganov GM, et al. Genome-wide profiling identifies epithelial cell genes associated with asthma and with treatment response to corticosteroids. Proc Natl Acad Sci USA 2007;104:15858-63.
35. Chung KF, Caramori G, Adcock IM. Inhaled corticosteroids as combination therapy with β-adrenergic agonists in airways disease: present and future. Eur J Clin Pharmacol 2009;65:853-71.
36. Adcock IM, Caramori G, Chung KF. New targets for drug development in asthma. Lancet 2008;372(9643):1073-87.
37. Barnes PJ, Adcock IM. Glucocorticoid resistance in inflammatory diseases. Lancet 2009;373(9678):1905-17.
38. Giembycz MA, Lindsay MA. Pharmacology of the eosinophil. Pharmacol Rev 1999;51:213-340.
39. Leckie MJ, ten Brinke A, Khan J, et al. Effects of an interleukin-5 blocking monoclonal antibody on eosinophils, airway hyperresponsiveness, and the late asthmatic response. Lancet 2000;356(9248):2144-8.
40. Haldar P, Brightling CE, Hargadon B, et al. Mepolizumab and exacerbations of refractory eosinophilic asthma. N Engl J Med 2009;360:973-84.
41. Nair P, Pizzichini MM, Kjarsgaard M, et al. Mepolizumab for prednisone-dependent asthma with sputum eosinophilia. N Engl J Med 2009;360:985-93.
42. Pavord ID, Korn S, Howarth P, et al. Mepolizumab for severe eosinophilic asthma (DREAM): a multicentre, double-blind, placebo-controlled trial. Lancet 2012;380(9842):651-9.
43. Uller L, Lloyd CM, Rydell-Tormanen K, Persson CG, Erjefalt JS. Effects of steroid treatment on lung CC chemokines, apoptosis and transepithelial cell clearance during development and resolution of allergic airway inflammation. Clin Exp Allergy 2006;36:111-21.
44. Hallett JM, Leitch AE, Riley NA, et al. Novel pharmacological strategies for driving inflammatory cell apoptosis and enhancing the resolution of inflammation. Trends Pharmacol Sci 2008;29:250-7.
45. Nakagawa M, Terashima T, D'yachkova Y, et al. Glucocorticoid-induced granulocytosis: contribution of marrow release and demargination of intravascular granulocytes. Circulation 1998;98:2307-13.
46. Rhen T, Cidlowski JA: Antiinflammatory action of glucocorticoids: new mechanisms for old drugs. N Engl J Med 2005;353:1711-23.
47. Eberhart K, Rainer J, Bindreither D, et al. Glucocorticoid-induced alterations in mitochondrial membrane properties and respiration in childhood acute lymphoblastic leukemia. Biochim Biophys Acta 2011;1807:719-25.
48. Psarra AM, Sekeris CE. Glucocorticoids induce mitochondrial gene transcription in HepG2 cells: role of the mitochondrial glucocorticoid receptor. Biochim Biophys Acta 2011;1813:1814-21.
49. Vasavda N, Eichholtz T, Takahashi A, et al. Expression of nonmuscle cofilin-1 and steroid responsiveness in severe asthma. J Allergy Clin Immunol 2006;118:1090-6.
50. Urry Z, Chambers ES, Xystrakis E, et al. The role of 1α,25-dihydroxyvitamin D_3 and cytokines in the promotion of distinct $Foxp3^+$ and $IL\text{-}10^+$ $CD4^+$ T cells. Eur J Immunol 2012;42:2697-708.
51. McKinley L, Alcorn JF, Peterson A, et al. TH17 cells mediate steroid-resistant airway inflammation and airway hyperresponsiveness in mice. J Immunol 2008;181:4089-97.
52. Zijlstra GJ, ten Hacken NH, Hoffmann RF, van Oosterhout AJ, Heijink IH. IL-17A induces glucocorticoid insensitivity in human bronchial epithelial cells. Eur Respir J 2012;39:439-45.

53. Holgate ST, Holloway J, Wilson S, et al. Understanding the pathophysiology of severe asthma to generate new therapeutic opportunities. J Allergy Clin Immunol 2006;117: 496-506.
54. Donnelly LE, Barnes PJ. Defective phagocytosis in airways disease. Chest 2012;141:1055-62.
55. Lambrecht BN, Hammad H. Lung dendritic cells in respiratory viral infection and asthma: from protection to immunopathology. Annu Rev Immunol 2012;30:243-70.
56. Martinon F, Mayor A, Tschopp J. The inflammasomes: guardians of the body. Annu Rev Immunol 2009:27:229-65.
57. Ito K, Chung KF, Adcock IM. Update on glucocorticoid action and resistance. J Allergy Clin Immunol 2006;117:522-43.
58. Hodrea J, Majai G, Doro Z, et al. The glucocorticoid dexamethasone programs human dendritic cells for enhanced phagocytosis of apoptotic neutrophils and inflammatory response. J Leukoc Biol 2012;91:127-36.
59. Amin K. The role of mast cells in allergic inflammation. Respir Med 2012;106:9-14.
60. Voehringer D. Basophils in allergic immune responses. Curr Opin Immunol 2011;23: 789-93.
61. Kato A, Schleimer RP. Beyond inflammation: airway epithelial cells are at the interface of innate and adaptive immunity. Curr Opin Immunol 2007;19:711-20.
62. Proud D, Leigh R. Epithelial cells and airway diseases. Immunol Rev 2011;242:186-204.
63. Chen Y, Watson AM, Williamson CD, et al. Glucocorticoid receptor and histone deacetylase-2 mediate dexamethasone-induced repression of MUC5AC gene expression. Am J Respir Cell Mol Biol 2012;47:637-44.
64. Sweet D, Bevilacqua G, Carnielli V, et al. European consensus guidelines on the management of neonatal respiratory distress syndrome. Working Group on Prematurity of World Association of Perinatal Medicine, European Association of Perinatal Medicine. J Perinat Med 2007;35:175-86.
65. Chung KF. The role of airway smooth muscle in the pathogenesis of airway wall remodeling in chronic obstructive pulmonary disease. Proc Am Thorac Soc 2005;2:347-54.
66. Clifford RL, Coward WR, Knox AJ, John AE. Transcriptional regulation of inflammatory genes associated with severe asthma. Curr Pharm Des 2011;17:653-66.
67. Chang PJ, Bhavsar PK, Michaeloudes C, Khorasani N, Chung KF. Corticosteroid insensitivity of chemokine expression in airway smooth muscle of patients with severe asthma. J Allergy Clin Immunol 2012;130:877-85.
68. Lee CG, Ma B, Takyar S, et al. Studies of vascular endothelial growth factor in asthma and chronic obstructive pulmonary disease. Proc Am Thorac Soc 2011;8:512-15.
69. Schmuth M, Watson RE, Deplewski D, et al. Nuclear hormone receptors in human skin. Horm Metab Res 2007;39:96-105.
70. Barnes PJ. Beta-adrenergic receptors and their regulation. Am J Respir Crit Care Med 1995; 152:838-60.
71. Holden NS, Bell MJ, Rider CF, et al. β_2-Adrenoceptor agonist-induced RGS2 expression is a genomic mechanism of bronchoprotection that is enhanced by glucocorticoids. Proc Natl Acad Sci USA 2011;108: 19713-18.
72. Johnson M. Interactions between corticosteroids and beta2-agonists in asthma and chronic obstructive pulmonary disease. Proc Am Thorac Soc 2004;1:200-6.
73. Usmani OS, Ito K, Maneechotesuwan K, et al. Glucocorticoid receptor nuclear translocation in airway cells after inhaled combination therapy. Am J Respir Crit Care Med 2005;172: 704-12.

Arachidonic Acid Metabolites

74. Back M, Dahlen SE, Drazen JM, et al. Leukotriene receptor nomenclature, distribution, and pathophysiological functions. International Union of Basic and Clinical Pharmacology. Pharmacol Rev 2011;63:539-84.
75. Dahlen SE. Treatment of asthma with antileukotrienes: first line or last resort therapy? Eur J Pharmacol 2006;533:40-56.
76. Serhan CN, Petasis NA. Resolvins and protectins in inflammation resolution. Chem Rev 2011;111:5922-43.
77. Schif-Zuck S, Gross N, Assi S, et al. Saturated-efferocytosis generates pro-resolving CD11b low macrophages: modulation by resolvins and glucocorticoids. Eur J Immunol 2011;41: 366-79.

Inflammatory Gene Expression

78. Perkins ND. Post-translational modifications regulating the activity and function of the nuclear factor-κB pathway. Oncogene 2006; 25:6717-30.
79. Perkins ND. The diverse and complex roles of NF-κB subunits in cancer. Nat Rev Cancer 2012;12:121-32.
80. Barnes PJ, Adcock IM, Ito K. Histone acetylation and deacetylation: importance in inflammatory lung diseases. Eur.Respir J 2005;25: 552-63.
81. Li B, Carey M, Workman JL. The role of chromatin during transcription. Cell 2007;128: 707-19.
82. Adcock IM, Ford P, Barnes PJ, Ito K. Epigenetics and airways disease. Respir Res 2006; 7:21.
83. Yang IV, Schwartz DA. Epigenetic control of gene expression in the lung. Am J Respir Crit Care Med 2011;183:1295-301.
84. Happel N, Doenecke D. Histone H1 and its isoforms: contribution to chromatin structure and function. Gene 2009;431:1-12.
85. De Bosscher K, Vanden Berghe W, Haegeman G. Cross-talk between nuclear receptors and nuclear factor-κB. Oncogene 2006;25(51): 6868-86.
86. Yao X, Zha W, Song W, et al. Coordinated regulation of IL-4 and IL-13 expression in human T cells: 3C analysis for DNA looping. Biochem Biophys Res Commun 2012;417: 996-1001.
87. Beck IM, Vanden Berghe W, Vermeulen L, et al. Crosstalk in inflammation: the interplay of glucocorticoid receptor-based mechanisms and kinases and phosphatases. Endocr Rev 2009;30:830-82.
88. Delmore JE, Issa GC, Lemieux ME, et al. BET bromodomain inhibition as a therapeutic strategy to target c-Myc. Cell 2011;146:904-17.

Mechanisms of Corticosteroid Action

89. Lu NZ, Cidlowski JA. Glucocorticoid receptor isoforms generate transcription specificity. Trends Cell Biol 2006;16:301-7.
90. Adcock IM, Gilbey T, Gelder CM, Chung KF, Barnes PJ. Glucocorticoid receptor localization in normal and asthmatic lung. Am J Respir Crit Care Med 1996;154(3 Pt 1):771-82.
91. Marwick JA, Caramori G, Stevenson CS, et al. Inhibition of PI3Kδ restores glucocorticoid function in smoking-induced airway inflammation in mice. Am J Respir Crit Care Med 2009;179:542-8.
92. Weigel NL, Moore NL. Steroid receptor phosphorylation: a key modulator of multiple receptor functions. Mol Endocrinol 2007;21: 2311-19.
93. Avenant C, Kotitschke A, Hapgood JP. Glucocorticoid receptor phosphorylation modulates transcription efficacy through GRIP-1 recruitment. Biochemistry, 2010;49:972-85.
94. Avenant C, Ronacher K, Stubsrud E, Louw A, Hapgood JP. Role of ligand-dependent GR phosphorylation and half-life in determination of ligand-specific transcriptional activity. Mol Cell Endocrinol 2010:327:72-88.
95. Verhoog NJ, Du Toit A, Avenant C, Hapgood JP. Glucocorticoid-independent repression of tumor necrosis factor (TNF)-α–stimulated interleukin (IL)–6 expression by the glucocorticoid receptor: a potential mechanism for protection against an excessive inflammatory response. J Biol Chem 2011;286:19297-310.
96. Wang C, Tian L, Popov VM, Pestell RG. Acetylation and nuclear receptor action. J Steroid Biochem Mol Biol 2011;123:91-100.
97. Ito K, Yamamura S, Essilfie-Quaye S, et al. Histone deacetylase 2-mediated deacetylation of the glucocorticoid receptor enables NF-κB suppression. J Exp Med 2006;203:7-13.
98. Davies L, Karthikeyan N, Lynch JT, et al. Cross talk of signaling pathways in the regulation of the glucocorticoid receptor function. Mol Endocrinol 2008;22:1331-44.
99. Geiss-Friedlander R, Melchior F. Concepts in sumoylation: a decade on. Nat Rev Mol Cell Biol 2007;8:947-56.
100. Zhou J, Cidlowski JA. The human glucocorticoid receptor: one gene, multiple proteins and diverse responses. Steroids 2005;70: 407-17.
101. Lu NZ, Cidlowski JA. The origin and functions of multiple human glucocorticoid receptor isoforms. Ann NY Acad Sci 2004;1024:102-23.
102. Kino T, Su YA, Chrousos GP. Human glucocorticoid receptor isoform β: recent understanding of its potential implications in physiology and pathophysiology. Cell Mol Life Sci 2009; 66:3435-48.
103. Charmandari E, Kino T, Ichijo T, Chrousos GP. Generalized glucocorticoid resistance: clinical aspects, molecular mechanisms, and implications of a rare genetic disorder. J Clin Endocrinol Metab 2008;93:1563-72.
104. Hew M, Chung KF. Corticosteroid insensitivity in severe asthma: significance, mechanisms and aetiology. Intern Med J 2010;40:323-34.
105. Maneechotesuwan K, Yao X, Ito K, et al. Suppression of GATA-3 nuclear import and phosphorylation: a novel mechanism of corticosteroid action in allergic disease. PLoS Med 2009;6:e1000076.
106. Savory JG, Hsu B, Laquian IR, et al. Discrimination between NL1- and NL2-mediated nuclear localization of the glucocorticoid receptor. Mol Cell Biol 1999;19:1025-37.
107. Freedman ND, Yamamoto KR. Importin 7 and importin α/importin β are nuclear import receptors for the glucocorticoid receptor. Mol Biol Cell 2004;15:2276-86.
108. Holaska JM, Black BE, Rastinejad F, Paschal BM. Ca^{2+}-dependent nuclear export mediated by calreticulin. Mol Cell Biol 2002;22: 6286-97.

109. Adcock IM, Caramori G. Cross-talk between pro-inflammatory transcription factors and glucocorticoids. Immunol Cell Biol 2001;79: 376-84.
110. Meijsing SH, Pufall MA, So AY, et al. DNA binding site sequence directs glucocorticoid receptor structure and activity. Science 2009; 324(5925):407-10.
111. Leung TH, Hoffmann A, Baltimore D. One nucleotide in a κB site can determine cofactor specificity for NF-κB dimers. Cell 2004;118: 453-64.
112. Reddy TE, Pauli F, Sprouse RO, et al. Genomic determination of the glucocorticoid response reveals unexpected mechanisms of gene regulation. Genome Res 2009;19:2163-71.
113. De Bosscher K, Vanden Berghe W, Haegeman G. Mechanisms of anti-inflammatory action and of immunosuppression by glucocorticoids: negative interference of activated glucocorticoid receptor with transcription factors. J Neuroimmunol 2000;109:16-22.
114. Biddie SC, John S, Sabo PJ, et al. Transcription factor AP1 potentiates chromatin accessibility and glucocorticoid receptor binding. Mol Cell 2011;43:145-55.
115. Biddie SC, Conway-Campbell BL, Lightman SL. Dynamic regulation of glucocorticoid signaling in health and disease. Rheumatology (Oxford) 2012;51:403-12.
116. Stavreva DA, McNally JG. Role of H1 phosphorylation in rapid GR exchange and function at the MMTV promoter. Histochem Cell Biol 2006;125:83-9.
117. Wiench M, John S, Baek S, et al. DNA methylation status predicts cell type-specific enhancer activity. EMBO J 2011;30:3028-39.
118. Surjit M, Ganti KP, Mukherji A, et al. Widespread negative response elements mediate direct repression by agonist-liganded glucocorticoid receptor. Cell 2011;145:224-41.
119. Hew M, Chung KF. Corticosteroid insensitivity in severe asthma: significance, mechanisms and aetiology. Intern Med J 2010;40:323–34.
120. Li LB, Leung DY, Martin RJ, Goleva E. Inhibition of histone deacetylase 2 expression by elevated glucocorticoid receptor beta in steroid resistant asthma. Am J Respir Crit Care Med 2010;182:877-83.
121. Bilodeau S, Vallette-Kasic S, Gauthier Y, et al. Role of Brg1 and HDAC2 in GR transrepression of the pituitary POMC gene and misexpression in Cushing disease. Genes Dev 2006;20:2871-86.
122. Nissen RM, Yamamoto KR. The glucocorticoid receptor inhibits NF-κB by interfering with serine-2 phosphorylation of the RNA polymerase II carboxy-terminal domain. Genes Dev 2000;14:2314-29.
123. Luecke HF, Yamamoto KR. The glucocorticoid receptor blocks P-TEFb recruitment by NF-κB to effect promoter-specific transcriptional repression. Genes Dev 2005;19: 1116-27.
124. Kovacs JJ, Murphy PJ, Gaillard S, et al. HDAC6 regulates Hsp90 acetylation and chaperone-dependent activation of glucocorticoid receptor. Mol Cell 2005;18:601-7.
125. Qiu Y, Stavreva DA, Luo Y, et al. Dynamic interaction of HDAC1 with a glucocorticoid receptor-regulated gene is modulated by the activity state of the promoter. J Biol Chem 2011;286:7641-7.
126. Jee YK, Gilmour J, Kelly A, et al. Repression of interleukin-5 transcription by the glucocorticoid receptor targets GATA3 signaling and involves histone deacetylase recruitment. J Biol Chem 2005;280:3243-50.
127. Hong W, Baniahmad A, Li J, et al. Bag-1M inhibits the transactivation of the glucocorticoid receptor via recruitment of corepressors. FEBS Lett 2009;583:2451-6.
128. Amat R, Solanes G, Giralt M, Villarroya F. SIRT1 is involved in glucocorticoid-mediated control of uncoupling protein-3 gene transcription. J Biol Chem 2007;282:34066-76.
129. Islam KN, Mendelson CR. Glucocorticoid/glucocorticoid receptor inhibition of surfactant protein-A (SP-A) gene expression in lung type II cells is mediated by repressive changes in histone modification at the SP-A promoter. Mol Endocrinol 2008;22:585-96.
130. Langlais D, Couture C, Balsalobre A, Drouin J. The Stat3/GR interaction code: predictive value of direct/indirect DNA recruitment for transcription outcome. Mol Cell 2012;47: 38-49.
131. O'Shea JJ, Plenge R. JAK and STAT signaling molecules in immunoregulation and immune-mediated disease. Immunity 2012;36:542-50.
132. Rincon M, Irvin CG. Role of IL-6 in asthma and other inflammatory pulmonary diseases. Int J Biol Sci 2012;8:1281-90.
133. Yamaya M. Virus infection–induced bronchial asthma exacerbation. Pulm Med 2012;2012: 834826.
134. Hawkins GA, Robinson MB, Hastie AT, et al. The IL6R variation Asp(358)Ala is a potential modifier of lung function in subjects with asthma. J Allergy Clin Immunol 2012;130: 510-15.
135. Smoak K, Cidlowski JA. Glucocorticoids regulate tristetraprolin synthesis and posttranscriptionally regulate tumor necrosis factor-α inflammatory signaling. Mol Cell Biol 2006: 26:9126-35.
136. Ishmael FT, Fang X, Galdiero MR, et al. Role of the RNA-binding protein tristetraprolin in glucocorticoid-mediated gene regulation. J Immunol 2008;180:8342-53.
137. Ariel D, Upadhyay D. The role and regulation of microRNAs in asthma. Curr Opin Allergy Clin Immunol 2012;12:49-52.
138. Kabesch M, Adcock IM. Epigenetics in asthma and COPD. Biochimie 2012;94(11): 2231-41.
139. Ledderose C, Mohnle P, Limbeck E, et al. Corticosteroid resistance in sepsis is influenced by microRNA-124–induced downregulation of glucocorticoid receptor-α. Crit Care Med 2012;40:2745-53.
140. Solberg OD, Ostrin EJ, Love MI, et al. Airway epithelial miRNA expression is altered in asthma. Am J Respir Crit Care Med 2012;186: 965-74.
141. Jardim MJ, Dailey L, Silbajoris R, Diaz-Sanchez D. Distinct microRNA expression in human airway cells of asthmatic donors identifies a novel asthma-associated gene. Am J Respir Cell Mol Biol 2012;47:536-42.
142. Clark MB, Mattick JS. Long noncoding RNAs in cell biology. Semin Cell Dev Biol 2011;22: 366-76.
143. Lanz RB, McKenna NJ, Onate SA, et al. A steroid receptor coactivator, SRA, functions as an RNA and is present in an SRC-1 complex. Cell 1999;97:17-27.
144. Kino T, Hurt DE, Ichijo T, Nader N, Chrousos GP. Noncoding RNA gas5 is a growth arrest- and starvation-associated repressor of the glucocorticoid receptor. Sci Signal 2010;3(107): ra8.

Steroid-refractory Asthma

145. Bel EH, Sousa A, Fleming L, et al. Diagnosis and definition of severe refractory asthma: an international consensus statement from the Innovative Medicine Initiative (IMI). Thorax 2011;66:910-17.
146. Woodruff PG, Modrek B, Choy DF, et al. T-helper type 2-driven inflammation defines major subphenotypes of asthma. Am J Respir Crit Care Med 2009;180:388-95.
147. Choy DF, Modrek B, Abbas AR, et al. Gene expression patterns of Th2 inflammation and intercellular communication in asthmatic airways. J Immunol 2011;186:1861-9.
148. Corren J, Lemanske RF, Hanania NA, et al. Lebrikizumab treatment in adults with asthma. N Engl J Med 2011;365:1088-98.
149. Irusen E, Matthews JG, Takahashi A, et al. p38 mitogen–activated protein kinase–induced glucocorticoid receptor phosphorylation reduces its activity: role in steroid-insensitive asthma. J Allergy Clin Immunol 2002;109: 649-57.
150. Goleva E, Li LB, Leung DY. IFN-γ reverses IL-2- and IL-4-mediated T-cell steroid resistance. Am J Respir Cell Mol.Biol 2009;40:223-30.
151. Galliher-Beckley AJ, Williams JG, Cidlowski JA. Ligand-independent phosphorylation of the glucocorticoid receptor integrates cellular stress pathways with nuclear receptor signaling. Mol Cell Biol 2011;31:4663-75.
152. Tchen CR, Martins JRS, Paktiawal N, et al. Glucocorticoid regulation of mouse and human dual specificity phosphatase 1 (DUSP1) genes. J Biol Chem 2010;285:2642-52.
153. Zhu QY, Liu Q, Chen JX, Lan K, Ge BX. MicroRNA-101 targets MAPK phosphatase-1 to regulate the activation of MAPKs in macrophages. J Immunol 2010;185:7435-42.
154. Pillai VB, Sundaresan NR, Samant SA, et al. Acetylation of a conserved lysine residue in the ATP binding pocket of p38 augments its kinase activity during hypertrophy of cardiomyocytes. Mol Cell Biol 2011;31:2349-63.
155. Kobayashi Y, Mercado N, Barnes PJ, Ito K. Defects of protein phosphatase 2A causes corticosteroid insensitivity in severe asthma. PLoS ONE 2011;6:e27627.
156. Li LB, Leung DY, Strand MJ, Goleva EA: TF2 impairs glucocorticoid receptor-mediated transactivation in human $CD8^+$ T cells. Blood 2007;110:1570-7.
157. Tsitsiou E, Williams AE, Moschos SA, et al. Transcriptome analysis shows activation of circulating $CD8^+$ T cells in patients with severe asthma. J Allergy Clin Immunol 2012;129: 95-103.
158. Traves SL, Donnelly LE. Th17 cells in airway diseases. Curr Mol Med 2008;8:416-26.
159. Kaminska M, Foley S, Maghni K, et al. Airway remodeling in subjects with severe asthma with or without chronic persistent airflow obstruction. J Allergy Clin Immunol 2009;124:45-51.
160. Jackson DJ, Sykes A, Mallia P, Johnston SL. Asthma exacerbations: origin, effect, and prevention. J Allergy Clin Immunol 2011;128: 1165-74.
161. Grunberg K, Sharon RF, Sont JK, et al. Rhinovirus-induced airway inflammation in asthma: effect of treatment with inhaled corticosteroids before and during experimental infection. Am J Respir Crit Care Med 2001; 164(10 Pt 1):1816-22.
162. Gustafson LM, Proud D, Hendley JO, Hayden FG, Gwaltney JM Jr. Oral prednisone therapy

in experimental rhinovirus infections. J Allergy Clin Immunol 1996;97:1009-14.
163. Hinzey A, Alexander J, Corry J, et al. Respiratory syncytial virus represses glucocorticoid receptor-mediated gene activation. Endocrinology 2011;152:483-94.
164. Adcock IM, Ford PA, Bhavsar P, Ahmad T, Chung KF. Steroid resistance in asthma: mechanisms and treatment options. Curr Allergy Asthma Rep 2008;8:171-8.
165. Bhandare R, Damera G, Banerjee A, et al. Glucocorticoid receptor interacting protein-1 restores glucocorticoid responsiveness in steroid-resistant airway structural cells. Am J Respir Cell Mol Biol 2010;42:9-15.
166. Barnes PJ. Intrinsic asthma: not so different from allergic asthma but driven by superantigens? Clin Exp Allergy 2009;39:1145-51.
167. Agache I, Duca L, Anghel M, Pamfil G. Antinuclear antibodies in asthma patients: a special asthma phenotype? Iran J Allergy Asthma Immunol 2009;8:49-52.
168. Zehn D, Bevan MJ, Fink PJ. Cutting edge: TCR revision affects predominantly Foxp3 cells and skews them toward the Th17 lineage. J Immunol 2007;179:5653-7.
169. Ou LS, Goleva E, Hall C, Leung DY. T regulatory cells in atopic dermatitis and subversion of their activity by superantigens. J Allergy Clin Immunol 2004;113:756-63.
170. Li LB, Goleva E, Hall CF, Ou LS, Leung DY. Superantigen-induced corticosteroid resistance of human T cells occurs through activation of the mitogen-activated protein kinase kinase/extracellular signal-regulated kinase (MEK-ERK) pathway. J Allergy Clin Immunol 2004;114:1059-69.
171. Guiducci C, Gong M, Xu Z, et al. TLR recognition of self nucleic acids hampers glucocorticoid activity in lupus. Nature 2010; 465(7300):937-41.
172. Gupta A, Sjoukes A, Richards D, et al. Relationship between serum vitamin D, disease severity, and airway remodeling in children with asthma. Am J Respir Crit Care Med 2011;184: 1342-9.
173. Rahman I, Adcock IM. Oxidative stress and redox regulation of lung inflammation in COPD. Eur Respir J 2006;28:219-42.
174. Adcock IM, Barnes PJ. Molecular mechanisms of corticosteroid resistance. Chest 2008;134: 394–401.
175. Brindicci C, Ito K, Barnes PJ, Kharitonov SA. Differential flow analysis of exhaled nitric oxide in patients with asthma of differing severity. Chest 2007;131:1353-62.
176. Osoata GO, Yamamura S, Ito M, et al. Nitration of distinct tyrosine residues causes inactivation of histone deacetylase 2. Biochem Biophys Res Commun 2009;384:366-71.
177. Nott A, Watson PM, Robinson JD, Crepaldi L, Riccio A. *S*-Nitrosylation of histone deacetylase 2 induces chromatin remodelling in neurons. Nature 2008;455(7211):411-15.
178. Barnes PJ. Targeting the epigenome in the treatment of asthma and chronic obstructive pulmonary disease. Proc Am Thorac Soc 2009; 6:693-6.
179. Bartling TR, Drumm ML. Loss of CFTR results in reduction of histone deacetylase 2 in airway epithelial cells. Am J Physiol Lung Cell Mol Physiol 2009;297:L35-43.
180. Ford PA, Durham AL, Russell RE, et al. Treatment effects of low-dose theophylline combined with an inhaled corticosteroid in COPD. Chest 2010;137:1338-44.
181. Spears M, Donnelly I, Jolly L, et al. Effect of theophylline plus beclometasone on lung function in smokers with asthma-a pilot study. Eur Respir J 2009;33:1010-17.
182. To Y, Ito K, Kizawa Y, et al. Targeting phosphoinositide-3-kinase-δ with theophylline reverses corticosteroid insensitivity in chronic obstructive pulmonary disease. Am J Respir Crit Care Med 2010;182:897-904.
183. Moore WC, Bleecker ER, Curran-Everett D, et al. Characterization of the severe asthma phenotype by the National Heart, Lung, and Blood Institute's Severe Asthma Research Program. J Allergy Clin Immunol 2007;119: 405-13.
184. Fleischmann R, Kremer J, Cush J, et al. Placebo-controlled trial of tofacitinib monotherapy in rheumatoid arthritis. N Engl J Med 2012;367: 495-507.
185. Wenzel SE, Barnes PJ, Bleecker ER, et al. A randomized, double-blind, placebo-controlled study of tumor necrosis factor-α blockade in severe persistent asthma. Am J Respir Crit Care Med 2009;179:549-58.
186. Woodruff PG, Boushey HA, Dolganov GM, et al. Genome-wide profiling identifies epithelial cell genes associated with asthma and with treatment response to corticosteroids. Proc Natl Acad Sci USA 2007;104:15858-63.
187. Goleva E, Hauk PJ, Hall CF, et al. Corticosteroid-resistant asthma is associated with classical antimicrobial activation of airway macrophages. J Allergy Clin Immunol 2008;122: 550-9.
188. Bellattato C, Adcock IM, Ito K, et al. Rhinovirus infection reduces glucocorticoid receptor nuclear translocation in airway epithelial cells. Eur Respir J 2003;22:565S.
189. Garn H, Mittermann I, Valenta R, Renz H. Autosensitization as a pathomechanism in asthma. Ann NY Acad Sci 2007;1107:417-25.

ADDITIONAL READINGS

Bhavsar P, Hew M, Khorasani N, et al. Relative corticosteroid insensitivity of alveolar macrophages in severe asthma compared to non-severe asthma. Thorax 2008;63:784-90.

Cole ZA, Clough GF, Church MK. Inhibition by glucocorticoids of the mast cell–dependent weal and flare response in human skin in vivo. Br J Pharmacol 2001;132:286-92.

Cream JJ. Prednisolone-induced granulocytosis. Br J Haematol 1968;15:259-67.

Lavker RM, Schechter NM. Cutaneous mast cell depletion results from topical corticosteroid usage. J Immunol 1985;135:2368-73.

Lou X, Sun S, Chen W, et al. Negative feedback regulation of NF-κB action by CITED2 in the nucleus. J Immunol 2011;186:539-48.

Mattes J, Collison A, Plank M, Phipps S, Foster PS. Antagonism of microRNA-126 suppresses the effector function of TH2 cells and the development of allergic airways disease. Proc Natl Acad Sci USA 2009;106:18704-9.

McNally JG, Muller WG, Walker D, Wolford R, Hager GL. The glucocorticoid receptor: rapid exchange with regulatory sites in living cells. Science 2000;287(5456):1262-5.

Pipkorn U, Andersson P. Budesonide and nasal mucosal histamine content and anti-IgE induced histamine release. Allergy 1982;37:591-5.

Schleimer RP, Freeland HS, Peters SP, Brown KE, Derse CP. An assessment of the effects of glucocorticoids on degranulation, chemotaxis, binding to vascular endothelium and formation of leukotriene B_4 by purified human neutrophils. J Pharmacol Exp Ther 1989;250:598-605.

Schacke H, Hennekes H, Schottelius A, et al. SEGRAs: a novel class of anti-inflammatory compounds. Ernst Schering Res Found Workshop 2002;40: 357-71.

Schacke H, Schottelius A, Docke WD, et al. Dissociation of transactivation from transrepression by a selective glucocorticoid receptor agonist leads to separation of therapeutic effects from side effects. Proc Natl Acad Sci USA 2004;101:227-32.

Simon HU. Eosinophil apoptosis–pathophysiologic and therapeutic implications. Allergy 2000;55: 910-15.

Woo PL, Ching D, Guan Y, Firestone GL. Requirement for Ras and phosphatidylinositol 3-kinase signaling uncouples the glucocorticoid-induced junctional organization and transepithelial electrical resistance in mammary tumor cells. J Biol Chem 1999;274:32818-28.

Antileukotriene Therapy in Asthma

SALLY E. WENZEL

CONTENTS

SUMMARY OF IMPORTANT CONCEPTS

» Leukotrienes are lipid mediators formed from arachidonic acid.
» Cysteinyl leukotrienes (LTC_4, LTD_4, and LTE_4) induce bronchoconstriction and eosinophilic inflammation, whereas LTB_4 enhances neutrophilic inflammation.
» Leukotriene modifiers (receptor antagonists and synthesis inhibitors) improve asthma symptoms and lung function, although their efficacy is less than that of inhaled corticosteroids.
» Leukotriene modifiers are, in general, less effective as add-on therapy to inhaled corticosteroids than long-acting beta agonists.
» In addition to asthma, leukotrine modifiers have efficacy in allergic rhinitis.

Introduction

Leukotrienes, are the first biologic substances to have confirmed importance in the clinical course and physiologic changes of asthma. Leukotrienes, both the cysteinyl leukotrienes (cysLTs)—LTC_4, LTD_4, and LTE_4—as well as leukotriene B_4 (LTB_4), have long been implicated in the pathogenesis of asthma. The cysLTs are potent bronchoconstrictors, with additional effects on blood vessels, mucociliary clearance and eosinophilic inflammation. LTB_4, whose role is less well defined in asthma, is a potent chemoattractant (and cell activator) for both neutrophils and eosinophils. Recent murine studies suggest leukotrienes may also play an active role in allergic sensitization. The cysLTs are formed from cells typically associated with asthma, including eosinophils and mast cells.

Clinical and physiologic studies of drugs that interfere with the leukotriene pathway (both CysLT1 receptor antagonists and synthesis inhibitors) confirm their activity as modest, short-acting bronchodilators and their ability to improve FEV_1, treat symptoms, and prevent exacerbations in adults and children over time. These drugs have demonstrated efficacy in preventing bronchoconstriction caused by leukotrienes, allergen, exercise, and other agents. Comparison studies with inhaled corticosteroids (ICS) consistently demonstrate that ICS are superior to antileukotriene (anti-LT) drugs, but also that variability exists in response to both drug classes. Studies also suggest anti-LT drugs can be effective when added to ongoing therapy with ICS, although the improvements are less than those seen with long-acting β-adrenergic agonists. Although a marginal effect on cellular inflammation is observed, longer-term, earlier interventional studies are needed to determine whether any effect on the natural history of the disease will be seen in responders to anti-LT therapy.

Inflammation is likely the most significant contributing factor to the symptoms and physiologic changes of asthma and imminently approachable with therapy. As part of this inflammatory process, activation of the arachidonic acid cascade leads to production of leukotrienes. These lipid mediators are formed from the enzymatic metabolism of arachidonic acid and play a role in the bronchoconstriction, edema, and increased mucus associated with the symptoms of asthma. Drugs that specifically interfere with the leukotriene pathway are the cysLT receptor antagonists and 5-lipoxygenase inhibitors. Although other pathways are actively being targeted, leukotriene modifiers remain the only drugs targeting a specific pathway involved in the complex pathobiology of asthma.

The Leukotriene Pathway

Leukotrienes are potent lipid mediators formed through multiple enzymatic steps (Fig. 100-1). Leukotrienes are downstream products of the metabolism of cell or nuclear membrane phospholipids. Phospholipids, ubiquitous elements of cellular membranes, can be enzymatically metabolized by the actions of phospholipases to arachidonic acid (AA). Although best understood is the cytosolic phospholipase A_2 (PLA_2), others play a significant role in AA production, such as the low-molecular-weight or secretory phospholipases.[1,2] The AA formed from these enzymes can be further metabolized down a variety of pathways, including the cyclooxygenase pathway, which leads to production of prostaglandins and thromboxane (and is inhibited by aspirin and other nonsteroidal antiinflammatory compounds), and a variety of lipoxygenase pathways, including the 5-lipoxygenase (5-LO) pathway. Which pathway is activated depends on the specific cell type and stimuli, with 5-LO being most abundant in cells of the myeloid lineage.[3] Activation of

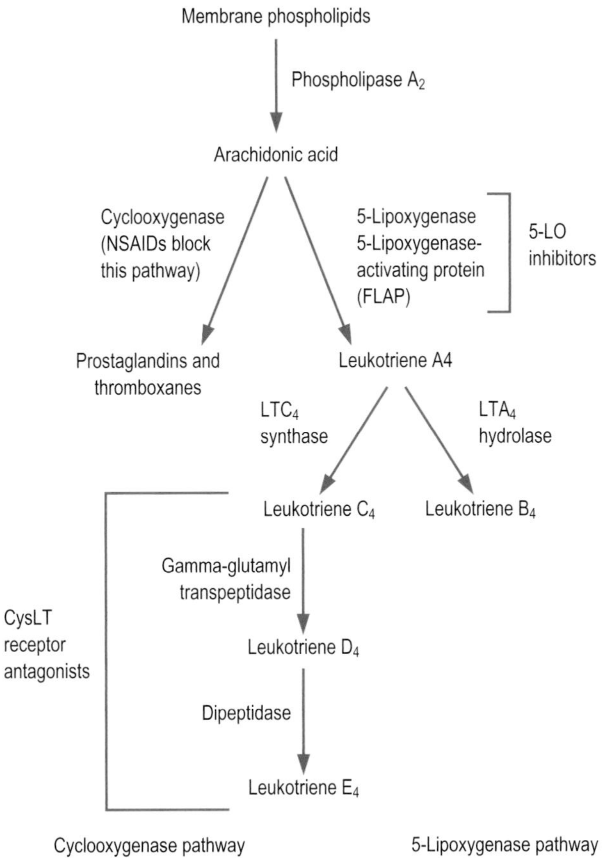

Figure 100-1 Arachidonic acid cascade. *CysLT*, Cysteinyl leukotriene; *NSAIDs*, nonsteroidal antiinflammatory drugs.

5-LO in these cells is thought to require generalized cellular activation with mobilization of calcium stores and availability of AA as substrate.

The activation also likely requires interaction with 5-LO–activating protein (FLAP), which is thought to channel AA to the enzyme 5-LO.[3] Although polymorphisms in the genes for both 5-LO (chromosome 10q) and FLAP (chromosome 13q) have been identified, these polymorphisms have not been consistently linked to general asthma end points.[4-6] In certain inflammatory cells (macrophages, eosinophils, and likely mast cells), this process occurs at the nuclear membrane rather than the cytoplasmic membrane, which may affect biologic functions of the leukotrienes, once formed.[7,8] The 5 LO activation at the cytoplasmic or nuclear membrane then leads to the production of an unstable intermediate known as leukotriene A_4, which can be further metabolized, depending on cell type, to LTB_4 or the cysteinyl leukotrienes LTC_4, LTD_4, and LTE_4 (formerly known as slow-reacting substance of anaphylaxis). LTC_4 synthase metabolizes LTA_4 to LTC_4 through a glutathione transferase. LTC_4 synthase resides on human chromosome 5q, a region associated with many other genes linked with asthma and atopy.[9] Although numerous studies have evaluated single-nucleotide polymorphisms (SNPs) in this gene, no consistently observed associations of SNPs with asthma outcomes have been seen across studies or populations.[4,10,11] LTC_4 is then rapidly metabolized to LTD_4 and LTE_4, through the enzymes γ-glutamyl transpeptidase and a dipeptidase. LTC_4 and LTD_4 both have a very short half-life, and LTE_4 appears to be the most stable of the three, with the longest half-life. Both LTB_4 and the cysLTs appear to be exported to the extracellular space, primarily through the transporter multidrug-resistant protein 1 (MRP-1).[12,13]

Based on the distribution of the necessary enzymes, leukotrienes are produced almost exclusively by cells of the myeloid lineage. LTC_4 is produced primarily by mast cells, basophils, and eosinophils, cells usually associated with asthma.[3] LTB_4 is produced primarily by neutrophils and monocytes/macrophages. Although these cells had not been closely linked to asthma, more recent studies of severe asthma and exacerbations of asthma suggest that LTB_4 could be important as well.[14-16]

LEUKOTRIENE RECEPTORS

Until recently, the production of the leukotrienes was more completely understood than were the interactions with the receptors that ultimately determine their biologic effects. However, four leukotriene receptors have now been cloned. The first to be cloned was the LTB_4 receptor (BLT1 receptor), which was found to be a single G protein–coupled receptor on mononuclear cells (monocytes and lymphocytes), neutrophils, and eosinophils.[17-19] The BLT1 receptor gene is localized to chromosome 14q11.[20] Shortly thereafter, a second LTB_4 receptor, also chromosome 14q, was cloned and identified (BLT2).[17,21] Unlike the BLT1 receptor, this lower-affinity receptor was also found to be expressed on structural cells, and in higher concentrations on lymphocytes.[17,21] Although they continue in development, currently no pharmacologic agents in clinical use antagonize either LTB_4 receptor.

Cysteinyl leukotrienes in humans also appear to function through at least two receptors, CysLT1 and CysLT2, both of which have been cloned and their general organ and cellular distribution mapped.[22-24] The CysLT1 receptor and its mRNA have been localized to airway smooth muscle cells, eosinophils, B lymphocytes, mast cells, and monocyte/macrophages.[23,25] The CysLT1 receptor gene maps to the X chromosome near a region of interest in asthma (Xq13-21).[26] However, no studies have yet shown associations with polymorphisms in this gene and asthma end points, although one study did suggest an association with atopy.[27,28] CysLT1, also identified on human mast cells, appears able to respond to pyrimidinergic ligands (e.g., uridine diphosphate) in addition to cysLTs.[29] CysLT2 was cloned in 2000.[22] It is not antagonized by any of the available leukotriene receptor antagonists (LTRAs), and there are currently no specific CysLT2 receptor antagonists.[30] Unlike CystLT1 receptor, LTC_4 and LTD_4 are of equal potency in activation of the receptor. CysLT2 receptor mRNA has been mapped to lung macrophages, airway smooth muscle, Purkinje cells, peripheral blood leukocytes, mast cells, and brain. Studies in human mast cells in which CysLT1 has been antagonized suggest that CysLT2 may be involved in activation of proneutrophilic pathways, possibly relevant to infection-related and more severe asthma.[31] Also, studies of cysLT2-deficient mice suggest that that this receptor pathway is likely to be important in lung fibrosis.[32] The gene for CysLT2 is on chromosome 13, also in a region linked to asthma (13q14), with Caucasian and Japanese population studies suggesting that several different polymorphisms are associated with asthma.[33,34] Whether CysLT2 distribution or amount varies in different disease states, or whether CysLT2 or other, more poorly defined receptors will prove to be important in human diseases, awaits further study.[35]

TABLE 100-1 **Leukotriene Antagonists and Pathway Inhibitors**

	Leukotriene Receptor Antagonists	Leukotriene Pathway Inhibitors
Mechanism of action	Block the actions of cysteinyl leukotrienes (cysLTs)	Block the production of leukotriene B_4 *and* cysLTs
Specific agents	Zafirlukast (Accolate) Montelukast (Singulair) Pranlukast (Onon)	Zileuton (ZyfloCR)

PHARMACOLOGIC ANTAGONISM AND INHIBITION

As the understanding of the biochemical pathways for the leukotrienes evolved, so did efforts to pharmacologically inhibit or antagonize this pathway, both at the enzyme and receptor levels. Well before the cloning of the CysLT1 or CysLT2 receptor, compounds based on pharmacologic studies were shown to be highly selective for CysLT1. These drugs, in fact, have become helpful in sorting out different types of cysLT receptors, as they are so specific for CysLT1. The compounds that antagonize CysLT1 currently available for clinical use include montelukast, pranlukast, and zafirlukast. Of these, montelukast appears to have the highest binding affinity to CysLT1 in biologic receptor-binding models.[23]

In addition to antagonism at the receptor level, multiple compounds were developed to inhibit leukotriene production. These strategies involved efforts to inhibit the 5-LO enzyme and the ability of FLAP to interact with 5-LO, preventing leukotriene production. 5-LO inhibitors have been developed that (oddly) demonstrate greater than 80% inhibition of the 5-LO enzyme in vitro (ionophore-stimulated LTB_4 production), although the in vivo level of inhibition may be less.[36] Currently, only one drug, zileuton, is available in the United States only for clinical use that works at this level.[37] These types of drugs have a broader range of activity because they inhibit the production of all the leukotrienes, including LTB_4. By so doing, these agents have the ability to decrease the activation of all the leukotriene receptors, including all the cysLT receptors and the two LTB_4 receptors. Although the clinical relevance of these different modes of action to the treatment of asthma and other allergic diseases remains unclear, these drugs have proved instrumental in improving the understanding of the biologic and clinical implications of leukotrienes in the airway diseases, particularly as related to allergic rhinitis and asthma (Table 100-1).

Biologic Properties of Leukotrienes

PHYSIOLOGIC PROPERTIES

Cysteinyl leukotrienes are potent bronchoconstrictors (100 to 1000 times more potent than histamine), with LTC_4 and LTD_4 appearing to be almost equipotent in this regard.[38] Asthmatic patients appear to be more sensitive to inhalational challenge with LTE_4, but increased responsiveness to LTD_4 has not always been described.[39-41] Recent studies have suggested that cysLTs significantly impact ventilation-perfusion mismatch and associated hypoxemia.[42] The currently available CysLT1 receptor antagonists (cysLTRAs) are all effective in dose-dependent reduction in the bronchoconstriction and ventilation-perfusion mismatch that occur after inhalation of LTD_4.

It is doubtful that cysLTs are capable of inducing airway hyperreactivity (AHR).[39,43] LTB_4 has no bronchoconstrictive or hyperresponsive qualities in humans.

INFLAMMATORY PROPERTIES

The discovery of the CysLT1 receptor on other cell types in addition to smooth muscle cells led to studies of other biologic effects.[25] Inhalation of LTE_4 resulted in increased numbers of eosinophils for up to 6 weeks into the lungs of asthmatic patients, but LTD_4 has been less impressive.[39,44-46] The mechanisms for these differences may relate to the ability to provide much larger molar amounts of LTE_4 than the more potent LTD_4, although preferential binding of LTE_4 to the newly described P2Y12 receptor in mice appears to control the eosinophilic response to cysLTs.[35] In vitro studies of the chemoattractant properties of the cysLTs have shown only marginal effects with LTD_4.[47] If present, chemoattractant activity may occur through secondary activation of the eosinophil chemoattractant and activator interleukin-5 (IL-5).[48,49] In addition, cysLTs may be important in prolonging eosinophil survival, explaining the increased numbers after inhalation; in this regard, LTD_4 appears to have similar potency as granulocyte-macrophage colony-stimulating factor (GM-CSF).[50] LTRAs and leukotriene synthesis inhibitors are able to abolish the effect on eosinophil apoptosis, possibly in an autocrine manner through the CysLT1 receptor. Also, cysLTs may be able to act as cofactors for the enhanced production of eosinophils from the bone marrow, when used in combination with the growth factor GM-CSF.[51]

Whether the leukotrienes have any role in the modulation of structural changes is not clear. Two studies showed that LTD_4 affects smooth muscle proliferation when added to epidermal growth factor (EGF).[52,53] No human data support a clinically important effect on smooth muscle proliferation in addition to the increased contractile effect. However, a study in rats suggested that a leukotriene synthesis inhibitor (MK-886) prevented the increase in smooth muscle area after chronic inhalation of allergen in a brown-rat model.[52] The relevance of this potential effect on structural elements (smooth muscle) of the airway in human asthma may be impossible to confirm.

The role of leukotrienes has also been studied in allergic sensitization and effector responses. In an ovalbumin model of allergic inflammation, LTC_4 synthase–knockout mice showed a marked effect to increase levels of IgE and type 2 helper T cytokine (Th2) mRNA expression both in the lung and in the parabronchial lymph nodes.[54] These effects on Th2 pathways suggest that further studies of the role of cysLTs in allergic sensitization should be pursued, with potential implications for early intervention studies in children.

A potent chemoattractant for neutrophils and eosinophils, LTB_4 is also an activator of neutrophils, which appears to enhance adhesion and migration of the cells through the endothelium.[55] LTB_4 seems to affect eosinophils less than do the cysLTs. Interestingly, murine studies supported a role for LTB_4 (as well as cysLTs) in the sensitization phase of allergic inflammation. $CD8^+$ T cells were recruited to inflammatory sites through an LTB_4/BLT1-dependent pathway after mast cell activation.[56] Later studies showed that $BLT1^{-/-}$ mice developed a blunted Th2/IgE response to ovalbumin, suggesting that LTB_4

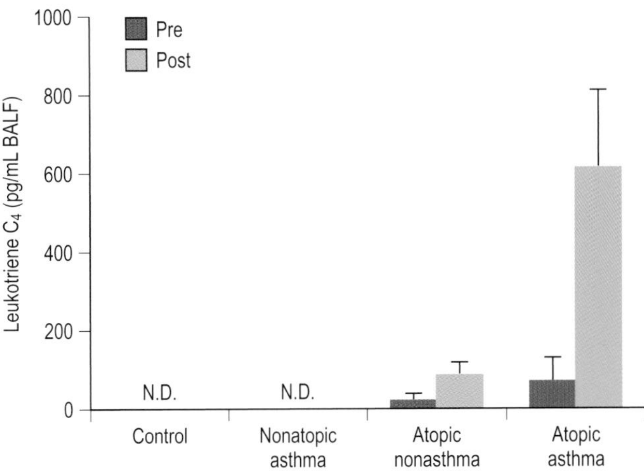

Figure 100-2 Concentrations of immunoreactive leukotriene C_4 (*LTC_4*) in bronchoalveolar lavage fluid (*BALF*) before (*Pre*) and after (*Post*) endobronchial allergen challenge. LTC_4 levels were low but measurable at baseline in atopic asthmatic subjects, but levels in nonatopic subjects and atopic nonasthmatic subjects were undetectable (*N.D.*). In addition, LTC_4 levels were significantly higher after allergen challenge in atopic asthmatic subjects than in prechallenge and control groups ($P < .05$). *(Reproduced from Wenzel SE, Larsen GL, Johnston K, et al. Elevated levels of leukotriene C_4 in bronchoalveolar lavage fluid from atopic asthmatics after endobronchial allergen challenge. Am Rev Respir Dis 1990;142:112-9. From the official journal of the American Thoracic Society. © American Thoracic Society.)*

is important to the sensitization response.[57] Finally, using a mast cell–dependent passive sensitization model (administration of antiovalbumin IgE followed by ovalbumin inhalation), AHR was abolished in the absence of $CD8^+$ cells, dependent on BLT1 expression.[58] These studies support an active role for both cysteinyl and LTB_4 leukotrienes in the early phases of allergic responses, as well as later effectors of bronchoconstriction. Application of these findings to human asthma awaits further study.

Fluid Measurement

Both cystLTs and LTB_4 have been measured in body fluids in asthma, including bronchoalveolar lavage (BAL) fluid, urine, and blood.[36,59-61] CysLTs are increased in BAL fluid after allergen and aspirin challenges at night in patients with nocturnal asthma (along with LTB_4) and in infants with persistent wheezing[36,60,62,63] (Fig. 100-2). The cysLTs have also been demonstrated in nasal fluid after allergen challenge and in respiratory syncytial virus (RSV) infection.[64] Importantly, leukotrienes increase in urine during an acute asthma exacerbation and decrease with resolution of the exacerbation.[59,61]

Leukotriene Inhibition/Antagonism and Asthmatic Inflammation

Modulation of leukotriene activity, as an initial "proof of concept" for the role of leukotrienes in asthma, centered on two components of the pathway. Both antagonists of the CysLT1 receptor and inhibitors of 5-LO have undergone proof of concept and large-scale clinical trials. The chief biologic difference between the LTRAs and the 5-LO inhibitors is that LTRAs inhibit the activity of cysLTs at CysLT1 only, whereas 5-LO inhibitors block the production and all downstream activity of both LTB_4 and cysLTs. Although animal and in vitro studies suggest important implications of blocking one or both pathways, whether this difference has clinical applications for asthma therapy remains unclear.

ALLERGEN-INDUCED INFLAMMATION

Early studies confirmed that bronchoconstriction from inhalation of LTD_4 could be almost completely inhibited by CysLT1 antagonists. Subsequent studies confirmed that cysLTs contributed to a large percentage of the bronchospasm occurring after allergen challenge. Studies using zafirlukast prior to allergen challenge demonstrated an inhibition of the immediate response by about 80% and the late response by 50%.[65,66] In addition to improvement in obstruction, the cysLTRA zafirlukast demonstrated a small but significant ability to limit the usual increase in airway reactivity after allergen exposure.[67] However, this effect has not been seen chronically and is not of the same magnitude as seen with ICS.[68] Of note, eosinophil numbers in sputum during the late phase response have not been reported to decrease (from placebo) after treatment with the LTRA montelukast, despite 50% inhibition of the airflow limitation associated with the late phase, suggesting that the inhibition of the late phase may occur through a different, non–eosinophilic-mediated mechanism.[69,70] Therefore, the mechanism behind the improvement in the late phase response with LTRAs is not clear.

The inflammation after allergen challenge has also been studied through BAL fluid and biopsy. Both LTRAs and 5-LO inhibitors may decrease the inflammatory cell influx into the airways after instillation of allergen.[71,72] Administration of zafirlukast for 1 week before instillation of allergen directly into the airways of asthmatic patients significantly decreased the influx of basophils and lymphocytes into the airways 48 hours after antigen exposure compared with placebo. However, similar to sputum studies, it only tended to decrease the numbers of eosinophils migrating into the airways.[71] There was an associated decrease in airway histamine and tumor necrosis factor-α levels, with the effect likely caused by direct antagonism of CysLT1 receptors on mast cells and alveolar macrophages.[25] Similar findings were seen with the 5-LO inhibitor zileuton.[72] Interestingly, one study suggested that the efficacy of leukotriene modifiers in allergen challenge may depend on leukotriene levels produced after allergen challenge, with the degree of modification of inflammation dependent on the degree of leukotriene production.[73] In that small study, 50% of the asthmatic patients studied were leukotriene producers, similar to percentages of "responders" described in clinical trials (see later discussion).

NOCTURNAL ASTHMA

Patients with nocturnal asthma have been described to have an increase in airway eosinophils at 4 AM.[74] In addition, subjects with nocturnal asthma have an increase in urinary excretion of LTE_4 at night, as well as increases in both LTB_4 and cysLTs in BAL fluid at night.[36] Using a nocturnal asthma model, zileuton, decreased BAL eosinophils, urinary and BAL leukotriene levels, and improved pulmonary function and symptoms in patients with nocturnal asthma. Of note, the improvement in forced expiratory volume in 1 second (FEV_1) correlated with the levels of LTB_4, but not cysLTs, in the airways.

EXERCISE

The role of inflammation and cysLTs in exercise-induced bronchospasm (EIB) has been controversial. Although one study showed no increase in urinary LTE_4 (as a marker of the cysLT pathway), a second study did show an increase in LTE_4 after exercise, and that the addition of an LTRA (montelukast) significantly inhibited EIB.[61,75] EIB appears to be consistently inhibited by cysLTRAs (and 5 LO inhibitors) in the range of 30% to 60%.[76-79] This inhibition compares favorably to pretreatment with cromolyn.[80] The effects in children may be less than the protective effects seen in adults, with inhibition of 30% to 40% seen.[81,82] However, in contrast, a study of the cold-air hyperventilation response in children age 3 to 5 years suggested almost 60% inhibition in this age group, with consistent prevention of bronchospasm across the subject groups, and no evidence for responders or nonresponders.[83] Whether this implies that the bronchoconstriction associated with cold-air hyperventilation is different from EIB (at least in children), or whether LTRAs have an increased effect in very young children, awaits further study.

In adults, a long-term study with the LTRA montelukast demonstrated sustained protection against EIB over 12 weeks, when montelukast was taken 16 to 18 hours before exercise.[77] These long-term effects were significantly better than outcomes with the long-acting β-agonist salmeterol administered in the same time frame before exercise in two long-term (8-week) studies.[84,85] Although the initial protection against EIB was similar between salmeterol and montelukast, the long-term use of salmeterol led to a reduction in the protection against EIB when given 8 to 10 hours before exercise. Other studies report similar data, with the bronchoprotective effect of salmeterol decreasing over time.[86,87] In contrast, the protection afforded by montelukast was maintained throughout both studies.[84,85]

ASPIRIN-INDUCED ASTHMA[88]

In the 10% of adult asthmatic patients sensitive to aspirin, the associated bronchoconstriction has been linked to increased production of cysLTs at baseline and after aspirin challenge.[89] The mechanism is not clear, although studies suggest that increases in mast cells, activated eosinophils, and expression of LTC_4 synthase and CysLT2 by these cells in aspirin-induced asthma (AIA) may play a role.[90-92] Whether the increase in LTC_4 synthase is the rate-limiting step for the excess cysLT production in AIA remains to be clarified.[10,93] Although initial studies suggested that the increase in LTC_4 synthase was caused by the $A_{-444}C$ promoter polymorphism, this effect has not been confirmed.[74,94,95]

Studies with both cysLTRAs and 5-LO inhibitors have verified the importance of leukotrienes in the aspirin reaction, with almost 100% inhibition of the bronchoconstriction associated with a "threshold aspirin dose."[96-98] Inhibition of the response is dose dependent, with loss of inhibition occurring when standard doses of aspirin are given.[99] Studies using 5-LO inhibitors in AIA patients have demonstrated an associated reduction in urinary LTE_4 excretion, as well as a reduction in nasal tryptase (primarily a mast cell product).[96,100] These data support an impact of these drugs on mast cells and their activation, but further study is required to determine the mechanism and clinical relevance.

Longer-term studies of aspirin-sensitive asthmatic patients support the clinical efficacy of chronic dosing in this population.[77,101] These patients tend to have more severe asthma and show incremental improvement in FEV_1 and symptom control with further addition of a 5-LO inhibitor or LTRA, despite treatment with ICS as well as oral corticosteroids. Studies with the 5-LO inhibitor zileuton also demonstrated improvement in nasal and sinus symptoms.[101] No studies yet support any greater efficacy of anti-LT therapy in patients with AIA than in the population as a whole.

ANTIINFLAMMATORY EFFECTS IN CHRONIC ASTHMA

Several studies support a "chronic" antiinflammatory effect of antileukotriene therapy, first observing that circulating blood eosinophils decreased over time after both cysLTRA and 5-LO inhibitor therapy.[102,103] A biopsy study evaluated the effect of pranlukast on airway tissue eosinophils and showed a reduction in EG2-positive cells in the tissue after 4 weeks of therapy.[104] Of note, there was no significant impact on FEV_1 in that study, despite the reduction in eosinophils. A biopsy study of the effect of montelukast on large-airway eosinophils demonstrated a decrease in tissue eosinophils compared to baseline; the decrease compared to placebo was not statistically significant.[105] In contrast, a second study showed no decrease in eosinophil numbers, while suggesting overall less antiinflammatory effects than with fluticasone.[106]

Sputum analysis revealed a significant decrease in eosinophils after 4 weeks of therapy with montelukast.[107] Participants were screened for inclusion into the study based on a baseline elevation in sputum eosinophils. In those with baseline eosinophilia, the improvement in morning peak flow with montelukast therapy may have been greater than the responses seen in a group of randomly selected patients. In contrast, no effect on sputum eosinophils was observed after 4 weeks of montelukast therapy in patients dependent on high-dose ICS, suggesting severity of disease affects the mechanism for sputum eosinophilia.[108]

Exhaled nitric oxide has also been used as a marker of airway inflammation. In three studies a small but significant decrease was seen with montelukast therapy versus placebo.[109-112] The effect in adults was similar to that seen with once-daily budesonide (400 μg).

Efficacy in Chronic Asthma

Oral preparations of antileukotriene drugs can induce a rapid and significant, immediate bronchodilating effect of 10% to 30%.[113] This effect has been seen with zileuton, high-dose zafirlukast, and montelukast[114-116] (Fig. 100-3). Interestingly, when montelukast was given orally or intravenously, with dosing based on matching blood levels, not only was the effect of montelukast more rapid using an IV formulation, but the maximal bronchodilating effect was also larger.[114] The IV dose of montelukast achieved greater than 15% improvement in FEV_1 at the first measurement (15 minutes after dose), a degree of effect not seen until 2 hours after the oral dose.

These results indicate that leukotrienes are continuously present in the airways in asthma and play an important role in maintaining baseline bronchoconstriction. In addition, concomitant treatment of these patients with a β-agonist induces

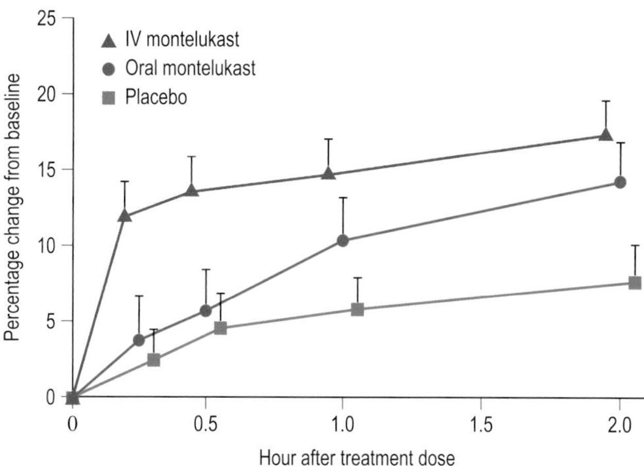

Figure 100-3 Mean percentage change from baseline in forced expiratory volume in 1 second (FEV_1) over 2-hour period after treatment. *(Reproduced from Dockhorn RJ, Baumgartner RA, Leff JA, et al. Comparison of the effects of intravenous and oral montelukast on airway function: a double blind, placebo controlled, three period, crossover study in asthmatic patients. Thorax 2000;55:260-5.)*

an additive effect on the bronchodilation, suggesting that the two types of compounds are working through different bronchodilating pathways.[113] These effects, as well as the known increase in LTE_4 excretion during acute asthma, suggest that anti-LT drugs may be useful in the treatment of status asthmaticus.[61] Two clinical trials evaluating IV montelukast (7 or 14 mg) in patients with acute asthma showed improved FEV_1 and a nonsignificant reduction in hospitalizations.[117,118] Although several studies have evaluated oral LTRAs, no consistent improvement was seen in outcomes. A recent Cochrane review recommended against the routine use of these agents in patients with acute asthma, while stating more studies were needed to determine any possible benefit from IV formulations.[119]

Multiple controlled trials of 3 to 6 months' duration evaluating the LTRAs zafirlukast and montelukast and the 5-LO inhibitor zileuton consistently showed both statistical and clinical efficacy in patients with asthma, generally of moderate severity.[75,103,120,121] Use of these compounds led to sustained and significant improvements in FEV_1 (7% to 15%), symptom scores, and β-agonist use for the duration of the trials versus placebo. Nocturnal asthma symptoms also were improved by 30% to 40%. No rebound effect seems to occur with LTRAs and 5-LO inhibitors after cessation of therapy.[75] Asthma quality-of-life scores have been clinically and significantly improved with both montelukast and zileuton.[75] Zafirlukast, montelukast, and zileuton all significantly decreased the number of times participants needed a steroid burst.[75,103,122] From an economic health perspective, statistically significant improvement was seen in days missed from work and school compared with the placebo group, as well as significantly decreased rates of asthma exacerbation.[102,103,120]

Chronic efficacy data in asthmatic children are also available. An 8-week study with oral montelukast (5 mg in the evening) demonstrated safety and efficacy compared to placebo in children 6 to 14 years old, 43% of whom were receiving concurrent ICS therapy.[123] Regardless of ICS use, improvement in FEV_1 was significantly greater in the montelukast (8.3%) versus placebo (3.6%) group.[124] Improvement in secondary outcomes, such as β-agonist use ($P = .01$), asthma exacerbations ($P = .002$), and pediatric quality of life, all support efficacy compared to placebo in this population. In a smaller study of 36 children 6 to 14 years old taking ICS, montelukast improved symptoms more than placebo and allowed for a lower dose of ICS when tapered.[125]

Wheezing in children younger than 6 years likely has many causes, with not all evolving into chronic asthma. Therapy is therefore often problematic and measurement of efficacy even more difficult. Children as young as 6 months have been treated with cysLTRAs in clinical trials. Montelukast (4 mg) in children 2 to 6 years old improved wheezing episodes compared with placebo, while an exploratory 6-week study in children 6 months to 2 years demonstrated safety but not efficacy compared to placebo.[126,127] However, a small study of 24 children age 10 to 26 months did suggest improvement in FEV_1, symptoms, and inflammation as measured by exhaled nitric oxide (FeNO).[128] A study to evaluate the impact on asthma exacerbations in young children 2 to 5 years of age with intermittent asthma demonstrated a significant reduction in the exacerbation rate (32%) versus placebo, while decreasing the need for ICS.[129] Although one study suggested montelukast improved the bronchiolitic syndrome after severe lower respiratory RSV infection, subsequent investigations have not shown efficacy.[130-132] Another study found no added benefit of montelukast in healthy children age 1 to 5 years in the prophylaxis of upper respiratory tract infections.[133]

Several small studies have addressed the impact of systemic therapy with montelukast on changes in the small airways, as assessed by lung function testing or computed tomography scans.[134,135] In corticosteroid-naïve adult patients, montelukast improved regional air trapping on CT scan compared with placebo.[134] This improvement was associated with improved quality of life and symptoms and marginally with improved FEV_1, but not lung volume. In contrast, in another study of asthmatic adults prescreened for increased residual volume (RV) on plethysmography, montelukast significantly improved physiologic measures of small-airway function such as RV. Interestingly, in both studies the changes in air trapping (on CT or plethysmography) correlated with improvements in symptom scores, whereas the changes in FEV_1 did not correlate. Also, a small study in 21 children with relatively preserved FEV_1 (mean predicted: 83% placebo group, 88% montelukast group) failed to show an effect of montelukast on FEV_1 but did note significant improvement in both RV% predicted and RV/total lung capacity ratio.[136] Whether similar changes would be seen in patients already treated with ICS, or as compared with ICS therapy versus systemic corticosteroids, is not clear. Thus the overall significance of these effects requires further study.

COMPARISON WITH INHALED CORTICOSTEROIDS

Double-blind comparison studies to ICS with the LTRAs zafirlukast, montelukast, and pranlukast (one with placebo control,[102] two not controlled[137,138]) have shown remarkably similar results and suggest that LTRAs are not as effective as low-dose beclomethasone in FEV_1 improvement (Fig. 100-4). There is consistently twice the improvement in FEV_1 with low-dose ICS (beclomethasone or fluticasone) compared to the LTRA. Less consistent differences were seen between ICS and LTRAs when evaluating other outcomes, such as symptoms and β-agonist use, although generally ICS are superior.[102,137] The differences in symptoms may not become significant until 2 to 3 weeks into

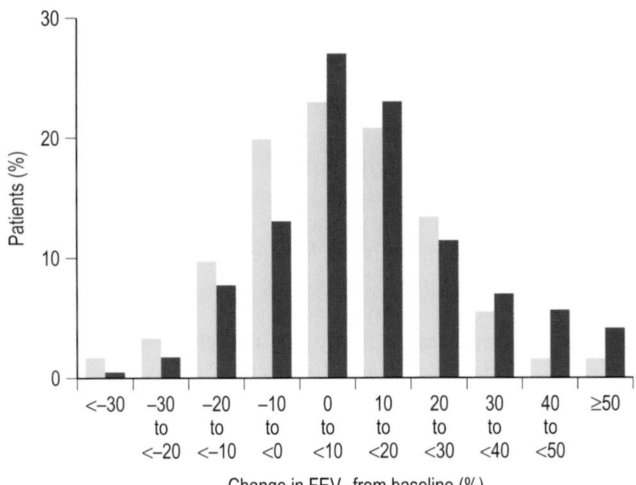

Figure 100-4 Distribution of responses in FEV_1 to treatment with montelukast, 10 mg once daily (*yellow bars*), or beclomethasone, 200 μg twice daily (*teal blue bars*). Distribution of response in FEV_1 favors beclomethasone. *(Reproduced from Malmstrom K, Rodriguez-Gomez G, Guerra J, et al. Oral montelukast, inhaled beclomethasone, and placebo for chronic asthma. Ann Intern Med 1999;130:487-95.)*

therapy.[137] The three studies did not show a statistically significant difference in exacerbation rates.[102,137,138] The effect of both classes of drugs on circulating eosinophils was similar.[102] Comparison studies in children 6 to 14 years of age have shown similar superiority of ICS (fluticasone) to montelukast in terms of pulmonary function, symptoms, and in contrast to adult studies, exacerbations.[139,140]

A Cochrane review evaluated 56 trials comparing LTRAs to ICS, generally given at low dose and concluded that ICS remain superior to LTRAs in all outcome parameters, including exacerbations, lung function, and symptoms.[141]

In all leukotriene-modulating studies, it has become clear that not all patients respond to this class of drugs. An analysis suggests that 40% to 55% of patients will have a "significant" clinical response, depending on the outcomes used.[102,142] In the study by Malmstrom and colleagues,[102] for example, 42% of the montelukast and 50% of the beclomethasone group had 11% or greater improvement in FEV_1 (see Fig. 100-4). In the study by DuBuske and associates,[142] 54% of patients treated with zileuton at standard doses achieved 10% or greater improvement in FEV_1. These studies suggest that generally there are fewer responders to anti-LT therapy than responders to ICS. A crossover study in children 6 to 17 years old reported a somewhat lower response rate (22%) when evaluating improvement in FEV_1 (≥7.5%, although response to inhaled fluticasone was lower as well (40%).[143] Interestingly, for both medications, increases in asthma control days occurred in a substantially larger percentage of the study population than improved FEV_1.[144] Unfortunately, no clinical or biomarkers are currently available to predict patients who will or will not respond to anti-LT therapy, although the two studies in children suggested that elevated urinary leukotrienes, particularly with lower FeNO levels, were associated with better response to montelukast.[143,145]

There has been increasing interest in the concept of efficacy of an intervention in clinical trials, versus "effectiveness" in a more real-world setting. Because LTRAs are oral compounds, data show greater adherence to these drugs than inhaled products. Thus, even though clinical trials confirm the superior efficacy of ICS in the treatment of asthma, LTRAs, with their greater associated adherence, might prove more beneficial in a clinical setting. A "pragmatic" study compared ICS with montelukast in a large outpatient population in the United Kingdom. Follow-up at 2 months showed that the treatments were equivalent; by 2 years, however, the ICS group showed small but significantly better outcomes, despite greater adherence in the montelukast group.[146] A similar effectiveness study in children suggested that ICS were no more effective than LTRAs in preventing hospitalizations, again likely reflected by a greater adherence to montelukast.[147] Also, retrospective cohort analyses of pharmacy and medical claims evaluated 12 months of zafirlukast or montelukast therapy compared to fluticasone.[148] However, no information was given on the initial severity of the patients' asthma, and no control was performed for physician involvement. In these studies, fluticasone was superior to either LTRA in fewer hospitalizations and emergency room visits as well as lower asthma-related health care costs. Thus, even the pragmatic effectiveness of LTRAs remains controversial.

Genetic factors also may play a role in the response to antileukotriene therapy. Several studies suggested that certain mutations in the promoter region of 5-LO or LTC_4 synthase enzymes contribute to the level of response.[10,149-151] With the 5-LO promoter, certain polymorphisms may decrease production of leukotrienes and thereby lessen the response to anti-LT therapy.[149] However, other studies have not supported those initial results; one small study found that the response to montelukast was greatest in patients (~36%) with the previously described mutant allele in the 5-LO promoter.[27] This same mutant allele has been associated with a greater risk for atherosclerotic disease, especially in individuals with high dietary intake of arachidonic acid.[152]

In a small study to evaluate polymorphisms in LTC_4 synthase, patients with the $A_{-444}C$ polymorphism had greater improvement in FEV_1 than a cysLTRA (pranlukast), and this polymorphism was an independent predictor of the response.[153] This greater response to a cysLTRA, when measured as a decrease in exacerbations, was also seen in C-allele carriers in a montelukast study.[27] The same study identified additional rare (<10% allele frequency) SNPs in the leukotriene transporter protein MRP-1 as influencing the response to montelukast. Although small, these studies support the concept that pharmacogenetics assumes a role in the response pattern to anti-LT therapy. Larger studies addressing both genotypic and phenotypic factors (e.g., heterogeneity of asthma) will be needed for a better understanding of the variable response to LTRAs.

COMPARISON WITH OTHER ASTHMA DRUGS

Few published studies compare antileukotrienes with other asthma medications. One study compared cromolyn, 1600 μg four times daily (qid) with zafirlukast, 20 mg twice daily (bid) for mild to moderate asthma.[154] Only patients with moderate peak flow variability (≥10%) at baseline showed improvement in pulmonary function. However, minimal difference was seen between the treatment groups, with cromolyn slightly superior numerically in most symptom parameters. Differences between active treatment groups were not statistically assessed. A double-blind, non–placebo-controlled study compared zileuton, 400 or 600 mg qid, with theophylline bid (titrated to therapeutic levels).[155] The theophylline group showed greater improvements over baseline in pulmonary function prior to dosing. However, within 60 minutes of dosing in the morning, there were no differences in pulmonary function among the three treatment groups. Although differences were seen at some time points between the zileuton treatment groups and the theophylline group, by the end of the study there were no significant differences in symptom scores or β-agonist use among the groups. Interestingly, zileuton had a greater effect on blood eosinophil levels than theophylline. No differences in adverse events or exacerbations suggests, with limited data, minimal difference between theophylline and one anti-LT drug, the 5-LO inhibitor zileuton. Further study is needed.

Efficacy as Add-on Therapy in Moderate to Severe Asthma

Studies with all the leukotriene-modulating drugs suggest additional benefits to these drugs versus ICS. LTRAs have been evaluated for efficacy, both "in addition" to ICS and as "steroid-sparing" agents, for their ability to allow the tapering of ICS. Cysteinyl LTRAs have not been evaluated for their ability to allow tapering of oral corticosteroids.

Numerous studies suggest that the addition of a long-acting β-agonist is more effective to control asthma than doubling the dose of ICS.[156-159] Similarly, studies have evaluated the addition of a cysLTRA to ICS, versus placebo or the long-acting β-agonist salmeterol. In the placebo comparison studies, montelukast improved clinical and physiologic outcomes when added to low doses of beclomethasone for 12 weeks in a double-blind, double-dummy placebo-controlled trial. Patients were required to be symptomatic despite therapy with low-dose beclomethasone.[160] The improvements seen were modest, with increases in FEV_1 of 5% with beclomethasone plus montelukast versus 1% with beclomethasone alone. However, all other parameters favored the combined therapy. There also were additive effects on peripheral blood eosinophil counts. In a double-blind controlled study of patients with severe asthma (baseline FEV_1 of 64% predicted) receiving high but not identical doses of ICS (average 1624 μg/day of beclomethasone or equivalent), the addition of high doses of zafirlukast (80 mg bid) improved pulmonary function, symptoms, and asthma exacerbations compared to placebo.[161] Exacerbations were reduced whether categorized as mild, moderate, or severe. Caution must be used with this study, however, because the dose of zafirlukast was four times the suggested dose and associated with increased risk of liver toxicity. In contrast, the addition of montelukast to patients still symptomatic while receiving 800 μg of budesonide, compared to doubling the dose of budesonide, demonstrated no superiority of one treatment over the other.[162] Although both groups had improved FEV_1 values and symptoms during the course of the study, no placebo group was included. A small study evaluated the short-term efficacy of adding montelukast to severely asthmatic patients, most of whom were taking at least three controller medications at baseline, with almost half taking oral corticosteroids.[163] This short-term study showed no added benefit with the addition of montelukast to therapy for patients with severe asthma.

Two double-blind placebo-controlled studies confirmed the ability of cysLTRAs to reduce high-dose ICS beyond that seen with placebo.[164,165] Concomitant use of the LTRA pranlukast in the first study allowed reduction in the beclomethasone dose of 1600 μg/day to 800 μg/day in patients with moderately severe asthma, without compromising disease control.[164] The addition of pranlukast maintained morning and evening peak flows, despite the reduced beclomethasone dose. Similarly, although patients taking the reduced dose of beclomethasone (with placebo) had increased peripheral blood eosinophils and FeNO, no increases were seen in patients taking pranlukast in addition to the reduced ICS dose. In the second study, ICS doses were tapered from about 1600 to 1000 μg/day in a single-blind, placebo run-in period. At that point, participants were treated with montelukast or placebo. The montelukast-treated group was able to reduce further ICS by another 47%, and the placebo group reduced these medications by 30% ($P < .05$).[165]

CYSTEINYL LEUKOTRIENE RECEPTOR ANTAGONISTS VERSUS LONG-ACTING β-AGONISTS

Several studies have compared add-on therapy to ICS with either a long-acting β-agonist (LABA) or a cysLTRA.[166-171] No study had a placebo arm, or even a corticosteroid doubling arm. In all cases, there were improvements in clinicophysiologic outcomes with the addition of both drugs. In the large studies, LABAs (all studies were done with salmeterol) are more potent in improving pulmonary function parameters and, in most cases, symptom scores compared to cysLTRAs. Peak flow improvement in the salmeterol groups ranged from 25 to 35 L/min, whereas improvements versus 15 to 25 L/min in the montelukast group (Fig. 100-5). However, all these studies incorporated the usual entry criteria for asthma (≥12% improvement in FEV_1 after short-acting bronchodilator), effectively screening patients for significant physiologic response to one of the study drugs (LABA). In most studies, asthma symptoms, including chest tightness, wheeze, and overall daytime

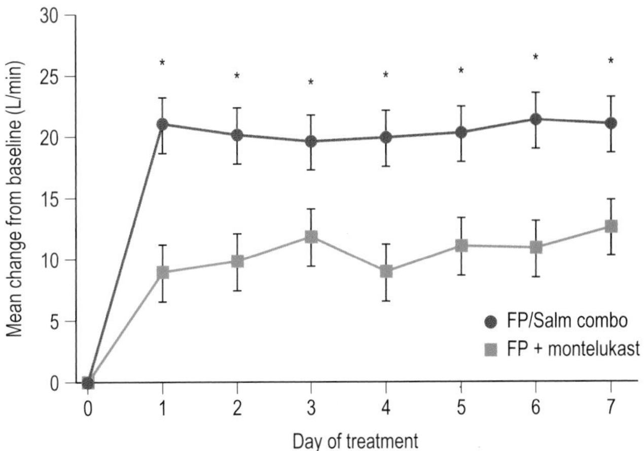

Figure 100-5 Mean percentage change from baseline in morning peak expiratory flow (PEF) during first 7 days of treatment with double-blind study medication. Baseline values were obtained during treatment with fluticasone propionate (*FP*), 100 μg twice daily. Comparable baseline morning PEFs were found in the FP/salmeteol (*Salm*) combination (398 L/min) and FP + montelukast (392 L/min) groups ($P \neq .021$) vs. FP + montelukast. *(Reproduced from Nelson HS, Busse WW, Kerwin E, et al. Fluticasone propionate/salmeterol combination provides more effective asthma control then low-dose inhaled corticosteroid plus montelukast. J Allergy Clin Immunol 2000;106:1088-95.)*

symptoms, improved more with the addition of a LABA versus the LTRA montelukast, although this has not always been the case.[166,167,169,170] In this group of more severe asthma, the effect on exacerbations may be the most important outcome. A Cochrane analysis compared the addition of LABAs versus cysLTRAs to ICS and concluded that LABAs were superior to LTRAs in reducing corticosteroid use in exacerbations (17% better with LABA versus LTRA).[172] In addition, LABAs were reported to be superior to LTRAs as adjunctive therapy in most other relevant end points, although no differences were reported for overall hospitalization rates, likely because of the overall low occurrence.

Comparative data in children are limited. A study by the National Heart, Lung and Blood Institute's Childhood Asthma Research and Education (CARE) network compared the addition of montelukast to that of LABA or a doubling of the ICS dose in children 6 to 17 years old not well controlled with low-dose ICS alone.[173] Of the three treatments, the addition of the LTRA was preferred significantly less often than the LABA in improved exacerbation rates, symptoms, and lung function. However, there was little difference between doubling the ICS dose and adding the LTRA, with a substantial percentage of children (~30%) responding more to the LTRA. Thus, although this study supports initial use of LABA in children not well controlled with ICS, substantial patient-to-patient variability in responses suggests that, as with any medication, continuous assessment of response is advised.

The effect on "inflammation" has not been carefully evaluated. However, three studies suggest that the addition of a cysLTRA to ICS may produce a greater antiinflammatory effect, as assessed by changes in peripheral blood eosinophils and a decrease in FeNO, than the addition of the LABA salmeterol or formoterol.[109,171,174] Further, the LTRA decreased the response to adenosine monophosphate (indirect measure of AHR) more than the LABA.[109] Although concerns remain about increased inflammation after long-term ICS tapering (in patients also receiving LABA), the clinical relevance is still uncertain.[175]

Use in Allergic Rhinitis and Atopic Dermatitis

Antileukotriene therapy is beneficial in both seasonal and perennial rhinitis,[176-179] and montelukast is approved by the U.S. Food and Drug Administration (FDA) for treatment of seasonal allergic rhinitis. Nasal challenge studies with LTD_4 demonstrated an increase in congestion and blood flow.[180] Although initial studies suggest that antihistamine combined with cysLTRA may be more efficacious than either agent alone, additional studies have not supported added benefit from the combination.[178] Numerous studies have compared the effect of LTRAs, alone or with antihistamines, to nasal corticosteroids, particularly fluticasone.[181-185] In every case the nasal corticosteroid was more efficacious in improving rhinitis symptoms than the LTRA. Interestingly, when montelukast versus fluticasone nasal spray was added to a salmeterol-fluticasone combination, fluticasone had greater impact on rhinitis symptoms, while neither therapy improved asthma outcomes.[181] No study has addressed the issue of response rate to LTRAs in the nose (as done for the lung), but responders and nonresponders likely exist in the allergic rhinitis population as well. Although one study supported overall efficacy of montelukast in patients with both allergic rhinitis and asthma, no studies have evaluated the overall effectiveness of LTRA therapy in patients with asthma who have concomitant allergic rhinitis versus those without rhinitis.[177]

Cysteinyl leukotrienes may also play a role in atopic dermatitis, although few trials exist. Two double-blind studies of montelukast in atopic dermatitis showed no efficacy over placebo.[186,187]

Dosing and Safety

The antileukotriene drugs are dosed orally one to four times daily. This oral dosing may lead to better compliance with these medications. Zafirlukast is dosed as 20 mg orally bid (without food) but can be safely increased to 40 mg/day; some reports suggest greater efficacy at higher doses.[161,179] Montelukast is dosed at 10 mg every evening in patients over 16 years of age. For children age 6 to 14 years, recommended dose is 5 mg/day, and for children 2 to 5 years, 4 mg/day. All the clinical trials with montelukast were done with bedtime dosing, with no information on dosing at other times of the day. There is no indication that higher doses of montelukast may be more effective. Zileuton (controlled release) is dosed at 1200 mg bid. Again, data suggest that compliance/adherence may be greater with these oral formulations.[188] Although improved adherence could affect long-term outcomes, it is not known whether adherence would offset the lesser clinical and physiologic efficacy noted with ICS.

In general, the antileukotriene class of drugs appears to be well tolerated. Zileuton has a 3% incidence of elevated alanine transaminase (ALT) levels versus placebo.[103] Higher doses of zafirlukast (80 mg bid) will likely have a similar effect on transaminases, although these data have not been published. No effect on liver function tests has been reported with montelukast beyond that seen with placebo.

All these compounds are metabolized by the liver, and thus the risk of significant interactions with other drugs metabolized by the cytochrome P-450 (CYP) enzyme system clearly exists. However, many such interactions, as could occur with antiepileptic drugs, have not yet been reported. Zafirlukast and less so zileuton have considerable interaction with warfarin, which will likely need to be reduced by up to 50%. Zileuton is also metabolized by the specific CYP system that metabolizes theophylline; recommendations for concurrent use suggest decreasing theophylline dose by 50% and then monitoring theophylline level. In addition, because food appears to interfere with its absorption, zafirlukast should be dosed 1 hour before or after meals. Montelukast has no known drug interactions.

A possible association of anti-LT therapy with Churg-Strauss syndrome, a rare eosinophilic vasculitis, has long been reported. Eight patients treated with zafirlukast with Churg-Strauss syndrome who previously received oral corticosteroids (OCS) and since had their OCS tapered.[189] Since that report, further reports of Churg-Strauss syndrome have involved patients receiving montelukast, pranlukast, and zileuton.[190-192] It remains unclear whether this is a direct causal effect, or whether the Churg-Strauss existed and was unmasked when OCS were tapered. Although most patients who developed Churg-Strauss syndrome were taking OCS, some were not. Also, Churg-Strauss syndrome has been reported with other medications, including ICS, in patients who had tapered systemic corticosteroids.[190] More information is needed before conclusions can definitively be drawn, but physicians should seriously consider complaints regarding new rashes, neurologic signs, or worsening respiratory symptoms.[189,191] All these symptoms require assessment with a minimum of a chest radiograph and a peripheral eosinophil count.

In 2009 the FDA concluded that there were sufficient reports of neuropsychiatric changes after initiation of therapy with leukotriene-modifying drugs that this was added as a precaution to consider when prescribing these agents.[193] However, this association remains controversial. Asthma itself is associated with a higher rate of suicide and other neuropsychiatric disorders, such that the true relevance of this observation remains poorly understood.[194]

Antileukotriene Therapy in Asthma Guidelines

Over the years that antileukotriene therapies have been available, our understanding of how to use them has improved. Current guidelines suggest that these drugs can be used as alternatives to ICS in the treatment of mild persistent asthma, primarily in those patients who do not respond or who choose not to take ICS.[195,196] In recent years, guidelines have also generally considered anti-LT therapy as an alternative add-on therapy to ICS in patients still symptomatic while taking single-controller therapy. However, LABAs are the preferred add-on therapy in all guidelines. There are no data to support the added benefit of triple-controller therapy (ICS + LABA + cysLTRA) in patients receiving two agents who are still symptomatic.

The anti-LT drugs should continue to be helpful in the treatment of aspirin-sensitive asthmatic patients. Although no data indicate these agents are more effective in this population of asthma patients, anecdotal experience suggests that some of the largest responses are seen in this asthma phenotype. Additionally, some patients with mild intermittent asthma, where exercise is a significant trigger, may benefit from anti-LT therapy. However, their position in this category of asthma severity is not currently listed in guidelines. Whether any clinically significant differences exist between the cysLT receptor antagonists and the 5-lipoxygenase inhibitors will likely require the development of better 5 LO inhibitors than the currently available zileuton.

In all cases, it is important to consider the individual patient, because there continue to be responders and nonresponders to all these therapies. Despite the recognition that some individuals respond better to antileukotriene therapy than others, no studies to date have (1) prospectively identified markers for response to these drugs or (2) targeted short-term or long-term efficacy trials to patients initially responsive to therapy. Whether such studies would demonstrate improved efficacy with these drugs as single-agent or add-on therapy in this responder population cannot be known; however, studies of the efficacy of LABA therapy as add-on therapy to ICS routinely target asthmatic patients with known responses to β-agonists. These more individualized approaches to the pharmacotherapy of asthma are likely to increase as additional selective pathway agents become available to treat patients with asthma.

REFERENCES

The Leukotriene Pathway

1. Sapirstein A, Bonventre JV. Specific physiological roles of cytosolic phospholipase A(2) as defined by gene knockouts. Biochim Biophys Acta 2000;1488:139-48.
2. Marshall LA, Bolognese B, Roshak A. Respective roles of the 14 kDa and 85 kDa phospholipase A_2 enzymes in human monocyte eicosanoid formation. Adv Exp Med Biol 1999;469:215-9.
3. Henderson J. The role of leukotrienes in inflammation. Ann Intern Med 1994;121: 684-97.
4. Kedda MA, Worsley P, Shi J, et al. Polymorphisms in the 5-lipoxygenase activating protein (ALOX5AP) gene are not associated with asthma in an Australian population. Clin Exp Allergy 2005;35(3):332-8.
5. Koshino T, Takano S, Kitani S, et al. Novel polymorphism of the 5-lipoxygenase activating protein (FLAP) promoter gene associated with asthma. Mol Cell Biol Res Commun 1999;2:32-5.
6. Sayers I, Barton S, Rorke S, et al. Promoter polymorphism in the 5-lipoxygenase (ALOX5) and 5-lipoxygenase-activating protein (ALOX5AP) genes and asthma susceptibility in a Caucasian population. Clin Exp Allergy 2003;33:1103-10.
7. Brock TG, Paine RI, Peters-Golden M. Localization of 5-lipoxygenase to the nucleus of unstimulated rat basophilic leukemia cells. J Biol Chem 1994;269:22059-66.
8. Woods JW, Coffey MJ, Brock TG, Singer II, Peters-Golden M. 5-Lipoxygenase is located in the euchromatin of the nucleus in resting human alveolar macrophages and translocates to the nuclear envelope upon cell activation. J Clin Invest 1995;95:2035-46.
9. Bigby TD, Hodulik CR, Arden KC, Fu L. Molecular cloning of the human leukotriene C_4 synthase gene and assignment to chromosome 5q35. Mol Med 1996;2:637-46.
10. Sanak M, Simon H-U, Szczeklik A. Leukotriene C_4 synthase promoter polymorphism and risk of aspirin-induced asthma. Lancet 1997;350 (9091):1599-600.
11. Sayers I, Barton S, Rorke S, et al. Allelic association and functional studies of promoter polymorphism in the leukotriene C_4 synthase gene (LTC_4S) in asthma. Thorax 2003;58:417-24.
12. Lam BK, Gagnon L, Austen KF, Soberman RJ. The mechanism of leukotriene B_4 export from human polymorphonuclear leukocytes. J Biol Chem 1990;265:13438-41.
13. Lam BK, Owen Jr WF, Austen KF, Soberman RJ. The identification of a distinct export step following the biosynthesis of leukotriene C_4 by human eosinophils. J Biol Chem 1989;264: 12885-9.
14. Wenzel SE, Szefler SJ, Leung DYM, et al. Bronchoscopic evaluation of severe asthma: persistent inflammation associated with high-dose glucocorticoids. Am J Respir Crit Care Med 1997;156:737-43.
15. Jatakanon A, Uasuf C, Maziak W, et al. Neutrophilic inflammation in severe persistent asthma. Am J Respir Crit Care Med 1999;160: 1532-9.
16. Fahy JV, Kim KW, Liu J. Prominent neutrophilic inflammation in sputum from subjects with asthma exacerbation. J Allergy Clin Immunol 1995;95:843-52.
17. Kamohara M, Takasaki J, Matsumoto M, et al. Molecular cloning and characterization of another leukotriene B_4 receptor. J Biol Chem 2000;275:27000-4.
18. Dasari VR, Jin J, Kunapuli SP. Distribution of leukotriene B_4 receptors in human hematopoietic cells. Immunopharmacology 2000;48: 157-63.
19. Yokomizo T, Izumi T, Chang K, Takuwa Y, Shimizu T. A G-protein-coupled receptor for leukotriene B_4 that mediates chemotaxis. Nature 1997;387:620-4.
20. Owman C, Nilsson C, Lolait SJ. Cloning of cDNA encoding a putative chemoattractant receptor. Genomics 1996;37:187-94.
21. Yokomizo T, Kato K, Terawaki K, Izumi T, Shimizu T. A second leukotriene B(4) receptor, BLT2: a new therapeutic target in inflammation and immunological disorders. J Exp Med 2000;192:421-32.
22. Heise CE, O'Dowd BF, Figueroa DJ, et al. Characterization of the human cysteinyl leukotriene 2 receptor. J Biol Chem 2000;275: 30531-36.
23. Lynch KR, O'Neill GP, Liu Q, et al. Characterization of the human cysteinyl leukotriene CysLT1 receptor. Nature 1999;399:789-93.
24. Kanaoka Y, Boyce JA. Cysteinyl leukotrienes and their receptors: cellular distribution and function in immune and inflammatory responses. J Immunol 2004;173:1503-10.
25. Figueroa DJ, Breyer RM, Defoe SK, et al. Expression of the cysteinyl leukotriene 1 receptor in normal human lung and peripheral blood leukocytes. Am J Respir Crit Care Med 2001;163:226-33.

26. Holroyd KJ, Martinati LC, Trabetti E, et al. Asthma and bronchial hyperresponsiveness linked to the XY long arm pseudoautosomal region. Genomics 1998;52:233-5.
27. Lima JJ, Zhang S, Grant A, et al. Influence of leukotriene pathway polymorphisms on response to montelukast in asthma. Am J Respir Crit Care Med 2006;173:379-85.
28. Hao L, Sayers I, Cakebread JA, et al. The cysteinyl-leukotriene type 1 receptor polymorphism 927T/C is associated with atopy severity but not with asthma. Clin Exp Allergy 2006; 36:735-41.
29. Mellor EA, Maekawa A, Austen KF, Boyce JA. Cysteinyl leukotriene receptor 1 is also a pyrimidinergic receptor and is expressed by human mast cells. Proc Natl Acad Sci USA 2001;98:7964-9.
30. Nothacker HP, Wang Z, Zhu Y, et al. Molecular cloning and characterization of a second human cysteinyl leukotriene receptor: discovery of a subtype selective agonist. Mol Pharmacol 2000;58:1601-8.
31. Mellor EA, Frank N, Soler D, et al. Expression of the type 2 receptor for cysteinyl leukotrienes (CysLT2R) by human mast cells: functional distinction from CysLT1R. Proc Natl Acad Sci USA 2003;100:11589-93.
32. Beller TC, Maekawa A, Friend DS, Austen KF, Kanaoka Y. Targeted gene disruption reveals the role of the cysteinyl leukotriene 2 receptor in increased vascular permeability and in bleomycin-induced pulmonary fibrosis in mice. J Biol Chem 2004;279:46129-34.
33. Pillai SG, Cousens DJ, Barnes AA, et al. A coding polymorphism in the CysLT2 receptor with reduced affinity to LTD_4 is associated with asthma. Pharmacogenetics 2004;14:627-33.
34. Fukai H, Ogasawara Y, Migita O, et al. Association between a polymorphism in cysteinyl leukotriene receptor 2 on chromosome 13q14 and atopic asthma. Pharmacogenetics 2004;14: 683-90.
35. Paruchuri S, Tashimo H, Feng C, et al. Leukotriene E4–induced pulmonary inflammation is mediated by the P2Y12 receptor. J Exp Med 2009;206:2543-55.
36. Wenzel S, Trudeau J, Kaminsky D, et al. Effect of 5-lypoxygenase inhibition on bronchoconstraction and airway inflammation in nocturnal asthma. Am J Respir Crit Care Med 1995;152: 897-905.
37. McGill KA, Busse WW. Zileuton. Lancet 1996; 348:519-24.

Biologic Properties of Leukotrienes

38. Adelroth E, Morris MM, Hargreave FE, O'Byrne PM. Airway responsiveness to leukotrienes C_4 and D_4 and to methacholine in patients with asthma and normal controls. N Engl J Med 1986;315:480-4.
39. Mulder A, Gauvreau GM, Watson RM, O'Byrne PM. Effect of inhaled leukotriene D_4 on airway eosinophilia and airway hyperresponsiveness in asthmatic subjects. Am J Respir Crit Care Med 1999;159(5 Pt 1):1562-7.
40. Arm JP, O'Hickey SP, Hawksworth RJ, et al. Asthmatic airways have a disproportionate hyperresponsiveness to LTE_4, as compared with normal airways, but not to LTC_4, LTD_4, methacholine, and histamine. Am Rev Respir Dis 1990;142:1112-8.
41. Drazen JM. Inhalation challenge with sulfidopeptide leukotrienes in human subjects. Chest 1986;89:414-9.
42. Casas A, Gomez FP, Dahlen B, et al. Leukotriene D_4-induced hypoxaemia in asthma is mediated by the cys-leukotriene1 receptor. Eur Respir J 2005;26:442-8.
43. Arm JP, Spur BW, Lee TH. The effects of inhaled leukotriene E_4 on the airway responsiveness to histamine in subjects with asthma and normal subjects. J Allergy Clin Immunol 1988;82:654-60.
44. Laitinen LA, Laitinen A, Haahtela T, et al. Leukotriene E_4 and granulocytic infiltration into asthmatic airways. Lancet 1993;341:989-90.
45. Diamant Z, Hiltermann JT, Van Resen ELJ, et al. The effect of inhaled leukotriene D_4 and methacholine on cell differentials in sputum from patients with asthma. Am J Respir Crit Care Med 1997;155:1247-53.
46. Laitinen A, Lindqvist A, Halme M, Altraja A, Laitinen LA. Leukotriene E(4)–induced persistent eosinophilia and airway obstruction are reversed by zafirlukast in patients with asthma. J Allergy Clin Immunol 2005;115:259-65.
47. Woodward DF, Krauss AH, Nieves AL, Spada CS. Studies on leukotriene D_4 as an eosinophil chemoattractant. Drugs Exp Clin Res 1991;17: 543-8.
48. Saito H, Morikawa H, Howie K, et al. Effects of a cysteinyl leukotriene receptor antagonist on eosinophil recruitment in experimental allergic rhinitis. Immunology 2004;113:246-52.
49. Underwood DC, Osborn RR, Newsholme SJ, Torphy TJ, Hay DW. Persistent airway eosinophilia after leukotriene (LT) D_4 administration in the guinea pig: modulation by the LTD_4 receptor antagonist, pranlukast, or an interleukin-5 monoclonal antibody. Am J Respir Crit Care Med 1996;154:850-7.
50. Lee E, Robertson T, Smith J, Kilfeather S. Leukotriene receptor antagonists and synthesis inhibitors reverse survival in eosinophils of asthmatic individuals. Am J Respir Crit Care Med 2000;161:1881-6.
51. Stenke L, Mansour M, Reizenstein P, Lindgrem JA. Stimulation of human myelopoiesis by leukotrienes B_4 and C_4: interactions with granulocyte-macrophage colony-stimulating factor. Am Soc Hematol 1993;81:352-6.
52. Wang CG, Du T, Xu LJ, Martin JG. Role of leukotriene D_4 in allergen-induced increases in airway smooth muscle in the rat. Am Rev Respir Dis 1993;148:413-7.
53. Panettieri RA, Tan EML, Ciocca V, et al. Effects of LTD_4 on human airway smooth muscle cell proliferation, matrix expression, and contraction in vitro: differential sensitivity to cysteinyl leukotriene receptor antagonists. Am J Respir Cell Mol Biol 1998;19:453-61.
54. Kim DC, Hsu FI, Barrett NA, et al. Cysteinyl leukotrienes regulate Th2 cell–dependent pulmonary inflammation. J Immunol 2006;176: 4440-8.
55. Lewis RA, Austen F, Soberman RJ. Leukotrienes and other products of the 5-lipoxygenase pathway. N Engl J Med 1990;323:645-55.
56. Ott VL, Cambier JC, Kappler J, Marrack P, Swanson BJ. Mast cell–dependent migration of effector $CD8^+$ T cells through production of leukotriene B_4. Nat Immunol 2003;4:974-81.
57. Terawaki K, Yokomizo T, Nagase T, et al. Absence of leukotriene B_4 receptor 1 confers resistance to airway hyperresponsiveness and Th2-type immune responses. J Immunol 2005;175:4217-25.
58. Taube C, Miyahara N, Ott V, et al. The leukotriene B_4 receptor (BLT1) is required for effector $CD8^+$ T cell–mediated, mast cell–dependent airway hyperresponsiveness. J Immunol 2006;176:3157-64.
59. Westcott JY, Johnston K, Batt RA, Wenzel SE, Voelkel NF. Measurement of peptidoleukotrienes in biologic fluid. J Appl Physiol 1990;68: 2640-8.
60. Wenzel SE, Larsen GL, Johnston K, Voelkel NF, Westcott JY. Elevated levels of leukotriene C_4 in bronchoalveolar lavage fluid from atopic asthmatics after endobronchial allergen challenge. Am Rev Respir Dis 1990;142:112-9.
61. Taylor IK, Wellings R, Taylor GW, Fuller RW. Urinary leukotriene E_4 excretion in exercise-induced asthma. J Appl Physiol 1992;73: 743-8.
62. Krawiec ME, Westcott JY, Chu HW, et al. Persistent wheezing in very young children is associated with lower respiratory inflammation. Am J Respir Crit Care Med 2001;163: 1338-43.
63. Szczeklik A, Sladek K, Dworski R, et al. Bronchial aspirin challenge causes specific eicosanoid response in aspirin-sensitive asthmatics. Am J Respir Crit Care Med 1996;154:1608-14.
64. Volovitz B, Welliver RC, De Castro G, Krystofik DA, Ogra PL. The release of leukotrienes in the respiratory tract during infection with respiratory syncytial virus: role in obstructive airway disease. Pediatr Res 1988;24:504-7.

Leukotriene Inhibition/Antagonism and Asthmatic Inflammation

65. Taylor IK, Fuller RW, Dollery CT. Effect of cysteinyl-leukotriene receptor antagonist ICI 204, 219 on allergen-induced bronchoconstriction and airway hyperreactivity in atopic subjects. Lancet 1991;337:690-4.
66. Findlay SR, Barden JM, Easley CB, Glass M. Effect of the oral leukotriene antagonist ICI 204,219 on antigen-induced bronchoconstriction in subjects with asthma. J Allergy Clin Immunol 1992;89:1040-5.
67. Hui KP, Barnes NC. Lung function improvement in asthma with a cysteinyl-leukotriene receptor antagonist. Lancet 1991;337:1062-3.
68. Bel EH, Timmers MC, Hermans J, Dijkman JH, Sterk PJ. The long-term effects of nedocromil sodium and beclomethasone dipropionate on bronchial responsiveness to methacholine in nonatopic asthmatic subjects. Am Rev Respir Dis 1990;141:21-8.
69. Diamant Z, Grootendorst C, Veselic-Charvat M, et al. The effect of montelukast (MK-0476), a cysteinyl leukotriene receptor antagonist, on allergen-induced airway responses and sputum cell counts in asthma. Clin Exp Allergy 1999;29:42-51.
70. Wenzel SE. Inflammation, leukotrienes and the pathogenesis of the late asthmatic response. Clin Exp Allergy 1999;29(1):1-3.
71. Calhoun WJ, Lavins BJ, Minkwitz MC, et al. Effect of zafirlukast (Accolate) on cellular mediators of inflammation. Am J Respir Crit Care Med 1998;157:1381-9.
72. Kane GC, Pollice M, Kim C-J, et al. A controlled trial of the effect of the 5-lipoxygenase inhibitor, zileuton, on lung inflammation produced by segmental antigen challenge in human beings. J Allergy Clin Immunol 1996; 97:646-54.
73. Hasday JD, Meltzer SS, Moore WC, et al. Anti-inflammatory effects of zileuton in a subpopulation of allergic asthmatics. Am J Respir Crit Care Med 2000;161:1229-36.

74. Martin RJ, Cicutto LC, Ballard RD. Factors related to the nocturnal worsening of asthma. Am Rev Respir Dis 1990;141:33-8.
75. Reiss TF, Chervinsky P, Dockhorn RJ, et al. Montelukast, a once-daily leukotriene receptor antagonist, in the treatment of chronic asthma. Arch Intern Med 1998;158:1213-20.
76. Meltzer SS, Hasday JD, Cohn J, Bleecker ER. Inhibition of exercise-induced bronchospasm by zileuton: a 5-lipoxygenase inhibitor. Am J Respir Crit Care Med 1996;153:931-5.
77. Leff JA, Busse WW, Pearlman D, et al. Montelukast, a leukotriene-receptor antagonist, for the treatment of mild asthma and exercise-induced bronchoconstriction. N Engl J Med 1998;339:147-52.
78. Reiss TF, Hill JB, Harman E, et al. Increased urinary excretion of LTE_4 after exercise and attenuation of exercise-induced bronchospasm by montelukast, a cysteinyl leukotriene receptor antagonist. Thorax 1997;52:1030-5.
79. Finnerty J, Wood-Baker R, Thomson H, et al. Role of leukotrienes in exercise-induced asthma inhibitory effect of ICI 204,219, a potent leukotriene D_4 receptor antagonist. Am Rev Respir Dis 1992;145(4 Pt 1):746-9.
80. Robuschi M, Riva E, Fuccella L, et al. Prevention of exercise-induced bronchoconstriction by a new leukotriene antagonist (SK&F 104353). Am Rev Respir Dis 1992;145:1285-8.
81. Kemp JP, Dockhorn RJ, Shapiro GG, et al. Montelukast once daily inhibits exercise-induced bronchoconstriction in 6- to 14-year-old children with asthma. J Pediatr 1998;133: 424-8.
82. Pearlman DS, Ostrom NK, Bronsky EA, Bonuccelli CM, Hanby LA. The leukotriene D_4-receptor antagonist zafirlukast attenuates exercise- induced bronchoconstriction in children. J Pediatr 1999;134:273-9.
83. Bisgaard H, Nielsen KG. Bronchoprotection with a leukotriene receptor antagonist in asthmatic preschool children. Am J Respir Crit Care Med 2000;162:187-90.
84. Edelman JM, Turpin JA, Bronsky EA, et al. Oral montelukast compared with inhaled salmeterol to prevent exercise- induced bronchoconstriction: a randomized, double-blind trial. Exercise Study Group. Ann Intern Med 2000; 132:97-104.
85. Villaran C, O'Neill SJ, Helbling A, et al. Montelukast versus salmeterol in patients with asthma and exercise-induced bronchoconstriction. J Allergy Clin Immunol 1999;104: 547-53.
86. Simons FE, Gerstner TV, Cheang MS. Tolerance to the bronchoprotective effect of salmeterol in adolescents with exercise-induced asthma using concurrent inhaled glucocorticoid treatment. Pediatrics 1997;99:655-9.
87. Nelson JA, Strauss L, Skowronski M, et al. Effect of long-term salmeterol treatment on exercise-induced asthma. N Engl J Med 1998; 339:141-6.
88. Sanderson N, Factor V, Nagy P, et al. Hepatic expression of mature transforming growth factor β1 in transgenic mice results in multiple tissue lesions. Proc Natl Acad Sci USA 1995; 92:2572-6.
89. Sladek K, Szczeklik A. Cysteinyl leukotrienes overproduction and mast cell activation in aspirin-provoked bronchospasm in asthma. Eur Respir J 1993;6:391-9.
90. Cowburn AS, Sladek K, Soja J, et al. Overexpression of leukotriene C_4 synthase in bronchial biopsies from patients with aspirin-intolerant asthma. J Clin Invest 1998;101: 834-46.
91. Nasser SMS, Christie PE, Pfister R, Sousa AR. Effect of endobronchial challenge on inflammatory cells in bronchial biopsy samples from aspirin-sensitive asthmatic subjects. Thorax 1996;51:64-70.
92. Corrigan C, Mallett K, Ying S, et al. Expression of the cysteinyl leukotriene receptors CysLT(1) and CysLT(2) in aspirin-sensitive and aspirin-tolerant chronic rhinosinusitis. J Allergy Clin Immunol 2005;115:316-22.
93. Sanak M, Pierzchalska M, Bazan-Socha S, Szczeklik A. Enhanced expression of the leukotriene C(4) synthase due to overactive transcription of an allelic variant associated with aspirin-intolerant asthma. Am J Respir Cell Mol Biol 2000;23:290-6.
94. Van Sambeek R, Stevenson DD, Baldasaro M, et al. 5′ flanking region polymorphism of the gene encoding leukotriene C_4 synthase does not correlate with the aspirin-intolerant asthma phenotype in the United States. J Allergy Clin Immunol 2000;106:72-6.
95. Kedda MA, Shi J, Duffy D, et al. Characterization of two polymorphisms in the leukotriene C_4 synthase gene in an Australian population of subjects with mild, moderate, and severe asthma. J Allergy Clin Immunol 2004;113: 889-95.
96. Fischer AR, Rosenberg MA, Lilly CM, et al. Direct evidence for a role of the mast cell in the nasal response to aspirin in aspirin-sensitive asthma. J Allergy Clin Immunol 1994;94:1046-56.
97. Israel E, Fischer AR, Rosenberg MA, et al. The pivotal role of 5-lipoxygenase products in the reaction of aspirin-sensitive asthmatics to aspirin. Am Rev Respir Dis 1993;148: 1447-51.
98. Christie P, Smith C, Lee TH. The potent and selective sulfidopeptide leukotriene antagonist, SK&F 104353 inhibits aspirin induced asthma. Am Rev Respir Dis 1991;144:957-8.
99. Stevenson DD, Simon RA, Mathison DA, Christiansen SC. Montelukast is only partially effective in inhibiting aspirin responses in aspirin-sensitive asthmatics. Ann Allergy Asthma Immunol 2000;85(6 Pt 1):477-82.
100. Kumlin M, Dahlen B, Bjorck T, et al. Urinary excretion of leukotriene E_4 and 11-dehydro-thromboxane B_2 in response to bronchial provocations with allergen, aspirin, leukotriene D_4, and histamine in asthmatics. Am Rev Respir Dis 1992;146:96-103.
101. Dahlen B, Nizankowska E, Szczeklik A, et al. Benefits from adding the 5-lipoxygenase inhibitor zileuton to conventional therapy in aspirin-intolerant asthmatics. Am J Respir Crit Care Med 1998;157:1187-94.
102. Malmstrom K, Rodriguez-Gomez G, Guerra J, et al. Oral montelukast, inhaled beclomethasone, and placebo for chronic asthma. Ann Intern Med 1999;130:487-95.
103. Liu MC, Dube LM, Lancaster J, Group ZS. Acute and chronic effects of a 5-lipoxygenase inhibitor in asthma: a 6-month randomized multicenter trial. J Allergy Clin Immunol 1996;98:859-71.
104. Nakamura Y, Hoshino M, Sim JJ, et al. Effect of the leukotriene receptor antagonist pranlukast on cellular infiltration in the bronchial mucosa of patients with asthma. Thorax 1998;53:835-41.
105. Ramsay CF, Li D, Wang D, et al. Bronchial biopsy specimen variability: requirement for large sample size and repeated measurements to improve reliability. Am J Respir Crit Care Med 1999;159:A655.
106. Overbeek SE, O'Sullivan S, Leman K, et al. Effect of montelukast compared with inhaled fluticasone on airway inflammation. Clin Exp Allergy 2004;34:1388-94.
107. Pizzichini E, Leff JA, Reiss TF, et al. Montelukast reduces airway eosinophilic inflammation in asthma: a randomized, controlled trial. Eur Respir J 1999;14:12-8.
108. Jayaram L, Duong M, Pizzichini MM, et al. Failure of montelukast to reduce sputum eosinophilia in high-dose corticosteroid-dependent asthma. Eur Respir J 2005;25: 41-6.
109. Wilson AM, Dempsey OJ, Sims EJ, Lipworth BJ. Evaluation of salmeterol or montelukast as second-line therapy for asthma not controlled with inhaled corticosteroids. Chest 2001;119: 1021-6.
110. Bisgaard H, Loland L, Anhoj J. NO in exhaled air of asthmatic children is reduced by the leukotriene receptor antagonist montelukast. Am J Resp Crit Care Med 1999;160:1227-31.
111. Sandrini A, Ferreira IM, Gutierrez C, et al. Effect of montelukast on exhaled nitric oxide and nonvolatile markers of inflammation in mild asthma. Chest 2003;124:1334-40.
112. Straub DA, Minocchieri S, Moeller A, et al. The effect of montelukast on exhaled nitric oxide and lung function in asthmatic children 2 to 5 years old. Chest 2005;127:509-14.

Efficacy in Chronic Asthma

113. Gaddy J, Margolskee D, Bush R, Williams VWB. Bronchodilation with a potent and selective leukotriene D_4 (LTD_4) receptor antagonist (MK-571) in patients with asthma. Am Rev Respir Dis 1992;146:303-29.
114. Dockhorn RJ, Baumgartner RA, Leff JA, et al. Comparison of the effects of intravenous and oral montelukast on airway function: a double blind, placebo controlled, three period, crossover study in asthmatic patients. Thorax 2000;55:260-5.
115. Bateman ED, Aitchison JA, Summerton L, Harris A. The early onset of action of zafirlukast (Accolate) in patients with asthma. Am J Respir Crit Care Med 1997;155:A663.
116. Israel E, Rubin P, Kemp J, et al. The effect of inhibition of 5-lipoxygenase by zileuton in mild-to-moderate asthma. Ann Intern Med 1993;119:1059-66.
117. Camargo Jr CA, Smithline HA, Malice MP, Green SA, Reiss TF. A randomized controlled trial of intravenous montelukast in acute asthma. Am J Respir Crit Care Med 2003;167: 528-33.
118. Camargo Jr CA, Gurner DM, Smithline HA, et al. A randomized placebo-controlled study of intravenous montelukast for the treatment of acute asthma. J Allergy Clin Immunol 2010; 125:374-80.
119. Watts K, Chavasse RJ. Leukotriene receptor antagonists in addition to usual care for acute asthma in adults and children. Cochrane Database Syst Rev Online 2012;(5):CD006100.
120. Suissa S, Dennis R, Ernst P, et al. Effectiveness of the leukotriene receptor antagonist zafirlukast for mild-to-moderate asthma: a randomized, double-blind, placebo-controlled trial. Ann Intern Med 1997;126:177-83.

121. Spector SL, Smith LJ, Glass M. Effects of 6 weeks of therapy with oral doses of ICI 204,219, a leukotriene D_4 receptor antagonist, in subjects with bronchial asthma. Am J Respir Crit Care Med 1994;150:618-23.
122. Barnes NC, Black B, Syrett N, Cohn J. Reduction of exacerbations of asthma in multinational clinical trials of zafirlukast (Accolate). Am J Respir Crit Care Med 1996;153:A802.
123. Meyers DA, Banks-Schlegel S, Bleecker ER, et al. A genome-wide search for asthma susceptibility loci in ethnically diverse populations. Am J Hum Genet 1996;59:A228.
124. Knorr B, Matz J, Bernstin JA, et al. Montelukast for chronic asthma in 6- to 14-year-old children: a randomized, double-blind trial. JAMA 1998;279:1181-6.
125. Phipatanakul W, Greene C, Downes SJ, et al. Montelukast improves asthma control in asthmatic children maintained on inhaled corticosteroids. Ann Allergy Asthma Immunol 2003; 91:49-54.
126. Van Adelsberg J, Moy J, Wei LX, et al. Safety, tolerability, and exploratory efficacy of montelukast in 6- to 24-month-old patients with asthma. Curr Med Res Opin 2005;21:971-9.
127. Knorr B, Franchi LM, Bisgaard H, et al. Montelukast, a leukotriene receptor antagonist, for the treatment of persistent asthma in children aged 2 to 5 years. Pediatrics 2001; 108:E48.
128. Straub DA, Moeller A, Minocchieri S, et al. The effect of montelukast on lung function and exhaled nitric oxide in infants with early childhood asthma. Eur Respir J 2005;25:289-94.
129. Bisgaard H, Zielen S, Garcia-Garcia ML, et al. Montelukast reduces asthma exacerbations in 2- to 5-year-old children with intermittent asthma. Am J Respir Crit Care Med 2005;171: 315-22.
130. Bisgaard H. A randomized trial of montelukast in respiratory syncytial virus postbronchiolitis. Am J Respir Crit Care Med 2003;167:379-83.
131. Bisgaard H, Flores-Nunez A, Goh A, et al. Study of montelukast for the treatment of respiratory symptoms of post-respiratory syncytial virus bronchiolitis in children. Am J Respir Crit Care Med 2008;178:854-60.
132. Proesmans M, Sauer K, Govaere E, et al. Montelukast does not prevent reactive airway disease in young children hospitalized for RSV bronchiolitis. Acta Paediatr 2009;98:1830-4.
133. Kozer E, Lotem Z, Elgarushe M, et al. RCT of montelukast as prophylaxis for upper respiratory tract infections in children. Pediatrics 2012;129:e285-90.
134. Zeidler MR, Kleerup EC, Goldin JG, et al. Montelukast improves regional air-trapping due to small airways obstruction in asthma. Eur Respir J 2006;27:307-15.
135. Kraft M, Cairns CB, Ellison MC, et al. Improvements in distal lung function correlate with asthma symptoms after treatment with oral montelukast. Chest 2006;130:1726-32.
136. Spahn JD, Covar RA, Jain N, et al. Effect of montelukast on peripheral airflow obstruction in children with asthma. Ann Allergy Asthma Immunol 2006;96:541-9.
137. Busse W, Raphael GD, Galant S, et al. Low-dose fluticasone propionate compared with montelukast for first-line treatment of persistent asthma: a randomized clinical trial. J Allergy Clin Immunol 2001;107:461-8.
138. Bleecker ER, Welch MJ, Weinstein SF, et al. Low-dose inhaled fluticasone propionate versus oral zafirlukast in the treatment of persistent asthma. J Allergy Clin Immunol 2000; 105:1123-9.
139. Ostrom NK, Decotiis BA, Lincourt WR, et al. Comparative efficacy and safety of low-dose fluticasone propionate and montelukast in children with persistent asthma. J Pediatr 2005;147:213-20.
140. Garcia Garcia ML, Wahn U, Gilles L, et al. Montelukast, compared with fluticasone, for control of asthma among 6- to 14-year-old patients with mild asthma: the MOSAIC study. Pediatrics 2005;116:360-9.
141. Chauhan BF, Ducharme FM. Anti-leukotriene agents compared to inhaled corticosteroids in the management of recurrent and/or chronic asthma in adults and children. Cochrane Database Syst Rev Online 2012;(5): CD002314.
142. DuBuske LM, Grossman J, Dube LM, Swanson LJ, Lancaster JF. Randomized trial of zileuton in patients with moderate asthma: effect of reduced dosing frequency and amounts on pulmonary function and asthma symptoms. Zileuton Study Group. Am J Manag Care 1997;3:633-40.
143. Szefler SJ, Phillips BR, Martinez FD, et al. Characterization of within-subject responses to fluticasone and montelukast in childhood asthma. J Allergy Clin Immunol 2005;115: 233-42.
144. Zeiger RS, Szefler SJ, Phillips BR, et al. Response profiles to fluticasone and montelukast in mild-to-moderate persistent childhood asthma. J Allergy Clin Immunol 2006; 117:45-52.
145. Rabinovitch N, Graber NJ, Chinchilli VM, et al. Urinary leukotriene E_4/exhaled nitric oxide ratio and montelukast response in childhood asthma. J Allergy Clin Immunol 2010; 126:545-51.
146. Price D, Musgrave SD, Shepstone L, et al. Leukotriene antagonists as first-line or add-on asthma-controller therapy. N Engl J Med 2011;364:1695-707.
147. Ducharme FM, Noya FJ, Allen-Ramey FC, et al. Clinical effectiveness of inhaled corticosteroids versus montelukast in children with asthma: prescription patterns and patient adherence as key factors. Curr Med Res Opin 2012;28:111-9.
148. Stempel DA, Meyer JW, Stanford RH, Yancey SW. One-year claims analysis comparing inhaled fluticasone propionate with zafirlukast for the treatment of asthma. J Allergy Clin Immunol 2001;107:94-8.
149. Drazen JM, Yandava CN, Dube L, et al. Pharmacogenetic association between ALOX5 promoter genotype and the response to anti-asthma treatment. Nat Genet 1999;22: 168-70.
150. Sampson AP, Siddiqui S, Buchanan D, et al. Variant LTC(4) synthase allele modifies cysteinyl leukotriene synthesis in eosinophils and predicts clinical response to zafirlukast. Thorax 2000;55(Suppl 2):28-31.
151. In KH, Asano K, Beier D, et al. Naturally occurring mutations in the human 5-lipoxygenase gene promoter that modify transcription factor binding and reporter gene transcription. J Clin Invest 1997;99:1130-7.
152. Dwyer JH, Allayee H, Dwyer KM, et al. Arachidonate 5-lipoxygenase promoter genotype, dietary arachidonic acid, and atherosclerosis. N Engl J Med 2004;350:29-37.
153. Asano K, Shiomi T, Hasegawa N, et al. Leukotriene C_4 synthase gene A(−444)C polymorphism and clinical response to a CYS-LT(1) antagonist, pranlukast, in Japanese patients with moderate asthma. Pharmacogenetics 2002;12:565-70.
154. Nathan RA, Minkwitz MC, Bonuccelli CM. Two first-line therapies in the treatment of mild asthma: use of peak flow variability as a predictor of effectiveness. Ann Allergy Asthma Immunol 1999;82:497-503.
155. Schwartz HJ, Petty T, Dube LM, Swanson LJ, Lancaster JF. A randomized controlled trial comparing zileuton with theophylline in moderate asthma. The Zileuton Study Group. Arch Intern Med 1998;158:141-8.

Efficacy as Add-on Therapy in Moderate to Severe Asthma

156. Woolcock A, Lundback B, Ringdal N, Jacques LA. Comparison of addition of salmeterol to inhaled steroids with doubling of the dose of inhaled steroids. Am J Respir Crit Care Med 1996;153:1481-8.
157. Greening AP, Ind PW, Northfield M, Shaw G. Added salmeterol versus higher-dose corticosteroid in asthma patients with symptoms on existing inhaled corticosteroid. Lancet 1994; 344:219-24.
158. Evans DJ, Taylor DA, Zetterstrom O, et al. A comparison of low-dose inhaled budesonide plus theophylline and high-dose inhaled budesonide for moderate asthma. N Engl J Med 1997;337:1412-8.
159. Pauwels RA, Lofdahl CG, Postma DS, et al. Effect of inhaled formoterol and budesonide on exacerbations of asthma. N Engl J Med 1997;337:1405-11.
160. Laviolette M, Malmstrom K, Lu S, et al. Montelukast added to inhaled beclomethasone in treatment of asthma. Montelukast/Beclomethasone Additivity Group. Am J Respir Crit Care Med 1999;160:1862-8.
161. Virchow J, Prasse A, Naya I, Summerton L, Harris A. Zafirlukast improves asthma control in patients receiving high-dose inhaled corticosteroids. Am J Respir Crit Care Med 2000;162:578-85.
162. Price DB, Hernandez D, Magyar P, et al. Randomised controlled trial of montelukast plus inhaled budesonide versus double dose inhaled budesonide in adult patients with asthma. Thorax 2003;58:211-6.
163. Robinson DS, Campbell D, Barnes PJ. Addition of leukotriene antagonists to therapy in chronic persistent asthma: a randomised double-blind placebo-controlled trial. Lancet 2001;357(9273):2007-11.
164. Tamaoki J, Kondo M, Sakai N. Leukotriene antagonist prevents exacerbation of asthma during reduction of high-dose inhaled corticosteroid. Am J Respir Crit Care Med 1997;155: 1235-40.
165. Lofdahl CG, Reiss TF, Leff JA, et al. Randomised, placebo controlled trial of effect of a leukotriene receptor antagonist, montelukast, on tapering inhaled corticosteroids in asthmatic patients. BMJ 1999;319:87-90.
166. Fish JE, Israel E, Murray JJ, et al. Salmeterol powder provides significantly better benefit than montelukast in asthmatic patients receiving concomitant inhaled corticosteroid therapy. Chest 2001;120:423-30.
167. Nelson HS, Busse WW, Kerwin E, et al. Fluticasone propionate/salmeterol combination

provides more effective asthma control than low-dose inhaled corticosteroid plus montelukast. J Allergy Clin Immunol 2000;106:1088-95.
168. Busse W, Nelson H, Wolfe J, et al. Comparison of inhaled salmeterol and oral zafirlukast in patients with asthma. J Allergy Clin Immunol 1999;103:1075-80.
169. Ilowite J, Webb R, Friedman B, et al. Addition of montelukast or salmeterol to fluticasone for protection against asthma attacks: a randomized, double-blind, multicenter study. Ann Allergy Asthma Immunol 2004;92:641-8.
170. Ringdal N, Eliraz A, Pruzinec R, et al. The salmeterol/fluticasone combination is more effective than fluticasone plus oral montelukast in asthma. Respir Med 2003;97:234-41.
171. Bjermer L, Bisgaard H, Bousquet J, et al. Montelukast and fluticasone compared with salmeterol and fluticasone in protecting against asthma exacerbation in adults: one year, double blind, randomised, comparative trial. BMJ 2003;327(7420):891.
172. Ram FSF, Cates CJ, Ducharme FM. Long-acting β_2-agonists versus anti-leukotrienes as add-on therapy to inhaled corticosteroids for chronic asthma. Cochrane Database Syst Rev 2005;1-74.
173. Lemanske Jr RF, Mauger DT, Sorkness CA, et al. Step-up therapy for children with uncontrolled asthma receiving inhaled corticosteroids. N Engl J Med 2010;362:975-85.
174. Lipworth BJ, Dempsey OJ, Aziz I, Wilson AM. Effects of adding a leukotriene antagonist or a long-acting β_2-agonist in asthmatic patients with the glycine-16 β_2-adrenoceptor genotype. Am J Med 2000;109:114-21.
175. McIvor RA, Pizzichini E, Turner MO, et al. Potential masking effects of salmeterol on airway inflammation in asthma. Am J Respir Crit Care Med 1998;158:924-30.

Allergic Rhinitis and Atopic Dermatitis

176. Van Adelsberg J, Philip G, Pedinoff AJ, et al. Montelukast improves symptoms of seasonal allergic rhinitis over a 4-week treatment period. Allergy 2003;58:1268-76.
177. Busse WW, Casale TB, Dykewicz MS, et al. Efficacy of montelukast during the allergy season in patients with chronic asthma and seasonal aeroallergen sensitivity. Ann Allergy Asthma Immunol 2006;96:60-8.
178. Meltzer EO, Malmstrom K, Lu S, et al. Concomitant montelukast and loratadine as treatment for seasonal allergic rhinitis: a randomized, placebo-controlled clinical trial. J Allergy Clin Immunol 2000;105:917-22.
179. Donnelly AL, Glass M, Minkwitz MC, Casale TB. The leukotriene D_4-receptor antagonist, ICI 204, 219, relieves symptoms of acute seasonal allergic rhinitis. Am J Respir Crit Care Med 1995;151:1734-9.
180. Naclerio RM, Baroody FM, Togias AG. The role of leukotrienes in allergic rhinitis: a review. Am Rev Respir Dis 1991;143(5 Pt 2):S91-5.
181. Nathan RA, Yancey SW, Waitkus-Edwards K, et al. Fluticasone propionate nasal spray is superior to montelukast for allergic rhinitis while neither affects overall asthma control. Chest 2005;128:1910-20.
182. Pullerits T, Praks L, Ristioja V, Lotvall J. Comparison of a nasal glucocorticoid, antileukotriene, and a combination of antileukotriene and antihistamine in the treatment of seasonal allergic rhinitis. J Allergy Clin Immunol 2002;109:949-55.
183. Di Lorenzo G, Pacor ML, Pellitteri ME, et al. Randomized placebo-controlled trial comparing fluticasone aqueous nasal spray in monotherapy, fluticasone plus cetirizine, fluticasone plus montelukast and cetirizine plus montelukast for seasonal allergic rhinitis. Clin Exp Allergy 2004;34:259-67.
184. Martin BG, Andrews CP, van Bavel JH, et al. Comparison of fluticasone propionate aqueous nasal spray and oral montelukast for the treatment of seasonal allergic rhinitis symptoms. Ann Allergy Asthma Immunol 2006;96:851-7.
185. Ratner PH, Howland 3rd WC, Arastu R, et al. Fluticasone propionate aqueous nasal spray provided significantly greater improvement in daytime and nighttime nasal symptoms of seasonal allergic rhinitis compared with montelukast. Ann Allergy Asthma Immunol 2003;90:536-42.
186. Veien NK, Busch-Sorensen M, Stausbol-Gron B. Montelukast treatment of moderate to severe atopic dermatitis in adults: a randomized, double-blind, placebo-controlled trial. J Am Acad Dermatol 2005;53:147-9.
187. Friedmann PS, Palmer R, Tan E, et al. A double-blind, placebo-controlled trial of montelukast in adult atopic eczema. Clin Exp Allergy 2007;37:1536-40.

Dosing and Safety

188. Kelloway JS, Wyatt RA, Adlis SA. Comparison of patients' compliance with prescribed oral and inhaled asthma medications. Arch Intern Med 1994;154:1349-52.
189. Wechsler ME, Garpestad E, Flier SR, et al. Pulmonary infiltrates, eosinophilia, and cardiomyopathy following corticosteroid withdrawal in patients with asthma receiving zafirlukast. JAMA 1998;279:455-7.
190. Weller PF, Plaut M, Taggart V, Trontell A. The relationship of asthma therapy and Churg-Strauss syndrome: NIH workshop summary report. J Allergy Clin Immunol 2001;108:175-83.
191. Wechsler ME, Pauwels R, Drazen JM. Leukotriene modifiers and Churg-Strauss syndrome. Drug Safety 1999;21:241-51.
192. Wechsler ME, Finn D, Gunawardena D, et al. Churg-Strauss syndrome in patients receiving montelukast as treatment for asthma. Chest 2000;117:708-13.
193. US Food and Drug Administration. Early communication about an ongoing safety review of montelukast (Singular). 2009. Available at http://www.fda.gov/drugs/drugsafety/postmarketdrugsafetyinfomrationforpatientsandproviders/drugsafteryinfmaitonaforhealthcareprofessionals/ucm070618.htm.
194. Kuo CJ, Chen VC, Lee WC, et al. Asthma and suicide mortality in young people: a 12-year follow-up study. Am J Psychiatry 2010;167:1092-9.

Antileukotriene Therapy in Asthma Guidelines

195. National Asthma Education and Prevention Program. Guidelines for the Diagnosis and Management of Asthma. Expert Panel Report 3. 2007. Available at www.nhlbi.nih.gov/guidelines/asthma.
196. Global Initiative for Asthma. Global Strategy for Asthma Management and Prevention (GINA). 2011. Available at www.ginasthma.org/guidelines-gina-report-global-strategy-for-asthma.html.

Unconventional Theories and Unproven Methods in Allergy

LEONARD BIELORY | ABBA I. TERR

CONTENTS

SUMMARY OF IMPORTANT CONCEPTS

» Optimal allergy practice requires scientifically based medical knowledge and procedures.
» Unconventional, unscientific methods of allergy diagnosis and treatment are widespread.
» Unorthodox medical theories lead to numerous unproven procedures.
» Allergy practitioners should be knowledgeable about both conventional and unconventional methods to provide optimal management of patients with allergic disease.

Certain practitioners use unconventional, unproven, and controversial procedures and theories for allergy diagnosis and therapy. These practices often are referred to collectively as "alternative" or "complementary."[1,2] Complementary and alternative medicine (CAM) and integrative medicine (IM) are frequently used terms, but the theories and methods embraced by CAM and IM neither replace nor assist those methods that are based on scientific principles and have been shown by proper clinical trials to be both effective and safe for allergic patients.[3]

The National Center for Complementary and Alternative Medicine (NCCAM) was established in 1998 to "define, through rigorous scientific investigation, the usefulness and safety of complementary and alternative medicine interventions and their roles in improving health and health care."[3a] Throughout this chapter, selected references to such trials in allergic disease are provided when applicable.

Several scholarly reviews and meta-analyses of unproven methods and theories are the source of additional references to primary studies for the interested reader.[4-18] These issues concern local and national medical societies, third-party payers of medical services, and certain governmental bodies. Some of these organizations have studied these procedures and have issued statements, position papers, or practice guidelines on dealing with unproven diagnostic and therapeutic methods in allergy.[19-26]

Introduction

This chapter reviews and critiques unproven diagnostic tests, treatment methods, theories, and diagnoses that have been used in "alternative" approaches to allergy. The physician who treats patients with allergic disease should be knowledgeable about both accepted and unproven techniques and theories in order to provide the best currently available care and to counsel the patient about the questionable benefits of and risks associated with unconventional methods.

Unproven methods of diagnosis and treatment include those subjected to clinical trials with negative results and those not evaluated. They frequently are referred to as *controversial methods* because they lack scientific credibility and have not been shown to have clinical efficacy. *Experimental methods* are those that show promise of effectiveness based on sound scientific principles or chance empirical observations, but for which the results of clinical trials are not yet available or are insufficient to recommend them for general use. Clinical trials must be performed in subjects fully informed of the experimental nature of the procedure or treatment, along with its potential benefit and associated potential risks. Subjects must give formal informed consent to participate in experimental trials. *Standard practice* encompasses the various methods of diagnosis and treatment used by most reputable physicians in a particular specialty who are knowledgeable about the disease. Trained and experienced allergists use methods that are scientifically based and have documented effectiveness and safety. They select procedures for each patient based on personal knowledge of that patient's history and examination. Within the range of acceptable methods, often more than one choice may be appropriate. Factors such as the patient's preference and lifestyle may be applicable in deciding among several options.

Unproven Diagnostic Tests

The diagnostic procedures discussed in this chapter fall into two categories: (1) those that have no diagnostic value for any disease under any circumstances and (2) those that are intrinsically capable of a valid measurement that may be effective and appropriate for diagnosing certain diseases but not for allergy. Also available are other scientifically valid procedures that are capable of giving diagnostic information relevant to an allergic disease, but they are not currently appropriate for use in clinical practice because of inadequate or untested sensitivity or specificity, cost, or lack of general availability.

The methods described in this section are not based on sound scientific principles. Although they may give the superficial appearance of a "test," they have not been shown by controlled clinical trials to be diagnostic for any condition, and the procedures used are not in accord with current knowledge of allergy pathophysiology.

SKIN END POINT TITRATION

The established prick and intradermal skin testing methods for diagnosis of immunoglobulin E (IgE) antibody–mediated diseases are discussed in Chapter 70.

Serial end point titration refers to a method of testing *and treatment* of inhalant allergy introduced by Rinkel[27] and later adopted for use with food allergens. It is a procedure used not only for diagnosis but also for establishing a "safe" dose for initiating immunotherapy and for the "neutralization" of symptoms.

Method

The method described by Rinkel[27] and its subsequent modifications are complicated and ritualistic, being based on uncontrolled empirical observations. Increasing fivefold serial concentrations of allergen are injected intradermally, usually in 0.01-mL doses. The test site is observed for the presence of a wheal after 10 minutes,[28,29] without regard for the presence or absence of erythema[27,28,30]; observed results are called "end points." In this context, *end point* is defined as a clinical pattern associated with the test dose that initiates serial 2-mm or greater incremental increases in wheal diameter with increasing fivefold concentrations. Test results that do not fit into this defined pattern are considered "bizarre."[27,30] "Hourglass" patterns (in which wheal diameter decreases and then increases with increasing concentrations of allergen), "flash responses" (characterized by a nonreproducible wheal), and "plateau" responses (marked by unchanging wheal diameters with increasing dose) are attributed to a variety of extraneous factors, such as infection, exposure to airborne pollen or food allergens, alteration by immunotherapy treatment, and peculiarities of specific allergens. Because every allergen is tested with up to nine serial intradermal injections, the total number of injections is high and the cost of the procedure is considerable. Furthermore, retesting is recommended to establish a new end point during the course of immunotherapy if the patient fails to improve.

In addition to establishing the initial dose of immunotherapy, the "optimal" dose—defined as the dose at which symptoms are eliminated—is said to be 25 to 50 times the quantity of allergen producing the end point, but this may vary with the particular allergen.[28,30]

The Rinkel method of serial end point titration evolved into the concept of symptom neutralization at a particular injected dose of allergen, as discussed in the next section.

Theory

Serial end point titration testing is based on empirical observations supported by case reports only, with no controlled objective measures for the test's claimed efficacy and safety. A critical fault of this method is the lack of attention to the presence of erythema at the test site. The mast cell–derived mediators of atopic and anaphylactic allergy produce localized pruritus, erythema, and wheal. Therefore objective evidence of erythema at the skin test site is a prerequisite for a specific diagnostic test in these diseases. Measuring wheal diameter with accompanying erythema is an efficient and accepted indication of the degree of skin test reactivity to an allergen, but in the absence of erythema, use of such determinations is likely to lead to clinically false-positive test results.

Evaluations of the Method

Several controlled clinical trials provide evidence that serial intradermal end point titration of pollen allergens produces increasing wheal diameter with increasing doses of the allergen, and that the end point as defined by Rinkel and others—but visualizing both wheal and erythema—is a safe method for establishing the starting dose for immunotherapy.[31-33] The method is too conservative, however, because it usually underestimates the safe starting dose, especially in patients who are highly sensitive to the allergen,[34] thereby prolonging the time required to reach the maintenance level for immunotherapy shown by numerous controlled studies to be effective for ameliorating allergic rhinitis or asthma. These studies further show that a calculated optimal immunotherapy dose based on the end point is almost always too low, and no more effective than placebo.[33-35]

Conclusions from Available Evidence

The technique of skin testing by intradermal serial end point titration using the method of Rinkel and his followers cannot be recommended as a reliable test for IgE-mediated skin sensitivity, because the test responses are read too early, and the presence or absence of concomitant erythema is not considered. In addition, the method requires an unnecessarily large number of intradermal injections. Frequently, use of the end point as the dose for initiating immunotherapy unnecessarily prolongs the course of treatment. Calculation of an optimal dose of immunotherapy based on the test end point is arbitrary, and controlled studies show that this approach results in ineffective treatment.

PROVOCATION-NEUTRALIZATION

"Provocation-neutralization" is a procedure that purports to test for allergy to foods, inhalants, and environmental chemicals by exposing the patient to test doses of these substances administered intradermally, subcutaneously, or sublingually, with the aim of either producing or preventing subjective symptoms.[4,5,36-43] It evolved from serial end point titration skin testing, initially to diagnose food allergy in patients with multiple subjective symptoms and later using inhalant[27] and chemical allergens. The method is based on the concept that extremely small quantities of allergen can make symptoms disappear (neutralization). The publications on this procedure frequently discuss testing and treatment as a single entity.

Procedure

Intracutaneous provocation testing is similar to skin end point titration. Increasing serial fivefold dilutions of allergen or chemical extracts are administered into the arm while the patient records subjective sensations in an unblinded manner. Neither the nature nor the intensity of the symptoms constituting a positive test result is standardized, nor are these measures necessarily the same as those reported by the patient for the illness being tested. Once a test result is considered positive, a progressive series of lower concentrations is administered until a dose is reached at which the patient reports no sensations. This dose is considered the neutralizing dose, which is then used for subsequent treatment.

Many variations of this testing procedure have been used. Some proponents believe that absence of symptoms constitutes a positive test result. Others lower the dose to provoke symptoms and then increase it to reach neutralization.[40,42] No consensus has been reached regarding the diagnostic significance of the wheal size or its relation to the subjective symptoms. Published protocols often are complex and uncontrolled.

Provocation-neutralization testing is used primarily by those physicians who subscribe to the concept of multiple food and chemical sensitivities. Because testing requires provoking and neutralizing symptoms one item at a time, and the theory is based on illness caused by multiple foods and environmental substances, the procedure could involve hundreds of individual tests, requiring weeks or months of full-day testing.

Theory

Provocation-neutralization testing is derived from empirical observations of fluctuating symptoms during serial titration testing. One theory assumes that the allergen is present within the intradermal wheal.[28] Depending on the size, shape, color, texture, and firmness of the wheal, the allergen is thought to remain within the wheal or to be released into the circulation, causing a "systemic reaction," defined as essentially any reported symptom. This theory, for which any proof is lacking, is contrary to well-established evidence that the skin test wheal in IgE-mediated allergy consists of localized edema fluid extravasated from postcapillary venules through the action of mast cell–derived mediators, not an accumulation of allergen.

Another theory proposes that administering the test dose induces antibody formation, resulting in circulating immune complexes, which then either provoke or eliminate symptoms, depending on the size of those complexes.[44] This theory is clearly inconsistent with the kinetics of antibody production and immune complex formation.

Other theories of neutralization involve either stimulation or suppression of lymphocyte function, depending on the test dose, but no experimental evidence is available to show that lymphocyte activation causes the reported symptoms.[19]

The procedure is intimately tied to concepts of delayed and cyclic food allergy, allergen overload, and the masking phenomenon. These are described later in the chapter.

Studies

Published reports on provocation-neutralization testing (not treatment) reached various conclusions, depending on methodology.[40-49] A variety of illnesses were investigated using different end point measurements, reflecting the lack of standardization for the procedure and the numerous diseases for which it is recommended. Rigorous evaluation using double-blind, placebo-controlled clinical trials showed conclusively that symptom provocation is a placebo effect. A more detailed analysis of these studies can be found elsewhere.[19]

Summary

Provocation-neutralization does not meet even the most rudimentary criteria for a diagnostic test in allergy. No standardized protocol has been established. Selection of test substances, doses, and route of administration can be altered during the course of the extensive procedure depending on how the results unfold. The test end point is entirely subjective, and no provision is made for spontaneous symptoms that may be unrelated to the administered test material. No limits on the type or severity of subjective sensations that constitute a positive test result have been designated. Those practitioners who use provocation-neutralization have not defined either the patient population or the disease being tested, so in practice it is applied to a wide range of allergic and nonallergic diseases. It is most often used in patients who have numerous subjective complaints without objective signs of illness.

The safety of provocation-neutralization has never been studied. Significant adverse reactions can result from sublingual testing.[36] A recognized danger is the potential for development of oral mucosa angioedema or systemic anaphylaxis from sublingual exposure in patients with extreme IgE sensitivity to the allergen.

A scientifically based theory for provocation-neutralization is lacking. No published reports have shown conclusively that provocation-neutralization can diagnose any disease, and good evidence indicates that symptoms that arise during the course of the testing are random and unrelated to the test itself.[42]

Provocation-neutralization testing must not be confused with the recognized forms of target organ provocative testing discussed elsewhere in this book. Bronchial provocation testing with allergens (Chapter 64); provocative nasal inhalation testing (Chapter 41); the oral, double-blind, placebo-controlled food challenge test (Chapter 83); and patch testing for contact dermatitis (Chapter 35) all are reliable, well-standardized techniques with defined, objective physical measurements or observations.

CYTOTOXIC TEST

The cytotoxic test (also known as the leukocytotoxic test) for food allergy was first described in 1956 and later modified.[50-55] It is based on an unsupported claim that morphologic changes in peripheral blood leukocytes exposed to allergen in vitro indicate allergy to that particular allergen. "Allergy" allegedly diagnosed by this method encompasses rhinitis, asthma, headache, gastrointestinal symptoms, skin disease, hearing disorders, genitourinary diseases, and obesity.

Procedure

Centrifuged leukocytes suspended in a mixture of sterile distilled water and autologous serum are placed on a siliconized microscope slide previously coated with a dried extract of the food to be tested. The unstained cells are viewed microscopically at room temperature for various intervals of up to 2 hours. Any lack of movement, rounding, vacuolization, flattening, fragmentation, or disintegration of cells is used as evidence of cytotoxicity. Typically, approximately 150 to 200 extracts of foods, drugs, chemicals, or aeroallergens are tested on each sample of blood.[50-54]

Theory

The cytotoxic test evolved from reports that leukopenia occurs during the course of symptomatic pollen allergy, found to be unsubstantiated.[56] Allergen-induced release of mediators from basophils in IgE-mediated allergy is not likely to be detected by this method.[57] IgG-, IgM-, and cell-mediated allergic responses can induce cytotoxic effects, but no clear evidence has established that ingestion of foods causes disease through any of these mechanisms. Therefore there is no theoretical foundation for a diagnostic test for food allergy based on immunologically induced cytotoxicity.

Diagnostic Efficacy

Reports of symptomatic improvement from a diet based on the cytotoxic test are anecdotal.[58-60] None used a double-blind, placebo-controlled food challenge. Various investigators have failed to confirm that the cytotoxic test results correlate with clinical illness.[61-66]

Summary

The cytotoxic test for food allergy has no scientific support as a procedure to diagnose allergy to foods. No proof has been found that leukocyte toxicity is even involved in food allergy. The procedure does not control for artifacts, such as changes in pH, osmolarity, time of incubation, or temperature, or even for contaminants in the food extract.[64]

ANTIGEN LEUKOCYTE CELLULAR ANTIBODY TEST

The antigen leukocyte cellular antibody test (ALCAT) is a modification of the cytotoxic test that uses electronic instrumentation and computerized data analysis to examine and monitor changes in leukocyte cell volumes. Like the cytotoxic test, it also has been promoted as a diagnostic test for food, inhalant, and chemical allergy or intolerance in a host of conditions, including arthritis, urticaria, bronchitis, gastroenteritis, childhood hyperreactivity, rhinitis, and atopic dermatitis. Typically, the results are used to establish elimination diets for these diseases.

The few reported experiences with this test are not properly controlled trials to establish diagnostic efficacy.[65-71]

ELECTRODERMAL TESTING

Electrodermal testing (electroacupuncture) is claimed to identify substances, especially foods, that cause allergy and to provide information about optimal dilution of treatment extracts in immunotherapy,[72,73] although these claims are often misrepresented.[74] It uses a device, often referred to as a Voll machine,[73] that measures the electrical impedance of the skin at designated acupuncture points in response to a 1.5-V electric current while the patient holds the negative electrode in one hand. Vials of food or inhalant extracts are placed in contact with an aluminum plate in the circuit. A change in impedance supposedly detects allergy to that particular food. The positive electrode is used to probe selected points on the skin. The lower extremities are said to relate to food allergy, the trunk and upper extremities to inhalant allergies, and the scalp to allergies that localize in the nose and sinuses.

Proponents of this procedure claim that it has been used successfully for many years in Europe to diagnose and treat allergy. They admit that the theory for the procedure is unknown and that results are empirical. The equipment is expensive, and the manufacturer warns that its use in the United States is for investigational purposes only.

A double-blind, randomized block design study of atopic patients and controls tested repeatedly showed that the procedure was unable to confirm the presence or absence of skin test reactivity, and the test could not distinguish atopic from nonatopic individuals.[75,76] Previous claims of diagnostic efficacy used unscientific study methods.[66,67,77-80]

APPLIED KINESIOLOGY

Applied kinesiology claims to identify specific allergies through measuring the patient's muscle strength by manual muscle testing in the presence of a putative allergen.[81] Practitioners assert that pathologic conditions in individual organ systems are reflected in corresponding muscle groups, known as viscerosomatic relationships, maintained through energy fields communicating throughout the body. In patients with allergy, especially food allergy, this communication presumably can be influenced by the allergen if present nearby.

Typically, allergens are placed in closed containers that the patient holds in one hand while a technician subjectively estimates muscle strength in the opposite arm. A decrease in muscle power is said to indicate a positive test result. Variations in the procedure include placing the allergen container on the chest while the patient is supine with the arms outstretched, or even testing while the allergen is placed near but not in actual contact with the body. For uncooperative infants, a surrogate is tested, first alone and then while holding the child's hand, with the results based on subtraction of the two results of subjectively measuring the muscle strength of the surrogate.

Proponents of applied kinesiology claim efficacy and reliability for this procedure without any support from properly controlled studies.[67-69,82] No credible theory has been advanced for this form of testing. A single published report of blinded testing to multiple foods in 20 subjects showed that results are random and not reproducible.[81] Reliability of the test is no greater than for random guessing.[83]

Inappropriate Diagnostic Tests

The methods discussed in this section are considered inappropriate for allergy diagnosis because they are ineffective when used for that purpose, although they may be validated, effective, and proper to diagnose other diseases. These modalities include both immunologic and nonimmunologic tests. Some of these methods promoted for allergy diagnosis are based on an incorrect concept of allergic disease pathogenesis; others were derived from unconfirmed observations of patients.

TOTAL SERUM IMMUNOGLOBULINS

Quantitative measurement of the total serum levels of IgG (and subclasses), IgA, and IgM is appropriate for patients with suspected functional antibody deficiency. Polyclonal increases in total serum immunoglobulins occur in some autoimmune diseases, hypersensitivity pneumonitis, and certain chronic infections. Monoclonal increase in a particular immunoglobulin characterizes the gammopathies, multiple myeloma, and Waldenstrom's macroglobulinemia. The quantitative levels of serum IgG, IgA, and IgM are not altered by allergic diseases, so their measurement in allergy diagnosis is irrelevant.

Normal levels of total serum IgE are extremely low. Total serum IgE is elevated in many patients with allergic rhinitis and allergic asthma, and very high levels occur in allergic bronchopulmonary aspergillosis and in some cases of atopic dermatitis and allergic fungal sinusitis. Considerable overlap within the atopic and normal populations has been documented, however, so the test is not a satisfactory screening test, especially because a normal level of total serum IgE does not exclude clinically significant atopy. Total serum IgE concentration usually is normal in patients with systemic anaphylaxis or urticaria. Furthermore, the test does not give any information about specific IgE antibodies.

SPECIFIC IMMUNOGLOBULIN G ANTIBODIES

Some clinical laboratories offer quantitative measurements of circulating IgG antibodies to food and mold allergens. Antibodies are measured by solid phase immunoassay methods, discussed in Chapter 74.

Low-level IgG antibodies to foods may circulate normally, but they are of no known pathogenic significance in atopic disease. Although some practitioners have postulated that these antibodies may be responsible for delayed symptoms or vague intolerance to foods, any proof of this claim remains lacking.[69,84]

Allergen immunotherapy induces IgG4 allergen-specific "blocking" antibodies. These are thus the result of the treatment, not the disease. Investigators who have studied blocking antibodies agree that with few exceptions, their quantification is not a useful measurement for the clinical management of immunotherapy.

High-level IgG antibodies, often sufficient for detection by the precipitin reaction, are involved in the pathogenesis of serum sickness and possibly in certain phases of hypersensitivity pneumonitis. Measurement of specific IgG antibodies to the relevant allergen may be diagnostically helpful in these particular diseases, especially to confirm that exposure to a suspect allergen has occurred.

LYMPHOCYTE SUBSET COUNTS

The circulating pool of lymphocytes comprises numerous functionally distinct subsets identified by specific cell surface (i.e., CD) markers (see Appendix A). Quantitative lymphocyte subset analysis is an accepted diagnostic test in cellular imunodeficiencies and in lymphocytic leukemias. Lymphocyte subset analyses must be interpreted with caution, because the normal range for many of the subsets is wide and variable, and the circulating levels may be subject to diurnal change, as well as to the effects of viral infections and certain drugs.

LYMPHOCYTE FUNCTION ASSAYS

Lymphocyte function can be assessed by the activation of lymphocytes with nonspecific mitogens, such as phytohemagglutinin (PHA), pokeweed mitogen (PWM), and concanavalin A (ConA) (see Chapter 74). These tests may offer help in the diagnosis of some immunodeficiency diseases, but not in allergic diseases.

CYTOKINE AND CYTOKINE RECEPTOR ASSAYS

Quantitative immunoassay of many of the known cytokines and circulating cytokine receptors is available in some clinical laboratories, but normal circulating levels are quite low and are subject to physiologic fluctuations. Although IgE antibody–induced inflammatory responses are associated with the helper T cell (Th2) cytokine profile, there is limited evidence that measurements of cytokine or cytokine receptor levels in blood is currently of diagnostic value.

CHEMICAL ANALYSIS OF BODY FLUIDS

The diagnosis of "chemical sensitivities" by those who subscribe to the concept of idiopathic environmental intolerance (IEI), discussed later in this chapter, may involve tests for the presence of environmental chemicals in samples of whole blood, serum, erythrocytes, urine, fat, and hair. IEI is a subjective illness marked by multiple nonspecific symptoms related to exposure to various chemicals, biologics, and physical agents. The most common chemicals measured are organic solvents, other hydrocarbons, pesticides, and metals.

Analytic techniques and instrumentation are available today to quantify almost any inorganic or organic chemical in exceedingly small amounts in samples of biologic material. These sensitive methods have revealed that many environmental chemicals are found in virtually everyone because of their ubiquitous presence in the environment of today's industrialized world. Under certain circumstances it may be proper and appropriate to diagnose a suspected chemical poisoning by the detection of potentially toxic quantities of a specific chemical, but widespread screening of large numbers of chemicals, as performed by some physicians, has not yielded any information that lends credence to the concept of chemical sensitivities.

In similar fashion, some physicians also recommend quantitative measurements of vitamins, minerals, and amino acids in blood and urine in a search for environmental chemical sensitivities. The rationale for doing so is obscure, because no evidence has been found for the involvement of nutrient deficiency in the pathogenesis of allergic disease.

FOOD IMMUNE COMPLEX ASSAY

Food intolerance causing delayed symptoms (i.e., more than 2 hours after ingestion) is a vexing problem, especially because patients presumably so affected often describe vague and subjective symptoms inconsistent with known allergic manifestations. With no supporting evidence, a few allergists suspect that such delayed food reactions may be immunologic, mediated by circulating complexes containing food antigen. Therefore the food immune complex assay (FICA) has been promoted for diagnosis of food allergy.[69,85-88]

Methods

The usual procedure is a radioimmunoassay in which an antibody to a food is coupled covalently to the solid phase immunosorbent and then incubated with the test serum to permit the insolubilized antibody to react with the food allergen in circulating immune complexes. Radiolabeled antiimmunoglobulin (usually anti-human IgE or anti-human IgG) is added; after washing, radiolabel remaining on the solid phase is quantitatively proportional to the amount of circulating immune complexes containing the food allergen.[85-88] Alternative methods to separate immune complexes from free antibody include ultracentrifugation[89] and polyethylene glycol precipitation.[90]

Theory

Absorption of ingested food antigen with deposition of immune complexes into tissues presumably causes these subjective symptoms. The theory is based on studies of experimental and human serum sickness.[91] Circulating immune complexes can be found in many autoimmune diseases, although a pathogenic role for these immune complexes probably is limited, correlating best with vasculitis.[92,93] In contrast with serum sickness, the antigens comprising the immune complexes in various autoimmune diseases have rarely been identified with certainty. Any test to detect circulating food immune complexes, therefore, is based on a theory of disease etiology that is currently speculative.

Studies

Several published studies indicate that circulating food proteins,[94-96] food antibodies,[90] and food immune complexes[97] are normal findings. Circulating food antigens have been detected in serum from normal individuals.[98,99] Other studies showed evidence of circulating immune complexes of several different antibody isotypes in the serum of normal and atopic persons.[89,100] Patients with food-induced symptoms have not yet been shown to differ from normal control subjects in the quantity or quality of these complexes.[87,89] High levels of immune complexes to a bovine antigen have been detected in patients with IgA deficiency.[101-103] In a single case of arthritis apparently provoked by food ingestion, circulating immune complexes were present, but the level of these complexes did not correlated with clinical symptoms elicited by oral food challenge.[104]

Conclusions from Available Evidence

Food immune complex assays based on the solid phase radioimmunoassay methodology have not yet been subjected to rigorous study of potential false-negative and false-positive results on diagnostic testing.[88] Clinical studies to date indicate that such immune complexes can be found in a normal population of people without food intolerance. No well-defined clinical disease has yet been identified as being causally linked to food immune complexes. The test must be considered experimental at this time.

PULSE TEST

A change in pulse rate—either an increase or a decrease—after the ingestion, injection, or sublingual application of an allergen has been claimed by some to indicate allergy to the substance.[105] It has been used as a diagnostic test most often in cases of suspected food allergy, in which a change in pulse rate—usually 10 beats per minute or more—occurring from 5 to 90 minutes after the allergen exposure, is declared to represent a positive test result.

No valid theory has been advanced to support this test. Changes in heart rate can occur from a variety of physiologic and pathologic conditions, but they are not a diagnostic feature of any allergic disease. A controlled clinical trial of pulse testing in allergy has yet to be conducted.

Unproven Treatment Methods

This section describes a group of procedures advocated for treatment of allergic diseases, some of which are directed specifically toward allergic conditions and others promoted for many chronic conditions, including allergy. All are without proven benefit, although many are widely used. Their perceived benefits usually can be shown to be based on a placebo effect, involving an improved sense of well-being unrelated to a pharmacologic action.

Experienced allergists use scientifically validated therapeutic practices supplemented by supportive measures appropriate to individual patients. This combined approach generally is recognized as the art of medicine. Other formalized methods such as relaxation, hypnosis, and biofeedback—albeit effective in some cases—have demonstrated no consistent superiority over placebo in clinical trials of allergic disease,[106] and a discussion of these modalities is not included in this chapter.

NEUTRALIZATION THERAPY

Neutralization therapy, also called "symptom-relieving" therapy[45] and "tolerance," is an extension of provocation-neutralization testing. Specified doses of allergen extracts are self-administered to relieve symptoms.

Description

After provocation-neutralization testing, neutralizing doses of one or more tested substances are self-administered by the intracutaneous,[40,107] subcutaneous,[31,45,77,108] or sublingual route.[109-111] No established protocols have been delineated; patients use the neutralizing solution whenever symptoms appear, or before anticipated exposure to the substance believed to cause illness. Treatment also can be given on a regular maintenance schedule, usually daily or twice weekly.

The published literature on neutralization therapy indicates that it has been used in a variety of conditions, including atopy, rheumatic diseases, premenstrual syndrome, viral infections,[112] headache, musculoskeletal complaints, and many others. Neutralizing substances include atopic allergens, environmental chemicals, hormones, viral vaccines, food extracts, histamine or serotonin, and even saline or distilled water.

Theory

The treatment supposedly induces immunologic tolerance. Use of the sublingual route to avoid gastrointestinal metabolism is claimed to facilitate lymphocyte desensitization. No testing by animal experiments or clinical studies supports these theories. Other concepts for neutralization were discussed previously in the section on provocation-neutralization testing.

Clinical Studies

The literature on this subject is confusing, because published reports do not usually separate provocation-neutralization testing from neutralization treatment. Support rests largely on a single reported double-blind, placebo-controlled, crossover study of daily subcutaneous injections of food extracts in eight patients.[108] Improvement occurred with both placebo and food extract, but more frequently with the latter. The study, labeled by the author as preliminary, has been criticized for inappropriate statistical analysis, and no final report has ever been published. A report that 20 patients with perennial rhinitis treated with sublingual dust extract improved both subjectively and objectively is suspect, because five of the patients did not have house-dust mite allergen sensitivity.[113] Other reports consist of single cases or uncontrolled series yielding both negative and positive results.

Risks

One patient with systemic mastocytosis experienced a potentially life-threatening reaction of flushing, palpitations, and syncope.[114]

Conclusions from Available Evidence

Neutralization therapy is an unproven procedure. Its advocates recommend its use for such a wide variety of illnesses and subjective conditions, using a large number of different substances administered by three different routes, that its efficacy defies critical evaluation. No scientific publication on neutralization treatment supports its use in any condition.

It is important not to confuse this form of treatment with allergen immunotherapy, in which extracts of specific allergens for defined atopic respiratory disease or Hymenoptera venom anaphylaxis are first selected by objective testing methods, after which injection therapy with sufficient dosages is given for a sufficient period to attenuate the allergic response to naturally occurring allergen (see Chapters 87 and 78).

ENZYME-POTENTIATED DESENSITIZATION

Enzyme-potentiated desensitization (EPD) is a procedure in which allergen is mixed with the enzyme β-glucuronidase immediately before injection. It is promoted as an improvement over conventional allergen immunotherapy because it requires fewer injections.

Method

A very low dose of allergen, approximately equivalent to the amount administered in a standard skin-prick test, is mixed with partially purified β-glucuronidase in a dose equivalent to the amount of enzyme present in 4 mL of human blood. Immediately after mixing, 0.125 mL of the mixture is injected intradermally. A single preseasonal dose is considered sufficient to produce a therapeutic effect lasting for an entire pollen season,[115] and a dose every 2 to 6 months for perennial allergy.

Proponents have claimed success in treating allergic rhinitis, asthma, sinusitis, nasal polyposis, eczema, urticaria, migraine headaches, ulcerative colitis, irritable bowel syndrome, rheumatoid arthritis, and petit mal seizures.

Theory

β-Glucuronidase is said to activate $CD8^+$ lymphocytes, thereby suppressing the immune response to the allergen.[116-120] Reports of such activation have not been verified.

Studies

The effectiveness of this form of treatment and the presumed effect of β-glucuronidase on the immune system has yet to be shown. In a double-blind study in which a single injection was given preseasonally to 44 patients allergic to grass pollen, significant improvement over a placebo effect was evident when measured by overall patient preference and reduced requirement for drug therapy, but daily symptom records showed no effect.[115] Several reports of double-blind studies in children with mite-allergic asthma and pollen-allergic rhinitis showed clinical improvement,[121-125] but a similar trial of grass pollen–allergic rhinitis in England showed no treatment effect.[126]

Conclusions from Available Evidence

EPD is based on a presumption that the enzyme suppresses the immune response to ambient allergen exposure. The minute amount of enzyme used is unlikely to have a pharmacologic effect at a dose much less than for the same enzyme at levels normally present in the body. It is extremely unlikely that any form of desensitization would be effective for the large number of allergic and nonallergic diseases claimed. EPD at this time must be considered experimental.

DETOXIFICATION

Chemical detoxification is recommended by a small group of practitioners to remove undesirable chemicals from patients believed to have IEI. The putative basis for this modality is that the sensitivity is caused by toxic effects of low-level synthetic chemicals in the body.[127]

Procedure

Treatment consists of several steps. Aerobic physical exercise is performed for 20 to 30 minutes, followed immediately by forced sweating in a sauna at 140° to 180° F for 2.5 to 5 hours and then physical exercise, a cooling shower, and additional exercise. Niacin is then given in increasing doses to produce a flush. Water and salts of sodium, potassium, calcium, magnesium, and other minerals are prescribed to correct for water and salt depletion from sweating. Polyunsaturated oils, as a mixture of soybean, walnut, peanut, and safflower oils, which are said to be "essential," are consumed orally. A planned schedule of balanced meals and adequate sleep is recommended, along with avoidance of medications and alcohol. This routine is repeated daily, usually for 30 days.

Theory

The enforced program of exercise and sweating with niacin-induced cutaneous vasodilation is believed to mobilize fat-soluble toxic chemicals, presumably into the circulation, followed by urinary excretion. The oil ingestion is to prevent reabsorption of chemicals through enterohepatic recirculation. The "essential oils" are believed to allow toxic substances mobilized into the gut to be excreted from the colon, but some toxic material is said to be excreted also through sweat.

Studies of Effectiveness

All reports to date by proponents of this detoxification procedure are anecdotal. Results are measured by the patient's self-report of symptomatic improvement. Accordingly, placebo effect, proper diet, elimination of unnecessary medications, aerobic exercise, and adequate sleep have not been ruled out as the reasons for subjective improvement.

Conclusions from Available Evidence

This form of detoxification has yet to be proved effective for the treatment of allergy, IEI, drug addiction, or any other illness. The ability of the procedure to remove chemicals from fat has not been confirmed. The theory of immunotoxicity as a cause of allergic disease is contrary to accumulated scientific knowledge. The potential dangers of this program have not yet been adequately evaluated.

AUTOGENOUS URINE THERAPY

A belief that human urine is therapeutic has existed since ancient times. In the early 1930s, several medical publications claimed that a specific substance called proteose, one of various water-soluble compounds produced during hydrolysis of proteins, is excreted in allergic disease.[128] Injections of extracts of this substance were recommended for treatment of allergy, with reports of successes in many other diseases as well. Other reports could not reproduce these findings. The practice subsided after several years but then resurfaced.[129]

Method

Several chemical extraction procedures have been recommended for obtaining proteose from the urine. The extracted protein is suspended in a buffered solution and then injected for intradermal testing and for subcutaneous injection treatments.

Theory

Proponents of this form of treatment believe that urinary proteose contains the allergen specific for that particular individual and that it is a superior source of allergen for therapy, having gone through unspecified and unproved processing by the body.

Studies

The published reports consist of uncontrolled anecdotal histories of apparently successful treatment of a variety of allergic conditions, including asthma, rhinitis, anaphylaxis, urticaria, angioedema, and serum sickness. Other reports have failed to prove efficacy. No properly controlled studies have been published to date.

Safety

No studies have been performed to address the question of long-term safety of urine therapy. This issue is critical, because small quantities of glomerular basement membrane antigens are found in normal urine. It is not unreasonable that chemical treatment of urine during the extraction process could lead to the production of altered renal proteins that might induce autoantibodies.

Conclusions from Available Evidence

The practice of injecting an extract of the patient's own urine for the diagnosis or treatment of allergy is clearly unacceptable and must be discouraged. It is not based on a rational theory, and no scientific investigations of efficacy or safety have been conducted. The potential for induction of autoimmune nephritis is a clear danger that precludes consideration of this procedure in humans, even on an experimental basis.

ACUPUNCTURE

Acupuncture is an ancient Oriental form of medical practice that is recommended for virtually any disease. Over the centuries, its popularity has waxed and waned. Today, some medical and nonmedical practitioners use acupuncture exclusively or in connection with other forms of treatment, including medications, Chinese herbal therapy, homeopathy, naturopathy, and psychotherapy. In moxibustion, heated ground mugwort plant is burned into the patient's skin with acupuncture needles.[130] Modern versions of acupuncture include the use of laser beams, electrical stimulation, and injections of medications or supplements at acupuncture sites.[131,132]

Acupuncture is commonly used to treat allergic diseases. Some proponents claim that needling of the skin activates or inhibits various cell mediators and enzymes, with no scientific proof. Randomized controlled clinical trials and meta-analyses on acupuncture treatment for various allergic diseases have been performed. Some trials use sham acupoints as placebo, but others use no treatment or "standard therapy." A few regimens have included adjunctive treatment when necessary. A wide variety of measures have been used to determine effectiveness, including symptom reports, pulmonary function testing, laboratory data, and quality of life questionnaires. A particularly vexing problem is the lack of uniformity in selection of skin sites, depth of penetration, and other factors in the placement of acupoints. Reported results include effectiveness in some measures to no improvement at all. Meta-analyses reflect these uncertainties, inadequate methodology, poor quality of data reporting, and evidence of selection bias.[106,133-138] Any reported beneficial effect is most likely to be attributable to suggestion.[139] Life-threatening complications, although not common, have been reported.[140]

HOMEOPATHY

Homeopathy is both a philosophy and an alternative medical practice. The theory that "like cures like" is translated into the administration of exceedingly minute quantities of substances believed to cause disease as a method of curing the disease. The substances are called "remedies" and usually consist of extensive dilutions of various plant and animal organ extracts. The exceedingly small quantities used for treatment are prepared by serial dilution of extracts through the violent shaking of a container of diluted extract. The remedies are given orally, and patients sometimes take as many as 50 different extracts daily. An alternative theory proposes that disease is cured by the induction of immunity.

On theoretical grounds, it is highly unlikely that these exceedingly minute quantities of ingested material would have any therapeutic effect. The materials used for treatment are unstandardized. Adverse effects are unlikely because of the small amount of material administered. The real dangers are psychological dependence and delay in the institution of effective therapy.

In common with other practitioners of "alternative" disease treatment, homeopathic practitioners claim to cure numerous diseases, including all forms of allergy. Several published controlled clinical trials have compared homeopathic treatment with placebo or standard therapy for allergic rhinitis and asthma. Both allergen extracts in vanishingly low concentrations and standard homeopathic remedies are used. These trials report both positive[141-145] and negative[146-151] results. Meta-analyses conclude that homeopathic treatment of respiratory allergy cannot be recommended.[106,132,133,152-154]

LASER THERAPY

Laser treatment for asthma delivers laser energy to specific targets, including endobronchial tissue, tympanic membrane, blood, and skin. These modalities are variously named laser ablation, photodynamic therapy, helium-neon laser irradiation, noninvasive hemolaserotherapy, low-intensity or low-energy laser radiation, pulsed- and continuous-wave low-energy infrared laser radiations, and laseropuncture (laser acupuncture).

In practice, the patient's tissue is exposed to a light energy source to induce a "stimulatory effect," based on the direct exposure, at acupuncture points, or indirect exposure of blood, to effect a specific change in pulmonary function, including bronchial hyperreactivity, immune status, and symptoms.[155]

Cochrane database reviews reflect the absence of common end point measurements and poor reporting quality, with little insight into the long-term efficacy and harm profiles of these treatments. Assessment of validity of laser therapy requires additional well-designed trials.[156] A single small pilot investigational study using laser acupuncture and probiotics, which according to Traditional Chinese Medicine associates the lung to the large intestine, demonstrated a beneficial effect on bronchial hyperreactivity in school-aged children with intermittent or mild persistent asthma.[132]

Inappropriate Therapy

Despite the availability of effective measures for the management of allergic diseases, some patients are being treated inappropriately. In some cases, legitimate procedures such as allergen avoidance are applied excessively. In others, treatments that would be indicated for a different disease are used to treat an allergic disease on the basis of an erroneous theory of allergic hypersensitivity.

The various unproven and controversial diagnoses described earlier in this chapter lead to inappropriate treatments that may be effective for other diseases. For example, intravenous immunoglobulin infusions, which are appropriately indicated for treatment of antibody deficiency or certain other diseases, are not appropriate therapy for allergy. Similarly, antifungal therapy is indicated for severe systemic fungal infection but not for presumed "*Candida* hypersensitivity syndrome."

VITAMIN AND NUTRIENT SUPPLEMENTS

Vitamins, minerals, amino acids, enzymes, and other nutritional supplements are recommended by some practitioners for numerous medical and psychiatric conditions, including allergy. These may be prescribed singly or in combination, often in very large doses, a form of therapy known as "orthomolecular."

Those physicians who recommend vitamin therapy believe that a deficiency of these substances causes allergic disease—a mechanism for which any scientific evidence is lacking. Antioxidant supplements, such as vitamin C, vitamin E, and glutathione, are recommended according to a theory that allergic inflammation generates free radicals, which cause oxidative damage to tissues.[157] Although toxic oxygen metabolites are activated during the course of certain inflammatory conditions, the kinetics and localization of these reactions make it unlikely that ingestion of these dietary supplements would be any more effective than the activity of normal endogenous antioxidants.

No clinical studies have documented a more favorable outcome with use of any dietary supplements for any allergic condition,[158] nor has any systematic study of safety been conducted. Of note, however, excessive intake of fat-soluble vitamins can result in their accumulation in the body and subsequent toxicity.

Vitamin C (ascorbic acid) is one of the most widely used supplements. Among its claimed effects is the ability to prevent allergen-induced bronchial obstruction. An initial report[159] that vitamin C inhibited histamine-induced bronchoconstriction in healthy subjects was not confirmed in a later study.[160] Pretreatment with vitamin C failed to protect asthmatic subjects from the effect of inhaled histamine[161] or ragweed allergens.[162]

Supplementation with specific vitamins, minerals, or other nutrients is standard treatment for the corresponding deficiency diseases. No credible information is available to support involvement of vitamin or nutritional deficiency in the pathogenesis of allergic conditions, and evidence for pharmacologic efficacy in allergy of supraphysiologic doses of vitamins is lacking. Epidemiologic evidence suggests a causal association between vitamin D deficiency and morbidity from asthma and other allergic diseases, but clinical trials are necessary to assess the role of vitamin D supplementation.[163]

ENVIRONMENTAL CHEMICAL AVOIDANCE

Avoiding allergens whenever possible is a cornerstone of allergy treatment. Patients who have experienced anaphylaxis on exposure to a specific drug or food or Hymenoptera venom must be particularly vigilant in avoiding contact with the inciting substance. Controlling exposure to indoor house-dust mite, indoor molds, and animal pets is the standard recommendation for patients with these specific allergies. Allergen avoidance is thus part of an overall management program, with the goal to reduce or eliminate allergic disease without undue disruption of the patient's daily activities.

In sharp contrast with these well-recognized and well-established principles of allergy management, physicians who subscribe to concepts such as those of IEI recommend extreme measures to eliminate environmental chemicals, especially plastic materials, synthetic clothing, perfumes, detergents, pesticides, synthetic carpeting, gasoline or diesel fumes, vehicle exhaust emissions, smoke, natural gas fuel, chlorine, alcohol, and virtually all synthetic chemicals. Many patients subjected to this form of treatment have been unable to continue employment[164-167] or to live in their homes. These environmental restrictions are often accompanied by extreme dietary restrictions. The physical and emotional dangers of such extraordinary but unproven avoidance measures are obvious, yet no controlled studies address the need for or efficacy of such treatment.

OTHER ENVIRONMENTAL TREATMENTS

Speleotherapy (Greek *speleos*, "cave") is treatment in underground environments said to be of benefit in cutaneous disorders, asthma, and other respiratory disorders. Spa treatments arose in northern Mediterranean and eastern European countries and later in the Dead Sea because of the high content of mineral salts in certain geologic formations and seawater, respectively. Treatment is carried out in specifically designated caves or mines, sometimes with patients performing physical or breathing exercises. Benefits are variously attributed to air quality (pressure, salts, humidity), underground climate, or radiation, which differ among the caves and mines. No evidence from randomized controlled trials has been found for these conditions.[1-3,168,169]

Halotherapy (Greek *halos*, "salt") is designed to replicate, in the clinic, the conditions of speleotherapy. Most trials are reported in Russian language journals, examining the impact of the treatment on asthma, chronic bronchitis, and other upper and lower respiratory tract diseases. Halotherapy also is recommended as adjuvant therapy to accompany conventional or "alternative" treatments.[170]

DIETARY THERAPY

Elimination of a food allergen is the only currently effective form of treatment for proven food allergy. Fortunately, in most documented cases, the number of foods to be avoided is small, so that highly restrictive diets are unnecessary. For infants or children with proven cow's milk allergy, suitable substitutes are available.

By contrast, the recommendation to eliminate multiple foods, resulting in excessive dietary restriction, has been a major component of certain unconventional allergy treatment programs. In general, two theories for multiple food eliminations are recognized: (1) the concept of multiple food allergy, based on incorrect testing, and (2) the concept that many foods inhibit the functioning of the immune system.[171] Both of these theories are unsupported by proper clinical investigation.

Treatment based on provocation-neutralization testing requires the elimination of all foods and environmental chemicals that provoke symptoms. Because such a diet is almost always inconsistent with proper nutrition, a "rotary diversified diet" is recommended,[171,172] in which the foods believed to cause sensitivity are permitted in the diet once every 4 or 5 days. This diet also is claimed to prevent the development of new food sensitivities. No studies showing efficacy of either of these diets have been published.

Many unsubstantiated theories claim that foods, food additives, and food contaminants can alter, disturb, or inhibit the normal functioning of the immune system. Highly restrictive diets, often accompanied by supplemental vitamins, minerals, amino acids, or other nutrients, have been recommended to boost the immune system. Diets and supplements, including Chinese herbs, also have been recommended as treatment for atopic diseases.[173] These theories and recommendations are not originally based on scientific evidence, some being thousands of years old.[15] Subjective beneficial effects of a diet that restricts multiple foods based on unproven diagnostic methods have been shown to be attributable primarily to suggestion.[174-176] Recent controlled trials have started to examine various Chinese herbal remedies for asthma and anaphylaxis.[177]

APITHERAPY

Apitherapy[178,179] is the use of bee stings to treat specific chronic inflammatory disorders[180] including rheumatism[181] neurologic disorders,[182] vascular disorders, gastrointestinal disorders,[183] or allergic disorders.[184] (This modality must not be confused with specific Hymenoptera venom immunotherapy to desensitize patients who have experienced anaphylaxis from the stings of these insects, discussed in Chapter 78.)

This therapy grew out of anecdotal reports of bee stings that cured bronchitis and arthritis. The treatment regimen consisted of live bee stings once daily or three times a week applied to the spine, presumably correlating with the involved joint or along acupuncture "trigger" points. Pressure was then applied by the thumb to the point of pain. After the first weeks of treatment, some patients experienced exacerbation of their disease in a so-called reactive stage, considered as essential and reflecting activation of the immune system. When a specific (unidentified) level of resistance is reached, therapy is commonly stopped. Treatment was individualized in accordance with clinical response and was stopped if anaphylaxis occurred.

In the 1930s, commercial forms of injectable bee venom (Apiven, Venapis, Lyovac, Imminin, Apicosan) became available, with 0.1 mg of pure dry bee venom equated to one bee sting. Active research in the United States and other countries stopped in the early 1950s with the advent of effective antibiotics and corticosteroids. A recent resurgence in studies on the beneficial effects of bee stings, however, has been attributed to the availability of water-soluble fractions, interaction with metalloproteinases, and mellitin (mellitinin),[180,185,186] an antiinflammatory agent known to be 100 times stronger than cortisone in suppression of cytokine production.[187] In clinical practice, adverse effects such as anaphylaxis have been one of the major issues, as well associated risk for development of other complications such as hepatotoxicity.[188]

Unconventional Theories of Allergic Disease

Many unconventional allergy practices are based on a theory that numerous physical, behavioral, cognitive, affective, and emotional symptoms and personality patterns are allergic diseases caused by environmental antigens.

Descriptions of these conditions are strikingly similar. Patients typically report a long-standing pattern of multiple symptoms suggesting the involvement of many different organ systems. They also have difficulties in their thought processes. Results of physical examinations are usually normal. Conventional tests of allergic sensitivities are claimed to be unreliable. Unproven diagnostic methods are used to confirm the existence of these diseases, although the patient's belief that the symptoms are caused by environmental exposures usually is sufficient for diagnosis. Extensive laboratory testing fails to reveal any consistent organ dysfunction, and there is no physical evidence of pathology.

The perceived allergens include foods, food additives, drugs, environmental chemicals, hormones, microorganisms, and even electromagnetic radiation. The reported sensitivities usually are multiple.

A succession of theories for the etiology and pathogenesis of these conditions based on alternative forms of hypersensitivity all lack experimental proof that the presumed sensitivity to environmental substances is immunologically mediated. Anecdotal case reports and clinical experience are cited as evidence.

ALLERGIC TOXEMIA OR TENSION FATIGUE SYNDROME

So-called allergic toxemia is the prototype for a certain category of sensitivity-related "diseases." This entity is difficult to define because descriptions vary in publications on the subject,[189] even though it is said to be associated with a "specific symptom complex."[171] The most commonly reported clinical manifestations are recurrent headache, abdominal pain, fatigue, musculoskeletal pain, various respiratory complaints, and pallor. Fatigue is the most prominent and frequent symptom. The term "allergic tension fatigue syndrome"[190] has been applied to the same condition, especially when diagnosed in children. Patterns of symptoms vary over time. Fatigue and listlessness may alternate with hyperactivity, and insomnia with hypersomnia. Pain may be referable at various times to muscles, joints, bones, the abdomen, the chest, and the head. Less frequent complaints are lymph node enlargement, low-grade fever, urinary frequency, bladder discomfort, excessive colds, tachycardia, hives, difficulty concentrating, and a bluish discoloration of the lower eyelids (so-called allergic shiners).

Etiology

The condition is almost always attributed to sensitivity to multiple foods, especially milk, chocolate, corn, and wheat. It is claimed that reactions to foods occur more commonly in the winter than in summer.

Diagnosis

The diagnosis is based solely on symptoms.[27] Findings on physical examination are said to be unrevealing, and even the reported clinical manifestations that could be verified objectively, such as lymphadenopathy, fever, and tachycardia, are rarely confirmed by examination. Routine laboratory testing shows no abnormalities.

The onset of symptoms and signs after ingestion of foods often is delayed by hours, days, or even weeks. Improvement from an elimination diet is at best temporary, leading to the elimination of additional foods. Lack of response to the elimination diet may be attributed to poor cooperation by the patient, trace quantities of food allergens in the diet, or intercurrent infections.

Studies

No definitive double-blind, placebo-controlled clinical trials supporting the existence of food-induced allergic toxemia have been published.

Conclusions from Available Evidence

The symptoms reported by patients with allergic toxemia are common in the general healthy population. In the absence of objective physical or pathologic signs, they do not suggest an allergic mechanism. The pattern of symptoms in these patients is variable, and it has yet to be shown that they are consistently reproduced by the ingestion of specific foods. Patients with active allergic rhinitis and asthma or other chronic diseases also may experience fatigue, difficulty in concentration, and other nonspecific symptoms, but the concept that these represent primary allergic manifestations is unproved. No evidence has emerged showing that elimination diets have successfully controlled the symptoms in so-called allergic toxemia.

MULTIPLE FOOD AND CHEMICAL SENSITIVITIES

Historical Overview

The concept that certain persons suffer a specific illness caused by multiple food and chemical sensitivities is the basis of a medical practice known as "clinical ecology,"[171,172,191] which evolved from the theory of food-induced allergic toxemia. The presumed illness was termed "environmental illness"; this entity also has been called environmentally induced disease,[101,192,193] chemical hypersensitivity syndrome,[156] multiple chemical sensitivities (MCS),[194] cerebral allergy,[195] chemically induced immune dysregulation,[196] "20th century disease,"[196,197] total allergy syndrome,[197,198] ecologic illness,[171,172] food and chemical sensitivities,[199] and toxic chemical encephalopathy.

The syndrome of IEI/MCS was first described in patients who attributed their illness to workplace exposures, as

> an acquired disorder characterized by recurrent symptoms, referable to multiple organ systems, occurring in response to demonstrable exposure to many chemically unrelated compounds at doses far below those established in the general population to cause harmful effects. No single widely accepted test of physiologic function can be shown to correlate with symptoms.[196]

A workshop of the International Programme on Chemical Safety of the World Health Organization[200] recommended the term *idiopathic environmental intolerances*, because the term *multiple chemical sensitivities* "makes an unsupported judgment on causation" (i.e., environmental chemicals), does not refer to a clinically defined disease, and is not based on "accepted theories of underlying mechanisms [or] validated clinical criteria for diagnosis." Furthermore, the "relationship between exposures and symptoms is unproven."

IEI is described by clinical ecologists as a polysymptomatic condition, which suggests pathologic changes in numerous areas and systems of the body. Nevertheless, no abnormal physical findings or laboratory test results, gross or microscopic evidence of inflammation, or other objective signs of a disorder can be found on appropriate investigations.[171,172,191] The most common complaints in IEI—fatigue, headache, nausea, malaise, pain, mucosal irritation, disorientation, and dizziness—are nonspecific[152,167,174] and commonly reported in the absence of physical illness. Some defined physical and psychiatric disorders also have been attributed by clinical ecologists to multiple food and chemical sensitivities.[164,165,192,193,195,201-208]

The methods used for diagnosing and treating IEI encompass many of the unproven and inappropriate procedures described in some detail previously. The clinical findings in and theories of IEI and the phenomenon of the clinical ecology movement have been critically scrutinized in recent years.[166,209-213]

Causes

The list of items purported to cause this condition is virtually unlimited: any naturally occurring food, including drinking water; artificial food additives; any synthetic product; specific chemicals such as formaldehyde, phenol, ethanol, ammonia, hydrocarbons, and petrochemicals; and sources of environmental chemicals, particularly cleaning solvents, paints, smoke, gasoline, vehicle exhaust fumes, fumes from office machines, perfumes, synthetic clothing, pesticides, structural plastics, building construction materials, and new carpeting.[164,167] Patients often complain of difficulty in tolerating exposure to certain buildings. Despite the emphasis on synthetic chemicals, causes of illness also have included natural gas, electromagnetic radiation, viruses, fungi, yeast, and wood dust.[202,213,214] In certain cases the presumed causative chemical is an endogenous hormone, especially progesterone.[202] Patients almost always attribute their illness to a combination of foods, environmental chemicals, and drugs.

The presumed causes are believed to act both in the induction of disease and in provoking symptoms once disease occurs. No consistent dose-response relationship in the provocation of symptoms is evident. The duration of exposure to environmental agents required to induce the disease has ranged from seconds to years, with no correlation of presumed dose and exposure duration with the severity of illness.[164,167]

The diagnostic procedure most commonly used by clinical ecologists is provocation-neutralization, as discussed earlier. After testing, many of these patients develop a new set of "causes" corresponding to the items used in the test.[164,167]

Theories of Environmental Illness

Initially Randolph and Moss[192] proposed a theory that failure of the human body to adapt to industrial synthetic chemicals produces a condition of hypersensitivity to these agents. The mechanism of the hypersensitivity is unexplained, and no supporting empirical evidence for the theory is available.

Various immunologic mechanisms have been proposed for IEI on the theory that environmental chemicals function as haptens to induce formation of IgG antibodies, IgE antibodies, or sensitized T cells.[192,214-217] The clinical illness in IEI, however, does not suggest immunologic hypersensitivity, and evidence of specific antibodies, or of a cellular immune response to any of the environmental agents identified by these patients as a cause of their illness, is lacking. An autoimmune theory was proposed from an unconfirmed report of circulating immune complexes or autoantibodies in some patients with IEI.[192] Immune response dysregulation also has been suggested,[196] but evidence for abnormal immune function or immune deficiency in IEI has not emerged.

Additional concepts unique to the field of clinical ecology are total body load, chemical overload, masked food sensitivity, and spreading phenomenon.[171] These concepts are used to explain the lack of a consistent dose-response relationship between the perceived chemical exposure and the symptoms, and they are inconsistent with modern concepts of immunology. *Total body load* and *chemical overload* assume that the immune system has a fixed capacity to handle a limited quantity of environmental antigen, and that exceeding this capacity provokes symptoms.[214] *Masked food sensitivity* is used to explain an adverse reaction to a food when it is eaten after several days of abstention, whereas frequent ingestion of the same food causes symptoms to disappear. These concepts sometimes are referred to collectively as "adaptation-deadaptation," but they have never been explained physiologically or even documented as in valid observations.[214] *Spreading phenomenon* is a putative mechanism whereby exposure to one substance induces or predisposes to immune responses to other, unrelated ones; it is used to explain periods of increasing symptoms in the absence of environmental changes.

Nonimmunologic theories include (1) deficiency of antioxidants induced by the generation of free radicals by environmental chemicals, drugs, and foods[156]; (2) neurotoxicity caused by endogenous β-endorphin "sensitization" induced by environmental stimuli,[218] odor-induced "kindling" of olfactory-limbic neural pathways,[219-221] or immunologic-to-neurogenic inflammation "switching" mediated by neuropeptides[222]; (3) end-organ dysesthesia involving the nasal mucosa,[223,224] the lung,[225] the entire respiratory tree,[226] or multiple organs[227]; and (4) hereditary coproporphyria.[228] None of these theories is supported by experimental proof or controlled clinical studies.

In contrast with theories of an organic basis for IEI, many physicians prefer a psychiatric explanation for the IEI phenomenon. This approach is discussed later under "Clinical Studies."

Diagnosis

The diagnosis of IEI most often rests on an environmental history and provocation-neutralization tests.[172] The patient's self-report of symptoms after presumed exposure to odors or fumes, or after eating certain foods, usually suffices. Many clinical ecologists supplement the provocation-neutralization testing with various laboratory tests, including quantification of serum immunoglobulins and complement components; detection of circulating autoantibodies and immune complexes; lymphocyte subset analysis; measurement of a variety of environmental chemicals in blood, urine, fat, and hair samples; and assays for circulating hormones, amino acids, and mediators.

Data from the clinical ecology literature and from independent reviews of series of patients with IEI lend no support to the diagnostic usefulness of any of these tests.[110,155,164,194-213] Levels of serum immunoglobulins and complement components, blood levels of total lymphocytes and various subsets, circulating hormones or other natural body constituents, and quantities of xenobiotics in various body fluids are not consistently abnormal.

Treatment Methods

Proponents of the IEI concept use three treatment modalities: avoidance of environmental chemical exposure, special elimination diets, and neutralization therapy. Drugs are regarded as harmful synthetic chemicals that cause environmental illness, yet patients are often instructed to take vitamin and mineral supplements. Some are treated with certain salts, such as sodium bicarbonate, to "neutralize" allergic reactions, and with amino acids, intravenous γ-globulin, or oxygen inhalation to relieve symptoms.

The rationale for the program is to eliminate or reduce symptoms and to "strengthen" the immune system. Complete avoidance of multiple environmental chemicals is invariably recommended,[171,190] often requiring a significant change in lifestyle. Many patients remodel their homes to make them safe from exposure to toxic chemicals,[213] or they relocate to isolated communities. They often wear masks in public, and even within their own homes.

The elimination diet typically includes avoidance of all food additives and a "rotary diversified diet" in which foods are rotated on a 4- to 5-day cycle.[171,190,218,229]

No prospective, controlled clinical trials have been performed to evaluate the effectiveness of the combination of food and chemical avoidance with neutralization therapy. An unblinded evaluation of 21 patients with a variety of illnesses treated by food and chemical avoidance and with neutralizing injections for food sensitivity showed improvement in both patients and control subjects.[108] A retrospective review of 50 cases showed that after an average of 2 years of treatment, the condition had been ameliorated in only 4% of the patients, whereas it was unchanged in 44% and had worsened in 52%.[164]

Clinical Studies

Published results of several critical evaluations of patients claiming to have IEI do not support a role for food and chemical sensitivities as a cause of the reported symptoms, nor do they indicate immunologic dysfunction. Instead, they provide evidence for a significant role for underlying psychiatric illness.

Patients with IEI are predominantly female and typically have consulted numerous physicians for their symptoms before their diagnosis of IEI. In the absence of objective findings, a case definition is limited to self-report. Most patients describe multiple symptoms, although some are asymptomatic and a few have a physical illness that had been undiagnosed and untreated.[164] There are no consistent physical findings or laboratory abnormalities. Evaluation of 90 patients claiming work-related IEI showed that illness was attributed to an extremely heterogeneous group of environmental substances of differing chemical composition within an extremely diverse group of occupations.[167] Their medical records revealed that two thirds of these patients had been treated for the same symptoms for many years before their occupational exposure, and three quarters had acquired a new set of symptoms after provocation-neutralization testing. Furthermore, the most common alternative diagnoses made by physicians who were not clinical ecologists were somatoform illness, anxiety disorder, depression, hyperventilation, and iatrogenic disease.

Psychiatric evaluations of patients with IEI confirm the impression that their perceived reactions to environmental chemicals and foods are manifestations of preexisting psychiatric disease.[165,197,201,209,211,230] These reports show that many patients with environmental illness fit the criteria of the American Psychiatric Association's *Diagnostic and Statistical Manual of Mental Disorders,* 4th edition (DSM-IV) for several psychiatric illnesses.[231,232] The predominance of women and the multisystemic polysomatic nature of the illness are suggestive of somatoform disorder, although not all patients meet the strict descriptive criteria. By including normal control subjects in their study, Black and colleagues[230] showed that the number of reported symptoms and the prevalence of mood disorder, anxiety disorder, and somatoform illness were all significantly higher in patients with IEI than in a population of normal people. Stewart and Raskin[197] pointed out that although somatoform illness is notoriously difficult to treat effectively, a majority of patients have had psychotic, affective, or anxiety disorders, all of which can be effectively treated with appropriate medications or psychotherapy, or both. Unfortunately, most patients with IEI are reluctant to accept a psychiatric diagnosis or treatment, opting instead for an extreme avoidant lifestyle, to which they may adhere for years.[233] Terr[164,167] showed that clinical ecology treatment is almost always ineffective or counterproductive. Brodsky[201] has studied the social consequences of extreme environmental chemical avoidance that leads to social isolation centered on the illness.

The importance of preexisting psychiatric illness is made particularly clear by the study of Simon and associates,[209] who evaluated 37 aircraft workers exposed to phenol-formaldehyde causing transient mucosal irritation that resolved on cessation of exposure. Thirteen of these workers had chronic disabling symptoms provoked by common environmental agents and were diagnosed by a clinical ecologist as having IEI. The prevalence of preexisting psychiatric morbidity caused by anxiety, depression, somatization, and medically unexplained symptoms was significantly higher in these patients than in the 24 patients who had transient symptoms only.

Patients who accept the concept of IEI for their somatic symptoms are psychologically diverse, although limited or extensive somatoform illness is the most common pattern. Other patients have features of posttraumatic stress disorder,[234,235] agoraphobia caused by conditioning,[236,237] panic disorder,[238] or the adult manifestation of childhood abuse.[239] The IEI phenomenon has been viewed in cultural terms[240] and has been called a "belief system"[241] and "illness and disability as lifestyle."[242]

Immunologic Evaluation

Two studies have examined the clinical and laboratory evidence for immunologic illness in patients with multiple food and chemical sensitivities. In 50 cases studied by Terr,[164] levels of circulating immunoglobulins, complement components, and lymphocyte subsets were mostly within the normal expected range and did not correlate with severity of reported illness or length of reported exposure to the foods or chemicals thought to cause the illness. None of the patients had clinical evidence of immunodeficiency or autoimmune disease, and the prevalence of allergic disease was similar to that found in the general population.

A review of the clinical ecology publications citing results of immunologic tests in patients with environmental illness failed to reveal a consistent pattern of abnormalities.[212]

Conclusions from Available Evidence

The diagnosis of multiple food and/or chemical sensitivities manifested by numerous symptoms in the absence of objective physical findings lacks a scientific foundation.[243] There is no evidence that such patients suffer from an allergic or other immunologic abnormality. The concept of the illness is based on anecdotal reports with no verification using properly controlled, blinded challenges. The diagnosis comes from the subjective history alone or in combination with provocation-neutralization testing, which has been shown to be unreliable. The treatment and theories underlying this presumed illness are not consistent with current immunologic knowledge and theory. Medical and psychiatric evaluations of these patients indicate instead that most probably suffer from psychiatric illness but prefer to interpret their symptoms as environmental sensitivities. Treatment by avoidance of environmental chemicals and foods and by the use of injections or sublingual drops to "neutralize" (i.e., reverse) ongoing symptoms is ineffective and is likely to lead to harmful social isolation. In some cases,[244] the diagnosis of IEI obscures a treatable psychiatric or physical disease.

CANDIDA HYPERSENSITIVITY SYNDROME

Candida hypersensitivity syndrome (also called candidiasis hypersensitivity syndrome and yeast hypersensitivity syndrome) is a proposed hypersensitivity to a toxin released from *Candida albicans.*[245-248] The illness, like IEI, is described in terms of numerous wide-ranging symptoms without specific physical findings or laboratory abnormalities. In fact, many patients are diagnosed with the combination of food, chemical, and *Candida* sensitivity. Popular books written for lay persons promote self-diagnosis.

C. albicans may be found normally on the skin and as a part of the normal flora of the mucosae of the respiratory, gastrointestinal, and female genitourinary tracts.[249] Because it is a commensal organism for humans, exposure to *Candida* antigens is virtually universal, and low levels of antibody- and cell-mediated immunity are usual in immunologically normal, healthy persons.

Opportunistic candidiasis is found in conditions involving impaired innate or acquired immunity.[250] Thrush or localized infection of the buccal mucosa is not unusual in infants. In children and adults it may result from antibiotic or topical inhaled corticosteroid therapy. Thrush or *Candida* vulvovaginitis can be a complication of diabetes mellitus, pregnancy, or progesterone therapy and may occur transiently during antibiotic therapy. Systemic candidiasis is seen most commonly in states of cell-mediated immunosuppression and in chronic granulomatous disease.[251] Chronic mucocutaneous candidiasis also accompanies certain states of impaired cell-mediated immunity.[252] These pathologic forms of candidiasis must not be confused with the unproven condition of "*Candida* hypersensitivity."[253]

Disease Description

As in IEI, proponents of so-called *Candida* hypersensitivity syndrome usually make the diagnosis in persons with numerous subjective symptoms, but they also claim that it is a cause of, or a potentiating factor for, numerous other diseases, including multiple sclerosis, arthritis, psoriasis, schizophrenia, cancer, acquired immunodeficiency syndrome (AIDS), depression, and various behavioral and emotional problems. The syndrome lacks a specific definition, and there are no diagnostic physical or laboratory test abnormalities or evidence of *C. albicans* overgrowth, either locally or systemically. Predisposing factors are said to include current or past use of antibiotics, corticosteroids, or birth control pills and diets of yeast (not *Candida*)-containing foods, sugars, and other carbohydrates. No evidence is available, however, to show that these patients differ from others in their exposure to any of these factors.[254]

Theory of Pathogenesis

Theoretical explanations include both hypersensitivity and toxicity. A presumed *C. albicans* toxin is claimed to have a suppressive effect on the immune system, although clinical or experimental data indicating immunotoxicity in these patients are lacking.

Diagnosis

The diagnosis is based entirely on history, often established by questionnaire. No published reports showing that antibody levels of any immunoglobulin isotype specific to *Candida* antigens are higher in patients with this diagnosis than in control subjects are available.

Treatment

The recommended treatment consists of diet, nutritional supplements, vitamins, minerals, and certain medications. The diet restricts intake of sugar, dietary yeast, and foods believed to contain mold. A rotary diet, as used in IEI, often is advised. Antifungal drugs are recommended, usually in exceedingly low oral doses.

To date, no clinical trials have been conducted to evaluate the effectiveness of diet or nutritional supplements. In a randomized, double-blind trial of nystatin for patients supposedly suffering from *Candida* hypersensitivity syndrome, oral or vaginal nystatin, or a combination of the two, was no different from placebo in altering symptoms.[254] No data are available on the natural course of the condition.

Conclusions from Available Evidence

Candida hypersensitivity syndrome has not been defined as a clinical entity. It is an unproven concept purporting that a wide range of subjective symptoms can be caused by immunologic toxicity from the normal reservoir of *C. albicans* resident in the gastrointestinal and genitourinary tracts.[255] A theoretical basis for the syndrome has not been identified. The efficacy of the diagnostic questionnaire and of serum antibody levels to *C. albicans* antigens is untested. The single reported therapeutic trial of nystatin indicates that any benefit is consistent with a placebo effect, and the other recommended therapeutic measures are untested.

FOOD ADDITIVE SENSITIVITY

Attention deficit–hyperactivity disorder (ADHD) in children and some adults was previously called hyperactivity, hyperkinesis, and minimal brain dysfunction. It is considered to be a psychiatric condition characterized by excessive activity, inattention that is inappropriate to the stage of development, increased level of impulsivity, difficulty in discipline, and poor school performance. It is not an uncommon problem of childhood. The natural history is unpredictable, with some children losing all symptoms during puberty and others continuing to exhibit some or all manifestations into adulthood. The cause is unknown, but the disorder is thought to encompass some combination of constitutional, genetic, environmental, and psychosocial factors.

The suggestion that ADHD is caused by sensitivity to aspirin and other salicylates was first made in 1973 by Feingold,[256] who recommended elimination of dietary salicylates as treatment for this and other psychiatric conditions, claiming improvement in up to 50% of children with ADHD. Because other investigators had reported that asthma attacks in patients with aspirin-sensitive asthma could be triggered by ingestion of the yellow food coloring dye tartrazine,[257,258] it was recommended that *all* food dyes and other additives, regardless of their chemical structure, toxicity, or pharmacologic properties, be eliminated. Thus the "Feingold diet" evolved as a salicylate-free, additive-free diet.

Virtually all plants contain some salicylate, making it unlikely that any plant food is truly salicylate-free. Small amounts of salicylates are found in certain animal products and even in drinking water. In fact, a true salicylate-free diet would be limited to plain meat, egg, and distilled water only.[259-261] In practice, adherents of the Feingold diet focus on eliminating food additives, particularly dyes and preservatives, so the role of natural salicylates in foods—the issue on which the diet was based—is no longer thought to be important.

Mechanism

Scientific evidence for direct effects on the central nervous system caused by toxicity, idiosyncrasy, or allergic hypersensitivity to food additives is lacking. Acute asthma attacks precipitated by the ingestion of aspirin and other nonsteroidal antiinflammatory drugs are discussed in Chapter 80.

Clinical Trials

Several published controlled clinical trials have used different protocols, with conflicting results.[262-265] A consensus conference by the Office of Medical Applications for Research of the National Institutes of Health concluded that only a few children might benefit by improvement in behavior from a defined diet.[266,267]

Conclusions from Available Evidence

The hypothesis that naturally occurring food salicylates and artificial food additives cause ADHD is unproved. An additive-free diet cannot be recommended as definitive therapy for children with this condition. No evidence is available at this time to confirm that any food additive affects behavior in children through an immunologic or allergic mechanism.

Remote Practice of Allergy

Managing allergy effectively requires an initial careful history and physical examination followed by relevant laboratory tests, including specific allergy testing based on the patient's exposure or environmental history. The selection of tests and their interpretation are the responsibility of the physician who has performed the history and examination personally, and who has the requisite knowledge of allergic diseases obtained through training and experience. Test results, especially of allergy tests, can be interpreted only with reference to the patient's history.

The basic elements of allergic disease management are (1) allergen avoidance, (2) medications to prevent or alleviate allergic inflammation, and (3) allergen immunotherapy. The selection of one or more of these modes of therapy, prescription of specific drugs, instruction on elimination of items from the environment, and decisions about allergen immunotherapy must be individualized to each patient's disease manifestations and physical and psychosocial environment. Finally, because most allergic diseases tend to be chronic and intermittent, monitoring of the results of therapy by the treating physician is necessary.

Decisions regarding diagnosis and treatment made by a physician or other person who has not personally examined the patient constitute the "remote practice of allergy." Remote practice may take several forms, such as use of a standardized questionnaire history for diagnosis and treatment without a personal history and appropriate physical examination, or diagnosis of specific allergies and recommendation of immunotherapy based on results of skin or in vitro testing without reference to the patient's history. These tests detect the presence of specific IgE antibody (or specific cellular hypersensitivity in the case of patch testing) but alone do not reveal the cause of the patient's illness. Positive test results may indicate past, future, or irrelevant sensitivities and may not necessarily identify the cause of the patient's current allergic illness.

The remote practice of allergy, therefore, refers to the diagnosis and management of allergy without personal knowledge and evaluation of the patient's history, physical examination, and relevant testing. Optimal treatment under these conditions is highly unlikely. The physician assuming responsibility for the management of an allergic patient should do so on the basis of direct observation and hands-on examination of the patient. This definition of the remote practice of allergy does not, of course, preclude the practice of giving and receiving consultative advice between a specialist and the primary physician.[268]

BOX 101-1 CURRENT STATUS OF UNORTHODOX AND UNPROVEN DIAGNOSTIC AND THERAPEUTIC PRACTICES IN ALLERGY IN THE UNITED STATES

PROCEDURES CURRENTLY BEING ACTIVELY PRACTICED

Diagnosis

- Skin end point titration
- Provocation-neutralization
- Antigen leukocyte cellular antibody test
- Electrodermal testing
- Applied kinesiology
- Various serum assays for immunoglobulins, cytokines, receptors, others
- Blood lymphocyte counts and functions
- Food immune complex assay

Treatment

- Acupuncture
- Homeopathic "remedies"
- Herbal medicine
- Chiropractic manipulation
- Diets and dietary supplements
- Neutralization (subcutaneous, intradermal) therapy and variations

NEWER VARIATIONS OF ESTABLISHED BUT UNPROVEN PRACTICES

Treatment

- Laser acupuncture (with or without medication or allergen insertion at acupoints)
- Electrical transcutaneous nerve stimulation (TNS)

PROCEDURES CURRENTLY OF MINOR INTEREST

Diagnosis

- Iridology

Treatment

- Enzyme-potentiated desensitization
- Detoxification

PROCEDURES OF LARGELY HISTORICAL INTEREST

Diagnosis

- Cytotoxic test
- Pulse test

Treatment

- Autogenous urine injection

PROCEDURES UNDERGOING CURRENT CONTROLLED CLINICAL TRIALS

Treatment

- Sublingual immunotherapy

Current Versus Historical Practices

A number of the unproven and controversial methods described and referenced in this chapter are currently being espoused by certain practitioners; other such methods now are of historical interest only, although they may be revived eventually in a similar or altered form. In some cases, notably that of sublingual immunotherapy (see Chapter 88), methods previously considered unproved may be undergoing intensive controlled trials that may or may not establish their usefulness in allergy practice.

Numerous studies and abundant anecdotal information attest to the interest in and use of unconventional diagnostic and therapeutic methodologies and theories in the United States and other countries. Some modalities are especially prevalent in Europe; Chinese medicine is undoubtedly widely practiced in Asia and has gained prominence elsewhere. The current status of these methods and theories in the United States is summarized in Box 101-1.

Perspective

Scientifically unproven and medically illogical methods of diagnosis and treatment that are controversial and unorthodox in the view of most practicing physicians are not unique to the fields of clinical allergy and immunology. The overview of such methods and concepts presented in this chapter provides a background against which relevant issues likely to be encountered in clinical practice can be identified. Allergists and immunologists must be familiar with these methods in order to counsel patients appropriately.

REFERENCES

Introduction

1. Ernst E. The role of complementary and alternative medicine. BMJ 2000;321:1133-5.
2. Druss BG, Rosenbeck RA. Association between use of unconventional therapies and conventional medical services. JAMA 1999;282:651-6.
3. Fentanarosa PB, Lunberg JD. Alternative medicine meets science. JAMA 1998;280:1618-9.

3a. National Center for Complementary and Alternative Medicine (NCCAM) website. Available at http://nccam.nih.gov/about/ataglance. Accessed May 11, 2013.

4. Golbert TM. A review of controversial diagnostic and therapeutic techniques employed in allergy. J Allergy Clin Immunol 1975;56:170-90.
5. Grieco MH. Controversial practices in allergy. JAMA 1982;247:3105-11.
6. Council on Scientific Affairs. In vivo diagnostic testing and immunotherapy for allergy. Report of the allergy panel. JAMA 1987;258:1363, 1505-8.
7. Council on Scientific Affairs. In vitro testing for allergy. Report II of the allergy panel. JAMA 1987;258:1639-43.
8. David TJ. Unorthodox allergy procedures. Arch Dis Child 1987;62:1060-2.
9. Sullivan-Fowler M, Austin T, Hofner AW. Alternative therapies, unproven methods, and health fraud. a selected annotated bibliography. Chicago: American Medical Association; 1988.
10. Van Arsdel PP, Larson EB. Review diagnostic tests for patients with suspected allergic disease. Utility and limitations. Ann Intern Med 1989;110:304-12.
11. Goldberg BJ, Kaplan MS. Controversial concepts and techniques in the diagnosis and management of food allergies. In: Anderson JA, editor. Food allergy. Immunology and Allergy Clinics of North America, vol 2. Philadelphia: WB Saunders; 1991.
12. Markham AW, Wilkinson JM. Complementary and alternative medicines (CAM) in the management of asthma: an examination of the evidence. J Asthma 2004;41:131-9.
13. Bielory L, Russin J, Zuckerman GB. Clinical efficacy, mechanisms of action, and adverse effects of complementary and alternative medicine therapies for asthma. Allergy Asthma Proc 2004;25:283-91.
14. Wuthrich B. Unproven techniques in allergy diagnosis. J Investig Allergol Clin Immunol 2005;15:86-90.
15. Passalacqua G, Bousquet PJ, Carlsen KH, et al. ARIA update. 1. Systematic review of complementary and alternative medicine for rhinitis and asthma. J Allergy Clin Immunol 2006;117:1054-62.
16. Xue CC, Li CG, Hugel HM, Story DF. Does acupuncture or Chinese herbal medicine have a role in the treatment of allergic rhinitis? Curr Opin Allergy Clin Immunol 2006;6:175-9.
17. Karkos PD, Leong SC, Arya AK, et al. "Complementary ENT": a systematic review of commonly used supplements. J Laryngol Otol 2007;121:779-82.
18. Altunc U, Pittler MH, Ernst E. Homeopathy for childhood and adolescence ailments: systematic review of randomized clinical trials. Mayo Clin Proc 2007;82:69-75.
19. American College of Physicians. Position paper: allergy testing. Ann Intern Med 1989;110:317-20.
20. National Center for Health Care Technology. Summary of assessments. JAMA 1981;246:1499.
21. Availability of compliance policy guide for cytotoxic testing for allergic diseases. Fed Regist 1985;50:27691-3.
22. Health Care Financing Administration. Medicare programs: exclusions from Medicare coverage of certain food allergy tests and treatments. Fed Regist 1983;46:37716-22.
23. Health Care Financing Administration. Medicare program; exclusion of certain food allergy tests and treatments from Medicare coverage. Fed Regist 1990;55:35466-9.
24. Kay AB, Lessof MH. Allergy: conventional and alternative concepts. A report of the Royal College of Physicians Committee on Clinical Immunology and Allergy. Clin Exp Allergy 1992;22(Suppl 3):1-44.
25. Bernstein IL, Li JT, Bernstein DI, et al. Allergy diagnostic testing: an updated practice parameter. Ann Allergy Asthma Immunol 2008;100:S1-48.
26. Allergy: conventional and alternative concepts. Summary of a report of the Royal College of Physicians Committee on Clinical Immunology and Allergy. J R Coll Physicians Lond 1992;26:260-4.

Unproven Diagnostic Tests

27. Rinkel HJ. Inhalant allergy. 1. The whealing response of the skin to serial dilution testing. Ann Allergy 1949;7:625-30.
28. Williams RJ. Skin titration: testing and treatment. Otolaryngol Clin North Am 1971;3:507-21.
29. Richardson GS. Titration: evaluation of an office system of allergy diagnosis and treatment. Its use in otolaryngology. Ann Otolaryngol Rhinol Laryngol 1961;70:344-66.
30. Willoughby JW. Serial dilution titration skin tests in inhalant allergy: a clinical quantitative assessment of biologic skin reactivity to allergenic extracts. Otolaryngol Clin North Am 1974;7:579-615.
31. Hirsch S, Kalbfleisch JH, Cohen SH. Comparison of therapy with standard immunotherapy. J Allergy Clin Immunol 1982;70:183-90.
32. Hirsch SR, Kalbfleisch JH, Golbert TM, et al. Rinkel injection therapy: a multi-center controlled study. J Allergy Clin Immunol 1981;68:133-55.
33. Van Metre TE, Adkinson NF, Amodio FJ, et al. A comparative study of the effectiveness of the Rinkel method and the current standard method of immunotherapy for ragweed pollen hay fever. J Allergy Clin Immunol 1980;66:500-13.
34. Van Metre TE, Adkinson NF Jr, Lichtenstein LM, et al. A controlled study of the effectiveness of the Rinkel method: immunotherapy for ragweed pollen hay fever. J Allergy Clin Immunol 1980;65:288-97.
35. Van Metre TE. Critique of controversial and unproven procedures for diagnosis and therapy of allergy disorders. Pediatr Clin North Am 1983;30:807.
36. Green M. Sublingual provocative testing for food and FD and C dyes. Ann Allergy 1974;33:274-81.
37. Lehman CW. A double-blind study of sublingual provocation food testing: a study of its efficacy. Ann Allergy 1980;45:144-9.
38. Morris DL. Use of sublingual antigen in diagnosis and treatment of food allergy. Ann Allergy 1971;27:289-94.
39. Breneman JC, Crook WG, Deamer W, et al. Report of the Food Allergy Committee on the sublingual method of provocation testing for food allergy. Ann Allergy 1973;31:382-5.
40. Kailin EW, Collier R. "Relieving" therapy for antigen exposure. JAMA 1971;217:78.
41. King DS. Can allergic exposure provoke psychological symptoms? A double-blind test. Biol Psychiatry 1981;16:3-19.
42. Jewett DL, Fein G, Greenberg MH. Double blind study of symptom provocation to determine food sensitivity. N Engl J Med 1990;323:429-33.
43. Dickey LD. Sublingual antigens. JAMA 1971;217:214.
44. Dolowitz DA. Theories of allergy brought up to date. Ann Allergy 1974;32:183-8.
45. Rea WJ, Podell RN, Williams M, et al. Elimination of oral food challenge reaction by injection of food extract. Arch Otolaryngol 1984;110:248-52.
46. Bronsky EA, Burkley DP, Ellis EF. Evaluations of provocative food skin test technique [abstract]. J Allergy 1971;47:104.
47. Draper WL. Food testing in allergy: intradermal provocation vs. deliberate feeding. Arch Otolaryngol 1972;95:169-71.
48. Caplin I. Report of the Committee on Provocative Food Testing. Ann Allergy 1973;31:375-81.
49. Crawford LV, Lieberman P, Hanfi HA, et al. A double-blind study of subcutaneous food testing, sponsored by the Food Committee of the American Academy of Allergy [abstract]. J Allergy Clin Immunol 1976;57:236.
50. Bryan WT, Bryan MP. Cytotoxic reactions in the diagnosis of food allergy. Otolaryngol Clin North Am 1971;4:523-34.
51. Bryan WT, Bryan M. Clinical examples of resolution of some idiopathic and other chronic disease by careful allergic management. Laryngoscope 1972;82:1231-8.
52. Bryan WT, Bryan MP. Allergy in otolaryngology. In: Paparella MM, Shumrick DA, editors. Otolaryngology, vol 3. Philadelphia: WB Saunders; 1973.
53. Bryan MP, Bryan WT. Cytologic diagnosis of allergic disorders. Otolaryngol Clin North Am 1974;7:637-66.
54. Bryan WT, Bryan MP. Cytotoxic reactions in the diagnosis of food allergy. In: Dickey LD, editor. Clinical ecology. Springfield, Ill.: Charles C Thomas; 1976.
55. Squier TL, Lee HJ. Lysis in vitro of sensitized leukocytes by ragweed antigen. J Allergy 1947;18:156-63.
56. Franklin W, Lowell FC. Failure of ragweed pollen extract to destroy white cells from ragweed-sensitive patients. J Allergy 1949;20:375-7.
57. Siraganian RP, Hook WA. Histamine release and assay methods for the study of human allergy. In: Rose NR, Friedman H, Fahey JC, editors. Manual of clinical laboratory immunology. Washington, D.C.: American Society of Microbiology; 1986.
58. Ulett GA, Perry SC. Cytotoxic testing and leukocyte increase: an index of food sensitivity. II. Coffee and tobacco. Ann Allergy 1975;34:150-60.
59. Updegraff TR. Food allergy and cytotoxic test. Ear Nose Throat J 1977;56:450-9.
60. Boyles JH. The validity of using cytotoxic food test in clinical allergy. Ear Nose Throat J 1977;56:168-73.

61. Lieberman P, Crawford L, Bjelland J, Connell B, Rice M. Controlled study of the cytotoxic food test. JAMA 1974;231:728-30.
62. Benson TE, Atkins JA. Cytotoxic testing for food allergy: evaluations of reproducibility and correlation. J Allergy Clin Immunol 1976;58: 471-6.
63. Lehman CW. The leukocytotoxic food allergy test: a study of its reliability and reproducibility. Effect of diet and sublingual food drops on this test. Ann Allergy 1980;45:150-8.
64. Terr AI. The cytotoxic test [editorial]. West J Med 1983;139:702-3.
65. Pasula MJ. The ALCAT test: in vitro procedure for determining food sensitivities. Folia Med Cracov 1993;34:153-7.
66. Buczyłko K, Obarzanowski T, Rosiak K, et al. Prevalence of food allergy and intolerance in children based on MAST CLA and ALCAT tests. Rocz Akad Med Bialymst 1995;40:452-6.
67. Wuthrich B. Unproven techniques in allergy diagnosis. J Investig Allergol Clin Immunol 2005;15:86-90.
68. Kleine-Tebbe J, Herold DA. Inappropriate test methods in allergy. Hautarzt 2001;61:961-6.
69. Senne G, Gani F, Leo G, Schiappoli M. Alternative tests in the diagnosis of food allergies. Recenti Prog Med 2002;93:327-34.
70. Mylek D. ALCAT rest results in the treatment of respiratory and gastrointestinal symptoms, arthritis, skin and central nervous system. Rocz Akad Med Bialymst 1995;40:625-9.
71. Mancini S, Fierimonte V, Iacovoni R, et al. [Food allergy: comparison of diagnostic techniques.] Minerva Pediatr 1995;47:159-63.
72. Tsuei JJ, Lehman CW, Lam FM, et al. A food allergy study utilizing the EAV acupuncture technique. Am J Acupuncture 1984;12:105.
73. Voll R. The phenomenon of medicine testing in electroacupuncture according to Voll. Am J Acupuncture 1980;8:87.
74. Lewith GT. Can we evaluate electrodermal testing? Complement Ther Med 2003;11: 115-7.
75. Lewith GT, Kenyon JN, Broomfield J, et al. Is electrodermal testing as effective as skin prick tests for diagnosing allergies? A double blind, randomised block design study. BMJ 2001; 322:131-4.
76. Semizzi M, Senna G, Crivellaro M, et al. A double-blind, placebo-controlled study on the diagnostic accuracy of an electrodermal test in allergic subjects. Clin Exp Allergy 2002;32: 928-32.
77. Fox A. Determination of neutralisation point for allergic hypersensitivity. Br Homeopathic J 1987;76:230-4.
78. Ali M. Correlation of IgE antibodies with specificity for pollen and mould allergy changes in electrodermal skin responses following exposure to allergens. Am J Clin Pathol 1989; 91:357.
79. Krop J, Sweisczck J, Wood A. Comparison of ecological testing with the Vegatest method in identifying sensitivities to chemicals, foods and inhalants. Am J Acupuncture 1985;13: 253-9.
80. Krop J, Lewith GT, Gziut W, Radulescu C. A double blind, randomized, controlled investigation of electrodermal testing in the diagnosis of allergies. J Altern Complement Med 1997;3:241-8.
81. Garrow JS. Kinesiology and food allergy. BMJ 1988;296:1573-4.
82. Schmitt WH Jr, Leisman G. Correlation of applied kinesiology muscle testing findings with serum immunoglobulin levels for food allergies. Int J Neurosci 1998;96:237-44.
83. Ludke R, Kunz B, Seeber N, Ring J. Test-retest-reliability and validity of the kinesiology muscle test. Complement Ther Med 2001;9: 141-5.

Inappropriate Diagnostic Tests

84. Mullin GE, Swift KM, Lipski L, Turnbull LK, Rampertab SD. Testing for food reactions: the good, the bad, and the ugly. Nutr Clin Pract 2010;25:192-8.
85. Sheffer AL, Lieberman PL, Aaronson DW, et al. Measurement of circulating IgG and IgE food-immune complexes. J Allergy Clin Immunol 1988;81:758-60.
86. Inganäs M, Johansson SG, Dannaeus A. A method for estimation of circulating immune complexes after oral challenge with ovalbumin. Clin Allergy 1980;10:293-302.
87. Haddad ZH, Vetter M, Friedman J, Sainz C, Brunner E. Detection and kinetics of antigen-specific IgE and IgG immune complexes in food allergy. Ann Allergy 1983;51:255.
88. Leary HL, Halsey JF. An assay to measure antigen-specific immune complexes in food allergy patients. J Allergy Clin Immunol 1984;74:190-5.
89. Brostoff J, Carini C. Production of IgE complexes by allergen challenge in atopic patients and the effect of sodium cromoglycate. Lancet 1979;1:1268-70.
90. Djurup R, Kappelgaard E, Stahl Skov P, Permin H, Nielsen H. Determination of IgE-containing immune complexes in human sera: evaluation of polyethylene glycol precipitation of monomeric and complex IgE and of the detectability of IgE in the complexes. Allergy 1984;39: 395-406.
91. Dixon FJ. The role of antigen-antibody complexes in disease. Harvey Lect 1963;58: 21-52.
92. Cochrane CG, Koffler D. Immune complex disease in experimental animals and man. Adv Immunol 1973;16:185-264.
93. Russell BA, Lockwood CM, Scott DM, Pinching AJ, Peters DK. Value of immune complex assays in diagnosis and management. Lancet 1978;2:359-64.
94. Dannaeus A, Inganäs M, Johansson SG, Foucard T. Intestinal intake of ovalbumin in malabsorption and food allergy in relation to serum IgE antibody and orally administered sodium cromoglycate. Clin Allergy 1979;9: 263-70.
95. Walker WA, Isselbacher KJ. Update and transport of macromolecules by the intestine: possible role in clinical disorders. Gastroenterology 1974;67:531-50.
96. Husby S, Oxellus VA, Teisner B, Jensenius JC, Svehag SE. Humoral immunity to dietary antigens in healthy adults: occurrence, isotype and IgG subclass distribution of serum antibodies to protein antigens. Int Arch Allergy Appl Immunol 1985;77:416-22.
97. Paganelli R, Levinsky RJ, Brostoff J, Wraith DG. Immune complexes containing food proteins in normal and atopic subjects after oral challenge and effect of sodium cromoglycate on antigen absorption. Lancet 1979;1:1270-2.
98. Paganelli R, Levinsky RJ, Atherton DJ. Detection of specific antigen within circulating immune complexes; validation of the assay and its application to food antigen-antibody complexes formed in healthy and food-allergic subjects. Clin Exp Immunol 1981;46:44-53.
99. Paganelli R, Atherton DJ, Levinsky RJ. The differences between normal and milk allergic subjects in their immune response after milk ingestion. Arch Dis Child 1983;58:201-6.
100. Paganelli R, Cavagni G, Pallone F. The role of antigenic absorption and circulating immune complexes in food allergy. Ann Allergy 1986; 57:330-6.
101. Cunningham-Rundels C, Brandeis WE, Good RA, Day NK. Milk precipitins, circulating immune complexes, and IgA deficiency. Proc Natl Acad Sci U S A 1978;75:3387-9.
102. Cunningham-Rundels C, Brandeis WE, Good RA, Day NK. Bovine proteins and the formation of circulating immune complexes in selective IgA deficiency. J Clin Invest 1979; 64:272-9.
103. Cunningham-Rundels C, Brandeis WE, Safai E, et al. Selective Ig A deficiency and circulating immune complexes containing bovine proteins in a child with chronic graft vs. host disease. Am J Med 1979;67:883-90.
104. Panush RS, Stroud RM, Webster EM. Food-induced (allergic) arthritis. Inflammatory arthritis aggravated by milk. Arthritis Rheum 1986;29:220-6.
105. Coca AF. The pulse test. New York: Carol Publishing Group; 1982.

Unproven Treatment Methods

106. Gyorik SA, Brutsche MH. Complementary and alternative medicine for bronchial asthma: is there new evidence? Curr Opin Pulm Med 2004;10:37-43.
107. Warren CM. Inhalant allergy: diagnosis and treatment by provocation intracutaneous method. Med Digest 1979;33:24.
108. Miller JB. A double-blind study of food extract injection therapy: a preliminary report. Ann Allergy 1977;38:185-91.
109. Rapp D. Double-blind confirmation and treatment of milk sensitivity. Med J Aust 1978;1: 571-2.
110. Morris DL. Treatment of respiratory disease with ultra-small doses of antigens. Ann Allergy 1970;28:494-500.
111. Morris DL. Treatment of atopic dermatitis with tolerogenic doses of antigen. Acta Dermatol Venereol (Stockh) 1980;92:97-8.
112. Miller JB, Lee CE, Binkley EL Jr, Hardt SM. Relief of influenza symptoms by the provocative-neutralizing method. A preliminary report. J Med Assoc State Ala 1972;41: 493-500.
113. Scadding GK, Brostoff J. Low dose sublingual therapy in patients with allergic rhinitis due to house dust mite. Clin Allergy 1986;16: 483-502.
114. Teuber SS, Vogt PJ. An unproven technique with potentially fatal outcome: provocation/neutralization in a patient with systemic mastocytosis. Ann Allergy Asthma 1999;82:61-5.
115. Fell P, Brostoff J. A single dose desensitization for summer hayfever: results of a double blind study—1988. Eur J Clin Pharmacol 1990;38: 77-9.
116. McEwen LM, Nicholson M, Kitchen I, White S. Enzyme-potentiated desensitization. 3. Control by sugars and diols of the immunological effect of beta glucuronidase in mice and patients with hay fever. Ann Allergy 1973;31:543-50.
117. McEwen LM, Nicholson M, Kitchen I, et al. Enzyme potentiated desensitization. IV. Effect of protamine on the immunological behavior of beta-glucuronidase in mice and patients with hay fever. Ann Allergy 1975;34:290-5.

118. McEwen LM. Enzyme potentiated desensitization. V. Five case reports of patients with acute food allergy. Ann Allergy 1975;35:98-103.
119. McEwen LM, Starr MS. Enzyme-potentiated desensitization. I. The effect of pre-treatment with β-glucuronidase, hyaluronidase, and antigen on anaphylactic sensitivity of guinea pigs, rats and mice. Int Arch Allergy 1972;42:152-8.
120. McEwen LM. Enzyme potentiated hyposensitization. Effects of glucose, glucosamine, N-acetylamino sugars and gelatin on the ability of β-glucuronidase to block the anamnestic response to antigen in mice. Ann Allergy 1973;31:79-83.
121. Cantani A, Ragno V, Monteleone MA, Lucenti P, Businco L. Enzyme-potentiated desensitization in children with asthma and mite allergy; a double-blind study. J Investig Allergol Clin Immunol 1996;6:270-6.
122. Astarita C, Scala G, Sproviero S, Franzese A. Effects of enzyme-potentiated desensitization in the treatment of pollinosis: a double-blind placebo-controlled trial. J Investig Allergol Clin Immunol 1996;6:248-55.
123. Di Stanislao C, Di Berardino L, Bianchi I, Bologna G. A double-blind, placebo-controlled study of preventive immunotherapy with EPD in the treatment of seasonal allergic disease. Allerg Immunol (Paris) 1997;29:39-42.
124. Caramia G, Franceschini F, Cimarelli ZA, et al. The efficacy of E.P.D., a new immunotherapy, in the treatment of allergic diseases in children. Allerg Immunol (Paris) 1996;28:308-10.
125. Galli E, Bassi MS, Mora E, et al. A double-blind randomized placebo-controlled trial with short-term beta-glucuronidase therapy in children with chronic rhinoconjunctivitis and/or asthma due to dust mite allergy. J Investig Allergol Clin Imunol 2006;16:345-50.
126. Radcliffe MJ, Lewith GT, Turner RG, et al. Enzyme-potentiated desensitization of seasonal allergic rhinitis: double-blind randomized controlled study. BMJ 2003;327:251-4.
127. Root DE, Katzin DB, Schnare DW. Diagnosis and treatment of patients presenting subclinical signs and symptoms of exposure to chemicals which bioaccumulate in human tissue. Proceedings of the National Conference on Hazardous Wastes and Environmental Emergencies, May 14-6, 1985, Cincinnati.
128. Liberman J, Bigland AD. Autogenous urinary proteose in asthma and other allergic conditions. BMJ 1937;1:62-5.
129. Plesch J. Urine therapy. Med Press 1994;218:128.
130. Park JE, Lee SS, Lee MS, Choi SM, Ernst E. Adverse events of moxibustion: a systematic review. Complement Ther Med 2010;18:215-23.
131. Stockert K, Schneider B, Porenta G, et al. Laser acupuncture and probiotics in school age children with asthma: a randomized, placebo-controlled pilot study of therapy guided by principles of Traditional Chinese Medicine. Pediatr Allergy Immunol 2007;18:160-6.
132. Li YL, Luo F, Zhang JY, Liu C. [Clinical study on effect of acupoint sticking of chuanfuling in dog-days in preventing and treating: children asthma [sic] in remission stage.] Zhongguo Zhong Xi Yi Jie He Za Zhi 2004;24:601-4.
133. McCarney RW, Lasserson TJ, Linde K, Brinkaus B. An overview of two Cochrane systematic reviews of complementary treatments for chronic asthma: acupuncture and homeopathy. Respir Med 2004;98:687-96.
134. Passalacqua G, Bousquet PJ, Carlsen KH, et al. ARIA update: 1. Systematic review of complementary and alternative medicine for rhinitis and asthma. J Allergy Clin Immunol 2006;117:1054-62.
135. Linde K, Vickers A, Hondras M, et al. Systematic reviews of complementary therapies—an annotated bibliography. Part 1: acupuncture. BMC Complement Altern Med 2001;1:4.
136. Linde K, Jobst K, Panton J. Acupuncture for chronic asthma. Cochrane Database Syst Rev 2004;(1):CD000008.
137. Martin J, Donaldson AN, Villarroel R, et al. Efficacy of acupuncture in asthma: systematic review and meta-analysis of published data from 11 randomised controlled trials. Eur Respir J 2002;20:846-52.
138. Kleijnen I, ter Riet G, Knipschild P. Acupuncture and asthma: a review of controlled trials. Thorax 1991;46:799-802.
139. Skrabanek P. Acupuncture and the age of unreason. Lancet 1984;1:1169.
140. Ernst E, White AR. Acupuncture may be associated with serious adverse events. BMJ 2000;320:513-4.
141. Reilly DT, Taylor MA, McSharry C, Aitchison T. Is homoeopathy a placebo response? Controlled trial of homoeopathic potency, with pollen in hayfever as model. Lancet 1985;2:881-6.
142. Weiser M, Gegenheimer LH, Klein P. A randomized equivalence trial comparing the efficacy and safety of Luffa comp.-Heel nasal spray with cromolyn sodium spray in the treatment of seasonal allergic rhinitis. Forsch Komplementarmed 1999;6:142-8.
143. Taylor MA, Reilly D, Llewellyn-Jones RH, et al. Randomised controlled trial of homoeopathy versus placebo in perennial allergic rhinitis with overview of four trial series. BMJ 2000;321:471-6.
144. Kim LS, Riedlinger JE, Baldwin CM, et al. Treatment of seasonal allergic rhinitis using homeopathic preparation of common allergens in the southwest region of the US: a randomized, controlled clinical trial. Ann Pharmacother 2005;39:617-24.
145. Wirt CM, Ludtke R, Baur R, Willich SN. Homeopathic medical practice: long-term results of a cohort study with 3981 patients. BMC Public Health 2005;35:115.
146. Wiesenauer M, Gaus W. Double-blind trial comparing the effectiveness of the homeopathic preparation Galphimia potentiation D6, Galphimia dilution 10(-6) and placebo on pollinosis. Arzneimittelforschung 1985;35:1745-7.
147. Aabel S. No beneficial effect of isopathic prophylactic treatment tor birch pollen allergy during a low-pollen season: a double-blind, placebo-controlled clinical trial of homeopathic Betula 30e. Br Homeopath J 2000;89:169-73.
148. Lewitt CT, Watkins AD, Hyland ME, et al. Use of ultramolecular potencies of allergen to treat asthmatic people allergic to house dust mite: double blind randomised controlled clinical trial. BMJ 2002;324:520.
149. White A, Slade P, Hunt C, Hart A, Ernst E. Individualised homeopathy as an adjunct in the treatment of childhood asthma: a randomised placebo controlled trial. Thorax 2003;58:317-21.
150. Brien S, Lewitt G, Bryant T. Ultramolecular homeopathy has no observable clinical effects. A randomized, double-blind, placebo-controlled proving trial of Belladonna 30C. Br J Clin Pharmacol 2003;56:562-8.
151. Taylor MA, Reilly D, Llewellyn-Jones RH, McSharry C, Aitchison TC. Randomised controlled trial of homoeopathy versus placebo in perennial allergic rhinitis with overview of four trial series. BMJ 2000;321:471-6.
152. Ernst E. Homeopathy: what does the "best" evidence tell us? Med J Aust 2010;192:458-60.
153. Linde K, Hondras M, Vickers A, ter Riet G, Melchart D. Systematic reviews of complementary therapies—an annotated bibliography. Part 3: homeopathy. BMC Complement Altern Med 2001;1:4.
154. Linde K, Jobst KA. Homeopathy for chronic asthma. Cochrane Database Syst Rev 2000;(2):CD000353.
155. Aimbire F, Ligeiro de Oliveira AP, Albertini R, et al. Low level laser therapy (LLLT) decreases pulmonary microvascular leakage, neutrophil influx and IL-1 beat levels in airway and lung from rat subjected to LPS-induced inflammation. Inflammation 2008;31:189-97.
156. Arnold E, Clark CE, Lasserson TJ, Wu T. Herbal interventions for chronic asthma in adults and children. Cochrane Database Syst Rev 2008;(1):CD005989.

Inappropriate Therapy

157. Levine SA, Reinhardt JH. Biochemical pathology initiated by free radicals, oxidant chemicals, and therapeutic drugs in the etiology of chemical hypersensitivity disease. Orthomol Psychiatry 1983;12:166-83.
158. Kershner J, Hawke W. Megavitamin therapy. J Nutr 1979;109:819-26.
159. Zuskin E, Lewis AJ, Bouhuys A. Inhibition of histamine-induced airway constriction by ascorbic acid. J Allergy Clin Immunol 1973;51:18-26.
160. Kreisman H, Mitchell C, Bouhuys A. Inhibition of histamine-induced airway constriction. Lung 1977;154:223-9.
161. Cockcroft DW, Killian DN, Mellon JJ, Hargreave FE. Protective effect of drugs on histamine-induced asthma. Thorax 1977;32:429-37.
162. Kordansky DW, Rosenthal RR, Norman PS. The effect of vitamin C on antigen-induced bronchospasm. J Allergy Clin Immunol 1979;63:61-4.
163. Paul GJ, Brehm JM, Alcorn JF, et al. Vitamin D and asthma. Am J Respir Crit Care Med 2012;185:124-32.
164. Terr AI. Environmental illness: a clinical review of 50 cases. Arch Intern Med 1986;146:145-9.
165. Sparks PJ, Simon GE, Katon WJ, et al. An outbreak of illness among aerospace workers. West J Med 1990;153:28-33.
166. Kahn E, Letz G. Clinical ecology: environmental medicine or unsubstantiated theory? Ann Intern Med 1989;111:104-6.
167. Terr AI. Clinical ecology in the workplace. J Occup Med 1989;31:257-61.
168. Nagy K, Berhes I, Kovacs T, et al. Study on endocrinological effects of radon speleotherapy on chronic respiratory diseases. Int J Radiat Biol 2009;85:281-90.
169. Beamon S, Falkenbach A, Fainburg G, Linde K. Speleotherapy for asthma. Cochrane Database Syst Rev 2001;(2):CD001741.
170. Gyorik SA, Brutsche MH. Complementary and alternative medicine for bronchial asthma: is there new evidence? Curr Opin Pulm Med 2004;10:37-43.

171. Bell IR. Clinical ecology: a new medical approach to environmental illness. Bolinas, Calif.: Common Knowledge Press; 1982.
172. Dickey LD, editor. Clinical ecology. Springfield, Ill.: Charles C Thomas; 1976.
173. Jaber R. Respiratory and allergic diseases: from upper respiratory tract infections to asthma. Prim Care 2002;29:231-61.
174. Ferguson A. Food sensitivity or self-deception? N Engl Med 1990;323:476-8.
175. Pearson DJ, Rix KJ, Bentley SJ. Food allergy: how much in the mind? A clinical and psychiatric study of patients with suspected food hypersensitivity. Lancet 1983;1:1259-61.
176. Pearson DJ. Food allergy, hypersensitivity and intolerance. J Ry Coll Physicians Lond 1985; 19:154-62.
177. Li XM. Treatment of asthma and food allergy with herbal interventions from traditional Chinese medicine. Mt Sinai J Med 2011; 78:697-716.
178. Cherniack EP. Bugs as drugs, part 1. Insects: the "new" alternative medicine for the 21st century? Altern Med Rev 2010;15:124-35.
179. Fisher RB. Bee venom and chronic inflammatory disease. N Z Med J 1986;99:639.
180. Li J, Ke T, He C, et al. The anti-arthritic effects of synthetic mellitin on the complete Freund's adjuvant-induced rheumatoid arthritis model in rats. Am J Chin Med 2010;38: 1039-49.
181. Branas P, Jordan R, Fry-Smith A, Burls A, Hyde C. Treatments for fatigue in multiple sclerosis: a rapid and systemic review. Health Technol Assess 2000;4:1-61.
182. Sel'tsovskii AP, Lazebnik LB, Vostikov GP, Nesterov AO. Apitherapy in gastroenterology. Eksp Klin Gastroenterol 2002;1:8-12.
183. Paunescu C. Apitherapy of chronic rhinopharyngolaryngitis and rhinosinusitis. Rev Chir Oncol Radiol O R L Oftalmol Stomatol Otorinolaringol 1982;27:137-42.
184. Beck BF. Bee venom therapy: bee venom, its nature, and its effect on arthritic and rheumatoid conditions. New York: Appleton-Century Company; 1935.
185. Cho HJ, Jeong YJ, Park KK, et al. Bee venom suppresses PMA-mediated MMP-9 gene activation via JNK/p38 and NK-kappa-B-dependent mechanisms. J Ethnopharmacol 2010;127:662-8.
186. Nah SS, Ha E, Mun SH, Won HJ, Chung JH. Effects of mellitin on the production of matrix metalloproteinase-1 and -3 in rheumatoid arthritic fibroblast-like synoviocytes. J Pharmacol Sci 2008;106:162-6.
187. Kim SJ, Park JH, Kim KH, et al. Bee vonom inhibits hepatic fibrosis through suppression of pro-fibrogenic cytokine expression. Am J Chin Med 2010;38:921-35.
188. Alqutub AN, Masoodi I, Alsayari K, Alomair A. Bee sting therapy-induced hepatotoxicity: a case report. World J Hepatol 2011;3:161-2.

Unconventional Theories of Allergic Disease

189. Crook WG. Nervous-system symptoms, emotional behavior, and learning problems: the allergic tension fatigue syndrome. In: Crook WG. Your allergic child. New York: Medcom Press; 1973.
190. Speer F. The allergic tension fatigue syndrome. Pediatr Clin North Am 1954;1:1029-37.
191. Randolph TG, Moss RW. An alternative approach to allergies. New York: Lippincott & Crowell; 1980.
192. Rea WJ. Environmentally triggered small vessel vasculitis. Ann Allergy 1977;38:245-51.
193. Rea WJ. Environmentally triggered cardiac disease. Ann Allergy 1978;40:243-51.
194. Cullen MR. The worker with multiple chemical hypersensitivities: an overview. State Art Rev Occup Med 1987;2:655-61.
195. Miller JB. Virus and hormone neutralization. In: Dickey LD, editor. Clinical ecology. Springfield, Ill.: Charles C Thomas, 1976; p. 597-605.
196. Levin AS, Byers VS. Environmental illness: a disorder of immune regulation. State Art Rev Occup Med 1987;2:669-81.
197. Stewart DE, Raskin J. Psychiatric assessment of patients with "20th-century disease" ("total allergy syndrome"). Can Med Assoc J 1985; 133:1001-6.
198. Green MA. 'Allergic to everything': 20th century syndrome. JAMA 1985;253:842.
199. Bell IR. A kinin model of mediation for food and chemical sensitivities: biobehavioral implications. Ann Allergy 1975;35:206-15.
200. International Program on Chemical Safety. Conclusions and recommendations of a workshop on multiple chemical sensitivities, Berlin, Germany, February 21-23. Reg Toxicol Pharmacol 1996;24:5188-9.
201. Brodsky CM. 'Allergic to everything': a medical subculture. Psychosomatics 1983;24:731.
202. Mabray CR, Burditt ML, Martin TL, et al. Treatment of common gynecologic-endocrinologic symptoms by allergy management procedures. Obstet Gynecol 1982;59:560.
203. Mandell M, Conte A. The role of allergy in arthritis, rheumatism, and polysymptomatic cerebral, visceral, and somatic disorders: a double-blind study. J Int Acad Preventive Med 1982;July 5-6.
204. Missal SC. Food allergy in ear, nose, and throat disease. Otolaryngol Clin North Am 1971;4: 479-90.
205. Missal SC. Allergy and the general otolaryngologist: the need for regional treatment. Otolaryngol Clin North Am 1974;7:681-702.
206. Monro JA. Food allergy in migraine. Proc Nutr Soc 1983;42:241-6.
207. Monro J, Carini C, Brostoff J. Migraine in an allergic disease. Lancet 1984;2:719-21.
208. O'Shea JA, Porter SF. Double-blind study of children with hyperkinetic syndrome treated with multi-allergen extract sublingually. J Learn Disabil 1981;14:189-91.
209. Simon GE, Katon WJ, Sparks PJ. Allergic to life: psychological factors in environmental illness. Am J Psychiatry 1990;147:901-6.
210. Brodsky CM. Psychological factors contributing to somatoform diseases attributed to the workplace: the case of intoxication. J Occup Med 1983;25:459-64.
211. Terr AI. Clinical ecology [editorial]. Allergy Clin Immunol 1987;79:423-6.
212. Terr AI. 'Multiple chemical sensitivities': immunologic critique of clinical ecology theories and practice. State Art Rev Occup Med 1987;3:683-94.
213. California Medical Association Scientific Task Force on Clinical Ecology. Clinical ecology: a critical appraisal. West J Med 1986;144:239-45.
214. Rea WJ, Bell IR, Suits CW, Smiley RE. Food and chemical susceptibility after environmental chemical overexposure: case histories. Ann Allergy 1978;41:101-9.
215. McGovern JJ Jr, Lazaroni JA, Hicks MF, Adler JC, Cleary P. Food and chemical sensitivity: clinical and immunologic correlates. Arch Otolaryngol 1983;109:292-7.
216. McGovern JJ, Lazaroni JA, Saifer P, et al. Clinical evaluation of the major plasma and cellular measures of immunity. J Orthomol Psychiat 1983;12:60-71.
217. Ashford NA, Miller CS. Clinical exposures. New York: Van Nostrand Reinhold; 1991.
218. Bell IR, Bootzin RR, Davis TP, et al. Time-dependent sensitization of plasma beta-endorphin in community elderly with self-reported environmental chemical odor intolerance. Biol Psychiatry 1996;40:134-43.
219. Miller CS. Possible models for multiple chemical sensitivity: conceptual issues and role of the limbic system. Toxicol Ind Health 1992;8: 181-202.
220. Rossi J III. Sensitization induced by kindling and kindling-related phenomena as a model for multiple chemical sensitivity. Toxicology 1996;111:87-100.
221. Bell IR, Miller CS, Schwartz GE. An olfactory-limbic model of multiple chemical sensitivity syndrome: possible relationships to kindling and affective spectrum disorders. Biol Psychiatry 1992;32:218-42.
222. Meggs WJ. Neurogenic switching: a hypothesis for a mechanism for shifting the site of inflammation in allergy and chemical sensitivity. Environ Health Perspect 1995;103: 54-6.
223. Dory RL. Olfaction and multiple chemical sensitivity. Toxicol Ind Health 1994;10: 359-68.
224. Meggs WJ, Cleveland CH Jr. Rhinolaryngoscopic examination of patients with the multiple chemical sensitivity syndrome. Arch Environ Health 1993;48:14.
225. Bascom R. Multiple chemical sensitivity: a respiratory disorder? Toxicol Ind Health 1992;8:221-8.
226. Meggs WJ. Multiple chemical sensitivities—chemical sensitivity as a symptom of airway inflammation. J Toxicol Clin Toxicol 1995;33: 107-10.
227. Cohn JR. Multiple chemical sensitivity or multi-organ dysesthesias? [editorial]. J Allergy Clin Immunol 1994;93:953-4.
228. Hahn M, Bonkovsky HL. Multiple chemical sensitivity syndrome and porphyria: a note of caution and concern. Arch Intern Med 1997;157:281-6.
229. Finn R, Battcock TM. A critical study of clinical ecology. Practitioner 1985;229:883-5.
230. Black DW, Rathe A, Goldstein RB. Environmental illness: a controlled clinical trial of 26 subjects with '20th century disease.' JAMA 1990;264:3166-70.
231. Diagnostic and statistical manual of mental disorders. 4th ed. Washington, D.C.: American Psychiatric Association; 1994.
232. Caccappolo-van Vliet E, Kelly-McNeil K, Natelson B, Kipen H, Fiedler N. Anxiety sensitivity and depression in multiple chemical sensitivities and asthma. J Occup Environ Med 2002;44:890-901.
233. Black DW, Okiishi C, Schlosser S. A nine-year follow-up of people diagnosed with multiple chemical sensitivities. Psychosomatics 2000;41: 253-61.
234. Schottenfeld RS, Cullen MR. Occupation-induced posttraumatic stress disorder. Am J Psychiatry 1985;142:198.
235. Friedman MJ. Neurobiological sensitization models of post-traumatic stress disorder: their possible relevance to multiple chemical sensitivity syndrome. Toxicol Ind Health 1994;10: 449-62.

236. Spyker DA. Multiple chemical sensitivities: syndrome and solution. J Toxicol Clin Toxicol 1995;33:95-9.
237. Guglielmi RS, Cox DJ, Spyker DA. Behavioral treatment of phobic avoidance multiple chemical sensitivity. J Behav Ther Exp Psychiatry 1994;25:197-209.
238. Kurt TL. Multiple chemical sensitivities: a syndrome of pseudotoxicity manifest as exposure perceived symptoms. J Toxicol Clin Toxicol 1995;33:101-5.
239. Staudenmayer H, Selner ME, Selner J. Adult sequelae of childhood abuse presenting as environmental illness. Ann Allergy 1993;71: 538-46.
240. Lipson JG. Multiple chemical sensitivities: stigma and social experiences. Med Anthropol Q 2004;18:200-13.
241. Staudenmayer H, Selner JC. Failure to assess psychopathology in patients presenting with chemical sensitivities. J Occup Environ Med 1995;37:704-9.
242. Goodman M. Illness as lifestyle. Can Fam Physician 1995;41:267-70.
243. American Academy of Allergy, Asthma and Immunology Board of Directors. Position statement: idiopathic environmental intolerances. J Allergy Clin Immunol 1999;103:36.
244. Moorhead JF, Smuda AJ. Occipital lobe meningioma in a patient with multiple chemical sensitivities. Am J Ind Med 2000;37:443-6.
245. Truss CO. Tissue injury induced by *Candida albicans*: mental and neurologic manifestations. J Orthomol Psychiatry 1978;7:17.
246. Truss CO. The role of *Candida albicans* in human illness. J Orthomol Psychiatry 1981; 10:228.
247. Truss CO. Metabolic abnormalities in patients with chronic candidiasis: the acetaldehyde hypothesis. J Orthomol Psychiat 1984;13:66.
248. Truss CO. The missing diagnosis. 2nd ed. Birmingham, Ala.: C. O. Truss; 1986.
249. Emmons CW, Binford CH, Utz JP, et al. Medical mycology. 3rd ed. Philadelphia: Lea & Febiger; 1977.
250. Edwards JE Jr, Lehrer RI, Stiehm ER, Fischer TJ, Young LS. Severe candidal infections: clinical perspective, immune defense mechanisms and current concepts of therapy. Ann Intern Med 1978;89:91-106.
251. Roberto RL, Stiehm ER. Phagocytic dysfunction diseases. In: Parslow TG, Stites DP, Terr AI, Imboden JB, editors. Human immunology. 10th ed. New York: Lange Medical Books; 2001.
252. Kirkpatrick CH, Sohnle PC. Chronic mucocutaneous candidiasis. In: Safai B, Good RA, editors. Immunodermatology. New York: Plenum Press; 1981.
253. Haas A, Stiehm ER. The 'yeast connection' meets chronic mucocutaneous candidiasis. [letter]. N Engl J Med 1986;314:854-5.
254. Dismukes WE, Wade JS, Lee JY, Dockery BK, Hain JD. A randomized, double-blind trial of nystatin therapy for the candidiasis hypersensitivity syndrome. N Engl J Med 1990;323: 1717-23.
255. Bennett JE. Searching for the yeast connection. N Engl J Med 1990;323:1766-7.
256. Feingold BF. Why your child is hyperactive. New York: Random House; 1975.
257. Lockey SD. Allergic reactions due to F D and C Yellow No. 5, tartrazine, an aniline dye used as a coloring and identifying agent in various steroids. Ann Allergy 1959;17:719-21.
258. Chafee FH, Settipane GA. Asthma caused by FD&C approved dyes. J Allergy 1967;40: 65-72.
259. South MA. The so-called "salicylate-free diet." Cutis 1976;18:183.
260. South MA. The so-called salicylate-free diet: part II. Cutis 1976;18:332, 339.
261. South MA. The so-called salicylate-free diet: part III. Cutis 1977;19:23, 35.
262. Conners CK, Goyette CH, Southwick DA, Lees JM, Andrulonis PA. Food additives and hyperkinesis: a controlled double-blind experiment. Pediatrics 1976;58:154-66.
263. Williams JI, Grain DM, Taussig FT, Webster E. Relative effects of drugs and diet on hyperkinetic behaviors: an experimental study. Pediatrics 1978;61:811-7.
264. Werry JS. Food additives and hyperactivity. Med J Aust 1976;2:281-2.
265. Swanson JM, Kinsbourne M. Food dyes impair performance of hyperactive children on a laboratory learning test. Science 1980;207:1485-7.
266. National Institutes of Health Consensus Development Panel. Defined diets in childhood hyperactivity. Bethesda, Md.: Office of Medical Applications for Research; 1982.
267. Consensus Conference. Defined diets and childhood hyperactivity. JAMA 1982;248: 290-2.

Remote Practice of Allergy

268. American Academy of Allergy, Asthma and Immunology. Position statement: the remote practice of allergy. J Allergy Clin Immunol 1986;77:651-2.

102 Complementary and Alternative Medicine

RENATA J.M. ENGLER | XIU-MIN LI

CONTENTS

SUMMARY OF IMPORTANT CONCEPTS

» Complementary and alternative medicine (CAM) comprises medical practices that are used to augment (complementary) or replace (alternative) allopathic or conventional medicine.
» Representing most of the global health care services, CAM therapies use natural products, mind-body techniques, mechanical body-based practices, and other methods to enhance wellness and healing.
» With a shift to evidence-based and personalized medicine, integrative medicine focuses on combining CAM and conventional medicine approaches when the evidence for safety and efficacy exists and outcomes support use.
» The 2007 U.S. National Health Interview Survey identified many CAM therapies (other than vitamins and minerals) commonly used by adults (e.g., natural products, breathing exercises) and children (e.g., herbals, chiropractic or osteopathic manipulation).
» CAM use by the U.S. population (4 of 10 adults, 1 of 9 children) accounts for 11.2% of the total out-of-pocket expenditures on health care ($33.9 billion in 2007).
» Use of CAM therapies and practitioners requires consideration of safety, efficacy, disease or drug interactions, and optimization of personalized medicine in the context of medical evidence-based practice and legal issues.

Background

Conventional, allopathic, or Western medicine (i.e., mainstream medicine, orthodox medicine, regular medicine, or biomedicine) includes health care delivered by licensed physicians or doctors of osteopathy, other providers (e.g., nurse practitioners, physician assistants), and allied health professionals (e.g., physical therapists, psychologists, registered nurses).[1] On a global basis, conventional medicine represents less than one half of available medical care delivery systems. Table 102-1 describes the complementary and alternative medicine (CAM) practitioners and therapies that were included in the 2007 National Health Interview Survey (NHIS). The selected listings represent the four major categories of CAM modalities: alternative medical systems with various forms of licensing for competency (e.g., acupuncture, Ayurveda, homeopathy, naturopathy); biologically based therapies (e.g., chelation therapy, natural products such as herbal and nutritional supplements); manipulation and body-based therapies (e.g., chiropractic and osteopathic manipulation, massage, movement therapies); and mind-body therapies (e.g., biofeedback, meditation, guided imagery, progressive relaxation, deep-breathing exercises, hypnosis, yoga). CAM use by the U.S. population represents 11.2% of their total out-of-pocket expenditures on health care ($33.9 billion in 2007).[2]

The use of CAM therapies presents major challenges for optimizing the quality of care and ensuring efficacy and safety when combined into complex care plans.[3] Table 102-2 details the frequencies and age-adjusted percentages of CAM use for children and adults by therapeutic modality. Among the most commonly used modalities are natural products (by 17.7% of adults and 3.9% of children), which constitute a vast array of nonvitamin, nonmineral herbals and supplements.[1] Dietary supplement use, including vitamins and minerals, is increasing. Multivitamins and multiminerals, particularly calcium and vitamin D, are the most commonly used supplements.[4] Approximately 34% of children (<18 years old) used vitamin and mineral supplements in the month before the survey, with underweight children reporting greater intake.[5]

A search of the peer-reviewed medical literature on PubMed with the English terms *complementary medicine*, *alternative medicine*, *integrative medicine*, or *complementary and alternative medicine* resulted in more than 190,000 citations, more than 80% of which were published between January 1990 and December 2011. According to the 2007 NHIS,[1] approximately 4 of every 10 U.S. adults use CAM. Use varies by age group (highest among those 60 to 69 years old), sex (females more than males), and race (highest among Alaska Natives or American Indians at 50.3%, followed by whites, Asians, blacks, and Hispanics).[1] Figure 102-1 details the frequencies and age-adjusted percentages of CAM use by adults and children. Children with parents or other relatives who use CAM therapies were almost five times more likely (23.9%) to use CAM than children whose parents did not use CAM (5.1%).[1]

With widespread access to and globalization of CAM therapies by the Internet, there is a growing need for education and reliable information about CAM therapies to avoid unnecessary harm and to balance benefits with risks, particularly in the context of an individual patient's disease and medical history.[6] CAM therapies are commonly used in low- and middle-income

TABLE 102-1 Complementary and Alternative Medicine Practitioners, Practices, and Therapies

Therapy	Description of Medical Practice or Therapy
PRACTITIONER REQUIRED	
Acupuncture	Procedures involve stimulation of anatomic points on the body by several techniques. American acupuncture incorporates medical traditions from China, Japan, Korea, and other countries. Classic acupuncture uses fine needles to penetrate the skin with manual or electrical stimulation, but newer approaches use direct cutaneous stimulation without a needle.
Ayurveda	Originating in India, the system of medicine focuses on prevention and treatment of health problems through integration and balance of body, mind, and spirit (i.e., holistic approach). Proposed treatments aim to cleanse the body of substances that cause disease, helping to reestablish harmony and balance.
Biofeedback	Simple electronic devices are used to teach clients how to consciously regulate body functions such as breathing, heart rate, and blood pressure to improve health and well-being. Applications include stress reduction, headache elimination, reconditioning of injured muscles, pain relief, and control of asthma attacks.
Chelation therapy	A chemical is used to bind molecules of a substance (e.g., metals, minerals) and remove them from the body. In conventional medicine, the process is used to remove toxic metals such as lead, and in complementary and alternative medicine, it is used to treat conditions such as cardiovascular and cerebrovascular disease.
Chiropractic manipulation	Adjustment of the spine and joints influences the body's nervous system and natural defense mechanisms to alleviate pain and improve general health. Chiropractic care is a form of health care that focuses on the relationship between the body's structure, primarily the spine, and function.
Osteopathic manipulation	Like doctors of chiropractic medicine, osteopathic physicians also use hands-on therapy (i.e., manipulation or adjustment) as their core clinical procedure. Osteopathic manipulation is a full-body system of hands-on techniques to alleviate pain, restore function, and promote health and well-being.
Energy healing therapy, Reiki	Reiki is an energy medicine practice that originated in Japan. The practitioner places his hands on or near the person receiving the treatment with the intent of transmitting *ki*, which is thought to be life-force energy.
Hypnosis	Induction of an altered state of consciousness is characterized by increased responsiveness to suggestion. The hypnotic state is attained by first relaxing the body and then shifting attention to a narrow range of objects or ideas suggested by the hypnotherapist or hypnotist. The procedure is used to effect positive changes and to treat conditions such as chronic pain, respiratory ailments, stress, and headache.
Massage	Massage therapists manipulate muscle and connective tissue to enhance the function of those tissues and promote relaxation and well-being.
Naturopathy	An alternative medical system, naturopathic medicine proposes that there is a healing power in the body that establishes, maintains, and restores health. Practitioners work with patients toward a goal of supporting this power through the use of nutrition and lifestyle counseling, dietary supplements, medicinal plants, exercise, homeopathy, and treatments from traditional Chinese medicine.
Traditional healing	Traditional healers employ ancient medical practices that are based on indigenous theories, beliefs, and experiences handed down through generations. Their methods reflect different philosophical backgrounds, cultural origins, and regional natural products adapted to healing.
Traditional Chinese medicine	Traditional Chinese medicine is the current name for a comprehensive, ancient system of health care from China that is based on the concept of a vital energy or life force, called *qi* or *chi*, that is flows throughout the body along channels known as *meridians*, regulating a person's spiritual, emotional, mental, and physical balance. This energy is influenced by the opposing forces of *yin* (negative energy) and *yang* (positive energy). Disease is thought to result from the disrupted flow of qi and imbalanced yin and yang. The focus is on the notion of harmony and balance, including ideas of moderation and prevention. It incorporates herbal (complex mixtures) and nutritional therapy, restorative physical exercises, meditation, acupuncture, and remedial massage.
PRACTITIONER NOT REQUIRED	
Deep-breathing exercises	Slow and deep inhalation through the nose, usually to a count of 10, is followed by slow and complete exhalation for a similar count. The process may be repeated 5 to 10 times for several times each day.
Diet-based therapies	These dietary practices are designed to promote health and wellness, and they have various degrees of evidence for efficacy and safety. The high-fiber, low-fat, vegetarian Ornish diet promotes weight loss and health by controlling what is eaten rather than counting calories. The South Beach diet distinguishes between good and bad carbohydrates, promoting low glycemic index foods and enhanced intake of vegetables and whole grains (without counting calories). The Atkins diet emphasizes a drastic reduction in daily intake of carbohydrates ($\leq$40 g) coupled with an increase in protein and fat. Others special approaches include the macrobiotic and Zone diets.
Guided imagery	A series of relaxation techniques is followed by visualization of detailed, usually peaceful images. If used for treatment, the individual visualizes his or her body free of the specific problem or condition. Sessions are usually 20 to 30 min long and practiced several times each week.
Homeopathic treatment	Homeopathy is a system of medical practices based on the theory that any substance that can produce disease symptoms in a healthy person can cure those symptoms in a sick person. For example, someone with insomnia may be given a homeopathic dose of coffee. Administered in diluted form, homeopathic remedies are derived from many natural sources, including plants, metals, and minerals. Toxic metals such as arsenic are diluted to a point at which the concentration is almost undetectable.
Meditation	Most of these techniques started in Eastern religious or spiritual traditions. During meditation, a person learns to focus his or her attention and suspend the stream of thoughts that normally occupy the mind. This practice is thought to result in a state of greater physical relaxation, mental calmness, and psychological balance. Practicing meditation can change how a person responds to the flow of emotions and thoughts in the mind.

Continued

TABLE 102-1 Complementary and Alternative Medicine Practitioners, Practices, and Therapies—cont'd

Therapy	Description of Medical Practice or Therapy
Movement therapies	Motion therapies and exercises are designed to promote health and well-being. Alexander technique teaches how to use muscles more efficiently to improve posture and overall function. It is used for low back pain and symptoms of Parkinson disease.
Natural products	Supplemental dietary ingredients other than vitamins and minerals include single ingredients or mixtures of herbal and botanical products (e.g., soy, flax seeds), enzymes, and glandular extracts. Among the most popular are echinacea, ginkgo biloba, ginseng, feverfew, garlic, kava kava, and saw palmetto.
Progressive relaxation	Tension and stress are relieved by systematically contracting and relaxing successive muscle groups.
Qi gong	The ancient Chinese discipline combines gentle physical movements, mental focus, and deep breathing directed toward specific parts of the body. Performed in repetitions, the exercises are normally performed alone or in a group for two or more times per week for 30 minutes each time.
Tai chi	The mind-body practice originated in China as a martial art. Tai chi involves slow, gentle, and controlled body movements while breathing deeply and meditating. Also known as *moving meditation*, tai chi is believed to help the flow throughout the body of a proposed vital energy called *qi*. The relaxed and graceful series of movements are done in sets called *forms* or *routines*, which are performed alone or in a group.
Yoga	Breathing exercises, physical postures, and meditation are combined to calm the nervous system and balance body, mind, and spirit. Sessions usually are 45 minutes long and are conducted one or more times each week alone or in a group.

Data from Barnes PM, Bloom B, Nahin RL. Complementary and alternative medicine use among adults and children: United States, 2007. Natl Health Stat Report 2008;12:1-24 Available at http://nccam.nih.gov/sites/nccam.nih.gov/files/news/nhsr12.pdf (accessed June 2, 2013); MedicineNet. Definitions of traditional Chinese medicine. Available at http://www.medterms.com/script/main/art.asp?articlekey=33520 (accessed June 1, 2014); Medical Free Dictionary. Traditional Chinese Medicine definition. Available at http://medical-dictionary.thefreedictionary.com/traditional+Chinese+medicine (accessed June 1, 2013); and the National Cancer Institute. NCI dictionary of cancer terms. Available at http://www.cancer.gov/dictionary?cdrid=449722 (accessed June 1, 2013).

TABLE 102-2 Frequencies and Age-Adjusted Percentages for U.S. Adults and Children Who Used Complementary and Alternative Medicine in 2007

Therapy	Adults (≥18 yr) *n* × 1000 (%, SE)*	Children (<18 yr) *n* × 1000 (%, SE)*
ALTERNATIVE MEDICAL SYSTEMS		
Acupuncture	3,141 (1.4%, 0.10)	150 (0.2%, 0.05)
Ayurveda	214 (†0.1%, 0.03)	79 (†0.1%, 0.04)
Homeopathic treatment	3,909 (1.8%, 0.11)	907 (1.3%, 0.22)
Naturopathy	729 (0.3%, 0.04)	237 (0.3%, 0.09)
Traditional healers	812 (0.4%, 0.06)	767 (1.1%, 0.18)
BIOLOGICALLY BASED THERAPIES		
Chelation therapy	111 (†0.0%, 0.02)	72 (0.1%, 0.04)
Natural products‡	38,797 (17.7%, 0.37)	2,850 (3.9%, 0.32)
Diet-based therapies§	7,893 (3.6%, 0.15)	565 (0.8%, 0.11)
MANIPULATION AND BODY-BASED THERAPIES		
Chiropractic or osteopathic manipulation	18,740 (8.6%, 0.27)	2,020 (2.8%, 0.25)
Massage	18,068 (8.3%, 0.23)	743 (1.0%, 0.13)
Movement therapies¶	3,146 (1.5%, 0.10)	299 (0.4%, 0.09)
MIND-BODY THERAPIES		
Biofeedback	362 (0.2%, 0.04)	119 (0.2%, 0.05)
Meditation	20,541 (9.4%, 0.27)	725 (1.0%, 0.12)
Guided imagery	4,866 (2.2%, 0.16)	293 (0.4%, 0.09)
Progressive relaxation	6,454 (2.9%, 0.15)	329 (0.5%, 0.09)
Deep-breathing exercises	27,794 (12.7%, 0.30	1,558 (2.2%, 0.22)
Hypnosis	561 (0.2%, 0.04)	67 (†0.1%, 0.04)
Yoga	13,172 (6.1%, 0.21)	1,505 (2.1%, 0.18)
Tai chi	2,267 (1.0%, 0.08)	113 (†0.2%, 0.05)
Qi gong	625 (0.3%, 0.04)	50 (—)
Energy healing therapy, Reiki	1,216 (0.5%, 0.06)	161 (0.2%, 0.05)

Data from Barnes PM, Bloom B, Nahin RL. Complementary and alternative medicine use among adults and children: United States, 2007. Natl Health Stat Report 2008;12:1-24. Available at http://nccam.nih.gov/sites/nccam.nih.gov/files/news/nhsr12.pdf (accessed June 2, 2013).

*Numbers for adults or children should be multiplied by 1000, and percentages of the total and standard errors (SE) are given parenthetically.

†Estimates preceded by a dagger have a relative standard error of greater than 30% and less than or equal to 50% and therefore do not meet the standard of reliability or precision.

‡Nonvitamin and nonmineral.

§Diets: vegetarian, macrolide, Atkins, Pritikin, Ornish, Zone, South Beach.

¶Movement therapies: Feldenkrais, Alexander technique, Pilates, Trager psychophysical integration.

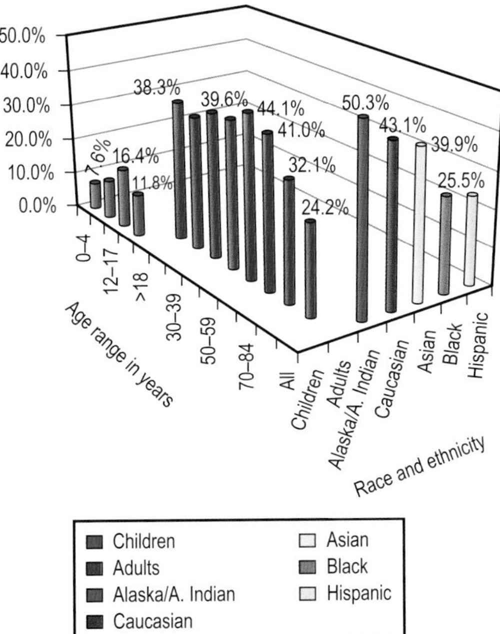

Figure 102-1 Rates of complementary and alternative medicine use in 2007. *(Adapted from National Center for Complementary and Alternative Medicine [NCCAM]: Statistics on Complementary and Alternative Medicine National Health Interview Survey. Available at http://nncam.nih.gov/news/camstats/NHIS.htm [accessed July 12, 2013].)*

countries because they are affordable and available. International surveys of CAM consumption among patients with allergies reported prevalence rates ranging from 18% to 65%.[6-11] In the 2007 NHIS, asthma, sinusitis, and other allergic disorders were ranked among the top 10 conditions treated with CAM for children younger than 18 years of age.[1] Studies of people with allergies show that CAM users usually are younger, are female, and have a higher level of education than those who do not use CAM.[9] Patients with allergies who seek out CAM treatments tend to have a better quality of life, are dissatisfied with conventional medications, have a perception of fewer side effects with CAM, and are influenced by social networks.[12,13] Few patients with allergies inform their physicians about the use of CAM.[8,10,14,15]

Natural (nonvitamin, nonmineral) products vary widely. Table 102-3 list products commonly used by adults and children as identified in the 2007 NHIS. This listing is a fraction of the more than 60,000 commercially available products on the open market and described in the Natural Medicines Comprehensive Database (naturaldatabase.therapeuticresearch.com). Table 102-4 outlines the top common medical conditions of adults and children that are associated with higher frequencies of CAM use.

Economic evaluations of complementary medicine that incorporate differences in health care systems, including estimates of cost-effectiveness and net health benefits, are needed.[16] Among those with chronic diseases such as asthma, a better understanding of CAM use patterns in subpopulations may improve provider recognition and management. In a study of behavioral risk factors for adult patients with asthma from 37 states and the District of Columbia, 56.6% of those with work-related asthma used CAM, compared with 27.9% of those who had non–work-related asthma.[17] Higher CAM use was associated with a greater likelihood of adverse asthma attacks in the preceding month, more emergency department visits and overnight hospital stays, and poorly controlled asthma.[17]

In counseling patients about CAM therapies, providers should use an evidence-based approach that considers the relevance and validity of the available literature on efficacy and safety. The Natural Medicines Comprehensive Database (NMCD), with independent health professional reviewers, has developed a level of evidence ranking as part of its editorial principles and processes, and it is incorporated in educational resources for consumers, patients, and medical professionals.[3] The categories for safety and efficacy (as tools for balanced risk-benefit communication) are detailed in Tables 102-5 and 102-6. The National Institutes of Health (NIH) Center for Complementary and Alternative Medicine (NCCAM) offers an online guide to common herbs that was adapted from the NMCD approach.[18]

The U.S. Food and Drug Administration (FDA) regulates herbal and other over-the-counter dietary supplements differently from conventional medicines. It has less oversight of good manufacturing practices and fewer evidence standards related to safety and efficacy. The standards for supplements are found in the Dietary Supplement Health and Education Act (DSHEA), a federal law that defines dietary supplements and sets product-labeling standards and health claim limits.[19] It continues to be a daunting task for conventional providers to incorporate the expanding information about CAM into patient management. Table 102-7 outlines a published approach to addressing and documenting CAM use in the context of a medical visit, along with consideration of medicolegal issues.[3]

Allergic rhinitis is commonly treated with antihistamines, decongestants, topical corticosteroids, mast cell stabilizers, leukotriene inhibitors, and immunotherapy. Within the NMCD, a March 2012 search for herbal and supplements used for allergic rhinitis identified 43 ingredients (in thousands of combination trade name products) marketed to the public for treating allergic rhinitis.[20] Commonly advertised product ingredients and their presumed mechanism of action are detailed in Table 102-8. The NMCD efficacy rating system (see Table 102-6) has listed the following products as *possibly effective* for allergic rhinitis: butterbur, milk thistle, nasal irrigation, *Phleum pratense* (Timothy grass), pycnogenol, thymus extract, and *Tinospora cordifolia* (an herbaceous vine). As of June 2012, no ingredients were listed with a rating of *likely effective* or *effective.*

An NMCD search in January 2012 identified 171 potential natural ingredients or practices marketed to the public for use in asthma.[21] Commonly used agents are detailed in Table 102-9. Using the NMCD efficacy rating system (see Table 102-6) within the database, the following products were listed as *possibly effective* for asthma: β-carotene (for exercise-induced asthma), caffeine, choline, fish oil, magnesium, pycnogenol, and thymus extract. As of June 2012, none of the ingredients in the database was listed with a rating of *likely effective* or *effective* for asthma.

Alternative therapies such as acupuncture, chiropractic manipulation, yoga, and movement therapies (e.g., Alexander technique) are advertised as potential asthma therapies. If all CAM modalities are considered, up to 89% of persons with asthma use some form of alternative medicine, and one fourth use herbal or natural medicine.[22] In a 2010 review of cases in which asthma was considered unresponsive to usual care, the following additional CAM therapeutic options were listed[23]: homeopathy, chiropractic care, acupuncture, hypnosis and

Text continued on page 1645

TABLE 102-3 Frequencies and Age-Adjusted Percentages for U.S. Adults and Children Who Used Nonvitamin, Nonmineral Natural Products during a 30-Day Period in 2007

Nonvitamin, Nonmineral Natural Products*	Adults (≥18 yr) n × 1000 (%, SE)[†]	Children (<18 yr) n × 1000 (%, SE)[†]
Omega-3 fatty acids (fish oil, DHA)	10,923 (37.4%, 1.13)	441 (30.5%, 4.88)
Echinacea	4,848 (19.8%, 1.01)	524 (37.2%, 4.94)
Flaxseed oil or pills	4,416 (15.9%, 0.87)	233 (16.7%, 4.85)
Ginseng	3,345 (14.1%, 0.87)	19 (‡)
Combination herb pill	3,446 (13.0%, 0.83)	296 (17.9%, 3.94)
Ginkgo biloba	2,977 (11.3%, 0.88)	24[‡]
Soy supplements or isoflavones	1,363 (5.0%, 0.53)	15[‡]
Cranberry (pills, gelatin capsules)	1,560 (6.0%, 0.63)	33 (§1.8%, 0.83)
Garlic supplements	3,278 (11.0%, 0.66)	84 (§5.9%, 1.85)
Melatonin	1,296 (4.6%, 0.48)	92 (§5.8%, 2.02)
Fiber or psyllium	1,791 (6.6%, 0.61)	33[‡]
Glucosamine	6,132 (19.9%, 0.91)	
Chondroitin	3,390 (11.2%, 0.82)	
Coenzyme Q-10	2,691 (8.7%, 0.60)	
Green tea pills	1,528 (6.3%, 0.65)	
Saw palmetto	1,682 (5.1%, 0.46)	
Grape seed extract	1,214 (4.3%, 0.43)	
Methylsulfonylmethane (MSM)	1,312 (4.1%, 0.37)	
Milk thistle	1,001 (3.7%, 0.49)	
Lutein	1,047 (3.4%, 0.38)	
Prebiotics or probiotics		199 (§13.6%, 4.49)
Goldenseal		143 (§8.6%, 3.83)
Creatine		24[‡]
Dehydroepiandrosterone (DHEA)		15[‡]

Data from Barnes PM, Bloom B, Nahin RL. Complementary and alternative medicine use among adults and children: United States, 2007. Natl Health Stat Report 2008;12:1-24. Available at http://nccam.nih.gov/sites/nccam.nih.gov/files/news/nhsr12.pdf (accessed June 2, 2013).

*Respondents might have used more than one nonvitamin, nonmineral natural product.

†Numbers for adults or children should be multiplied by 1000, and percentages of the total and standard errors (SE) are given parenthetically. The denominator used in the calculation of percentages was the number of adults or children who used nonvitamin, nonmineral, natural products within the past 30 days, excluding persons without usable information. Estimates are based on household interviews of a sample of the civilian, noninstitutionalized population.

‡Estimates with a relative standard error greater than 50% are indicated with a double dagger but are not shown.

§Estimates preceded by a section mark have a relative standard error of greater than 30% and less than or equal to 50% and do not meet the standard of reliability or precision.

TABLE 102-4 Frequencies and Age-Adjusted Percentages for U.S. Adults and Children Who Used Complementary and Alternative Medicine for Various Conditions in 2007

Condition for Which Alternative Medicine Was Used	Adults (≥18 yr) n × 1000 (%, SE)*	Children (<18 yr) n × 1000 (%, SE)*
Back pain or problem	14,325 (17.1%, 0.54)	705 (6.7%, 0.87)[†]
Neck pain or problem	5,031 (5.9%, 0.33)	
Insomnia or trouble sleeping	1,191 (1.4%, 0.16)	158 (1.8%, 0.50)
Head or chest cold	1,693 (2.0%, 0.17)	515 (6.6%, 1.24)
Depression	962 (1.2%, 0.16)	110 (1.0%, 0.27)
Anxiety	2,293 (2.8%, 0.23)	427 (4.8%, 0.87)[‡]
Stress	1,124 (1.3%, 0.15)	
Arthritis	3,057 (3.5%, 0.23)	
Joint pain or stiffness	4,537 (5.2%, 0.27)	
Sprain or strain	605 (0.7%, 0.10)	
Fibromyalgia	755 (0.8%, 0.11)	

TABLE 102-4 Frequencies and Age-Adjusted Percentages for U.S. Adults and Children Who Used Complementary and Alternative Medicine for Various Conditions in 2007—cont'd

Condition for Which Alternative Medicine Was Used	Adults (≥18 yr) n × 1000 (%, SE)*	Children (<18 yr) n × 1000 (%, SE)*
Other musculoskeletal	1,498 (1.8%, 0.19)	378 (4.2%, 0.83)
Stomach or intestinal illness	974 (1.2%, 0.14)	75 (§0.8%, 0.30)‖
Severe headache or migraine	1,359 (1.6%, 0.16)	
Regular headaches	813 (1.0%, 0.15)	
Cholesterol	1,827 (2.1%, 0.17)	
Hypertension	842 (0.9%, 0.12)	
Coronary heart disease	586 (0.7%, 0.10)	
Diabetes	650 (0.7%, 0.12)	
Attention deficit hyperactivity disorder		237 (2.5%, 0.54)
Influenza or pneumonia		123¶
Sore throat other than strep or tonsillitis		97 (§1.1%, 0.43)
Asthma		137 (§1.6%, 0.49)
Sinusitis		117 (§1.5%, 0.62)
Respiratory allergy		95 (§1.3%, 0.62)
Other allergies		114 (§1.4%, 0.46)
Other conditions	2,733 (3.3%, 0.23)	625 (8.3%, 1.14)

Data from Barnes PM, Bloom B, Nahin RL. Complementary and alternative medicine use among adults and children: United States, 2007. Natl Health Stat Report 2008;12:1-24. Available at http://nccam.nih.gov/sites/nccam.nih.gov/files/news/nhsr12.pdf (accessed June 2, 2013).

*Numbers for adults or children should be multiplied by 1000, and percentages of the total and standard errors (SE) are given parenthetically.

†Combined figure for back and neck pain.

‡Combined figure for anxiety and stress.

§Estimates preceded by a section mark have a relative standard error of greater than 30% and less than or equal to 50% and do not meet the standard of reliability or precision.

‖For abdominal pain only.

¶Estimates with a relative standard error greater than 50% are indicated with a paragraph symbol but are not shown.

TABLE 102-5 Criteria for Evidence-Based Safety Ratings

Rating	Definition	Criteria for the Rating
Likely safe	Very high level of reliable clinical evidence shows it is safe when used appropriately. Products rated likely safe are generally considered appropriate to recommend.	Safety data are available from two or more randomized clinical trials, a meta-analysis, or large-scale postmarketing surveillance that includes several hundred patients (level of evidence = A),* or the product has undergone a safety review consistent with or equivalent to passing a review by the U.S. Food and Drug Administration (FDA), Health Canada, or a similarly rigorous approval process. Studies have a low risk of bias and a high level of validity by meeting stringent assessment criteria (quality rating = A).† Studies adequately measure and report safety and adverse outcomes data and consistently show no significant serious adverse effects without valid evidence to the contrary.
Possibly safe	Some clinical evidence shows it is safe when used appropriately; however, the evidence is limited by quantity, quality, or contradictory findings. Products rated possibly safe appear to be safe but do not have enough high-quality evidence to recommend for most people.	Safety data are available from one or more randomized clinical trials, a meta-analysis (level of evidence = A or B), case series, two or more population-based or epidemiologic studies (level of evidence = B), or limited postmarketing surveillance data. Studies have a low to moderate risk of bias and moderate to high level of validity by meeting or partially meeting assessment criteria (quality rating = A or B). Studies adequately measure and report safety and adverse outcomes data and show no significant serious adverse effects without substantial evidence to the contrary. Some contrary evidence may exist; however, valid evidence supporting safety outweighs contrary evidence.
Possibly unsafe	Some clinical evidence shows safety concerns or significant adverse outcomes; however, the evidence is limited by quantity, quality, or contradictory findings. People should be advised not to take products with a possibly unsafe rating.	Safety data are available from one or more randomized clinical trials, meta-analysis (level of evidence = A or B), two or more population-based or epidemiologic studies (level of evidence = B), or limited postmarketing surveillance data, or multiple, reliable case reports show a potential causal relationship between a product and serious adverse outcome. Studies have a low to moderate risk of bias and moderate to high level of validity by meeting or partially meeting assessment criteria (quality rating = A or B). Studies adequately measure and report safety and adverse outcomes data and show significant serious adverse effects without substantial evidence to the contrary. Some contrary evidence may exist; however, valid evidence supporting potential safety concerns outweighs contrary evidence.

Continued

TABLE 102-5 Criteria for Evidence-Based Safety Ratings—cont'd

Rating	Definition	Criteria for the Rating
Likely unsafe	Very high level of reliable clinical evidence shows safety concerns or significant adverse outcomes. People should be discouraged from taking products with a likely unsafe rating.	Safety data are available from two or more randomized clinical trials, a meta-analysis, or large-scale postmarketing surveillance that include several hundred to several thousand patients (level of evidence = A). Studies have a low risk of bias and high level of validity by meeting stringent assessment criteria (quality rating = A). Studies adequately measure and report safety and adverse outcomes data and consistently show significant serious adverse effects without valid evidence to the contrary.
Unsafe	Very high level of reliable clinical evidence shows safety concerns or significant adverse outcomes. People should be discouraged from taking products with an unsafe rating.	Safety data are available from two or more randomized clinical trials, a meta-analysis, or large-scale postmarketing surveillance that includes several hundred to several thousand patients (level of evidence = A). Studies have a low risk of bias and high level of validity by meeting stringent assessment criteria (quality rating = A). Studies adequately measure and report safety and adverse outcomes data and consistently show significant serious adverse effects without valid evidence to the contrary.

Adapted from Natural Medicines Comprehensive Database. Safety ratings. Available at http://naturaldatabase.therapeuticresearch.com/Content.aspx?cs=&s=ND&page=edprinciples&xsl=generic (accessed June 2, 2013).

*Level of evidence is assessed using the following scale: *A*, high-quality, randomized, controlled trial (RCT) or high-quality meta-analysis (quantitative systematic review); *B*, nonrandomized clinical trial, nonquantitative systematic review, lower-quality RCT, clinical cohort study, case-control study, historical control, or epidemiologic study; *C*, consensus or expert opinion; *D*, anecdotal evidence, in vitro research, or animal research.

†Study quality is assessed using the following scale: A, meets assessment criteria and has a low risk of bias; B, partially meets assessment criteria and has a low to moderate risk of bias; C, does not meet assessment criteria and has a moderate to high risk of bias.

TABLE 102-6 Criteria for Evidence-Based Efficacy Ratings

Rating	Definition	Criteria for the Rating
Effective	Very high level of reliable clinical evidence supports its use for a specific indication. Products rated effective generally are considered appropriate to recommend.	Evidence is consistent with or equivalent to passing a review by the U.S. Food and Drug Administration (FDA), Health Canada, or similarly rigorous approval process. Evidence from two or more randomized clinical trials or a meta-analysis that includes several hundred to several thousand patients (level of evidence = A).* Studies have a low risk of bias and high level of validity by meeting stringent assessment criteria (quality rating = A).† Evidence consistently shows positive outcomes for a given indication without valid evidence to the contrary.
Likely effective	Very high level of reliable clinical evidence supports its use for a specific indication. Products rated likely effective generally are considered appropriate to recommend.	Evidence from two or more randomized clinical trials or a meta-analysis that includes several hundred patients (level of evidence = A). Studies have a low risk of bias and high level of validity by meeting stringent assessment criteria (quality rating = A). Evidence consistently shows positive outcomes for a given indication without significant valid evidence to the contrary.
Possibly effective	Some clinical evidence supports its use for a specific indication; however, the evidence is limited by quantity, quality, or contradictory findings. Products rated possibly effective may be beneficial but do not have enough high-quality evidence to recommend for most people.	One or more randomized clinical trials or a meta-analysis (level of evidence = A or B) or two or more population-based or epidemiologic studies (level of evidence = B). Studies have a low to moderate risk of bias and moderate to high level of validity by meeting or partially meeting assessment criteria (quality rating = A or B). Evidence shows positive outcomes for a given indication without substantial valid evidence to the contrary. Some contrary evidence may exist; however, valid positive evidence outweighs contrary evidence.
Possibly ineffective	Some clinical evidence shows ineffectiveness for a specific indication; however, the evidence is limited by quantity, quality, or contradictory findings. People should be advised that the product is possibly ineffective.	One or more randomized clinical trials or a meta-analysis (level of evidence = A or B) or two or more population-based or epidemiologic studies (level of evidence = B). Studies have a low to moderate risk of bias and moderate to high level of validity by meeting or partially meeting assessment criteria (quality rating = A or B). Evidence shows positive outcomes for a given indication without substantial valid evidence to the contrary. Some contrary evidence may exist; however, valid positive evidence outweighs contrary evidence.

TABLE 102-6 Criteria for Evidence-Based Efficacy Ratings—cont'd

Rating	Definition	Criteria for the Rating
Likely Ineffective	Very high level of reliable clinical evidence shows ineffectiveness for its use for a specific indication. People should be warned about a product that is likely ineffective.	Evidence from two or more randomized clinical trials or a meta-analysis that includes several hundred to several thousand patients (level of evidence = A). Studies have a low risk of bias and high level of validity by meeting stringent assessment criteria (quality rating = A). Evidence consistently shows negative outcomes for a given indication without valid evidence to the contrary.

Adapted from Natural Medicines Comprehensive Database. Effectiveness ratings. Available at http://naturaldatabase.therapeuticresearch.com/Content.aspx?cs=&s=ND&page=edprinciples&xsl=generic (accessed June 2, 2013).

*Level of evidence is assessed using the following scale: *A*, high-quality, randomized, controlled trial (RCT) or high-quality meta-analysis (quantitative systematic review); *B*, nonrandomized clinical trial, nonquantitative systematic review, lower-quality RCT, clinical cohort study, case-control study, historical control, or epidemiologic study; *C*, consensus or expert opinion; *D*, anecdotal evidence, in vitro research, or animal research.

†Study quality is assessed using the following scale: *A*, meets assessment criteria and has a low risk of bias; *B*, partially meets assessment criteria and has a low to moderate risk of bias; *C*, does not meet assessment criteria and has a moderate to high risk of bias.

TABLE 102-7 Best Practice Principles for Integrating Complementary and Alternative Therapies into Management Plans

Step	Physician-Patient Interactions	Actions and Special Considerations
1	Explore factors driving interest in complementary and alternative medicine (CAM) therapy or therapist. Document instigating factors: current use, intent for future use, considering future use, seeking information, and desire to access alternative provider. Discuss reasons for choice, such as desire for greater efficacy and safety and the acceptability of CAM compared with traditional approaches.	Explore whether to engage or not. Support request for CAM but indicate limitations of that support, payment issues, and time limits. Refer to another provider for in-depth consultation (if possible).
2	Document clinical reasons for seeking CAM, such as exhausted conventional medicine options with unsatisfactory outcomes, disease with bad prognosis or disability impact, and fear of conventional therapies.	Physician-patient perceptions can be shared, including clinical status, options, and understanding; need for enhanced care or diagnostics; and need for other therapeutic options.
3	Assess current disease and health status and the previous therapies used. Use a symptom diary or validated quality-of-life survey tools. Use an objective measure of disease control such as blood pressure or peak expiratory flow Consider duration of treatment trial.	Educate the patient about options. Discuss efficacy and safety data (if available), disease evaluation, and treatment options and risks. Address acceptance or refusal of partnership (may refer elsewhere if possible).
4	Document the patient's preferences, factors in CAM therapy choice (if defined by patient), attitude toward CAM and conventional medicine, level of trust in exploring all therapeutic options.	Consider caveats that influence patient's comfort with discussion and disclosure. Evaluate neutrality of questions asked. Assess for a caring, supportive, and respectful atmosphere.
5	Assess and document the adequacy of the medical evaluation. Consider the need for additional testing or consultation. Explain all options to optimize diagnosis and treatment. Assess quality-of-life impact of medical concerns.	Consider provider options or recommendations. Discuss overall risks and benefits of using treatments for which data are limited. Provide an opportunity for questions and a dialogue.
6	Define a plan for follow-up visits, including provider-patient agreement regarding therapeutic partnership (with referral rather than refusal of care). Consider providing a fact sheet that includes reliable information and other resources about CAM therapy. Provider may opt out of further involvement when available evidence indicates serious risk or lack of efficacy of product. The patient may agree but continue use anyway.	Out-of-pocket costs for patient care may be required. Visits may not be covered by existing health insurance plan; future visits may be required at nonreimbursed payment rates (per hour rate). The patient's choice may result in the provider suggesting a move to a new provider. Avoiding patient abandonment is a challenge.
7	Provide good communication by defining respectfully and clearly what the physician can do about the patient's request, including additional visit options. Determine whether insurance will cover the therapy or time for consultation on CAM therapy. Define the provider's perception of liability risk concerns.	Communication is optimized if the physician is honest and caring about the patient's issues. Explain limitations such as time, the need for separate visits, cost and time needed for imparting information, and risks for the provider. Review alternatives for how to proceed, and build a consensus plan.
8	Acknowledge evolving expectations. At each visit, review shared goals for disease or symptom control, detail shared responsibility to gather more information, establish the provider's ability to support a request or validate the safety and efficacy of the CAM therapy of interest, and clarify the roles of the therapy team involved in care management.	Consider the level of the patient's suffering, fear, and trust. Assess psychological factors such as depression and the need for validation. Share and document disclaimers that are needed in the context of ethical considerations in the care plan.

Continued

TABLE 102-7 Best Practice Principles for Integrating Complementary and Alternative Therapies into Management Plans—cont'd

Step	Physician-Patient Interactions	Actions and Special Considerations
9	Educate about new safety and efficacy issues. Monitor the patient and literature concerning specific CAM therapy. Define guidelines for stopping the trial and any ethical concerns about supporting continuation of treatment. Consider an ethics committee consultation for complex benefit-risk analyses if controversial. Document the patient's preferences and understanding.	Explain safety and efficacy levels of evidence. Communicate balanced clinical considerations, including defined and undefined risks and the levels of evidence and uncertainty. Educate the patient about evaluating individualized benefit-risk ratio versus alternatives.
10	Discuss factors in choosing a CAM-qualified provider, and address questions of suitability, licensure, and competencies. Document how provider or practice was identified by the patient. Educate patient about questions for a CAM therapy consultation. Support the patient seeking input for an informed choice, and empower the patient to critically assess a treatment trial. Communicate and document the referring provider's responsibilities, permission to release medical information, and disclaimer regarding any conflict of interest. The patient's choice is tempered by risk-benefit considerations and the concept of "do no harm"; discuss reporting of adverse events and unethical or untested practices.	Resources are available to assess providers, including state certification requirements for CAM therapists, objective reviews, and checklists for patients during a CAM visit. Before starting unconventional treatment, educate about patient choice and establish ground rules for appointments and the level of continued physician engagement Discuss reporting adverse events for CAM through MedWatch (www.fda.gov/Safety/MedWatch/default.htm)

Adapted from Engler RJ, With CM, Gregory PJ, Jellin JM. Complementary and alternative medicine for the allergist-immunologist: where do I start? J Allergy Clin Immunol 2009;123:309-16.

TABLE 102-8 Herbal or Food-Derived Ingredients Found in Products Used for Allergic Rhinitis

Mechanisms of Action	Common Name	Botanical Name
Antihistamine	Grape seed extract	*Vitis vinifera*
Decongestants	Ephedra	*Ephedra* spp.
Mast cell stabilizers	Quercetin	
	Spirulina	*Spirulina* spp.
	Stinging nettle	*Urtica dioica*
Leukotriene modifiers	Butterbur	*Petasites hybridus*
Potential immunomodulators	Echinacea	*Echinacea* spp.
	Thymus extract	*Tinospora cordifolia*
Vitamin C	Bitter orange	*Citrus aurantium*
Other natural therapies	Capsaicin	
	Cat's claw	*Uncaria guyanensis, Uncaria tomentosa*
	Goldenseal	*Hydrastis canadensis*
	Methylsulfonylmethane	

TABLE 102-9 Herbal or Food-Derived Ingredients Found in Products Used for Asthma

Mechanism of Action	Common Name	Botanical Name
Mast cell stabilizers	Indian frankincense	*Boswellia serrata*
	Picrorhiza	*Picrorhiza kurroa*
	Quercetin	
	Spirulina	
	Stinging nettle	*Urtica dioica*
Leukotriene modifiers	Butterbur	*Petasites hybridus*
	Fish oil	
	Indian frankincense	*Boswellia serrata*
	New Zealand green-lipped mussel	*Perna canaliculus*
	Perilla	*Perilla frutescens*
	Pycnogenol	*Pinus pinaster*
Antioxidants	Grapefruit	*Citrus paradisi*
	Kiwi	*Actinidia chinensis*
	Noni juice	*Morinda citrifolia*
	Sweet orange	*Citrus sinensis*
	Vitamin C, E	

TABLE 102-9 Herbal or Food-Derived Ingredients Found in Products Used for Asthma—cont'd

Mechanism of Action	Common Name	Botanical Name
Other agents	Choline	
	Eucalyptus	*Eucalyptus globulus*
	Magnesium	
	Pyridoxine (vitamin B_6)	
	Soybean	*Glycine max*

relaxation, herbal medicine, Chinese medicine, Ayurvedic medicine, and supplements such as vitamin E, magnesium, and fish oil. None of these CAM options has sufficient evidence to merit routine use in clinical practice at this time, although some modalities merit further study and are perceived as beneficial for some patients. What role these diverse therapies may have in personalized medicine and how to validate efficacy and safety for individual patients remains an ongoing challenge for clinicians.

Hypertonic saline nasal irrigations are listed as a CAM therapy, and there is considerable literature supporting a *possibly effective* and *likely safe* classification of this modality in allergic rhinitis and sinusitis.[22,24-26] There is evidence that hypertonic saline nasal irrigations reduce oral antihistamine use and markers of inflammation (e.g., histamine, leukotriene) and that they improve quality of life.[26] Results of a 2012 study indicate that buffered hypertonic saline irrigations are more effective than normal saline in reducing symptoms in children with allergic rhinitis.[27] This therapeutic modality is increasingly incorporated in care plans within conventional medicine.

Although vitamin and mineral supplements, including antioxidants, are not always included in reviews of CAM, these agents further complicate and challenge the practice of evidence-based integrative medicine. Often considered safe and effective in the absence of objective data, these health adjuvants and their widespread use have raised concerns described in the peer-reviewed literature. An example is β-carotene supplementation beyond standard dietary intake. Some evidence indicates that mixtures of β-carotene isomers prevent exercise-induced asthma,[28] but there are growing concerns that as little as 20 mg/day for 5 to 8 years may increase the risk of lung and prostate cancer, cardiovascular mortality, and total mortality for individuals who smoke or have exposure to asbestos.[29,30]

Vitamin E supplementation ranging between 50 and 600 IU (daily or every other day, depending on sex) has been promoted as beneficial for preventing strokes, improving heart and lung health, and decreasing health care costs. A meta-analysis of nine randomized, controlled trials (RCTs) reported that vitamin E supplementation increased the risk of hemorrhagic stroke by 22% and decreased the risk of ischemic stroke by 10%.[31] A second meta-analysis of 13 RCTs that included more than 166,000 subjects found no benefit from vitamin E supplementation at any dose (i.e., less than or greater than 300 IU/day) for any stroke type, nor for any preparation type (i.e., synthetic or natural source).[32] A 2012 Cochrane review of 78 RCTs with more than 296,000 participants found no evidence to support antioxidant supplements for primary or secondary prevention of stroke.[33] This meta-analysis suggested that a small increase in the overall mortality rate was associated with β-carotene and vitamin E and with higher doses of vitamin A. The report suggested that antioxidant supplements be considered medicinal products that should undergo "evaluation before marketing" and that no recommendations could be made for their use in "the general population or patients with various diseases." Dietary supplementation use, even with a placebo, may encourage other health-risk behaviors (e.g., smoking) by creating an illusion of invulnerability.[34]

The Second National Report on Biochemical Indicators of Diet and Nutrition in the U.S. population indicates that no more than 10% of the general population have nutritional deficiencies of selected vitamins and minerals.[35] Fewer than 1% of them have deficiencies of vitamin E, vitamin A (with 2% to 4%, depending on age, at risk for excess vitamin A and associated hepatotoxicity risk), or folate. Vitamin C deficiency (i.e., serum levels of ascorbic acid <11.4 mmol/L) is estimated at 6%, with a higher incidence in men (7%) than in women (5%). The incidence of vitamin D deficiency (with levels <12 ng/mL) is relatively high at 8.1%. Vitamin D insufficiency (with levels of 12 to 20 ng/mL) is not rare (24%) and occurs at higher rates among non-Hispanic blacks (31%) and Mexican Americans (12%) compared with non-Hispanic whites (3%).

Iron deficiency remains a significant issue; it affects 6.7% of the population, and its rates are high among women between the ages of 12 and 29 years (9.5%), children between the ages of 1 and 5 years (6.7%), and non-Hispanic black women (16%) and Mexican-American women (13%) of childbearing age (12 to 49 years old). In the setting of poverty and poor nutrition, these rates may be much higher and have secondary impacts on wellness and quality of life. Few men are at risk for iron deficiency, but 29% are at risk for iron excess.

Deficiencies in vitamin B_6 (10.5%) and vitamin B_{12} (2% overall and 4% of older adults) may also present a significant health issue that is amenable to corrective nutrition. Women of childbearing age have iodine levels bordering on insufficiency, a concern because iodine is necessary for optimal fetal brain development.

The Childhood Asthma Management Program (1024 subjects) identified higher rates of vitamin D insufficiency (using ≤30 ng/mL rather than ≤20 ng/mL as the cutoff point) among African Americans (35%).[36] In an analysis adjusted for age, sex, body mass index (BMI), income, and treatment group, vitamin D insufficiency was associated with higher odds of severe asthma exacerbation over a 4-year period.[37] Definitive studies incorporating biodiversity considerations are needed to define the optimal use of supplements and complementary foods as modulators of allergic and immunologic disease in different populations.[38]

Alternative Medical Systems

The remainder of this chapter focuses on specific CAM therapies that are most likely to have an impact on patients seen in an allergy-immunology practice.

ACUPUNCTURE

Acupuncture has several described forms: acupuntura, auricular acupuncture, Chinese acupuncture, ear acupuncture, foot acupuncture, hand acupuncture, Japanese acupuncture, Korean acupuncture, needle moxibustion, single point acupuncture, trigger point acupuncture, and Western acupuncture. Acupressure uses some of the principles of acupuncture but does not use needles. Acupuncture is part of Kampo medicine and traditional Chinese medicine (TCM). Acupuncture is used for a wide variety of medical conditions and is most commonly used to treat pain in the forms of neuropathy, low back pain, labor pain, temporomandibular joint dysfunction, and migraine headache.[39] Acupuncture is used for a broad range of conditions (e.g., depression, anxiety, insomnia) and has been the focus of well-controlled clinical studies of its use for allergic rhinitis, asthma, and skin itching (i.e., eczema).[39]

Allergic Rhinitis

A study of 5237 allergic rhinitis included 487 patients randomly assigned to acupuncture and 494 to control therapy, and 4256 were in a nonrandomized acupuncture group (i.e., two groups receiving acupuncture).[36] The results of this and other trials suggest that treating patients with allergic rhinitis in routine care with acupuncture may enhance clinically relevant quality-of-life parameters.[36,40,41] In a 2011 prospective, randomized, sham-controlled trial of semi–self-administered ear acupressure for persistent allergic rhinitis, acupressure resulted in beneficial changes in global symptom scores, sneezing scores, and activities related to quality of life.[42] These preliminary results support further investigation to determine the efficacy, cost-effectiveness, and safety of this modified approach to acupuncture-like therapy. Other than some ear discomfort, the ear acupressure was considered safe.

Asthma

As acupuncture use grows in Europe and the United States, there are increasing numbers of publications addressing its use in asthma (>180 articles cited in PubMed with English language and human limits as of April 12, 2012). Scheewe and colleagues[43] conducted an RCT to evaluate the immediate effects of acupuncture as an add-on therapy to inpatient rehabilitation of children and adolescents with bronchial asthma. The intervention group ($n = 46$) received acupuncture; the control group ($n = 47$) did not. Both groups received asthma sports, climate therapy, and behavioral training. In the acupuncture group, peak expiratory flow measurement variability improved significantly ($P < .01$) more than that of the control patients. Moreover, the acupuncture group had significant reduction of perceived anxiety. However, the lung function tests did not show differences between the groups. A similar finding was reported by Choi and coworkers[44] in a randomized pilot study.

Ngai and colleagues[45] examined the effect of transcutaneous electrical nerve stimulation applied over acupoints (Acu-TENS) on forced expiratory volume in patients with asthma, after exercise. Adjunctive Acu-TENS therapy appeared to reduce the decline of forced expiratory volume in 1 second (FEV_1) after exercise training in patients with asthma. A 2011 sham-acupuncture controlled study did not show any significant benefit for acupuncture, but many questions were raised about technique, and this study did not address the applicability of these findings to variations of acupuncture-like methods.[46]

Atopic Dermatitis

Itch is a major symptom of atopic dermatitis. In 2010, Pfab and colleagues reported results of a blinded, randomized, placebo-controlled, crossover trial of 30 subjects with atopic eczema showing that acupuncture significantly reduced the mean itch intensity and mean wheal and flare size in response to house-dust mite or grass pollen skin-prick testing compared with the control group.[47] In 2012, the same group conducted a patient- and examiner-blinded, randomized, placebo-controlled, crossover trial of acupuncture compared with oral antihistamine for type I hypersensitivity itch and skin response in 20 adults with atopic dermatitis. The mean itch intensity and flare size after acupuncture was significantly lower compared with the antihistamine group receiving sham acupuncture ($P < .05$ versus $P < .001$).[48] Additional studies with large samples size are warranted, and the possible impact on skin testing results must be considered.

Mechanism of Action

Acupuncture involves stimulation, traditionally with fine-needle insertion but also with pressure or electrical stimulation, of specific parts or points on the body along pathways called *meridians*. The goal is to stimulate points that correspond to specific organs, emotions, or sensory feelings. In TCM, it is described as a procedure that stimulates energy flow to unblock and rebalance energy (i.e., *qi*) for the purpose of healing.[37,49] Numerous attempts to find evidence for stimulation-induced release of natural endorphins, opioids, or other inflammatory biomarkers such as prostaglandins in urine have produced conflicting results, and this topic is beyond the scope of this chapter.[37,49] Studies showing measurable changes in biomarkers tend to be associated with the combination of acupuncture plus electrical stimulation.[44,50] One study showed that the mean itch intensity was significantly lower in the 3-week acupuncture group than in the control group of patients with atopic dermatitis. This effect was associated with suppression of basophil activation as indicated by a reduced percentage of CD63-positive basophils.[51]

Dosage

Acupuncture therapy can be applied daily or every other day for various durations (e.g., 10 to 15 treatments initially and then adjusted based on disease response or need).[39] There are no well-characterized, evidence-based guidelines uniformly applied by all practitioners. The use of noninvasive stimulation of acupuncture sites with the potential for self-treatment, similar to TENS, introduces further variability in the frequency of use. There are no data indicating that more frequent use increases safety risks.[52]

Side Effects

Acupuncture, when used appropriately, usually is well tolerated. Side effects occur rarely and include dizziness, nausea, vomiting, pain, fainting, and infection of the needle insertion sites. Jindal and coworkers[52] reviewed 31 published journal articles, including 23 RCTs and 8 meta-analyses with systematic reviews addressing the safety and efficacy of acupuncture in children. Serious adverse event risks are very low (1 in 10,000 to 100,000), with the pediatric risk estimated at 1.55 events per 100 treatments.[49,52]

Disposable acupuncture needles are classified by the FDA as a class II medical device and are the standard of care for acupuncture therapy. Reuse of contaminated needles is a deviation from best practice and can be associated with transmission of viral infections such as hepatitis B.

Indications and Contraindications

Acupuncture has been rated as possibly effective for back pain, chemotherapy-induced nausea and vomiting, labor pain, and osteoarthritis. Although preliminary clinical reports suggest potential benefits, there is insufficient reliable evidence to rate acupuncture as an effective therapy for allergic disease and asthma or for a broad range of other conditions There are no known interactions with herbs, supplements, other drugs, foods, laboratory tests, or specific diseases.[39,49,52]

AYURVEDA

Ayurveda, also known as Ayurvedic medicine, traditional Asian medicine, or traditional Indian medicine, is an ancient medical system that uses a variety of methods for diagnosing and treating various medical conditions.[53-55] Yoga and Shirodhara are practices frequently included with Ayurveda. Shirodhara is a relaxation-stimulation method that involves pouring liquids (e.g., oil, milk, buttermilk, coconut water, plain water) over the forehead and is often combined with different massage techniques in spas. Shirodhara and has been used to treat symptoms of eye disease, allergic rhinitis, sinusitis, insomnia, and fatigue. The method has also been used for relieving symptoms of allergic rhinitis, sinusitis, insomnia, tinnitus, vertigo, Ménière disease, hearing impairment, memory loss, diabetes, and other conditions.[56]

Mechanism of Action

Ayurveda means "the science of life." It was developed as a platform for holistic healing (i.e., harmonizing body, mind, and spirit) in India more than 2000 years ago. Ayurveda incorporates meditation and yoga practices and has parallels with Chinese medicine.[57-59] Treatments commonly used in Ayurveda include meditation with controlled breathing, exercise, diet, herbs, and massage. This ancient system of viewing the body and affecting function is built on several concepts:

- Tridosha: Ayurvedic theory that the body's physiologic processes are regulated by three integrated doshas (bodily humors that regulate bodily function), each of which is responsible for a particular physiologic area. Disease occurs when there is imbalance in the doshas.
- Kapha: the dosha that governs structure, cohesion, and lubrication, located primarily in the upper torso
- Pitta: the dosha that governs energy, located in the middle of the body
- Vata: dosha that governs movement, including in the mind, located primarily in the lower abdomen
- Prakriti: refers to nature or a person's nature and is the name for a person's physiology or physiologic processes

Ayurveda uses herbal products in fixed combinations or formulations to help balance physiologic processes.[56] Many of the herbs commonly used in TCM are also used in Ayurvedic practices.

Dosage

Most therapies are administered orally without standardized dosing. Evidence-based pediatric and adult dosing information remains unclear given the individualized approaches to therapy in this system of health care.

Side Effects

Ayurveda uses a variety of treatments, such as specific combinations of herbal ingredients. Safety information and possible drug or disease interactions must be considered in the context of the specific ingredients. Some products may be contaminated with prescription drugs such as corticosteroids and nonsteroidal antiinflammatory drugs or have high concentrations of heavy metals, including mercury, arsenic, and lead.[56,60] With all medications, efficacy and safety data related to specific products and manufacturing practices should be assessed. Information related to pregnancy and lactation is frequently limited.

Indications and Contraindications

There is insufficient reliable evidence to rate the efficacy of Ayurvedic practices for allergic disease and asthma or other conditions. Contraindications and potential interactions among drugs, herbs, supplements, diseases, foods, and laboratory tests must be considered in the context of the individual therapy and must use independent, reliable, evidence-based resources.

HOMEOPATHY

Although the terms *holistic* and *natural medicine* are often confused with homeopathic medicine, homeopathy and homeopathic medicine represent a distinct formal system of medicine that uses natural products. The NCCAM web site reports that over-the-counter products labeled homeopathic represent a $2.9 billion industry annually. An additional $170 million is spent for visits to homeopathic practitioners. It is estimated that 3.9 million adults and 910,000 children used homeopathy in the year before the 2007 NHIS was published.[61,62]

Starting in eighteenth-century Germany, homeopathy was built on two theories: *like cures like*, meaning that a substance that produces symptoms similar to the disease in healthy people can cure if given in very dilute amounts, and the *law of minimum dose* (i.e., law of infinitesimals), which states that lower doses have greater efficacy and makes an assumption of greater safety for the lower doses.[61,62] Dilutions are recorded by a number with an X (1X = 1/10, 2X = 1/100, progressing to 6X = 1/1,000,000 and beyond) or by a number with a C (1C = 1/100, 2C = 1/10,000, 3C = 1/1,000,000, and so on). Remedies are derived from substances that come from plants (e.g., poison ivy, deadly nightshade as a source of belladonna), minerals (including poisons such as arsenic), or animals (e.g., crushed whole bees). Regulatory oversight of and evidence-based support for homeopathic therapies and products are lacking.[57,63]

Mechanism of Action

Within the context of Western scientific inquiry, evidence-based information supporting a mechanism of action beyond a placebo effect is lacking.

Dosage

Pediatric and adult dosing information remains limited given the individualized approaches to therapy development and presumed lack of measurable concentrations. Most therapies are administered in concentrations dilute enough to be considered equivalent to nonmedication dosing. Anthroposophic and homeopathic medicines are administered orally (frequently formulated in sugar pellets to be placed under the tongue or as tablets and drops, usually in alcohol), topically (e.g., ointments, gels, creams), or by injection (particularly outside the United States).[61] Evidence-based data to support effective dosing recommendations are lacking.

Side Effects

Systematic evidence addressing concerns about safety risks remains limited and fragmented. Although many homeopathic remedies are highly dilute, some products may not be dilute and may contain ingredients that can cause side effects and drug interactions.[61,62] Some zinc gluconate spray used for the common cold are marketed as a homeopathic product despite a 2X dilution (1/100). Containing 2.1 mg of elemental zinc per dose (i.e., two intranasal sprays), this measurable amount of zinc has pharmacologic effects and potential adverse effects. Several of these products were removed from the market in 2009 because of reports of anosmia after regular use.[58] Homeopathic remedies may have a higher concentration of alcohol than allowed in conventional drugs (10% maximum).

A German pharmacovigilance database review evaluated the safety data for more than 303 million ampoules for homeopathic use sold between 2000 and 2009.[59] Of 486 adverse event cases reported (representing 1180 adverse drug reactions [ADRs]), 71.8% were listed in the package leaflet (primarily local reactions including pain, erythema, swelling, and inflammation), and 9.5% were classified as serious. The most frequently reported ADRs were pruritus, angioedema, diarrhea, and erythema. The overall rate of ADRs with injections was less than 4 cases per 1 million sold (i.e., very rare). Unlike Europe, standardized training and licensure for homeopathic practitioners does not exist in the United States.

There are growing concerns that homeopathic immunizations have been promoted as substitutes for conventional immunizations, even though no data support this use and the lack of evidence-based immunization could leave patients vulnerable to diseases such as measles and pertussis.[61] For asthma and allergic diseases, there continues to be concern that avoidance of conventional therapies may increase the risk of morbidity and mortality.

Indications, Contraindications, and Interactions

Clinical trials and systematic reviews of research on homeopathy have not provided evidence-based support for disease-specific efficacy.[57,64] Given the lack of systematic studies, some independent reviewing groups have classified the evidence as insufficient to rank efficacy. Contraindications and potential interactions among drugs, herbs, supplements, diseases, foods, and laboratory tests must be considered in the context of the individual therapy and must use independent, reliable, evidence-based resources.

Manipulation and Body-Based Therapies

CHIROPRACTIC AND OSTEOPATHIC MANIPULATION

Chiropractic and osteopathic manipulation, also known as chiro therapy, chirotherapy, chiropratique, manipulative therapy, physical medicine, quiropráctica, spinal manipulative therapy (SMT), or subluxation. It is a widely used alternative system of medicine that is used for a broad range of medical conditions, particularly pain syndromes (e.g., low back pain, neck pain, fibromyalgia, headaches, otitis media), and for conditions such as asthma.

Chiropractic manipulation was founded as an alternative healing discipline by Daniel David Palmer in 1895 in Davenport, Iowa. Chiropractors represent the third largest primary contact health profession in North America, and licensing exists in 46 states in the United States and in dozens of countries around the world.[65] The growth of this profession has been attributed to increased public acceptance due to positive results and recognition in international guidelines of evidence-based benefits of manipulation. In particular, benefits for low back pain have been shown, although chiropractic manipulation has not been shown to be superior to other medical management approaches.

Mechanism of Action

In chiropractic medicine, most illness is thought to be caused by malpositioned vertebrae interfering with the nervous system and the body's innate healing ability.[66] Studies, including seven RCTs and one observational study applying cranial osteopathic manipulation, reported outcome measures on pain, sleep, quality of life, motor function, cerebral oxygenation, and autonomic nervous system function.[67-71] Positive clinical outcomes were reported for pain reduction and improved sleep patterns in addition to objective measures of autonomic nervous system function.[67,68] Given the role of the autonomic nervous system in bronchospasm, it has been suggested that this mode may benefit some patients with asthma. However, available evidence on clinical efficacy of manipulation therapy for treating asthma is insufficient to draw definitive conclusions. Whether subsets of asthma patients could benefit from some types of manipulations requires further research with careful characterization of phenotypes and objective responses to sham versus applied therapy.

Dosage

Regimens of manipulation types and frequencies vary from a series of treatments over weeks and months to a limited set of treatment. There are no published, standardized, evidence-based schedules for treatments, and health insurance policies may not cover services provided.

Side Effects

The preponderance of evidence and clinical experience indicates that chiropractic therapy is safe when used appropriately by trained practitioners. Inappropriate use, such as neck manipulation or use of excessive force in some settings, has been linked with serious and potentially life-threatening reactions, including stroke, artery dissection, spinal hematoma, and esophageal tearing.[69-75] Reported adverse events occur in approximately 30% to 56% of patients receiving treatment for neck pain, and approximately 13% of reported side effects are classified as severe.[76,77] Several cases of vertebral artery dissection have been reported after neck manipulation.[72] In most cases, symptoms developed within 12 hours of receiving treatment. Death resulted in one case. Several instances of spinal epidural hematoma after cervical manipulation have been reported.[73] In some cases, spinal epidural hematoma occurred in patients receiving oral anticoagulation therapy with warfarin. The risk of stroke after spinal manipulation is estimated at 1 case per 400,000 to 3 to 6 cases per 10 million manipulations.[74,75]

Upper spinal manipulation has been linked to at least 14 reports of ophthalmologic side effects.[77] These adverse events include loss of vision, diplopia, Horner syndrome, and ophthalmoplegia. In many cases, the cause of the adverse outcome was arterial wall dissection due to chiropractic manipulation.

Chiropractic manipulation may not be safe in children. Chiropractic manipulation in children has been linked to at least nine cases of subarachnoid hemorrhage and several cases of less severe side effects such as headache and back pain.[78]

Safety of spinal manipulation in the pregnant and postpartum periods was reviewed by Stuber and coworkers in March of 2012.[79] There are few reported cases of adverse events, and they included increasing pain, fracture, stroke, and epidural hematoma. Although the need for improved reporting was cited, the Canadian perspective was that injuries were rare.

Indications, Contraindications, and Interactions

Despite case reports of benefit, the efficacy of chiropractic manipulation in asthma and allergic disease remains undefined. The Natural Standard Database system, an independent expert consensus review process, rated the level of scientific evidence for using chiropractic manipulation for asthma as "unclear or conflicting" (grade C).[80] This rating is consistent with that of the NMCD, which uses a category definition of *insufficient reliable evidence to rate* given the mixed published results and despite preliminary clinical trial data indicating that chiropractic manipulation in children can "improve subjective measures of asthma severity and quality of life."[65] Bleeding disorders, anticoagulation therapy (e.g., warfarin), and underlying disease states predisposing to strokes are potential contraindications for chiropractic manipulations. Children may be at increased risk for certain types of manipulations leading to serious adverse events. Side effects, including severe headaches, should be considered in the communication of risk before initiating procedures.

MASSAGE THERAPY

Many patients want more time to interact with physicians and desire a "healing touch." A Google search with the term *healing touch* found more than 23 million potential links in May of 2012, up from less than 1 million in November of 2008.

Massage has been defined as the systematic manipulation of soft tissues of the body for therapeutic effect. Classic (i.e., Swedish) massage consists of stroking and gliding (i.e., effleurage), kneading (i.e., pétrissage), and percussion (i.e., tapotement), but other forms of massage have originated in different parts of the world.[81] Between 1990 and 1997, the 1-year prevalence of use of massage by the U.S. general population increased from 6% to 12%, and it continues to be one of the three most popular CAM therapies in the United States and the United Kingdom.[82]

Adding parental massage therapy to traditional medical management for children with asthma has been linked with improvement in quality of life and trends toward reduced medication requirements and improved pulmonary function.[83,84] Because massage techniques are low risk, they are appealing as an adjunct to holistic management strategies. Although a 2005 updated Cochrane review[85] concluded there was insufficient evidence to support the use of manual therapies for patients with asthma, the report acknowledged that there was a need to conduct adequately sized RCTs examining the effects of manual therapies on clinically relevant outcomes (review not updated since 2008).

Mechanism of Action

Positive effects of massage therapy, such as decreased levels of cortisol in saliva or urine and increased levels of the activating neurotransmitters serotonin and dopamine, have been measured in a variety of medical conditions and stressful experiences.[85,86] However, in a comprehensive literature review with a meta-analysis (2010 cutoff), it was concluded that cortisol changes were small and could not explain all the clinical benefits observed with massage therapy.[87]

Dosage

In one study of young asthma patients, 20 minutes of massage at bedtime by parents was associated with measurable benefit.[83] In a study of breast cancer pain management, 30-minute massage sessions twice each week were associated with measurable reductions in stress cortisol levels.[88]

Side Effects

Massage therapy is considered safe. In a comprehensive literature review, 16 case reports of adverse effects and 4 case series were identified.[75,76,78] Most adverse effects were associated with untrained layman; adverse effects associated with massage therapists were rare. The reported adverse events included cerebrovascular accidents, displacement of a ureteral stent, embolization of a kidney, hematoma, leg ulcers, nerve damage, posterior interosseous syndrome, pseudoaneurysm, pulmonary embolism, ruptured uterus, strangulation of neck, thyrotoxicosis, and various pain syndromes.

Cause-and-effect relationships were suggested, but mostly with the use of non-Swedish massage techniques. Although not entirely risk free, massage was only rarely associated with serious adverse events, which were mostly linked to forceful techniques such as shiatsu, urut, and Rolfing.[75] Bruising, discomfort, and bleeding into tissues, particularly in patients with bleeding disorders or on blood thinners, can occur with deep tissue massage. Underreporting of adverse events remains a significant challenge to the accurate collection of safety data.

Indications, Contraindications, and Interactions

Evidence to support definitive statements about indications, contraindications, or interactions is limited for massage therapy. For deep tissue massage or other methods using more force than Swedish massage, bleeding disorders, anticoagulation therapies, and underlying conditions producing enhanced tissue sensitivity should be considered possible risk factors for adverse events. No data regarding safety during pregnancy or lactation are available.

Mind-Body Therapies

MEDITATION AND RELAXATION

The various forms of meditation include concentrative meditation, méditation, mindfulness, mindfulness meditation, mindfulness training, and transcendental meditation. Meditation is a mind-body technique used for inducing relaxation or reducing the symptoms of fatigue, depression, anxiety, fibromyalgia, anger, hypertension, rheumatoid arthritis, diabetes, tinnitus, congestive heart failure, back pain, and many other chronic medical conditions.[89,90] Relaxation therapies[91] used for asthma include the following approaches:

- Jacobsonian progressive relaxation: routine of exercises that involve tensing, relaxing, and attending to the sensations of each of the 15 muscle groups
- Hypnotherapy: induction of a trancelike state of heightened suggestibility or compliance, with the subject passively receiving ideas, images, or instructions from the hypnotist
- Autogenic training: like self-hypnosis, involves a series of visual and sensory exercises focused on achieving deep relaxation states
- Biofeedback training: a technique for monitoring and gaining control over automatic, reflex-regulated body functions by using information obtained from an objective monitoring device (e.g., blood pressure, oxygen saturation)
- Transcendental meditation: mental repetition of a *mantra* (Sanskrit word meaning "tool or instrument of thought"), a sound, syllable, word, or group of words provided by an instructor or self-help resource that can create a positive transformation for inducing deep relaxation

Stress and anxiety may precipitate or exacerbate acute and chronic asthma. Although there is no evidence to support stress as a primary cause of asthma, stress and anxiety as a confounder to disease management continue to be a focus of mind-body medicine and integrative, holistic care approaches.

Meditation is usually combined with breathing exercises, relaxation exercises (e.g., yoga, qi gong, tai chi), or guided imagery, but the techniques vary, and it is difficult to separate meditation from other modalities.[89,90] Meditation is a mental practice used to clear the mind of distracting thoughts and create a relaxed mental and physical state.

Mechanism of Action

During meditation, the brain is thought to switch from resting brain waves (alpha) to relaxing brain waves (theta). This switch may be associated with increased release of endorphins, slowed breathing and heart rate, decreased blood pressure, and decreased metabolism. Researchers theorize that psychological stress and fatigue significantly contribute to many disease processes. By reducing stress and fatigue, meditation coupled with breathing and physical exercises may help to treat and prevent a variety of conditions. In an RCT of Shaja yoga used by individuals with moderate to severe asthma, airway hyperresponsiveness (measured by responses to a methacholine dose), asthma-related quality of life (AQLQ) mood subscale values, and profiles of mood states improved, but overall AQLQ measures did not significantly improve.[92] Meta-analysis reviews have not consistently indicated that meditation has a benefit in asthma.[91]

Dosage and Route of Administration

In studies evaluating meditation, the frequency and duration of regimens, the type of breathing exercises, and the training times varied. It is often recommended that patients perform daily exercises after they undergo reinforced training several times per week for a few weeks. Incorporating meditation with daily conditioning exercise seems to be the norm. Yoga, meditation, and relaxation exercises are learned in classes or by self-study. After initial training, individuals continue to practice yoga on their own.[89]

Side Effects

When used appropriately, meditation and relaxation techniques are likely safe unless they result in treatment delays or worsening of disease status Two serious adverse events occurred with yoga training and breathing exercises. A 40-year-old man developed subcutaneous emphysema after aggressive pranayama yoga breathing, which involves Valsalva maneuvers, and a 29-year-old woman experienced pneumothorax after an aggressive yoga breathing technique called Kapalabhati pranayama, also known as breath of fire or skull shining breath.[93,94] No safety data for pregnancy and lactation exist, but there is no reason to expect adverse reactions. A review of hypnosis and the potential risks of adverse events is beyond the scope of this chapter.

Indications, Contraindications, and Interactions

Although some studies suggest muscle relaxation improves lung function, there is a lack of consistent evidence suggesting that relaxation therapies are effective in managing asthma.[89,90,92] The Natural Standards Database ranks meditation as grade C because of "unclear or conflicting scientific evidence." However, the same database ranks the scientific evidence for yoga as grade A (i.e., strong scientific evidence) and psychotherapy as grade B (i.e., good scientific evidence), which is not consistent with the rankings given by other independent reviews. There are no reported interactions with drugs, herbals, or supplements or risks associated with pregnancy or specific disease states. There are limited reports of adverse reactions, particularly when considering the many variations of this therapy.

BREATHING TRAINING

Breathing retraining techniques have been popular with the public and have elicited renewed therapeutic interest.[95-103] As of April 2012, data from seven RCTs indicate that certain techniques, specifically the Buteyko breathing technique and Papworth Method, tend to improve asthma symptoms.[95-103] The Buteyko breathing technique was developed by Konstantin Buteyko, a Russian physician who postulated that asthma was caused by hyperventilation due to secondary low tension of carbon dioxide. Several studies indicated benefits, but the studies were uncontrolled or only showed trends toward improvement. Three of four RCTs produced data favorable to the Buteyko method, but in one, the benefit was no greater than with the Pink City Lung Exerciser,[103] and it indicated that the mechanism of action might not depend on carbon dioxide alone. The latest study designs for the Buteyko and Papworth methods follow:

- The Buteyko breathing technique[100] is a patented method of instruction for breathing that involves techniques to reduce hyperventilation. The techniques include breath holding at functional residual capacity, avoidance of breathing through the mouth, mouth taping at night, and a series of exercises for daily use.
- The Papworth Method[101] is integrated diaphragmatic breathing with relaxation that includes five major components:
  - Breathing training includes teaching of appropriate minute and tidal volume breathing and the development of a pattern of breathing suitable to current

metabolic activity. A method diaphragmatic breathing technique is taught to replace the use of inappropriate accessory muscles of respiration. Emphasis, when relaxed, is placed on calm, slow nasal expiration. Patients are encouraged to breathe through the nose rather than the mouth.

- Education emphasizes the recognition and physical management of stress responses.
- Patients receive specific and general relaxation training.
- Appropriate breathing and relaxation techniques are integrated into daily living activities. Initially, the techniques are taught in a semirecumbent position, and they are then progressively done while sitting, when standing, during daily living activities, and while integrating breathing and relaxation techniques with speech.
- Home exercises are performed with an audiotape or CD containing reminders of the breathing and relaxation techniques that is supplied at the third treatment.

The Papworth Method study[101] demonstrated significant amelioration of respiratory symptoms, dysfunctional breathing, and adverse mood compared with usual care in a primary care setting, but there were no significant differences in objective measures of respiratory function except for relaxed breathing rates. Of 612 adults with asthma who were approached for participation, only 142 responded positively, 109 attended the assessment, and 85 were included in the study.

The Buteyko breathing technique study[100] showed substantial and similar improvements, with a high level of asthma control 6 months after completion of the intervention (40% to 79% versus 44% to 72% in the control group). The Buteyko group had a significant reduction in inhaled corticosteroid use compared with the control group, but none of the differences between groups at 6 months was significant. The study did not define the functional differences between approaches that might have accounted for different reductions in corticosteroid use.

Mechanism of Action

It has been postulated that respiratory muscle training is a beneficial mechanism in breathing training exercises.[96]

Dosage and Route of Administration

Because types and frequencies of training dosage are diverse, it is difficult to define an evidence-based, unifying prescription for breathing retraining. Daily training is often required, and this creates a challenge in maintaining patient compliance.

Side Effects

No serious adverse effects have been reported with the breathing training exercises addressed in this section. However, as outlined previously, when yoga has been combined with intense breathing exercises, serious adverse events have occurred.

Indications, Contraindications, and Major Interactions

Breathing techniques, yoga, and respiratory muscle training have showed some benefit in asthma treatment. Well-designed studies with adequate power and length of follow-up remain limited. Provided that prescribed medications are continued, it is reasonable for clinicians to support asthma patients intending to undertake such techniques under the supervision of a qualified instructor. Given the rising popularity of CAM in asthma, further studies of breathing retraining are warranted so that clinicians and patients have access to safe, cost-effective, and time-efficient methods.

Biologically Based Therapies

TRADITIONAL CHINESE MEDICINE FOR ASTHMA AND ALLERGY

TCM has a long history of use in China and other Asian countries, such as Japan and Korea. TCM is part of mainstream medicine in these countries and is frequently used by Americans who have roots in these traditions of healing.[104-106] Herbal therapy and acupuncture are the main components of TCM.[104] TCM substances are considered dietary supplements in the United States and are therefore not regulated by the FDA. The quality and concentrations of individual ingredients in complex herbal mixtures, which are common in TCM, are not regulated, and no herbals are covered by traditional health insurance plans. The FDA has provided guidance for investigating botanical drug products, including complex formulas, and the NIH and NCCAM are providing grants to support clinical and basic research on botanical drug products.[106]

TCM practices focus on correcting energy flow and restoring balance.[104,107] In the TCM tradition, four qualities are considered important in determining effects:

- Action: Herbs are often described based on their primary action, such as tonic (meaning to strengthen) or astringent.
- Affinity: Herbs can be described according to which organ system they have an affinity for.
- Nature: The herb's nature usually refers to whether it has cooling or heating effects or has energizing or relaxing effects.
- Taste: Herbs can have different effects based on tastes such as sweet, sour, bitter, spicy, salty, or bland. Bitter herbs such as goldenseal are often described as having a drying effect and are used for upper respiratory tract infections.

Herbs usually are prescribed as fixed formulas or combinations. Individual herbs within the combinations presumably address a particular imbalance in the patient. The mixtures usually contain a main ingredient with other supportive agents. Mixtures with unique and potentially novel therapeutic effects for asthma and peanut anaphylaxis are the focus of this section.

The following concepts and terminology provide an understanding of the core hypotheses used in TCM practices, and they are not a part of allopathic medical practice or evidence-based medicine mechanisms of action.[104,107,108]

- Meridian: Twelve meridians form a continuous pathway throughout the body. Qi (i.e., energy) circulates through the body on these meridians.
- Pulse diagnosis: The radial pulse is taken on each side and in three different positions.[109]
- Qi: Pronounced *chee*, qi refers to the total energy of the body.[108,109]
- Tongue diagnosis: The appearance of the tongue, such as moistness, coloring, or coating, is used to assess certain conditions.[109]
- Yin and yang: In China, yin and yang are two forces that control the universe. Medical problems are considered to be rooted in imbalances within and between these forces, and the goal of therapy is correction of the imbalances.

TABLE 102-10 Chinese Medicine–Derived Herbal Medicine Mixtures Used for Asthma

Characteristic	ASHMI	mMMDT	Ding Chuan	STA-1
Study type and date	RCT, 2005	RCT, 2006	RCT, 2006	RCT, 2006
Number of herbs	3	5	9	10
Sample sizes	*n* = 45ASHMI *n* = 46 prednisone	*n* = 40 mMMDT (80 mg) *n* = 40 mMMDT (40 mg) *n* = 20 placebo	*n* = 28 DCT *n* = 24 placebo	*n* = 50 STA-1* *n* = 50 STA-2 *n* = 20 placebo
Age range (yr)	18-65	5-18	8-15	8-15
Indication	Moderate to severe, persistent asthma	Mild to moderate, persistent asthma	Mild to moderate, persistent asthma	Mild to moderate, persistent asthma
Length of study	4 wk	4 mo	3 mo	6 mo
Herbal components	1. Radix glycyrrhizae† 2. Radix *Sophorae flavescentis* 3. *Ganoderma*	1. Radix glycyrrhizae 2. Radix *Ophiopogon japonicus* 3. Radix *Panacis quinquefolii* 4. Tuber *Pinellia* 5. Herba *Tridacis procumbentis*	1. Radix glycyrrhizae 2. Tuber *Pinellia* 3. Gingko biloba 4. Herba *Ephedra* 5. Flos *Tussilaginis farfarae* 6. Cortex *Mori albae radicis* 7. Fructus *Perilla frutescens* 8. Semen *Prunus armeniaca* 9. Radix *Scutellariae baicalensis*	Combined formula of mMMDT (without *Tussilaginis farfarae*) and Lui Wei Di Huang Wan, which contains six herbs
Improved FEV_1	Yes	Yes	Yes	Yes
Improved symptom score	Yes	Yes	Yes	Yes

Adapted from Li XM. Traditional Chinese herbal remedies for asthma and food allergy. J Allergy Clin Immunol 2007;120:25-31.

ASHMI, Antiasthma herbal medicine intervention; *DCT*, Ding Chuan Tang formula; *FEV_1*, forced expiratory volume in 1 second; *mMMDT*, modified Mai-Men-Dong-Tang formula; *RCT*, randomized, placebo-controlled, double-blind, clinical trial.

*STA-1 is a combination of the mMMDT and Lui-Wei-Di-Huang Wan.(LWDHW) formulas. For STA-1, the six herbs of LWDHW were milled to a powder. For STA-2, the herbs were extracted with boiling water.

†All of the herbals contain radix glycyrrhizae, or licorice root, which is derived from *Glycyrrhiza uralensis*, also known as Chinese licorice.

Yin, the feminine side of nature, includes tranquility, darkness, cold, wetness, and depth. Yang, the masculine, represents light, heat, activity, dryness, and height. Yin and yang are considered necessary and complementary forces, not dichotomous.[108]

Several TCM herbal medications have been reported as being effective in treating asthma.[110] Table 102-10 summarizes information on four classic and modified formulas reported to produce some beneficial effects in clinical trials. These mixtures are available as food supplements and do not require FDA approval; however, efforts to standardize and validate efficacy and safety of mixtures require approved investigational new drug (IND) status so that organized clinical research data can be compiled and used for future licensing through the FDA. Information presented does not represent a recommendation for use but is intended to inform clinicians about the pharmacologic data to consider if patients want to use herbs found in these mixtures. Given the steroid-sparing effects described, some of these mixtures may become fully licensed therapeutics in the future.

- Antiasthma simplified herbal medicine intervention (ASHMI): ASHMI is an approved IND for asthma. Derived from the original 14-herb Chinese formula, it is composed of three herbs (i.e., radix glycyrrhizae [licorice root], radix *Sophorae flavescentis*, and *Ganoderma*) (see Table 102-10).[110-112] Several studies investigating efficacy and tolerability suggest that ASHMI is associated with increased lung function, lowered clinical symptom scores, reduced rescue medication use, and increased interferon-γ (IFN-γ) levels but not with significant adverse effects.[111-115]
- Modified Mai-Men-Dong-Tang (mMMDT): In a study of a 5-herb modified mixture of MMDT used in children, two separate doses led to greater increases in FEV_1 (without a dose-response effect) and improved symptom scores relative to placebo.[116]
- Ding Chuan Tang (DCT): In an RCT in children (18 to 15 years old) with mild to moderate, persistent asthma, a 9-herb DCT mixture used in addition to conventional therapy reduced the severity of airway hyperreactivity and improved clinical and medication scores compared with placebo.[117]
- STA-1: Composed of Mai-Men-Dong-Tang (MMDT, 4 herbs) and Lui-Wei-Di-Huang Wan (LWDHW, 6 herbs), STA-1 represents the originally formulated TCM mixtures developed by Zhang Zhong-Jing (Han Dynasty, 150-219 AD) and Qian Yi (Song Dynasty, 1035-1117 AD), respectively. STA-1 reportedly had clinical benefits in children with mild to moderate asthma; in an RCT of 120 patients between 5 and 20 years of age, twice-daily treatment with STA-1 for 6 months resulted in improved FEV_1 for lung function and reduced symptom scores, systemic corticosteroid dose, and serum total immunoglobulin E levels.[118]

Although herbal medications are lawfully used as dietary supplements, until high-level RCTs are conducted on ASHMI and other herbal medicines, clinicians should continue to follow current pharmaceutical guidelines, possibly with incorporation of herbal therapeutics.

Mechanism of Action

Pharmacologic activity of TCM herbal mixtures targeting allergic inflammation has been described in several studies demonstrating immunomodulation without immunosuppression, suggesting a unique mechanism of action distinct from corticosteroids. With the 3-herb preparation described earlier, studies demonstrate suppression of interleukin-5 (IL-5) production (without affecting IFN-γ or cell viability) and increasing interleukin-10 (IL-10) production after antigen stimulation, consistent with earlier reports by Wen and colleagues.[113,118-120] In the murine model of chronic asthma, the antiinflammatory effect appears to persist after stopping therapy, and this effect is distinct from that of dexamethasone, whose benefits disappear after it is stopped.[119,121] Chang's study of STA-1 in a murine challenge model showed a reduction in the influx of eosinophils and neutrophils in bronchioalveolar lavage fluids and of Dp-induced airway hyperreactivity when treated with the herbal mixture.[122] Other studies suggest STA-1 has an inhibitory effect on early phase airway responses and causes reductions in plasma and bronchoalveolar lavage fluid histamine and leukotriene C_4 levels.[120] Late phase responses are inhibited and airway eosinophils, collagen content, goblet cells, and helper T cell type 2 (Th2) cytokines (e.g. IL-4, IL-5, IL-13) are reduced. However, IFN-γ, IL-10, and transforming growth factor-β levels are increased.

Dosage

The preparations are administered by the oral route in divided doses given two to three times per day. Dosing ranges for selected mixtures are summarized in Table 102-10. However, these specific preparations are not commercially available, and there are no data enabling extrapolation of their dosing to commercially available herbal products.

Side Effects

The herbal mixtures described may cause gastric discomfort. In one study, approximately 5% of patients receiving ASHMI had gastric discomfort compared with 15% of patients receiving prednisone.[113] No clinically significant adverse effects were observed, and no changes in body weight or laboratory study results were identified during more than 3 months of treatment, although the total number of patients in the study was probably too small for identifying rare adverse events.[115]

The market for TCM herbal mixtures is expanding but is poorly regulated. Globally, there are concerns about quality control in manufacturing and whether package labeling accurately depicts contents. In an analysis of the components of 15 Chinese medicine preparations seized by Austrian customs, the herb *Ephedra sinica* was identified, as was the woody vine of *Aristolochia* species, which contains aristolochic acid, a known carcinogen (bladder cancer) and a toxin that can cause liver and kidney damage.[123,124] The medicinal use of this herb may explain reportedly high rates of bladder cancer in Taiwan.[124]

Because of the growing concerns about herb product safety, in April of 2011, the European Commission for Public Health (European Union) launched the Traditional Herbal Medicinal Products Directive (THMPD), requiring more stringent quality control in manufacturing.[125] The stricter rules aim to ensure a better understanding of the products' active ingredients and eliminate those containing potentially harmful or undesirable substances. More than 350 herbal medicines have been licensed for sale under the THMPD requirements. The first product manufactured in China was approved in 2012 and involved a single herb, an extract of rhizomes from Japanese yam (Diao Xin Xue Kang, used for relief of headaches, pain, and cramps) rather than a mixture of herbs.[126]

Indications, Contraindications, and Interactions

Although there is a growing body of evidence to suggest some herbal mixtures may become valuable therapies for asthma and food allergy in the future, there are still safety concerns about some of the products on the market. Patients considering the use of such products should consult with their physicians and obtain trusted information (e.g., NCCAM, FDA MedWatch, NMCD, Natural Standard Database) about any product, including its manufacturing quality controls, ingredients, and potential drug-disease interactions.

HERBAL SUPPLEMENTS

Natural supplements, including herbs, minerals, and vitamins, constitute an expanding market of CAM therapies, and more than 17% of adults and almost 4% of children use them (see Table 102-2). Thousands of herbs and more than 30,000 supplements are on the market, and sales accounted for an estimated \$20 billion in 2006.[127] The DSHEA requires manufacturers to label products as supplements and to include a full list of ingredients. In 2006, the FDA seized \$3 million worth of products containing ephedrine alkaloids from Hi-Tech Pharmaceuticals, a Georgia company that was manufacturing three dietary supplements containing ephedrine, which was banned in 2004 because of health concerns related to its cardiovascular effects (i.e., high blood pressure and irregular heart rhythms). The death of Baltimore Orioles pitcher Steve Belcher due to ephedra intake added to the level of concern.

Ephedra and its variants were the first dietary supplement banned for sale by the FDA under the 1994 DSHEA. Under this law, dietary supplements do not need FDA approval before manufacturing, labeling, distribution, and marketing. The regulation primarily focuses on postmarketing surveillance. For supplements that do not contain a new dietary ingredient (i.e., sold before October 15, 1994), there is no requirement for manufacturers to provide the FDA with evidence about safety of the product before or after marketing.

A 2002 Harris Poll survey of perceptions about regulation and quality control of supplement manufacturing highlighted the public's poor understanding about the levels of safety and efficacy oversight for supplements[127]:

- About 68% of American adults believe the federal government requires supplements to carry warning labels about potential side effects, but this is not true.
- About 59% believe supplements must be approved by a government agency, such as the FDA, before they can be sold, but this is not true.
- About 55% believe supplement manufacturers are not permitted to make claims regarding safety without solid scientific evidence, but this is not true.

TABLE 102-11 Level of Evidence Supporting Efficacy in Allergies and Asthma

Therapy	Latin and Other Names	Evidence Grade for Asthma*	Evidence Grade for Allergies*
Borage seed oil	*Borago officinalis*	C	—
Boswellia	*Boswellia serrata*	B	B
Bromelai	*Ananas comosus, Ananas sativus*	C	B
Buteyko breathing		B	—
Butterbur	*Petasites hybridus*	C	B
Choline		B	C
Coleus	*Coleus forskohlii*	B	Insufficient
Ephedra	*Ephedra sinica*, ma huang	B	C
Grape seed	*Vitis vinifera, Vitis coignetiae*	—	D
Magnesium		B	—
Nasal irrigation		—	B
Omega-3 fatty acids	Fish oil, α-linolenic acid	C	—
Psychotherapy		B	—
Pycnogenol	*Pinus pinaster* subsp. *atlantica* Villar	B	Insufficient
Yoga		A/B	—

Adapted from Natural Standard Database. Review of consensus evidence ratings for CAM therapies for asthma and allergies. Available at www.naturalstandard.com (accessed June 2, 2013).

A, Strong scientific evidence; *B*, good scientific evidence; *C*, unclear or conflicting scientific evidence; *D*, fair to negative scientific evidence; *insufficient*, traditional or theoretical uses lack sufficient evidence.

*The Natural Medicines Comprehensive Database (see Table 102-6) uses different terms and definitions for rating evidence and may be discordant to some degree with the Natural Standard Database ratings.

In 2005, the *Washington Post* purchased five dietary supplements that were labeled as muscle builders and were available over the Internet. All preparations were tested by the independent University of California a Los Angeles Olympic Analytical Laboratory for anabolic steroids, and all five tested positive for designer steroids.

The challenges presented to clinicians and patients searching for unregulated alternative or complementary therapies are immense. Every product recommends that patients discuss the use with their health care provider or physician, but the truth is that providers lack knowledge and time for such consultations, and nondisclosure continues to be common for adults and parents of children with asthma.[15,128]

As shown in Table 102-11, the Natural Standard Database listed *Boswellia* and pycnogenol as having good scientific evidence for the treatment of asthma and allergic disease. The NMCD gave them a lower rating and, only for pycnogenol (derived from pine bark), a possible evidence-based efficacy rating. However, reviews and meta-analyses of the existing literature remain conservative and recommend further study and caution with the use of dietary supplements.[129-131] For patients with asthma who need a nonsteroidal antiinflammatory drug (NSAID) but cannot tolerate them, *Boswellia* may be good option because of its unique mechanism of action and gastrointestinal tract–sparing activity.[129] Figures 102-2 and 102-3 are examples of patient handouts providing information relevant to the use of the herbs *Boswellia* and pycnogenol.[131-133]

Table 102-12 outlines the U.S. government and private independent agencies involved in oversight and quality assurance initiatives for CAM therapies. Trusted resources available to health care professionals and consumers are identified. Navigating these resources to answer patient-specific issues takes some time but can significantly improve the efficacy and safety of integrative medicine care.

Other products of potential interest are outlined in Table 102-10. There is a growing interest in herbs that act as adaptogens. Defined as a new class of metabolic regulators that increase the ability of the organism to adapt to environmental factors and to avoid damage from such agents,"[121] certain herbs are considered powerful immune modulators and of interest for treating a broad range of diseases and symptoms, particularly chronic fatigue.

Summary

Although a growing body of evidence suggests that CMA will enable better quality of care in the future, particularly when considered as a part of integrative personalized medicine, large gaps remain in the high-quality evidence needed to build guidelines for its use in asthma and allergic disease. The challenge for clinicians is navigating in an environment in which patients and their advocates do not want to wait years before accessing therapies that may improve disease control, quality of life, and well-being. Ignoring CAM therapies is no longer an option. The call for personalized medicine that focuses on outcomes requires specialists and primary care physicians to objectively evaluate information and tailor therapy for individual patients. There is an urgent need for better safety surveillance and adverse reaction reporting, particularly in the allergy-immunology community.

INDIAN FRANKINCENSE

What is it?

Indian frankincense is a tree that is native to India and Arabia. It is commonly used in the traditional Indian medicine Ayurveda.

Olibanum is another word for frankincense. It refers to a resin or "sap" that seeps from openings in the bark of several *Boswellia* species, including *Boswellia serrata*, *Boswellia carterii*, and *Boswellia frereana*. Of these, *Boswellia serrata* is most commonly used for medicine.

Indian frankincense is used for osteoarthritis, rheumatoid arthritis, joint pain (rheumatism), bursitis, and tendonitis. Other uses include ulcerative colitis, abdominal pain, asthma, hay fever, sore throat, syphilis, painful menstruation, pimples, and cancer. Indian frankincense is also used as a stimulant, to increase urine flow, and for stimulating menstrual flow.

In manufacturing, Indian frankincense resin oil and extracts are used in soaps, cosmetics, foods, and beverages.

Is it Effective?

Natural Medicines Comprehensive Database rates effectiveness based on scientific evidence according to the following scale: *Effective, Likely Effective, Possibly Effective, Possibly Ineffective, Likely Ineffective, Ineffective,* and *Insufficient Evidence to Rate.*

The effectiveness ratings for **INDIAN FRANKINCENSE** are as follows:

Possibly Effective for...

- **Osteoarthritis.** Some studies show that taking certain extracts of Indian frankincense (5-Loxin, Aflapin) can reduce pain and improve mobility in people with osteoarthritis in joints. Research shows that it might decrease joint pain by 32% to 65%.
- **Ulcerative colitis.** Taking Indian frankincense seems to improve symptoms of ulcerative colitis in some people. For some people, Indian frankincense seems to work as well as the prescription drug sulfasalazine. Some research shows that it can induce disease remission in 70% to 82% of people.

Insufficient Evidence to Rate Effectiveness for...

- **Asthma.** Developing evidence suggests that taking Indian frankincense extract might help asthma.
- **Rheumatoid arthritis (RA).** Research results are mixed so far about the effectiveness of Indian frankincense in the treatment of RA.
- **Crohn's disease.** There is some evidence that taking Indian frankincense extract might reduce symptoms of Crohn's disease, but research findings have been inconsistent.
- **Other conditions.**

More evidence is needed to rate Indian frankincense for these uses.

How does it work?

The resin of Indian frankincense contains substances that may decrease inflammation.

Are there safety concerns?

Indian frankincense is **LIKELY SAFE** for most adults.

Indian frankincense usually doesn't cause important side effects. However, some people who took it reported stomach pain, nausea, and diarrhea. When applied to the skin, it can cause allergic rash.

Special Precautions & Warnings:

Pregnancy and breast-feeding: Indian frankincense is **LIKELY SAFE** when used in amounts commonly found in foods. But don't use it in the larger amounts needed for medicinal effects. Not enough is known about the safety of using Indian frankincense in these amounts during pregnancy or breast-feeding.

Are there any interactions with medications?

It is not known if this product interacts with any medicines.Before taking this product, talk with your health professional if you take any medications.

Are there any interactions with Herbs and Supplements?

There are no known interactions with herbs and supplements.

Are there interactions with Foods?

There are no known interactions with foods.

Figure 102-2 *Boswellia* (Indian frankincense) consumer information and education. *(Adapted from the Natural Medicines Comprehensive Database. Indian frankincense monograph. Available at http://naturaldatabase.therapeuticresearch.com/nd/Search.aspx?cs=&s=nd&pt=100&id=63 [accessed May 30, 2013].)*

Continued

What dose is used?

The following doses have been studied in scientific research:

BY MOUTH:

- **Osteoarthritis:** 100–250 mg daily of a specific extract (5-Loxin); 100 mg daily of another specific extract (Aflapin); 333 mg daily of another specific extract.
- **Ulcerative colitis:** 300–350 mg three times daily.

What other names is the product known by?

Arbre à Encens, Arbre à Oliban Indien, Boswella, Boswellia, Boswellia serrata, Boswellie, Boswellin, Boswellin Serrata Resin, Encens Indien, Franquincienso, Gajabhakshya, Indian Olibanum, Oliban Indien, Resina Boswelliae, Ru Xiang, Salai Guggal, Salai Guggul, Sallaki Guggul, Shallaki.

This monograph was last reviewed on 04/13/2012 and last updated on 04/13/2012. Monographs are reviewed and/or updated multiple times per month and at least once per year.

Figure 102-2, cont'd

TABLE 102-12 Agencies and Resources Supporting Independent Review of Complementary and Alternative Therapies

Resource	Link	Description
American National Standards Institute (ANSI)	www.ansi.org	Since 1918, private, not-for-profit organization that provides accreditation of globally recognized programs (used by NSF certification program)
ConsumerLab	www.consumerlab.com/aboutcl.asp	Subscription fee–based private testing and certification of health products; affiliated with PharmacyChecker.com, MedicareDrugPlans.com
Food and Drug Administration (FDA) MedWatch	www.fda.gov/Safety/MedWatch/SafetyInformation/default.htm	Department of Health and Human Services; national passive adverse event reporting system databases that are searchable by the public; gateway for clinically important safety information with human products
DailyMed (National Library of Medicine)	dailymed.nlm.nih.gov/dailymed/about.cfm	Current drug prescribing information for licensed products only; FDA-approved safety information
National Center for Complementary and Alternative Medicine (NCCAM)	nccam.nih.gov	National Institutes of Health (NIH) based; provides information, education, and research support for improved evidenced-based complementary and alternative medicine (CAM) use
National Sanitation Foundation (NSF) International	www.nsf.org	Not-for-profit; since 1944, provides standards for development, product certification, auditing, education, and risk management services; developed more than 75 public health and safety American national standards plus international standards
Natural Medicines Comprehensive Database (NMCD)	naturaldatabase.therapeuticresearch.co	Nonprofit, evidence-based educational database supporting rapid access to most recent information on safety, efficacy, and commercial product quality assessments with standardized ratings; professional monographs targeting health care providers and workers issued by editors of *Prescriber's Letter*
NMCD Consumer Version	naturaldatabaseconsumer.therapeuticresearch.com	Provides product information in a language and format supporting lay public and patient education about CAM therapies
Natural MedWatch (NCMD and FDA partnership)	naturaldatabase.therapeuticresearch.com/nd/adverseevent.asp	Public access for facilitated and improved quality reporting of CAM adverse events under a private-government partnership
FDA medication guides	www.fda.gov/Drugs/DrugSafety/ucm085729.htm	Paper handouts that come with prescription drugs; NMCD provides comparable tools for CAM therapies
Natural Standard Database	www.naturalstandard.com	Nonprofit founded by a group of physicians at Harvard Medical School to provide decision-support tools for providers, insurers, and consumers; different standardized rating classification from that of NCMD

PYCNOGENOL

What is it?

Pycnogenol is the US registered trademark name for a product derived from the pine bark of a tree known as *Pinus pinaster*. The active ingredients in pycnogenol can also be extracted from other sources, including peanut skin, grape seed, and witch hazel bark.

Pycnogenol is used for treating circulation problems, allergies, asthma, ringing in the ears, high blood pressure, muscle soreness, pain, osteoarthritis, diabetes, attention deficit-hyperactivity disorder (ADHD), a disease of the female reproductive system called endometriosis, menopausal symptoms, painful menstrual periods, erectile dysfunction (ED), and an eye disease called retinopathy.

It is also used for preventing disorders of the heart and blood vessels, including stroke, heart disease, and varicose veins.

Pycnogenol is used to slow the aging process, maintain healthy skin, improve athletic endurance, and improve male fertility.

Some people use skin creams that contain pycnogenol as "anti-aging" products.

Is it Effective?

Natural Medicines Comprehensive Database rates effectiveness based on scientific evidence according to the following scale: *Effective, Likely Effective, Possibly Effective, Possibly Ineffective, Likely Ineffective, Ineffective,* and *Insufficient Evidence to Rate.*

The effectiveness ratings for **PYCNOGENOL** are as follows:

Possibly Effective for...

Allergies. Some research in people with allergies to birch shows that taking pycnogenol starting before allergy season begins might reduce allergy symptoms.
Circulation problems. Taking pycnogenol by mouth seems to significantly reduce leg pain and heaviness, as well as fluid retention in people with circulation problems. Some people use horse chestnut seed extract to treat this condition, but pycnogenol alone appears to be more effective.
Disease of the retina in the eye. Taking pycnogenol daily for two months seems to slow or prevent further worsening of retinal disease caused by diabetes, atherosclerosis, or other diseases. It also seems to improve eyesight.
Improved endurance in athletes. Young people (age 20-35) seem to be able to exercise on a treadmill for a longer time after taking pycnogenol daily for about a month.
High blood pressure. Pycnogenol seems to lower systolic blood pressure (the first number in a blood pressure reading) but does not significantly lower diastolic blood pressure (the second number).
Asthma in children.
Varicose veins.

Possibly Ineffective for...

Attention deficit-hyperactivity disorder (ADHD).

Insufficient Evidence to Rate Effectiveness for...

Blood clots in the vein (deep vein thrombosis, DVT). There is some evidence that taking a specific combination product (Flite Tabs) might help to prevent DVT during long-haul plane flights. The product combines a blend of 150 mg of pycnogenol plus nattokinase. Two capsules are taken 2 hours before the flight and then again 6 hours later.
High cholesterol. Pycnogenol seems to lower "bad cholesterol" (low-density lipoprotein (LDL) cholesterol).
Pelvic pain in women. There is preliminary evidence that pycnogenol might help reduce pelvic pain in women with endometriosis or severe menstrual cramps.
Pain in late pregnancy. Preliminary research suggests that taking 30 mg of pycnogenol daily reduces lower back pain, hip joint pain, pelvic pain, and pain due to varicose veins or calf cramps in the last three months of pregnancy.
Erectile dysfunction (ED). Limited research suggests pycnogenol, used alone or in combination with L-arginine, might improve sexual function in men with ED. It seems to take up to three months of treatment for significant improvement.
Aging.
Heart disease.
Stroke prevention.
Muscle soreness.
Leg cramps.
Circulation problems in diabetes.
Osteoarthritis.
Menopausal symptoms.
Ringing in the ears (tinnitus).
Other conditions.

More evidence is needed to rate pycnogenol for these uses.

Figure 102-3 Pycnogenol consumer information and education. *(Adapted from the Natural Medicines Comprehensive Database. Pycnogenol monograph. Available at http://naturaldatabase.therapeuticresearch.com/nd/Search.aspx?cs=&s=nd&pt=100&id=1019 [accessed May 30, 2013].)*

Continued

How does it work?

Pycnogenol contains substances that might improve blood flow. It might also stimulate the immune system and have antioxidant effects.

Are there safety concerns?

Pycnogenol is **POSSIBLY SAFE** when taken in doses of 50 mg to 450 mg daily for up to 6 months. Pycnogenol can cause dizziness, gut problems, headache, and mouth ulcers.
Special Precautions & Warnings: Pregnancy and breast-feeding: Preliminary research suggests pycnogenol might be safe in late pregnancy. But until more is known, pycnogenol should be avoided by women who are pregnant or breast-feeding.

"Auto-immune diseases" such as multiple sclerosis (MS), lupus (systemic lupus erythematosus, SLE), rheumatoid arthritis (RA), or other conditions: Pycnogenol might cause the immune system to become more active, and this could increase the symptoms of auto-immune diseases. If you have one of these conditions, it's best to avoid using pycnogenol.

Are there any interactions with medications?

Medications that decrease the immune system (Immunosuppressants)
Interaction Rating = Moderate be cautious with this combination.
Talk with your health provider.

Pycnogenol seems to increase the immune system. By increasing the immune system, pycnogenol might decrease the effectiveness of medications that decrease the immune system.

Some medications that decrease the immune system include azathioprine (Imuran), basiliximab (Simulect), cyclosporine (Neoral, Sandimmune), daclizumab (Zenapax), muromonab-CD3 (OKT3, Orthoclone OKT3), mycophenolate (CellCept), tacrolimus (FK506, Prograf), sirolimus (Rapamune), prednisone (Deltasone, Orasone), corticosteroids (glucocorticoids), and others.

Are there any interactions with Herbs and Supplements?

There are no known interactions with herbs and supplements.

Are there interactions with Foods?

There are no known interactions with foods.

What dose is used?

The following doses have been studied in scientific research:

BY MOUTH:

For allergies: 50 mg twice daily.
For asthma in children: 1 mg per pound of body weight given in two divided doses.
For poor circulation: 45–360 mg daily, or 50–100 mg three times daily.
For diseases of the retina, including those related to diabetes: 50 mg three times daily.
For mild high blood pressure: 200 mg of pycnogenol daily.
For improving exercise capacity in athletes: 200 mg daily.

What other names is the product known by?

Condensed Tannins, Écorce de Pin, Écorce de Pin Maritime, Extrait d'Écorce de Pin, French Marine Pine Bark Extract, French Maritime Pine Bark Extract, Leucoanthocyanidins, Maritime Bark Extract, Oligomères de Procyanidine, Oligomères Procyanidoliques, Oligomeric Proanthocyanidins, OPC, OPCs, PCO, PCOs, Pine Bark, Pine Bark Extract, Pinus pinaster, Pinus maritima, Proanthocyanidines Oligomériques, Procyanidin Oligomers, Procyanodolic Oligomers, Pycnogénol, Pygenol, Tannins Condensés.

This monograph was last reviewed on 08/15/2011 and last updated on 08/15/2011. Monographs are reviewed and/or updated multiple times per month and at least once per year.

Figure 102-3, cont'd

REFERENCES

Background

1. Barnes PM, Bloom B, Nahin RL. Complementary and alternative medicine use among adults and children: United States, 2007. Natl Health Stat Rep 2008;12:1-24. Available at http://nccam.nih.gov/sites/nccam.nih.gov/files/news/nhsr12.pdf (accessed June 2, 2013).
2. Nahin RL, Barnes PM, Stussman BA, Bloom B. Costs of complementary and alternative medicine (CAM) and frequency of visits to CAM practitioners: United States, 2007. Natl Health Stat Report 2009;18:1-15. Available at http://nccam.nih.gov/news/camstats/costs/nhsrn18.pdf (accessed June 2, 2013).
3. Engler RJ, With CM, Gregory PJ, Jellin JM. Complementary and alternative medicine for the allergist-immunologist: where do I start? J Allergy Clin Immunol 2009;123:309-16.
4. Gahche J, Bailey R, Burt V, et al; National Center for Health Statistics (NCHS). Dietary supplement use among U.S. adults has increased since NHANES III (1988-1994). Data Brief 2011;61:1-8. Available at http://www.cdc.gov/nchs/data/databriefs/db61.pdf (accessed June 2, 2013).
5. Shaikh U, Byrd RS, Auinger P. Vitamin and mineral supplement use by children and adolescents in the 1999-2004 National Health and Nutrition Examination Survey: relationship with nutrition, food security, physical activity, and health care access. Arch Pediatr Adolesc Med 2009;163:150-7. Available at www.ncbi.nlm.nih.gov/pmc/articles/PMC2996491/?tool=pubmed (accessed June 2, 2013).
6. World Health Organization. Guidelines on developing consumer information for the proper use of traditional, complementary, and alternative medicine, 2004. Available at http://apps.who.int/medicinedocs/pdf/s5525e/s5525e.pdf (accessed June 2, 2013).
7. Yakirevitch A, Bedrin L, Migirov L, Wolf M, Talmi YP. Use of alternative medicine in Israeli chronic rhinosinusitis patients. J Otolaryngol Head Neck Surg 2009;38:517-20.
8. Newton JR, Santangeli L, Shakeel M, Ram B. Use of complementary and alternative medicine by patients attending a rhinology outpatient clinic. Am J Rhinol Allergy 2009;23:59-63.
9. Schäfer T. Epidemiology of complementary alternative medicine for asthma and allergy in Europe and Germany. Ann Allergy Asthma Immunol 2004;93:S5-10.
10. Ko J, Lee JI, Muñoz-Furlong A, Li X-m, Sicherer SH. Use of complementary and alternative medicine by food-allergic patients. Ann Allergy Asthma Immunol 2006;97:365-9.
11. Sibbritt D, Adams J, Lui CW, Broom A. Health services use among young Australian women with allergies, hay fever and sinusitis: a longitudinal analysis. Complement Ther Med 2012;20:135-42.
12. Freidin B, Timmermans S. Complementary and alternative medicine for children's asthma: satisfaction, care provider responsiveness, and networks of care. Qual Health Res 2008;18:43-55.
13. Schäfer T, Riehle A, Wichmann HE, Ring J. Alternative medicine and allergies: life satisfaction, health locus of control and quality of life. J Psychosom Res 2003;55:543-6.
14. Shaw A, Noble A, Salisbury C, et al. Predictors of complementary therapy use among asthma patients: results of a primary care survey. Health Soc Care Community 2008;16:155-64.
15. Sidora-Arcoleo K, Yoos HL, Kitzman H, McMullen A, Anson E. Don't ask, don't tell: parental nondisclosure of complementary and alternative medicine and over-the-counter medication use in children's asthma management. J Pediatric Health Care 2008;22:221-9.
16. Ostermann T, Krummenauer F, Heusser P, Boehm K. Health economic evaluation in complementary medicine: development within the last decades concerning local origin and quality. Complement Ther Med 2011;19:289-302.
17. Knoeller GE, Mazurek JM, Moorman JE. Complementary and alternative medicine use among adults with work-related and non-work-related asthma. J Asthma 2012;49:107-13.
18. U.S. Department of Health and Human Services, National Institutes of Health, National Center for Complementary and Alternative Medicine. Herbs at a glance: a quick guide to herbal supplements. Available at http://nccam.nih.gov/sites/nccam.nih.gov/files/herbs/NIH_Herbs_at_a_Glance.pdf (accessed June 2, 2013).
19. US Food and Drug Administration (FDA). Dietary Supplement Health and Education Act of 1994. Available at www.fda.gov/RegulatoryInformation/Legislation/FederalFoodDrugandCosmeticActFDCAct/SignificantAmendmentstotheFDCAct/ucm148003.htm?utm_campaign=Google2&utm_source=fdaSearch&utm_medium=website&utm_term=DSHEA&utm_content=1 (accessed June 2, 2013).
20. Natural Medicines Comprehensive Database. Clinical review series: natural medicines in the clinical management of allergic rhinitis. Available at http://naturaldatabase.therapeuticresearch.com (accessed June 2, 2013).
21 Natural Medicines Comprehensive Database. Clinical review series: natural medicines in the clinical management of asthma. Available at http://naturaldatabase.therapeuticresearch.com (accessed June 2, 2013).
22. Garavello W, DiBerardino F, Romagnoli M, et al. Nasal rinsing with hypertonic solution: an adjunctive treatment for pediatric seasonal allergic rhinoconjunctivitis. Int Arch Allergy Immunol 2005;137:310-14.
23. Slader CA, Reddel HK, Jenkins CR, et al. Complementary and alternative medicine use in asthma: who is using what? Respirology 2006;11:373-87.
24. Chapman KR, McIvor A. Asthma that is unresponsive to usual care. CMAJ 2010;182:45-52.
25. Garavello W, Romagnoli M, Sordo L, et al. Hypersaline nasal irrigation in children with symptomatic seasonal allergic rhinitis: a randomized study. Pediatr Allergy Immunol 2003;14:140-3.
26. Rabago D, Zgierska A, Mundt M, et al. Efficacy of daily hypertonic saline nasal irrigation among patients with sinusitis: a randomized controlled trial. J Fam Pract 2002;51:1049-55.
27. Satdhabudha A, Poachanukoon O. Efficacy of buffered hypertonic saline nasal irrigation in children with symptomatic allergic rhinitis: a randomized double-blind study. Int J Pediatr Otorhinolaryngol 2012;76:583-8.
28. Neuman I, Nahum H, Ben-Amotz A. Prevention of exercise-induced asthma by a natural isomer mixture of beta-carotene. Ann Allergy Asthma Immunol 1999;82:549-53.
29. Food Standards Agency. Medicines and Healthcare Products Regulatory Agency (MHRA) expert group on vitamins and minerals. Available at http://www.foodstandards.gov.uk (accessed June 2, 2013).
30. Bjelakovic G, Nikolova D, Gluud LL, et al. Mortality in randomized trials of antioxidant supplements for primary and secondary prevention: systematic review and meta-analysis. JAMA 2007;297:842-57.
31. Schürks M, Glynn RJ, Rist PM, Tzourio C, Kurth T. Effects of vitamin E on stroke subtypes: meta-analysis of randomised controlled trials. BMJ 2010;341:c5702.
32. Bin Q, Hu X, Cao Y, Gao F. Feng Gao, The role of vitamin E (tocopherol) supplementation in the prevention of stroke. A meta-analysis of 13 randomised controlled trials. Thromb Haemost 2011;105:579-85.
33. Bjelakovic G, Nikolova D, Gluud LL, Simonetti RG, Gluud C. Antioxidant supplements for prevention of mortality in healthy participants and patients with various diseases. Cochrane Database Syst Rev 2012;(3):CD007176.
34. Chiou WB, Yang CC, Wan CS. Ironic effects of dietary supplementation: illusory invulnerability created by taking dietary supplements licenses health-risk behaviors. Psychol Sci 2011:22: 1081-6.
35. National Center for Environmental Health Division of Laboratory Sciences. Second national report on biochemical indicators of diet and nutrition in the U.S. Population, 2012: executive summary. Available at http://www.cdc.gov/nutritionreport/pdf/ExeSummary_Web_032612.pdf#zoom=100 (accessed June 2, 2013).
36. Ng DK, Chow PY, Ming SP, e al. A double-blind, randomized, placebo-controlled trial of acupuncture for the treatment of childhood persistent allergic rhinitis. Pediatrics 2004;114:1242-7.
37. Brehm JM, Schuemann B, Fuhlbrigge AL, et al; Childhood Asthma Management Program Research Group. Serum vitamin D levels and severe asthma exacerbations in the Childhood Asthma Management Program study. J Allergy Clin Immunol 2010;126:52-8.e5.
38. Prescott S, Nowak-Węgrzyn A. Strategies to prevent or reduce allergic disease. Ann Nutr Metab 2011;59(Suppl 1):28-42.

Alternative Medical Systems

39. Natural Medicines Comprehensive Database. Monograph on acupuncture. Available at http://naturaldatabase.therapeuticresearch.com (accessed June 2, 2013).
40. Witt CM, Brinkhaus B. Efficacy, effectiveness and cost-effectiveness of acupuncture for allergic rhinitis—an overview about previous and ongoing studies. Auton Neurosci 2010;157:42-5.
41. Brinkhaus B, Witt CM, Ortiz M, et al. Acupuncture in seasonal allergic rhinitis (ACUSAR)—design and protocol of a randomised controlled multi-centre trial. Forsch Komplementmed 2010;17:95-102.
42. Xue CC, Zhang CS, Yang AW, et al. Semi-self-administered ear acupressure for persistent allergic rhinitis: a randomised sham controlled trial. Ann Allergy Asthma Immunol 2011;106:168-70.

43. Scheewe S, Vogt L, Minakawa S, et al. Acupuncture in children and adolescents with bronchial asthma: a randomised controlled study. Complement Ther Med 2011;19:239-46.
44. Choi JY, Jung HJ, Kim JI, et al. A randomized pilot study of acupuncture as an adjunct therapy in adult asthmatic patients. J Asthma 2010;47:774-80.
45. Ngai SP, Jones AY, Hui-Chan CW, Ko FW, Hui DS. Effect of Acu-TENS on post-exercise expiratory lung volume in subjects with asthma—a randomized controlled trial. Respir Physiol Neurobiol 2009;167:348-53.
46. Wechsler ME, Kelley JM, Boyd IO, et al. Active albuterol or placebo, sham acupuncture, or no intervention in asthma. N Engl J Med 2011; 365:119-26.
47. Pfab F, Huss-Marp J, Gatti A, et al. Influence of acupuncture on type I hypersensitivity itch and the wheal and flare response in adults with atopic eczema—a blinded, randomized, placebo-controlled, crossover trial. Allergy 2010;65:903-10.
48. Pfab F, Kirchner MT, Huss-Marp J, et al. Acupuncture compared with oral antihistamine for type I hypersensitivity itch and skin response in adults with atopic dermatitis: a patient- and examiner-blinded, randomized, placebo-controlled, crossover trial. Allergy 2012;67:566-73.
49. National Center for Complementary and Alternative Medicine, National Institute of Health. Acupuncture for pain. Available at http://nccam.nih.gov/health/acupuncture/acupuncture-for-pain.htm (accessed June 2, 2013).
50. Leung WW, Jones AY, Ng SS, Wong CY, Lee JF. Electroacupuncture in reduction of discomfort associated with barostat-induced rectal distension–a randomized controlled study. J Gastrointest Surg 2011;15:660-6.
51. Pfab F, Athanasiadis GI, Huss-Marp J, et al. Effect of acupuncture on allergen-induced basophil activation in patients with atopic eczema: a pilot trial. J Altern Complement Med 2011;17:309-14.
52. Jindal V, Ge A, Mansky PJ. Safety and efficacy of acupuncture in children: a review of the evidence. J Pediatr Hematol Oncol 2008;30: 431-42.
53. National Center for Complementary and Alternative Medicine. Ayurvedic medicine: an Introduction. Available at http://nccam.nih.gov/sites/nccam.nih.gov/files/D287_BKG.pdf (accessed June 2, 2013).
54. Hankey A. The scientific value of Ayurveda. J Altern Complement Med 2005;11:221-5.
55. Patwardhan B, Warude D, Pushpangadan P, Bhatt N. Ayurveda and traditional Chinese medicine: a comparative overview. Evid Based Complement Alternat Med 2005;2:465-73.
56. Sridharan K, Mohan R, Ramaratnam S, Panneerselvam D. Ayurvedic treatments for diabetes mellitus. Cochrane Database Syst Rev 2011;(12):CD008288.
57. Ernst E. Homeopathy: what does the "best" evidence tell us? Med J Aust 2010;192:458-60.
58. US Food and Drug Administration (FDA). Loss of sense of smell with intranasal cold remedies containing zinc. Public health advisory, June 16, 2009. Available at: http://www.fda.gov/Drugs/DrugSafety/PublicHealthAdvisories/ucm166059.htm (accessed June 2, 2013).
59. Jong MC, Jong MU, Baars EW. Adverse drug reactions to anthroposophic and homeopathic solutions for injection: a systematic evaluation of German pharmacovigilance databases. Pharmacoepidemiol Drug Saf 2012;21:1295-301.
60. Gunturu KS, Gunturu KS, Nagarajan P, et al. Ayurvedic herbal medicine and lead poisoning. J Hematol Oncol 2011;4:51.
61. National Center for Complementary and Alternative Medicine. Homeopathy: an introduction. Available at http://nccam.nih.gov/health/homeopathy (accessed June , 2013).
62. Natural Medicines Comprehensive Database. Monograph on homeopathy. Available at http://naturaldatabase.therapeuticresearch.com (accessed June2, 2013).
63. Borneman JP, Field RI. Regulation of homeopathic products. Am J Health Syst Pharm 2006;63:86-91.
64. Walach H, Jonas WB, Ives J, et al. Research on homeopathy: state of the art. J Altern Complement Med 2005;11:813-29.

Manipulation and Body-Based Therapies

65. Natural Medicines Comprehensive Database. Monograph on chiropractic. http://naturaldatabase.therapeuticresearch.com/nd/Search.aspx?cs=DOD&s=ND&pt=100&id=1211&ds=&name=CHIROPRACTIC&lang=0&searchid=35441264 (accessed June 2, 2013).
66. Balon JW, Mior SA. Chiropractic care in asthma and allergy. Ann Allergy Asthma Immunol 2004;93(Suppl 1):S55-60.
67. Henley CE, Ivins D, Mills M, Wen FK, Benjamin BA. Osteopathic manipulation treatment and its relationship to autonomic nervous system activity as demonstrated by heart rate variability: a repeated measures study. Osteopath Med Prim Care 2008;2:7-15.
68. Jäkel A, von Hauenschild P. Therapeutic effects of cranial osteopathic manipulative medicine: a systematic review. J Am Osteopath Assoc 2011;111:685-93.
69. Shi X, Rehrer S, Prajapati P, et al. Effect of cranial osteopathic manipulative medicine on cerebral tissue oxygenation. J Am Osteopath Assoc 2011;111:660-6.
70. Hurwitz EL, Morgenstern H, Vassilaki M, Chiang LM. Frequency and clinical predictors of adverse reactions to chiropractic care in the UCLA neck pain study. Spine 2005;30: 1477-84.
71. Rubinstein SM, Leboeuf-Yde C, Knol DL, et al. The benefits outweigh the risks for patients undergoing chiropractic care for neck pain: a prospective, multicenter, cohort study. J Manipulative Physiol Ther 2007;30:408-18.
72. Reuter U, Hämling M, Kavuk I, et al. Vertebral artery dissections after chiropractic neck manipulation in Germany over three years. J Neurol 2006;253:724-30.
73. Whedon JM, Quebada PB, Roberts DW, Radwan TA. Spinal epidural hematoma after spinal manipulative therapy in a patient undergoing anticoagulant therapy: a case report. J Manipulative Physiol Ther 2006;29:582-5.
74. Klougart N, Leboeuf-Yde C, Rasmussen LR. Safety in chiropractic practice. Part I: the occurrence of cerebrovascular accidents after manipulation to the neck in Denmark from 1978-1988. J Manipulative Physiol Ther 1996; 19:371-7.
75. Hurwitz EL, Aker PD, Adams AH, et al. Manipulation and mobilization of the cervical spine. A systematic review of the literature. Spine 1996;21:1746-59.
76. Dvorak J, Orelli F. How dangerous is manipulation of the cervical spine: case report and results of a survey. Manual Med 1985;2:1-4.
77. Ernst E. Ophthalmological adverse effects of (chiropractic) upper spinal manipulation: evidence from recent case reports. Acta Ophthalmol Scand 2005;83:581-5.
78. Vohra S, Johnston BC, Cramer K, Humphreys K. Adverse events associated with pediatric spinal manipulation: a systematic review. Pediatrics 2007;119:e275-83.
79. Stuber KJ, Wynd S, Weis CA. Adverse events from spinal manipulation in the pregnant and postpartum periods: a critical review of the literature. Chiropr Man Therap 2012; 8:20. Full article can be accessed free at http://www.ncbi.nlm.nih.gov/pmc/articles/PMC3348005/.
80. Natural Standard Database. Review of evidence ratings for CAM therapies for asthma and allergies. Available at www.naturalstandard.com (accessed June 2, 2013).
81. Geiringer SR, deLateur BJ. Physiatric therapeutics. 3. Traction, manipulation, and massage. Arch Phys Med Rehabil 1990;71: S264–6.
82. Ernst E. The safety of massage therapy. Rheumatology 2003;42:1101-6.
83. Field T, Henteleff T, Hernandez-Reif M, et al. Children with asthma have improved pulmonary functions after massage therapy. J Pediatr 1998;132:854-8.
84. Fattah MA, Hamdy B. Pulmonary functions of children with asthma improve following massage therapy. J Altern Complement Med 2011;17:1065-8.
85. Hondras MA, Linde K, Jones AP. Manual therapy for asthma. Cochrane Database Syst Rev 2005;(2):CD001002.
86. Field T, Hernandez-Reif M, Diego M, Schanberg S, Kuhn C. Cortisol decreases and serotonin and dopamine increase following massage therapy. Int J Neurosci 2005;115: 1397-413.
87. Listing M, Krohn M, Liezmann C, et al. The efficacy of classical massage on stress perception and cortisol following primary treatment of breast cancer. Arch Womens Ment Health 2010;13:165-73.
88. Crane JD, Ogborn DI, Cupido C, et al. Massage therapy attenuates inflammatory signaling after exercise-induced muscle damage. Sci Transl Med 2012;4:119ra13. doi:10.1126/scitranslmed.3002882. PubMed PMID: 22301554.

Mind-Body Therapies

89. Natural Medicines Comprehensive Database. Monograph on meditation. Available at http://naturaldatabase.therapeuticresearch.com/nd/Search.aspx?cs=DOD&s=ND&pt=9&Product=Meditation (accessed June 2, 2013).
90. National Center for Complementary and Alternative Medicine. Meditation: an introduction. Available at http://nccam.nih.gov/health/meditation/overview.htm (accessed June 2, 2013).
91. Huntley A, White AR, Ernst E. Relaxation therapies for asthma: a systematic review. Thorax 2002;57:127-31.
92. Manocha R, Marks GB, Kenchington P, Peters D, Salome CM. Sahaja yoga in the management of moderate to severe asthma: a randomised controlled trial. Thorax 2002;57: 110-15.
93. Singh V, Wisniewski A, Britton J, et al. Effect of yoga breathing exercises (pranayama) on airway reactivity in subjects with asthma. Lancet 1990;335:1381-3.

94. Johnson DB, Tierney MJ, Sadighi PJ. Kapalabhati pranayama: breath of fire or cause of pneumothorax? A case report. Chest 2004;125: 1951-2.
95. National Center for Complementary and Alternative Medicine. Clinical digest: asthma and complementary health practices, 2012. Available at nccam.nih.gov/health/providers/digest/asthma-science (accessed June 2, 2013).
96. Burgess J, Ekanayake B, Lowe A, et al. Systematic review of the effectiveness of breathing retraining in asthma management. Expert Rev Respir Med 2011;5:789-807.
97. Thomas M, McKinley RK, Mellor S, et al. Breathing exercises for asthma: a randomised controlled trial. Thorax 2009;64:55-61.
98. Slader CA, Reddel HK, Spencer LM, et al. Double blind randomised controlled trial of two different breathing techniques in the management of asthma. Thorax 2006;61:651-6.
99. Holloway EA, West RJ. Integrated breathing and relaxation training (the Papworth method) for adults with asthma in primary care: a randomised controlled trial. Thorax 2007;62: 1039-42.
100. Cowie RL, Conley DP, Underwood MF, Reader PG. A randomised controlled trial of the Buteyko technique as an adjunct to conventional management of asthma. Respir Med 2008;102:726-32.
101. Bowler SD, Green A, Mitchell CA. Buteyko breathing techniques in asthma: a blinded randomised controlled trial. Med J Aust 1998;169: 575-8.
102. Berlowitz D, Denehy L, Johns DP, Bish RM, Walters EH. The Buteyko asthma breathing technique. Med J Aust 1995;162:53.
103. Opat AJ, Cohen MM, Bailey MJ, Abramson MJ. A clinical trial of the Buteyko breathing technique in asthma as taught by a video. J Asthma 2000;37:557-64.

Biologically Based Therapies

104. Natural Medicines Comprehensive Database. Monograph on traditional Chinese medicine. Available at http://naturaldatabase.therapeuticresearch.com/nd/Search.aspx?pt=100&id=1202&ds=&name=TRADITIONAL+CHINESE+MEDICINE&lang=0&searchid=35463131&cs=dod&s=ND (accessed June 2, 201).
105. National Center for Complementary and Alternative Medicine. Traditional Chinese medicine: an introduction. Available at http://nccam.nih.gov/health/whatiscam/chinesemed.htm (accessed June 2, 2013.).
106. US Food and Drug Administration (FDA), Center for Drug Evaluation and Research. Guidance for industry botanical drug products, 2004. Available at http://www.fda.gov/downloads/Drugs/GuidanceCompliance RegulatoryInformation/Guidances/ucm070491.pdf (accessed June 2, 2013).
107. Lu AP, Jia HW, Xiao C, Lu QP. Theory of traditional Chinese medicine and therapeutic method of diseases. World J Gastroenterol 2004;10:1854-56.
108. Huang KC. The pharmacology of Chinese herbs. 2nd ed. Boca Raton, Fla.: CRC Press; 1999.
109. Ernst E, Pittler MH, Stevinson C, White A, editors. The desktop guide to complementary and alternative medicine: an evidence-based approach. New York: Mosby; 2001.
110. Li XM, Huang CK, Zhang TF, et al. The Chinese herbal medicine formula MSSM-002 suppresses allergic airway hyperreactivity and modulates TH1/TH2 responses in a murine model of allergic asthma. J Allergy Clin Immunol 2000;106:660-8.
111. Li XM. Traditional Chinese herbal remedies for asthma and food allergy. J Allergy Clin Immunol 2007;120:25-31.
112. Busse PJ, Schofield B, Birmingham N, et al. The traditional Chinese herbal formula ASHMI inhibits allergic lung inflammation in antigen-sensitized and antigen-challenged aged mice. Ann Allergy Asthma Immunol 2010;104: 236-46.
113 Wen MC, Wei CH, Hu ZQ, et al. Efficacy and tolerability of anti-asthma herbal medicine intervention in adult patients with moderate-severe allergic asthma. J Allergy Clin Immunol 2005;116:517-24.
114. Li XM, Brown L. Efficacy and mechanisms of action of traditional Chinese medicines for treating asthma and allergy. J Allergy Clin Immunol 2009;123:297-306.
115. Kelly-Pieper K, Patil SP, Busse P, et al. Safety and tolerability of an antiasthma herbal formula (ASHMI™) in adult asthmatics: a randomized, double-blinded, placebo-controlled, dose escalation phase I study. J Altern Complement Med 2009;15:735-43.
116. Hsu CH, Lu CM, Chang TT. Efficacy and safety of modified Mai-Men-Dong-Tang for treatment of allergic asthma. Pediatr Allergy Immunol 2005;16:76-81.
117. Chan CK, Kuo ML, Shen JJ, et al. Ding Chuan Tang, a Chinese herb decoction, could improve airway hyper-responsiveness in stabilized asthmatic children: a randomized, double-blind clinical trial. Pediatr Allergy Immunol 2006; 17:316-22.
118. Chang TT, Huang CC, Hsu CH. Clinical evaluation of the Chinese herbal medicine formula STA-1 in the treatment of allergic asthma. Phytother Res 2006;20:342-7.
119. Srivastava K, Sampson H, Li X. The anti-asthma Chinese herbal formula ASHMI provides more persistent benefits than dexamethasone in a murine asthma model. J Allergy Clin Immunol 2011;127:AB261.
120. Zhang T, Srivastava K, Wen MC, et al. Pharmacology and immunological actions of a herbal medicine ASHMI on allergic asthma. Phytother Res 2010;24:1047-55.
121. Panossian A, Wikman G, Wagner H. Plant adaptogens. III. Earlier and more recent aspects and concepts on their mode of action. Phytomedicine 1999;6:287-300.
122. Chang TT, Huang CC, Hsu CH. Inhibition of mite-induced immunoglobulin E synthesis, airway inflammation, and hyperreactivity by herbal medicine STA-1. Immunopharmacol Immunotoxicol 2006;28:683-95.
123. Coghlan ML, Haile J, Houston J, et al. Deep sequencing of plant and animal DNA contained within traditional Chinese medicines reveals legality issues and health safety concerns. PLoS Genet 2012;8:e1002657.
124. Chen CH, Dickman KG, Masaaki M, et al. Aristolochic acid-associated urothelial cancer in Taiwan. Proc Natl Acad Sci U S A 2012;109: 8241-6.
125. European Commission for Public Health, European Medicines Agency. Traditional herbal medicinal products directive (THMPD). Available at http://ec.europa.eu/health/human-use/herbal-medicines/index_en.htm (accessed June 2, 2013).
126. Nature News. Chinese herbal medicine licensed in Europe. Available at http://blogs.nature.com/news/2012/04/chinese-herbal-medicine-breaks-into-eu-market.html (accessed June , 2013).
127. Committee on Government Reform, House of Representatives, 109th Congress. Hearing on the regulation of dietary supplements: a review of consumer safeguards, March 9, 2006, serial no. 109-35. Available at http://www.gpo.gov/fdsys/pkg/CHRG-109hhrg27187/pdf/CHRG-109hhrg27187.pdf (accessed June 2, 2013).
128. Shelley BM, Sussman AL, Williams RL, Segal AR, Crabtree BF; Rios Net Clinicians. 'They don't ask me so I don't tell them': patient-clinician communication about traditional, complementary, and alternative medicine. Ann Fam Med 2009;7:139-47. http://www.ncbi.nlm.nih.gov/pmc/articles/PMC2653970/pdf/0060139.pdf
129. Abdel-Tawab M, Werz O, Schubert-Zsilavecz M. Boswellia serrata: an overall assessment of in vitro, preclinical, pharmacokinetic and clinical data. Clin Pharmacokinet 2011;50:349-69.
130. Clark CE, Arnold E, Lasserson TJ, Wu T. Herbal interventions for chronic asthma in adults and children: a systematic review and meta-analysis. Prim Care Respir J 2010;19:307-14.
131. Schoonees A, Visser J, Musekiwa A, Volmink J. Pycnogenol® for the treatment of chronic disorders. Cochrane Database Syst Rev 2012;(2): CD008294.
132. Natural Medicines Comprehensive Database. Indian frankincense monograph. Available at http://naturaldatabase.therapeuticresearch.com/nd/Search.aspx?cs=&s=nd&pt=100&id=63 (accessed May 30, 2013).
133. Natural Medicines Comprehensive Database. Pycnogenol monograph. Available at http://naturaldatabase.therapeuticresearch.com/nd/Search.aspx?cs=&s=nd&pt=100&id=1019 (accessed May 30, 2013).

WITHDRAWN

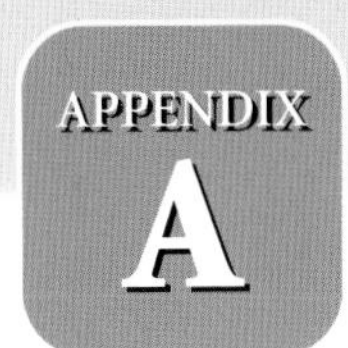

CD Molecules

STEPHAN VON GUNTEN | VIVIANE GHANIM | PETER VALENT | BRUCE S. BOCHNER

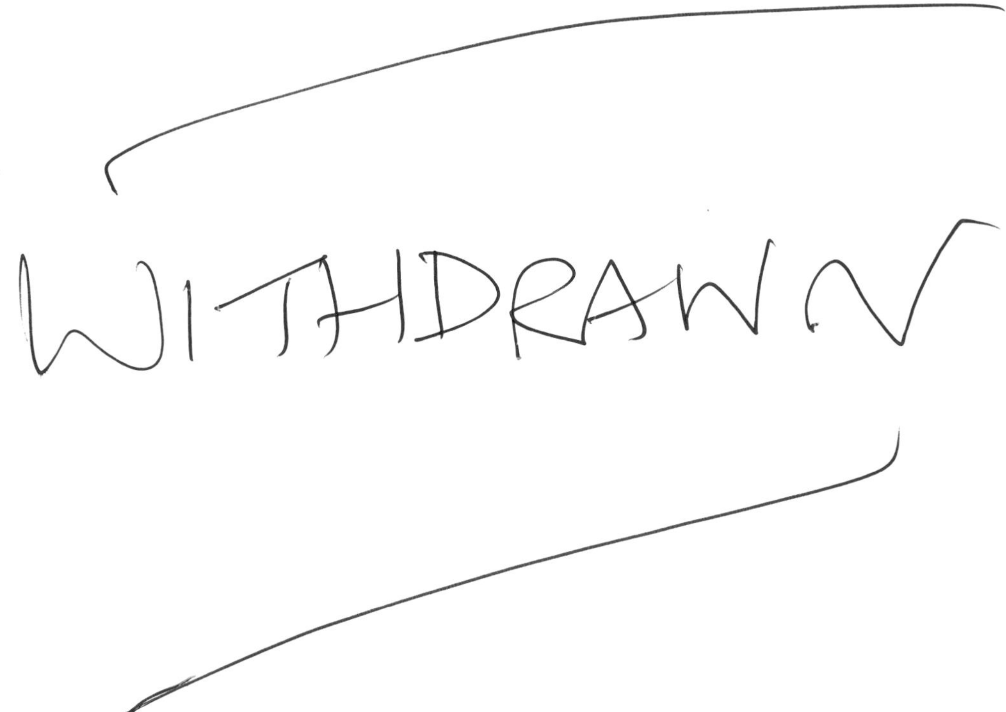

CD Molecule (Common Name)	Molecular Weight (kD, Unreduced), Family	Neutrophil	Eosinophil	Basophil	Mast Cell	Monocyte	Dendritic Cell	T Cell	B Cell	NK Cell	Platelet	Erythrocyte	Thymocytes	Stem Cell/Precursor	Endothelial Cell	Epithelial Cell	Known or Proposed Function	Binding Partner(s)
CD1a	49, Ig	–	–	–	–	a	+	a	a	–	–	–	s		–		Non-peptide antigen presentation	Glycolipids, lipopeptides; associates with β2-microglobulin
CD1b	45, Ig	–	–	–	–	a	+	a	a	–	–	–	s		–		Non-peptide antigen presentation	Glycolipids, lipopeptides; associates with β2-microglobulin
CD1c (BDCA-1)	43, Ig	–	–	–	–	a	s	a	s	–	–	–	s		–		Non-peptide antigen presentation	Glycolipids, lipopeptides; associates with β2-microglobulin
CD1d	49, Ig	–	–	–	–	+	s	a	s	–	–	–				c	Non-peptide antigen presentation	Glycolipids, lipopeptides; associates with β2-microglobulin
CD1e	28, Ig	–	–	–	–		+	a		–	–	–					Non-peptide antigen presentation	Glycolipids, lipopeptides; associates with β2-microglobulin
CD2 (LFA-2)	50, Ig	–	–	–	–	s	s	+	+	+	–	–	+		–		Costimulation, adhesion, regulation of apoptosis, immunoregulation	CD58, CD48, CD59, CD15; associates with CD45
CD3 (d,e,g)	d,e-20 kD, g-25-28 kD, Ig	–	+	–	–	–	–	+	–	–	–	–	s	–	–	–	Recognition of peptide antigen presented by MHC molecules, T cell activation	MHC classes I and II, CD38; associated in TCR complex; associates with CD45
CD4	55, Ig	–	w	–	s	+	s	s	–	–	–	–	s	–	–	–	MHC class II antigen-restricted T-cell activation, thymic differentiation, receptor for HIV-1	MHC class II, IL-16, HIV-1 gp120; associates with CD45, CD82
CD5	58, SR	–	–	–	–	–		+	s	–	–	–	s		–		Modulates signaling through TCR and BCR; regulates T-B lymphcyte interaction	CD72; associates with TCR or BCR, CD2
CD6	100-120 [reduced], SR	–	–	–	–	–		+	s		–	–	+		–	w/s	Adhesion, costimulation, regulation of apoptosis	CD166
CD7	38, Ig	–	–	–	–	–		+	–	+	–	–		s	–		Costimulation, immunoregulation	Galectin-1, SECTM1 (K12)
CD8a	32-34 [reduced], Ig	–	–	–	–	–	s	s		s	–	–	s	–	–	–	MHC class I restricted T-cell activation	MHC class I; forms dimers with CD8a, CD8b

CD8b	30-32 [reduced], Ig	–	–	–	–	–		s		s	–	–	s	–	–	–	MHC class I restricted T-cell activation	MHC class I; forms dimers with CD8a, CD8b
CD9	24 [reduced], TM4	w	+	+	+	w	+	a	+	+	+			s	+	s	Adhesion, activation	Associates with CD63, CD81, CD82, CD171, CD315, CD316
CD10 (Neutral endopeptidase)	100, metalloproteinase	+	+	–	–		–	s	s	–	–	–	s	s		s	Enzymatic activity, differentiation	Unknown
CD11a (LFA-1 α)	170, integrin	+	+	+	–	+	+	+	+	+		–		s	s	s	Adhesion, migration	CD54, CD102, CD50; possibly CD242, CD321, ICAM-5
CD11b (Mac-1α, CR3)	165, integrin	+	+	+	–	+	+	s	s	+		–		s	–	s	Adhesion, migration	CD54, extracellular matrix proteins, C3bi, LPS/LBP complex, microbial proteins
CD11c (p150,95α)	145, integrin	+	+	+	+	+	+	s	s	+		–			–		Adhesion, migration	iC3b, fibrinogen, CD23, CD87, LPS/LBP complex
CD11d	125, integrin	w	w	w	+	w	w	w	w	w							Adhesion	CD50, CD106
CDw12	120, unknown	+	+	–	–	+		–	–	+	+	–		–			Unknown	Unknown
CD13 (Aminopeptidase N)	150, metalloproteinase	+	+	+	+	+	s	–	–	–	+	–		s	s	s	Enzymatic activity	Small peptides, encephalins, MIP-1, Coronavirus, CMV
CD14 (LPS receptor)	53, leucine-rich repeat	w	–	w	–	+	s	–	w		w			–	w		Activation	LPS/LBP complex, LTA, phosphatidyl inositol
CD15 (Lewis x, Le[x])	Branched trisaccharide	+	+	w	–	+		–	–	–	–	–		–	–		Adhesion	CD62E, CD62P
CD15s (Sialyl-Lewis X, sLe[x])	Terminal tetrasaccharide	+	w	+	+	+		+	a	+				s		+	Adhesion	CD62E, CD62P
CD15su (6-sulfo sLex, L-selectin ligand)	Sulfated CD15	+	+	+		+		+	a	+					–	+	Adhesion	CD62L
CD16a (FcγRIIIa)	50-65, Ig	+	–	–	s	+	s	–	–	s	–	–		+	–		Phagocytosis and antibody-dependent cytotoxicity	Aggregated IgG
CD16b (FcγRIIIb)	48, Ig	+	a	–	s	+	s	s		s		–			–	+	Phagocytosis and antibody-dependent cytotoxicity	Aggregated IgG
CD17 (Lactosylceramide)	150-160, ceramide	+	+	+		+	+	+	+	–	+	–			+	+	Homotypic adhesion, phagocytosis, intracellular trafficking, granule exocytosis	GM3 gangliosides, bacteria
CD18 (β2 integrin subunit)	120, integrin	+	+	+	w	+	+	+	+	+		–		s	–		Adhesion	See CD11a,b,c,d
CD19	90, Ig	–	–	–	–	–	s	–	+	–	–	–		s	–	–	B cell maturation, proliferation and activation; germinal center formation	CD77; associates with CD21, CD81

Continued

CD Molecule (Common Name)	Molecular Weight (kD, Unreduced), Family	Neutrophil	Eosinophil	Basophil	Mast Cell	Monocyte	Dendritic Cell	T Cell	B Cell	NK Cell	Platelet	Erythrocyte	Thymocytes	Stem Cell/Precursor	Endothelial Cell	Epithelial Cell	Known or Proposed Function	Binding Partner(s)
CD20	33/35/37, TM4	–	–	–	–	–	–	s/w	+	–	–	–		–	–	–	B cell activation and proliferation	
CD21 (CR2)	130-145, RCA	–	–	–	+	–	s	–	+	–	–	–		s	–	+	B cell activation and proliferation; on interaction with CD23 regulates synthesis of IgE	C3d, C3dg, iC3b, CD35, Epstein-Barr virus; associates with CD19, CD23 and CD81
CD22 (Siglec-2)	140, Ig	–	–	–	s	–	–	–	+	–	–	–		s	–	–	B cell adhesion, immunoregulation, signal transduction	Sialylated glycans, CD45RO, CD75
CD23 (FcεRII)	45, lectin	–	–/w	–	–	+	+	–	+	–	+	–			–	–	Low-affinity IgE receptor; mediates cytotoxicity and phagocytosis; soluble form has multiple functions, including B cell differentiation	IgE
CD24	35-45, selectin	+	+	–	–	–	–	–	+	–	–	–		s	–	s	Regulation of B cell proliferation and differentiation, reactive oxygen species production in neutrophils, eosinophils	CD171
CD25 (IL-2R α chain)	55, CCP-like	–	a	+	–	a	–	a/s	a	+	–	–		–	–	w/s	Activation/costimulation	IL-2; associates with CD122, CD132
CD26 (dipeptidyl peptidase IV)	110, peptidase	–	–	+	–	+	–	+	+	+	–	–		–	–	s	Activation/costimulation, adhesion; enzymatic activity	Adenosine deaminase, collagen, fibroblast activation protein, Tat protein of HIV
CD27	110-120, TNFR	–	–	–	–	–	–	+	a	a	–	–	s	s	–	–	Activation/costimulation, cell differentiation	CD70, TRAF2, TRAF5
CD28	90, Ig	–	+	–	–	–	–	+	–	–	–	–		–	–	–	Activation/costimulation, signal transduction	CD80, CD86
CD29 (β1 integrin subunit)	110, integrin	+	+	+	+	+	+	+	+	+	+			s	+	s	Adhesion, migration	Associates with CD49a-f
CD30	120, TNFR	–	+	–		+		a	a	a	–	–			–	–	Cell death, immunoregulation	CD153
CD31 (PECAM-1)	130-140, Ig	+	+	+	–	+		s	s	+	+	–		s	+		Adhesion, migration	CD31 (homophilic binding), CD38

CD32a (FcγRIIA)	40, Ig	+	+	+	s	+		–	–	–	+	–		s	–	+	Activation, phagocytosis	Aggregated IgG or complexes with antigen
CD32b (FcγRIIB)	40, Ig	+		+	s	+	s		+	–		–					Immunoregulation	Aggregated IgG or complexes with antigen
CD32c (FcγRIIC)	40, Ig					+		a		+							Activation, ADCC	Aggregated IgG or complexes with antigen
CD33 (Siglec-3)	150, Ig	+	+	+	+	+	+	–	–	–	–	–	–	s	–	–	Adhesion, regulation of cell growth	Sialylated glycans
CD34	105-120, sialomucin	–	–	–	–	–	–	–	–	–	–	–		+	+	–	Adhesion	CD62L, CD62E
CD35 (CR1)	165-255, RCA	+	+	+	–	+	s	s	+	–		+			+		Phagocytosis, regulation of complement	C3b, iC3b, C3dg, C4b, iC3, iC4
CD36	88-113, SR	–	–	–		+	+	–	–	–	+	+		s	+	–	Adhesion, pathogen recognition	Collagen, thrombospondin, oxidized LDL, bacterial diacyl glycerides
CD37	40-52, TM4	w	w	w		w		w	+	–	–	–			–		Immunoregulation	Associates with CD53, CD81, CD82, MHC class II
CD38	45, ectoenzyme	–	–	+	–	+	+	s/a	s/a	+	+			s	–	+	Adhesion, activation/costimulation, enzymatic activity	CD31, hyaluronic acid
CD39	78, ectoapyrase	+	+	+		+	+	a	s	a	+				+	+	Platelet aggregation, enzymatic activity	ADP, ATP
CD40	85 (dimers), TNFR	–	+	+	+	+	s	a	+	–		–		s	+	w/s	Activation/costimulation, differentiation, isotype switching of B-cells	CD154
CD41 (GPIIb)	120/23, integrin	–	–	–	–	–	–	–	–	–	+	–		s	–	–	Adhesion	Fibrinogen, von Willebrand factor, fibronectin, vitronectin, thrombospondin; associates with CD61
CD42a (GPIX)	22, leucine-rich repeat	–	–	–	–	–	–	–	–	–	+	–		s	–	–	Adhesion, CD42 a-d complex serves as von Willebrand factor receptor	Von Willebrand factor, thrombin
CD42b (GPIbα)	160, leucine-rich repeat	–	–	–	–	–	–	–	–	–	+	–		s	–	–	Actual binding site for von Willebrand factor and thrombin lies on CD42b	See CD42a
CD42c (GPIbβ)	160, leucine-rich repeat	–	–	–	–	–	–	–	–	–	+	–		s	–	–	See CD42a	See CD42a
CD42d (GPV)	82, leucine-rich repeat	–	–	–		–	–	–	–	–	+	–		s	–	–	See CD42a	See CD42a
CD43	95-135, sialomucin	+	+	+	+	+		+	a	+	+	–		+		+	Adhesion, signal transduction	CD54, CD169, MHC class I, CD62P, hyaluronic acid

Continued

CD Molecule (Common Name)	Molecular Weight (kD, Unreduced), Family	Neutrophil	Eosinophil	Basophil	Mast Cell	Monocyte	Dendritic Cell	T Cell	B Cell	NK Cell	Platelet	Erythrocyte	Thymocytes	Stem Cell/Precursor	Endothelial Cell	Epithelial Cell	Known or Proposed Function	Binding Partner(s)
CD44	85, core/link proteoglycan	+	+	+	+	+		+	+	+	–	+		+	+	s	Adhesion, activation/ costimulation	Hyaluronan, MIP-1b, osteopontin, ankyrin, fibronectin
CD44R	85-200, core/link proteoglycan					a						+				s	See CD44	See CD44
CD45	180-240, RPTP	+	+	+	+	+	+	+	+	+	–	–	+	+	–	w/s	Activation/ costimulation, differentiation, apoptosis	Galectin-1, CD206; associates with CD2, CD3, CD4, LPAP
CD45RA	205-220, RPTP	–	–			+	+	s	+	+	–	–	+	+	–	–	Activation/ costimulation, differentiation, apoptosis	See CD45
CD45RB	190-220, RPTP	+	+			+	+	s	+	+	–	+	+	+	–	–	Activation/ costimulation, differentiation, apoptosis	See CD45
CD45RC	220, RPTP	+	+			+	+	s	+	+	–	–	+	+	–	–	Activation/ costimulation, differentiation, apoptosis	See CD45
CD45RO	180, RPTP	+	+			+	+	s	+	+	–	–	+	+	–	w/s	Activation/ costimulation, differentiation, apoptosis	See CD45; CD22
CD46	52-58, RCA	+	+	+		+	+	+	+	+	+	–			+	+	Regulation of complement, pathogen recognition	C3b, C4b, many pathogens including measles virus, Herpes virus, Streptococcus pyogenes, and pathogenic Neisseria sp.
CD47	45-60, Ig	+	+	+	+	+		+	+	+	+	+			+	+	Adhesion, activation/ costimulation, cell death, hemostasis	Thrombospondin-1, CD172a, CD172g; associates with integrins; part of the Rhesus antigen complex (see CD240CE)
CD47R (Formerly CDw149)	120, Ig	+	+	+		+		+	+	+	+				+	+	See CD47	See CD47

CD48 (SLAMF2)	45, Ig	–	+		+	+		+	+	+	–		+	s	–	+	Activation/ costimulation, immunoregulation, pathogen recognition	CD2, CD244, FimH
CD49a (VLA-1α)	200, integrin	–	–	–	–	+	+	a	–	a	–	–			s		Adhesion, costimulation	Laminin, collagen type IV; associates with CD29
CD49b (VLA-2α)	160, integrin	–	–	–	+	+		a	+	+	+	–		s	+	+	Adhesion, costimulation	Laminin, collagen type I, VLA-3, E-cadherin, echovirus; associates with CD29
CD49c (VLA-3α)	150, integrin	–	–	–	+	+		+	+	–		–			+	+	Adhesion	Laminin, collagen, fibronectin, entactin, CD151; associates with CD29, CD63
CD49d (VLA-4α)	150/180, integrin	–	+	+	+	a	+	+	+	+	–	–		s	+		Adhesion	CD53, CD160, fibronectin, MAdCAM-1; associates with CD29
CD49e (VLA-5α)	155, integrin	+	–	+	+	+	+	a/s	a/s	+		+	+	s	+	+	Adhesion	Fibronectin, CD171; associates with CD29
CD49f (VLA-6α)	140, integrin	+	+	+	–	+		+	w		+		+	s	+	+	Adhesion	Laminin, invasin, merosin, CD151; associates with CD29, CD63
CD50 (ICAM-3)	110-170, Ig	+	+	+		+	s	+	+	+	–	–		s	+	–	Adhesion, costimulation	LFA-1 (CD11a/CD18), αdβ2 (CD11d/CD18), CD209
CD51 (Vitronectin-Ra)	150, integrin	–	+	–	+	a			s		+				+		Adhesion	ECM proteins
CD52	25-29, CD24/HSA/ CD52	+	+	+		+	s	+	+	+	–	–	+		–	+	Costimulation	
CD53	32-42, TM4	+	+	+		+	–	+	+	+	–	–	+	s	–	–	Activation/ costimulation, signal transduction	VLA-4 (CD49d/CD29), HLA-DR
CD54 (ICAM-1)	80-114, Ig	+	a	+	+	w		a	a	w	–			s	+/a	+/a	Adhesion	LFA-1 (CD11a/CD18), Mac-1 (CD11b/CD18), fibrinogen, hyaluronan, CD227, rhinovirus, *Plasmodium falciparum*-infected erythrocytes
CD55 (decay accelerating factor)	50/70, RCA	+	+	+	+	+	+	+	+	+	+	+		+	+	+	Complement regulation, activation	C3b/C3bBb convertase, C4b/C4b2a convertase, CD97, coxsackie virus, echovirus, enterovirus, *E.coli*
CD56 (NCAM)	130/140/180, Ig	–	–	–		–	–	s	–	+					–		Adhesion, differentiation/ development	CD56 (homotypic binding), CD155, CD171, heparin sulfate, chondroitin sulfate, proteglycans
CD57	110, carbohydrate	–	–	–				s		s					–	s	Adhesion	Laminin
CD58 (LFA-3)	40-70, Ig	+	+	+	+	+	+	+	+	+		+	+		+	+	Adhesion, activation/ costimulation	CD2

Continued

CD Molecule (Common Name)	Molecular Weight (kD, Unreduced), Family	Neutrophil	Eosinophil	Basophil	Mast Cell	Monocyte	Dendritic Cell	T Cell	B Cell	NK Cell	Platelet	Erythrocyte	Thymocytes	Stem Cell/Precursor	Endothelial Cell	Epithelial Cell	Known or Proposed Function	Binding Partner(s)
CD59	18-25, Ly-6	+	+	+		+	+	+	+	+		+		s	+	s	Complement regulation, activation, cell survival	Complement components C8a and C9
CD60a (GD3)	Glycolipid	+	+	+		+		s	+	+	+	–	+				Apoptosis, costimulation	Siglec-7
CD60b (9-O-acetyl-GD3)	Glycolipid					+		s	a		+			s		+	Costimulation	
CD60c (7-O-acetyl-GD3)	Glycolipid							+									Costimulation	
CD61 (b3 integrin subunit)	90, integrin	–	–	–	s	+			s		+			s	+		Adhesion	Vitronectin, fibrinogen, von Willebrand factor, CD9; associates with CD41 and CD51
CD62E (E-selectin)	107-115, lectin	a	–	–	–	–	–	–	–	–	–	–	–	s	a/s	–	Rolling and adhesion	CD15, CD62L, CD65, CD66a, CD162, CD163, CD227, ESL-1, myeloglycans
CD62L (L-selectin)	65, lectin	+	+	+	–	+	+	+	+	+	–	–		s	–	–	Rolling and adhesion	CD15su, CD34, CD62E, CD227, MAdCAM-1, GlyCAM-1
CD62P (P-selectin)	120, lectin	–	–	–	–	–	–	+	–	–	a	–	–	s	a	–	Rolling and adhesion	CD15s, CD24, CD162, CD227
CD63	40-60, TM4	+	+	+	+	+	+	+	s	+	a				a	s	Adhesion	Associates with VLA-3 (CD49c/CD29), VLA-6 (CD49f/CD29), CD9, CD81
CD64 (FcγRI)	72, Ig	a	–	–	–	+	s	–	–	–	–	–		s	–	s	ADCC, phagocytosis of immune complexes	Monomeric IgG
CD65 (Ceramide-dodecasaccharide)	Carbohydrate	+	+	–	–	+		+	+					s	–		Adhesion	CD62E
CD65s (sialylated-CD65)	Carbohydrate	+	+		–	+		–	–	–	–	–			–		Adhesion	Possibly CD62E or CD62P
CD66a (CEA-related cell adhesion molecule 1, CEACAM1)	140-180, Ig	+	+			+		a	–	+	–	–		–	–	+	Multifunctional, adhesion, signal transduction, inhibition, tumor suppression	CD62E, CD66a,c,e, microbial proteins
CD66b	95-100, Ig	+	+	–				–	–	–	–	–		–	–		Adhesion, signal transduction, activation	CD66c
CD66c	90 [reduced], Ig	+	+					–	–	–	–	–			–	+	Adhesion, signal transduction, activation	CD66a,b,c,e, microbial proteins

CD66d	35, Ig	+	+					–	–	–	–	–			–		Adhesion, signal transduction, activation	Microbial proteins
CD66e (Carcinoembryonic antigen, CEA)	180-200 [reduced], Ig		+					–	–	–	–	–			–	+	Adhesion, possibly tumor metastasis	CD66a,c,e, microbial proteins
CD66f	54-72, Ig							–	–	–	–	–			–	+	Essential for successful pregnancy, may protect fetus from maternal immune system	Unknown
CD68	110, sialomucin	c	c	c	c	c	c	a	a		–	–		c	–		Atherosclerosis (foam cell formation)	Oxidatively modified LDL
CD69	60, lectin	a	a	a	a	a		a	a	a	+		a		–		Signal transduction, activation	Unknown
CD70	170 [trimeric], TNF	–	–	–		–	–	a	a	a	–	–		–	–	–	Activation/ costimulation	CD27
CD71 (transferrin receptor)	190	–	+	w		+	–	+	+	+		–	+	+	+	+	Metabolism, cell growth	Transferrin, IgA
CD72	43, lectin	–	–	–		w	+	–	+	–	–	–		s	–		Differentiation, immunoregulation	CD5, CD100
CD73	69-72	–	–	–		–	s	s	s	–	–	–	w	w	+	+	Enzymatic activity	Unknown
CD74 (Invariant chain)	33-41	–	–	–		w	+	a	+						a	a	Antigen presentation, activation, differentiation	HLA-DR heterodimers, MIF, CD44
CD75	Carbohydrate	–	–	–		+		s	+	–	–	+		–	–	s	Adhesion	CD22
CD75s	α2,6 sialylated CD75	+				+		s	+	–	–	+		–	+	+	Adhesion	CD22
CD77	Carbohydrate	–	–	–		–		–	a/s	–	–	–		–	+	+	Apoptosis	CD19, Shiga toxin, verotoxin 1
CD79a (Iga)	33, Ig	–	–	–		–		–	+	–	–	–		s	–	–	Part of the BCR, activation, differentiation	Associates with membrane Ig (mIgM), CD179b, CD5, CD19, CD22
CD79b (Igb)	31, Ig	–	–	–		–		–	+	–	–	–		s	–	s	Part of the BCR, activation, differentiation	Associates with membrane Ig (mIgM), CD179a, CD5, CD19, CD23
CD80 (B7-1)	60, Ig	–	+	–		+	+	a	a	–	–	–		–	–	–	Activation/ costimulation, immunoregulation	CD28, CD152
CD81 (TAPA-1)	26, TM4	–	+	w		+	+	+	+	w	–	–		s	+	+	Associates with CD19 and CD21 for signalling complex, B cell activation, regulation of cell growth	Hepatitis C virus; associates with CD9, CD19, CD21, CD63, CD82, CD315, CD316
CD82	45-90, TM4	+	+	+		+		+	+	+	+	–		s	+	+	Activation/ costimulation	Associates with MHC molecules, integrins, CD4, CD8, CD20, CD37, CD53, CD81

Continued

CD Molecule (Common Name)	Molecular Weight (kD, Unreduced), Family	Neutrophil	Eosinophil	Basophil	Mast Cell	Monocyte	Dendritic Cell	T Cell	B Cell	NK Cell	Platelet	Erythrocyte	Thymocytes	Stem Cell/Precursor	Endothelial Cell	Epithelial Cell	Known or Proposed Function	Binding Partner(s)
CD83	43 [reduced], Ig	+	–	–		–	+	–	s	–	–	–		–	–	–	Possibly activation, differentiation	Unknown
CD84 (SLAMF5)	68-80, Ig	+	+	+	+	+	+	+	+	+	+	–		–	–	–	Immunoregulation	CD84 [homotypic adhesion]
CD85a	110, Ig	+	+			+	+	s	–	+	–	–		s	–	–	Immunoregulation	HLA class I molecules
CD85d	110, Ig	w	+			+	s			+		–					Immunoregulation, differentiation	HLA class I molecules
CD85j	110, Ig		+			+	+	+	w	+							Immunoregulation	HLA class I molecules, CMV
CD85k	60, Ig					+	+					–			a		Immunoregulation, differentiation	Unknown
CD86 (B7-2)	80 [reduced], Ig	–	a	–		+	+	a	a/s	–	–	–		–	+	–	Activation/ costimulation, immunoregulation	CD28, CD152
CD87 (uPAR, urokinase plasminogen activator receptor)	35-68, Ly-6	+	+	+		+	+	a	–	+	–	–		–	+	–	Adhesion, migration, tumor metastasis	uPA, Vitronectin, integrins, kininogen
CD88 (C5a receptor)	43, TM7	+	+	+	s	+	+	–	–	–	–	–		–	+	+	Activation	C5a, anaphylatoxin
CD89 (IgA receptor)	45-100, Ig	+	w	–		+	+	–	–	–	–	–			–	–	Activation, signal transduction	Serum and secretory IgA1 and IgA2; associates with common Fc receptor γ-chain, Mac-1 (CD11b/CD18)
CD90 (Thy-1)	25-35, Ig	–	–	–		–		–	–	–	–	–		+	+	–	Activation/ costimulation, adhesion, differentiation	Mac-1 (CD11b/CD18)
CD91 (LDL receptor)	600, LDLR	–	–	–		+		–	–	–	–	–		+	–	+	Antigen presentation, phagocytosis, metabolism	Plasminogen activator, lipoproteins, lipoprotein lipase, β-amyloid precursor protein, heat shock proteins, various toxins and drugs
CD92	70, choline transporter-like	+	w	+	+	+		w	w	w	–	–			w	w	Metabolism, possibly immunoregulation	Choline
CD93	110, lectin	+	+	–		+	s	–	–	+	+	–		–	+	–	Possibly phagocytosis	C1q
CD94	30 [reduced], lectin	–	–	–		–		s	–	+	–	–			–	–	Immunoregulation	Heterodimer formation with CD159a, CD159c
CD95 (Fas)	45, TNFR	+	+	+	+	+	+	+	+	+	–	–	+	+	w/a	+	Apoptosis, immunoregulation	CD178
CD96	160, 180, 240, Ig	–	–	–		–		+	–	+	–	–			–		Adhesion	CD155

CD97	28, 74-89,TM7	+	+	+		+	+	a	a	a	–	–			–	–	Adhesion, migration, tumor metastasis	CD55, chondroitin sulphate
CD98	125	+	+	+		+		+	+	+	+	–			+	+	Adhesion, metabolism	Integrins, associates with actin, CD147
CD99	32	+	+	+	+	+	+	+	+	+	+	+	+	+	+	+	Adhesion, apoptosis, activation/ costimulation	CD99 [homophilic adhesion]
CD100	300, Ig	+	+	+		+	–	+	+	+	–	–		–	–		Activation/ costimulation	CD45, CD72, plexin B
CD101	240, Ig	+	+	–		+	+	a	–	–	–	–			w		Activation/ costimulation, immunoregulation	Unknown
CD102 (ICAM-2)	55-65 kD, Ig	–	–	+		+	s	+	+	+	+	–			+		Adhesion, costimulatin	LFA-1 (CD11a/CD18), CR3 (CD18/CD11b)
CD103 (Integrin αE)	175, integrin	–	–	–		–		a	–	–	–	–			–		Adhesion, lymphocyte homing to epithelia	CD324
CD104 (β4 Integrin)	205, integrin	–	–	–		–		–	–	–	–	–	+	s	+	+	Adhesion, activation	Laminins, keratin filaments
CD105 (Endoglin)	180, TGFR	+	–	–		a	s	–	–	–	–	–		s	+		Angiogenesis, signal transduction	TGF-β1, TGF-β3 isoforms
CD106 (VCAM-1)	110, Ig	–	–	–		–	s	–	–	–	–	–			a		Adhesion, costimulation, differentiation	VLA-4 (CD49d/CD29), α4β7 integrin
CD107a (LAMP-1)	100-120, LAMP	a	–	a		a		a	–	–	a	–			a	s	Possibly adhesion, metabolism	Galectins, CD62L,E,P
CD107b (LAMP-2)	100-120, LAMP	a	–	–		a		a	–	–	a	–			a	s	Possibly adhesion, metabolism	Galectins, CD62L,E,P
CD108	80, Ig	–	–	–				+	+		–	+	+	s	w		Activation	CD232
CD109	170	–	–			–		a	–	–	a	–		+	+	+	Possibly differentiation	Unknown
CD110	85-92, CR, Ig	–	–	–		–	–	–	–	–	+	–		+			Differentiation	Thrombopoietin
CD111	75 [reduced], Ig	+	–	–		+		–	–		+	+		+	+	+	Adhesion	CD111 [homophilic binding], CD112, CD113, CD155, HSV-1, HSV-2, PRV
CD112	64 -72, Ig	+	+	–	w	+		–			+	–		+	+	+	Adhesion	CD111, CD112 [homophilic binding], CD113, CD155, CD226, HSV-1, PRV
CD113	83, Ig	–	–	–	–	–	–	–	–	–	–	–	–	–	–	+	Adhesion	CD111, CD112, CD113 [homophilic binding], CD155
CD114 (G-CSF receptor)	130 [reduced], CR, Ig	+	–	–		+	+	–	–	–	+	–	–	s	+		Signal transduction, differentiation, survival	G-CSF
CD115 (M-CSF receptor)	150, RTK, Ig	–	–	–		+	+	–		–	–	–	–	s	–		Signal transduction, differentiation, survival	M-CSF
CD116 (GM-CSF receptor α)	80-85, CR, Ig	+	+	+	–	+	+	–	–	–	–	–	–	s	–	+	Signal transduction, differentiation, survival	GM-CSF; associates with CD131

Continued

CD Molecule (Common Name)	Molecular Weight (kD, Unreduced), Family	Neutrophil	Eosinophil	Basophil	Mast Cell	Monocyte	Dendritic Cell	T Cell	B Cell	NK Cell	Platelet	Erythrocyte	Thymocytes	Stem Cell/Precursor	Endothelial Cell	Epithelial Cell	Known or Proposed Function	Binding Partner(s)
CD117 (stem cell factor receptor, KIT)	145, RTK, Ig	–	w	w/–	+	–	–	–	–	–	–	–	+	+	–	–	Signal transduction, differentiation, survival	SCF
CD118	190, CR	+	+	–	–	+										+	Signal transduction	LIF, oncostatin M, IFN-a and -b; associates with CD130
CD119 (IFN-g receptor)	90, CR, Ig	+	+	+		+		+	+	+		–			+	+	Signal transduction	IFN-g
CD120a (TNF receptor 1)	55, TNFR	+	+	+		+	+	+	+	+		–			+	+	Signal transduction	TNF-a, TNF-b
CD120b (TNF receptor 2)	75, TNFR	+	+	+		+	+	+	+	+		–			+	+	Signal transduction	TNF-a, TNF-b
CD121a (IL-1 receptor, type 1)	75-85, Ig	–	–	–		–	–	+	–	–	–	–			+	–	Signal transduction	IL-1
CD121b (IL-1 receptor, type 2)	60-68, Ig	+	–	+		+		+	+		–	–			–	s	Decoy receptor	IL-1
CD122 (IL-2 receptor, β chain)	70-75, CR, Ig	–	–	a		+		+	+	+	–	–	+		–		Signal transduction	IL-2, IL-15, associates with CD25, CD132
CD123 (IL-3 receptor, α chain)	70, CR, Ig	+	w	+	+	+	s	–	s					+	s		Signal transduction	IL-3, associates with CD131
CD124 (IL-4 receptor, α chain)	140, CR, Ig	w	+	a	+	+	–	+	+	–	–	–		s	–	+	Signal transduction	IL-4, IL-13, associates with CD132
CD125 (IL-5 receptor, α chain)	60, CR, Ig	–	+	+	+	–		–	s	–	–	–		s	–		Signal transduction	IL-5, associates with CD131
CD126 (IL-6 receptor, α chain)	80, CR, Ig	+	+	+		+	–	+	+	–				s	+		Signal transduction	IL-6, associates with CD130
CD127 (IL-7 receptor, α chain)	80, CR, Ig	–	w	–		+		+	–		–	–	+	s	–		Signal transduction	IL-7, associates with CD132
CD129 (IL-9 receptor, α chain)	65-90, CR, Ig		+	–	+			+	+					s		+	Signal transduction	IL-9, associates with CD132
CD130 (common β chain of IL-6, IL-11 and LIF receptors)	130-140, CR, Ig	–	–	+		+	–	+	+	+	–			+	+		Signal transduction	IL-6, IL-11, oncostatin M, LIF; associates with CD126
CD131 (common β chain of IL-3, IL-5 and GM-CSF receptors)	120-140, CR, Ig	+	+	+		+		–	–	–				+			Signal transduction	IL-3, IL-5, GMCSF, associates with CD116, CD123, CD125
CD132 (common γ chain of IL-2, IL-4, IL-7, IL-9, IL-15 receptors)	65-70, CR, Ig	+	+	+		+		+	+	+	+	–					Signal transduction	IL2, IL4, IL7, IL9, IL15, associates with CD25, CD122, CD124, CD127, CD129

CD133	120, TM5	–	–	–	–	–	–	–	–	–	–	–	+	+	s	+	Unknown, mutation of gene responsible for retinal degeneration	Unknown
CD134 (OX40)	35-50, TNFR	+	+			–	+	a	+					+			Activation/ costimulation, survival	CD252
CD135	130, RTK	–	–	–		–	–	–	–	–	–	–		+			Differentiation	FLT3 ligand
CD136	180, RTK					+										+	Migration, proliferation, differentiation	MSP
CD137	83, TNFR	–	+			+	s	a	a	–						+	Activation/ costimulation	CD137L
CD138 (Syndecan-1)	70-92, glycosaminoglycan	–	–	–	–	–		–	a	–	–	–		s	+	+	Adhesion, marker of plasma cells and Reed-Sternberg cells	Collagen, fibronectin, thrombospondin, basic fibroblast growth factor
CD139	209-238 [reduced]	+	+			+	s	–	+	–		+		–			Unknown	Unknown
CD140a (PDGF receptor α)	160-180, RTK, Ig	–	–	–		+		–	–	–	+	–		s	+		Signal transduction	PDGF isoforms
CD140b (PDGF receptor β)	170-190, RTK, Ig	–	–	–		–		–	–	–	–	–	–	–	+	–	Signal transduction	PDGF isoforms
CD141 (BDCA-3, Thrombo-modulin)	105, lectin, BDCA-3	w	–	–	–	w	s	–	–	–	+	–	–	–	+	+	Hemostasis	Thrombin, protein C
CD142 (Thromboplastin, tissue factor)	45-47, CR	–	–	–	–	a		–	–	–	–	–	–	–	a	+	Hemostasis, possibly angiogenesis, tumor metastasis	Factor VII/ VIIa
CD143 (Angiotensin-converting enzyme)	90 or 170, peptidase	–	–	–		a		s	–	–	–	–			+	s	Enzymatic activity	Angiotensins I and II, bradykinin, substance P
CD144 (VE-cadherin)	135, cadherin	–	–	–	–	–	–	–	–	–	–	–	–	–	+	–	Adhesion, angiogenesis	CD144 [homotypic binding]
CDw145	25,90,110	–	–	–	–	–				–	–	–			+	+	Unknown	Unknown
CD146	118, Ig	–		–		–	s	a	–	–	–	–			+	s	Possibly adhesion, development, tumor metastasis	Unknown
CD147 (Neurothelin)	54, Ig	+	+	+	+	+	+	+	+	+	+	+	+	+	+	+	Adhesion	Possibly integrins; associates with CD98
CD148	240-260, RPTP	+	+			+	+	+	w	+	+				–		Signal transduction, immunoregulation	Unknown
CD150 (SLAM,SLAMF1)	65-85, Ig	–	–	w	–	–	+	a/s	a/s	–	+	–	+		+		Activation, signal transduction	CD150 (homotypic binding), measles virus (H), Gram-negative OmpC and OmpF
CD151	32, TM4	–	+	+	+	–	–	a	–		+			+	+	+	Adhesion, signal transduction	Integrins
CD152 (CTLA-4)	50, Ig	–	–	–		–	–	a/s	a(s)	–	–						Immunoregulation	CD80, CD86
CD153	40, TNF	+	+			a	–	a	+					+			Activation/ costimulation, immunoregulation	CD30

Continued

CD Molecule (Common Name)	Molecular Weight (kD, Unreduced), Family	Neutrophil	Eosinophil	Basophil	Mast Cell	Monocyte	Dendritic Cell	T Cell	B Cell	NK Cell	Platelet	Erythrocyte	Thymocytes	Stem Cell/Precursor	Endothelial Cell	Epithelial Cell	Known or Proposed Function	Binding Partner(s)
CD154 (CD40 ligand)	28-33, TNF	+	+	a	+	–	+	a/s	+	+	+	–			–	–	Activatin/ costimulation	CD40
CD155 (poliovirus receptor)	60-90, Ig	–	–	–	–	+	–	–	–	–	–	–	–	–	+	+	Adhesion	Integrins, poliovirus, CMV, possibly CD56, CD111, CD112, CD226, vitronectin; associates with CD113
CD156a (ADAM8)	89, metalloproteinase	+	+			+		–	w								Adhesion, enzymatic activity	Unknown
CD156b (TACE, TNF-α converting enzyme)	130, metalloproteinase	+				+	+	+	–	–	–	–		–	+	s	Enzymatic activity	Membrane TNFα and TGFα
CD156c	65, metalloproteinase					+											Enzymatic activity	Membrane TNFα and Ephrin A2
CD157	42-50, ADP-ribocyclase	+	a	+		+	s							+	+		Enzymatic activity, signal transduction, differentiation	NAD, cyclic ADP-ribose
CD158a (KIR2DL1)	58, Ig	–	–	–	–	–	–	s	–	+	–	–	–	–	–	–	Immunoregulation	HLA-C
CD158b1	58, Ig	–	–	–	–	–	–	+	–	+	–	–	–	–	–	–	Immunoregulation	HLA-C
CD158b2	58, Ig	–	–	–	–	–	–	+	–	+	–	–	–	–	–	–	Immunoregulation	HLA-C
CD158c	58, Ig	–	–	–	–	–	–	+	–	+	–	–	–	–	–	–	Immunoregulation	HLA-C
CD158d (KIR2DL4)	41, Ig	–	–	–	–	–	–		–	+	–	–	–	–	–	–	Activation	HLA-B
CD158e1/e2	70, Ig	–	–	–	–	–	–	+	–	+	–	–	–	–	–	–	Immunoregulation	HLA-B
CD158f	58, Ig	–	–	–	–	–	–	+	–	+	–	–	–	–	–	–	Immunoregulation	See CD158a
CD158g	50, Ig	–	–	–	–	–	–	+	–	+	–	–	–	–	–	–	Activation	See CD158a
CD158h (KIR2DS1)	50, Ig	–	–	–	–	–	–	+	–	+	–	–	–	–	–	–	Activation	HLA-C (low affinity)
CD158i	50, Ig	–	–	–	–	–	–	+	–	+	–	–	–	–	–	–	Activation	HLA-C
CD158j (KIR2DS1)	50, Ig	–	–	–	–	–	–	+	–	+	–	–	–	–	–	–	Activation	HLA-C
CD158k (KIR3DL2)	70, Ig	–	–	–	–	–	–	+	–	+	–	–	–	–	–	–	Immunoregulation	HLA-A
CD159a (NKG2A [CD94/ CD159a])	43, lectin							s		+							Immunoregulation	HLA-E; associates with CD94
CD159c	36, lectin							s		+							Immunoregulation	HLA-E; associates with CD94
CD160 (BY55)	80, Ig	–	–	–	+	–	–	s	–	s	–	–	–	–	–	–	Activation/ costimulation	HLA-C
CD161 (NKR-P1A)	80, lectin	–	+				–	s	–	+	–	–			–	–	NK cell activation, TH17 lymphocytes	LLT1
CD162 (PSGL1)	160/250, sialomucin	+	+	+	+	+	+	+	+		–	–		s	–	–	Adhesion	CD62E,L,P, CD169
CD162R	220-240, sialomucin									+							Adhesion	CD62L

CD163	110, SR	–	–	–	–	+	–	–	–		–	–		–	–	–	Endocytosis, possibly immunoregulation	CD62L
CD164	170-180, sialomucin	–		a		+		+	+			–		+	s	+	Adhesion, possibly development	Unknown, *Plasmodium falciparum* gametocytes
CD165	37		+			+		s			+	–		–		+	Adhesion, cell cycle, tumorogenesis	Hyaluronan
CD166 (ALCAM)	100-105, Ig	–	–	–		a		a	+					+	+	+	Adhesion, differentiation/ development, costimulation	CD6, CD166 [homophilic binding]
CD167a	125, RTK						s		w							+	Adhesion, signal transduction, possibly tumor metastasis	Collagen type I-IV and VIII
CD167b	130, RTK															+	Adhesion, signal transduction	Collagen type I-III and V
CD168	80-88			–	–	+	+	a/s	a				+	+	+	s	Adhesion, tumorogenesis	Hyaluronan
CD169 (Siglec-1, sialoadhesin)	180, Ig	–	–	–	–	–	a	–	–	–	–	–	–	–	–	–	Adhesion, differentiation of macrophages	Sialylated glycans, CD43, CD206, CD227, *Neisseria* sp.
CD170 (Siglec-5)	140, Ig	+	–	+	+	+	+		s	–	–	–	–	–	–	–	Immunoregulation, adhesion	Sialylated glycans
CD171	200-230, Ig					+	s	s	s						+	s	Adhesion, activation/ costimulation	CD171 (homophilic binding), CD9, CD24, CD56, laminin, integrins
CD172a	85-90, Ig, SIRP-α	+	+	+	+	+	+							+			Immunoregulation, cell death	CD47, SP-A, SP-D
CD172b	110-120, Ig, SIRP-β	+		–	s	+	+										Activation	Unknown
CD172g	55, Ig	–	–	–	–	–	–	+	s	a	–	–	–	–	–	–	Immunoregulation, cell death	CD47
CD173	Carbohydrate									–		+		+	+	+	Adhesion	Unknown
CD174 (Lewis Y)	Carbohydrate	+	+							–				+		+	Angiogenesis, hemostasis	Unknown
CD175 (Tn)	Carbohydrate	–	–	–	–	–	–	–	+	–	–	+	–	+	–	+	Unknown	Unknown
CD175s (sialylTn)	Carbohydrate							–	+	–		+		+	+	+	Possibly immunoregulation and tumor metastasis	CD22, CD33, CD170 and Siglec-6
CD176	Carbohydrate								–			+		+	+	+	Tumor metastasis	Unknown
CD177	49-55, Ly-6	+		w	–									s			Unknown	Unknown
CD178 (Fas ligand)	40 [monomer], TNF	+	+	–	–	+	s	a	–	+	–	–			+	+	Apoptosis, immunoregulation	CD95
CD179a	16-18, Ig			–	–									s			Differentiation	Associates with CD179b, mIgM, CD79a/CD79b to form pre-BCR
CD179b	22, Ig				s									s			Differentiation	Associates with CD179a, mIgM, CD79a/CD79b to form pre-BCR

Continued

CD Molecule (Common Name)	Molecular Weight (kD, Unreduced), Family	Neutrophil	Eosinophil	Basophil	Mast Cell	Monocyte	Dendritic Cell	T Cell	B Cell	NK Cell	Platelet	Erythrocyte	Thymocytes	Stem Cell/Precursor	Endothelial Cell	Epithelial Cell	Known or Proposed Function	Binding Partner(s)
CD180	95-105, TLR					+	+		+								Activation, signal transduction	LPS
CD181 (CXCR1)	39, TM7	+	+	+	–	+		s		+		–			+		Signal transduction	CXCL6,8
CD182 (CXCR2, IL-8 receptor)	40, TM7	+	+	s	+	+		s		+		–		s	+	s	Signal transduction	CXCL1-3,5,6, CXCL8 (IL-8)
CD183 (CXCR3)	40, TM7		+		+			+		a		–		s	+		Signal transduction	CXCL9-11
CD184 (CXCR4)	45, TM7		+	+	+	+	+	+	+	+		–		s	+		Signal transduction	CXCL12, HIV-1 X4
CD185 (CXCR5)	42, TM7		–	–	–	+	+	s	+	+		–					Signal transduction	CXCL13
CDw186 (CXCR6)	40, TM7		–	–	–			s	s	s		–					Signal transduction	CXCL16, strains of HIV and SIV
CD191 (CCR1)	42, TM7	+	+	s	–	+	+	+	+	+		–		s			Signal transduction	CCL3,5,7,14
CD192 (CCR2)	40, TM7	+	+	+	–	+	s	s	+			–			+		Signal transduction	CCL2,7,8,13,16, HIV
CD193 (CCR3)	45, TM7	–	+	+	+	–	s	s	–	–	+	–	–	–	–	+	Signal transduction	CCL5,7,8,11,13, HIV
CD194 (CCR4)	41, TM7	–	–	+		w		s	+	a	+	–					Signal transduction	CCL17,22, HIV
CD195 (CCR5)	62, TM7	+	–	s	s	+	s	+	–	–	–	–			–		Signal transduction	CCL3,4,5,11,14,16, HIV
CD196 (CCR6)	45, TM7	a	+	s	s	–	s	s	s	–		–					Signal transduction	CCL20
CD197 (CCR7)	45, TM7	+	–	s	s		+	+	+	+		–					Signal transduction	CCL19,21
CDw198 (CCR8)	41, TM7		+			+	+	s		+		–	+				Signal transduction	CCL1
CDw199 (CCR9)	43, TM7		–	s	–			+				–	+	s			Signal transduction	CCL25
CD200 (OX-2)	40-45, Ig	–	–	–		–	s	+	+	–	–	–	+	s	+		Immunoregulation	OX-2 receptor, Herpes virus
CD201	50 [reduced], Ig		–	–	+										+		Hemostasis	Protein C, proteinase 3, unidentified phospholipid
CD202b	140, RTK		–											s	+		Angiogenesis, development, survival	Angiopoietins Ang-1, Ang-2, Ang-4
CD203c	270, E-NNP		–	+	+									+			Enzymatic activity	Extracellular nucleotides
CD204	220, SR		–	–	–	+	s										Endocytosis	Lipoproteins, LDL, collagen type IV, β-amyloid, AGEs, apoptotic cells, LPS, LTA
CD205	205, lectin		–			+	+	w	+					s			Endocytosis	Carbohydrates
CD206	162-175, lectin					+	s							s	s		Endocytosis	Mannosylated glycoproteins and antigens, CD45, CD169

CD207 (Langerin)	40, lectin	–	–	–	–	–	s	–	–	–	–	–	–	–	–	–	Endocytosis	Mannosylated glycoproteins, glycolipids and antigens, HIV
CD208 (DC-LAMP)	70-90, LAMP	–	–	–	–	–	s	–	–	–	–	–	–	–	–	s	Endocytosis	Unknown
CD209 (DC-SIGN)	44, lectin	–	–	–	–	–	+	–	–	–	–	–	–	–	–	–	Adhesion, activation/ costimulation, endocytosis	CD50, CD102, mannosylated glycoproteins and antigens, HIV
CDw210a	90-110, Ig					+	s	+	+	+							Signal transduction	IL-10
CDw210b	90-110, Ig					+	+	+	+	+							Signal transduction	IL-10, IL-22, IL-26, IL-28A,B, IL-29
CD212 (IL-12R β1-chain)	110 [reduced], Ig	–		–	–	–		s	–	+							Signal transduction	IL-12
CD213α1 (IL-13R α1-chain)	65, Ig	–		–	–	+	s	–	+	–				s	+		Signal transduction	IL-13
CD213α2 (IL-13R α2-chain)	65, Ig			–	s	+	s	s	+								Signal transduction	IL-13
CD215 (IL15RA)		–				–	–	a/s	s	a							Signal transduction	IL-15
CD217 (IL-17 receptor)	130-158					+	+	+	+	+			+			+	Signal transduction	IL-17
CD218a (IL-18Rα)	70, Ig	+		+	–	+	+	+	+	+					+		Signal transduction	IL-18; associates with CD128b
CD218b (IL-18Rβ)	70, Ig	+		+	–	+	+	+	+	+					+		Signal transduction	Associates with CD128a
CD220 (Insulin receptor)	400, RTK	+				+	+	+	+	+				+	+	+	Signal transduction	Insulin, IGF-II
CD221 (IGF1R, Insulin-like growth factor R)	90/135 [reduced], RTK	+		–	–	+	+	+	+	+				+			Signal transduction	IGF-I (high affinity), IGF-II, Insulin
CD222	250, lectin	+		–	–	+	+	+	+	+		+					Endocytosis, signal transduction	Mannose-6 phosphate, IGF-II, TGF-b, LAP, LIF, proliferin, plasminogen, retinoic acid, HSV
CD223	70, Ig	–				–	–	a	–	a							Immunoregulation, activation	MHC class II molecules
CD224 (γ-glutamyltransferase)	100, peptidase	–				+		+	+	–				s	+	+	Enzymatic activity	Glutathione
CD225	17, IFITM	–				–		+	+	+				s	+	–	Unknown	Associates with CD81
CD226	65, Ig, DNAM-1		+		+	a		a/s		a	a	–			–		Adhesion, activation	CD112, CD155
CD227 (MUC.1)	220-700, mucin					a	+	a	+					+		+	Adhesion, signal transduction	CD54, CD169, CD62E,L,P
CD228	97, transferrin	–				–	–	–	–					w	+		Metabolism, migration	Plasminogen and pro-UPA
CD229 (Ly9, SLAMF3)	120, Ig	–	–	–	–	–	+	+	+	w	–	–	+	s			Adhesion, possibly immunoregulation	CD229 (homophilic binding)
CD230	35, prion	+				+	+	+	+	+				+			Signal transduction	CD230 (homophilic binding)
CD231	150, TM4			–	–										+		Neuronal function	Unknown
CD232	200, plexin					+	+		+	+							Immunomodulation	CD108, poxvirus semaphorin-like protein A39R
CD233	95-110, anion exchanger	–	–	–	–	–	–	–	–	–	–	+		–	–	s	Metabolism	Associates with CD235a

Continued

CD Molecule (Common Name)	Molecular Weight (kD, Unreduced), Family	Neutrophil	Eosinophil	Basophil	Mast Cell	Monocyte	Dendritic Cell	T Cell	B Cell	NK Cell	Platelet	Erythrocyte	Thymocytes	Stem Cell/Precursor	Endothelial Cell	Epithelial Cell	Known or Proposed Function	Binding Partner(s)
CD234 (Duffy)	35-43, TM7	–	–	–	–	–	–	–	–	–	–	+		s	+	+	Immunoregulation	CXCL1,5,8, CCL2,5,7, *Plasmodium vivax* and *knowlesi*
CD235a (Glycophorin A)	36 [reduced], glycophorin	–	–	–	–	–	–	–	–	–	–	+		s	–		Possibly prevention of cell aggregation	CD170, influenza virus, *Plasmodium falciparum*
CD235b (Glycophorin B)	20 [reduced], glycophorin	–	–	–	–	–	–	–	–	–	–	+		–	–	–	Possibly prevention of cell aggregation	Unknown
CD236 (Glycophorin C/D)	40, glycophorin	–	–	–	–	–	–	–	–	–	–	+		s	–	–	Mechanical stability	*Plasmodium falciparum*
CD236R (Glycophorin C)	30, glycophorin	–	–	+	s	–	–	–	–	–	–	+		s	–	–	Mechanical stability	*Plasmodium falciparum*
CD238 (Kell)	115-200, metalloproteinase	–	–	–	–	–	–	–	–	–	–	+		s	–	–	Enzymatic activity	Big endothelin-3
CD239 (B-CAM)	78-85 [reduced], Ig	–	–	–	–	–	–	–	–	–	–	+			+	+	Adhesion	Laminin
CD240CE	30-32, TM12	–	–	–	–	–	–	–	–	–	–	+		s			Red cell skeleton	Associates with CD47, CD235b, CD241, CD242 to form Rhesus antigen complex
CD240D	30, TM12	–	–	–	–	–	–	–	–	–	–	+		s			Red cell skeleton	See CD240CE
CD240DCE	30, TM12	–	–	–	–	–	–	–	–	–	–	+		s			Red cell skeleton	See CD240CE
CD241	50, TM12	–	–	–	–	–	–	–	–	–	–	+		s			Mechanical stability	Part of the Rhesus antigen complex (see CD240CE)
CD242 (ICAM-4)	42, Ig	–	–	–		–	–	–	–	–	–	+		s	+		Adhesion	Integrins, platelet fibrinogen receptor, endothelial cell vitronectin receptor; part of the Rhesus antigen complex (see CD240CE)
CD243	170, ABC	–	–	–	–	–		–	–	–	–	–		+	+	+	Metabolism	Certain drugs and toxins
CD244 (2B4, SLAMF4)	70, Ig		+	+		+	+	a/s	–	+							Costimulation, immunoregulation	CD48
CD245	220-250	+				+		+	+	+	+	–	w				Costimulation	Unknown
CD246	200, RTK														+		Signal transduction	Possibly pleiotrophin, midkine
CD247 (CD3 ζ chain)	16 [reduced]	–	–	–	–	–	–	+		s							Signal transduction	Associates with TCR α/β and γ/δ, and CD3g, d and e to form TCR-CD3 complex
CD248 (Endosialin)	175, lectin			–	–			+									Tumor angiogenesis	Unknown

CD249 (aminopeptidase A)	160, peptidase			–											+	+	Enzymatic activity, regulation of angiogenesis	Angiotensin II
CD252 (OX40 ligand)	34, TNF				+		+	a	a						+		Activation/ costimulation, survival	CD134 (OX40)
CD253 (TRAIL)	33-34, TNF	+	+	–	+	a	a	a	a	a							Apoptosis	CD261, CD262, CD263, CD264
CD254 (TRANCE, RANKL)	35, TNF			s	s			a	–								T cell–B cell and dendritic cell interaction, lymph node development, differentiation, survival, bone remodelling	CD265, Osteoprotegerin
CD256 (APRIL)	28, TNF	a		–		a	+									+	Activation/ costimulation, development/ differentiation, apoptosis	CD267, CD269
CD257 (BAFF, TNF13b)	45, TNF	a		–		a	+		+	+						+	Activation/ costimulation, development/ differentiation	CD267, CD268, CD269
CD258 (LIGHT)	29, TNF			s		a	s	a	s	–							Activation/ costimulation, apoptosis	CD270, LTbR
CD261 (TRAIL-R1)	57, TNFR		+	s	s	+	–	+	+	+							Apoptosis	CD253
CD262 (TRAIL-R2)	60, TNFR	+	+	w	+	+	–	+	+	+							Apoptosis	CD253
CD263 (TRAIL-R3)	65, TNFR	+	+			+		+	+	+							Decoy receptor	CD253
CD264 (TRAIL-R4)	35, TNFR		+			+	–	+	+	+							Decoy receptor	CD253
CD265 (TRANCER)	97, TNFR	+	+	s	s	+	+	+	+	+	+		+	s			T cell–B cell and dendritic cell interaction, lymph node development, differentiation, survival, bone remodelling	CD254
CD266 (TWEAK-R)	14, TNFR			–											+	+	Angiogenesis, inflammation	TWEAK
CD267 (TACI)	32, TNFR			s		+	–	a	+								Immunoregulation	CD256, CD257
CD268 (BAFF-R)	25, TNFR					+	–	s	+	–							Survival	CD257
CD269	27, TNFR			–					+								Survival	CD256, CD257
CD270 (HVEM, TNFRSF14)		+				+	+	+	+	+								
CD271 (NGFR, NGF receptor)	75, TNFR			–	–		s										Apoptosis, signal transduction	NGF, BDNF, neurotrophin-3, neurotrophin-4, β-amyloid, CD230

Continued

CD Molecule (Common Name)	Molecular Weight (kD, Unreduced), Family	Neutrophil	Eosinophil	Basophil	Mast Cell	Monocyte	Dendritic Cell	T Cell	B Cell	NK Cell	Platelet	Erythrocyte	Thymocytes	Stem Cell/Precursor	Endothelial Cell	Epithelial Cell	Known or Proposed Function	Binding Partner(s)
CD272 (BTLA)	33, Ig					+	s	+	+	–				s			Immunoregulation	CD272 (homotypic binding), CD258, CD270
CD273	25, Ig					a	+	a									Activation/ costimulation, immunoregulation	CD279
CD274 (B7-H1)	40, Ig					a	+	a	+	+							Costimulation, immunoregulation	CD279
CD275 (ICOS-L; B7-H2)	60, Ig			s	s	a	+		+	–					+		Costimulation, immunoregulation	CD278
CD276 (B7-H3)	40-45/110, Ig					a	+	a	+	+							Costimulation, immunoregulation	Unknown
CD277	56, Ig					+	+	+	+	+				s			Possibly activation/ costimulation	Unknown
CD278 (ICOS, inducible T-cell co-stimulator)	56, Ig							a									Costimulation, differentiation/ development	CD275
CD279 (PD1, programmed cell death 1)	55, Ig					a		a	a				s				Immunoregulation	CD273, CD274
CD280	180, lectin			–	–	s				+				s	s		Adhesion, extracellular matrix degradation	Gelatin, collagen types I, II, IV, V; associates with uPA and CD87
CD281 (TLR1)	90, TLR	+			+	+	+										Pathogen recognition, activation	*M. leprae* lipopeptide, *Borrelia* outer surface protein
CD282 (TLR2)	85, TLR	+	+	+	+	+		a/s									Pathogen recognition, activation	Peptidoglycan, LTA, bacterial lipoprotein, *Mycoplasma* lipopeptide, zymosan, CMV, *M. leprae*, lipoarabinomannans
CD283 (TLR3)	100-120, TLR		+		+	–	s		–	–						+	Pathogen recognition, activation, apoptosis	Double-stranded RNA
CD284 (TLR4)	85, TLR	+	+	+	–	+	+	a/s			w	+					Pathogen recognition, activation	Endotoxin (LPS), HSP60, β-glucan, elastase, heparan sulfate
CD286 (TLR6)	85, TLR				+	+	s					s					Pathogen recognition, activation	Flagellin, diacyl-lipoproteins
CD288 (TLR8)	83, TLR		+			+	s										Pathogen recognition, activation	Single-stranded RNA

CD289 (TLR9)	115-120, TLR		+	+		+	s		+	–							Pathogen recognition, activation	Unmethylated CpG DNA
CD290 (TLR10)	91-100, TLR		+	+			+		+					s			Pathogen recognition, activation	Unkown
CD292	50-58, RTK			–	s											+	Endochondral bone formation, embryogenesis	Bone morphogenetic proteins (BMPs)
CDw293	50-58, RTK			s	–											+	Endochondral bone formation, embryogenesis	Bone morphogenetic proteins (BMPs)
CD294 (CRTH2)	55-70, TM7		+	+	+			s									Activation	Prostaglandin D2
CD295 (leptin receptor)	130-150, Ig	+	+	s		+	+	+	+	+	+			+	+	+	Regulation of fat metabolism, activation, survival	Leptin (LEP)
CD296	37, ADP-ribosyltransferase	+						+		+						+	Enzymatic activity, differentiation, inflammation, immunoregulation	NAD, integrins, defensin-1
CD297	38, ADP-ribosyltransferase			s	s	a		+				+			+	s	Enzymatic activity	Possibly integrins
CD298	32, Na/K-ATPase	+	+	+		+	+	+	+	+	+			+			Ion transport	Na, K
CD299 (L-SIGN)	40, lectin			s	s										+	s	Pathogen recognition, adhesion	Mannose bearing ligands, CD50, lentiviruses, CMV, hepatitis C virus, SARS coronavirus, *Mycobacterium tuberculosis*
CD300a	60, Ig	+	+	+	+	+	+	+	+	+							Immunoregulation	Unknown
CD300c	23, Ig					+	+	+	+								Immunoregulation	Unknown
CD300e	Ig					+	s										Immunoregulation	Unknown
CD301	38-42, lectin					+	s										Adhesion, endocytosis	Galactose and N-acetylgalactosamine bearing ligands
CD302	30, lectin	+	+	+		+	+										Endocytosis	Unknown
CD303 (BDCA-2)	38, lectin	–	–	s	–	–	s	–	–	–	–	–	–	–	–	–	Endocytosis, immunoregulation	Unknown
CD304 (BDCA-4, Neuropilin 1)	140, neuropilin	–	–	–	–	–	s	s	–	–	–	–	–	–	+	–	Angiogenesis, survival, tumor metastasis	VEGF, Semaphorin-3A
CD305 (LAIR-1)	31, Ig			+	+	+	+	+	+	+							Immunoregulation	CD326, collagen
CD306 (LAIR-2)	16, Ig			–		+											Unknown	CD326
CD307a (FCRL1)	100, Ig	–				–	–		+	–							Possibly immunoregulation	Unknown
CD307b (FCRL2)	100, Ig	–				–	–		+	–							Possibly immunoregulation	Unknown
CD307c (FCRL3)	100, Ig	–				–	–	s	+	–							Possibly immunoregulation	Unknown
CD307d (FCRL4)	100, Ig	–				–	–		+	–							Possibly immunoregulation	Unknown

Continued

CD Molecule (Common Name)	Molecular Weight (kD, Unreduced), Family	Neutrophil	Eosinophil	Basophil	Mast Cell	Monocyte	Dendritic Cell	T Cell	B Cell	NK Cell	Platelet	Erythrocyte	Thymocytes	Stem Cell/Precursor	Endothelial Cell	Epithelial Cell	Known or Proposed Function	Binding Partner(s)
CD307d (FCRL5)		–				–	–			–							Possibly immunoregulation	Unknown
CD309	230, RTK			w							+			s	+		Angiogenesis	VEGF
CD312	90, TM7	+		+	+	a	s	a	a								Adhesion, inflammation	Glycosaminoglycans, chondroitin sulphate, dermatan sulphate
CD314 (NKG2D)	42, lectin			–	–	s	–	s	w	+							Immune surveillance	ULBP, MICA, MICB
CD315 (prostaglandin F2 receptor negative regulator)	135, Ig					a			s							s	Cell polarity, motility	Associates with CD9, CD81
CD316	63, Ig							+	+	+							Cell polarity, motility	Associates with CD9, CD81
CD317	29-33					+	+	+	s	+							Possibly differentiation/ development	Unknown
CD318	140			–	–									s		s	Differentiation/ development	Unknown
CD319 (SLAMF7/8, CRACC)	66, Ig			–		+	s	s	a	+		–					Activation, adhesion	CD319 [homophilic binding]
CD320	29, LDL-R			–	–		s										Follicular dendritic cell-B-cell interaction	Unknown
CD321 (JAM-1, junctional adhesion molecule)	32-35, Ig	+	+	+	+	+	+	+	+	+	+	+		+		+	Adhesion, embryogenesis	CD321 (homophilic binding), CD11a, Reovirus
CD322 (JAM-2, junctional adhesion molecule)	45, Ig			+		+		s	s						+	+	Adhesion, embryogenesis	CD322 [homophilic binding], JAM-3
CD324 (E-cadherin)	120, cadherin			s	–							+		+	+	+	Adhesion, embryogenesis	CD103, catenins, PS1
CD325 (N-cadherin)	140, cadherin													+	+		Adhesion, embryogenesis	CD325 [homophilic binding]
CD326 (Ep-CAM)	40			–										s		+	Adhesion, development	CD326 [homophilic binding], CD306
CDw327 (Siglec-6)	49, Ig	–	–	w	s	–	–	–	+	–	–	–	–	–	–	–	Immunoregulation	Sialylated glycans
CDw328 (Siglec-7)	75, Ig	–	–	–	–	+		s	s	+	–	–	–	–	–	–	Immunoregulation	Sialylated glycans
CDw329 (Siglec-9)	50, Ig	+	–	–	–	+	+	s	s	s	–	–	–	–	–	–	Immunoregulation, apoptosis, autophagy-like cell death	Sialylated glycans

CD331 (FGFR1, FGF receptor 1)	130, RTK			s	–										+	+	Embryogenesis, angiogenesis, tissue repair	FGF
CD332 (FGFR2, FGF receptor 2)	115-135, RTK			s	s											+	Embryogenesis, angiogenesis, tissue repair	FGF
CD333 (FGFR3, FGF receptor 3)	115-135, RTK			s												+	Embryogenesis	FGF
CD334 (FGFR4, FGF receptor 4)	110-140, RTK			s	s	+		+	+	+						+	Embryogenesis, tissue repair	FGF
CD335 (NKp46)	46, Ig			–	–					+							NK cell activation	Heparan sulfate proteoglycans, viral hemagglutinins, neuraminidase of the Sendai virus
CD336 (NKp44)	46, Ig			–	–					+							NK cell activation	Viral hemagglutinins
CD337 (NKp30)	30, Ig			–	–					+							NK cell activation	BAT-3, heparan sulfate proteoglycans, glycosaminoglycans
CD338 (ABCG2)	72, ABC transporter			–		+			w	–				s			Transport of xenobiotics	Xenobiotics
CD339 (Jagged1)	150, jagged ligands			s	s											+	Hematopoiesis, differentiation/ development	Notch 1,2,3
CD340 (HER-2)	185, RTK	–	–	–	–	–	–	–	–	–	–	–	–	–	–	s	Signal transduction, cancer marker	Associates with ERBB family members, plexin-B1
CD344 (Frizzled-4)	60 [unprocessed precursor], TM7	–	–	–	–	–	–	–	–	–	–	–	–	S	–	–	Tissue homeostasis, polarity, embryogenesis	Wnt proteins, norrin
CD349 (Frizzled-9)	65 [unprocessed precursor], TM7	–	–	–	–	–	–	–	–	–	–	–	–	S	–	–	Tissue homeostasis, polarity, embryogenesis	Wnt proteins
CD350 (Frizzled-10)	65 [unprocessed precursor], TM7	–	–	–	–	–	–	–	–	–	–	–	–	–	–	–	Tissue homeostasis, polarity, embryogenesis	Wnt proteins
CD351 (Fcα/μ receptor)		–				+	–	+	+	–							Alternative IgM and IgA receptor	IgM and IgA
CD352 (SLAMF6; human: NTB-A; mouse: Ly108)		+	+			+	w	+	+	+							Positive regulation, Immunoglobulin SF (SLAM Family)	CD352 (homotypic binding)
CD353 (SLAMF8, NTBA)		–				+	–	–	+	+							Immunoglobulin SF (SLAM Family)	Unknown
CD354 (TREM1)		+				+	s	–	–	+							Immunoglobulin SF	Unknown
CD355 (CRTAM)		–				–	–	s	s	+							Immunoglobulin SF	Unknown
CD357 (GITR, TNFRSF18)						+	+	+	+	+							TNF Receptor SF	GITR-L
CD358 (TNFRSF21)						+	–	+	+	–							TNF Receptor SF	
CD359 (IL15RA)						–			+	–							Human IL-15Rα	IL-15

Continued

CD Molecule (Common Name)	Molecular Weight (kD, Unreduced), Family	Neutrophil	Eosinophil	Basophil	Mast Cell	Monocyte	Dendritic Cell	T Cell	B Cell	NK Cell	Platelet	Erythrocyte	Thymocytes	Stem Cell/Precursor	Endothelial Cell	Epithelial Cell	Known or Proposed Function	Binding Partner(s)
CD360 (IL21R)		+				+	+	+	+	+							Type I Cytokine Receptor	IL-21
CD361 (EVI2B)		+				+	+	+	+	+								Unknown
CD362 (SDC2)		+				+		+	+	–							syndecan proteoglycan family	Unknown
CD363 (S1PR1)						–		+	+	+							G protein-coupled receptor	Sphingosine 1 phosphate

Symbols:
+ present
– negative
a activated
c cytosolic
s subset
w weak

List of abbreviations used:

ABC ATP-binding cassette
ADCC Antibody-dependent cellular cytotoxicity
AGEs Advanced glycation end products
BAT-3 HLA-B associated transcript 3
BCR B cell receptor
BDNF Brain-derived neurotrophic factor
CCP Complement control protein
CD Cluster of differentiation
CMV Cytomegalovirus
CR Cytokine receptor
ECM Extracellular matrix
E-NNP Ectonucleotide pyrophosphatase/phosphodiesterase
ESL E-selectin ligand
FGF Fibroblast growth factor
HIV Human immunodeficiency virus
HLA Human leukocyte antigen
HSA Heat stable antigen
HSV Herpes simplex virus
HVEM Herpes virus entry mediator
ICAM Intercellular adhesion molecule
IFITM Interferon-induced transmembrane protein
IFN Interferon
Ig Immunoglobulin
IGF Insulin-like growth factor
IL Interleukin
ITAM Immunoreceptor tyrosine-based activation motif
ITIM Immunoreceptor tyrosine-based inhibition motif
kD kiloDaltons
LAMP Lysosomal associated membrane protein
LAP Latency-associated peptide

LBP	LPS binding protein
LDL	Low density lipoprotein
LIF	Leukemia inhibitory factor
LFA	Lymphocyte function associated antigen
LLT1	Lectin-like transcript 1
LPAP	Lymphocyte phosphatase-associated phosphoprotein
LPS	Lipopolysaccharide
LTA	Lipoteichoic acid
Ly-6	Lymphocyte antigen 6
Mac	Macrophage antigen
MAdCAM	Mucosal addressin cellular adhesion molecule
MDR	Multi-drug resistance
MSP	Macrophage-stimulating protein
MHC	Major histocompatibility complex
MIC	MHC class I polypeptide-related sequence
NGF	Nerve growth factor
PTPase	Protein tyrosine phosphatase
PRV	Pseudorabies virus
RCA	Regulators of complement activity
RPTP	Receptor-like protein tyrosine phosphatase
RTK	Receptor tyrosine kinase
SECTM1	Secreted and transmembrane 1
SLAM(F)	signaling lymphocyte activation molecule (family)
SP	Surfactant protein
SR	Scavenger receptor
TCR	T cell receptor
TGFR	Transforming growth factor
TGFR	Transforming growth factor receptor
TLR	Toll-like receptor
TM4	Transmembrane 4
TM7	Transmembrane 7
TNF	Tumor necrosis factor
TNFR	Tumor necrosis factor receptor
ULBP	UL16 binding protein
uPA	Urokinase type plasminogen activator
uPAR	Urokinase type plasminogen activator receptor
VCAM	Vascular cell adhesion molecule
VLA	Very late antigen

References:

Zola H, Swart, B, Nicholson I, Voss E. Leukocyte and Stromal Cell Molecules: The CD Markers. Wiley-Liss, 2007. ISBN-13:978-0-471-70132-3
OMIM: http://www.ncbi.nlm.nih.gov:80/entrez/query.fcgi?db=OMIM
Pubmed: http://www.ncbi.nlm.nih.gov/Entrez/
http://www.vetmed.wsu.edu/tkp/search.aspx
http://hcdm.org/HLDA9Workshop/tabid/60/Default.aspx

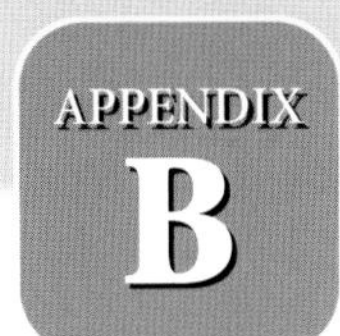

Internet Resources for Allergy and Immunology Professionals

N. FRANKLIN ADKINSON, JR.

Organization/Resource	Internet Address
PROFESSIONAL ORGANIZATIONS	
American Academy of Allergy, Asthma and Immunology	www.aaaai.org
American Academy of Pediatrics	www.aap.org
American Association of Immunologists	www.aai.org
American College of Allergy, Asthma and Immunology	www.acaai.org
American College of Chest Physicians	www.chestnet.org
American College of Physicians	www.acponline.org
American College of Rheumatology	www.rheumatology.org
American Medical Association	www.ama-assn.org
American Thoracic Society	www.thoracic.org
Asian Pacific Association of Allergy Asthma and Clinical Immunology (APAAACI)	www.apaaaci.org
Australasian Society for Clinical Immunology and Allergy (ASCIA)	www.allergy.org.au
British Society for Allergy and Clinical Immunology (BSACI)	www.bsaci.org
Clinical Immunology Society	www.clinimmsoc.org
International Eosinophil Society	www.eosinophil-society.org
European Academy of Allergology and Clinical Immunology (EAACI)	www.eaaci.net
International Association of Asthmology	www.interasma.org
World Allergy Organization	www.worldallergy.org
GOVERNMENT AGENCIES	
Centers for Disease Control and Prevention (U.S.)	www.cdc.gov
Clinical Trials registry	www.clinicaltrials.gov
Food and Drug Administration (U.S.)	www.fda.gov
Global Initiative for Asthma	www.ginasthma.com
National Institute of Allergy and Infectious Disease (U.S.)	www3.niaid.nih.gov
National Heart, Lung, and Blood Institute (U.S.)	www.nhlbi.nih.gov
National Institutes of Health (U.S.)	www.nih.gov
World Health Organization	www.who.org
LAY SUPPORT ORGANIZATIONS	
Allergy and Asthma Network/Mothers of Asthmatics	www.aanma.org
American Partnership for Eosiniphilic Disorders (APFED)	www.apfed.org
American Latex Allergy Association (A.L.E.R.T., Inc.)	www.latexallergyresources.org
American Lung Association	www.lung.org
Asthma and Allergy Foundation of America	www.aafa.org
European Federation of Allergy and Airways Diseases Patients Association (EFA)	www.efanet.org
The Food Allergy and Anaphylaxis Network (FAAN)	www.foodallergy.org
Immune Deficiency Foundation	www.primaryimmune.org
The Mastocytosis Society, Inc. (TMS)	www.tmsforacure.org
MEDICAL RESOURCES	
Adverse Drug Reaction Reporting (USFDA)	www.fda.gov/medwatch
Allergic Rhinitis and its Impact on Asthma (ARIA)	www.whiar.org
Asthma and Allergic Disease Management Center	www.aaaai.org
Asthma Prevention Program and Guidelines	www.nhlbi.nih.gov/about/naepp/index.htm
American Partnership for Eosinophilic Disorders	apfed.org
International Food Information Council Foundation	www.ific.org
NLM Literature Searches (Pubmed)	www.ncbi.nlm.nih.gov/sites/entrez?db=PubMed
Clinical Trials	clinicaltrials.gov
SCIENTIFIC RESOURCES	
Allergome Database (allergenic molecules)	www.allergome.org
The International Cell Death Society	www.celldeath-apoptosis.org
Cytokines and Cells Online Pathfinder Encyclopedia (COPE)	www.copewithcytokines.de/cope.cgi
IUIS Allergen Nomenclature Subcommittee	www.allergen.org/Allergen.aspx
National Center for Biotechnology Information	www.ncbi.nlm.nih.gov
Web-based Protein Resources (NCBI)	http://www.ncbi.nlm.nih.gov/guide/proteins/
The Cytokines Web	cmbi.bjmu.edu.cn/cmbidata/cgf/CGF_Database/cytweb
Biocompare Buyer's Guide for Antibodies	http://www.biocompare.com/Antibodies/
Human Cell Differentiation Molecules	http://hcdm.org
Mouse Genomic Informatics	www.informatics.jax.org
Genetic Association Database	geneticassociationdb.nih.gov
CREDENTIALING ORGANIZATIONS (U.S.)	
Accreditation Council for Graduate Medical Education	www.acgme.org
American Board of Allergy and Immunology	www.abai.org
American Board of Internal Medicine	www.abim.org
American Board of Medical Specialties	www.abms.org
American Board of Pediatrics	www.abp.org

INDEX

Pages followed by *f* indicate figures; *t*, tables; *b*, boxes.

D

F

H

J

P

Q

R

S

T

W

X

Y

Z

WITHDRAWN